drug information

A GUIDE FOR PHARMACISTS

D1559828

Notice

Medicine is an ever-changing science. As new research and clinical experience broaden our knowledge, changes in treatment and drug therapy are required. The authors and the publisher of this work have checked with sources believed to be reliable in their efforts to provide information that is complete and generally in accord with the standards accepted at the time of publication. However, in view of the possibility of human error or changes in medical sciences, neither the authors nor the publisher nor any other party who has been involved in the preparation or publication of this work warrants that the information contained herein is in every respect accurate or complete, and they disclaim all responsibility for any errors or omissions or for the results obtained from use of the information contained in this work. Readers are encouraged to confirm the information contained herein with other sources. For example and in particular, readers are advised to check the product information sheet included in the package of each drug they plan to administer to be certain that the information contained in this work is accurate and that changes have not been made in the recommended dose or in the contraindications for administration. This recommendation is of particular importance in connection with new or infrequently used drugs.

drug
information

A GUIDE FOR PHARMACISTS

sixth edition

Editors

Patrick M. Malone, PharmD, FASHP
Associate Dean of Internal Affairs and
   Professor of Pharmacy Practice
The University of Findlay
College of Pharmacy
Findlay, Ohio

Meghan J. Malone, PharmD, BCPS, CACP, BCACP
Clinical Pharmacist
ProMedica
Toledo, Ohio

Sharon K. Park, PharmD, MEd, BCPS
Associate Professor
Department of Clinical and Administrative Sciences
School of Pharmacy
Notre Dame of Maryland University
Baltimore, Maryland

Mc
Graw
Hill
Education

New York • Chicago • San Francisco • Athens • London • Madrid • Mexico City • Milan
New Delhi • Singapore • Sydney • Toronto

Drug Information: A Guide for Pharmacists, Sixth Edition

1 2 3 4 5 6 7 8 9   LCR   22 21 20 19 18 17

ISBN   978-1-259-83797-5
MHID   1-259-83797-1

This book was set in Century Old Style by MPS Limited.
The editors were Michael Weitz, Brian Kearns, and Peter J. Boyle.
The production supervisor was Catherine H. Saggese.
Project management was provided by Vivek Khandelwal, MPS Limited.

This book is printed on acid-free paper.

Cataloging-in-publication data for this book is on file at the Library of Congress.

Contents

**Chapter Six. The Application of Statistical Analysis
in the Biomedical Sciences .289**
Ryan W. Walters

Chapter Seven. Pharmacoeconomics 397
James P. Wilson and Karen L. Rascati

Chapter Eight. Evidence-Based Clinical Practice Guidelines 435
Kevin G. Moores and Jeanine P. Abrons

Chapter Nine. Journal Clubs 477
Benjamin A. Witt

Chapter Ten. Legal Aspects of Drug Information Practice 489
Martha M. Rumore

Chapter Eleven. Ethical Aspects of Drug Information Practice 557
Elyse A. MacDonald and Linda K. Ohri

Chapter Twelve. Professional Communication
of Drug Information. 595
Patrick M. Malone and Meghan J. Malone

Chapter Thirteen. Pharmacy and Therapeutics Committee 641
*Patrick M. Malone, Mark A. Malesker, Indrani Kar, Jason E. Glowczewski
and Devin J. Fox*

Chapter Eighteen. Medication Misadventures II:
Medication and Patient Safety 849
Kathryn A. Crea

Appendices 1171

Contributors

Jeanine P. Abrons, PharmD, MS
Clinical Assistant Professor
Director of Student Pharmacist International
  Activities
College of Pharmacy
The University of Iowa
Iowa City, Iowa
Chapter 8

Robert D. Beckett, PharmD, BCPS
Associate Professor of Pharmacy Practice
Director, Drug Information Center
Manchester University College of Pharmacy,
  Natural and Health Sciences
Fort Wayne, Indiana
Chapter 23

Kelly Besco, PharmD, FISMP, CPPS
Medication Safety Officer
OhioHealth Pharmacy Services
Dublin, Ohio
Chapter 17

Patrick J. Bryant, PharmD, FSCIP, CCIF
Director, Drug Information Center
Clinical Professor, Pharmacy Practice and
  Administration
School of Pharmacy
University of Missouri—Kansas City
Kansas City, Missouri
Chapter 5

Sabrina W. Cole, PharmD, BCPS, CPHIMS
Medication Policy and Outcomes Director
Intermountain Healthcare, Pharmacy
  Services
Taylorsville, Utah
Chapters 19, 20

Kathryn A. Crea, PharmD, BCPS, CPPS
Director of Quality, Accreditation and Patient
  Safety
Riverside Methodist Hospital—OhioHealth
Columbus, Ohio
Chapter 18

Brent I. Fox, PharmD, PhD
Associate Professor, Department of Health
  Outcomes Research and Policy
Harrison School of Pharmacy, Auburn
  University
Auburn University, Alabama
Chapter 26

Devin J. Fox, MD
VP – Medical Operations
Creighton University Medical Center-Bergan
  Mercy
Assistant Dean for Patient Safety and Quality
Creighton University School of Medicine
Omaha, NE
Chapters 13, 14

Erin R. Fox, PharmD, BCPS, FASHP
Director, Drug Information Service
University of Utah Health
Adjunct Associate Professor
Department of Pharmacotherapy
University of Utah College of Pharmacy
Salt Lake City, Utah
Chapter 15

Maisha Kelly Freeman, PharmD, MS, BCPS, FASCP
Director, Center for Healthcare Innovation
    and Outcomes Research
Professor, Samford University
McWhorter School of Pharmacy
Birmingham, Alabama
Chapter 4

Jason Glowczewski, PharmD., MBA, FASHP
Chief Operating Officer
University Hospitals Conneaut and Geneva
    Medical Centers
Conneaut and Geneva, Ohio
Clinical Assistant Professor of Pharmacy
    Practice
Northeast Ohio Medical University College
    of Pharmacy
Rootstown, Ohio
Chapters 13, 14

Bambi Grilley, RPh, RAC, CIP, CCRC, CCRP
Associate Professor, Pediatrics
Director, Clinical Research and Early Product
    Development
Center for Cell and Gene Therapy
Baylor College of Medicine
Houston, Texas
Chapter 21

Conor Hanrahan, PharmD, BCPS, CPHIMS, CPPS
Manager, Drug Information Services
Intermountain Healthcare Pharmacy
    Services
Sorenson Research Park
Taylorsville, Utah
Chapters 19, 20

Amy Heck Sheehan, PharmD
Drug Information Specialist, Indiana
    University Health
Associate Professor of Pharmacy Practice
Purdue University College of Pharmacy
Indianapolis, Indiana
Chapter 2

Gregory Heindel, PharmD, BCPS
Drug Information Specialist
Intermountain Healthcare, Pharmacy
    Services
Taylorsville, Utah
Chapter 19

Joshua C. Hollingsworth, PharmD, PhD
Assistant Professor of Pharmacology
Edward Via College of Osteopathic
    Medicine—Auburn Campus
Auburn, Alabama
Chapter 26

Peter J. Hughes, PharmD, BCPS
Director, Continuing Professional
    Development
Associate Professor
Samford University
McWhorter School of Pharmacy
Birmingham, Alabama
Chapter 4

Joseph K. Jordan, Pharm, BCPS
Drug Information Specialist, Indiana
  University Health
Associate Professor of Pharmacy Practice
Butler University College of Pharmacy and
  Health Sciences
Indianapolis, Indiana
Chapter 2

Indrani Kar, PharmD
Drug Policy/Formulary Specialist
System Pharmacy Services
University Hospitals
Cleveland, Ohio
Chapters 13, 14

Michael Kendrach, PharmD, FASHP
Associate Dean Academic Affairs
Professor, Samford University
McWhorter School of Pharmacy
Birmingham, Alabama
Chapter 4

Genevieve Lynn Ness, PharmD
Director, Christy Houston Foundation Drug
  Information Center
Assistant Professor of Pharmaceutical, Social
  and Administrative Science
Belmont University College of Pharmacy
Nashville, Tennessee
Chapter 23

Elyse A. MacDonald, PharmD, MS, BCPS
Drug Information Specialist
Drug Information Services
University of Utah Health
Salt Lake City, Utah
Chapter 11

**Mark A. Malesker, Pharm.D., FCCP,
FCCP, FCCM, FASHP, BCPS**
Professor of Pharmacy Practice
  and Medicine
Creighton University
2500 California Plaza
Omaha, NE 68178
Chapters 13, 14

**Meghan J. Malone, PharmD, BCPS,
CACP, BCACP**
Clinical Pharmacist
ProMedica
Toledo, Ohio
Chapter 12

Patrick M. Malone, PharmD, FASHP
Associate Dean of Internal Affairs and
  Professor of Pharmacy Practice
The University of Findlay
College of Pharmacy
Findlay, Ohio
Chapters 12, 13, 14

Dianne May, PharmD, FCCP, BCPS
Clinical Professor
College of Pharmacy
University of Georgia
Augusta, Georgia
Chapter 1

J. Russell May, PharmD, FASHP
Clinical Professor
College of Pharmacy
University of Georgia
Augusta, Georgia
Chapter 1

Michelle W. McCarthy, PharmD, FASHP
Coordinator, Pharmacy Education, Training,
  and Development Programs
Director, PGY1 Pharmacy and PGY2 Drug
  Information Residency Programs
University of Virginia Health System
Charlottesville, Virginia
Clinical Assistant Professor
Virginia Commonwealth University
  Medical College of Virginia School of
  Pharmacy
Department of Pharmacotherapy and
  Outcomes Science
Richmond, Virginia
Chapter 27

Cydney E. McQueen, PharmD
Clinical Associate Professor, Pharmacy
  Practice and Administration
School of Pharmacy
University of Missouri – Kansas City School
  of Pharmacy
Kansas City, Missouri
Chapter 5

Kevin G. Moores
Clinical Associate Professor
College of Pharmacy
The University of Iowa
Iowa City, Iowa
Chapter 8

David P. Nau, RPh, PhD, FAPhA
Assistant Dean, Assessment & Accreditation
  Professor
College of Pharmacy
Nova Southeastern University
Fort Lauderdale, FL
Chapter 16

Linda K. Ohri, PharmD, MPH
Associate Professor of Pharmacy Practice
Creighton University
School of Pharmacy & Health Professions
Omaha, Nebraska
Chapter 11

Heather A. Pace, PharmD
Assistant Director, UMKC Drug Information
  Center
Clinical Associate Professor, Division of
  Pharmacy Practice and Administration
University of Missouri—Kansas City School
  of Pharmacy
Kansas City, Missouri
Chapter 25

Bhavini T. Parikh, PharmD
Senior Medical Information Manager
AstraZeneca Pharmaceuticals LP
Wilmington, Delaware
Chapter 22

Sharon K. Park, PharmD, MEd, BCPS
Associate Professor
Department of Clinical and Administrative
  Sciences
School of Pharmacy
Notre Dame of Maryland University
Baltimore, Maryland
Chapter 3

Karen L. Rascati, PhD
Professor
College of Pharmacy
University of Texas
Health Outcomes and Pharmacy Practice
  Division
Austin, Texas
Chapter 7

**Martha M. Rumore, PharmD, JD, MS
LLM, FAPhA**
Clinical Pharmacist
Monefiore Medical Center & Of Counsel,
 Sorell, Lenna & Schmidt, LLP
New York, New York
Chapter 10

Kelly M. Shields, PharmD
Associate Dean and Associate Professor
Pharmacy Practice
Raabe College of Pharmacy
Ohio Northern University
Ada, Ohio
Chapter 3

Rachel M. Slaton, PharmD, BCPS
Associate Professor
Samford University
McWhorter School of Pharmacy
Birmingham, Alabama
Chapter 4

Morgan L. Sperry, PharmD
Assistant Director, UMKC Drug Information
 Center
Clinical Associate Professor, Division of
 Pharmacy Practice and Administration
University of Missouri—Kansas City School
 of Pharmacy
Kansas City, Missouri
Chapter 25

Suzanne M. Surowiec, PharmD, BCACP
Assistant Professor, Pharmacy Practice
The University of Findlay
College of Pharmacy
Findlay, Ohio
Chapter 24

Jennifer K. Thomas, PharmD, CSSGB
Sr. Pharmacist
Delmarva Foundation
Quality Improvement Organization,
 District of Columbia
Columbia, Maryland
Chapter 16

Ryan W. Walters, PhD
Assistant Professor
Division of Clinical Research and Evaluative
 Sciences
Department of Medicine
CHI Health Creighton University Medical
 Center
Omaha, Nebraska
Chapter 6

James P. Wilson, PharmD, PhD
Associate Professor
College of Pharmacy
University of Texas
Health Outcomes and Pharmacy Practice
 Division
Austin, Texas
Chapter 7

Benjamin A. Witt, PharmD, BCPS
Drug Information Specialist
Drug Information Service
University of Utah Health
Salt Lake City, Utah
Chapter 9

Candice Burns Wood, PSM
Professional Scrum Master
Clearwater, Florida
Chapter 20

Preface

It sometimes seems that the one constant in life is change. However, it has become more evident that change is not a constant—it is increasing rapidly. In a recent book, the Captain of Moonshots (yes, this is the official title) at Google X was quoted as showing how the rate of change has been increasing exponentially. For centuries, change was very slow, but now the rate of change seems to be increasing straight up, to the extent that society cannot currently adapt to changes quickly enough.[1]

Change has happened rapidly in this book. In the first edition, there were only two pages about the World Wide Web, which was very new at that point. The reason for such little information was that there was nearly no information on the topic. The number of useful websites for medical information could easily be counted on one hand. By the second edition, there was enough information to have a whole chapter on the topic. Of course, since then, the use of information sources on the Internet has exploded and permeates the whole book. Many other changes have been seen, and the book has grown to be more than twice as long as the first edition with 50% more chapters.

Change continues to happen in the book. Perhaps the most obvious upon picking up the book is the change in editors. While one of the original editors left after the second edition, the other three have remained until now. However, John Stanovich and Karen Kier have retired from editing the book. We wish them a long and enjoyable retirement. In recognition of the previous editors, an editor emeritus page has been added to the book, starting with this edition. John had brought on Meghan Malone as his replacement, starting with the fifth edition. Sharon Park has now been added to this edition—welcome Sharon!

One constant in the book has been that it was originally written to provide training in drug information management. It has been tested and refined continuously, based on experience in both practice and the classroom. In this sixth edition, the

---

[1] Friedman TL. *Thank You for Being Late: An Optimist's Guide to Thriving in the Age of Accelerations*. New York, NY: Farrar, Straus and Giroux; 2016.

goal of this book continues to be to educate both students and practitioners on how to efficiently research, interpret, evaluate, collate, and disseminate information in the most usable form. While there is no one right method to perform these professional responsibilities, proven methods are presented and demonstrated. Also, seldom-addressed issues are covered, such as the legal and ethical considerations of providing drug information.

However, other significant changes have been made to the sixth edition that allow it to continue to expand, updating information from previous editions, and go into new areas. This includes new chapters on journal clubs and counterfeit drugs/drugs shortages. In addition, the chapter on Policy Development, Project Design and Implementation from the fifth edition has been expanded to be two separate chapters.

As in the past, the book begins by introducing the concept of drug information, including its history, and providing information on various places drug information specialists may be employed. This is followed by information on how to answer a question, from the process of gathering necessary background information, through determining the actual information need, to answering the question. The chapter on drug information resources includes descriptions of the most commonly used references and contains information on apps available for practitioners. The drug literature evaluation chapters have been updated and expanded to cover newer concepts, such as adaptive clinical trials. Chapters from the previous edition have been updated and rearranged in a way to make the subjects flow better. As always, numerous practical examples are provided through the chapters and in the appendices. As with the previous edition, the following features are provided:

- A series of Key Concepts at the beginning of each chapter are then identified throughout the chapter using circled numbers placed within the text.
- The main areas outlined in the Learning Objectives have been highlighted throughout the chapter using vertical rules placed in the margins alongside the relevant passages of text.
- Most chapters have cases, where a situation that might be faced by a practitioner is described, with a series of discussion points presented.
- A series of multiple-choice questions are included and many chapters provide suggested readings for further information on topics.

With the veritable Niagara Falls of drug, medical, and pharmacy information available, much of which is complex, health care professionals have an increasing need for information management skills. This book will assist health care professionals and students with improvement in drug information skills and allow individuals to evolve into new roles for the advancement of the profession and patient care. The authors and editors of this book hope the readers enjoy their journey toward expertise in drug information management.

Editors Emeriti

The following individuals have each been editors for at least two editions. Their contributions have been valuable and greatly appreciated.

- Karen L. Kier, PhD, MSc, RPh, BCPS, BCACP (editions 1 to 5)
- Kristen Wilkinson Mosdell, PharmD, BCPS (editions 1 and 2)
- John E. Stanovich, RPh (editions 1 to 5)

Chapter One

Introduction to the Concept of Drug Information

J. Russell May • Dianne May

Learning Objectives

After completing this chapter, the reader will be able to

- Define the term drug information and how it has changed as practiced currently.
- Identify the services provided by drug information specialists.
- Describe the skills needed to perform drug information responsibilities.
- Identify major factors that have influenced the ability to provide drug information.
- Describe how the expanding integration of information technology has changed the methods of searching, analyzing, and providing drug information to patients and health care professionals.
- Describe practice opportunities for a drug information specialist.

Key Concepts

❶ Drug information may be patient-specific or developed for a given patient population.

❷ Drug information provision has evolved over the last 50 years as focus has shifted to medication safety, advances in pharmacy informatics, evidence-based medicine, formulary management, medication policy development, and new environments of care.

❸ With computerized medical records and order entry systems, drug information specialists can take a leadership role in incorporating automated interventions that improve safety and provide education at the point of prescribing.

❹ Drug information specialists and clinical specialists must keep abreast of advances in information technology.

❺ Biomedical literature evaluation skills are essential for all health care professionals.

❻ Leadership and career opportunities exist in a variety of settings for a drug information specialist.

Introduction

The United States (U.S.) health care system is undergoing important changes, which is offering challenges and opportunities for health care professionals, insurers, caregivers, and consumers. Several factors are driving these changes including new regulations in health care, continued pressure to reduce health care costs, and need to improve efficiency, quality, and safety of care.[1-3] The appropriate use of medications continues to be an essential element in this process because it represents a significant portion of the health care dollars spent in the United States. Total health care system spending on medications reached $2.23 trillion in 2015. Within nonfederal hospitals and clinics, medication expenditures exceeded $56 billion.[2] The use of "specialty drugs" such as those for hepatitis C, cancer, cystic fibrosis, rheumatoid arthritis, and pulmonary arterial hypertension have contributed greatly to the increased medication expenditures. The availability of patient-, disease-, and medication-specific information, and a knowledgeable decision maker are integral components of providing a system that supports the safe and appropriate use of medications.

The provision of **drug information** is among the most fundamental responsibilities of all pharmacists. ❶ *Drug information may be patient-specific, or developed for a given patient population*, such as development of therapeutic guidelines, communication of a national quality initiative, coordination of an adverse drug event reporting and monitoring program, publication of newsletters, or updating websites. The pharmacist can serve as a resource for issues regarding cost, medication selection and use, medication policy decisions, medical and drug information resource selection, or medication information and education.

Changes in health care drive increased opportunities for providing drug information, which include national efforts to expand access to care while reducing health care costs, the rise in the self-care movement, and the integration of new health information technologies (e.g., electronic health record [EHR], telemedicine, social media, computerized provider order entry [CPOE], and changes in environment of care). Opportunities for provision of drug information are growing in several areas within the health care environment including managed care organizations, pharmaceutical industry, medical and specialty care clinics, scientific writing and medical communication companies, and the insurance industry.

The term drug information may have different meanings to different people depending on the context in which it is used. It is sometimes used interchangeably with the term medication information. If asked to define this term, one could describe it as information found in a reference or verbalized by an individual that pertains to medications. In many cases, individuals put this term in different contexts by associating it with other words which include (1) specialist/practitioner/pharmacist/provider; (2) center/service/practice; and (3) functions/skills. The first group of words implies a specific individual, the second group implies a place, and the third implies activities and abilities of individuals. These terms may refer to either the provision of information for a specific patient or in the context of addressing medication use issues for a population (i.e., individuals defined by a set of common characteristics, such as a policy on medication use developed by health care professional working in the emergency department of a hospital).

Pharmacy informatics emphasizes the use of technology and automation as an integral tool in effectively organizing, analyzing, managing, and communicating information on medication use in patients.[4] It refers to the management and integration of medication-related data, information, and knowledge that spans across systems and supports the medication-use process.[4] With the mandated integration of EHR and CPOE, there is greater opportunity to provide medication information on to individual patients at the point of care, and be able to assess outcomes more readily.[5] The impact of new technologies and opportunities in pharmacy informatics in current and future practice will be discussed later (see Chapter 26 for more details). The goals of this chapter are to describe how the role of the pharmacist has evolved in providing drug information, to discuss factors contributing to that evolution, and to describe opportunities to use drug information skills, either as a generalist or in a specialty practice.

The Beginning

The term "drug information" was developed in the early 1960s and used in conjunction with the word "center" and "specialist." In 1962, the first drug information center was opened at the University of Kentucky Medical Center.[6] This center desired to be a source of comprehensive drug information for staff physicians, dentists, and nurses. Another goal was to take an active role in the education of health professional students including medicine, dentistry, and nursing, and specifically influence pharmacy students in developing their role as medication consultants. Several other drug information centers were established shortly thereafter. The first formal survey, conducted in 1983, identified 54 pharmacist-operated centers in the United States.[7]

The individual responsible for operating the center was called the drug information specialist. The expectation was that drug information would be stored in the center and retrieved, selected, evaluated, and disseminated by the specialist. As practice progressed, some drug information centers evolved to drug information services where drug information activities were provided outside a formalized center. In addition, other specific functions evolved over time as listed in Table 1-1.[8] A drug information center or specialist may be involved in one or all of these functions. Detailed information regarding these activities is provided in subsequent chapters.

In the 1960s, the availability of new medications (e.g., neuromuscular blockers, first-generation cephalosporins) provided challenges for practitioners to keep abreast and make appropriate decisions for their patients. Part of the problem was finding a way to effectively communicate the wealth of information to those needing it. The information environment relied heavily on the print medium for storage, retrieval, and dissemination of information. MEDLARS® (Medical Literature Retrieval and Analysis System) was developed by the National Library of Medicine in the early 1960s.[9] While it provided a computerized form of searching, requests for searches were submitted by mail and results returned by mail. The ability to transmit such information over telephone lines (online technology) was not available until 1971 when MEDLINE® was introduced and

TABLE 1–1. DRUG INFORMATION SERVICES[8]

- Supporting clinical services with drug information
- Answering questions regarding medications from patients and health care professionals
- Coordinating pharmacy and therapeutics committee activity
- Developing and educating health care professionals on medication-use policies
- Critically evaluating the literature to make formulary and patient-specific decisions (e.g., drug monograph, class review)
- Providing poison information
- Publishing or editing information on appropriate medication use through newsletters, journal columns, websites, e-mail, social media, etc.
- Providing education (e.g., in-services, classes, experiential education, journal club) for health care professionals, students, and patients
- Participating in health outcome initiatives
- Coordinating formulary management initiatives
- Developing criteria/guidelines for medication use
- Analyzing the clinical and economic impact of drug policy decisions
- Managing medication-use evaluation and other quality assurance/improvement activities
- Managing drug shortages
- Managing investigational medication use (e.g., Institutional Review Board activities, information for practitioners—see Chapter 21)
- Coordinating of adverse drug event reporting and monitoring programs (e.g., adverse medication reactions and medication errors)
- Consulting on pharmacy informatics projects in the health care system setting
- Ensuring and implementing changes to medication-use policies and formulary decisions via informatics system

was limited to libraries. During this time, the drug information specialist was viewed as a person who could bridge the gap and effectively communicate drug information.[10] Direct access by other health care professionals was allowed in 1981, if they completed a week-long training class offered only in three cities. Of course, methods for accessing information have evolved tremendously with the creation of the Internet, mobile technologies and applications (apps), and the integration of EHR.

Early reports that examined the requirements for training of a drug information specialist recommended the following courses be added or strengthened in the pharmacy school curricula: biochemistry, anatomy, physiology, pathology, biostatistics, and experimental design (with some histology, embryology, and endocrinology incorporated into other courses).[11] In today's pharmacy curricula, most of these topics receive considerable emphasis. In addition to these subjects, progress has been made to incorporate evidence-based practice and patient-centered care into curricula.[12] Pharmacists today use knowledge and skills to make clinical decisions about medication use in specific patients or a group of patients in conjunction with other health care professionals. Training and expertise in evidence-based practice have led pharmacists to take a leadership role in publishing in the area of therapeutic guidelines, drug policies, and outcome analyses. These activities illustrate how pharmacists play a major role in meeting the needs of individual patients and large patient groups.

The Evolution

It is useful to look at the evolution of drug information practice from the perspective of drug information centers and from the perspective of practicing pharmacists. Calculating accurate numbers of drug information centers nationally or internationally (e.g., Puerto Rico, Japan, Saudi Arabia, Africa) is difficult, because no agency or organization is responsible for maintaining a list. Well-defined criteria are not established for using the titles of drug information center/service. Some centers specialize in a particular area of drug information, and their name may reflect that specific function (e.g., Center for Drug Evaluation and Research, Center for Clinical Outcomes Research and Education, Center for Drug Policy, Drug Information Center, Poison Control Center). Some centers limit their practice to a subset of clients (e.g., pharmacists, physicians, nurses, attorneys, faculty, consumers) based on their source of funding (e.g., pharmaceutical manufacturer, government, college of pharmacy, managed care organization, law firm, law enforcement agencies, fee-for-service). Some drug information centers are available for all consumers, 7 days a week, 24 hours a day, as is the case for a poison control center. The center may provide services via telephone, website, face-to face, e-mail, or other methods.

IMPACT OF DRUG INFORMATION SERVICE

One study examined 89 drug information centers for changes in number or type of questions, and time spent on activities compared to 5 years earlier.[13] Eighty-four percent of the drug information centers were still in existence in 2009 when the paper was published. There was an increase in time spent educating students (53%) and supporting adverse drug reaction reporting initiatives (44%). Seventy-six reported an increase in the number of complex questions, with 53% documenting an increase in the time required to answer questions.

When studying the availability of a drug information center specifically in the hospital setting, a 2013 survey examining over 1,400 U.S. general and children's medical-surgical hospitals found that 54.5% of surveyed hospitals with more than 600 beds had a formal drug information center.[14] Formal drug information centers were found in 1.6% to 17.6% of hospitals with less than 600 beds.[14] Regardless of hospital size, 97.2% of hospitals reported having a pharmacist available to answer drug information questions as the most frequent method for providing objective drug information to precribers.[14] In an earlier survey of 1,950 hospitals in 2010, 96.6% of hospitals reported that having a pharmacist available to provide drug information was the most frequent method for providing objective drug information.[15]

There have been a few studies that have described the economic benefit of maintaining a drug information center or related activity in an academic institution or hospital. One such study examined the economic impact of drug information services responding to patient-specific requests.[16] The resultant cost-benefit ratio was found to be 2.9:1 to 13.2:1. Most of the cost savings resulted from decreased need for monitoring (e.g., laboratory tests) or decreased need for additional treatment related to an adverse effect. Another study examined the drug cost avoidance and revenue associated with the provision of investigational drug services, which was not part of drug information center in this study, but may be the responsibility of a drug information center.[17] The annualized drug cost avoidance plus revenue was 2.6 million dollars. Studies of this nature are becoming increasingly important in an era of cost containment. Although these studies were completed several years ago, the basic premise of the design and results are applicable today and can be used to assess the value of a particular center or service based on location, clientele, and funding. Other literature also exists that evaluates the economic return on investment for clinical services, which can help provide a framework for how to assess the value of a drug information service.[18]

DRUG INFORMATION SERVICE—FROM CENTERS TO PRACTITIONERS

The responsibilities of individual pharmacists providing drug information have changed substantially over the years. The impetus for this change was provided not only by the development of drug information centers and the clinical pharmacy concept, but also by the Study Commission on Pharmacy.[19] This external group was established to review the state of the practice and education of pharmacists and report its findings. One of the findings and recommendations stated that:

> "... among deficiencies in the health care system, one is the unavailability of adequate information for those who consume, prescribe, dispense, and administer drugs. This deficiency has resulted in inappropriate drug use and an unacceptable frequency of drug-induced disease. Pharmacists are seen as health care professionals who could make an important contribution to the health care system of the future by providing information about drugs to consumers and health care professionals. Education and training of pharmacists now and in the future must be developed to meet these important responsibilities."

The report of the Commission was issued in 1975, and since that time, drug information practice has changed both for drug information centers and individual pharmacists. The development of clinical pharmacy has helped move pharmacy forward in recognizing its capabilities to contribute to the care of patients. Clinical pharmacy was thought of primarily as an institutional patient care process and did not gain widespread acceptance outside of hospitals.

EVOLVING ROLE OF PHARMACISTS AS MEDICATION EXPERTS IN HEALTH CARE

Pharmacists are now involved in many patient care areas (e.g., hospitals, primary care and specialty clinics, long-term care, home health care) where they frequently answer drug information questions, participate in evaluating a patient's medication therapy, conduct medication-use evaluation activities, and coordinate medication policy and formulary management activities. Over time, the activity of the pharmacist as a medication expert for patients has gained acceptance and span the continuum of care. There is much emphasis on pharmacists in community and ambulatory settings to counsel patients, answer drug information questions, review patient medication regimens for potential problems (medication therapy management), and assist patients in managing their chronic diseases. The **patient-centered medical home** (PCMH) philosophy has become a widely accepted model for how primary care should be organized and delivered throughout the health care system. While not a particular building or place, the PCMH model is considered to be comprehensive, team-based, coordinated, and accessible. As a component, the health care team helps improve the quality of care through access to information technology and other tools, to help make sure that both patients and families are making informed choices about their health. Drug information should be provided when needed, and in a culturally and linguistically appropriate manner. Proficiency in finding and evaluating the literature helps the pharmacist become an integral part of the patient-centered care model.[20]

Other organizations, including the Joint Commission of Pharmacy Practitioners (JCPP), have formalized the concept of patient-centered care with the adoption of the Pharmacists' Patient Care Process (PPCP) which is now widely accepted by pharmacy organizations and accrediting bodies including those charged with training future pharmacists (e.g., Accreditation Council for Pharmacy Education and American Society of Health-System Pharmacy Post-Graduate Year 1 [PGY-1] Residency Standards).[21] In fact, Standard 10 in the Accreditation Council for Pharmacy Education (ACPE) Accreditation Standards and Key Elements for the Professional Program in Pharmacy Leading to the Doctor of Pharmacy Degree has a Key Element (10.8) specifically stating that "the curriculum must prepare students to provide patient-centered collaborative care as described in the PPCP model endorsed by the Joint Commission of Pharmacy Practitioners."[12]

PHARMACISTS AS EDUCATORS OF MEDICATION INFORMATION

Providing drug information may be on a one-on-one basis or may occur using a more structured approach, such as a presentation to a class of patients with diabetes or a group of nurses in the practice facility. In either case, the pharmacist educates those who are the beneficiaries of the drug information. There is a well-described systematic approach to answering drug information questions (see Chapter 2). It is important to obtain the necessary background information including pertinent patient factors, disease factors, and medication-related factors to determine the true question. Good problem-solving skills are required to fully assess the situation, develop a search strategy (see Chapter 3), evaluate the information (see Chapters 4 and 5), then formulate and communicate a response. Good communication skills are essential to respond in a clear and concise manner, using terminology that is consistent with the patients', caregivers', or health care professionals' level of understanding. Table 1-2 lists the drug information skills that a pharmacist should possess when confronted with a drug information question.

TABLE 1–2. DRUG INFORMATION SKILLS

1. Access available information (e.g., drug information database, patient's medical records) and gather situational data needed to characterize question or issue
2. Assess the level of urgency, detail, and extent of the needs for information
3. Formulate appropriate question(s)
4. Use a systematic approach to find needed information
5. Evaluate information critically for validity and applicability
6. Develop, organize, and summarize response for question or issue
7. Communicate clearly and effectively when speaking or writing, at an appropriate level of understanding
8. Anticipate other information needs and follow-up

Pharmacists may also participate in precepting students in patient care or pharmacy environments. In any of these roles, the pharmacist must use appropriate information retrieval and evaluation skills to make sure that the most current and accurate information is provided to make decisions about medication use for those they are serving. This role of the pharmacists as a drug information provider continues to be an important component of the Center for the Advancement of Pharmaceutical Education (CAPE) educational outcomes. These outcomes are initiated and maintained by the American Association of Colleges of Pharmacy (AACP) to help transform the pharmacy curriculum to support education of the future.[22]

FACTORS INFLUENCING THE EVOLUTION OF THE PHARMACIST'S ROLE AS A DRUG INFORMATION PROVIDER

❷ *Drug information provision has evolved in the last 50 years as focus has shifted to medication safety, advances in pharmacy informatics, evidence-based medicine, formulary management, medication policy development, and new environments of care.*

Medication Safety: Adverse Drug Events (ADEs)

An estimated 700,000 emergency room visits and 120,000 hospitalizations annually are attributed to ADEs, with an extra cost of 3.5 billion dollars annually to the health care system.[23,24] Forty percent of these events are considered to be preventable.[24] These numbers are probably even higher in the elderly population because of age-related physiological changes, coexisting conditions, and polypharmacy.[25] Pediatrics is another population of concern. A medication-related cause was found in approximately 8% of emergency department visits by pediatric patients with 67% of them deemed preventable.[26] The prevention of ADEs is important today, and will continue to be a significant health care issue in the future.[27]

One of the primary roles for drug information specialist in the beginning was collecting and evaluating ADEs.[6] This role will continue to expand due to an anticipated increase in the number of ADEs in the future. Reasons for this increase include (1) the availability of new medications and new indications, (2) the growing elderly population, (3) increased use of medications for disease prevention, and (4) improved insurance coverage for medications.[28] Pharmacists perform this function in institutional health systems, managed care, or the pharmaceutical industry. To illustrate how a central area for reporting ADEs, such as a drug information center in an institutional health system, can be beneficial, consider the following unpublished example from an academic medical center.

The drug information center received three reports of patients developing methemoglobinemia within a two-week period. The offending agent was suspected to be benzocaine spray. Upon investigation, the drug information pharmacist recognized that all reports had one thing in common, the administering nurse. The pharmacist witnessed the administration of the medication by the nurse the next time it was ordered for a patient. Instead of a single brief spray as directed by the prescribing information, several sprays were used resulting in a potentially toxic dose of medication. A series of in-services for nurses was developed by the drug information pharmacist. No reports of benzocaine-induced methemoglobinemia have occurred since then.

The role of the drug information specialist in the pharmaceutical industry, as it relates to reporting ADEs, is especially important in postmarketing surveillance activities. Because of the specific definition of a study population using inclusion and exclusion criteria in a new medication trial, many ADEs go undetected until the agent is commercially available and used in a broader population. By quickly identifying potential problems and communicating them to health care professionals, patient safety may be improved. The training and expertise of the drug information specialist qualifies them to play a major role in this process.

The importance of maintaining a comprehensive, multidisciplinary, ongoing program for monitoring, reporting, and resolving drug-related problems, and developing mechanisms to prevent future ADEs will continue to be an important element of managing medication use. The drug information specialist can provide leadership and innovative techniques to improve the overall ADE monitoring and reporting program (e.g., establishment of a multidisciplinary adverse drug reaction conference was an innovative way to increase awareness and reporting of adverse drug reactions at one health system).

Integration of New Health Information Technologies

There is a massive effort nationally to modernize health care by making all medical records standardized and electronic.[29] This is considered to be the cornerstone for improvements in quality of care, patient safety, and efficiencies, all leading to an economic benefit.[30]

Pharmacy Informatics

Pharmacy informatics emphasizes the use of technology and automation as an integral tool in effectively organizing, analyzing, managing, and communicating information on medication use in patients. It refers to the management and integration of medication-related data, information, and knowledge that spans across systems and supports the medication-use process.

Several key advancements in health information technologies include the use of CPOE, electronic order sets with clinical decision support, smart pumps, and barcoding. With the mandated integration of EHR and CPOE, there is greater opportunity to provide information on medications for individual patients at the point of care, and be able to assess outcomes more readily.[5] In fact, the Joint Commission of Pharmacy Practitioners' PPCP takes full advantage of advancements in health information technologies to make communication between health care professionals more efficient and effective. Pharmacists can use the electronic medical record to document progress notes and patient education encounters and review patient-specific data.[21] A properly configured medical record provides decision support, facilitates workflow, and enables the routine collection of data for performance feedback in an effort to help improve efficiency and quality of care, including patient safety.[31]

❸ *With computerized medical records and order entry systems, drug information specialists can take a leadership role in incorporating automated interventions that improve safety and provide education at the point of prescribing.* The use of **computer-based clinical decision support systems** (CDSS) (see Chapter 26) that provide patient information with recommendations based on the best evidence have shown to be valuable in the patient care setting, including a reported decrease in length of hospital stay.[32,33] In one study that examined the value of using a decision support program to assist physicians in using anti-infective agents, the length of hospital stay of patients who used the recommendations was compared with a group of patients who did not always use the recommendations, and compared against a group of patients who were admitted to the unit 2 years before the intervention program.[32] The length of hospital stay was statistically different with an average of 10 days, 16.7 days, and 12.9 days, respectively. Drug information pharmacists can also play an instrumental role in developing and maintaining electronic order sets to be used within CPOE and medication libraries used with smart pump technology.

Although technology affords remote-site access to drug information resources, it is critical that pharmacists have the skills to perceive, assess, and evaluate the information, and apply the information to the situation. One of the most rapidly changing technologies in health care is information technology. ❹ *Drug information specialists and clinical specialists must keep abreast of advances in information technology* in an effort to integrate new and valuable systems in a timely and efficient manner. The need for this type of training is emphasized in an Institute of Medicine (IOM) report.[34]

Drug Information Resources and Apps

Even though the amount of literature is much larger today than in the past, it is more manageable (see Chapter 3). The Internet allows the user to easily access the scientific literature, government publications, news reports, clinical guidelines, and other useful items, frequently without cost to the health care professional or the consumer. Handheld devices (e.g., smartphones, tablets) allow health care professionals to have a full range of applications (e.g., decision support tools, medical references) available at the point of care.[35] These offer the convenience of collecting and accessing information from a device that can be carried in a user's pocket. These systems can be used more conveniently than a desktop computer for online searching, calculations, patient tracking, laboratory order entry, and results. They are also convenient for providing medication profiles, setting up appointments, and searching drug information databases. Patients and health care professionals can find information on nearly every disease and treatment, and virtual health communities and forums provide a mutually supportive environment for patients and their families, and friends. The use of social media (e.g., Twitter®, Facebook®, LinkedIn®), web forums, and blogs has simplified the way in which peers can exchange news and share opinions. Several professional organizations (e.g., American Society of Health-System Pharmacists [ASHP]) have used technology to maintain awareness of important news affecting pharmacy and the health care environment (e.g., regulatory and health policy issues), drug shortages, and meeting notifications. Live continuing education is offered at a health care professional's computer desktop through webinars.

Drug Information Availability

There is an increasing need by health care professionals, as well as consumers, to get more information about medications sooner. Information is needed quickly when a new medication becomes commercially available because of the potential for health and cost implications, when a product is withdrawn from the market for safety reasons, or when data from a new study is released that could have an impact on how a common disease is treated. The lag time that occurs with the print format may not be acceptable for many direct patient care issues. The Internet allows medical information to be available sooner to both health care professionals and the public. The availability of electronic journals and texts has minimized the need to travel to a library. Online repositories for articles, such as BioMed Central (http://www.biomedcentral.com) and PubMed Central® (http://www.pubmedcentral.nih.gov) have allowed individuals to access millions of articles quickly, easily, and free of charge. The majority of printed medical textbooks with an online version require a subscription; however, there are exceptions (e.g., http://www.merckmanuals.com) where two editions of Merck Manuals can be viewed and searched for free: one for health care professionals and one for patients, parents, or care givers. Registries of ongoing clinical trials, such as ClinicalTrials.gov (http://www.ClinicalTrials.gov), provide information on the purpose and criteria for participation in an ongoing clinical trial. This has allowed pharmacists to anticipate new therapies, and perhaps help their patients receive medications not yet FDA-approved through enrollment in a clinical trial.

Accuracy of Drug Information on the Internet

In addition to health care professionals, patients are also accessing information from the web, using sites that are sponsored by a variety of companies and individuals with diverse interests. In a recent survey, 85% of physician respondents had experienced a patient bringing Internet information to a visit.[36] Information that is either incomplete or inaccurate may result in harmful behavior.[37] In one study, medication information on Wikipedia was found to be more narrow in scope and had more errors of omission than the comparator database on the web (i.e., Medscape Drug Reference which is a free, online, evidence-based, peer-reviewed database).[38]

There is some effort toward helping consumers accurately assess the quality of information on the Internet. Health on the Net (http://www.hon.ch) is a nonprofit, nongovernment organization that uses criteria to assess the quality of a website. The organization will give a seal of approval to those sites that apply and meet the quality criteria. If misinformation or inaccurate information is found on the web, organizations exist to monitor fraud (e.g., Quackwatch®, www.quackwatch.com).

Some drug information centers have created their own websites to (1) post information about their center and services; (2) provide links to related sites considered to be of acceptable quality; (3) accept adverse drug reaction reports; (4) serve as a convenient means of receiving and answering drug information questions; and (5) provide information regarding formulary changes, institution-specific therapeutic guidelines, and medication policy initiatives.[39,40]

Focus on Evidence-Based Medicine and Drug Policy Development

The pharmacist's ability to apply their drug information skills to medication policy decisions will be of growing importance in this changing health care environment. This includes identifying trends of inappropriate medication use and providing supporting scientific evidence to help change behavior. Continued growth in national health expenditures has raised the interest of government, insurance agencies, health care professionals, and the public in identifying strategies to control spending while maintaining access to quality health care. The United States spent greater than $419.4 billion on prescription medications in 2015.[2] This was an 11.7% increase from 2014.[2] For 2015 to 2025, health spending is projected to grow at an average rate of 5.8% per year.[41] Because drug expenditures are the largest component of the pharmacy operating budget and a significant portion of the entire health system budget, the pharmacy budget frequently attracts significant attention from leadership. In recent years, there has been a shift from a fee-for-service, inpatient focus, to a capitated, managed care, ambulatory focus.[42]

Managed care, a process seeking to manage the delivery of high-quality health care in order to improve cost effectiveness, is an ever-increasing portion of health care delivery. Today, providers are relying less on impressions of what may be happening in a practice setting and more on data that is actually being collected in that same group of patients (e.g., number of patients receiving appropriate dose of medications). Goals are set for a particular group of patients (e.g., all patients receive beta-blocker therapy after a myocardial infarction) based on evidence found in the scientific literature.

Evidence-Based Outcomes

The connection of applying the scientific information to the patient care setting is made through evidence-based medicine. Evidence-based medicine (see Chapter 8) is an approach to practice that integrates current clinical research evidence with pathophysiological rationale, professional expertise, and patient preferences to make decisions for a population.[43] ❺ *Biomedical literature evaluation skills are essential for all health care professionals.* Pharmacists, for example, need to have a solid understanding of drug information concepts and skills, be able to evaluate the medication-use issues for a group of patients, be able to search, retrieve, and critically evaluate the scientific literature, and apply the information to the targeted group of patients. Evidence-based medicine techniques are used in health care organizations to develop and implement various quality assurance tools (e.g., therapeutic guidelines, clinical pathways, medication-use evaluations) in an effort to improve patient outcomes and decrease costs across the health care system. The goal is to support the appropriate use of medications including correcting the overuse, underuse, or misuse of medicines. In the United States, the IOM designated evidence-based patient-centered health care delivery as a key feature of high-quality medical care.[44] The process of evidence-based medicine requires that systems be developed to measure and report processes and outcomes that can be used to drive quality improvement efforts. Data can be collected and analyzed by a drug information specialist using scientific methods to support the decision-making process in a managed care organization.[45]

Outcomes research is a type of investigation that uses scientific rigor to determine which interventions are most effective for certain types of patients and under certain circumstances. This contrasts with traditional randomized controlled studies to determine *efficacy*, which examines the success of treatments in controlled environments. Outcomes research, taking place in real-life settings, is called *effectiveness* research. A branch of outcomes research, pharmacoeconomics, provides tools to assess cost, consequences (e.g., quality of life, patient functionality, patient preferences), and efficiency (see Chapter 7).[46,47] These types of publications can help guide the health care professional in developing guidelines on appropriate medication use in their practice setting.

Sophistication of Medication Therapy

The sophisticated level of medication therapy that occurs today provides pharmacists much more opportunity to:

- lend their expertise in assessing drug information needs of health care professionals, patients, or family members
- provide literature to help choose the best medication to use within a class

- convey the appropriate information to help patients correctly and safely use the more potent medications
- address administration and delivery issues.

Keeping up with new developments in medication therapy is increasingly difficult for health care professionals. Over 5,400 compounds are in various stages of clinical drug development.[48] Nearly 78% of the projects in the clinical-study pipeline involve medications that attack a disease in a way that is unique to any other existing medicine. Several of the medications in the different stages of development could have a substantial impact on clinical practice and drug expenditures once they are commercially available. For instance, it is anticipated that at least 3,400 of these medications are anticancer agents, which could have an impact on life expectancy, quality of life, and the related expenses associated with the potential need for increased ancillary care, additional physician office visits, or hospitalization.[48] Pharmacists need to proactively monitor these pipeline medications to provide adequate time to identify the patient population that will most benefit from the new medication and to help anticipate the cost of treating these patients compared with traditional therapy.[2] See Chapter 19 for more information on medication policy, procedure, and guideline development.

The use of pharmacogenomic profiling is expanding with approximately 20 genes affecting about 80 medications now recognized as actionable in the clinic setting.[49] As the types and sophistication of medication therapy continues to evolve, this will present challenges for patients, family members, and health care providers seeking information on these emerging therapies. The ability to assess drug information needs, search, analyze and retrieve appropriate literature, and apply the information to patients will be important.

Rise in the Self-Care Movement

Consumers have a continually growing desire for information about their medications (see Chapter 25). The growth of the self-care movement, the increased focus on health care costs, and the improved accessibility of health information are some of the factors that have influenced patients to participate more fully in health care decisions, including the selection and use of medications. Direct-to-consumer advertising (DTCA) campaigns have appeared in virtually all mediums including magazines, television ads, web-based ads (e.g., through e-mail, search engine marketing, or banner style ads on specific websites), and radio reports (see Chapter 23). Patients will need assistance interpreting this DTCA to determine what information is applicable to their medical condition. While DTCA may be beneficial to patients by helping them feel empowered to have a more active role in their health care, it may lead to patients requesting medications that are more expensive or that are not the best choice for them.

Health information is one of the most frequently searched topics on the Internet. A recent report from the Pew Research Center stated approximately 60% of Americans sought health information online in the past year.[50] Nearly two-thirds of Americans own a smartphone and 62% of these owners used their phone to look up health information in 2015.[51] When a patient finds information about medications that they are either considering to start taking or are currently taking, from either the Internet, through the lay press, or by DTCA, a pharmacist can help patients critically assess the drug information that they find and add to the information based on specific patient-related needs (see Chapter 25).

Growing Use of Complementary and Alternative Medicine

The need to critically assess information regarding **complementary and alternative medicine** (CAM) has become increasingly important, with approximately 38% of U.S. adults aged 18 years and over and approximately 12% of children using some form of CAM.[52] Use of CAM (e.g., herbal or dietary supplements, meditation, chiropractic care, and acupuncture) is widespread. The 2007 National Health Interview Survey (NHIS), a nationwide government survey, found that 38% of U.S. adults reported using CAM in the previous 12 months, with the highest rates among people aged 50 to 59 (44%).[53] The NHIS data also revealed that approximately 42% of adults who used CAM in the past 12 months disclosed their use of CAM to their health care providers.[53] In a more recent survey, 42% of responding hospitals indicated that they offer one or more complementary or alternative medicine therapies.[54]

Because many adults also use nonprescription medications, prescription drugs, or other conventional medical approaches to manage their health, communication between patients and health care professionals about CAM and conventional therapies is vital to ensuring safe, integrated use of all health care approaches. The changing environment affords the pharmacist many opportunities to use the full spectrum of drug information skills. Factors such as the integration of new technologies, the focus on evidence-based medicine and drug policy development, the sophistication of medication therapy, and the rise in self-care movement require that all health care providers have a strong foundation in drug information concepts.

EDUCATING STUDENTS ON DRUG INFORMATION CONCEPTS

The education of pharmacists continues to evolve in scope and depth. Many of the areas identified earlier as needed by the drug information specialist are now incorporated into pharmacy curricula and taught to all student pharmacists. In 1991, a consensus conference in New Mexico was held to define a set of objectives for didactic and experiential training in drug information for the year 2000.[55] Twenty-three educators and practitioners participated in the conference. There were several key concepts that were developed including (1) drug information should be a required component of the pharmacy curriculum and include both didactic and competency-based experiential components, (2) drug information concepts and skills should be spread throughout the curriculum, beginning the day the students enter pharmacy school, and (3) problem solving should be a major technique in drug information education, with the goal of developing self-directed learners. Developing these skills should provide the foundation for the pharmacist to be a life-long learner and problem solver. Based upon the work of this conference, as well as changes in the health care system and the movement toward outcome-based education, many colleges of pharmacy have redesigned their curricula to provide a more comprehensive and integrated approach to teaching drug information concepts and skills.[56,57] The CAPE outcomes, which are guidelines used for pharmacy education, continue to include drug information skills for all student pharmacists.[22] In one survey, all pharmacy schools offered didactic drug information education to first professional year students either as a stand-alone course (70%) or integrated throughout the professional curriculum.[57] Fifty-one of the 60 colleges offered an advanced pharmacy practice experience (APPE) in drug information, and 62% of these had it as an elective. However, 58% of respondents felt that they had an inadequate number of drug information training sites. Communication skills are taught formally to facilitate the pharmacist's ability to transmit information to both health care professionals and patients.

In 2009, the American College of Clinical Pharmacy (ACCP) Drug Information Practice and Research Network (DI PRN) published an opinion paper that provided recommendations regarding the curriculum and instructional methods for teaching drug information in both colleges of pharmacy and advanced training to help meet the needs of the changing health care environment and the changing culture of drug information practice.[58] In a follow-up survey examining which recommendations were included in U.S. pharmacy college curricula in the areas of drug information, literature evaluation, and biostatistics, only 47% (9/19) of the core concepts outlined in the opinion paper were included in curricula of all responding institutions.[59]

This supports the need to continually reevaluate and update the curriculum that focuses on drug information concepts because of changes in the health care environment. Of note, many respondents identified the areas of evidence-based medicine, medication safety, and pharmacy informatics as areas of expanded focus. Technology (e.g., Twitter® in a pharmacy management course, use of e-portfolios) is also being integrated in the education process within the colleges of pharmacy.[60,61] The evolution in technology and social media has changed the way faculty teach, how students learn, and the way faculty and students communicate in colleges of pharmacy. An academic technologist can support the college faculty and staff in the use of learning management systems, distance education programs, and classroom technology.

Upon graduation, a pharmacist can choose to enter the workforce or continue their education in a practice-based mentorship in a residency or fellowship. Postgraduate training through residencies and fellowship experiences can help prepare a pharmacist to be a skilled clinical practitioner, researcher, educator, and leader in the profession of pharmacy. Drug information and medication policy development are integrated throughout the postgraduate year 1 (PGY-1) residency standards. Currently, there are 14 ASHP-accredited specialty practice (PGY-2) residencies in drug information with a total of 18 available positions (https://accred.ashp.org/aps/pages/directory/residency ProgramDirectory.aspx?pageno=1). These were designed for those who practice in health systems. Individuals who specialize in drug information can practice in a variety of different areas (e.g., scientific writing and medical communications). See Chapter 27 for more information.

Opportunities in Drug Information Specialty Practice

As the role of the practicing pharmacist has changed regarding drug information activities, so has the role of the specialist. The role of the drug information specialist has changed from an individual who specifically answers questions to one who focuses on development of medication policies and provides information on complex drug information questions. ❻ *Leadership and career opportunities exist in a variety of settings for drug information specialists,* including health system pharmacies (e.g., hospital pharmacy), a contract drug information center, pharmacy informatics, managed care organizations (e.g., health maintenance organizations [HMOs]/pharmacy benefit management organizations [PBMs]), scientific writing and medical communications, poison control, pharmaceutical industry, and academia. A drug information specialist can be involved in multiple activities in practice settings listed below.

INSTITUTIONAL HEALTH-SYSTEM DRUG INFORMATION SERVICES

Opportunities exist for drug information specialists in most health-system pharmacies. For example, roles covered by a drug information specialist in health systems often include managing the formulary system, medication safety programs, medication usage evaluation, and medication policy development and management.

Drug information practitioners are in an enviable position to provide a service that will improve patient outcomes and decrease health care costs through the provision of unbiased information that supports rational, cost-effective, and patient- and disease-specific medication therapy. With formulary management, more emphasis will be needed on evaluating nontraditional medications such as herbal and natural products, compounded products, and biosimilars to determine if they have a place on the formulary. Formulary management software will need to be evaluated and implemented, and automated formulary restrictions and decision support will need to be developed. In addition, drug shortages and counterfeit medications will need to be addressed (see Chapter 15). Drug information practitioners will also be tasked with deciding what drug information resources to be used by health care professionals in the health system, publishing drug information newsletters, and managing websites.

CONTRACTED DRUG INFORMATION CENTER (FEE-FOR-SERVICE)

Another way to deliver evidence-based drug information services is by contracting with a drug information service with formally trained drug information specialists. Potential clients include managed care groups, contract pharmacy services, federal or state government, pharmacy benefits managers, buying groups, attorneys, pharmaceutical industry, small hospitals, chain pharmacies, independent pharmacies, and nursing home chains. In one survey, 31% of managed care organizations contracted with a drug information center.[62] Several different fee structures have been used. A client may be charged a simple fee per question or may be offered a detailed menu of services (e.g., written medication evaluations) with the final cost dependent on the number and types of services chosen by the contracting party.

Services provided within these contracts may include:

- providing answers to medication information requests
- preparing new drug evaluation monographs or class reviews
- developing medication-use evaluation criteria
- preparing pharmacoeconomic evaluations
- developing guidelines for a particular disease
- writing a pharmacotherapy publication (e.g., website, blog, newsletter)
- providing continuing education programming.[63]

Additional services that the center may make available are access to in-house question files for sharing of information on commonly asked questions, and direct access to the center's Internet home page for review of medication-use evaluations, formulary reviews, and newsletters. One center reports providing information on drug shortages to ASHP through a grant.[64] Frequently, the contracting drug information center also has responsibilities for pharmacy services (e.g., drug information, medication policy) as part of an entire health system or is based in a college of pharmacy.

PHARMACY INFORMATICS IN A HEALTH SYSTEM

The majority (92%) of recently published articles on health information technology's effect on outcomes (quality, efficiency, and provider satisfaction) reached positive conclusions.[65] There are tremendous opportunities for a **pharmacy informatics specialist**—an individual who has advanced drug information skills with a keen understanding of computer and information technology. This individual can help support patient care activities by improving the efficiency of workflow, by increasing access to patient-specific information and the medical literature through technology by remote-site availability. This individual may also be involved in the area of institutional medication policy management. As the integration of EHRs and CPOE continues to expand, data that were only accessible through a paper record will be available for those health care professionals who understand the type of data that is needed for quality improvement efforts, and are able to get information efficiently out of the system and into the hands of health care professionals at the point of care.[66] The role of a pharmacist as an informatics specialist has been clearly described in the successful implementation of CPOE system in an academic medical center.[67] The role goes beyond the implementation phase and includes system maintenance (e.g., formulary updates, revised clinical decision support as new guidelines and medical evidence are published, developing specialized libraries such as customized cancer chemotherapy regimen library).[68]

MANAGED CARE PHARMACY

With total U.S. drug expenditures for pharmaceuticals increasing annually, there are tremendous opportunities for the drug information specialist to provide leadership in the development and implementation of mechanisms to support the cost-effective selection and use of medications in managed pharmacy organizations.[2] With the appropriate training (e.g., specialized residency in drug information practice or managed care pharmacy) and expertise, opportunities are growing for the drug information specialists in the insurance industry, HMOs, PBM companies, state and national government agencies (e.g., Medicaid, Medicare), as well as other groups interested in the cost-efficient use of medications. A list of residencies in managed care pharmacy is available through the Academy of Managed Care Pharmacy (AMCP; http://www.amcp.org). A drug information specialist may be involved in several activities which include providing medication-use evaluation assessments, encouraging the use of cost-effective alternatives, providing medication and practice-related information, managing formularies, providing information to support formulary guidelines, and developing disease management program.

Practice guidelines are becoming an increasingly important part of the biomedical literature. These clinical guidelines are systematically developed to assist health care professionals and patients with decisions about health care in an effort to improve the quality and consistency of health care while minimizing costs and liability.[69] Evidence-based practice guidelines are developed through systematic reviews of the literature appropriately adapted to local circumstances and values. Key questions to consider when reviewing a practice guideline have been proposed.[69] These questions primarily rely on how accurately the guideline reflects the research used to produce it. More information on clinical practice guidelines can be found in Chapter 8.

POISON CONTROL

Poison information is a specialized area of drug information with the practitioner typically practicing in an accredited poison information center or an emergency room. In drug information centers, health care professionals generate most consultations, whereas, in a poison control center, most are generated from the public. Poison control centers must be prepared to provide information on management of any poison situation, including household products, poisonous plants and animals, medications, and other chemicals. Because of the type of information that the specialist provides, nearly all requests for information to a poison control center are urgent. A specialist in poison information requires expertise in clinical toxicology to be able to obtain a complete history that correctly assesses the potential severity of exposure. They need to know where and how to search for this type of information and be able to develop an appropriate plan for intervention. They also need to be able to communicate the plan in a comprehensive, concise, and accurate manner to a consumer at an appropriate level of understanding.

PHARMACEUTICAL INDUSTRY

The pharmaceutical industry provides many career opportunities for pharmacists in a variety of areas including information technology, training and development, scientific communications, post-marketing research, regulatory affairs, professional affairs, medical information services, medical liaison, drug discovery, product development, and clinical research.[70] Each position listed above requires a different skill set, which may differ between companies, depending on the infrastructure and mission of the individual companies.

A pharmacist with specialized drug information expertise or training can answer drug information questions, report and monitor adverse drug reactions, and provide information support to other departments within the pharmaceutical industry. A pharmacist, who is often referred to as a medical science liaison, can help educate health care professionals about a particular group of products or provide academic support or partnership for educational initiatives. They may interact with sales and marketing, participate with regulatory affairs issues, and handle product complaints. Regulatory affairs specialists help ensure that medications under development meet the state and federal regulations that have been developed to protect the public. Pharmacists may be called on to review adverse effects identified in clinical studies and communicate this and other information to the appropriate research and development team.

In addition to providing written information on the medication product produced by the manufacturer, there are opportunities to provide additional information at pharmacy and therapeutics committees or state's drug use review (DUR) boards. Pharmaceutical companies have extensive scientific data on their products; some of which are not available through other published sources or may require a formal FOI (freedom of information) request.

Pharmacists with specialized drug information training can take a leadership role in evaluating current research, serving as an associate in managing ongoing research, or designing studies to help answer questions about new indications for future use of the product. The area of postmarketing research is a growing area that offers tremendous opportunity for pharmacists to share their knowledge of the health care environment, research design, technology, and economics from the perspective of the pharmaceutical industry. As the sophistication of medication products and information management (e.g., electronic **new drug application**—NDA) has increased, so have the opportunities for pharmacists to practice in the pharmaceutical industry and focus on using the skills of a drug information specialist and clinical specialist. Postgraduate residencies and fellowships, which are typically shared with a college of pharmacy, are available to help strengthen some of the drug information skills needed to work in the pharmaceutical industry. Other positions (e.g., drug discovery, product development, clinical research) require an advanced degree of study (MBA, PhD). See Chapter 22 for more information.

ACADEMIA

The drug information specialist has the opportunity to provide leadership in the pharmacy curriculum, including both didactic and experiential training. In addition to teaching drug information skills that are required across practice sites, the specialist also serves as collaborator with other faculty on cases and activity designed to reinforce drug information skills for students. Approximately one-third of drug information centers are funded by a college of pharmacy.[71] This environment allows the student to be prepared to efficiently and accurately provide information to the appropriate audience, while emphasizing both didactic and competency-based experiential training. New academic opportunities for drug information training include the ACPE-required introductory pharmacy practice experiences or IPPEs (http://www.acpe-accredit.org). In this experience, students that are in their first 3 years of pharmacy school are now required to gain exposure to patient care services prior to the last year of APPEs. Answering real questions from patients and about patients may be one way to satisfy this requirement and prepare students for the more challenging mediation questions they will receive in the future.

As the prevalence of evidence-based practice increases, the importance of teaching drug literature evaluation skills increases. Courses incorporating biomedical literature evaluation, formulary management, and the development and management of medication-use policies will be best taught by drug information specialists in academia. See Chapter 27 for more information.

SCIENTIFIC WRITING AND MEDICAL COMMUNICATION

Medical education and communications companies, separate from the pharmaceutical industry, may provide educational programming for health care professionals and consumers to meet continuing education needs (e.g., symposia, workshops, monographs), or nonaccredited or promotional activities (e.g., sales training, publication planning, journal articles).[72,73] These individuals may write, edit, or develop medication-related materials by gathering, organizing, interpreting, and presenting information for either health care professionals or the public. Examples of these materials include patient education materials, journal articles, regulatory documents, poster presentations, grant proposals, sales and marketing of pharmaceuticals, drug evaluation monographs for health care systems.

In addition to having good writing skills, the pharmacist also needs to have scientific expertise and literature evaluation skills. More than 77% of medical education and communication companies employ at least one licensed health care professional. These professionals may have several positions including director and scientific writer. Pharmacists in this capacity would work closely with editors, graphic designers, website strategists, meeting planners, and scientists. This type of information may be communicated in a variety of ways including orally, in print format, and electronically on the web. Medical communication fellowships are available to help provide a solid foundation through experiences to various aspects of the medical communication industry.

Summary and Direction for the Future

All pharmacists must be effective drug information providers regardless of their practice site. It is one of the most fundamental responsibilities of a practitioner. Developing the skills of an effective drug information provider is the foundation for the pharmacist to be a life-long learner and problem solver. The literature is a valuable component of both of these processes and will allow the individual pharmacist to adapt to the needs of a continually changing health care system.

Opportunities abound for pharmacists to use drug information skills in all practice settings either as a generalist or a specialist practitioner. Drug information specialists will still be needed to operate the drug information centers, to provide leadership in the area of pharmacy informatics, managed care organizations, poison control, pharmaceutical industry, scientific writing and medical communications, and academia.

Self-Assessment Questions

1. The first drug information center was opened in 1962 at:
   a. The University of Iowa
   b. The Ohio State University
   c. The University of Kentucky
   d. Misr International University in Cairo, Egypt
   e. None of the above

2. Formal drug information centers are found more often in hospitals of the following size:
   a. Less than 100 beds
   b. 100–150 beds
   c. 200–300 beds
   d. 301–400 beds
   e. >600 beds

3. In current practice, the term drug information is used:
   a. To convey the management and use of information on medication therapy
   b. To prevent confusion with information on drugs of abuse
   c. To signify the broader role that all pharmacists take in information provision
   d. a and b
   e. a and c

4. There is evidence that the cost-benefit ratio of drug information services ranges from:
   a. 1:1 to 1.5:1
   b. 1.6:1 to 2:1
   c. 2.9:1 to 13.2:1
   d. 14:1 to 20:1
   e. More than 25:1

5. The cost-benefit ratio of a drug information services related to patient-specific requests largely resulted from savings by:
   a. Decreasing the books in the library by increasing the use of electronic sources
   b. Decreasing the need for drug monitoring
   c. Decreasing the need for additional treatment related to an adverse event
   d. Preventing adverse drug reactions
   e. Both b and c are correct

6. What was the approximate cost for total health care spending on medications in the United States in 2015?
   a. $100 billion
   b. $200 million
   c. $300 billion
   d. $2.23 trillion
   e. $10.21 trillion

7. Which of the following are essential drug information skills in contemporary practice?
   a. Evaluate the medical literature critically for validity and applicability
   b. Use a systematic approach to find needed information
   c. Communicate clearly when writing and/or speaking at an appropriate level for understanding
   d. Anticipate drug information needs
   e. All of the above

8. What percentage of adverse drug events is considered to be preventable?
   a. 1%
   b. 2%
   c. 40%
   d. 95%
   e. 99%

9. The drug information pharmacist's role in pharmacy informatics should include:
   a. Incorporating automated interventions at the point of physicians' order entry
   b. Writing code for CPOE systems
   c. Developing and maintaining electronic order sets
   d. a and b
   e. a and c

10. With pharmacogenomics profiling, approximately how many medications are now recognized as actionable in the clinic setting?
   a. 80
   b. 10
   c. 1,000
   d. 25
   e. 500

11. What percentage of pharmacy schools offers didactic drug information education as either a stand-alone course or integrated throughout the curriculum?
    a. 100%
    b. 80%
    c. 75%
    d. 60%
    e. 50%

12. According to the Pew Research Center, approximately what percentage of smartphone owners used their smartphones to access health information?
    a. 10%
    b. 25%
    c. 51%
    d. 62%
    e. 99%

13. Which of the following changes have influenced the role of the drug information specialist?
    a. Rise in self-care movement
    b. Development of evidence-based medicine
    c. Expansion of social media
    d. Focus on medication safety
    e. All of the above

14. For pharmacies in organized health care settings, the largest component in the pharmacy operating budget is:
    a. Personnel
    b. Drugs
    c. Clerical supplies
    d. The drug information center
    e. Intravenous (IV) room equipment

15. Which of the following is true regarding complementary and alternative medicine (CAM)?
    a. Not used in children
    b. The use of CAM has been growing nationally
    c. Only 5% of hospitals have some sort of CAM option for patients
    d. It is easy to find complete and accurate information on CAM
    e. Drug information centers do not typically answer questions regarding CAM

REFERENCES

1. U.S. Department of Health and Human Services. Compilation of patient protection and affordable care act [Internet]. 2010 May [cited 2016 Dec 1]. Available from: www.healthreform.gov/law/full/index.html%20

2. Shumock GT, Li EC, Suda KJ, Wiest MD, Stubbings J, Matusiak LM, Hunkler RJ, Vermeulen LC. National trends in prescription drug expenditures and projections for 2016. Am J Health Syst Pharm. 2016;73:e357-72.

3. IMS Institute for Healthcare Informatics. The use of medicines in the United States: review of 2011 [Internet]. 2012 Apr [cited 2016 Dec 1]. Available from: http://www.environmentalhealthnews.org/ehs/news/2013/pdf-links/IHII_Medicines_in_U.S_Report_2011-1.pdf

4. American Society of Health System Pharmacist. Section of pharmacy informatics and technology's glossary of informatics terms [Internet]. [cited 2016 Oct 15]. Available from: https://www.ashp.org/Pharmacy-Practice/Pharmacy-Topics/Informatics/Other-Resources

5. Hing HS, Burt CW, Woodwell DA. Electronic health record use by office-based physicians and their practices: United States, 2006. Advanced Data from Vital and Health Statistics No. 393. DHHS Publication no. (PHS) 2008-1250. Hyattsville, MD: National Center for Health Statistics; October 26, 2007:1-7.

6. Parker PF. The University of Kentucky drug information center. Am J Hosp Pharm. 1965;22:42-7.

7. Amerson AB, Wallingford DM. Twenty years' experience with drug information centers. Am J Hosp Pharm. 1983;40:1172-78.

8. Ghaibi S, Ipema H, Gabay M. ASHP guidelines on the pharmacist's role in providing drug information. Am J Health Syst Pharm. 2015;72:573-7.

9. Mehnert RB. A world of knowledge for the nation's health: the U.S. National Library of Medicine. Am J Hosp Pharm. 1986;43:299-307.

10. Walton CA. Education and training of the drug information specialist and clinical specialist. Drug Intell. 1967;1:133-7.

11. Francke DE. The role of the pharmacist as a drug information specialist and clinical specialist. Am J Hosp Pharm. 1966;23:49.

12. Accreditation Council for Pharmacy Education. Accreditation standards and key elements for the professional program in pharmacy leading to the doctor of pharmacy degree [Internet]. [cited 2016 Oct 15]. Available from: www.acpe-accredit.org/pdf/Standards2016FINAL.pdf

13. Rosenberg JM, Schilit S, Nathan JP, Zerilli T. Update on the status of 89 drug information centers in the United States. Am J Health Syst Pharm. 2009;66:1718-22.

14. Pedersen CA, Schneider PJ, Scheckelhoff DJ. ASHP national survey of pharmacy practice in hospital settings: prescribing and transcribing—2013. Am J Health Syst Pharm. 2014;71:924-42.

15. Pedersen CA, Schneider PJ, Scheckelhoff DJ. ASHP national survey of pharmacy practice in hospital settings: prescribing and transcribing—2010. Am J Health Syst Pharm. 2011;68:669-88.

16. Kinky DE, Erush SC, Laskin MS, Gibson GA. Economic impact of a drug information service. Ann Pharmacother. 1999; 33:11-6.

17. LaFleur J, Tyler LS, Sharma RR. Economic benefits of investigational drug services at an academic institution. Am J Health Syst Pharm. 2004;61:27-32.

18. Perez A, Doloresco F, Hoffman JM, Meek PD, Touchette DR, Vermeulen LC, Schumock GT. ACCP: economic evaluations of clinical pharmacy services: 2001–2005. Pharmacotherapy. 2008;28(11)285e-323e.

19. Study Commission on Pharmacy. Pharmacists for the future. Ann Arbor, MI: Health Administration Press; 1975:139.

20. American Society of Health-System Pharmacists. ASHP guidelines on the provision of medication information by pharmacists. Am J Health Syst Pharm. 1996;53:1843-5.

21. Bonner L. Pharmacists' patient care process gains traction. Pharmacy Today [Internet]. [cited 2016 Oct 15]. Available from: http://www.pharmacist.com/pharmacists-patient-care-process-gains-traction

22. Medina MS, Plaza CM, Stowe CD, Robinson ET, DeLander G, Beck DE, Melchert RB, Supernaw RB, Roche VF, Gleason BL, Strong MN, Bain Am, Meyer GE, Dong BJ, Rochon J, Johnston P. Center for the advancement of pharmacy education 2013 educational outcomes. Am J Pharm Educ. 2013;77(8):Article 162, 1-10.

23. Budnitz DS, Pollock DA, Weidenbach KN, Mendelsohn AB, Schroeder TJ, Annest JL. National surveillance of emergency department visits for outpatient adverse drug events. *JAMA*. 2006;296:1858-66.

24. Institute of Medicine. Committee on Identifying and Preventing Medication Errors. Preventing medication errors. Washington, DC: The National Academies Press; 2006.

25. Budnitz DS, Lovegrove MC, Shehab N, Richards CL. Emergency hospitalizations for adverse drug events in older Americans. N Engl J Med. 2011;365:2002-12.

26. Zed PJ, Black KJL, Fitzpatrick EA, Ackroyd-Stolarz S, Murphy NG, Curran JA, MacKinnon NJ, Sinclair D. Medication-related emergency department visits in pediatrics: a prospective observational study. Pediatrics. 2015;135(3):435-43.

27. Wachter RM. The end of the beginning: patient safety five years after 'To err is human'. Health Aff [Internet]. 2004 Nov 30 [cited 2009 Aug 22]. Available from: http://content.healthaffairs.org/cgi/content/full/hlthaff.w4.534/DC1

28. Centers for Disease Control and Prevention, National Center for Emerging and Zoonotic Infectious Diseases (NCEZID), Division of Healthcare Quality Promotion (DHQP). Medication safety basics [Internet]. 2012 Aug 14 [cited 2016 Oct 15]. Available from: http://www.cdc.gov/medicationsafety/basics.html

29. Centers for Medicare and Medicaid Services. An introduction to the Medicare EHR Incentive Program for eligible professionals [Internet]. 2013 Mar 20 [cited 2016 Dec 1]. Available from: http://www.cms.gov/Regulations-and-Guidance/Legislation/EHRIncentivePrograms/Downloads/beginners_guide.pdf

30. Bond CA, Raehl CL. 2006 national clinical pharmacy services survey: clinical pharmacy services, collaborative drug management, medication errors, and pharmacy technology. Pharmacotherapy. 2008;28:1-13.

31. Elson RB, Connelly DP. Computerized medical records in primary care. Their role in mediating guideline-driven physician behavior change. Arch Fam Med. 1995;4:698-705.

32. Evans RS, Pestotnik SL, Classen DC, Clemmer TP, Weaver LK Orme JF, Lloyd JF, Burke JP. A computer-assisted management program for antibiotics and other anti-infective agents. N Engl J Med. 1998;338:232-8.

33. Hunt DL, Haynes RB, Hanna SE, Smith K. A computer-assisted management program for antibiotics and other anti-infective agents. JAMA. 1998;280;1339-46.

34. Institute of Medicine. Health professions education: a bridge to quality. Washington, DC: National Academy Press; 2003.

35. Ozdalga E, Ozdalga A, Ahuja N. The smartphone in medicine: a review of current and potential use among physicians and students. J Med Internet Res. 2012;14:e128.

36. Murray E, Pollack L, Donelan K, Catania J, Lee K, Zapert K, Turner R. The impact of health information on the Internet on health care and the physician-patient relationship: national U.S. survey among 1,050 U.S. physicians. J Med Internet Res. 2003;5:e17.

37. Berland GK, Elliott MN, Morales LS, Algazy JI, Kravitz RL, Broder MS, Kanouse DE, Muñoz JA, Lara M, Watkins KE, Yang H, McGlynn EA. Health information on the Internet: accessibility, quality, and readability in English and Spanish. JAMA. 2001;285:2612-21.

38. Clauson KA, Polen HH, Boulos MN, Dzenowagis JH. Drug information: scope, completeness, and accuracy of drug information in Wikipedia. Ann Pharmacother. 2008;42:1814-21.

39. Belgado BS. Drug information centers on the Internet. J Am Pharm Assoc. 2001;41:631-2.

40. Costerison EC, Graham AS. Developing and promoting an intranet site for a drug information service. Am J Health Syst Pharm. 2008;65:639-43.

41. Centers for Medicare and Medicaid Services. National Health Expenditure Projections 2015–2025 [Internet]. [cited 2016 Dec 1]. Available from: https://www.cms.gov/Research-Statistics-Data-and-Systems/Statistics-Trends-and-Reports/NationalHealthExpendData/Downloads/Proj2015.pdf

42. Opportunities for the community pharmacist in managed care. Special Report. Washington, DC: American Pharmaceutical Association; 1994.

43. Ellrodt G, Cook DJ, Lee J, Cho M, Hunt D, Weingarten S. Evidence-based disease management. JAMA. 1997;278:1687-92.

44. Committee on Quality of Health Care in America, Institute of Medicine. Crossing the quality chasm: a new health system for the 21st century. Washington, DC: National Academy Press; 2001.

45. Avorn J. In defense of pharmacoepidemiology—embracing the yin and yang of drug research. N Engl J Med. 2007;357(22):2219-21.

46. Vermeulen LC, Beis SJ, Cano SB. Applying outcomes research in improving the medication-use process. Am J Health Syst Pharm. 2000;57;2277-82.

47. Top 10 areas of research: report on the most popular fields of drug development. Med Ad News. 2003;137:S22.

48. Long G, Works J. Innovation in the biopharmaceutical pipeline: a multidimensional view. A report from the Analysis Group, Inc [Internet]. 2013 Jan [cited 2013 Mar 13]. Available from: http://www.analysisgroup.com/uploadedFiles/Publishing/Articles/2012_Innovation_in_the_Biopharmaceutical_Pipeline.pdf

49. Relling MV, Evans WE. Pharmacogenomics in the clinic. Nature. 2015;526(7573):343-50.

50. Pew Research Center. Majority of adults look online for health information [Internet]. 2013 Feb 1 [cited 2016 Dec 1]. Available from: www.pewresearch.org/daily-number/majority-of-adults-look-online-for-health-information

51. Pew Research Center. U.S. smartphone use in 2015 [Internet]. 2015 Apr 1 [cited 2016 Dec 1]. Available from: http://www.pewinternet.org/2015/04/01/us-smartphone-use-in-2015/

52. Barnes PM, Bloom B, Nahin R. Complementary and alternative medicine use among adults and children: United States, 2007. Natl Health Stat Report. December 10, 2008;(12):1-23.

53. Complementary and alternative medicine: what people aged 50 and older discuss with their healthcare providers. AARP and NCCAM Survey Report 2010 [Internet]. 2013 Mar 9 [cited 2016 Dec 1]. Available from: http://nccam.nih.gov/news/camstats/2010

54. American Hospital Association. More hospitals offering complementary and alternative medicine services. Washington, DC [Internet]. 2011 Sept 15 [accessed 2016 Oct 16]. Available from: http://www.aha.org/presscenter/pressrel/2011/110907-pr-camsurvey.pdf

55. Troutman WG. Consensus-derived objectives for drug information education. Drug Inf J. 1994;28:791-6.

56. Gora-Harper ML, Brandt B. An educational design to teach drug information across the curriculum. Am J Pharm Ed. 1997;61:296-302.

57. Wang F, Troutman WG, Seo T, Peak A, Rosenberg JM. Drug information in doctor of pharmacy programs. Am J Pharm Ed. 2006;70:51.

58. Bernknopf AC, Karpinski JP, McKeever AL, Peak AS, Smith KM, Smith WD, Timpe EM, Ward KE. Drug information: from education to practice. Pharmacotherapy. 2009;29:331-46.

59. Phillips JA, Gabay MP, Ficzere C, Ward KE. Curriculum and instructional methods for drug information, literature evaluation, and biostatistics: survey of US pharmacy schools. Ann Pharmacother. 2012;46:793-801.

60. Fox BI, Varadarajan R. Use of Twitter to encourage interaction in a multi-campus pharmacy management course. Am J Pharm Ed. 2011;75:88.

61. Lopez TC, Trang DD, Farrell NC, DeLeon MA, Villarreal CC, Maize DF. Development and implementation of a curricular-wide electronic portfolio system in a school of pharmacy. Curricular-wide use of ePortfolios. Am J Pharm Ed. 2011;75:1-6.

62. McCloskey WW, Vogenberg FR. Drug Information resources in managed care organizations. Am J Health Syst Pharm. 1998;55:2007-9.

63. Foresster LP, Scoggin JA, Valle RD. Pharmacy management company-negotiated contract for drug information services. Am J Health Syst Pharm. 1995;52:1074-7.

64. Fox ER, Tyler LS. Managing drug shortages: seven years' experience at one health-system. Am J Health Syst Pharm. 2003;60:245-53.

65. Buntin BM, Burke MF, Hoaglin MC, Blumenthal D. The benefits of health information technology: a review of the recent literature shows predominately positive results. Health Aff. 2011:30(3):464-71.

66. Woodruff AE, Hunt CA. Involvement in medical informatics may enable pharmacists to expand their consultation potential and improve the quality of healthcare. Ann Pharmacother. 1992;26:100-4.

67. Cooley TW, May D, Alwan M, Sue C. Implementation of computerized prescriber order entry in four academic medical centers. Am J Health Syst Pharm. 2012;69:2166-73.

68. Traynor K. Pharmacy informatics aids cancer center care. Am J Health Syst Pharm. 2012;69:2125.

69. Field JM, Lohr KN, editors. Guidelines for clinical practice: from development to use. Washington, DC: National Academy Press; 1992.

70. Riggins JL. Pharmaceutical industry as a career choice. Am J Health Syst Pharm. 2002;59:2097-8.

71. Rosenberg JM, Kournis T, Nathan JP, Cicero LA, McGuire H. Current status of pharmacist-operated drug information centers in the United States. Am J Health Syst Pharm. 2004;61:2023-32.

72. Overstreet KM. Medical education and communication companies: career options for pharmacists. Am J Health Syst Pharm. 2003;60:1896-97.

73. Moghadam RG. Scientific writing: a career for pharmacists. Am J Health Syst Pharm. 2003;60:1899-1900.

SUGGESTED READINGS

1. Shumock GT, Li EC, Suda KJ, Wiest MD, Stubbings J, Matusiak LM, Hunkler RJ, Vermeulen LC. National trends in prescription drug expenditures and projections for 2016. Am J Health Syst Pharm. 2016;73:e357-72.

2. Ghaibi S, Ipema H, Gabay M. ASHP guidelines on the pharmacist's role in providing drug information. Am J Health Syst Pharm. 2015;72:573-7.

3. Fox BI, Flynn AJ, Fortier CR, Clauson KA. Knowledge, skills and resources for pharmacy informatics education. Am J Pharm Educ. 2011;75(5):Article 93.

4. Pedersen CA, Gumpper KF. ASHP national survey on informatics: assessment of the adoption and use of pharmacy informatics in U.S. hospitals—2007. Am J Health Syst Pharm. 2008;65(23):2244-64.

5. Bernknopf AC, Karpinski JP, McKeever AL, Peak AS, Smith KM, Smith WD, Timpe EM, Ward KE. Drug information: from education to practice. Pharmacotherapy. 2009;29:331-46.

6. Costerison EC, Graham AS. Developing and promoting an intranet site for a drug information service. Am J Health Syst Pharm. 2008;65:639-43.

7. Wang F, Troutman WG, Seo T, Peak A, Rosenberg JM. Drug information in doctor of pharmacy programs. Am J Pharm Ed. 2006;70:51.

8. Zeind CS, Blagg JD, Amato MG, Jacobson S. Incorporation of Institute of Medicine competency recommendations with doctor of pharmacy curricula. Am J Pharm Ed. 2012;76(5):Article 83.

9. Shiffman S, Gerlach KK, Sembower MA, Rohay JM. Consumer understanding of prescription drug information: illustration using an antidepressant medication. Ann Pharmacother. 2011;45:452-8.

Chapter Two

Formulating an Effective Response: A Structured Approach

Amy Heck Sheehan • Joseph K. Jordan

Learning Objectives

After completing this chapter, the reader will be able to

- Develop strategies to overcome the impediments that prevent health care professionals from providing effective responses and recommendations.
- Outline the steps that are necessary to identify the actual drug information needs of the requestor.
- List and describe the four critical factors that should be considered and systematically addressed when formulating a response.
- Define analysis and synthesis, and describe their application in the process of formulating responses and recommendations.
- List the elements and characteristics of effective responses to medication-related queries.

Key Concepts

❶ Rational pharmacotherapy can be promoted by ensuring that drug information is correctly interpreted and appropriately applied.

❷ The absence of sufficient background information and pertinent patient data can greatly impair the process of information synthesis and the ability to formulate effective responses.

❸ Critical information that defines the problem and elucidates the context of the question is not readily volunteered, but must be expertly elicited.

❹ Providing responses and offering recommendations without knowledge of pertinent patient information, the context of the request, or how the information will be applied can be potentially harmful.

❺ Formulating the response requires the use of a structured, organized approach whereby critical factors are systematically considered and thoughtfully evaluated.

❻ Approaching a question haphazardly, or prematurely fixating on isolated details, can misdirect even the most skilled clinician.

❼ Responses to drug information queries often must be synthesized by integrating data from diverse sources through the use of logic and deductive reasoning.

Introduction

Health care professionals are asked to provide responses to a variety of drug information questions every day. Although the type of requestor, query, and setting can vary, the process of formulating responses remains consistent. This chapter introduces an organized, structured approach for formulating effective responses and recommendations to drug information questions.

As the medical literature expands, access to drug information resources by health care professionals and the public continues to grow. Yet many professionals and consumers lack the necessary skills to use this information effectively. ❶ *Rational pharmacotherapy can be promoted by ensuring that drug information is correctly interpreted and appropriately applied.* This presents an opportunity and a challenge for pharmacists who are true drug therapy experts and play a broader role in patient care.

Regardless of specialty or practice site, health care professionals with the responsibility for overseeing the safe and rational use of medications must strive to develop expertise in applied pharmacotherapy. Whether working in a community setting, nursing home, outpatient clinic, hospital, or in any other practice site, pharmacists and other health care professionals can apply their skills and knowledge for the optimal care of patients. Pharmacists should not be relegated to the role of information dispenser or gatekeeper, but they should instead extend their knowledge of drugs and therapeutics to the clinical management of individual patients or the care of large populations.

Steps for Answering a Question

ACCEPTING RESPONSIBILITY AND ELIMINATING BARRIERS

Health care professionals should recognize that their responsibility extends beyond simply providing an answer to a question. Rather, it is to assist in resolving therapeutic dilemmas or managing patients' medication regimens for their entire therapeutic outcome. Knowledge of pharmacotherapy alone does not ensure success. Moreover, isolated information is not sufficient for formulating responses to questions or ensuring proper patient management. In fact, it is uncommon to find comprehensive answers in the literature that completely and effectively address specific situations or circumstances that clinicians encounter in their daily practices. Responses and recommendations must often be thoughtfully synthesized using information and knowledge gathered from a number of diverse sources. To effectively manage the care of patients and resolve complex situations, added skills and competence in problem solving and direct patient care are also necessary.

In order to provide meaningful responses and effective recommendations to drug information questions, real or perceived impediments must first be overcome. One such impediment is the false perception that many drug information questions do not pertain to specific patients. Another is the perception that the seemingly casual interactions with requestors and the lack of formal, written consultation somehow preclude the need for in-depth analysis and extensive involvement in patient management. Oversimplification of these interactions with requestors and failure to identify the context of the question or recognize its significance can jeopardize the clinical management of patients. ❷ *The absence of sufficient background information and pertinent patient data can greatly impair the process of information synthesis and the ability to formulate effective responses.*

IDENTIFYING THE GENUINE AND PRECISE NEED

Evolution of the Systematic Approach

Historically, the approach to answering drug information queries has centered on the use of a systematic method first described by Watanabe and Conner and subsequently modified by others.[1,2] This simple approach relied on the collection of basic information to document and categorize the request and to subsequently develop an organized strategy for formulating cogent responses. Although this structure remains theoretically useful from a training standpoint, if strictly applied without proper context and guidance, it has the potential to artificially fragment the process and disrupt the natural exchange of information. A documentation form (see Appendix 2-1) may be useful to guide the process of data collection and ensure that all relevant information is considered. More recently, the Pharmacists' Patient Care Process (PPCP) has been used as a model by colleges and schools of pharmacy to provide students with a systematic, patient-centered approach to improving medication outcomes.[3] This approach is similar to Watanabe's method and includes collection of all necessary information in order to understand the clinical status of the patient; followed by analysis of data, development and implementation of an evidence-based plan, and appropriate follow-up.

Eliminating Potential Barriers

Ultimately, the success of providing an effective response will depend largely on maintaining the flow of information with minimal distractions and unnecessary or ill-timed questions. The goal should be to remove obstacles, such as those provided by lack of background or situational information, when communicating with clinicians so as to reveal the actual informational needs. This is particularly relevant in clinical settings where most queries are not purely academic or general in nature. In fact, it is rational to assume that queries from health care providers will invariably involve specific patients and unique clinical circumstances. For example, a physician who asks about the association of liver toxicity with atorvastatin is probably not asking this question whimsically or out of curiosity. The physician most likely is caring for a patient who has developed signs or symptoms of hepatic impairment possibly associated with the use of this medication. Although other reasonable scenarios, albeit less likely, could have prompted this question, it would be most prudent nonetheless to consider the possibility of a patient-specific drug-induced liver injury.

Eliciting Critical Information

Even questions that are not related to patient care (refer to Case Study 2-1 as an example) must be viewed in their proper context. Requestors of information are typically vague in verbalizing their needs and generally provide adequate information only when specifically asked and/or thoughtfully prompted. Although these requestors may seem confident about their perceived needs, they may be less certain after further probing. Requestors, regardless of background, are often uncertain about the nature and extent of information that should be disclosed in order to derive the most optimal assistance. ❸ *Critical information that defines the problem and elucidates the context of the question is not readily volunteered, but must be expertly elicited.* This can be accomplished through the use of effective questioning strategies (asking logical questions in a logical sequence) and other means of information gathering that are essential for formulating informed responses. Failure of the requestor to disclose critical information or clarify the question does not obviate the need for such information or relieve the pharmacist of the duty to collect it.

Although it is easy to assign blame to the requestor for failing to disclose all of the necessary information, it is ultimately the responsibility of the provider of the response to obtain this information completely and efficiently.

Case Study 2–1

■ INITIAL QUESTION

What is the molecular weight of fosamprenavir calcium?

■ POTENTIAL RESPONSE IN THE ABSENCE OF RELEVANT BACKGROUND INFORMATION

Fosamprenavir is an oral antiretroviral agent that is indicated for the treatment of human immunodeficiency virus (HIV-1) infection in combination with other antiretroviral agents.[5,6] The molecular weight of fosamprenavir is 623.7 g/mol.[6]

■ PERTINENT BACKGROUND INFORMATION

The requestor is a basic scientist who is conducting an *in vitro* experiment to evaluate the pharmacologic effects of fosamprenavir. She would like to know the molecular weight of fosamprenavir so that she can perform appropriate calculations specified for this experiment.

■ PERTINENT PATIENT FACTORS

N/A

■ PERTINENT DISEASE FACTORS

N/A

■ PERTINENT MEDICATION FACTORS

Fosamprenavir is a prodrug that is converted *in vivo* to the pharmacologically active form, amprenavir.[5,6] Fosamprenavir is available for prescription use in the United States as 700-mg oral tablets and 50 mg/mL oral suspension. Amprenavir has been discontinued and is no longer commercially available in the United States.

ANALYSIS AND SYNTHESIS

Considering that fosamprenavir is a prodrug that must be converted to a pharmacologically active compound *in vivo*, and given that this researcher wishes to conduct an *in vitro* study, the researcher should use the active form of the drug in the experiment. Therefore, they should have requested the molecular weight of amprenavir.

RESPONSE AND RECOMMENDATIONS

Fosamprenavir is an oral antiretroviral agent indicated for the treatment of human immunodeficiency virus (HIV-1) infection in combination with other antiretroviral agents.[5,6] Because fosamprenavir is a prodrug that requires conversion to the active form, the requestor was advised to consider using amprenavir in the experiment. The molecular weight of amprenavir is 505.6 g/mol, and is available for purchase from several chemical vendors.[7]

CASE MESSAGE

This example illustrates the importance of collecting pertinent background information, even for seemingly uncomplicated questions. Failure to understand exactly how the information that is provided will be used could result in an inaccurate or misleading response. In this case, providing the molecular weight without alerting the requestor that *in vitro* fosamprenavir is pharmacologically inactive would have resulted in wasted time and money, and the results of the experiment would likely have been invalid.

Good communication skills (both listening and questioning) are essential for gathering relevant information, discerning the real question, and identifying the genuine needs of the requestor. ❹ *Providing responses and offering recommendations without knowledge of pertinent patient information, the context of the request, or how the information will be applied can be potentially harmful.* For assistance in identifying some of the questions that should be posed, please refer to Appendix 2-2. Even well-equipped drug information centers with trained staff are not immune to this problem. A study of the quality of pharmacotherapy consultations provided by drug information centers in the United States found that the centers generally failed to obtain pertinent patient data, thereby risking incorrect responses and inappropriate recommendations.[4]

Verifying the Context of Question

Some health care professionals may be quick to attempt to answer questions without adequately understanding the context or unique circumstances from which they evolved. They focus exclusively on the answer and ignore or fail to obtain key information needed to establish the framework of the question. In essence, this can result in a correct response being provided to address an incorrect question. For example, in a question about the dose of an antibiotic, an incorrect response can be formulated and inappropriate recommendations made if one fails to consider such factors as the patient's age, sex, condition being treated, end-organ function, weight and body composition, concomitant diseases (e.g., cystic fibrosis), possible drug interactions, site of infection, spectrum of activity of the antimicrobial, resistance patterns, or other factors such as pregnancy or dialysis.

Before attempting to formulate responses, one must consider several important questions to ensure that they understand the context of the query and the scope of the issue or problem (see Table 2-1). Without this information, there is a risk of providing general responses that do not address the needs of the requestor. More concerning, however, is that the information provided can be misinterpreted or misapplied. This not only compromises one's credibility, but also can jeopardize patient care. Pharmacists must recognize the value and potential benefits of their contributions as members of the health care team. Lack of confidence in communicating with requestors can be a limiting factor. Because a telephone call from another health care provider or even a face-to-face

---

TABLE 2-1. QUESTIONS TO CONSIDER BEFORE FORMULATING A RESPONSE

Is the requestor's name, profession, and affiliation known?

Does the question pertain to a specific patient?

Is there a clear understanding of the question or problem?

Is the correct question being asked?

Why is the question being asked? Why now?

Are the requestor's expectations understood?

Has pertinent patient history and background information been obtained?

What are the unique circumstances that generated the query?

What information is actually needed?

When is the information needed and in what format (e.g., verbal, written)?

How will the information provided be used or applied?

How has the problem or situation been managed to date?

Are there alternative explanations or management options that should be explored?

How can the requestor be contacted (e.g., pager, e-mail, cellphone)?

interaction may not be perceived as a formal request for a consult, the significance of such apparently informal daily interactions can easily be overlooked. Interactions with physicians and other health care providers present valuable opportunities for direct involvement in patient care. The lesson often missed is that there is a fine line between a simple, seemingly general drug information question and a meaningful pharmacotherapy consult. Knowing the context of the question, obtaining the pertinent patient data and background information, and understanding the true needs of the requestor often can be the difference.

Case Study 2-2

■ INITIAL QUESTION

Can you tell me the recommended dose of azithromycin for gastroparesis?

■ POTENTIAL RESPONSE IN THE ABSENCE OF RELEVANT BACKGROUND INFORMATION

Azithromycin is structurally similar to erythromycin, a macrolide that has been used historically for short-term management of gastroparesis. While erythromycin is noted to reduce symptoms from delayed gastric emptying in either the IV or oral formulation, current guidelines from the American Gastroenterology Association do not address the role of azithromycin.[8] A search of tertiary and secondary sources did note a few reports of using IV or oral formulations of azithromycin at doses of 250 to 500 mg daily.[9-13]

■ PERTINENT BACKGROUND INFORMATION

The requestor is an internal medicine physician who is managing a patient with diabetic gastroparesis. A nurse recently informed the internal medicine team of a nationwide erythromycin shortage. The physician would like to know if azithromycin is an alternative to erythromycin, and if so what the appropriate dose would be for this specific patient.

■ PERTINENT PATIENT FACTORS

CD is a 53-year-old female. She is presenting today to the office with a reported history of abdominal pain, persistent nausea, occasional vomiting, decreased appetite, and flatulence for the past 2 months. Currently the patient is receiving as-needed metoclopramide 10 mg PO 10 minutes after meals.

Past Medical History

- Type 2 diabetes mellitus × 13 years
- Peripheral neuropathy × 5 years
- Diabetic gastroparesis × 2 years
- Hypertension × 8 years

Social History

- Negative for ethanol
- Negative for tobacco or illicit drugs

Current Medications and Supplements

- Insulin Glargine 15 units subcutaneously at bedtime
- Insulin Lispro 5 units subcutaneously 15 minutes before each meal
- Lisinopril 10 mg PO daily
- Hydrochlorothiazide 50 mg daily
- Metoclopramide 10 mg PO 10 minutes after meals PRN
- Atorvastatin 40 mg PO QPM
- Acetaminophen 1,000 mg PO Q6H PRN pain
- Centrum Women daily multivitamin
- Fish oil supplement

Allergies and Intolerances

- Morphine

Laboratory Results

- T 98°F, BP 151/84 mmHg, P 91 BPM, RR 18/min, O_2 sat 93%
- SCr 1.3 mg/dL, BUN 22 mmol/dL
- WBC 5.4 × 10^9 per liter
- Glucose 88 mg/dL, $A1_C$ 9.4% (3 months ago)
- LDL 126 mg/dL, HDL 44 mg/dL, TG 155 mg/dL

■ PERTINENT DISEASE FACTORS

Gastroparesis is characterized by delayed gastric emptying and is most commonly associated with diabetes mellitus. The incidence increases with the duration of diabetes and the presence of complications such as retinopathy, neuropathy, or nephropathy. Common symptoms of this condition include nausea, vomiting, abdominal pain, and fullness. Treatment of gastroparesis generally involves modifications to diet and pharmacotherapy with prokinetics, antiemetics, and non-opiate analgesics.[8]

◼ PERTINENT MEDICATION AND SUPPLEMENT FACTORS

Erythromycin is a macrolide antibiotic with known prokinetic effects resulting from stimulation of motilin receptors in the gut. Azithromycin is also a macrolide antibiotic but is more commonly used for infection-related conditions as opposed to gastrointestinal motility. As compared with erythromycin, azithromycin has less drug interactions and a longer half-life. While large trials comparing erythromycin and azithromycin for the treatment of gastroparesis were not located, there are some smaller trials comparing manometry results with both agents.[10-12] The administration of IV azithromycin 250 mg infused over 30 minutes was found to have a greater effect in the postprandial period than a dose of IV erythromycin 250 mg infused over 20 minutes.[10,11] Due to the long half-life of the agent, the authors argue that the product can be given once daily compared with the four times daily regimen of erythromycin. In addition, at higher doses of 500 mg of IV azithromycin infused over 30 minutes, a greater effect on manometry readings was noted.[12] A case report describing the effectiveness of azithromycin in an elderly woman with diabetic gastroparesis notes successful resolution of symptoms after a 3-day regimen of 500 mg IV azithromycin followed by a 14-day regimen of 500 mg PO azithromycin.[13]

◼ ANALYSIS AND SYNTHESIS

As CD is already on the first-line agent for gastroparesis (i.e., metoclopramide) and is still symptomatic, erythromycin would be an option to improve gastric emptying and symptoms from delayed gastric emptying. However, CD is not optimally taking the metoclopramide since she is taking it after meals instead of the recommended before meals. This should be pointed out since this may be contributing to symptoms. Since erythromycin is unavailable at the present time, azithromycin is an additional option based on similar effects seen in manometry studies.

◼ RESPONSE AND RECOMMENDATIONS

Metoclopramide is a first-line agent for treatment of diabetic gastroparesis at a dose of 10 mg up to four times daily before meals and at bedtime.[8] Taking the medication after meals, instead of the recommended 30 minutes before meals, will decrease the efficacy of the prokinetic agent. Before making additional changes to CD's regimen, it is worth adjusting the metoclopramide dosing.

■ CASE MESSAGE

This question highlights the importance of skillful problem solving. As always, collecting appropriate background information and patient data is critical. Analyzing this information before synthesizing a logical response is paramount for effective patient management. In this case, failure to recognize that the patient was inappropriately taking metoclopramide could lead to potentially unnecessary addition of therapy for her diabetic gastroparesis.

In the absence of information that provides the proper context, a question about the half-life of a medication appears rather simple. However, if the question was posed for the purpose of assisting the requestor in determining a sufficient washout period for a crossover study, one would be remiss if factors, other than the half-life of the parent compound, were not considered. Proper determination of a washout period also would mandate consideration of other factors such as the activity and half-lives of known metabolites; the presence of potentially interacting medications; the effects of age, illness, or end-organ function; the persistence of pharmacodynamic effects of the medication beyond its detection in the plasma (e.g., omeprazole); and the effect of administration route on the apparent half-life (e.g., transdermally administered fentanyl).

The case studies in this chapter emphasize the importance of looking beyond the initial question and recognizing that the requestor's needs often go well beyond a superficial answer to the primary question. Pharmacists should always anticipate additional questions or concerns, including those that are not directly asked or addressed by the requestor. These questions nonetheless must be considered if a clinical situation is to be managed optimally. In Case Study 2-3, as an example, a question is posed about antibiotics as a possible cause of tooth discoloration. Although the requestor may neglect to provide clarifying information or pose insightful questions that further inform the case, additional related issues and complementary questions should nonetheless be considered, as these will likely be critical in determining the ultimate success of the response (see Table 2-2). Failure to address such questions will undoubtedly result in either an incorrect or inadequate response.

TABLE 2–2. IMPORTANT QUESTIONS NOT POSED BY THE REQUESTOR

Initial query posed by requestor: Do any of the following antibiotics cause tooth discoloration?—amoxicillin, nitrofurantoin, and sulfamethoxazole-trimethoprim?

What is the incidence of antibiotic-induced tooth discoloration?

Are specific antibiotic agents (i.e., amoxicillin, nitrofurantoin, or sulfamethoxazole-trimethoprim) more likely to cause tooth discoloration than others?

Are there any known predisposing factors?

Is the pathogenesis of this adverse effect understood?

How does the tooth discoloration typically present?

Are there any characteristic subjective or objective findings?

Does tooth discoloration caused by antibiotics differ from that caused by other medications, or other etiologies?

Is the tooth discoloration dose related?

How severe can it become?

Is antibiotic tooth discoloration reversible?

How is antibiotic-induced tooth discoloration usually managed?

Are there other antibiotics available that can be used in place of the patient's current agents?

Are there alternative explanations for the tooth discoloration in this patient (including other medications, medication combinations, or underlying medical conditions)?

What complications, if any, can be expected?

Case Study 2–3

■ INITIAL QUESTION

Do any of the following antibiotics cause teeth discoloration—amoxicillin, nitrofurantoin, and sulfamethoxazole-trimethoprim?

■ POTENTIAL RESPONSE IN THE ABSENCE OF RELEVANT BACKGROUND INFORMATION

An extensive search of tertiary and secondary literature sources noted that tooth discoloration has been seen rarely with amoxicillin.[14] However, with dental hygiene practices such as brushing or professional cleaning, this discoloration may be reversible. No documentation was found of tooth discoloration with nitrofurantoin or sulfamethoxazole-trimethoprim.

■ PERTINENT BACKGROUND INFORMATION

The requestor is a urology nurse practitioner who is caring for a patient with vesicoureteral reflux. The patient had been receiving ½ teaspoon of sulfamethoxazole-trimethoprim for about 8 months when his parent noticed darkening of his two teeth. The clinician would like to use an antibiotic prophylaxis for vesicoureteral reflux, but wants to make sure that tooth discoloration is unlikely with choice.

■ PERTINENT PATIENT FACTORS

AB is a 10-month-old male with vesicoureteral reflux.

Past Medical History

- N/A

Social History

- N/A

Current Medications and Supplements

- Trimethoprim/sulfamethoxazole (40–200 mg/5 mL) 2.5 mL daily × 8 months [stopped]
- Patient is currently breastfed
- Liquid multivitamin supplement (Poly-Vi-Sol® with iron) 0.5 mL by mouth once daily

Allergies and Intolerances

- N/A

■ PERTINENT DISEASE FACTORS

Vesicoureteral reflux (VUR) involves the retrograde passage of urine from the bladder into the upper urinary tract. Patients with VUR who develop bladder infection are at increased risk for febrile urinary tract infections (UTI) compared with patients without VUR. The management of VUR involves preventing recurring febrile UTIs, preventing renal injury from potential kidney infections (e.g., acute pyelonephritis), and minimizing morbidity of treatment.[15-17] Antibiotic prophylaxis has been given for several decades under the idea that sterilizing the urine will lead to less kidney infections and in turn, less kidney scarring. Children younger than 1 year of age are recommended to receive antibiotic prophylaxis since they are more likely to suffer morbidity with acute kidney infections than older children.[17]

Tooth discoloration is described as either extrinsic (i.e., outer surface) or intrinsic (i.e., within enamel). Extrinsic discoloration can be seen with tea, coffee, tobacco, and some medications such as mouth rinses and iron salts. In contrast to intrinsic stains, extrinsic stains can usually be removed with tooth brushing or dental scaling and polishing.[14]

■ PERTINENT MEDICATION AND SUPPLEMENT FACTORS

Reports of tooth discoloration with amoxicillin, but not trimethoprim-sulfamethoxazole or nitrofurantoin, were found in the primary and tertiary literature. A review of the patient's current medication and supplements reveals an iron-containing multivitamin. Iron-containing products have more reports of tooth discoloration than amoxicillin.[14]

Trimethoprim-sulfamethoxazole and nitrofurantoin have traditionally been used for VUR prophylaxis at one-half to one-fourth of the usual therapeutic doses for treating acute infections. Amoxicillin is not traditionally used secondary to concerns of increased likelihood of resistant organisms.[15-17]

■ ANALYSIS AND SYNTHESIS

As AB is less than 1 year of age and has a history of febrile UTI, it is recommended to receive antibiotic prophylaxis. Trimethoprim-sulfamethoxazole and nitrofurantoin are the most common antibiotics recommended. While AB has been on trimethoprim-sulfamethoxazole for 8 months, there is no record of having received dental cleaning during this time. Amoxicillin and nitrofurantoin are other options for VUR prophylaxis although amoxicillin has reports of tooth discoloration. A more likely causative factor is the liquid multivitamin containing iron. Iron supplements are usually not needed in children who are breastfed or who get iron-fortified infant formula. Since AB is still being breastfed, there is likely not a need for the iron supplement.

■ RESPONSE AND RECOMMENDATIONS

A review of AB's current medications reveals one agent, a liquid multivitamin containing iron, which has been reported to cause extrinsic tooth discoloration. This discoloration is usually reversible with tooth brushing and polishing.[14] Trimethoprim-sulfamethoxazole has not previously been reported to cause tooth discoloration but it cannot be ruled out as a possible cause. The practitioner was advised to consult a dentist for cleaning of the extrinsic discoloration and to discuss discontinuing the iron-containing multivitamin supplement with the parents. If the staining returns after discontinuation of the iron supplement, then transition to nitrofurantoin could be considered.

■ CASE MESSAGE

This question highlights the importance of skillful problem solving. As always, collecting appropriate background information and patient data is critical. Analyzing this information before synthesizing a logical response is paramount for effective patient management. In this case, failure to recognize that the patient was receiving a liquid multivitamin with iron could have led to possible suboptimal antibiotic prophylactic therapy for VUR.

To expertly address requests for drug information, pharmacists also must depend on their patient care skills, problem-solving skills, insight, and professional judgment. Computer databases and other specialized information sources can assist in identifying critical data, but overreliance on such resources without careful attention to pertinent background information and patient data can mislead even the most experienced clinician.

Formulating the Response

BUILDING A DATABASE AND ASSESSING CRITICAL FACTORS

Formulating a response comprises a series of steps that must be performed completely, objectively, and in a logical sequence. The steps in the process include assembling and organizing a database of the patient information, gathering information about relevant disease states, collecting medication information, obtaining pertinent background information, and identifying other relevant factors and unique or special circumstances. ❺ *Formulating the response requires the use of a structured, organized approach whereby critical factors are systematically considered and thoughtfully evaluated.* Table 2-3 outlines in detail the specific types of information that may need to be considered for each factor depending on the nature of the query. A more thorough list of possible background questions is found in Appendix 2-2. It should be noted that only some of this information might be pertinent for a given query or case scenario.

For patient-related questions, development of a patient-specific database is one of the first steps in preparing a response. This requires the collection of pertinent information from the patient, caregivers, health care providers, medical chart, and other patient records. A comprehensive medication history also is essential. This database would invariably include information that overlaps with the medical and nursing databases. Because physicians, nurses, patients, and others often lack a clear understanding of the type of information needed for effective pharmacotherapy consultations, pharmacists must be able to identify and efficiently extract pivotal patient information from diverse sources.

TABLE 2–3. FACTORS TO BE CONSIDERED WHEN FORMULATING A RESPONSE

Patient Factors

Demographics (e.g., name, age, height, weight, gender, race/ethnic group, and setting)

Primary diagnosis and medical problem list

Allergies/intolerances

End-organ function, immune function, nutritional status

Chief complaint

History of present illness

Past medical history (including surgeries, radiation exposure, immunizations, psychiatric illnesses, and so forth)

Family history and genetic makeup

Social history (e.g., alcohol intake, smoking, substance abuse, exposure to environmental or occupational toxins, employment, income, education, religion, travel, diet, physical activity, stress, risky behavior, and compliance with treatment regimen)

Review of body systems

Medications (prescribed, nonprescription, and complementary/alternative)

Physical examination

Laboratory tests

Diagnostic studies or procedures

Disease Factors

Definition

Epidemiology (including incidence and prevalence)

Etiology

Pathophysiology (for infectious diseases consider site of infection, organism susceptibility, resistance patterns, and so forth)

Clinical findings (signs and symptoms, laboratory tests, diagnostic studies)[a]

Diagnosis

Treatment (medical, surgical, radiation, biologic and gene therapies, other)

Prevention and control

Risk factors

Complications

Prognosis

Medication Factors

Name of medication or substance (proprietary, nonproprietary, other)

Status and availability (investigational, nonprescription, prescription, orphan, foreign, complementary/alternative)

Physicochemical properties

Pharmacology and pharmacodynamics

continued

TABLE 2–3. FACTORS TO BE CONSIDERED WHEN FORMULATING A RESPONSE (*CONTINUED*)

Medication Factors (*continued*)

Pharmacokinetics (liberation, absorption, distribution, metabolism, and elimination)

Pharmacogenomics

Indications (Food and Drug Administration [FDA] approved and unlabeled)

Uses (diagnosis, prevention, replacement, or treatment)

Adverse effects

Allergy

Cross-allergenicity or cross-reactivity

Contraindications and precautions

Effects of age, organ system function, disease, pregnancy, extracorporeal circulation, or other conditions or environments

Mutagenicity and carcinogenicity

Effect on fertility, pregnancy, and lactation

Acute or chronic toxicity

Drug interactions (drug–drug or drug–food)

Laboratory test interference (analytical or physiologic effects)

Administration (routes, methods)

Dosage and schedule

Dosage forms, formulations, preservatives, excipients, product appearance, delivery systems

Monitoring parameters (therapeutic or toxic)

Product preparation (procedures, methods)

Compatibility and stability

Pertinent Background Information, Special Circumstances, and Other Factors

Setting

Context

Sequence and time frame of events

Rationale for the question

Event(s) prompting the question

Unusual or special circumstances (including medical errors)

Acuity and time constraints

Scope of question

Desired detail or depth of response

Limitations of available information or resources

Completeness, sufficiency, and quality of the information

Applicability and generalizability of the information

[a]Factors such as disease or symptom onset, duration, frequency, and severity must always be carefully assessed.

Case Study 2–4

◼ INITIAL QUESTION

What is the maximum dose of rizatriptan?

◼ POTENTIAL RESPONSE IN THE ABSENCE OF RELEVANT BACKGROUND INFORMATION

Rizatriptan is an oral selective serotonin 5-HT$_{1B/1D}$ receptor agonist indicated for the acute treatment of migraine headache.[18] The recommended dose for acute migraine is 5 to 10 mg. If the migraine resumes or symptoms have not subsided within 2 hours, a second dose may be administered. The maximum daily dose is 30 mg in a 24-hour time period.[18]

◼ PERTINENT BACKGROUND INFORMATION

The requestor is a medical resident who is caring for a patient with migraine headaches. The patient has experienced an increased intensity and frequency of migraines over the last several months. She reports that she has experienced two to three migraines per week over the last month. The patient uses 5 mg of rizatriptan for treatment of acute migraine attacks. This has worked in the past. However, recently she has required a second dose for complete resolution of symptoms. The medical resident would like to know if higher doses of rizatriptan have been studied. He is planning to increase the patient's dose of rizatriptan to provide more rapid relief to the patient.

◼ PERTINENT PATIENT FACTORS

EF is a 27-year-old woman who has suffered from migraine headaches for the last 7 years. She presents today complaining of increased frequency and intensity of migraine headaches over the last month. The migraines are now affecting her job performance as a teacher, and she has recently missed several days of work.

Past Medical History

- Recurrent migraine headaches
- Depression

Social History

- EF is a kindergarten teacher and lives with her husband
- EF denies alcohol and tobacco use

Current Medications

- Rizatriptan 5 mg orally for acute migraine
- Bupropion 150 mg twice daily
- Loratadine 10 mg daily

Allergies/Intolerances

- NSAIDs (anaphylaxis)

■ PERTINENT DISEASE FACTORS

Migraine is characterized by episodic attacks of severe headaches that are associated with throbbing pain, nausea, vomiting, and photophobia, with or without aura.[19] If not treated, the duration of a migraine headache can range from 4 hours to several days. Recommended treatments for the management of acute migraine include acetaminophen, nonsteroidal anti-inflammatory drugs (NSAIDs), selective serotonin 5-HT$_{1B/1D}$ receptor agonists, anti-emetics, and dihydroergotamine.[20] For patients who experience greater than six migraines per month or have very severe symptoms that are not relieved by acute treatment, use of preventive treatments are recommended.[21] First-line preventive treatments with established efficacy include antiepileptic drugs (e.g., valproate, topiramate) and beta-adrenergic blocking agents (e.g., metoprolol, propranolol).[22]

■ PERTINENT MEDICATION FACTORS

The recommended dose of rizatriptan for treatment of migraine in adults is 5 to 10 mg. If the migraine resumes or symptoms have not subsided within 2 hours, a second dose may be administered. The maximum daily dose is 30 mg in a 24-hour time period.[18] A dose of 10 mg may provide greater efficacy over a dose of 5 mg. However, adverse events of selective serotonin 5-HT$_{1B/1D}$ receptor agonists have been shown to be dose-related. In clinical trials, patients who received 40 mg of rizatriptan reported dizziness and somnolence.[18]

■ ANALYSIS AND SYNTHESIS

Although increasing EF's dose of rizatriptan to 10 mg may provide greater efficacy for acute migraine relief, doses above this level are associated with a higher incidence of adverse effects. Review of EF's migraine history reveals that she is a candidate for preventive treatment. Addition of a preventive treatment will likely have a greater clinical impact than increasing the rizatriptan dose by reducing the frequency of migraine headaches that she has been experiencing.

■ RESPONSE AND RECOMMENDATIONS

The practitioner was advised that the maximum dose of rizatriptan during a 24-hour period is 30 mg. Although it may be reasonable to increase EF's dose for acute migraine relief to 10 mg, EF should also be started on a preventive treatment, such as valproate, to minimize the frequency of migraine headaches that she has been experiencing.

■ CASE MESSAGE

This example demonstrates the importance of understanding the proper context of the query. In this case, the pharmacist must collect critical background information to determine the actual drug information needed. Had the pharmacist failed to collect pertinent patient information, the physician may have increased the dose of the medication after being told that the maximum dose is of 30 mg in a 24-hour time period. Given this patient's migraine history, it would be more important to also consider the addition of a preventive treatment in order to minimize the total number of migraine attacks. Moreover, larger doses of this medication are associated with a higher incidence of adverse effects.

Once these data are collected and carefully assembled, they must be critically analyzed and evaluated in the proper context before final responses and recommendations are synthesized. Background reading on topics related to the query (e.g., diseases, medications, laboratory tests) is often essential. This process also often involves careful evaluation of the literature (see Chapters 4 and 5). To effectively perform the steps outlined previously, one must begin with a broad perspective (i.e., observing the big picture) to avoid losing sight of important information. ❻ *Approaching a question haphazardly, or prematurely fixating on isolated details, can misdirect even the most skilled clinician.*

ANALYSIS AND SYNTHESIS

Analysis and **synthesis** of information are among the most critical steps in formulating responses and recommendations. Together, they assist in forming opinions, arriving at judgments, and ultimately drawing conclusions. Analysis is the critical assessment of the nature, merit, and significance of individual elements, ideas, or factors. Functionally, it involves separating the information into its isolated parts so that each can be critically assessed. Analysis requires thoughtful review and evaluation of the quality and overall weight of available evidence. Although this process requires consideration of all relevant positive findings, pertinent negative findings should not be overlooked.

Once the information has been carefully analyzed, synthesis can begin. Synthesis is the careful, systematic, and orderly process of combining or blending varied and diverse elements, ideas, or factors into a coherent response. ❼ *Responses to drug information queries often must be synthesized by integrating data from diverse sources through the use of logic and deductive reasoning.* This process relies not only on the type and quality of the data gathered, but also on how the data are organized, viewed, and evaluated. Synthesis, as it relates to pharmacotherapy, involves the careful integration of critical information about the patient, disease, and medication along with pertinent background information to arrive at a judgment or conclusion. Synthesis can give existing information new meaning and, in effect, create new knowledge. The use of analysis and synthesis to formulate a response is similar to assembling a jigsaw puzzle. If the pieces are identified and then grouped, organized, and assembled correctly, the image will be comprehensible. However, if too many of the pieces are missing—as may be the case if patient information or if supporting evidence is incomplete or absent—or are not arranged logically (e.g., when information is not evaluated, interpreted, or applied correctly), formulating a cogent response may prove difficult or altogether impossible.

RESPONSES AND RECOMMENDATIONS

An effective response obviously must adequately address and answer the question. Other characteristics of effective responses and recommendations are outlined in Table 2-4. The response to a question must include a restatement of the request and clear identification of the problems, issues, and circumstances. The response should begin with an introduction to the topic and systematically present the specific findings. Pertinent background information and patient data should be succinctly addressed. Conclusions and recommendations are also included in the response along with pertinent reference citations from the literature. In formulating responses, one should disclose the available information that is most relevant to the question and present all reasonable options and alternatives along with an explanation and evaluation of each. Specific recommendations must be scientifically sound, clearly justified, and well documented. A carefully written record of the response must be maintained for follow-up and legal reasons. The records may be confidentially maintained in a patient's chart or in the provider's secure files.

TABLE 2–4. DESIRED CHARACTERISTICS OF A RESPONSE

Timely

Current

Accurate

Complete

Concise

Supported by the best available evidence

Well-referenced

Clear and logical

Objective and balanced

Free of bias or flaws

Applicable and appropriate for specific circumstances

Answers important related questions

Addresses specific management of patients or situations

FOLLOW-UP

When recommendations are made, follow-up always should be provided in a timely manner. Follow-up is required for assessment of outcomes and, when necessary, to reevaluate the recommendations and make appropriate modifications; it is also a hallmark of a true professional and demonstrates a commitment to patient care. Furthermore, follow-up allows the provider of the information to know if their recommendations were accepted and implemented. Finally, follow-up also allows the provider to receive valuable feedback from other clinicians and to learn from the overall experience.

Conclusion

Formulating effective responses and recommendations requires the use of a structured, organized approach whereby critical factors are systematically considered and thoughtfully evaluated. The steps in this process include organizing relevant patient information, gathering information about the disease states and affected body systems, collecting medication information, obtaining pertinent background information, and identifying other relevant factors that can potentially influence outcomes. Once these data are collected and carefully assembled, they must be critically analyzed and evaluated in the proper context. Responses and recommendations are synthesized by integrating information from diverse sources through the use of logic and deductive reasoning.

Self-Assessment Questions

1. Which of the following best describes the role of the pharmacist in providing responses to drug information requests?
   a. Ensuring availability of drug information resources for clinicians
   b. Serving as a gate-keeper for information resources
   c. Ensuring correct interpretation and application of information
   d. Providing all clinicians with ready-access to electronic resources

2. Which of the following are necessary for pharmacists when formulating responses to drug information questions?
   a. Knowledge of pharmacotherapy
   b. Problem-solving skills
   c. Sufficient background and patient-specific information
   d. All of the above

3. Which of the following represents an impediment for pharmacists to overcome when collecting pertinent patient information for drug information responses?
   a. Access to adequate library resources
   b. Perception that most requests are general
   c. Excellent pharmacotherapy knowledge-base
   d. Appropriate use of a systematic method

4. Which of the following factors can greatly impair a pharmacists' ability to formulate an effective response for a drug information request?
   a. Absence of sufficient background information
   b. Lack of specialty training in drug information
   c. Absence of specialty board certification
   d. Lack of dedication to patient care

5. Which of the following represents a common reason why requestors fail to provide pertinent patient-specific information?
   a. Uncertainty about the extent of background information needed
   b. Lack of time to provide detailed background information
   c. Poor relationship between pharmacy and medical staff
   d. Lack of interpersonal communication skills

6. Which of the following can improve the process of data collection when a pharmacist is receiving a drug information request?
   a. Minimizing distractions to information flow
   b. Using a standard data collection form for all requests

    c. Using effective questioning strategies

    d. All of the above

7. What patient-specific factors would be MOST important to consider when responding to a drug information request regarding the dosage of an oral antibiotic?

    a. The patient's dietary and ethanol habits

    b. The patient's age, weight, and end-organ function

    c. The patient's gender and occupation

    d. All of the above

8. Which of the following is the first step in preparing an effective response to a patient-specific drug information request?

    a. Development of a patient-specific database

    b. Critical analysis of relevant literature

    c. Synthesis of information from diverse resources

    d. Use of deductive reasoning and logic

9. Which of the following skills requires thoughtful review and evaluation of the quality and overall weight of available evidence?

    a. Clinical experience

    b. Synthesis

    c. Resourcefulness

    d. Analysis

10. Which of the following steps is critical for assessment of the outcomes of a patient-specific drug information request?

    a. Analysis

    b. Research

    c. Follow-up

    d. Documentation

11. Which of the following statements is true regarding the process of eliciting critical background information from a requestor?

    a. The requestor should be blamed for failure to disclose critical information

    b. Communication skills are essential for gathering relevant information

    c. It is the requestor's responsibility to provide relevant background information

    d. Gathering background information is not essential to formulation of a response

12. Which of the following are potential consequences of providing responses and offering recommendations without knowledge of pertinent patient information?

    a. General response that does not meet the needs of the requestor

    b. Damage to the pharmacist's reputation

   c. Patient harm or death

   d. All of the above

13. Which of the following involves integration of information about the patient, disease, and medication to arrive at a judgment or conclusion?

   a. Synthesis

   b. Analysis

   c. Research

   d. Integration

14. Which of the following are desired characteristics of a well-formulated drug information response?

   a. Timely, accurate, and complete

   b. Applicable and appropriate for specific circumstance

   c. Supported by best available evidence

   d. All of the above

15. Which of the following assumptions is appropriate when receiving a drug information question from health care professional?

   a. Question is usually academic or general in nature

   b. Commonly prompted by drug company representatives

   c. Likely involves specific patients and unique clinical circumstances

   d. All of the above

REFERENCES

1. Watanabe AS, Conner CS. Principles of drug information services. Hamilton, IL: Drug Intelligence Publications Inc.; 1978.
2. Galt KA, Calis KA, Turcasso NM. Clinical skills program: module 3 drug information. Bethesda, MD: American Society of Health-System Pharmacists Inc.; 1995.
3. The Joint Commission of Pharmacy Practitioners. The Pharmacists' Patient Care Process [Internet]. c2014 [cited 2017 Feb 9]. Available from: https://jcpp.net/patient-care-process/
4. Calis KA, Anderson DW, Auth DA, Mays DA, Turcasso NM, Meyer CC, Young LR. Quality of pharmacotherapy consultations provided by drug information centers in the United States. Pharmacotherapy. 2000;20(7):830-6.
5. McEvoy GK, editor. AHFS drug information 2016. Bethesda, MD: American Society of Health-System Pharmacists; 2016.
6. Lexiva [package insert]. Cambridge, MA: Vertex Pharmaceuticals Inc.; 2016.
7. National Center for Biotechnology Information. PubChem Open Chemistry Database CID=65016 [Internet]. Bethesda, MD: U.S. National Library of Medicine; c2005-2017 [cited 2017 Feb 9]. Available from: https://pubchem.ncbi.nlm.nih.gov/compound/65016

8. Camilleri M, Parkman HP, Shafi MA, Abell TL, Gerson L. Clinical guideline: management of gastroparesis. Am J Gastroenterol. 2013;108:18-37.

9. Potter TG, Snider KR. Azithromycin for the treatment of gastroparesis. Ann Pharmacother. 2013;47:411-5.

10. Larson JM, Tavakkoli A, Drane WE, Toskes PP, Moshiree B. Advantages of azithromycin over erythromycin in improving the gastric emptying half-time in adult patients with gastroparesis. J Neurogastroenterol Motil. 2010;16:407-13.

11. Chini P, Toskes PP, Waseem S, Hou W, McDonald R, Moshiree. Effect of azithromycin on small bowel motility in patients with gastrointestinal dysmotility. Scand J Gastroenterol. 2012;47:422-7.

12. Moshiree B, McDonald R, Hou W, Toskes PP. Comparison of the effect of azithromycin versus erythromycin on antroduodenal pressure profiles of patients with chronic functional gastrointestinal pain and gastroparesis. Dig Dis Sci. 2010;55:675-83

13. Sutera L, Domingues LJ, Belvedere M, Putignano E, Vernuccio L, Ferlisi A, Fazio G, Costanza G, Barbagallo M. Azithromycin in an older woman with diabetic gastroparesis. Am J Therapeut. 2008;15:85-8.

14. Kumar A, Kumar V, Singh J, Hooda A, Dutta S. Drug-induced discoloration of teeth: an updated review. Clin Pediatr. 2012;51:181-5.

15. Subcommitee on Urinary Tract Infection, Steering Committee on Quality Improvement and Management. Urinary tract infection: clinical practice guideline for the diagnosis and management of the initial UTI in febrile infants and children 2 to 24 months. Pediatrics. 2011;128:595-610.

16. Peters CA, Skoog SJ, Arant BS, Coop HL, Elder JS, Hudson RG, Khoury AE, Lorenzo AJ, Pohl HG, Shapiro E, Snodgrass WT, Diaz M. Summary of the AUA guideline on management of primary vesicoureteral reflux in children. J Urol. 2010;184:1134-44.

17. Tullus K. Vesicoureteral reflux in children. Lancet. 2015;385:371-9.

18. Maxalt [package insert]. Whitehouse Station, NJ: Merck & Co Inc.; 2011.

19. Charles A. The evolution of a migraine attack—a review of recent evidence. Headache. 2013;53(2):413.

20. Marmura MJ, Silberstein SD, Schwedt TJ. The acute treatment of migraine in adults: the American Headache Society Evidence Assessment of Migraine Pharmacotherapies. Headache. 2015;55(1):3-20.

21. Lipton RB, Bigal ME, Diamond M, Freitag F, Reed ML, Steward WF. The American Migraine Prevalence and Prevention Advisory Group. Migraine prevalence, disease burden, and the need for preventive therapy. Neurology. 2007;68:343-9.

22. Silberstein SD, Holland S, Freitag F, Dodick DW, Argoff C, Ashman E. Evidence-based guideline update: pharmacologic treatment for episodic migraine prevention in adults: report of the Quality Standards Subcommittee of the American Academy of Neurology and the American Headache Society. Neurology. 2012;78(17):1337-45.

3

Chapter Three

Drug Information Resources

Kelly M. Shields • Sharon K. Park

Learning Objectives

● *After completing this chapter, the reader will be able to*

- Differentiate among primary, secondary, and tertiary sources of biomedical information.
- Select appropriate resources for a specific information request.
- Describe the role of Internet- and mobile-based resources in the provision of drug information.
- Explain the advantage and disadvantage of print- versus Internet- or mobile-based resources for drug information.
- Evaluate tertiary resources to determine appropriateness of information.
- Describe appropriate search strategy for identification of drug information.
- Recognize alternative resources for provision of drug information.
- Describe reliable health information resources for patients and consumers.
- Explain the role and progress of drug information resource retrieved from mobile applications and their potential impact on patient care.

Key Concepts

❶ There are three types of information resources in biomedical literature: primary, secondary, and tertiary resources.

❷ Tertiary resources provide information that has been filtered and summarized by an author or editor to provide a quick and easy summary of a topic.

❸ Secondary resources are mainly in the form of searchable database that enables location and retrieval of primary or tertiary resources.

4 There are several types of publications considered primary, including controlled trials, cohort studies, case series, and case reports.

5 Knowing the most appropriate resource for information retrieval is the first step in the provision of quality drug information.

6 Secondary electronic resources will index and possibly abstract information from different types and numbers of journals, meetings, publications, or sources; therefore in order to perform a comprehensive search for an article, multiple resources must be used.

7 Drug or health information retrieved from Internet-based or online media needs to be evaluated for its accuracy, comprehensiveness, and recent update.

Introduction

The quantity of medical information and medical literature available is growing at an astounding rate. Every year, 2.5 million articles are published from 28,100 active scholarly peer-reviewed English-language journals.[1] This number of articles published grows by about 3% each year. The U.S. National Library of Medicine (NLM) processes about 1 billion online searches per year from users seeking medical and health-related information via PubMed.[2]

The introduction of tablets, smartphones, and Internet resources has radically changed the methods by which information is accessed. Mobile devices may provide faster and more convenient access to information for answering drug information (DI) questions by increasing accessibility to information at the point of care.[3,4] They can also help health care providers access information via a large number of downloadable mobile applications (apps) instead of relying on access to the Internet.

These technology changes impact not only health care provider access to information but also patient access to medical information. Based on data from 2000 to 2015, 84% of American adults use the Internet to access information;[5] 35% of them access the Internet for medical and health information.[6] It was estimated that about 500 million smartphone owners use a health care app worldwide in 2015 and 50% of the more than 3.4 billion smartphone and tablet users will have downloaded mobile health applications, including health care professionals, consumers, and patients.[7]

Due to this access and trend in using online information by patients, health care professionals are faced with not only answering health- and medication-related questions as they occur, but also to stay current and vigilant on the latest information regarding medical practice and treatment. They also must realize that not all published information is accurate or reliable, and some resources are more accurate, more current, and easier to use than others.

As new therapies become available to treat many conditions, health care professionals, especially pharmacists, are daily being asked to provide responses to numerous DI requests for a variety of people. It is tempting just to select the easiest, most familiar resources to find information without ensuring or checking the original source of the information; however, doing so may increase the possibility of missing new resources, limiting the comprehensiveness of the information found, or potentially finding incorrect or outdated information. In clinical practice, providing inaccurate and outdated information may lead to suboptimal patient outcomes and harm, thus, caution should be used when using information from various online or mobile-enabled media (see Chapter 10 for more information on legal aspects of DI practice). Current standards and regulations on mobile application for DI are not adequate. Until there are tighter regulations over all medical- and health-related mobile apps, clinicians must be vigilant at choosing and using high-quality apps for patient care.

The systematic approach to answering DI questions discussed in Chapter 2 is helpful in order to streamline and use the most effective search process. While the amount of DI and the means of accessing such information have changed dramatically over the years, the process of evaluating and providing accurate DI have not changed. Thus, this chapter discusses many of the various DI resources that are reliable, current, and professionally prepared for everyday practice by clinicians.

Types of Biomedical Resources

Health care professionals must be knowledgeable about the different types of biomedical resources and be proficient at using them to tailor their search and find useful information in an efficient manner. Without this skill, they may not be able to use resources to their advantage, may waste time and energy, and not obtain appropriate information. ❶ *There are three types of information sources in biomedical literature: primary, secondary, and tertiary resources.* They are also synonymously referred to as primary, secondary, or tertiary literature or references. Typically, the most appropriate and efficient first step to finding information is to first consult **tertiary resources** before searching in other types of resources. ❷ *Tertiary resources provide information that has been filtered and summarized by the author or editor to provide a quick and easy summary of a topic.* Some examples of tertiary resources include textbooks, compendia, review articles in journals, clinical guidelines, and other general information (see below for more detail). Some tertiary resources are available via online access as electronic books (eBooks) or electronically searchable online application (e.g., Micromedex®, Clinical Pharmacology®, Lexicomp®). These resources will provide the practitioner with general information needed to familiarize the reader with the topic. This is also an opportunity for the practitioner to gain general information about the disease or drug in question, which will ultimately result in a more structured and productive search. The types and usability of tertiary resources will be discussed later.

After evaluation of the information found in tertiary resources, a **secondary resource** may be employed to search additional resources that might provide more insight on the topic. ❸ *Secondary resources are mainly in the form of searchable database that enables location and retrieval of primary or tertiary resources.* This category of resources is similar to an old cataloging system. There are various secondary resources available either as paid (e.g., EBSCOhost, Excerpta Medica, CINAHL) or free (e.g., PubMed) subscription to many health care professionals. Using a secondary resource allows more efficient and expedient search for either primary literature (e.g., a clinical trial) or tertiary literature (e.g., a review) for a given topic. More information is provided in the section "Secondary Resources" of this chapter.

Primary resources include clinical research studies and reports, both published and unpublished. ❹ *There are several types of publications considered primary, including controlled trials, cohort studies, case series, and case reports.* Primary resources often provides the most recent and in-depth information about a topic, and allows the reader to analyze and critique the study methodology to determine if the conclusions are valid (see Chapters 4 and 5 for more information on critiquing the primary literature). Typically, primary resources require a longer time commitment and a skilled expertise in literature evaluation to accurately assess the value and application to health care. They may be available freely (e.g., open-access articles) or by paid subscription (e.g., New England Journal of Medicine).

Often a search for information does not require the use of all three types of resources. ❺ *Knowing the most appropriate resource for information retrieval is the first step in the provision of quality drug information.* For example, a question regarding commercial availability of a product formulation or mechanism of action could quickly be found in a tertiary resource, such as the product's prescribing information (i.e., package insert). The information found there may be sufficient to conclude the search and provide a response. However, a question regarding the clinical trials supporting off-label use in a specific population will likely require a search of primary literature.

The type of requestor may also substantially influence the resources used to respond to a question. Generally, a request from a consumer or patient could more appropriately be answered from available tertiary resources than from a stack of clinical trials. However, if the requestor is a prescriber requesting detailed information about the management of a specific disease state and role of investigational therapies, provision of primary literature may be appropriate.

Tertiary Resources

BENEFITS OF TERTIARY RESOURCES

Tertiary sources provide information that has been filtered and summarized by the author or editor to provide a quick and easy summary of a topic. Thus, these resources are convenient, easy to use, as well as being familiar to most practitioners. As mentioned earlier, some examples of tertiary resources include textbooks, compendia, review articles in journals, clinical guidelines, and other general information. Some tertiary resources are available via online access as eBooks or electronically searchable online application (e.g., Micromedex®, Clinical Pharmacology®, Lexicomp®). These resources will provide the practitioner with general information needed to familiarize the reader with the topic and these references may often serve as an initial place to identify information, since they provide a fairly complete and concise overview of information available on a specific topic. Most of the basic information needed by a practitioner can be found in these sources, making these excellent first-line resources when dealing with a DI question.

LIMITATIONS OF TERTIARY RESOURCES

Many tertiary resources are available in both hard copy (print) and electronic formats (e.g., eBooks, electronically searchable DI databases). The major drawback to print copy tertiary resources, however, is the lag time associated with updating information. Medical information changes very rapidly; thus, it is possible that information may be out of date before a text is even published. Electronically available tertiary resources, such as eBooks and DI databases (e.g., Micromedex®, Lexicomp®), have helped this situation in some cases; however, the requirement for information to be reviewed and summarized requires an inherent delay in communicating new information. It is also possible that information in a tertiary resource may be incomplete, due either to space limitations of the resource or incomplete literature searches by the author. Some types of questions that should be considered when evaluating tertiary literature are listed in Table 3-1.

Other problems that can be seen with tertiary information include errors in transcription, human bias, incorrect interpretation of information, or a lack of expertise by authors. It is also important to note that DI databases (e.g., Lexicomp®, Micromedex®, Facts & Comparison® eAnswers, Clinical Pharmacology®) may contain different information for

TABLE 3–1. EVALUATION OF TERTIARY LITERATURE

Does the author have appropriate experience/expertise to publish in this area?
Is the information likely to be timely, based on publication date?
Is information supported by appropriate citations?
Does the resource contain relevant information?
Does the resource appear free from bias and blatant errors?
Is the information most updated version of the resource?

a particular question. An example might be a drug's indications for use; some references and databases show the exact same language as the drug's prescribing information (e.g., package insert), whereas some contain more in-depth literature evaluation pertaining to off-label uses. One resource may be favored over the other depending on the question asked. Therefore, it is important to become familiar with the expertise, scope, and other characteristics of each database before using them, as discussed below. Over time, practitioners get familiar with and comfortable at using one or two resources only; however, because of their inherent differences in the extent and quality of information, it is critical to always review the contents carefully and consult more than one resource when possible before providing clinical recommendations.

SELECTING TERTIARY RESOURCES

It is impossible to acquire all available resources that are useful in all areas of clinical practice. It is also difficult to choose only one resource for a practice setting, because each resource may possess different level of accuracy, comprehensiveness, currency, and ease of use. Differences in practice setting, available funding, patient populations seen, and types of information most commonly needed all impact which tertiary resources should be available at a specific practice site. The legal requirements for information sources available at a practice setting vary from state to state, but rarely will the minimally required texts be sufficient to meet all information needs in a practice.

Another important factor in the selection of appropriate tertiary resources includes selecting a resource focused on the type of information needed for a specific request or situation. For example, a very well written and comprehensive therapeutics text may have very limited use in providing information regarding pharmacokinetics of a specific drug. For this reason, it is important to consider the type of information most commonly needed in a particular practice setting to ensure that appropriate tertiary resources are available.

FORMAT OF TERTIARY RESOURCES

Electronic resources are often preferred because they may be easier to use (a keyword search and an instant return of search results), allow quicker access to information, allow multiple searches to be performed simultaneously, and often contain more recent information available regarding a topic than is found in the hard copy version of a reference. Additionally, many electronic networked resources allow use of the same resource at more than one location. This lets many practitioners access information from a variety of physical locations rather than being restricted to only medical libraries or DI centers. Mobile apps have no geographic restriction to accessing and retrieving information once downloaded.

Many textbooks are now being combined into electronic packages, for example, the McGraw-Hill Professional product AccessPharmacy® (http://www.accesspharmacy.com). The combination of multiple resources in one package may make selection of resources for a practice site much easier, but also more costly. As these combination packages increase in popularity with students and universities, the expectations that practitioners have for access to resources in work settings will also likely continue to increase.

TERTIARY RESOURCES FOR MOBILE DEVICES

The increasing incorporation of mobile devices into clinical practice settings has prompted an expanding choice of DI databases for that medium. Many of the major compendia available electronically also offer a product for a mobile device. A study investigating the preferences of community pharmacists using apps found that approximately 80% of participants felt confident when using medical apps and found them useful with patient consultations (55%) and health care education (80%).[5] However, these devices and apps are not without limitations. Johnson and colleagues[7] evaluated six mobile point-of-care tools (Medscape®, UpToDate®, DynaMed Plus®, EvidencePlus®, DynaMed®, and Epocrates®) for breadth of coverage, ease of use, and quality; they found that some of these tools were ranked substandard for one or more of the criteria. It is also important to recognize that the information available in a mobile app version of a database may differ from that available in the online or hardcopy forms. One study looking specifically at various DI databases highlighted some of the variations that may exist between different forms of the same resource.[8] The study demonstrated that some online databases provided more scope and completeness of information than their mobile versions. While the specific functionality of an app and the way that one accesses information for an app may change, the information is generally similar.

A summary of selected tertiary resources is listed below to provide examples of some resources that may be useful in the general pharmacy practice. Information is provided about the features of the resource as well as the publisher and publisher website. While specific electronic resources may be hosted at a different website, the publisher site will direct users toward the appropriate link.

This list is not comprehensive and reflects only a limited number of resources available because it is impossible to compile a comprehensive list of all resources that are useful in all areas of practice. The Basic Resources for Pharmacy Education listing distributed by the American Association of Colleges of Pharmacy (AACP)[9] and Doody's Core Titles (https://www.doody.com/dct/) are helpful compilation of available resources for clinicians and students.

GENERAL MEDICATION INFORMATION

Below is a list of tertiary resources that are commonly used by DI specialist and health care professionals. Descriptions of each resource have been briefly provided only for a select list. More comprehensive and inclusive list of resources and their categories are available in Table 3-2.

AHFS® Drug Information

Published by the American Society of Health-System Pharmacists (www.ashp.org) and found at http://www.ahfsdruginformation.com. This DI resource is organized by monographs containing information on both the Food and Drug Administration (FDA)-approved and off-label uses of medications. Information about dosing in specific populations is also included, as is a wide variety of general information about medications. Some information is also available about compatibility and stability of injectable formulations. AHFS® is available in paper format (updated annually) and an excerpted paper format (*AHFS DI® Essentials™*), a mobile drug reference version, and as a part of subscription in databases, such as Lexicomp®.

Clinical Pharmacology®

Elsevier's Gold Standard, http://www.clinicalpharmacology.com. This electronic database contains monographs of prescription and nonprescription products as well as some dietary supplements. Tools within the database allow users to screen for drug interactions, create comparison tables for drug products, determine intravenous (IV) compatibility (based on Trissel's 2™ Clinical Pharmaceutics Database), and search for tablets by description or imprint codes. Patient education information is available in English and Spanish. It is available online or as a mobile application, however, it is not available in print.

ClinicalTrials.gov

This website (http://www.clinicaltrials.gov) is maintained by the National Institutes of Health and serves as a main registry for publicly and privately supported clinical studies of human participants conducted in the world. Health care professionals can locate clinical researches currently ongoing or to be conducted in the future, and register their research as investigators. The trial results are not always fully added to the database and require an additional search via secondary resources such as PubMed. Since not all

TABLE 3–2. USEFUL RESOURCES FOR COMMON CATEGORIES OF DRUG INFORMATION

Category	Resource
General, Product-Related	Major compendia,[a] prescribing information, PDR[b], MPR[c]
Adverse Effects	Meyler's Side Effects of Drugs,[10] Side Effects of Drugs Annual,[11] major compendia,[a] prescribing information, PDR,[b] FDAble (Medwatch)
Compatibility, Stability	Handbook of Injectable Drugs,[12] King Guide to Parenteral Admixtures,[13] Trissel's 2 Clinical Pharmaceutics Database,[14] Extended Stability for Parenteral Drugs,[15] Trissel's Stability of Compounded Formulations,[16] Remington: The Science and Practice of Pharmacy,[17] USP–National Formulary (NF)[18]
Compounding, Formulations	Remington: The Science and Practice of Pharmacy,[17] Merck Index,[19] A Practical Guide to Contemporary Pharmacy Practice,[20] USP/NF,[18] Trissel's Stability of Compounded Formulations,[16] Extemporaneous Formulations[21]
Dietary Supplements, Herbal Supplements	Natural Medicines,[22] Natural Medicines Comprehensive Database,[23] NIH's Dietary Supplement Label Database,[24] MedlinePlus,[25] AltMedDex,[26] Review of Natural Products[27]
Diseases, Diagnoses	Pharmacotherapy: A Pathophysiologic Approach,[28] Pharmacotherapy Principles and Practice,[29] Applied Therapeutics: The Clinical Use of Drugs,[30] The Merck Manual of Diagnosis and Therapy,[31] Harrison's Principles of Internal Medicine,[32] Goldman's Cecil Medicine,[33] Textbook of Therapeutics,[34] Conn's Current Therapy,[35] Medscape[36]
Drug Availability, Price	RED BOOK,[37] Clinical Pharmacology (Elsevier),[38] Lexi-Drugs,[39] Medi-Span Price Rx[40]
Drug Identification	Identidex,[41] Clinical Pharmacology,[38] Drugs.com, Ident-A-Drug Reference (Pharmacist's Letter Online),[42] Lexi-Drug ID,[39] Facts & Comparisons® eAnswers,[43] American Drug Index,[44] The Merck Index[19]
Drug Interactions	Hansten and Horn's Drug Interaction Analysis and Management,[45] Drug Interaction Facts,[46] Stockley's Drug Interactions,[47] major compendia[a]
Drug Use in Renal Dysfunction	Major compendia,[a] Drug Prescribing in Renal Failure: Dosing Guidelines for Adults (Aronoff)[48]
Geriatric Pharmacotherapy	Geriatric Dosage Handbook,[49] major compendia[a]
International Drugs	Drug Information Handbook with International Trade Names Index,[50] Martindale: The Complete Drug Reference,[51] Index Nominum International Drug Directory,[52] Drugdex,[53] Clinical Pharmacology[38]
Investigational Drugs	FDA website (http://www.fda.gov), Clinicaltrials.gov, MedlinePlus,[25] manufacturer websites
Laboratory Tests	Basic Skills in Interpreting Laboratory Data (ASHP),[54] Mosby's Manual of Diagnostics and Laboratory Test (Pagana),[55] Pocket Guide to Diagnostic Tests (Nicoll),[56] Laboratory Tests and Diagnostic Procedure[57]
Method/Rate of Administration	FDA prescribing information, Handbook on Injectable Drugs,[12] major compendia[a]
Nonprescription Drugs	Handbook of Nonprescription Drugs,[58] Nonprescription Product Therapeutics,[59] FDA product labeling, major compendia[a]

continued

TABLE 3–2. USEFUL RESOURCES FOR COMMON CATEGORIES OF DRUG INFORMATION (*CONTINUED*)

Category	Resource
Pediatric Pharmacotherapy	The Harriet Lane Handbook,[60] Pediatric and Neonatal Dosage Handbook,[61] Nelson Textbook of Pediatrics,[62] Neofax,[63] Red Book: Report of the Committee on Infectious Diseases,[64] major compendia[a]
Pharmaceutical Calculations	Pharmaceutical Calculations (Zatz),[65] Pharmaceutical Calculations (Ansel),[66] Lexi-Calc[39]
Pharmaceutical Manufacturers	Clinical Pharmacology,[38] RED BOOK,[37] major compendia,[a] PDR[b]
Pharmacokinetics	Basic Clinical Pharmacokinetics,[67] Applied Biopharmaceutics and Pharmacokinetics,[68] Martindale: The Complete Drug Reference,[51] major compendia[a]
Pharmacology	Goodman & Gilman's: The Pharmacological Basis of Therapeutics,[69] Basic & Clinical Pharmacology (Katzung and Trevor),[70] Brody's Human Pharmacology: Molecular to Clinical,[71] Principles of Pharmacology (Golan)[72]
Pharmacotherapeutics	Pharmacotherapy: A Pathophysiologic Approach (DiPiro),[28] Applied Therapeutics: The Clinical Use of Drugs,[30] Textbook of Therapeutics,[34] Pharmacotherapy Principles and Practice[29]
Pharmacy Law	Pharmacy Practice and the Law,[73] Guide to Federal Pharmacy Law,[74] State Board of Pharmacy websites
Pregnancy, Lactation	Briggs Drugs in Pregnancy and Lactation,[75] LactMed,[76] Medications and Mother's Milk,[77] Catalog of Teratogenic Agents, Drugs During Pregnancy and Lactation,[78] REPRORISK,[79] major compendia[a]
Toxicology	TOXNET,[80] LiverTox,[81] POISINDEX,[82] Lexi-Tox, Goldfrank's Toxicologic Emergencies,[83] Casarett & Doull's Toxicology: The Basic Science of Poisons,[84] Poisoning and Toxicology Handbook[85]
Veterinary Medicine	Textbook of Veterinary Internal Medicine,[86] Veterinary Pharmacology and Therapeutics (Riviere),[87] The Merck Veterinary Manual (MVM),[88] Plumb's Veterinary Drug Handbook,[89] Exotic Animal Formulary,[90] FDA Center for Veterinary Medicine,[91] Animal Drugs@FDA,[92] Pet Education,[93] Pet Place,[94] Pets with Diabetes,[95] USP Veterinary Medicine[96]

[a]Major compendia include Clinical Pharmacology, Drugdex (Micromedex), Lexi-Drugs (Drug Information Handbook), Drug Facts and Comparisons, Martindale: The Complete Drug Reference, and AHFS Drug Information.
[b]Prescribers' Digital Reference (online).
[c]Monthly Prescribing Reference (online).

clinical trials, particularly those with negative results, are published, this can be a valuable source for professionals to try to locate unpublished data.

DailyMed

The U.S. National Library of Medicine, https://dailymed.nlm.nih.gov/. This electronic resource contains over 95,000 drugs in its monograph format as approved for marketing by the FDA (i.e., prescribing information). It is current and cross-references with FDA's website to provide FDA guidance, new DI, and updated warnings. DI can be searched with keywords or by drug class. This resource includes DI for both human and animals.

Drugs.com

Drugs.com, http://www.drugs.com. This online resource includes drug monographs, tablet/capsule identifier, interactions checker, and news related to medication approvals or recalls. The professional version provides more detailed information sourcing from reliable sources such as AHFS® DI, Micromedex®, Stedman's Medial Dictionary, and FDA. Drugs are searchable either as a keyword or choosing one from an alphabetical list. It is also available as a mobile application. One limitation of this resource is inclusion of commercial advertisements on each page of website.

Epocrates®

Epocrates, https://online.epocrates.com This family of electronic resources includes both mobile and online products. These resources include information about drugs (e.g., monographs, interaction checker, safety data, tablet identification) and diseases (epidemiology, prognosis, treatment). It is also available as a mobile application.

Facts and Comparisons®

Wolters Kluwer Health, Inc., http://www.factsandcomparisons.com. This reference is available both in print (updated quarterly) and online (Facts & Comparisons® eAnswers), and contains monographs for prescription and nonprescription drugs organized by drug class. The online database version includes a suite references such as drug comparison tables, immunization resources, manufacturer index, orphan drugs, patient assistance programs, toxicology guidelines, Review of Natural Products, and pregnancy and lactation warnings. The database also includes interactive tools such as drug identifier, drug interactions, Trissel's IV Check™, and clinical calculators. There are comparative monographs of drug classes to help discern differences between agents of the same class. This resource is also available as a mobile app, based on the subscription and availability. The database platform is available either in the current or the newer model with a similar appearance to Lexicomp®.

Handbook of Nonprescription Drugs: An Interactive Approach to Self-Care

American Pharmacists Association®, http://www.pharmacist.com. This text is organized by body system, focusing on those disease states for which self-care may be appropriate. Information is provided about FDA-approved dosing information, comparative efficacy of various over-the-counter (OTC) agents, as well as contraindications for self-treatment, drug interactions, and other safety information. It also includes information on herbal supplements and nondrug preventive measures. Use of treatment algorithms and patient care cases make this resource especially helpful for students and new practitioners. The text is also available as an e-book.

Index Nominum: International Drug Directory

Medpharm Scientific Publishers GmbH, http://www.medpharm.de. This DI reference contains information on over 4,500 drugs available in over 130 countries, with generic names, synonyms, and proprietary names as well as their chemical formulas, chemical structures, and therapeutic class. It is also available online as part of Micromedex®'s suite of references (subscription dependent).

Lexicomp®

Wolters Kluwer Health, Inc., http://online.lexi.com/action/home. This searchable database allows for integrated searches of various products (depending on subscription purchased) and includes a variety of references such as Lexi-Drugs, Geriatric Lexi-Drugs, Pediatric and Neonatal Lexi-Drugs, Lexi-Tox, Drug Allergy and Idiosyncratic Reactions, and Trissel's™ 2 Clinical Pharmaceutics Database. Lexicomp® has also partnered with AHFS® (described above) to offer an electronic subscription combining their two databases in a seamless search. The print version of Lexi-Drugs, Drug Information Handbook, is a monograph-based DI and available in multiple patient- and profession-specific references such as Geriatric Dosage Handbook, Pediatric and Neonatal Dosage Handbook, Drug Information Handbook for Nursing, and Drug Information Handbook for Oncology. Lexi-Drugs includes information on drug's product availability, price, clinical practice guideline references, and pharmacogenomics. Lexi-Drugs and its companion resources are available via mobile applications but require an additional subscription for them. Additional subscriptions include another useful resource, UpToDate, and allow for cross-referencing between the two databases.

Martindale: The Complete Drug Reference/MedicinesComplete

Pharmaceutical Press, http://www.pharmpress.com. This reference is considered one of the most comprehensive and trusted information sources on a variety of domestic and international drugs, including over 6,000 drug monographs in print and over 7,500 online, covering over 40 countries. It also includes treatment reviews, with references from published articles. Proprietary names and manufacturer contact information are available for a variety of countries. Some information is provided about common herbal products as well as diagnostic agents, radioactive pharmaceuticals, and some veterinary products. This information is available in hardcopy and via online (MedicinesComplete) subscription.

Medscape

Medscape, http://www.medscape.com. This electronic research is published by WebMD® that references over 125 medical journals and textbooks. It is a free subscription service that allows the health care professional to register their information preferences and it will send you the latest information within a particular specialty area. It also provides a free weekly e-mailed newsletter with the latest highlights with the field. It includes clinical information as well as financial, managed care, and medical practice information, and provides simplified monographs for DI as well as dose calculation. This resource is also available as a mobile application.

Micromedex®

Truven Health Analytics, http://www.micromedex.com. This electronic resource contains multiple references within the database including monograph-based DI both in the short (i.e., DrugPoint) and in-depth (i.e., Drugdex) platform providing FDA-approved indications, off-label uses, pharmacokinetic data, safety information, and pharmacology. Multiple interactive tools are available to assess for drug–drug/food/supplement interactions, IV incompatibilities (via Trissel's IV Compatibility), and pharmacokinetic adjustments. It includes a toxicology-related tool that allows identification of drugs based on imprint codes and discussion of overdose management. Patient-education materials are available via its CareNote reference. Micromedex® is available online and as a suite of multiple mobile applications (e.g., Micromedex® IV Compatibility, Micromedex® Drug Interactions).

MPR®

Haymarket Media, Inc., http://www.empr.com. This resource (also known as the *Monthly Prescribing Reference*) is available in print, online, and as a mobile app. The online and mobile versions are freely available; however, the print version requires a subscription. In the online version, DI is searchable by brand name, generic name, therapeutic category, and manufacturer. It also includes updates on new drugs and medical devices. The online version, however, includes several commercial advertisements on each page of website as well as pushed to the screen during search.

Physicians' Desk Reference/Prescribers' Digital Reference (PDR)

PDR, http://www.pdr.net. This resource is one of the oldest DI references and a compilation of prescription product's official prescribing information (i.e., package insert). It is available online or as mobile application (mobilePDR) and is available without subscription after a free registration via the website. The reference includes contact information for manufacturers and a list of poison control centers. It also publishes a patient-friendly version called PDR+ for Patients (http://www.pdr.net/browse-by-consumer-monograph-name/) for viewing and printing information on over 2,300 medications. In addition to the original PDR, there are a variety of focused editions, including the PDR® for Herbal Medicines, PDR® for Nutritional Supplements, PDR® for Ophthalmic Medicines, PDR® for Nonprescription Drugs, and the newest, PDR Drug Information Handbook.

U.S. Food and Drug Administration (FDA)

This website (http://www.fda.gov) provides very comprehensive information regarding drugs, food and dietary supplements, medical devices, vaccines, biologics, veterinary products, cosmetics, and tobacco products. It provides updates on drug recalls, medication safety information and adverse drug events, drug approvals, changes to the drug labeling, medication guides, and documents exchanged between the manufacturer and FDA during drug approval process. FDA-approved DI is searchable at Drugs@FDA by using brand, generic, or application number. The Orange Book is a helpful resource within the website that lists approved drug products with therapeutic equivalent evaluations. The website is also available in 15 different languages and for consumer use. Information such as drug shortages and drug recalls are also available via mobile apps.

USP Dictionary of United States Adopted Names (USAN) and International Drug Names

U.S. Pharmacopeial Convention, http://www.usp.org. This is the official resource for determining generic and chemical names of over 5,000 drugs as well as the international nonproprietary name. Additionally, useful information such as chemical structure, molecular weight, Chemical Abstracts Services (CAS) registry number, and a pronunciation guide are provided. This resource is available in print and online (subscription required).

ADVERSE EFFECTS

FDAble

FDAble, LLC, http://www.fdable.com. This online resource allows a search for adverse drug events reported to the FDA's MedWatch, FDA Adverse Event Reporting System (FAERS), Manufacturer and User Facility Device Experience (MAUDE), and Vaccine Adverse Event Reporting System (VAERS). The resource contains over 8 million adverse drug event cases, about 95,000 vaccine adverse event cases, and over 4.6 million medical device adverse event cases. It provides up to 30 events specific to a drug, device, or vaccine for free; obtaining more than 30 events requires a user to send a request with a fee. An event report includes suspected drug, adverse reaction, patient outcomes, patient's age and gender, and event date.

Meyler's Side Effects of Drugs

Elsevier Science, http://www.elsevier.com. As one of the most comprehensive information on adverse drug effects, this reference provides a critical review of international literature in the area of adverse events with thorough referencing. Chapters are organized by drug classification; adverse events are organized by drug name and then by organ system within each drug. Information is provided about adverse events and management.

It is published every 4 years, and complementary issues are published every year as Side Effects of Drugs Annual. It is available in print and as an eBook. Note that the books are not comprehensive. In any particular edition, it may refer you back to previous editions for further information on a topic.

Side Effects of Drugs Annual

Elsevier Publishing, http://www.elsevier.com. This reference is updated annually and serves as a companion to the text Meyler's Side Effects of Drugs. A team evaluates international literature published each year to identify new information and summarize that information in this resource. It is available in print and as an eBook.

DIETARY AND HERBAL SUPPLEMENTS

Dietary Supplement Label Database

The NIH Office of Dietary Supplements, http://www.dsld.nlm.nih.gov. This free online database is published and maintained by the Office of Dietary Supplements. It is one of the most comprehensive and unbiased resources on dietary and natural supplements, and includes the proprietary names, formulations, dietary claims made, and target consumer of available supplements. The online search feature makes it easy to navigate and find products containing particular ingredients.

Natural Medicines

Therapeutic Research Center, https://naturalmedicines.therapeuticresearch.com. This online resource uses a similar platform as that of Natural Medicines Comprehensive Database and includes detailed information on over 1,400 monographs with evidence-based ratings and references. It also includes information on drug–herb and drug–food interactions and safety during pregnancy and lactation.

Natural Medicines Comprehensive Database

Therapeutic Research Faculty, http://naturaldatabase.therapeuticresearch.com. This resource is available in a text, online, and mobile device formats, and is one of the most comprehensive resources on dietary and herbal supplements. It is also available as part of other publications. The database provides a summary of the information available for various dietary supplements and rates the relative safety and efficacy of those products. The electronic version includes an interaction checker and disease state/condition search, and can be accessed as a suite of references via Pharmacist's Letter. The electronic resource has also partnered with the USP-Verified program to indicate which supplements have been certified to contain a quality product by USP Verified.

Review of Natural Products

Facts and Comparisons Publishing Group, http://www.factsandcomparisons.com. This resource provides information about the chemistry, pharmacology, and toxicology of a number of natural products, based on references to primary literature. A summary of relevant clinical trials is also available. There is also limited patient counseling information, but the strength of this resource is in the chemistry and pharmacology information. Recent revisions have dramatically increased the amount of information included in patient counseling sections. This is available in loose-leaf, bound, online, and mobile device formats.

DRUG IDENTIFICATION (U.S. AND FOREIGN)

Ident-A-Drug

Therapeutic Research Faculty, http://www.indentadrug.com. This resource is organized by imprint codes and provides identification of drugs based on those codes. Descriptions of medications as well as NDC and Canadian DIN numbers are provided. This resources is accessed through Pharmacist's Letter Online.

Identidex

Truven Health Analytics, http://www.micromedex.com. This electronic resource can be accessed via Micromedex® and allows search by either description (e.g., color, shape, pattern) or imprint code. It provides information on dosage form, color, shape, active and inactive ingredients, manufacturer, NDC numbers, and available containers.

Lexi-DrugID

Wolters Kluwer, www.lexi.com. This resource is accessed through Lexicomp® and allows search by using one or more descriptors such as imprint, dosage form, color, or shape. It includes a picture of the product.

DRUG INTERACTIONS

Drug Interactions Analysis and Management (Hansten and Horn)

Wolters Kluwer, http://www.hanstenandhorn.com. This print resource provides summaries, mechanism, and management of reported drug interactions. The authors also provide information regarding severity of interaction and any risk factors that might predispose patients to this event. The reference is updated annually. Both provide rapid information regarding severity and likelihood of an interaction and actions needed to minimize this risk based on the case studies and primary literature available. Some of this content is integrated into other electronic Facts and Comparisons® products.

Drug Interaction Facts

Wolters Kluwer Health, Inc., http://www.factsandcomparisons.com. This resource provides information about drug–drug or drug–food interactions. Discussions of significance of the interaction as well as suggestions for management are included. This is available in both print and electronic formats as part of the Facts & Comparisons® eAnswers suite.

Stockley's Drug Interactions

Pharmaceutical Press, http://www.pharmpress.com. This print resource includes in-depth information on interactions among drugs, herbal medicines, foods, and drinks. It includes an assessment of the clinical importance of interactions and guidance on managing the interaction in practice. The online version is available via the MedicinesComplete database (http://www.medicinescomplete.com).

Case Study 3–1

A 15-year-old patient has recently been started on atomoxetine for treatment of attention deficit/hyperactivity disorder. He is taking no other medications. He has noted recently that his hair is thinning and wants to know if this might be drug related.

• *What are appropriate tertiary resources to consult for a response to this request?*

DRUG PRICE

RED BOOK Drug Topics

Truven Health Analytics, http://www.redbook.com. This resource primarily contains data regarding prescription and OTC product availability and pricing. There are also a number of tables listing information such as sugar-free, lactose-free, or alcohol-free preparations. Additionally, information such as National Drug Code (NDC) numbers, routes of administration, dosage form, size, and strength are included. This resource is available in paper copy and electronically within Micromedex®.

PHARMACOKINETICS

Applied Biopharmaceutics and Pharmacokinetics

McGraw-Hill Professional, https://www.mheducation.ca/professional/products/ 9780071830935/applied+biopharmaceutics+%7C%7C+pharmacokinetics,+seventh+ edition/. This text describes the role of pharmacokinetics as it relates to drug development and to patient care. This covers the clinical application of pharmacokinetics and addresses the impact of pharmacogenetics on drug metabolism. This text is also included in the AccessPharmacy™ electronic subscription.

Applied Clinical Pharmacokinetics

McGraw-Hill Education, https://www.mhprofessional.com/9780071794589-usa-applied-clinical-pharmacokinetics-3e-group. This print resource emphasizes the practical issues of drug dosing for patients with changes in pharmacokinetics and pharmacodynamic parameters, especially antibiotic drugs, anticonvulsants, and immunosuppressants. It is available as part of the AccessPharmacy™ suite of electronic textbooks.

Concepts in Clinical Pharmacokinetics

American Society of Health-System Pharmacists Publishing, https://store.ashp.org/ Store/ProductListing/ProductDetails.aspx?productId=153117615. This print resource includes clinical cases and topics in pharmacogenetics in addition to other pharmacokinetics concepts. It is also available as an eBook.

PHARMACOLOGY

Goodman & Gilman's: The Pharmacological Basis of Therapeutics

McGraw-Hill Professional, http://www.mcgraw-hill.com. This classic pharmacology text also provides information about pharmacokinetics and pharmacodynamics of a number of drugs. The focus of the resource is to provide a correlation between principles of pharmacology and contemporary clinical practice. The text makes extensive use of charts and tables to convey information. This text is also included in the AccessPharmacy™ electronic subscription.

Basic & Clinical Pharmacology (Katzung and Trevor)

McGraw-Hill Professional, http://www.mcgraw-hill.com. This text, organized by therapeutic class of agents, provides general discussion of pharmacology principles as well as more detailed discussion of specific agents. Figures and tables are frequently used to illustrate difficult material. This text is also included in the AccessPharmacy™ electronic subscription.

Brody's Human Pharmacology: Molecular to Clinical

Elsevier, http://www.elsevier.com. This text is designed with a student focus and emphasizes therapeutic impact of pharmacology. Students can use Student Consult which provides exam question, animations, and colorful illustrations. The text is organized by organ system impacted. The text also has accompanying mobile device downloads and is available as an eBook.

Principles of Pharmacology (Golan)

Wolters Kluwer, http://www.lww.com. This textbook is designed for students with clinical vignettes illustrating therapeutic problems and discussions. Chapters are listed by organ systems with highlighted key points and drug summary tables. This resource is also available as an eBook.

PHARMACY LAW

Information about individual state pharmacy law is best obtained through the individual state boards of pharmacy. A listing of state board website URLs is available at http://www.nabp.net/boards-of-pharmacy. Often the board will have this information available in PDF format on the website. The Code of Federal Regulations containing aspects of federal law is available at http://www.ecfr.gov. One general text about federal law is listed below.

Pharmacy Practice and the Law

Jones and Bartlett Publishers, http://www.jblearning.com. This print resource contains information about federal laws and regulations impacting pharmacy practice. Additional implications for pharmacy practice are provided for some legislation. Information is provided about federal and state regulations of product development, dispensing, and development. Various summaries of case law are provided.

PREGNANT AND LACTATING WOMEN

Drugs in Pregnancy and Lactation (Briggs)

Lippincott Williams & Wilkins, http://www.lww.com. This reference (often referred to as Briggs) focuses exclusively on the use of medications in pregnant or lactating women. Fetal risk summaries are provided via evaluation of the literature regarding the safety of fetal exposure *in utero* or exposure through breast milk. Animal literature is provided in cases where human literature is lacking. The online version is incorporated into tertiary databases such as Lexicomp® and Fact & Comparisons® eAnswers.

Drugs and Lactation Database (LactMed)

The U.S. National Library of Medicine (NLM), http://www.nlm.nih.gov. A peer-reviewed and fully referenced database of drugs to which breastfeeding mothers may be exposed; accessible through TOXNET database (http://toxnet.nlm.nih.gov/cgi-bin/sis/htmlgen?LACT) hosted by NLM. Among the included data are maternal and infant levels of drugs, possible effects on breastfed infants and on lactation, and alternate drugs to consider. This database is available as a mobile app for both Android and iOS devices.

Reprotox, Reprorisk System

Truven Health Analytics, http://truvenhealth.com. Retrieved through Micromedex® system, it provides comprehensive information on general toxicity, fertility, genetic influences, and teratogenic agents, and helps clinicians to evaluate human reproductive risks of drugs, chemicals, and physical/environmental agents. It is updated quarterly and available only online.

Catalog of Teratogenic Agents

Johns Hopkins University Press, http://www.press.jhu.edu. This print resource covers pharmaceuticals, chemicals, environmental pollutants, food additives, household products, and viruses and their possible teratogenicity. Special attention has been paid to including the international as well as domestic information.

SPECIAL POPULATIONS (GERIATRIC, PEDIATRIC)

Geriatric Dosage Handbook

Wolters Kluwer Health, Inc., http://www.lexi.com. The monographs in this resource contain traditional sections of DI, but focus on dosing recommendations for geriatric patients. There is a special section of each monograph addressing concerns specific to the geriatric population. Limited references to primary literature are provided. This reference is also available online and as a mobile app.

The Harriet Lane Handbook

Elsevier, http://www.us.elsevierhealth.com. This resource, assembled by medical residents, contains a succinct discussion of common diseases and conditions of newborn to adolescent patients. A significant portion of the book is dedicated to medication dosing, specifically pediatrics. This resource also contains information about common side effects and dosage forms available and includes a variety of topic areas, such as palliative care and toxicology. There is a separate publication that focuses on antimicrobial therapy. This resource is also available for mobile devices and as part of a supplemental reference in online databases such as Clinical Pharmacology.

Pediatric and Neonatal Dosage Handbook

Wolters Kluwer Health, Inc., http://www.lexi.com. The monographs in this resource contain traditional sections of DI, but focus on detailed dosing recommendations for pediatrics. It also includes information about common extemporaneous preparations for pediatric use. Limited references to primary literature are provided. This reference is also available online and for mobile devices.

Red Book: Report of the Committee on Infectious Diseases

American Academy of Pediatrics, http://www.aap.org. Written by the Committee on Infectious Diseases of the organization, this reference provides recommendations for care of pediatric patients from immunizations to summaries of infectious diseases and treatment. It is updated every 3 years and available in print and online.

_____ Case Study 3-2

A new mother has been breastfeeding her child for 3 months. The mother has recently been prescribed levofloxacin for treatment of an infection.

- *What sources should be consulted to determine the appropriateness of this choice?*
- *Is it safe for her to continue breastfeeding during this therapy?*
- *What additional information is needed to help shape your search strategy?*

STABILITY/COMPATIBILITY/COMPOUNDING

Handbook on Injectable Drugs

American Society of Health-System Pharmacists, https://www.ashp.org/marketing/handbookLP1.html. This resource, commonly called Trissel's, includes information regarding the compatibility and stability of various parenteral medications. Information is primarily provided in the form of charts and tables, making finding information relatively quick. This resource also provides information about routes of administration and commercially available strengths. This information is available in a print resource as well as being included in major compendia such as Facts & Comparisons® eAnswers and Clinical Pharmacology.

King Guide to Parenteral Admixtures

King Guide Publications, http://www.kingguide.com. This resource is one of the most comprehensive and oldest references covering over 450 IV drug monographs, focused on compatibility information for parenteral medications. Stability information is also included, although limited. This resource is available in loose-leaf, bound copy, online, and via database incorporation such as Facts & Comparisons® eAnswers.

Trissel's Stability of Compounded Formulations

American Pharmacists Association Publications, http://www.pharmacist.com. This reference is only available in print and provides stability information on medications that are compounded or mixed as oral, enteral, topical, ophthalmic, and other special formulations. It summarizes the literature regarding the stability for efficient evaluation and provides proper storage and packaging information.

Extemporaneous Formulations for Pediatric, Geriatric, and Special Needs Patients

American Society of Health-System Pharmacists, https://store.ashp.org/Store/ProductListing/ProductDetails.aspx?productId=484090199. This resource is a compilation of published formulations with stability data. Most products are oral formulations to reflect the unique needs of some pediatric patients. Information is also provided about legal and technical issues in compounding practices. It is available in print and as an electronic copy.

Merck Index

Merck & Co., Inc., https://www.rsc.org/merck-index. This resource is one of the oldest resources focusing on information on chemicals and drug ingredients. It provides descriptions of the chemical and pharmacological information about a variety of chemicals, drugs, and biologicals. Data include CAS number, chemical structure, molecular weight, and physical data, including solubility, which may be especially useful in compounding. This reference is available in print and online (The Merck Index Online).

Remington: The Science and Practice of Pharmacy

Pharmaceutical Press, http://www.pharmpress.com. This classic text contains information about all aspects of pharmacy practice. There is discussion of social issues impacting pharmacy as well as information about the basics of pharmaceutics, manufacturing, pharmacodynamics, nuclear pharmacy, and medicinal chemistry. Information is provided regarding common compounding techniques and ingredients. The paper text is divided into two volumes for print copy and is also available online.

USP/NF

U.S. Pharmacopeial Convention, http://www.usp.org. This resource, available in print and online formats, contains the official substance and product standards. Also, official preparation instructions are given for a limited number of commonly compounded products.

THERAPY EVALUATION/DRUG OF CHOICE

Applied Therapeutics (Koda-Kimble and Young's)

Lippincott Williams & Wilkins, http://www.lww.com. This text includes information about disease states and treatment options. Information is presented in the form of cases with follow-up discussion. Its focus is on clinical case-based presentation of information. It is available in both print and as an eBook.

Centers for Disease Control and Prevention (CDC)

A division of the Department of Health and Human Services, the CDC (http://www.cdc.gov) is the frontline information medium for any diseases of interest affecting a large patient population such as infectious disease and other epidemics of interest. It includes data and statistics regarding various diseases and conditions and practice recommendations for emergency preparedness and natural disasters. CDC also publishes *Morbidity and Mortality Weekly Report* (MMWR) which is CDC's main scientific publication of public health information and recommendation. MMWR is available free of charge via e-mail as it is published, simply by signing up for it. CDC-INFO on Demand includes valuable information that can be shared with patients. The resource is also available as a mobile app.

Goldman-Cecil Medicine

Saunders, http://www.us.elsevierhealth.com. As one of the oldest and most respected textbooks in internal medicine, this resource is available in print, online as eBook, and as mobile application, as well as incorporated in databases such as ClinicalKey (Elsevier). Information is organized by disease state and color-coded to speed usage. Information about etiology, manifestations, diagnosis, treatment, and prognosis is provided.

Harrison's Principles of Internal Medicine

McGraw-Hill Professional, http://www.mcgraw-hill.com. This text serves as a fairly comprehensive introduction to clinical medicine. It is available in text and electronic formats. Comprehensive information is presented including pathophysiology, differential diagnosis, and disease management. This text is also included in the AccessPharmacy™ electronic subscription.

The Merck Manual of Diagnosis and Therapy

Merck & Co. Inc., http://www.merck.com. This source provides a quick summary of disease state information, including pathology, symptoms, diagnosis, and treatment. It is also available online as a free resource at http://www.merckmanuals.com and as a mobile device app.

Medscape

WebMD, http://www.medscape.com. This electronic resource provides extensive information about disease states and conditions. It includes news and updates on treatment as well as clinical briefs, patient cases, slideshows, drug updates, and continuing education for health care providers. In addition, it includes basic monographs about prescription and OTC medications. It is available online and as a mobile app.

Pharmacotherapy: A Pathophysiological Approach (DiPiro)

McGraw-Hill Professional, http://www.mcgraw-hill.com. This textbook focuses on the management of a variety of disease states. Information provided about disorders include epidemiology, etiology, presentation of disease, treatment, and treatment outcomes. This is available in text and electronic formats. This resource also has accompanying texts: Pharmacotherapy Casebook: A Patient-Focused Approach and Pharmacotherapy Handbook. These resources are also included in the AccessPharmacy™ electronic subscription.

Pharmacotherapy Principles and Practice

McGraw-Hill Professional, http://www.mcgraw-hill.com. This text focuses on the management of a variety of disease states, centering on the diseases most likely to be seen by pharmacists, nurse practitioners, and physician assistants. It is somewhat more concise than Pharmacotherapy: A Pathophysiological Approach; it also contains various features to help student learning. Information provided about disorders include epidemiology, etiology, presentation of disease, treatment, and treatment outcomes. This is available in text and electronic formats. This resource also has accompanying text, Pharmacotherapy Principles and Practice Study Guide. It is also available as an add-on reference for AccessPharmacy™.

Textbook of Therapeutics

Lippincott Williams & Wilkins, http://www.lww.com. This text is available in print and as an eBook. While the resource focuses on treatment of disease states and development of a therapeutic plan, sections regarding pathophysiology and clinical presentation are also provided.

TOXICOLOGY

Casarett & Doull's Toxicology: The Basic Science of Poisons

McGraw-Hill Medical, http://www.mheducation.com. This resource provides a broad coverage of a basic approach to toxicology and presents information from general principles to organ-specific toxicology. This resource is available online as part of the AccessMedical™ or AccessPharmacy™ suite of resources.

Goldfrank's Toxicologic Emergencies

McGraw-Hill Education, http://www.mheducation.com. The text is one of the most comprehensive resources focusing on poisoning and overdose. It discusses clinical application of toxicology and poisoning and provides a case study approach to medical toxicology and poison management. It is available in print and through the AccessMedical™ or AccessPharmacy™ suite of resources.

Lexi-Tox®

Wolters Kluwer, http://www.lexi.com. This resource is accessed through Lexicomp® and contains information on agents of toxicity including chemical, pharmaceutical, nuclear, biologic, and terrorism agents, along with toxic bite information (i.e., envenomation). It also includes information on nontoxic agents, antidotes and decontaminants, household products, toxicology-specific calculations, and a drug identification tool.

Poisoning and Toxicology Handbook

CRC Press, http://www.crcpress.com. This print resource covers the uses, mechanism of action, adverse reactions, and pregnancy implications of over 900 drugs and poisons, and supplies Chemical Abstract Services Number and the United Nations/United States Department of Transportation number. This resource is also available as an eBook.

ToxFacts Treatment Guidelines

Facts and Comparison Publishing, http://www.factsandcomparisons.com. This resource is accessed through Facts & Comparisons® eAnswers and compiles toxicology-related information from human data published in primary biomedical journals and texts. Each guideline is well referenced and covers a comprehensive list of chemicals and ingredients.

TOXNET

U.S. National Library of Medicine, http://www.nlm.nih.gov. This free online resource is published and maintained by the NLM and includes a suite of databases such as LactMed, HSDB (Hazardous Substances Data Bank), TOXLINE, DART (Developmental

Toxicology Literature), and CTD (Comparative Toxicogenomics Database). It provides a search option to include all of the various available databases or to use one database for a more focused search.

Case Study 3–3

A pharmacy student is working on a presentation involving illicit drugs. She knows that there have been recent news stories about adolescents using Coricidin™ products for recreational use, and she is curious at what doses these products are toxic.

- *Which resources would be useful for her project?*
- *What search terms might she utilize?*

VETERINARY MEDICINE

Veterinary medicine as a specialty practice is a growing area in the United States, and pharmacists are interested in obtaining veterinary-specific knowledge and skills. The growth in veterinary medicine has allowed health care professionals, especially pharmacists, to apply their drug knowledge resources to veterinary situations.

Supporting the growth of veterinary medicine is the concept of "One Medicine," a blending of veterinary medicine and human medicine for the benefit of public health, and to better serve human and animal patients alike. From a pharmacy perspective, veterinary medicine and human medicine complement each other, with the human-trained pharmacist being uniquely positioned to educate and serve veterinarians and animal owners.

Opportunities for the practical application of One Medicine can occur in community pharmacy settings as most pharmacists practicing in a community setting have been presented with prescriptions for animal patients at some time during their career. Veterinarians outsource prescriptions to community pharmacists to help control inventory, high drug costs, and the need for compounded drug therapies. The use of human-labeled pharmaceuticals prescribed in an off-label manner to treat companion animal's disease states is a viable option for veterinary medicine. These factors contribute to a situation where pharmacists who receive veterinary prescriptions can be challenged in their knowledge of veterinary drugs, indications, dosages, disease states, and therapeutic monitoring parameters.

American Veterinary Medical Association

American Veterinary Medical Association (AVMA), http://www.avma.org. This website has a wealth of information for pharmacists and veterinarians alike. There is a collection of valuable veterinary compounding guidelines, brochures, federal regulations, frequently asked questions, definitions of compounding, and the AVMA compounding position statements (http://www.avma.org/KB/Resources/Reference/Pages/Compounding.aspx). This information is an excellent starting point for any health care professional wishing to prescribe, provide, or utilize compounded drug products for animal patients.

Animal Poison Control Center

American Society for the Prevention of Cruelty to Animals (ASPCA), https://www.aspca.org/pet-care/animal-poison-control. This website focuses on animal toxicology and safety and is the premier resource for pharmacists in a community setting who may receive poisoning questions about animals. A toll-free number is available for immediate assistance when faced with a toxicology problem (888-426-4435), and a fee is required. The center has extensive experience in assisting veterinarians in poison management by providing immediate and specific treatment recommendations. The site also provides useful information on poison prevention, human medications that are poisonous to pets, and guidance on what to do if a pet is poisoned. References to toxicology publications and general consultation are listed in this website.

Compendium of Veterinary Products (CVP)

North American Compendiums, http://naccvp.com. This online reference is similar to the human PDR in terms of information provided and format. The resource contains the product monographs for over 5,000 FDA-approved pharmaceuticals, USDA-approved biologicals, diagnostic, feed additive, and Environmental Protection Agency (EPA)-approved pesticide products that are currently available. The reference contains indexes of manufacturers and distributors, brand name/ingredient indexes, and product category indexes.

FDA/CVM Homepage

FDA Center for Veterinary Medicine, http://www.fda.gov/AnimalVeterinary. This website provides information about the legal or regulatory issues that affect the practice of veterinary pharmacy or veterinary medicine. It is useful for regulatory issues pertaining to animal health. The compliance policy guide (CPG 608.400) "Compounding of Drugs for Use in Animals" and the Animal Medicinal Drug Use Clarification Act (AMDUCA) can be found at this site. Center for Veterinary Medicine (CVM) updates are available that detail the prohibited use of drugs in certain animal populations. Updates on the judicious use of antibiotics in food producing animals are posted at this site. A listing of all FDA-approved animal drug products, also known as the "Green Book," is available and searchable at this site. Patent information, manufacturer lists, indications, approval numbers, general DI, code of regulations, and trade/generic names are just a few pieces of information that can be gathered from this website. Practitioners can also access the FDA Veterinarian Newsletter from this site.

Pet Place

The website (http://www.petplace.com) has pet centers focusing on different species (dog, cat, bird, horses, fish, reptiles, and small mammals) and is written for laypersons. The database includes articles on veterinary disease states and preventative medicine. The drug library search tool allows the user to find DI on a specific pharmaceutical. There are also text and graphics describing medication administration techniques for dogs and cats.

Pets with Diabetes

The website (http://www.petdiabetes.com) contains information on diabetes in small animals particularly dogs and cats. The website offers general diabetes education and DI and is written for laypersons. The site also offers insight into and information on home testing and complications. There are also resources to support owners of diabetic animals.

Plumb's Veterinary Drug Handbook

Wiley-Blackwell Publishing, www.wiley.com/wiley-blackwell. This resource is considered one of the most useful references for extra-label drug dosages, indications, and specific DI on human- and veterinary-labeled pharmaceuticals. Monographs are listed in alphabetical order, and categorize the drugs' chemistry, pharmacology, indications, species dosing, contraindications, and interactions into an easily identifiable format. It is often referred to as "The Virus" in veterinary medicine because it is everywhere. A client information booklet is also available. This resource is available in print, online, and as mobile application.

Small Animal Clinical Pharmacology and Therapeutics

Saunders Ltd., www.elseiver.com. A useful pharmacology reference textbook focusing on pharmaceuticals for the prevention and treatment of small animal diseases. The book is divided into three sections detailing principles of drug therapy with special attention to clinical relevancy, the use of drugs from a categorical basis, and pharmaceutical use from a body systems approach. It is available in print and eBook either as an electronic publication or as a downloadable PDF file.

Textbook of Veterinary Internal Medicine

Saunders, http://www.us.elsevierhealth.com. This is a practical, valuable, and informative two-volume resource, focusing on internal medicine topics in canines and felines.

The text provides extensive coverage of pathophysiology, diagnosis, and treatment of diseases affecting dogs and cats. This resource is available in print and eBook that allows a search using keywords and includes clinical video clips.

The Merck Veterinary Manual (MVM)

Merck & Co., Inc., http://www.merck.com. The manual has served veterinarians and other health care professionals as a concise and reliable animal health reference for over 45 years. The full-text electronic version is available for free online (http://www.merck-vetmanual.com). A guide to abbreviations used in veterinary medicine is also included.

Veterinary Pharmacology and Therapeutics

Wiley-Blackwell, http://www.wiley.com. This textbook provides comprehensive information on the basic and applied principles of veterinary pharmacology and therapeutics. Information on mechanisms of action, pharmacodynamics, and pharmacokinetics is detailed. This reference is also available as an eBook.

Case Study 3-4

You have an appointment to discuss compounding services with a local veterinarian. Your pharmacy has just begun offering these services and, in the conversation, the veterinarian references AMDUCA. You have not heard of this.

- *What is your strategy to find the meaning and relevance of this term?*

Secondary Resources

Secondary resources refer to the literature that indexes the primary (e.g., clinical trial) or some tertiary (e.g., a review) literature found in journals, with the goal of directing the user to relevant literature. This type of resource can be used for multiple purposes; it can help a practitioner keep abreast of recently published information or help to find more recent or detailed information on a specific topic. When discussing secondary resources, there are two commonly used terms, indexing and abstracting; the two terms differ slightly. **Indexing** consists of providing bibliographic citation information (e.g., title, author, and citation of the article), while **abstracting** also includes a brief description (or abstract) of the information provided by the article or resource cited. ❻ *Secondary electronic resources will index and possibly abstract information from different types and numbers of journals, meetings, publications, or sources; therefore in order to perform a comprehensive search for an article, multiple resources must be used.* For example, PsychINFO predominantly indexes and abstracts the primary and tertiary resources that focus on psychology-related topics and psychiatric illnesses and treatments.

In searching most databases, a user will follow a similar search strategy, with small changes to reflect differences in database systems. There are several challenges in searching secondary database systems. Systems do not index all terms the same and so it is necessary to determine what terms a database is using in order to conduct a successful search. For example, a disease known to most people as cystic fibrosis was once officially indexed by a system under the official term, fibrocystic disease of the pancreas. So, a person not consulting the indexing terms of that disease might have missed a number of references. Most computerized databases also include a free-text search option, which is very useful when the defined index terms are not identifying relevant data. This option may also be helpful when the term is newly emerging or before an official index term is defined.

The need to utilize a variety of terms for the search strategy is illustrated in the following sample question: "Is clonidine effective in the treatment of attention deficit hyperactivity disorder (ADHD) in adolescents?" It is first important to identify the key terms. These terms might include clonidine, attention deficit hyperactivity disorder, and adolescents. However, some databases may not recognize the term adolescent and instead use the term pediatric or child. Additionally, the use of the term pediatric may just refer to the medical specialty caring for pediatric in some resources, rather than treatment of a pediatric patient population. Therefore, it is important to recognize that different databases may require different search terms to be used.

Electronic searches generally use the Boolean operators AND, OR, and NOT (Figure 3-1), although natural language searching is becoming more available, as is seen in a typical Google search. The operator AND will combine two terms, returning only citations containing both of those concepts or terms. Combining two terms with the operator OR will result in an equal or greater number of returns since it will include any citation

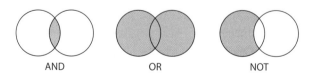

Figure 3–1. Boolean operators.

where either term is used. Use of the term NOT should be used with caution, as it will always decrease the number of returns. Since it eliminates any references having that term, it may eliminate appropriate articles simply because the term happens to appear somewhere in the article.

For example, in the earlier clonidine for the treatment of ADHD question, the appropriate search terms (clonidine AND attention deficit hyperactivity disorder) may be used with the AND operator. However, if the requestor wanted information regarding use of either clonidine or guanfacine in this disease state, then the operator OR might be used. See Figure 3-2 for a graphic presentation of this search. A search using OR will return a number of results equal to or greater than a search using the term AND. The operator OR might also be useful when searching for a term with synonyms, for example, attention deficit disorder OR attention deficit hyperactivity disorder. The operator NOT would be helpful if a user wants to exclude certain topics, for example, a specific disease state. In this case, a search might be performed for attention deficit hyperactivity disorder NOT Tourette's disorder. Since the use of the operator NOT will exclude any article mentioning Tourette's disease, an article focused on treatment of ADHD with a small section about Tourette's disease would also be excluded, so care is necessary in using that search strategy. Parentheses can also be used to further streamline a search. In this example, a search may be performed for clonidine AND (attention deficit disorder OR attention deficit hyperactivity disorder). This would retrieve articles that contain the drug of interest as well as either of the two disease states of interest. An additional example of search strategy using Boolean operators is provided in Appendix 3-1.

Some databases will also use the terms WITH or NEAR. These operators are similar to AND; however, they require the terms to be within a set number of words of each other. These terms may be useful when other searches are identifying a large number of articles where both terms are mentioned, but not in conjunction with each other.

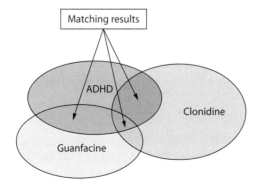

Figure 3–2. ADHD AND (clonidine OR guanfacine).

Most databases allow results to be restricted via use of limit fields. For example, this may include language of publication, year of publication, type of article (e.g., human study, review, case report), or type of journal where publication is found. Many more such limits are available in some databases, such as those based on the Medline database. This is most helpful when the initial search terms return a large number of possible matches. Using too many limits with the initial search may eliminate articles or citations that would be helpful.

One additional point to bear in mind when performing electronic searches is that the same search phrase could be indexed under a variety of search terms or spellings; thus, in order to provide a comprehensive search, it is important to address all of those. For example, if looking for information regarding the herbal product ginkgo, it may be helpful to search under the botanical name, common name(s), as well as common alternative spellings. Thus, a possible search strategy may be to use the terms "ginkgo," "ginkgo biloba," the Latin name "Ginkgoaceae," as well as the misspelled word "gingko." This same principle holds true when considering disease states whose names may have changed over time. As databases and resources continue to modify search features, there are more Google-like search engines that allow for a natural language search helping to minimize some of these concerns.

When trying to improve the overall quality of searching secondary references, DI specialists have looked at the use of filters to provide better searching strategies. The two most prominent types of filters are content filters and validity filters. The content filters are specific to the drug or disease state being searched. For this type of search, it helps to look at the **Medical Subject Heading (MeSH) terms** to make sure that the search has the most appropriate content. MeSH terms are a set of specific medical words that the NLM uses to define or categorize a topic for the purpose of indexing articles in PubMed, based on automatic mapping of the words to the topic. For example, when one enters a keyword "heart attack" using MeSH, the automatic mapping will know that it was supposed to mean myocardial infarction, instead of "heart" and "attack" as two separate terms. This automatic mapping capability of MeSH is quite helpful when a keyword can be interpreted in multiple ways and may pull too many articles. For example, when one enters the keyword "cold" in the search box, it will generate a large list of articles that interpreted the word as temperature OR an ailment. Using MeSH, the search will be more streamlined because there will be two specific topics from which to select articles, instead of mixing the two.

It is best to use the advanced searching features in these secondary databases versus the simple searching features because advanced searching allows for filters to be utilized. The second type of filter is known as a validity filter, which is a way to narrow the search to only the highest quality studies. Search terminology such as randomized controlled trial or double-blind can be used to eliminate studies of weaker/poorer methodology.

Listed below are some examples of secondary databases and types of literature that they index. Detailed information about PubMed (http://www.pubmed.gov) is found in Appendix 3-1.

BIOSIS PREVIEWS

Thompson Reuters Medical, http://www.thomsonreuters.com. This is a comprehensive database of biological information, covering biological and biomedical information. BIOSIS also covers abstracts from conferences relating to basic sciences. This is most helpful when seeking more basic science information about activity of compounds on a cellular level.

COCHRANE LIBRARY

Cochrane Library, http://www.cochrane.org. This database has three components: indexes of Cochrane reviews about a variety of medical treatments, conditions, and alternative therapies; abstracts of international systematic reviews; and a bibliography of systematic reviews in worldwide literature. These evidence-based medicine reviews are based on extensive analysis of current literature and provide treatment recommendations (see Chapter 8 on evidence-based medicine).

CUMULATIVE INDEX TO NURSING AND ALLIED HEALTH LITERATURE (CINAHL)

EBSCOhost, http://www.ebscohost.com. This is an indexing service that covers primarily literature in the fields of nursing and allied health. This database is useful when seeking information about patient care from the perspective of allied health professionals. It is updated monthly.

CURRENT CONTENTS CONNECT

Clarivate Analytics, http://wokinfo.com/training_support/training/current-contents-connect/. This electronic service offers an overview of very recently published literature as it relates to scientific information. There are multiple subsets; the clinical medicine and life science subgroups are likely the most useful for practitioners and focus on useful information about recent drug research or developments.

EMBASE®

Elsevier, http://www.embase.com. Embase is a comprehensive abstracting service covering biomedical literature worldwide. This database covers material similar to that covered by MEDLINE but with greater coverage of international publications. Additionally, there is less lag time between publication and inclusion in the database. This database is useful when seeking information about dietary supplements or medications that may be available in other countries.

GOOGLE SCHOLAR

Google, http://scholar.google.com. An Internet search engine that is designed to target scholarly materials available online, in a variety of professional areas including health care. In fact, it does contain all of the article indexes from Medline. Information from a variety of scholarly journals and publications is able to be searched, based on the keyword match. Google Scholar is different from Google search engine because it provides only scholarly publications. Because of its powerful search capability, it is useful when other secondary resources have not provided much success in finding an article of interest. The results of searched topics via Google Scholar are listed by how many times a particular article was cited on other publications whether scholarly or not. This can be troublesome when looking for recently published articles on a particular topic or when searching for scholarly publications only. It also allows connections to article retrieval systems, such as Open WorldCat or OhioLink.

INTERNATIONAL PHARMACEUTICAL ABSTRACTS (IPA)

Clarivate Analytics, http://clarivate.com. Coverage includes drug-related information, including drug use and development. This database also abstracts a variety of meeting presentations. The main focus of this database is pharmacy information, including pharmacy administration and clinical services, making it the most comprehensive global database for pharmacy-specific information.

JOURNAL WATCH®

Massachusetts Medical Society, http://www.jwatch.org. Journal Watch is an abstracting service, including recent information, summarized by physicians, from a variety of medical literature. A general newsletter covering major medical stories of interest to generalists is published as well as additional newsletters in specific specialty areas. This is most helpful when monitoring for new clinical trials involving specific medications.

LexisNexis®

LexisNexis Academic & Library Solutions, http://www.lexisnexis.com. This indexing and abstracting service provides coverage of a variety of types of information, including medical, legal, and business news. Some publications are available full text through this service. This resource is helpful when attempting to locate information about recent medical news or research.

MEDLINE®

National Library of Medicine, http://www.nlm.nih.gov. MEDLINE is part of the NLM PubMed program; about 5,600 medical journals are processed for MEDLINE to extract information from publications in 40 different languages. Coverage includes basic and clinical sciences as well as nursing, dentistry, veterinary medicine, and many other health care disciplines. This database is available through a variety of publishers; free access to content is available via PubMed (http://www.ncbi.nlm.nih.gov/pubmed). A sample search is provided in Appendix 3-1.

TRIP DATABASE

Trip Database Ltd., http://www.tripdatabase.com. This website provides advertisement-free, unbiased search results using the online searching capabilities through millions of articles. It allows literature search based on the PICO (patients, intervention, comparator, outcome; see Chapter 8 for more information) format or using an advanced search. Its search results are listed by evidence type (e.g., clinical trials, guidelines, systematic reviews) and include many guidelines sorted by the country of publication. It is one of the most comprehensive and evidence-based resources for retrieving medical literature. It is available free online.

Case Study 3–5

A physician requests information about the use of sildenafil for treatment of female sexual arousal disorder. She also requests information about use of any of the other phosphodiesterase-5 inhibitors.

- *What resources might be good places to look for this information?*
- *What search terms should be used?*
- *Should limits be utilized?*

Primary Resources

Primary literature includes clinical research studies and reports, both published and unpublished. Not all literature published in a journal is classified as primary literature, for example, review articles or editorials are not primary literature. There are several types of publications considered primary, including controlled trials, cohort studies, case series, and case reports. Additional information about study designs commonly found in medical literature and how to evaluate them is provided in Chapters 4 and 5.

Advantages to the use of primary literature include access to detailed information about a topic and the ability to personally assess the validity and applicability of study results. Additionally, primary literature is more recent than tertiary or secondary literature. However, there are several disadvantages to the use of primary literature alone, which include (1) misleading conclusions based on only one trial without the context of other research, (2) the need to have good skills in evaluating the literature (e.g., clinical trial evaluation) discussed in Chapters 4 and 5, and (3) the time needed to evaluate the potentially large volume of literature available.

Due to the rapidly increasing number of specialty journals being published, it is difficult to determine which journals are most essential in a pharmacy practice setting. Appendix 3-2 provides a listing of core holdings for a college of pharmacy assembled by the AACP and several commonly mentioned journals in medicine. While this list may be more extensive than what is required in most practice settings, it does provide a core listing of journals. Each practice setting requires slightly different primary literature based on the specific areas that are of greatest importance to that facility and the patients cared for in that location.

OBTAINING THE PRIMARY RESOURCES

Once literature has been identified in a secondary searching system, the actual articles can be obtained in various ways. Many electronic secondary resources link users directly to the article of interest. For example, PubMed links users to open access journal publications and articles resulting from NIH-funded research through PubMed Central (http://www.pubmedcentral.nih.gov). Some resources, such as Google Scholar, may link into other article retrieval systems, such as Open WorldCat or OhioLink.

However, many articles are not available via open access routes; in those cases alternative techniques may be needed. Once a citation is identified, utilizing a local library catalog is a good next step. Often a local library may carry the journal needed, or may be affiliated with other facilities that can provide that article. Articles are often available for a fee via the publisher website. If neither of these options is available, then the Loansome Doc ordering system might be used. This system is available through the NLM and offered for a fee to any user. Articles identified in PubMed can be easily ordered from that database through this system. Additional information about this program is available at http://www.nlm.nih.gov/pubs/factsheets/loansome_doc.html.

Alternative Resources

INTERNET SEARCHES

At times, even well-designed searches of standard medical literature do not yield sufficient information to make clinical decisions or recommendations. In these cases, alternative resources may need to be employed. One such method to identify relevant resources might be a general Internet search for information. This can be especially helpful to serve as a starting point for questions about uncommon diseases, new terms, drugs in development, or marketed OTC products and combination dietary supplements. For example, if a requestor asked about use of a dietary supplement product called GABA Plus in ADHD, it would be difficult to search for information, unless the requestor was able to provide a list of ingredients contained in the product. Often requestors may not have that information; therefore, it may be necessary to search for a manufacturer website to identify the specific individual ingredients and then look for information on the individual components. This is also helpful in identifying information or specific product claims provided by the manufacturer. Additionally, Internet searches may be useful for topics that have recently been in the news, where information is changing more rapidly than standard medical resources can be updated.

It is important to remember that different search engines use different techniques to identify webpages, and that no search engine identifies all websites. Some search engines are geared toward scholarly content (e.g., Google Scholar, http://scholar.google.com) or scientific research, rather than general information. In order to efficiently perform a search, it is important to consider which search engine would most likely index the desired materials.

There are, however, several caveats to finding information on the Internet. The first is to carefully evaluate the quality of all information provided. There are millions of websites and there is no true quality assurance measures in place to evaluate the reliability of information available. ❼ *Drug or health information retrieved from Internet-based or online media needs to be evaluated for its accuracy, comprehensiveness, and recent update.* There are some general tenets to keep in mind when evaluating this type of literature. Generally, sites maintained by educational institutions, not-for-profit medical organizations, or a division of the U.S. government are likely to contain high-quality information, whereas information maintained by a company selling and promoting a specific product may be more questionable. Some websites are maintained by individuals or organizations with questionable viewpoints and may be very questionable at best.

In order to assess quality of online information several standards and programs now exist. These include those from organizations such as the Health on the Net (HON code, http://www.hon.ch), which clearly define standards to evaluate the quality of information available via a website. These organizations do not evaluate every website available, but only those who request evaluation. Since many websites do not request evaluation, the lack of an organization's quality seal does not necessarily indicate that the information is of low quality.

The following criteria should be used when determining quality of online material:

- Is the source credible, without a vested interest in promoting one particular treatment or product?
- Is the information accurate and current?
- Does the site link to other nonaffiliated sites that provide consistently good information?
- Is the information appropriately detailed and referenced?
- Is it possible to identify the author of the site to contact with additional questions or comments?

Information on evaluating health-related contents on websites is discussed further in Chapter 5. In addition, the NLM posted a video and frequently asked questions to help determine high-quality sites (https://medlineplus.gov/evaluatinghealthinformation .html).

OTHER INFORMATION SOURCES

Occasionally, sufficient information to address a DI request cannot be obtained from standard resources and may require the use of some alternative sources of information. If a question involves, for example, a recent news story reporting the removal of a medication from the market, a logical first place to find initial information would be to identify the original news story. This can be done by searching various newswire services such as PR Newswire or even major news network websites such as CNN (Table 3-3). LexisNexis, http://www.lexisnexis.com, indexes a variety of newswire stories as well as transcripts of news reports. While this news story may not provide all the information needed, it might at least serve as a point from which to search for additional information.

In some cases, there may be such limited information available that it would be wise to seek out an expert in the field, for example, a question about the use of heparin in a troche dosage form. In these cases, it may be prudent to contact persons performing research in this area or practitioners who are currently using that therapy to identify information that might have been missed in an initial search or may not have been published.

TABLE 3–3. MAJOR ONLINE NEWS SOURCES

News Source	Website Address
ABC News	www.abcnews.go.com
The Associated Press (AP)	www.ap.org
BBC	www.bbc.com
Bloomberg	www.bloomberg.com
CBS News	www.cbsnews.com
The Chicago Tribune	www.chicagotribune.com
CNN	www.cnn.com
The Economist	www.economist.com
Fox News	www.foxnews.com
The Guardian	www.theguardian.com/us
Google News	https://news.google.com/
MSNBC	www.msnbc.com
The New York Times	www.nytimes.com
NPR	www.npr.org
PBS	www.pbs.org
Pink Sheet	https://pink.pharmamedtechbi.com/
Reuters	www.reuters.com
The Wall Street Journal	www.wsj.com
The Washington Post	www.washingtonpost.com
USA Today	www.usatoday.com
Yahoo News	www.yahoo.com/news/

Some experts may be identified via medical organizations focusing on specific disease states, leadership of medical societies, or persons who have authored numerous papers on a specific medication or medical condition.

When looking for recent recommendations regarding treatment of a specific disease state, it may be helpful to identify an organization affiliated with that disease state. For example, when looking for treatment recommendations for management of irritable bowel syndrome it might be appropriate to contact the International Foundation for Functional Gastrointestinal Disorders (http://www.iffgd.org/) to obtain information about current practice standards as well as possible emerging therapies.

Additionally, when seeking information about a specific drug therapy, it may be helpful to contact the product manufacturer via their medical information department to identify information that may be available in-house. This resource could be especially helpful for obtaining difficult to access literature, if a product is newly approved or for identifying a possible rare adverse drug reaction (Case Study 3-6).

Case Study 3–6

A patient tells you she saw a news story on NBC that said all patients should stop taking their Coumadin™ and switch to the "new Coumadin™." She tells you she is not planning to take it anymore and wants the physician to find a different medication. She is indignant that you as a health care professional did not know this was going on.

- *Where might you find a copy of the news story that this patient saw to help her better understand what the news reporter was trying to convey?*

CONSUMER HEALTH INFORMATION

Consumers may also benefit from some text resources available at a local library. Some resources are published by organizations that produce references for health care professionals, while lay press companies publish others. There is great variation in the quality of information provided from resource to resource. Some of the most popular resources may not be written at an appropriate level for a consumer to understand or may not provide helpful information for the patient. For this reason, it is important to discuss with patients what other resources they are using to find additional drug and medical information. Opening a dialog with patients about this topic is fairly simple and can consist open-ended questions such as "Where else have you found information on your disease state?" or "What other material have you read about your medication/ disease state?"

If being asked to recommend a source of online information for a patient, one can confidently recommend health care organizations or disease societies, both of which usually provide helpful, high-quality disease-specific information geared for the average consumer. The NLM also publishes information targeting patients and consumers about how to evaluate health information appropriately. One example is via MEDLINE Plus (https://medlineplus.gov/evaluatinghealthinformation.html). NIH also published via several of its offices information regarding how to find and evaluate online resources. One example of this is from the National Center for Complementary and Integrative Health (https://nccih.nih.gov/health/webresources).

In addition to these resources aimed at consumers, there are consumer-specific sections of many tertiary resources discussed earlier. Electronic resources such as

Micromedex®, Lexicomp®, Facts&Comparisons® eAnswers, ASHP's SafeMedication.com, or Clinical Pharmacology have subsections dedicated to consumer-level information available for a practitioner to print and provide to the patient. Of note, online resources such as Wikipedia and blogs are not appropriate and reliable sources for health- and medical-related topics for consumers; they lack scientific rigor and review for accuracy, comprehensiveness, and updates. In addition, information contained in such sources can be easily changed or manipulated by anyone who read them.

Below is a brief explanation of most widely used and reliable online information specifically designed for patients and consumers.

Centers for Disease Control and Prevention (CDC)

A division of the Department of Health and Human Services, the CDC (http://www.cdc.gov) is the frontline information medium for any diseases of interest affecting a large patient population such as infectious disease and other epidemics of interest. It includes information about diseases, conditions, and other special topics listed in the "Health Topics A-Z," and "Travelers' Health," with health recommendations for travelers in and out of the United States and other countries. Information is also available in Spanish and various health-related and educational publications are available in 26 different languages.

ClinicalTrials.gov

This website (http://www.clinicaltrials.gov) is maintained by the National Institutes of Health and serves as a main registry for publicly and privately supported clinical studies of human participants conducted in the world. Patients can find clinical researches currently ongoing or to be conducted in the future, and register themselves as participants. The trial results are not always fully added and requires health care professionals to effectively search for them using secondary resources discussed above.

Healthfinder.gov

This website (https://healthfinder.gov/FindServices/) is hosted and maintained by the Office of Disease Prevention and Health Promotion within the U.S. Department of Health and Human Services. It contains health topics that may be relevant to any consumers, including nutrition, parenting, healthy living tips, and directories for health care providers near consumers. It is also available in Spanish.

Informedhealth.org

Published by the German Institute for Quality and Efficiency in Health Care, this website (https://www.informedhealth.org/) provides an evidence-based consumer and patient health information free of bias and advertisement. The website is available in English and German and includes diverse topics including men's health, skin and hair, reproductive health and birth, and evidence-based medicine.

KidsHealth.org

This website (http://www.kidshealth.org) provides doctor-approved health information about children from before birth through adolescence. Created by The Nemours Foundation's Center for Children's Health Media, KidsHealth covers diverse topics including information specifically for kids, teens, parents, and educators.

Mayo Clinic

Mayo Clinic publishes and maintains this website (http://www.mayoclinic.org) which covers a wide variety of topics for general public, including health-related concerns, education for patients and medical professionals, research information, and Mayo's services. The information is of high quality and free of biases and advertisements.

MedlinePlus

Supported by reliable information generated from the NLM, this website (https://medlineplus.gov/) is one of the most highly regarded information medium for consumer seeking health information. It is available in Spanish as well. The information includes drugs, supplements, latest news, and clinical trials.

U.S. Food and Drug Administration (FDA)

This website (http://www.fda.gov/ForConsumers/default.htm) provides very comprehensive information regarding drugs, adverse effects, women's and minority health, and major recalls of drugs and food. It also provides information on veterinary medicine, vaccines, cosmetics, and tobacco products.

More resources to assist patients and consumers with questions related to medical information can be found in Table 3-4 of this chapter and in Chapter 25.

TABLE 3–4. ONLINE CONSUMER INFORMATION SOURCES

Title	Author/Owner	Website	Features
Centers for Disease Control and Prevention	Centers for Disease Control and Prevention	www.cdc.gov	Contains information about the treatment and prevention of infectious diseases. It also contains a listing of public health hoaxes.
Cleveland Clinic Health Library	Cleveland Clinic Health Information Center	http://my.clevelandclinic.org/health	Provides access to thousands of health articles, videos, and tools for patients, searchable by topic.
Complementary and Integrative Health	National Center for Complementary and Integrative Health	https://nccih.nih.gov	A government-maintained resource describing ongoing research in the area of dietary supplements, as well as detailing efficacy information currently available.
DailyMed	U.S. National Library of Medicine	https://dailymed.nlm.nih.gov/dailymed/	Contains about 95,000 drug listings as submitted to the Food and Drug Administration. Includes drug information based on drug classes and drug identification tool.
Dietary Supplements Fact Sheets	National Institute of Health Office of Dietary Supplements	http://ods.od.nih.gov	Compiles accurate and current information about the efficacy and safety of dietary supplements including scientific facts.
FamilyDoctor.org	American Academy of Family Physicians	https://familydoctor.org/	Provides information on various topics related to disease prevention and wellness, ranging from puberty to nutrition.
Healthfinder.gov	National Health Information Center	www.healthfinder.gov	Provides information on a variety of health topics, maintained by the Office of Disease Prevention and Health Promotion. Also provides information in Spanish.
HealthyChildren.org	American Academy of Pediatrics	www.healthychildren.org	Provides unbiased, accurate information focused on children from newborn to young adults. Information is available also in Spanish.
Informedhealth.org	Institute for Quality and Efficiency in Health Care	www.informedhealth.org	Established in Germany in 2004, provides independent and evidence-based health information.
KidsHealth	The Nemours Foundation	http://kidshealth.org	Provides health information about children from before birth through adolescence for parents.
Mayo Clinic	Mayo Foundation for Medical Education and Research	www.mayoclinic.org	Provides quality health information written for the general public.
Merck Manual Consumer Version	Merck	www.merckhomeedition.com	A consumer-based version of the Merck Manual. It includes a variety of medical topics and interactive features such as videos and self-assessment tools.

continued

TABLE 3-4. ONLINE CONSUMER INFORMATION SOURCES *(CONTINUED)*

Title	Author/Owner	Website	Features
MedlinePlus	U.S. National Library of Medicine	http://medlineplus.gov	Contains information about various medications as well as disease states and conditions.
Mental Health Information	National Institute of Mental Health	www.nimh.nih.gov/health/topics/index.shtml	Provides information regarding a variety of mental health topics, clinical trial information, and educational resources.
National Cancer Institute	National Cancer Institute/National Institutes of Health	www.cancer.gov	Provides helpful and accurate information regarding cancer research, diagnoses, prevention, and treatment.
NetWellness	University of Cincinnati, The Ohio State University, Case Western Reserve University	www.netwellness.org/	A global, community service providing quality unbiased health information from university faculty. The site is commercial free and has no advertising.
NIH Senior Health	National Institute on Aging and the National Library of Medicine	https://nihseniorhealth.gov/	Contains information on a variety of health topics focused on geriatric consumers and patients including tips on healthy aging and short videos.
Pillbox	U.S. National Library of Medicine	https://pillbox.nlm.nih.gov/pillimage/search.php	Helps identify or search for an unknown, typically oral solid dosage form medication, for patients or health care providers
SafeMedication	American Society of Health-System Pharmacists	www.safemedication.com	Provides a patient version of AHFS® Drug Information Resource, as well as tips about medication administration and resources to empower patients to better track/manage their own health care.
St. Jude Children's Research Hospital	St. Jude Children's Research Hospital	www.stjude.org	Contains information for caregivers of pediatric patients, medications, and infection control. Includes information about ongoing clinical research.
U.S. Food and Drug Administration	U.S. Food and Drug Administration	www.fda.gov/ForConsumers/default.htm	Contains information about new drugs as well as dietary supplements. Also contains information about recalls of drug or food.
WebMD	WebMD	http://www.webmd.com/	Provides information on a variety of topics and conditions including diet, nutrition, and medications. Contains interactive videos and self-assessment tools.
Womenshealth.gov	Office on Women's Health, U.S. Department of Health and Human Services	www.womenshealth.gov	Contains information about conditions and diseases of special interest to women, including drug use during pregnancy and lactation.

Case Study 3-7

A physician is seeking information about the use of chondroitin in the management of osteoarthritis. He sees a large number of patients in his practice and is seeking information about efficacy, safety, and appropriate dosing of this product.

- *What are the advantages and disadvantages of tertiary resources in responding to this request?*
- *What are the advantages and disadvantages of primary literature in this scenario?*

Conclusion

Medical information is changing rapidly and the amount of information is growing at a faster rate than health care professionals can keep pace in this digital technology era. More DI resources are becoming available online or via mobile access in addition to or replacing print versions. The information in this chapter helps provide guidance as to where specific types of DI might be found and how to begin a search for DI, targeting the tertiary and secondary resources.

Practitioners must not, however, be satisfied with merely identifying sources for DI. Understanding where to access information is only the first step in the provision of quality DI. Information must be interpreted and evaluated to become knowledge. It is this unique knowledge that will enable practitioners to optimize patient care. Therefore, health care professionals need to stay current and vigilant about the effective methods of retrieving and evaluating medical information for efficient patient care. The next several chapters will provide additional guidance on how to interpret and apply the information that is gathered.

As technological advances continue and more information becomes available regarding medications and their appropriate place in therapy, the need for pharmacists' expertise in DI would continue to grow. With the increased emphasis on interprofessional practice in all clinical settings, all health care professionals should develop skills in retrieving and interpreting medical literature in order to provide optimal patient care.

Self-Assessment Questions

1. A physician asks for a tertiary reference that discusses the results of a new drug's efficacy and safety in treating multiple sclerosis. Which of the following is a tertiary resource in biomedical literature?
   a. A research article describing a clinical trial
   b. A case report of one patient's experience
   c. A review paper describing several clinical trials
   d. MEDLINE

2. A pharmacy technician calls you and asks the following: "A patient is asking if it is okay to take oxycodone, aspirin, omeprazole, and ibuprofen together." Which of the following categories of drug information resources is most appropriate for an efficient search of references?
   a. Drug interaction
   b. Drug stability
   c. Adverse drug reaction
   d. Indication

3. A physician calls and asks "my patient takes ginkgo biloba supplements every day. Does that interact with his warfarin?" What would be the most appropriate DI reference to use for this question, given the product of interest?
   a. Facts & Comparisons® eAnswers
   b. Geriatric Dosage Handbook
   c. Natural Medicines
   d. Briggs Drugs in Pregnancy and Lactation

4. A nurse calls and asks "can I mix gentamicin and ampicillin in one bag for IV administration?" What would be the most appropriate DI reference to answer this question?
   a. Merck Index
   b. Lexi-Drugs
   c. Neofax
   d. Trissel's IV Compatibility

5. Which of the following is NOT a drug information resource that can answer the following question? "Are there any major warnings that I should know about gabapentin before using it?"
   a. DrugPoint
   b. AHFS DI

    c. Lexi-Drug ID

    d. Clinical Pharmacology

6. Which of the following is NOT a secondary resource that can assist in finding original research papers?

    a. MEDLINE

    b. Micromedex®

    c. PubMed

    d. EMBASE

7. A patient walks up to your pharmacy counter and asks "My doctor told me to take over-the-counter Benadryl for allergy. How much should I take?" Which of the following is the most appropriate tertiary resource for this question?

    a. Handbook of Nonprescription Drugs

    b. USP/NF

    c. Natural Medicines Comprehensive Database

    d. The Merck Manual

8. Which of the following online databases is not available as a print resource?

    a. Facts & Comparison® eAnswers

    b. Clinical Pharmacology®

    c. AHFS® DI

    d. RED BOOK

9. Which of the following electronic databases would provide the largest international biomedical journal coverage?

    a. EMBASE

    b. MEDLINE

    c. International Pharmaceutical Abstracts

    d. PsychINFO

10. A pregnant woman is concerned about potential adverse effects of her current medication to her baby. She is currently taking fexofenadine and sertraline. Which of the following is the most appropriate resources to determine if the medications are not teratogenic to the fetus?

    a. Briggs Drugs in Pregnancy and Lactation

    b. Meyler's Side Effects of Drugs

    c. Remington: The Science and Practice of Pharmacy

    d. Identidex

11. When evaluating the quality of tertiary biomedical resources, which of the following is NOT an appropriate questions to consider?
    a. Is the information likely to be timely based on publication date?
    b. Are there enough photos and animations to assist in understanding?
    c. Is information supported by appropriate citations?
    d. Does the resource appear free from bias and blatant errors?

12. A patient was admitted to your emergency department (ED) with chest pain while visiting his daughter in the United States. He brought with him a few medications from his home country and your ED team is trying to find similar therapy here. Which of the following resources would be most appropriate to help the ED team?
    a. TOXNET
    b. The Harriet Lane Handbook
    c. Martindale: The Complete Drug Reference
    d. Lexi-Drugs

13. Ms. Jones comes to your pharmacy and asks about how to manage her joint pain and insomnia at home. She wants to learn more about the conditions and her medications by searching them online. Which of the following is NOT a reliable patient resource that you can share with her?
    a. DailyMed
    b. Wikipedia
    c. Healthfinder.gov
    d. Safemedication.com

14. Which of the following is true when considering drug information (DI) resources for mobile devices?
    a. Current standards and regulations on mobile application for DI are not adequate.
    b. Mobile application versions of DI database are identical to their online databases.
    c. Health care providers rarely use mobile devices for retrieving DI.
    d. There are too few mobile applications available to use for patient care.

15. Which of the following is a benefit of using tertiary resources?
    a. They are quickly outdated.
    b. They provide a comprehensive and quick overview of a topic.
    c. Their contents are filtered by other experts and therefore are not biased.
    d. They are typically shorter than primary resources.

REFERENCES

1. Slomski A. The National Library of Medicine: 175 years of advancing biomedical knowledge. JAMA. 2011;305(21):2158-61.
2. International Association of Scientific, Technical and Medical Publishers. The STM report: an overview of scientific and scholarly journal publishing. 2015 [cited 2017 Mar 1]. Available from: http://www.stm-assoc.org/2015_02_20_STM_Report_2015.pdf. Accessed March 1, 2017.
3. Aungst TD. Medical applications for pharmacists using mobile devices. Ann Pharmacother. 2013;47(7-8):1088-95.
4. Aungst TD, Clauson KA, Misra S, Lewis TL, Husain I. How to identify, assess and utilise mobile medical applications in clinical practice. Int J Clin Pract. 2014;68(2):155-62.
5. Perrin A, Duggan M. Americans' Internet access: 2000-2015. June 26, 2015. Available from: http://www.pewinternet.org/2015/06/26/americans-internet-access-2000-2015/. Accessed March 1, 2017.
6. Fox S, Duggan M. Health online 2013. January 15, 2015. Available from: http://www.pewinternet.org/2013/01/15/health-online-2013/. Accessed March 1, 2017.
7. U.S. Food and Drug Administration. Mobile medical applications. 2015 [cited 2017 Mar 3]. Available from: https://www.fda.gov/MedicalDevices/DigitalHealth/MobileMedicalApplications/ucm255978.htm. Accessed March 3, 2017.
8. Clauson KA, Polen HH, Peak AS, Marsh WA, DiScala SL. Clinical decision support tools: personal digital assistant versus online dietary supplement databases. Ann Pharmacother. 2008;42(11):1592-9.
9. American Association of Colleges of Pharmacy. Basic resources for pharmacy education 2014 [Internet]. Alexandria, VA: American Association of Colleges of Pharmacy. June 2014 [cited 2017 Mar 1]; [53 pp.]. Available from: http://www.aacp.org/governance/SECTIONS/libraryinformationscience/Documents/Basic%20Resources%20for%20Pharmacy%20Education/2014%20June%20Basic%20Resources%20for%20Pharmacy%20Education.pdf. Accessed March 1, 2017.
10. Aronson JK. Meyler's side effects of drugs: the international encyclopedia of adverse drug reactions and interactions. 16th ed. Amsterdam: Elsevier; 2015.
11. Aronson JK. Side effects of drugs annual 38: a worldwide yearly survey of new data and trends in adverse drug reactions. 38th ed. Amsterdam: Elsevier; 2016.
12. Trissel LA. Handbook of injectable drugs. 19th ed. Bethesda, MD: American Society of Health-System Pharmacists; 2016.
13. King JC, Catania PN. King guide to parenteral admixtures. King Guide Publications. 1971-2016 [cited 2017 Apr 7]. Available from: https://www.kingguide.com. Accessed April 7, 2017.
14. Trissel's 2 Clinical Pharmaceutics Database [Internet]. Cashiers: TriPharma Communications [cited 2013 Mar 1]. Available from: http://www.wolterskluwercdi.com/. Accessed March 1, 2013.

15. Bing CD, Nowobilski-Vasilios A. Extended stability for parenteral drugs. 6th ed. Bethesda, MD: American Society of Health-System Pharmacists; 2017.

16. Trissel LA. Trissel's stability of compounded formulations. 5th ed. Washington, DC: American Pharmacists Association; 2012.

17. Allen LV, Adejare A, Desselle SP, Felton LA. Remington: the science and practice of pharmacy. 22nd ed. Philadelphia, PA: Lippincott Williams & Wilkins; 2012.

18. USP 40/NF 35: the official compendia of standards. Rockville, MD: U.S. Pharmacopeial Convention; 2017.

19. O'Neil MJ. Merck Index: an encyclopedia of chemicals, drugs and biologicals. 15th ed. Whitehouse Station, NJ: Royal Society of Chemistry; 2013.

20. Thompson JE. A practical guide to contemporary pharmacy practice. 3rd ed. Philadelphia, PA: Lippincott Williams & Wilkins; 2009.

21. Jew RK, Soo-Hoo W, Erush SC, Amiri E. Extemporaneous formulations. 3rd ed. Bethesda, MD: American Society of Health-System Pharmacists; 2016.

22. Natural Medicines [Internet]. Stockton: Therapeutic Research Faculty. Updated 2017 [cited 2017 Apr 7]. Available from: www.trchealthcare.com/solutions/natural-medicines. Accessed April 7, 2017.

23. Natural Medicines Comprehensive Database [Internet]. Stockton: Therapeutic Research Faculty. Updated 2017 [cited 2017 Apr 7]. Available from: https://naturalmedicines.therapeuticresearch.com/. Accessed April 7, 2017.

24. Dietary Supplement Label Database [Internet]. Bethesda, MD: National Institutes of Health Office of Dietary Supplements and the U.S. National Library of Medicine. Updated 2017 [cited 2017 Apr 7]. Available from: https://www.dsld.nlm.nih.gov/dsld/index.jsp. Accessed April 7, 2017.

25. MedlinePlus [Internet]. Bethesda, MD: U.S. National Library of Medicine. Updated 2017 [cited 2017 Apr 7]. Available from: https://medlineplus.gov/druginformation.html. Accessed April 7, 2017.

26. AltMedDex® [Internet]. Ann Arbor, MI: Truven Health Analytics. 2017 [cited 2017 Apr 7]. Available from: www.micromedexsolutions.com. Accessed April 7, 2017.

27. DerMarderosian A, Beutler JA. The review of natural products. 7th ed. St. Louis, MO: Wolters Kluwer; 2012.

28. DiPiro JT, Talbert RL, Yee GC, Matzke GR, Wells BG, Posey LM. Pharmacotherapy: a pathophysiologic approach. 10th ed. New York, NY: McGraw-Hill; 2016.

29. Chisholm-Burns MA, Schwinghammer TL, Wells BG, Malone PM, Kolesar JM, DiPiro JT, et al. Pharmacotherapy principles and practice. 4th ed. New York, NY: McGraw-Hill; 2016.

30. Alldredge BK, Corelli RL, Guglielmo BJ, Kradjan WA, Williams BR, Ernst ME, Jacobson PA. Koda-Kimble & Young's applied therapeutics: the clinical use of drugs. 10th ed. Philadelphia, PA: Lippincott Williams & Wilkins; 2012.

31. Porter RS. The Merck manual of diagnosis and therapy. 19th ed. Whitehouse Station, NJ: Merck Research Laboratories; 2011.

32. Kasper DL, Fauci AS, Braunwald E, Longo DL, Hauser SL, Jameson JL, Loscalzo J. Harrison's principles of internal medicine. 19th ed. New York, NY: McGraw-Hill; 2016.

33. Goldman L, Schafer AI. Goldman's Cecil medicine. 25th ed. Philadelphia, PA: Saunders Elsevier; 2011.

34. Helms RA, Quan DJ. Textbook of therapeutics: drug and disease management. 8th ed. Philadelphia, PA: Lippincott Williams & Wilkins; 2006.

35. Bope ET, Kellerman RD. Conn's current therapy 2017. Philadelphia, PA: Saunders Elsevier; 2017.

36. Medscape [Internet]. New York, NY: Medscape, LLC [cited 2017 Apr 7]. Available from: http://www.medscape.com/. Accessed April 7, 2017.

37. Red Book Online [Internet]. Ann Arbor, MI: Truven Health Analytics [cited 2017 Apr 7]. Available from: https://truvenhealth.com/products/micromedex/product-suites/clinical-knowledge/redbook. Accessed April 7, 2017.

38. Clinical Pharmacology [Internet]. Tampa, FL: Gold Standard, Inc. Updated 2017 [cited 2017 Apr 7]. Available from: www.clinicalpharmacology.com. Accessed April 7, 2017.

39. Lexicomp [Internet]. St. Louis, MO: Wolters Kluwer [cited 2017 Apr 7]. Available from: http://www.wolterskluwercdi.com/lexicomp-online/. Accessed April 7, 2017.

40. Medi-Span [Internet]. St. Louis, MO: Wolters Kluwer [cited 2017 Apr 7]. Available from: http://www.wolterskluwercdi.com/medispan-clinical/. Accessed April 7, 2017.

41. Identidex® [Internet]. Ann Arbor, MI: Truven Health Analytics [cited 2017 Apr 7]. Available from: http://truvenhealth.com/our-solutions/products#alphaTab7. Accessed April 7, 2017.

42. IDENT-A-DRUG REFERENCE [Internet]. Stockton, CA: Therapeutic Research Center. 1995-2013. Available from: www.indentadrug.com. Accessed April 7, 2017.

43. Facts & Comparisons® eAnswers [Internet]. St. Louis, MO: Wolters Kluwer Health. Updated 2017 [cited 2017 Apr 7]. Available from: http://www.wolterskluwercdi.com/facts-comparisons-online/. Accessed April 7, 2017.

44. Billups NF, Billups SM. American drug index 2016. 550th ed. (final). St. Louis, MO: Wolters Kluwer; 2016.

45. Hansten PD, Horn JR. Drug interaction analysis and management 2014. St. Louis, MO: Wolters Kluwer; 2014.

46. Drug Interaction Facts [Internet]. St. Louis, MO: Wolters Kluwer Health. Updated 2017 [cited 2017 Apr 7]. Available from: http://www.wolterskluwercdi.com/facts-comparisons-online/. Accessed April 7, 2017.

47. Baxter K. Stockley's drug interactions. 11th ed. London: Pharmaceutical Press; 2016.

48. Aronoff GR, Bennett WM, Berns JS, Brier ME, Kasbekar N, Mueller BA, Pasko DA, Smoyer WE. Drug prescribing in renal failure. 5th ed. Philadelphia, PA: American College of Physicians; 2007.

49. Semla TP, Beizer JL, Higbee MD. Geriatric dosage handbook. 21st ed. Hudson, OH: Lexicomp; 2015.

50. American Pharmacists Association. Drug information handbook with international trade names index. 26th ed. Hudson, OH: Lexicomp; 2017.

51. Brayfield A. Martindale: the complete drug reference. 39th ed. London: Pharmaceutical Press; 2017.

52. Swiss Pharmaceutical Society. Index Nominum: international drug directory. 19th ed. Stuttgart: Medpharm Scientific Publishers; 2008.
53. Drugdex [Internet]. Ann Arbor, MI: Truven Health Analytics [cited 2017 Apr 7]. Available from: http://www.micromedexsolutions.com/micromedex2/4.85.0/WebHelp/Document_help/Drug_Eval_document.htm. Accessed April 7, 2017.
54. Lee M. Basic skills in interpreting laboratory data. 6th ed. Bethesda, MD: American Society of Health-System Pharmacists; 2017.
55. Pagana KD, Pagana TJ. Mosby's manual of diagnostic and laboratory tests. 5th ed. Amsterdam: Elsevier; 2014.
56. Nicoll D, Lu CM, Pignone M, McPhee SJ. Pocket guide to diagnostic tests. 6th ed. New York, NY: McGraw-Hill; 2012.
57. Chernecky CC, Berger BJ. Laboratory tests and diagnostic procedures. 6th ed. Philadelphia, PA: Saunders; 2013.
58. Krinsky DL, Ferreri SP, Hemstreet B, Hume AL, Newton GD, Rollings CJ, et al. Handbook of nonprescription drugs. 18th ed. Washington, DC: American Pharmacists Association; 2015.
59. Pray WS. [eBook]. Nonprescription product therapeutics. 2nd ed. St. Louis, MO: Wolters Kluwer Health; 2010.
60. Engorn B, Flerlage J. The Harriet Lane handbook. 20th ed. Philadelphia, PA: Mosby; 2015.
61. Taketomo CK, Hodding JH, Kraus DM. Pediatric and neonatal dosage handbook. 23rd ed. Hudson, OH: Lexicomp; 2016.
62. Kliegman R, Stanton B, St. Geme J, Schor N. Nelson textbook of pediatrics. 20th ed. Amsterdam: Elsevier; 2015.
63. NeoFax [Internet]. Ann Arbor, MI: Truven Health Analytics [cited 2017 Apr 7]. Available from: http://neofax.micromedexsolutions.com/neofax/neofax.php. Accessed April 7, 2017.
64. American Academy of Pediatrics Committee on Infectious Diseases. Red Book. 30th ed. Elk Grove Village, IL: American Academy of Pediatrics; 2015.
65. Teixeira MG, Zatz JL. Pharmaceutical calculations. 5th ed. Hoboken, NJ: Wiley; 2017.
66. Ansel HC, Stockton SJ. Pharmaceutical calculations. 15th ed. St. Louis, MO: Wolters Kluwer; 2016.
67. Winter ME. Basic clinical pharmacokinetics. 5th ed. Philadelphia, PA: Lippincott Williams & Wilkins; 2009.
68. Shargel L, Yu AB. Applied biopharmaceutics and pharmacokinetics. 7th ed. New York, NY: McGraw-Hill; 2016.
69. Brunton LL, Chabner B, Knollman B. Goodman & Gilman's: the pharmacological basis of therapeutics. 12th ed. New York, NY: McGraw-Hill; 2010.
70. Katzung BG, Masters SB, Trevor AJ. Basic & clinical pharmacology. 13th ed. New York, NY: McGraw-Hill; 2015.
71. Wecker L, Crespo L, Dunaway G, Faingold C, Watts S. Brody's human pharmacology: molecular to clinical. 5th ed. Philadelphia, PA: Elsevier; 2010.
72. Golan DE, Armstrong EJ, Armstrong AW. Principles of pharmacology: the pathophysiologic basis of drug therapy. 4th ed. Philadelphia, PA: Lippincott Williams & Wilkins; 2016.

73. Abood RR, Burns KA. Pharmacy practice and the law. 8th ed. Sudbury, MA: Jones and Bartlett Publishers; 2017.

74. Reiss BS, Hall GD. Guide to federal pharmacy law. 9th ed. Delmar, NY: Apothecary Press; 2016.

75. Briggs GG, Freeman RK. Drugs in pregnancy and lactation: a reference guide to fetal and neonatal risk. 10th ed. Philadelphia, PA: Lippincott Williams & Wilkins; 2014.

76. LactMed [Internet]. Bethesda, MD: U.S. National Library of Medicine. Updated 2017 [cited 2017 Apr 7]. Available from: https://toxnet.nlm.nih.gov/newtoxnet/lactmed.htm. Accessed April 7, 2017.

77. Hale TW, Rowe HE. Medications and mother's milk 2017. 17th ed. New York, NY: Springer Publishing Co.; 2017.

78. Shepard TH, Lemire RJ. Catalog of teratogenic agents. 13th ed. Baltimore, MD: Johns Hopkins University Press; 2010.

79. REPROTOX [Internet]. Washington, DC: The Reproductive Toxicology Center [cited 2017 Apr 7]. Available from: https://reprotox.org/. Accessed April 7, 2017.

80. TOXNET [Internet]. Washington, DC: U.S. National Institutes of Health [cited 2017 Apr 7]. Available from: http://toxnet.nlm.nih.gov/. Accessed April 7, 2017.

81. LiverTox [Internet]. Bethesda, MD: U.S. National Library of Medicine. Updated 2017 [cited 2017 Apr 7]. Available from: https://livertox.nih.gov/. Accessed April 7, 2017.

82. POISINDEX® [Internet]. Ann Arbor, MI: Truven Health Analytics [cited 2017 Apr 7]. Available from: http://truvenhealth.com/our-solutions/products#alphaTab7. Accessed April 7, 2017.

83. Hoffman RS, Howland MA, Lewin NA, Nelson LS, Goldfrank LR. Goldfrank's toxicologic emergencies. 10th ed. New York, NY: McGraw-Hill; 2015.

84. Klaassen C. Casarett & Doull's toxicology: the basic science of poisons. 8th ed. New York, NY: McGraw-Hill; 2013.

85. Leikin JB, Paloucek FP. Poisoning and toxicology handbook. 4th ed. Boca Raton, FL: CRC; 2007.

86. Ettinger SJ, Feldman EL, editors. Textbook of veterinary internal medicine. 8th ed. Philadelphia, PA: W.B. Saunders; 2017.

87. Riviere JE, Papich MG. Veterinary pharmacology and therapeutics. 9th ed. Stockholm, WI: Wiley-Blackwell; 2009.

88. Merck Veterinary Manual [Internet]. Whitehouse Station, NJ: Merck & Co, Inc. [cited 2017 Apr 7]. Available from: http://www.merckvetmanual.com/. Accessed April 7, 2017.

89. Plumb DC. Plumb's veterinary drug handbook. 8th ed. Stockholm, WI: Wiley-Blackwell; 2015.

90. Carpenter JW, Mashima TY, Rupier DJ, editors. Exotic animal formulary. 4th ed. Philadelphia, PA: W.B. Saunders; 2012.

91. U.S. Food and Drug Administration Center for Veterinary Medicine [Internet]. Animal and Veterinary. Rockville, MD [cited 2017 Apr 7]. Available from: https://www.fda.gov/AnimalVeterinary/. Accessed April 7, 2017.

92. U.S. Food and Drug Administration [Internet]. Animal Drugs@FDA. Rockville, MD [cited 2017 Apr 7]. Available from: https://animaldrugsatfda.fda.gov/adafda/views/#/search. Accessed April 7, 2017.
93. PetEducation.com [Internet]. Drs. Foster & Smith Inc.; c1997-2013 [cited 2017 Apr 7]. Available from: http://www.petplace.com. Accessed April 7, 2017.
94. PetPlace.com [Internet]. Weston, FL: Intelligent Content Corp.; c1999-2013 [cited 2017 Apr 7]. Available from: http://www.petplace.com. Accessed April 7, 2017.
95. Pets with Diabetes [Internet]. Petdiabetes.com; c2000-2013 [cited 2017 Apr 7]. Available from: http://www.petdiabetes.com. Accessed April 7, 2017.
96. USP Veterinary Medicine [Internet]. Rockville, MD: United States Pharmacopeia 1 Convention; c1997-2017 [cited 2017 Apr 7]. Available from: http://www.usp.org/usp-healthcare-professionals/compounding/veterinary-compounding-monographs. Accessed April 7, 2017.

SUGGESTED READINGS

- National Center for Biotechnology Information (NCBI). Databases. Available from: https://www.ncbi.nlm.nih.gov/guide/all/#databases
- National Library of Medicine. Broad subject terms for indexed journals. Available from: https://wwwcf.nlm.nih.gov/serials/journals/index.cfm
- National Library of Medicine. Drug information from the National Library of Medicine. Available from: https://www.nlm.nih.gov/learn-about-drugs.html
- National Library of Medicine. Electronic databases and directories: alphabetical list. Available from: https://www.nlm.nih.gov/services/databases_abc.html
- National Library of Medicine. Medline Plus. Available from: https://medlineplus.gov/
- PubMed. National Library of Medicine catalog: journals references in the NCBI databases. Available from: https://www.ncbi.nlm.nih.gov/nlmcatalog/journals

Chapter Four

Drug Literature Evaluation I: Controlled Clinical Trial Evaluation

Maisha Kelly Freeman • Michael Kendrach • Peter J. Hughes • Rachel M. Slaton

Learning Objectives

After completing this chapter, the reader will be able to

- List the skills practitioners need to locate and evaluate current information for pharmacy practice activities.
- Explain the skills practitioners need to locate and evaluate current information for pharmacy practice activities.
- Describe special characteristics of a controlled clinical trial that distinguish this research design as the prototype for clinical research.
- Prepare a null hypothesis (H_0) based upon the clinical trial objective(s) and endpoint(s).
- Differentiate between the types of data, measures of central tendency, and measures of variability.
- Differentiate between Type I and Type II errors; discuss methods to reduce the possibility of either of these errors occurring.
- Interpret p-values and 95% confidence interval (CI); discuss whether to reject or fail-to-reject the H_0 by using these clinical trial results.
- Calculate and interpret relative risk (RR), relative risk reduction (RRR), absolute risk reduction (ARR), and number needed to treat (NNT).
- State whether a statistical significance and clinical difference are present using the clinical trial results.
- Explain the purpose and usage of editorials, letters to the editor, and secondary journals in critiquing clinical trials and in the decision-making process of applying the results into practice.

Key Concepts

1 Practitioners need to efficiently locate, critically analyze, and effectively communicate data from the primary literature in daily activities of patient care and the medication use process.

2 A controlled clinical trial is the premier study design to measure and quantify differences in effect between the intervention versus control.

3 Decision making should not rely solely on reading abstracts; the entire published study should be read and thoroughly evaluated.

4 The results of a controlled clinical trial should be extrapolated to the type of patient enrolled in the study and readers should be aware of the limitations of surrogate endpoints and subgroup analysis results.

5 Randomization is an essential component of controlled clinical trials and a significant differentiator from other study designs.

6 The controlled clinical trial primary endpoint should be appropriate for the study purpose and measured using valid techniques and methods.

7 An appropriate sample size in a controlled clinical trial is vital for the study results to have any significant meaning; conducting a power analysis is important to determine a suitable sample size.

8 Correctly interpreting the p-values is crucial in evaluating a controlled clinical trial; not all statistically significant p-values are clinically important. The magnitude of difference in effect between the intervention and control cannot be determined solely with the p-value.

9 The use of 95% confidence interval (CI) can assist the reader in assessing the magnitude of difference in effect between the intervention and control to apply to the population.

10 Calculating measures of association (relative risk, absolute risk reduction, relative risk reduction, number needed to treat) for nominal data provides further information to evaluate the meaning of controlled clinical trial results.

11 Nonstatistically significant results do not equate to the intervention and control being the same or equal.

12 All controlled clinical trial results need to be assessed to determine the clinical relevance (i.e., meaningfulness) of the intervention versus control.

13 Controlled clinical trial investigators and authors should disclose any funding sources and potential conflicts of interest.

14 Editorials, letters to the editor, and commentary publications can assist in interpreting controlled clinical trial results.

Introduction

Practitioners continuously rely upon the biomedical/pharmacy literature for many day-to-day activities. The practice of medicine and pharmacy are dynamic, and drug facts acquired during formal education cannot sustain a health care provider in future practice. In 2012 alone, 28,100 peer-reviewed journals were responsible for publishing 1.8 to 1.9 million articles.[1] Changes include new medications, dosage formulations and uses approved by the Food and Drug Administration (FDA), revised drug safety information (i.e., adverse drug effects, drug interactions), and updated disease state therapeutic guidelines. During 2016, greater than 37 new molecular entities/biological agents were approved by the FDA,[2,3] and over 3,000 published articles classified as human practice guidelines were added to the National Library of Medicine database.[4] Practitioners must employ methods to keep current with these advances in order to remain competent, trustworthy health care professionals.[5] ❶ *Practitioners need to efficiently locate, critically analyze, and effectively communicate data from the primary literature in daily activities of patient care and the medication use process.* Therefore, skills, such as drug literature evaluation, are necessary to prepare the health care provider for practice.

Multiple resources are available for practitioners to provide answers to questions, care for patients, make decisions, and solve problems. But practitioners need to recognize both the advantages and limitations of the information resources to meet the challenges encountered during their daily practice activities (see Chapter 3). Advantages include ready access and electronic formats. Potential disadvantages include biases, costs, and lag time (i.e., lack of current content) that hinder the usefulness of some references. In addition, misinterpretation of the information can lead to improper patient care.

Although access to information for both health care professionals and laypersons has increased exponentially, not all information can be deemed accurate. In a recent study of medical students' interpretation of the literature, almost 25% of students had trouble interpreting number needed to treat (NNT) and other numeracy questions.[6] As a result, practitioners are repeatedly relied upon to clarify, explain, defend, and/or refute information[7] because pharmacy practitioners have skills in efficiently locating and critically analyzing drug information to appropriately formulate and effectively communicate a response. In addition, practitioners are frequently consulted by other health care providers to assist in individual patient care regarding appropriate drug use.[8–10] Also, practitioners are in a position to select drugs for use in a multitude of patients (e.g., third-party health care plans, drug formulary decisions).[11,12] Furthermore, practitioners are expected to be providers of direct patient care in the new U.S. health care reform activities. All these activities require practitioners to carefully review and critique the literature instead of accepting the authors' conclusions. Many studies have very positive conclusions, but include study design errors that limit the clinical usefulness of the results. Also, medical/pharmacy continuing education presentations may contain biases and/or inaccuracies, while textbooks/review articles may contain misinterpreted, outdated, and/or noncomprehensive information. Due to the important contribution pharmacy practitioners have in patient care, they need to have skill in identifying the strengths and limitations of the biomedical literature. This chapter is devoted to explaining and discussing core concepts for critiquing one essential type of biomedical literature, a **controlled clinical trial.**

Biomedical/Pharmacy Literature

Three types of literature serve as information resources for practitioners: tertiary, secondary, and primary (Table 4-1).[13] Readers are referred to Chapter 3 in this textbook for more in-depth discussions of these three literature types.

Primary literature, specifically controlled clinical trials, serves as the foundation for clinical practice by providing the documentation for using therapy. Although vast amounts of primary literature articles are published each year, individuals can efficiently locate information specific and useful to their needs by incorporating appropriate search techniques.[14,15] Clinical trials are one particular type of primary literature that can be a reliable source of new information to change health care practices.[16-18] ❷ *A controlled clinical trial is the premier study design to measure and quantify differences in effect of the intervention versus control.* New information may either counter or serve as the root for altering existing practice regimens; as a result, practitioners need to critique clinical trials. The special features of clinical trial design allow investigators to determine which therapeutic interventions should be used in practice.[19,20] In fact, the FDA requires clinical trials to be

TABLE 4–1. THREE TYPES OF LITERATURE

Literature Type	Description	Examples
Tertiary	Established knowledge	Textbooks, review articles, Up-to-Date, WebMD, Lexicomp
Secondary	Indexing/abstracting services (i.e., databases)	PubMed® or MEDLINE® (National Library of Medicine), Embase® (Elsevier), International Pharmaceutical Abstracts (Wolters Kluwer Health)
		CINAHL (Cumulative Index to Nursing and Allied Health Literature)
		InfoTrac OneFile (Gale CENGAGE Learning), Academic LexisNexis® (Reed Elsevier)
Primary	Original research	Controlled clinical trials, case-control studies, crossover trials, case reports

conducted and the results submitted before a new molecular entity (i.e., medication) can be marketed and/or receive new indications for use.[21] Proper interpretation of clinical trials is vital to providing appropriate health care. Chapter 5 reviews evaluating publications using the other types of research designs.

In general, a controlled clinical trial consists of an investigational (intervention) group being directly compared to a control group (e.g., standard therapy, placebo).[19,20,22] The intervention under investigation may be a new medication, different medication dosing regimen, diet, surgery, behavioral process, exercise program, diagnostic procedure, or something else. The goal of the clinical trial is to measure and quantify the difference in effect (e.g., efficacy, safety) between the investigational and control groups. The results then can allow decisions to be made regarding proper care for patients (i.e., to use or not use the investigational therapy).[19] Although the origins of a controlled trial date back to the eighteenth century,[23] a formalized process of conducting controlled clinical trials was not implemented until the late 1940s.[24] However, poorly designed clinical trials are still published and the existence of a clinical trial may not translate into clinically useful information. Research has reported that results of well-designed clinical trials are considered to be of better quality and are usually more clinically relevant than clinical trials that are poorly designed (see Chapter 8).[25]

The published clinical trial is presented in a manner that explains the research process in an orderly format to improve the readers' comprehension of the study, results, and conclusions. Table 4-2 displays the style in which a clinical trial usually appears in printed resources.[26,27] This chapter discusses the information presented in these sections according to the CONSORT (Consolidated Standards of Reporting Trials) format. The CONSORT format was formulated to improve the quality of reporting clinical trials in the published literature, since inadequate reporting methods hinder the interpretation of results produced by clinical trials. CONSORT has been supported by an increasing number of medical and health care journals (e.g., Journal of the American Medical Association [JAMA]) and editorial groups (e.g., International Committee of Medical Journal Editors [ICMJE]).[27] Some further information about CONSORT may be found in Chapter 12. Other research types (e.g., case-control study) may use a publishing style similar to a controlled clinical trial.[28] Therefore, one should not assume all publications using this format are controlled clinical trials.

Evidence from clinical trials is used by health care providers to base their patient care decisions.[16,17,29,30] A controlled clinical trial is the most robust method to measure and quantify differences in effects between a therapy under study and the control group.[19,20,31] Many clinical studies are published annually, but not every study initiated is reported in the published literature.[32–34] Primary reasons for not publishing trials are lack of time, incomplete studies, manuscript in preparation or review, unimportant or negative result, poor study quality or design, fear of rejection, etc.[33] In order to treat patients most appropriately, all relevant information and data, both positive and negative, are needed in the

TABLE 4-2. FORMAT AND CONTENT OF CONTROLLED CLINICAL TRIALS

Controlled Clinical Trial Section	Type of Information Presented
Abstract	Brief overview of the research project
Introduction	Research background
	What is already known
	Needs for the study/rationale
	Objective/hypotheses
Methods	Study design
	Study Setting
	Population to be sampled
	Inclusion and exclusion criteria
	Intervention and control groups
	Randomization
	Blinding
	Endpoints/outcomes
	Follow-up procedure
	Sample size calculations/Power analysis
	Statistical analysis
Results	Subject characteristics
	Subject dropouts/adherence
	Endpoints quantified
	Statistical significance
	Safety assessments
Discussion	Result interpretations
	Clinical significance
	Other study results compared
	Limitations
	Conclusion/Application to practice
Acknowledgments	Other contributors
	Funding source
	Peer-review dates/Manuscript acceptance date (not all trials)
References/Bibliography	Citations for information included from other resources (e.g., trials and reports)

decision-making process.[33,35,36] In a recent study of registered trials (n = 585), 171 (29%) were unpublished. These unpublished studies enrolled 299,763 patients and those that were not published commonly received industry funding (150/468; 32%).[37]

Readers of the biomedical literature need to consider the issues of selective reporting (i.e., publishing positive study results, but not negative studies). In addition, usually one clinical trial is not sufficient to adopt a therapy under investigation as the first choice to treat patients. Results of multiple trials are usually combined together to serve as the evidence for either incorporating a newly developed therapy into practice or changing the existing method of treating a disease (see Chapter 8 on evidence-based clinical practice guidelines).[38,39] Journal editors have an obligation and should publish negative studies. In fact, more journal editors are publishing negative results. The Journal of Negative Results in BioMedicine was initiated to discuss "non-confirmatory and 'negative' data."[40] Results of these studies are important in formulating practice patterns based upon the available evidence. Failure by investigators, authors, and journal editors to publish negative studies contributes to publication bias.[35,41,42]

The intent of this chapter is for readers not to be misled by the literature, but to correctly critique the controlled clinical trial, then properly use the results and conclusions in health care practice settings. In addition to the discussions of critiquing clinical trials from this chapter, readers should use the principles of the evidence-based medicine (Chapter 8) of this textbook in providing patient care.

Approach to Evaluating Research Studies (True Experiments)

Many different research designs are published, but the most common of these are prospective studies in which an intervention (e.g., drug therapy) is directly compared to a control and differences between these are measured. A prospective study measures the effect of an intervention and control as the study progresses forward in time. Examples of prospective studies include clinical trials (e.g., evaluation of drug A versus drug B in humans); stability of compounded drug formulation (e.g., suspension made from drug tablets), compatibility of intravenous (IV) drug admixtures, and drug pharmacokinetic interactions. Regardless of the study design and objective, fundamental elements should be present in all studies, including appropriate qualifications of the researchers conducting the research; valid investigational methods; proper research techniques; and appropriate analysis as well as interpretation of the results. A similar process is used to evaluate prospective studies. A checklist for pertinent information to be included in a clinical trial is located in Appendix 4-1. Answering the questions contained in Appendix 4-1 can allow readers to determine the strengths and limitations of a clinical trial. The remainder of this chapter discusses the questions presented in the appendix plus techniques for critiquing a clinical trial.

JOURNAL, PEER REVIEW, AND INVESTIGATORS

Numerous journals are published covering the biomedical literature, including the professions of medicine, nursing, and pharmacy. Health care practitioners need to regularly access professional journals (either print or electronic) to assist them in keeping current in their practice responsibilities.[43] Misleading information may be presented to health care providers by pharmaceutical industry representatives (see Chapter 23).[44] As a result, prescribers' perception of the safety and efficacy of the drug product may be over and underemphasized, respectively, and use of these products can affect patient outcomes and increase the cost of care.[45,46] In addition, not all studies will be published in reliable journals.[47,48] Reliable journals typically employ some type of peer-review process. The peer-review process provides another step to reduce erroneous research from reaching the health care community. Simply defined, peer-reviewed articles are evaluated by someone who has expertise on the topic or in the field being evaluated and who is not one of the editorial staff.[41,49] Most journals incorporate the peer-review process in selecting articles for publication. Briefly, manuscripts submitted to the journal for publication consideration are screened by the editor; those deemed as potential publications are sent to individuals with expertise in the appropriate area. These individuals read the manuscript and comment upon the strengths and limitations, plus offer a recommendation to the journal editor regarding accepting or rejecting the manuscript for publication. The peer-reviewers' comments are sent to the authors for the manuscript to be revised and, if necessary, resubmitted for publication consideration. In some cases, manuscripts may be rejected as being too flawed or inappropriate for the journal. However, predatory journals have changed the face of publishing in which publishers send a large number of spam e-mails to potential authors with false claims of peer review. After the review is submitted, publishers charge a large publication fee.[50]

Although the peer-review process increases the time required before publication, the goal is to reduce the publication of manuscripts that have inappropriate methods/design, are poorly written, and/or do not meet the needs of the journal's readership.[47,51] However, the peer-review process does not always prevent publication of articles without deficiencies, and readers should assess the quality and critique of each published article.[51,52] Although the value of peer-review process has been debated, studies have been conducted demonstrating improved quality of journal article features after the peer-review process.[41,53,54] Two journal sections can be checked for information addressing whether the peer-review process is used: instructions for authors and journal's scope/purpose. Regardless of whether a clinical trial is published in a peer-reviewed or non-peer-reviewed journal, the article needs to be evaluated closely for biases and interpreted appropriately.

As readers become more familiar with the professional literature, they will find certain journals have a reputation for good quality publications, such as New England Journal of Medicine and Annals of Pharmacotherapy. This too can be considered in the evaluation of literature, although poor articles can still be found in well-respected journals and excellent articles are published in other journals.[52,53]

PUBLICATION TYPES

Research results can be published in other venues besides journals. A very common publication type is meeting abstracts. Research presented during a professional organization's meeting, whether as platform or poster, requires an abstract to be available for meeting attendees to review. These abstracts usually undergo the peer-review process to be selected, but readers should be cautious of the abstract content. The peer-review process may not be as thorough as that of a full manuscript because the entire study details are not available to the reader on the abstract. Another common publication type for research is journal supplements. The purpose of such supplements is to publish a collection of articles related to a specific topic in a separate journal issue.[41] Many, but not all, supplements are sponsored by an outside entity (e.g., pharmaceutical company), which serves as another source of revenue for the journal. The articles should undergo peer review using the same rigorous process, but readers should refer to the journal's website to obtain the policies regarding the peer-review process for journal supplements. However, not all articles published in journal supplements should be automatically discarded or classified as inferior information. Journal supplements can serve as a venue for organizations to publish their disease state practice guidelines. An example of a very informative journal supplement is the American College of Chest Physicians' supplement addressing antithrombotic therapy.[55] Many of the articles in this supplement are authored by recognized leaders and researchers in their field of practice.

The Internet is also a common venue to publish medical and pharmacy information. This resource is ideal for rapid communications of breaking news (e.g., contamination of drug product, study results) to better care for patients. But as many Internet users know, unreliable information is also posted and can influence some attitudes. The Health on the Net (HON) Foundation is an organization that is dedicated to disseminating quality health information to health care professionals and patients. This organization certifies Internet websites that apply for certification if they are able to demonstrate that the information contained within the website is of quality and meets the eight principles that the organization embodies, also known as the HON Code of Conduct. Typically, websites that have the HON Code logo included are reliable, trustworthy sites that cater to the health-related needs of patients and/or health care providers.[56]

Other factors to evaluate in a published study are the investigators' credentials and the practice site of these individuals. Investigators need to be properly trained and have active practice experience in the area of study. The site where the clinical trial was conducted should not immediately endorse or condemn the quality of the research, other than it should be a site that has the capability to perform the study (i.e., have the resources to properly and completely perform the necessary study methods). The quality of the research must be evaluated because even prestigious institutions can conduct poor clinical trials. Also, persons involved with the study need to be ethical and responsible to protect patients enrolled in the study.[57] Persons with specialized credentials in biostatistics need to contribute with statistical analysis of the data. Furthermore, all authors listed should have made substantial contributions to the research and/or publication. The Recommendations for the Conduct, Reporting, Editing, and Publication of Scholarly Work in Medical Journals, prepared by journal editors, explicitly outlines the criteria for persons to be listed as authors for a published article. According to this publication, an author has to meet four criteria. In addition, authors should be able to identify other authors and have confidence in other author's work (see Chapter 12 for more information about authorship).[41]

Articles by authors who are employees of a pharmaceutical company should be more selectively analyzed, since there may be concern about potential bias or conflicts of interest. The pharmaceutical industry must conduct research for new therapies to be introduced to the marketplace and many companies are collaborating with academic researchers.[44,58] The concern regarding influence from the pharmaceutical industry on health care providers has not gone unnoticed, particularly involving practitioners conducting research for the pharmaceutical industry. In response, many journals now are requiring article authors to declare any conflicts of interest with the research and outside interests.[41,55] A **conflict of interest** is possible even though investigators may not consider that their relationship affects their scientific judgment.[41] Authors need to state they have received honorariums and/or research grants, and/or are members of the speaker's bureau for pharmaceutical companies. Readers should be informed of potential bias of the investigators. However, immediately discarding or discounting clinical trials in which investigators declare relationships with the pharmaceutical industry may be premature. Many investigators are required to obtain external funding for research projects and academic promotion. Clinical trials that have researchers with relationships with multiple pharmaceutical companies may not be considered to be overtly biased. Investigators have an ethical obligation to submit credible research results for publication.[41] Biases may be present, but readers having the skills of identifying study strengths and limitations can still use the clinical trial results appropriately.

TITLE

The clinical trial title is important and should be carefully evaluated by the reader. A title should be reflective of the work, unbiased, specific, and concise (i.e., usually less than or equal to 10 words or 40 characters), but not too general or detailed. This is done in an effort to make the retrieval easier and for the title to be reflective of the work conducted. Declarative sentences, which tend to overemphasize a conclusion, are not preferred for scientific articles.[59] In addition, the title should not be phrased as a question and randomized clinical trials should be identified in the title; however, depending on the journal, the study design must be included in the title.[41] Furthermore, the title should include key words that are both sensitive (easing the task of locating the appropriate articles) and specific (excluding those not being searched for) that allow easier electronic retrieval of the article.[34]

The following is an example of a biased study title: "Improved bronchodilation with levalbuterol compared with racemic albuterol in patients with asthma."[60] The title implies levalbuterol to be better than racemic albuterol. Although the average change in lung function parameters was slightly greater with levalbuterol, no significant differences were reported.[58] Thus, one could have been misled by reading only the title, believing levalbuterol to be a superior agent. A suggested unbiased title for this trial is: "Comparison of levalbuterol and racemic albuterol bronchodilation in patients with asthma: a randomized clinical trial."

ABSTRACT

An abstract is considered to be a concise overview of the study or a synopsis of the major principles of the article. ❸ *Decision making should not rely solely on reading abstracts; the entire manuscript is to be read and thoroughly evaluated.* Abstracts include information addressing the article objective, methods, results, and conclusions. A primary use of abstracts is for readers to obtain an immediate overview of the article to determine if the entire article should be read.[61,62] Another use is publishing the abstract in secondary resources (e.g., PubMed®, International Pharmaceutical Abstracts [IPA]) for individuals conducting literature searches.

Although unique for each journal, authors are required to follow specific requirements while preparing an abstract. Many journals now require abstracts to be prepared in an organized format (i.e., structured abstract) and usually contain less than or equal to 500 words. The structured abstract includes the following sections: objective, research design, clinical setting, participants, interventions, main outcome measurements, results, and conclusions.[41,59] Structured abstracts, compared to unstructured abstracts, do have some advantages, including being more informative, easier to read, and generally preferred by readers.[63,64] However, structured abstracts usually require more journal space. Informative abstracts may entice some individuals to read the study; thus, abstracts should be thorough, complete, and unbiased in wording selection.[62]

Abstracts should be consistent with the manuscript and should not present biased and/or inaccurate information.[59,60,61] For further information regarding abstracts and preparation, refer to Appendix 12-2. Regardless of the abstract presentation style, readers should not make decisions based upon abstract information only. Results of published studies illustrate the dangers of reading only the abstract.[65–68] These studies provided evidence of omissions and discrepancies between the abstract and the manuscript in medical, psychology, and pharmacy journals.

INTRODUCTION

The introduction section serves two specific purposes: discussing the study rationale and study purpose.[27,69] The introduction section should capture the readers' interest. Scientific writing should be direct and straightforward. Usually, readers are first briefly educated on the issues that were the basis for conducting the study. The study investigators may state that the reason the research was conducted was due to the lack of data to answer a question or because available data are conflicting regarding an issue. Every clinical trial is designed to answer one or more research questions. The investigators should explain how the clinical trial will overcome the shortcomings of the prior research, if applicable. The study objective is often stated within the last paragraph, if not the last sentence, of this section. Well-written studies present a clearly stated research purpose and this statement should be understood by the reader before continuing with the remaining article content. Studies with a well-written purpose statement enable the reader to better comprehend and assess the research methods.

Once the clinical trial objective is determined, the investigators need to formulate a research and **null hypothesis**. A **research hypothesis** (also known as the alternative hypothesis) states that there is a difference between the therapy under investigation and the control, while the null hypothesis (H_0) states that there is no difference between these two groups (see next paragraph for an example). After the study is completed, the researchers analyze the data and the research hypothesis is either accepted (which also includes rejecting H_0) or rejected (which then means H_0 is accepted). Readers should recognize that not all clinical trials will include the specific research and null hypotheses in the introduction section. While this can be considered a deficiency in the paper, it does not necessarily indicate that the paper contains incorrect information.

An example to explain some of the material thus far included in this chapter is the trial that assessed whether ezetimibe added to statin therapy is associated with a reduction in cardiovascular mortality in patients who had an acute coronary syndrome and whose LDL cholesterol values were within guideline recommendations. The Improved Reduction of Outcomes: Vytorin Efficacy International Trial (IMPROVE-IT) compared simvastatin 40 mg plus ezetimibe 10 mg or simvastatin 40 mg plus placebo.[70] The investigators expressed in the introduction section that the rationale for conducting this clinical trial was that no evidence has been published that determines whether ezetimibe (a drug that reduces absorption of cholesterol from the intestine) added to simvastatin can improve cardiovascular events. The research hypothesis of IMPROVE-IT was: "There is a difference in the incidence of cardiovascular events in patients receiving combination therapy with ezetimibe and simvastatin compared to simvastatin monotherapy. The H_0 for this clinical trial was: "There is no difference in the incidence of cardiovascular outcomes between combination therapy with ezetimibe and simvastatin compared to simvastatin monotherapy."[68] After reading the IMPROVE-IT introduction, the reader has a clear understanding of the study rationale and purpose: the results of this trial should provide health care providers with evidence to prescribe combination therapy with ezetimibe and simvastatin or simvastatin monotherapy after acute coronary syndrome in patients with LDL cholesterol levels within the guideline recommendations.

As with all sections of a clinical trial, this section needs to be carefully read. Authors may set the stage by presenting only selective (i.e., not comprehensive) information and/ or weak references (to be discussed later in the chapter) to support the rationale for conducting the study. Also, the information may be presented using biased wording, which predisposes the reader to believing the prior research was insignificant in providing evidence applicable to practice.

METHODS

Following a well-designed plan is essential for the clinical trial results to be acceptable and useful to practitioners. The design of a study (i.e., methods) is important for the results to be valid, just as abiding by the blueprints is vital to building a house. The methods section of a clinical trial contains a large amount of information that includes the type of subjects enrolled, the comparative therapy description, outcome measures, and planned statistical analyses. Flaws within the design of a clinical trial limit the application and significance of the results. Poor study design leads to reduced study **internal validity**, thus resulting in limited external study validity (Table 4-3).[23,71] The methods section needs to be thorough in describing to the reader the process in which the study was conducted. The methods section should be written in such detail so that if another investigator wanted to duplicate the study, the study could be replicated with ease. A reader should devote the majority of time used to assess the trial in this section.

TABLE 4–3. INTERNAL VERSUS EXTERNAL VALIDITY OF CLINICAL TRIALS

Term	Meaning	Application
Internal validity	Quality of the study design	Strong design should translate into reliable results
External validity	Ability to apply results into practice	Study results meaningful to practitioners and can be used for patient care

Clinical trials follow a pattern in presenting the information within the methods section.[27] This standardized format allows study details to be in an orderly fashion and quickly located. The methods section should include the trial design, participants, interventions, outcomes, sample size, randomization sequence generation, allocation concealment mechanisms (e.g., mechanisms used to generate random allocation sequence), blinding, and statistical methods. Readers of the biomedical literature should have an understanding of the overall design to appropriately critique clinical trials and use the study results for patient care activities.

Study Design

Several study designs are available for investigators to select from when conducting research. The study questions that the researchers wish to answer dictates which study design is selected to conduct the research.[72,73] Both investigators and readers of the literature need to identify the strengths and limitations of the research designs. Although many study designs are available, this chapter only discusses controlled clinical trials. For additional information on other study designs, the reader is referred to Chapter 5.

Case Study 4–1

A controlled clinical trial was designed to assess the comparative effectiveness of trimethoprim-sulfamethoxazole (TMP-SMX) to clindamycin for the treatment of uncomplicated skin infections with cellulitis, abscesses >5 cm in diameter, or both in adults and children in the outpatient setting. All abscesses underwent incision and drainage and the subjects underwent randomization and were prescribed to receive TMP-SMX or clindamycin at an age-appropriate dose for 10 days in a double-blinded manner. The primary endpoint was clinical cure 7 to 10 days following treatment cessation. The study was designed with an 80% power to detect an absolute difference of 10 percentage points in cure rates between treatment groups at an alpha value of 0.05.

In total, 524 subjects (including 155 children) were enrolled in the study with even distribution of subjects receiving TMP-SMX (n = 260) and clindamycin (n = 264). Of the qualifying events for entry in the study protocol, 160 had an abscess, 208 had cellulitis, and 82 had a mixed infection. *Staphylococcus aureus* was a common isolate in the lesions (41.4%) and of those 77% were methicillin-resistant *S. aureus* (MRSA). Overall, there was similarity in treatment effectiveness between subjects receiving TMP-SMX (77.7% cure rate) and clindamycin (80.3% cure rate) with a difference of −2.6% in favor of clindamycin; 95% CI, −10.2 to 4.9; p = 0.52. Cure rates did not differ on the basis of gender, age, or based upon clinical features of disease (i.e., abscess versus cellulitis).

1. Does this study need IRB approval?
2. What is the type of data being evaluated for the primary endpoint? What is a potential advantage of this data type?
3. Which measures of central tendency are appropriate to present the primary endpoint?
4. Interpret the primary endpoint's p-value in terms of probability.
5. Interpret the 95% confidence interval for the primary endpoint.

A simple description of a controlled clinical trial is that it prospectively measures a difference in effect between two or more interventions (e.g., drug therapy). The groups are similar and treated identically with the exception of the interventions that are being investigated. The subjects in the study are assigned to one of the groups and monitored.[19,20,29,71] This study type, called parallel design, is the primary study design encountered in the literature.

Controlled clinical trials offer investigators the most rigorous method of establishing a cause and effect relationship between treatment and outcome.[20] Simply explained, the treatment under study is the cause and the result of giving the treatment is measured as the effect. The effect of the treatment being studied is compared to the effect of the other group(s). As a result, investigators can use a clinical trial to claim that a treatment has some effect that may be important in modifying disease outcomes. In addition, the magnitude (i.e., size) of the difference in the effect between the groups can be estimated.[20]

An example of a controlled clinical trial measuring a cause and effect is a study that compared simvastatin 80 mg plus placebo or with ezetimibe 10 mg in patients with familial hypercholesterolemia. The study objective was to compare simvastatin plus ezetimibe (cause) to simvastatin plus placebo and measure the change in intima-media thickness of the walls of the carotid and femoral arteries.[74] The study results documented that simvastatin plus ezetimibe did not result in a significant difference in changes in intima-media thickness, as compared with simvastatin alone.

A clinical trial also quantifies the differences in the effect, such as atorvastatin compared to simvastatin in lowering LDL-C.[75] Atorvastatin 10 mg was compared to simvastatin 20 mg (both once daily) to measure how much (if any) difference the average LDL-C level was lowered by these two agents. After 6 weeks of therapy, the average LDL-C level was lowered slightly more with atorvastatin than simvastatin (−37% versus −35%). Thus, the results of this study can be used to determine the magnitude of difference in LDL-C lowering by atorvastatin 10 mg daily (compared to simvastatin) and make the decision to use, or not, this medication instead of simvastatin 20 mg daily in practice.

Patient Inclusion/Exclusion Criteria

❹ *The results of a controlled clinical trial should be extrapolated to the patient type enrolled in the study and readers should be aware of the limitations of* **surrogate endpoints** *and subgroup analysis results.* The **inclusion criteria** lists subject demographics that must be present in order for the subject to be enrolled into the trial, while **exclusion criteria** are characteristics that prevent a subject from enrollment into the trial or necessitates withdrawal from the study, if they are later determined to be present.[27] Diagnostic criteria for conditions under study and definitions of the inclusion/exclusion criteria must be included in an article reporting study results. For instance, if subjects with hypertension are the target group to be enrolled in a trial, hypertension needs to be defined in terms of the minimal and maximum systolic blood pressure (SBP) and diastolic blood pressure (DBP). The study participant features should reflect the disease under investigation, but the existence of complex and/or extensive comorbid conditions (e.g., terminal cancer, pregnancy, numerous other disease states) in the study patients may not allow the researchers to accurately measure the differences in effect between the groups. The presence of these complex and/or extensive comorbid conditions can make for difficult decisions regarding including subjects representative of real patients versus excluding typical persons whose complicating conditions will make it impossible to accurately assess a new treatment. Whenever possible and appropriate, typical individuals with the condition being assessed, who in all probability will receive the therapy in real practice, should be represented in the trial. This includes ensuring a realistic representation of the gender, race, and other demographics. Subjects with one or more (but not numerous) other disease states and taking other medications are usually entered into the clinical trial, so the typical patients in which the therapy under investigation is intended are represented.

The inclusion/exclusion criteria are pertinent to the extrapolation of the study results (i.e., applying the study results into practice [**external validity**]).[69] Trial results are only applicable to the type of subject included in the study. The investigators of IMPROVE-IT enrolled men and women with acute coronary syndrome (an acute myocardial infarction [MI], with or without ST-segment elevation on electrocardiography, or high-risk unstable angina).[68] Additionally, patients were at least 50 years of age and were required to have an LDL-cholesterol level of 50 mg/dL. Thus, the results of IMPROVE-IT cannot be extrapolated to all patients who are younger than 50 years of age since only those who were at least 50 years of age with acute coronary syndrome were included in this clinical trial.

Researchers are careful in deciding which subjects to include and exclude in the clinical trial. Standard types of subjects disqualified are pregnant and lactating females or children; also, most clinical trials will not enroll subjects with severe conditions that may alter the medication's pharmacokinetics and/or pharmacodynamics (e.g., renal and/or hepatic dysfunction). Generally, the inclusion criteria attempts to include subjects that are homogeneous and are similar to the common type of patients in practice.[67] However, one criticism of clinical trials is that the patient population in the clinical trial does not match the ones that are encountered in clinical practice. There are inherent advantages and disadvantages to have stringent criteria for inclusion in studies. Tight criteria may reduce the number of people who will be able to participate in the trial or exclude patients who may be at risk for treatment complications. In other scenarios, subjects most likely to receive benefit may be selected or the patient population may be restricted to those with advanced disease, or who are more compliant, etc. If the criteria for inclusion is loose, more patients reflective of those encountered in clinical practice may be recruited; however, if a diverse patient population is included that has various disease states, it may be difficult to determine which intervention works the best in the heterogeneous population.[76]

During the process of the investigators selecting subjects to be included into a study, readers of clinical trials need to be conscious of the potential for a **selection bias** that may be present. A selection bias can occur due to various reasons, but can seriously affect the study results in a negative fashion. In general, a selection bias occurs after subjects meet the inclusion and exclusion criteria, but are not enrolled into the study.[77] The investigators may prevent a subject from being enrolled since this person may either positively or negatively alter the results.[19,29,75,78]

Although it is difficult for the reader to detect the above form of selection bias, the following paragraphs describe selection biases that can be more readily identified, but are not present in all clinical trials. One common form of a selection bias is requiring the subjects to complete a **run-in** phase (also called lead-in phase) before being officially enrolled in the study. This phase is usually short in duration (usually 2 to 4 weeks) in which the subjects may take a placebo or the therapy being investigated. The investigators should inform the reader of the intent of the run-in phase. Typical reasons include identifying subjects that may or may not adhere with the therapy regimen, experience side effects from the therapy, or did not meet prespecified criteria (e.g., blood pressure less than a set value). Afterwards, these identified subjects are excluded from participating in the study even though they met the original inclusion criteria. The run-in phase produces a bias by selecting a group of subjects who do not completely represent the population, since a selected group of the subjects meeting the study inclusion criteria are not included in the study and their run-in phase results are not included in the final analysis.[79] In addition, a run-in phase can delay the time from identifying candidates to actually enrolling into the clinical trial, which can increase the chance of patients withdrawing from the study.[80]

The following examples explain a selection bias by a run-in phase. Subjects meeting the hypothetical trial inclusion criteria complete a 4-week run-in phase in which a new therapy under investigation is given to all these persons. Those persons experiencing side effects to the new therapy during the run-in phase are not allowed to be enrolled into the study. By excluding those persons eliminated after the run-in phase, the incidence and severity of the side effects of the therapy is not accurately measured during the actual study since subjects experiencing the side effects during the run-in phase were not enrolled in the study. A second example is where researchers may include a run-in phase in which only those persons achieving a preset goal are allowed to be included in the study. For instance, only subjects achieving at least a 25% reduction in LDL-C after a 4-week phase with a new therapy are enrolled in the 12-week study comparing the new therapy to placebo. By only including those with a favorable response, the final average reduction in LDL-C with the new therapy is falsely elevated since only selected subjects were allowed into the study. Those persons with less than a 25% reduction in LDL-C were excluded from the 12-week trial; if these individuals were included in the 12-week trial, the final average reduction in LDL-C most likely would have been substantially lower than actually measured.

Trials including a run-in phase are not always considered to be a study limitation.[76] The investigators may stop a therapy previously prescribed to the subjects and give a placebo during the run-in phase. This allows the effects of the prior therapy to diminish and not interfere with the effects of the therapy under investigation. Furthermore, a clinical trial may be designed in which the investigators enroll a very specific type of subject, which can be considered a selection bias in the inclusion criteria. The purpose of this type of selection bias is to evaluate a therapy in a very unique group of individuals, usually those who met some predetermined criteria. For instance, a trial was designed so that only subjects who experienced a gastrointestinal (GI) bleed with aspirin alone were enrolled.[81] The investigators were specifically selecting a unique group of subjects (having a GI bleed due to aspirin). The combination of aspirin plus esomeprazole was compared to clopidogrel to determine which therapy had a lower recurrence of GI bleeding. Even though the trial results indicated that the aspirin plus esomeprazole combination has a lower GI bleeding recurrence rate, this does not mean this drug combination should be used instead of aspirin alone in those people needing aspirin therapy. The results of this trial can only be used for selected patients, those who had a GI bleed while taking aspirin and need to continue antiplatelet therapy.

Investigators also should explain the process of recruiting subjects and define the time period of which the recruitment occurred.[27] Sponsors of clinical trials and investigators typically recruit subjects for clinical trials by four main strategies: (1) sponsors may offer financial and other incentives to investigators to increase enrollment; (2) investigators may target their own patients as potential subjects; (3) investigators may seek additional subjects from other sources (e.g., physician referrals and disease registries); or (4) sponsors and investigators may advertise and promote their studies. The most common means for advertising for recruitment to clinical trials is through newspapers, radio, Internet, or television, or as posters on public transportation and in hospitals.[82] The methods in which investigators recruit subjects may have implications on the generalizability of the research results to the population (i.e., external validity). Newspaper and Internet advertisements are common; however, there are inherent problems with this form of advertisement. Survey results indicate that the majority of persons who read the newspapers are older in age, Caucasian, wealthier, more educated, and own more upscale homes than the average American. **Gender bias** also can affect recruitment rates as it has been documented that female readers consider newspaper advertising to be more important than do male readers.[83] Lack of representation by ethnic minorities, elders, and females represent a significant health burden as health care disparities are predominant in these patient populations. These disparities may persist if adequate clinical trial recruitment strategies are not developed. Community partnered research efforts may help increase clinical trial recruitment in these critical patient populations.[84]

Internet recruitment is not without similar problems. Typically, minority and elderly individuals are less familiar and have less access to the Internet. A study described the process of registering persons with cancer for clinical trials via the Internet and telephone call center. Most of the subjects registered via the Internet compared to the telephone call center (88% versus 12%). The majority of subjects who registered were female (73% versus 27% male; $p < 0.001$), Caucasian (88.9%), and received colorectal cancer screening (59%); the median age was 49 years. No differences with respect to ethnicity or gender were observed for patients registering via the Internet compared to the call center; however, subjects registering via the Internet were significantly younger than those registering through the call center. Recruitment via newspapers and the Internet may offer some benefits in terms of recruitment, although the lack of uniformity with respect to access to newspapers and the Internet for elderly and minority subjects may increase the difficulty of applying the clinical trial results to these under-represented populations because this subject type was not included in the trials.[85] In addition, other areas of significant concern with Internet recruitment are the potential for security lapses for personal data and ensuring a representative sample. However, when conducted appropriately, Internet recruitment can be an efficient and a cost saving method for clinical trial recruitment.[86]

Another important issue that affects the recruitment of patients is the increasing number of clinical studies that are outsourced to other countries due to costs associated with conducting clinical trials in the United States. Although outsourcing clinical trials to other countries may decrease the problems associated with insufficient recruitment of patients who enroll in clinical trials, other issues may occur as a result of including a large number of foreign patients in clinical trials.[87] Potential ethnic differences may affect the way drugs are handled in the body (e.g., overall response, drug distribution, metabolism, excretion). Therefore, readers of clinical studies that have included foreign patients need to ensure that the results of the study are generalizable to the patient population in which they serve. However, clinical trials including a majority of foreign patients should not be viewed with a bias. Various factors have led to more clinical research conducted in foreign countries, which includes governments competing for clinical research to be conducted in their country, increased number of health care specialists plus improving medical infrastructure in these countries, and changes in regulations.[88]

Intervention and Control Groups

Once the subjects are enrolled in the clinical trial, they are assigned to either the intervention or control group. The intervention group consists of the therapy under investigation (e.g., medication, procedure). The intervention is compared to a control so that the fundamental principle of a controlled clinical trial can be accomplished, measuring cause and effect. The control group can consist of no therapy (e.g., placebo), another therapy (a.k.a. **active control**) (e.g., drug, exercise), or compared to existing data (i.e., historical data). Both the intervention and control groups are to be as similar as possible in all respects (e.g., average age, number of males/females, medication use, existing disease states) other than the treatment received. Afterwards, the investigators will measure and quantify a difference in effect between the group assigned to the intervention with those in the control group. Any identified differences in the measured effect can be attributed to intervention rather than other factors (i.e., **confounders**).[19,89,90]

A key term in the phrase "controlled clinical trial" is the word control, indicating another therapy is serving as the measuring point for the effect of the intervention to be assessed. Reports have been published documenting placebo effects (i.e., measured change even though no therapy was given).[91] Without a control, the effects measured by the intervention may be by chance or falsely quantified. For example, investigators of a study reported that oxandrolone caused an average increase in body weight in patients with chronic obstructive pulmonary disease (COPD).[92] However, all the subjects were treated with oxandrolone and no control group was included in the study. Although these patients gained weight, oxandrolone may not be the sole reason for this effect. Weight gain may have occurred naturally, even without the medication or by some unidentified reason. The results of this noncontrolled clinical trial may be the rationale for a clinical trial being conducted to evaluate the weight-gaining effects of oxandrolone. However, a noncontrolled clinical trial cannot be used as evidence that weight gain was solely attributed to this drug. The results of studies designed without a control can be useful, but since no control group was present, readers cannot be certain that oxandrolone caused the weight gain, even if caloric intake and exercise were held constant.

Researchers can select from a few different types of controls, including historical, placebo, or active. Historical controls are described as data that have been collected prior to the beginning of a clinical trial. Investigators conduct the study with only the intervention group and then compare the results to the existing data.[93] One advantage of using historical controls is that only one group is needed to be enrolled, which may result in less time, expense, etc. Another advantage is the usefulness of studying a disease with a low occurrence or a disease with high incidence of death or other serious sequelae in which some form of therapy should not be denied.[91] Disadvantages include usually over-estimating the effect of the intervention,[25] lack of homogeneity between patients in the trial and historical controls, and differences in therapeutic procedures or techniques from one study period to the next.[91]

Historical controls are not used very often in published clinical trials, but are accept-able in selected situations. For example, the use of a placebo group is not considered ethical in clinical trials evaluating new therapies in patients with epilepsy. Due to the mor-bidity and/or mortality associated with an uncontrolled seizure disorder, this patient type should not be denied therapy in order to investigate a new therapy. Thus, investigators may assess a new therapy in these patients and compare the research results to historical data (obtained from prior research).[94]

An intervention under investigation is compared to a placebo in many clinical trials to document and measure the pharmacological effect of the intervention. These studies are generally conducted as a requirement by the FDA to document that drug therapy is better than no therapy (placebo) for a given disease state.[89] Those trials reporting a significant difference in effect of the intervention compared to placebo could be used to support the use of the intervention in treating patients. Simvastatin was compared to placebo to determine if the incidence of death would be lower in subjects with a history of angina pectoris or MI.[95] Before this study was conducted, health care providers did not have any information indicating that simvastatin would benefit or harm this subject type. At the time this trial was designed and initiated, persons with angina pectoris or history of MI were not routinely treated with a HMG-CoA reductase inhibitor (i.e., statins); thus, a placebo was selected as the control. However, the place in therapy for the intervention may be difficult to determine when a placebo is the control, since other drugs may be found to be better than the drug in question, upon further research. For example, in this case, although simvastatin lowers LDL-C greater than placebo,[96] it is not directly known how simvastatin compares to other drugs that also lower LDL-C, based solely on these trial results.

Not all clinical trials will have a placebo as the control group for various valid rea-sons. For example, including a placebo as one of the groups in a trial may decrease the willingness of subjects to participate; some may not wish to be treated with a placebo.[97] But more importantly, denying therapy that has been documented to reduce morbidity and/or mortality to patients with selected diseases may be unethical. These studies would not include a placebo as the control, but instead may use active control (i.e., standard therapy).[89,98] Patients with cancer enrolled in a clinical trial are prime examples of trials that will not include a placebo as the control.

Usually after the new therapy is compared to a placebo, a trial using an active therapy as the control is used to assess the difference in effect between the groups. Readers should be aware that clinical trials with a placebo as the control, particularly those funded by the pharmaceutical industry, yield a larger treatment effect than if an active therapy was selected as the control group.[99,100] For instance, the difference in the LDL-C lowering effect is expected to be significantly greater with a new statin versus placebo instead of another statin or other lipid-lowering agent. The treatment effect may appear to be substantial versus placebo, but could be minimally different from another active drug that was used as the control. Also, the possibility exists that the new treatment, in fact, may be inferior in efficacy and/or safety compared to an active drug, even though the new treatment appears better in comparison to a placebo. An appropriate control needs to be included in the study for the results to be applicable for practice. The use of historical or placebo as the control is acceptable in some clinical studies (as described above). Some studies may be designed with a control that may no longer be the preferred treatment after the trial results are published. The study may have been designed and initiated based upon either recommendations of the FDA or before new therapy recommendations were available.

Investigators need to not only choose an appropriate medication as the control, but also choose an appropriate dosing regimen (i.e., dose, frequency) suitable to the study.[97] Standard references should be consulted to ensure appropriate dosing regimens were included in the trial to reduce the chance of obtaining biased results. A trial concluding a new analgesic relieved pain better than morphine dosed 0.05 mg IV every 24 hours postsurgery in otherwise healthy adult subjects is biased because an appropriate morphine regimen was not used. However, at times investigators may not know the equivalent dosing regimen of the intervention relative to the control. Investigators directly comparing rosuvastatin to atorvastatin, both 10 mg once daily for 12 weeks, reported a greater lowering of mean LDL-C with rosuvastatin (43% versus 35%).[101] Other studies comparing these two medications have reported average LDL-C levels are similar with atorvastatin doses two times that of the rosuvastatin dose.[102] Thus, concluding rosuvastatin is a superior LDL-C lowering agent to atorvastatin, based solely upon the results of a single trial evaluating both agents dosed 10 mg once daily, is incorrect. A more appropriate conclusion is that these two agents do not have an equivalent pharmacological effect at this dose (Case Study 4–2).

Case Study 4–2

The AIM-HIGH study evaluated whether addition of extended-release niacin (niacin ER) to simvastatin therapy would raise persistently low levels of HDL cholesterol in subjects with established cardiovascular disease who have reached LDL goals with statin therapy. Eligible subjects were those who were 45 years of age or older, who had established cardiovascular disease, low baseline HDL levels (<40 mg/dL for men; <50 mg/dL for women) and elevated triglyceride levels (150 to 400 mg/dL).

After providing informed consent and completing a 4- to 8-week open-label run-in phase, subjects were randomized to receive niacin ER at a range of 1,500 to 2,000 mg/day, or an identical placebo. Additionally, all subjects in both groups received 40 to 80 mg of simvastatin per day plus ezetimibe 10 mg/day if needed to maintain desired LDL levels of 40 to 80 mg/dL. The primary endpoint was the first event occurrence of a composite end-point including fatal and nonfatal events: death from coronary heart disease, nonfatal MI, ischemic stroke, hospitalization for acute coronary syndrome, or coronary or cerebral revascularization due to cardiovascular disease.

In total, 3,414 subjects were included in the study, of which 1,718 received niacin ER and 1,696 received placebo. Ezetimibe therapy was received by 163 (9.5%) of subjects in the intervention group and 365 (21.5%) of subjects in the control group. The trial was halted prematurely due to lack of efficacy associated with the intervention therapy. At 2 years, the intervention therapy significantly improved all cholesterol and triglyceride values compared to control using the intention-to-treat principle. The primary composite endpoint occurred in 282 subjects in the niacin group (16.4%) and 274 subjects in the control group (16.2%) (HR = 1.02; 95% CI, 0.87 to 1.21; p = 0.79).

1. Evaluate the use of ezetimibe in this study. Is it considered ancillary or adjunctive therapy? Was use of this therapy appropriate?
2. The study included an open-label run-in phase. What is the purpose of the run-in phase and is it appropriate in this study?
3. This study used intention-to-treat principle in its statistical analysis. What is the benefit of using this method of analysis in this particular study?
4. Define the term "composite endpoint." What is a potential benefit and drawback of this endpoint type?

Institutional Review Board (IRB)/Subject Consent

Research projects that use humans as study subjects must be approved before investigators begin enrolling subjects into the trial. The IRB is the committee charged with ensuring that the study subjects are protected and not exposed to unnecessary harm or unethical medical procedures,[103,104] including vulnerable populations (e.g., pediatrics, pregnant women, impaired persons[105]). The name of the actual committee may differ from place to place (e.g., local ethics committee), although the purpose of the committee remains to protect the study subjects. This committee consists of both health care and non-health care professionals; people specialized in ethics also need to be included.[103]

The rules and regulations of human research require the study to be assessed prior to the initiation of the project.

Another primary responsibility of the IRB is to approve the informed consent form.[104,105] Before agreeing to participate in a trial, each subject is presented with an informed consent form that notifies the subjects of the study procedures, their rights and responsibilities of participating in the study, plus at least eight major points that include risks, benefits, compensation, voluntary participation, and right to withdraw from the study without any penalty. In addition to the content of the informed consent form, the IRB provides investigators with suggestions on how to write the form in language that laypersons can comprehend.[104–110] Additional information regarding the role of the IRB and investigator in clinical trial research can be obtained at http://phrp.nihtraining. com/users/login.php. Also, the reader may refer to Chapter 21 on investigational drugs. According to the Uniform Requirements, articles describing clinical trials using humans as research subjects are required to include a statement that the research was approved by the IRB (or other committee that protects subjects) and consent was obtained from the subject to participate in the research project.[41] Over the past several years, more medical journals include IRB/ethics approval information within the published studies.[106] Trials not including the IRB/informed consent information should be questioned.

Blinding

Since clinical trials measure differences in effect between groups, outside influences (i.e., biases) should be minimized. This is especially important in studies measuring subjective outcomes (e.g., pain, depression scores). **Blinding** is a technique in which subjects and/ or the investigators are unaware of who is in the intervention or control group. Blinding techniques are incorporated to reduce possible bias (defined as "differences between the true value and that actually obtained [are] due to all causes other than sampling variability").[29] Patients knowing they are taking a placebo to reduce depression symptoms are likely to report no change or worsening of the disease. The results are biased since subjects knowingly are taking a substance that does not reduce symptoms. Therefore, blinding techniques are important to reduce the influence of bias on measuring a difference in effect between the intervention and control. Four types of blinding can be used in a clinical trial (Table 4-4). The specific blinding type usually is dictated by the effect being measured during the trial.

Single- and non-blinding techniques are primarily incorporated in clinical trials that have study objectives not conducible to blinding (e.g., surgery versus medication). Some trials may include a procedure that is difficult to blind (e.g., surgery) and it may not be ideal to include a placebo procedure because sham surgery is not without risks as death or infection-related complications are possible.[111] The use of placebo/sham procedures

TABLE 4-4. TYPES OF BLINDING

Type of Blinding	Definition
No blinding (open-label)	Investigators and subjects are aware of the assignment of subjects to the intervention or control group
Single-blinding	Either investigators or subjects, but not both, are aware of the assignment of subjects to the intervention or control group
Double-blinding	Both investigators and subjects are not aware of the assignment of subjects to the intervention or control group
Triple-blinding	In addition to both investigators and subjects not being aware of the assignment of subjects to the intervention or control group, trial personnel involved with data analysis and interpretation are not aware of subject assignment

for blinding may increase the risk of adverse effects or other dangers, and is controversial and possibly unethical if the investigators do not thoroughly discuss the rationale for including and/or not using other methods to blind the trial.[112] A clinical trial designed to compare surgery to a medication is an example of using non-blinding methods since both the investigators and subjects know which group the subjects have been assigned.

An example of single-blinding of investigators is when one group of subjects is administered a medication subcutaneously once daily versus the other group who took an oral anticoagulation medication. The subjects would not be subjected to blinding since the risk of injecting a saline solution subcutaneously (i.e., bleeding complications may develop in persons taking an anticoagulant agent plus unnecessary injections) may outweigh the benefit. The investigators would measure the occurrence of a blood clot, an objective outcome that cannot be biased or influenced by the subjects. Therefore, the subjects' knowledge of which therapy they were receiving cannot influence the incidence of the blood clots. Since the investigators do not know which therapy is administered, the potential for the results to be biased is minimized. There are also cases in which the subjects were blinded, but not the investigator.

Double-blinding, where neither the investigator or patient knows who is receiving which treatment, is considered the gold-standard blinding technique and is most commonly used in clinical trials.[30] As a general rule, and regardless of whether the outcome is a subjective or an objective measure, the study should be double-blinded. A clinical trial measuring an objective outcome usually assesses other study outcome measures, such as the incidence and severity of side effects, which may be biased if double-blinding was not incorporated into the trial. For instance, double-blinding was used in IMPROVE-IT[68] to minimize biases in not only objective measurements (liver enzyme levels and creatine kinase levels) and also subjective assessments (side effects) in patients assigned to intervention or control.

In order to ensure that blinding remains intact, the therapy each group receives should be exact in frequency of administration, appearance, size, taste, smell, and other variables. Studies that compare regimens taken once daily to twice daily will require the once-daily group to take a placebo as the second dose (i.e., double-dummy).[19] Double-dummy methods are included in clinical trials when two therapies being compared are not the same (e.g., different routes of administration, different formulations). Patients receive two formulations, one active and one control, to ensure that blinding is maintained.[19] For example, investigators of a clinical trial evaluating the blood pressure lowering effects of amlodipine (a tablet) and the combination product of amlodipine plus benazepril (a capsule) should administer amlodipine tablets plus placebo capsules to those subjects randomized to amlodipine therapy and amlodipine/benazepril capsules plus placebo tablets to the other subjects. A similar situation may present in clinical trials in which the formulations being compared are administered via different routes. Investigators evaluating the efficacy of a once-daily oral contraceptive tablet to an intramuscular contraceptive agent administered every 3 months may allocate an intramuscular placebo to those patients randomized to once-daily oral contraceptives and a once-daily placebo tablet to those patients randomized to the intramuscular contraceptive. Each patient receives a formulation that represents each therapy and both subjects and investigators would be less likely to determine which formulation is active.

Sometimes it is necessary to triple-blind a study. In addition to the trial investigators and subjects, other personnel involved with the trial (e.g., data collection, analysis, or monitoring; drug administration or dispensing) can have opinions regarding the outcome of the therapy being studied based on their interaction with the subjects involved in the trial or their experience with the intervention and/or control being assessed. These opinions may cause inappropriate data collection, measurement, analysis, and/or interpretation of the results by the study personnel. Also, data collection personnel having a bias for or against the intervention may not be as consistent in their data collection procedures if they know which group the subjects were assigned. This may result in an inappropriate interpretation (e.g., overestimation of the treatment effects) of the study results.[19,25,30] Therefore, it is often necessary to blind these other individuals (i.e., triple-blinding).

Randomization

Randomization is a distinguishing study attribute that separates controlled clinical trials from other study designs (e.g., case-control, cohort). ❺ *Randomization is an essential component of all controlled clinical trials and a significant differentiator from other study designs.* Simple randomization can be described as all persons in a clinical trial have an equal chance to be in the intervention or control group.[113,114] Research has indicated that the results obtained from randomized trials are more dependable than nonrandomized trials. An analysis of randomized versus nonrandomized trials reported that, on average, investigators of nonrandomized trials overestimated the treatment effects of the intervention compared to the control primarily due to bias.[25] Even though including randomization in a clinical trial is important for more reliable results, it is necessary to remember that not all randomized trials are without faults.

Subject Eligibility

Subjects are eligible for randomization after meeting the trial inclusion criteria.[19] Subjects are randomized so the investigators cannot purposely assign selected persons to one group over another (i.e., individuals with more comorbidities in the control versus healthier individuals in the intervention group). Randomization minimizes bias by lowering the potential for an imbalance of risk factors or prognostic variations between the intervention and control groups.[29] A difference in effect measured by a clinical trial may result from many causes, and treatment may be just one of these. Disparities between the groups at baseline may cause a false result instead of measuring differences in effect between the intervention and control.[115] Therefore to be assured that the difference is truly due to the intervention, the groups need to be as similar as possible to control for any confounding variables.[87] Besides reducing bias,[116] an additional reason to include randomization in a clinical trial is so statistical tests are valid. Most statistical tests require subjects to be randomized so that similar groups are being compared and selected statistical tests can determine whether certain subject characteristics are equivalent between groups.[29]

Measuring differences in the effect between the intervention and control groups requires the groups to be as similar in as many characteristics as possible (e.g., age, gender, severity of illness) so that outside factors (i.e., confounders) do not influence the results.[114] Baseline discrepancies between the groups do not allow the true difference in effect between the intervention and group to be measured and quantified. If unbalanced factors are present between the two groups, the outcome measure is biased, and the treatment effect may be either under- or overestimated.[113]

Randomization Techniques

Many randomization techniques are available and range from very simple to complex processes. The nature of the study and outcomes measured influence the randomization procedure. Various methods are available that include random number tables and computer programs. The randomization procedures should be unbiased and unpredictable by not allowing the subjects or investigators to know in advance to which group the subject will be assigned.[19,114]

Specific randomization methods include from simple (i.e., coin toss) to more advanced techniques (i.e., **stratification**). Simple randomization is an easy technique to implement and includes assigning subjects according to some criteria (e.g., day of the week, subject birthday, or subject medical record number). But this method is not considered a proper randomization method since the number of subjects in the groups can be imbalanced due to the technique. If investigators assign all subjects with an office visit on a specific day of the week to one group (i.e., control), then these subjects did not have equal opportunity to be assigned to either group. These may lead to a reduction in the ability of the investigators to detect differences in effects between the two groups. Few trials use simple randomization techniques due to the limitations of this randomization method.[29] Although the mentioned simple randomization techniques do have limitations, a random number table can be considered useful since the table allows for each study subject to have equal opportunity to be assigned to either group.

One of the more sophisticated randomization procedures, stratification, is designed to achieve similarities in both known and unknown baseline patient characteristics between the groups. Selected factors are identified (e.g., age, smoking, presence of other disease states) and used in determining which group the subjects will be assigned so significant imbalances of these factors are not present among the groups, while all subjects with any specific factor have an equal chance of being in each group.[117] Since these patient factors can affect the outcome being measured, stratified randomization is a technique that enables these factors to be comparable between the study groups.[29] For example, the risk of developing a venous thrombosis is greater in cancer patients who are immobilized and/or receiving hormonal therapy.[53] Thus, a study comparing two agents (e.g., low-molecular-weight heparin versus unfractionated heparin) to prevent a venous thrombosis in this patient type would use stratified randomization to ensure a similar number of patients with these two risk factors are assigned in each of the two study groups. If one group had significantly more patients taking hormonal therapy, this factor could be the reason more patients had a venous thrombosis instead of the drug not being effective as the other drug. Thus, a false study result could occur due to the two patient groups not being similar at the beginning of the study.

The person randomizing study participants should receive only the participant information used for the randomization process. Extra and unnecessary patient information could bias the randomization process. Unduly influencing the randomization sequence by randomizing subjects to either therapy based on some preference can occur with the extra personal information.[29] Thus, to minimize these issues, investigators should only provide the pertinent subject information that will allow randomization of the subject to either the intervention or control group.

Patients may also be allocated to groups via a blocked randomization process. Block randomization allows for a balance of groups between the intervention and control. For instance, if there are four patients in each group, the group will be balanced every time the fourth patient is enrolled in the study. There are six ways in which four patients can be allocated to a group so that two subjects get two As and two Bs. The allocation sequence could look like this: (1) AABB; (2) ABAB; (3) ABBA; (4) BBAA; (5) BABA; and

(6) BAAB. Block randomization is helpful when interim analyses are planned because it ensures an equal balance between groups.[112] The disadvantage to this allocation is that the person who is responsible for treatment allocation can predict every fourth sample. To counter this effect, the allocator may hide the block size from the executor and use randomly mixed block sizes (e.g., 2, 4, 6).[118]

Although the majority of trials have an equal allocation of subjects, there are times when an unequal allocation (e.g., 2:1 ratio of treatment to control) is used.[119] If cost is a factor, an unequal allocation will allow for randomization to favor the least expensive trial arm and allows more patients to be included in the study. There are also times in which unequal randomization is favored when a new technology or treatment is available. Allocating more patients to the new treatment/technology will allow clinicians to find out more about the newer technology in relation to the existing technology. If additional adverse events are observed in one group over another, investigators may use an unequal randomization allocation to spare one group from additional adverse effects due to the study. In addition, if a higher dropout rate is expected in one group versus another, an investigator may opt to have more subjects in one group compared to another.[120] Allocating more subjects to the intervention group also allows for additional subjects to receive the presumed "beneficial" treatment option. Readers should keep in mind that unequal allocation of subjects in studies may predispose the evaluation to bias and may reduce statistical power.[117] Investigators should provide an explanation of the rational for unequal allocation of study subjects in the groups.

Endpoints

Clinical trials measure some effect caused by the intervention and control in order to compare these groups.[20,30,121] All trials specify one effect caused by the intervention and control as the **primary endpoint**, which can be referred to as what the investigators measured to achieve the study objective. Since significant time, money, and effort are devoted to conduct a clinical trial, researchers usually measure a primary and **secondary endpoints**. These secondary endpoints are important, but not considered to be the primary purpose of the study. The selected primary endpoint should be a routine and useful measure for the study.[30,119] For example, a trial evaluating the cholesterol lowering effect of an HMG coenzyme A reductase inhibitor compared to placebo selected a change in average LDL-C value, an appropriate measure, as the primary endpoint to satisfy the study objective. However, measuring a change in serum creatinine between losartan and captopril to improve heart failure (HF) symptoms[122] is not ideal, since serum creatinine is not the predominate parameter used in practice to monitor the progression or improvement in HF status.

❻ *The controlled clinical trial primary endpoint should be appropriate for the study purpose and measured using valid techniques and methods.* Investigators may combine a group of endpoint measures into one primary endpoint, referred to as a composite endpoint. The group usually consists of clinical outcomes directly related to morbidity and mortality as opposed to a pharmacological action (e.g., reduction in any incidence of stroke/MI/cardiovascular-related death versus lowering cholesterol levels). The investigators select a group of endpoints that can occur during therapy that are considered clinically important. For example, after experiencing an MI, a therapy is prescribed to reduce the occurrence of multiple adverse outcome (e.g., reinfarction, death, chest pain), not just one clinical outcome. The rationale for measuring composite endpoints is to measure an overall effect of therapy, since one specific outcome cannot be deemed to be the most important for the study subjects.[97,122,123]

The use of composite endpoints is not without debate.[97,121,122,124,125] The results of the individual components of the composite should be reported separately and analyzed.[121,122,126] Investigators may claim the investigational therapy is better than the control based upon the overall result of the composite endpoint, even though the investigational therapy was shown to significantly affect only one or a few (but not all) of the composite endpoint components. Also, the most important component of the composite may not be affected by the intervention under study. Due to the issues of using composite endpoints, researchers are in the process of designing new methods to assess the individual components of the composite endpoint (e.g., assigning weights to each endpoint) to better gauge the clinical trial results.[122,124]

The following example explains composite endpoints and issues encountered with these. The investigators of the Efficacy and Safety of Subcutaneous Enoxaparin in Non-Q-Wave Coronary Events (ESSENCE) trial used a composite primary endpoint, which consisted of death, MI (or reinfarction), or recurrent angina after 14 days of follow-up.[127] The incidence of the primary endpoint was lower with enoxaparin (intervention) than unfractionated heparin (control) (16.6% versus 19.8%, respectively; p = 0.02) in patients with angina at rest or non-Q-wave MI. However, only one of the three components of the composite endpoint was significantly different with enoxaparin, recurrent angina (12.9% versus 15.5%, respectively; p = 0.03).[125] As seen by the percentages, the majority of primary endpoint composite (~78%) consisted of this single event, which is the least robust of the three outcomes.[128] Although lowering the incidence of recurrent angina is clinically important, this outcome is not as severe as death or reinfarction. The composite endpoint effect of enoxaparin appears to be superior to heparin, even though the incidence of two of the three components of the composite endpoint indicates no difference between these two drugs. Enoxaparin was considered to be a useful therapy in this patient type, but further research was recommended to determine if the therapy reduces the occurrence of death and MI in these patients.[129]

The primary and other endpoint definitions, plus valid measuring techniques, need to be determined prior to the start of the clinical trial and incorporated in the study design.[19,30] By doing so, the investigators can be consistent throughout the trial in measuring the endpoints, thereby reducing study variances or biases. To illustrate, IMPROVE-IT primary endpoint was "a composite of cardiovascular death, nonfatal MI, unstable angina requiring rehospitalization, coronary revascularization ($\geq$30 days after randomization), or nonfatal stroke." If the reader is informed of the measurement types and methods under investigation, judgment may be made whether practical methods were used to measure the endpoints and can determine if the study can be replicated by future investigators or by individuals wanting to implement the trial results into practice to actual patients. Endpoints involving human judgment (e.g., cause of stroke) also can contribute to the complexity of analyzing and interpreting the study results if strict criteria or a blinded clinical events committee designed to produce valid recommendations are not incorporated and utilized during the trial.[121] Sponsors of clinical studies may elect to establish a blinded clinical events committee. This committee is responsible for reviewing endpoints in a clinical trial and determines whether or not the endpoints meet the criteria that was determined before the study began.[130]

A final type of endpoint that may be seen is a surrogate endpoint. This will be discussed later in the chapter.

Follow-Up Schedule/Data Collection/Adherence

A few important issues are considered here. A study should be conducted for an appropriate duration and data need to be consistently collected throughout the entire trial. A magical number of weeks or months has not been established as a rule for all clinical trials, but the length of the study (i.e., follow-up time) should be an ideal representation to answer the question being researched.[30] Statins usually exert the maximum cholesterol lowering effect after approximately 6 weeks of stable dosing.[131] Thus, the results of a study directly comparing the effects of atorvastatin 10 mg once daily to simvastatin 20 mg once daily for 6 weeks on the LDL-C level lowering differences between these two agents would be considered acceptable.[73]

A number of trials do not have an extensive follow-up time and the reader may have difficulty in interpreting the results for clinical practice. For example, in one study, the efficacy and safety of liraglutide versus placebo in patients with poorly controlled type 1 diabetes was evaluated.[132] The investigators of the clinical trial detected a reduction in body weight and insulin requirements, but the clinical effects and tolerability of the medication beyond this time period (e.g., 12 weeks) could not be assessed due to the short duration of the trial. Since diabetes is a chronic disease and the duration of drug therapy will exceed 12 weeks,[133] the trial should have been longer so investigators could determine the long-term clinical effects of this drug in practice.

Monitoring of the trial results at predetermined intervals is important throughout the duration of the trial. The Code of Federal Regulations and good clinical practice guidelines for clinical research state subject monitoring is required during the clinical investigation.[30] Larger trials may have a clinical trial investigator subgroup who serves as the data and safety monitoring board members. These individuals are blinded to the subject groupings and are responsible for reviewing the results obtained while the trial is ongoing. Interim analyses of the study results may indicate that the intervention produces either a favorable outcome or increased risk over the control before the established duration of the study has been completed. Typically, the protocol for discontinuing the clinical trial early is established prior to enrolling study subjects.[42]

If the study were discontinued because patients in the intervention group were experiencing significant harm compared to the control group, subjects randomized to the intervention would be at a greater risk for experiencing the harmful events if the trial was allowed to continue. Conversely, if the intervention was shown to be more beneficial than the control, the investigators would be denying useful therapy to those subjects randomized to the control if the trial continued.

Prior to the start of the study, data collection methods are established. These should be reasonable in that extensive time and/or procedures are not required, so that incomplete follow-up by trial personnel and subjects at each follow-up time can be minimized. In addition, investigators should ensure that trial personnel are properly trained and that they have sufficient resources to complete data collection.[134]

Another data collection and follow-up issue is measuring the adherence of therapy in the study participants.[30] This includes medication dosage unit counts, serum drug levels, or regular follow-up communications (i.e., telephone conversations). Subjects not complying with the therapy regimen may cause inaccuracies and less reliable data. Insufficient and/or inappropriate data collection methods and nonadherence usually lead to biased results that may make the extrapolation of results to clinical practice difficult.

Sample Size

❼*An appropriate* **sample** *size for a controlled clinical trial is vital for the study results to have any significant meaning; conducting a* **power** *analysis is important to determine a suitable sample size.* Sample size (denoted by the letter n) refers to the number of subjects randomized into a study and is of considerable importance to the validity of the study results. Financial and logistical limitations prevent all subjects with the specific inclusion criteria from being enrolled into the study.[30,133] For example, investigators may want to evaluate a new drug to treat hypertension. It would be virtually impossible to enroll all people with hypertension into this clinical trial. In response, investigators will draw a representative group (i.e., sample) of individuals from all those with hypertension (i.e., population). Researchers do not wish to include too few or too many subjects in the trial. Obviously, having only one subject in each group is insufficient to determine differences in effect between groups since chance alone may be the reason for a difference found (if any) between the two groups. On the other hand, having too many subjects can be excessive, costly, and may expose some subjects to unnecessary treatment. The sample size should not be determined on the basis of convenience, arbitrarily, or by the number of easily recruited subjects.[135]

The number of subjects to enroll in a clinical trial is dependent on the expected magnitude of difference in the endpoint effect between the intervention and control. The expected magnitude of difference in effect between groups is estimated based on the results of previously conducted trials or other research results assessing the intervention. In general, an inverse relationship exists between the sample size and the effect size. A large sample size is needed to detect a small difference in effect between the intervention and control outcomes, while a smaller sample size can detect larger differences between groups.[24,134] A large sample size is needed to detect differences in blood pressure between two antihypertensive therapies (small difference in blood pressure reductions), while a smaller sample size is needed to measure the difference in relieving postoperative pain between morphine and placebo (large difference in pain relief).

Researchers use various procedures, from table/charts to manual calculations, in estimating the necessary sample size for a particular trial.[88,134] Regardless of the method selected to determine the appropriate sample size, it must be calculated prior to initiating the clinical trial. A study lacking a sample size calculation may be biased since the reader is not informed of the basis on which the investigators determined the number of subjects to enroll. Also, another important issue is that the sample size is calculated based upon the estimated differences in the primary endpoint effect between the intervention and control groups. Investigators use existing data and information about the intervention and/or disease state to estimate the amount of difference between the effect in outcome by the intervention and control. The specific amount of difference in effect between the intervention and control is not known, thus the reason the study is conducted; but some estimate in the difference in effect is needed to determine a legitimate sample size. For example, IMPROVE-IT investigators[68] used a statistical model approach based on pooled blinded endpoint rates in previous trials; they assumed that a mean absolute reduction of 15 mg/dL in LDL-C in the combination group (ezetimibe/simvastatin) would result in a 9.375% reduction in the primary endpoint incidence of CV death, major coronary events, or nonfatal stroke at 2 years.[136]

Investigators intending to measure differences in effect for other endpoints besides the primary endpoint need to include this in the process of calculating the sample size. Clinical trials consisting of larger sample sizes can be considered more reliable in measuring and detecting true difference in the effect (if it exists) between the intervention and control.[137] Consequences of a clinical trial not having a sufficient sample size (i.e., too small or too large) are discussed later in the **Type I** and **II errors/Power Analysis** section of this chapter and in Chapters 5 and 6.

The importance of an appropriate sample size is exemplified in the following example. Investigators conducted a small study (51 patients) to evaluate fenoldopam mesylate compared with 0.45% sodium chloride infusion in enhancing renal plasma flow in patients undergoing contrast angiography. Fewer subjects receiving the fenoldopam developed a specific adverse event (radiocontrast-induced nephropathy [RCN]) at 48 hours than those treated with 0.45% sodium chloride infusion (21% versus 41%, respectively).[138] One primary contributor to the large difference in the results was the small number of subjects enrolled; the incidence of RCN is increased by 4% for each subject developing this outcome. Even though the difference was 20% (41% − 21%), this represents a difference of only five subjects developing RCN. After the results of this large difference in reducing RCN incidence were released, fenoldopam was frequently used in these patients.[139] However, the CONTRAST study (Evaluation of Corlopam in Patients at Risk for Renal Failure—A Safety and Efficacy Trial) was designed to determine if fenoldopam reduces RCN in patients after receiving iodine-based dye during cardiac angioplasty,[138] but this study had a much larger sample size (157 patients in the fenoldopam group and 158 in the placebo) compared to the previous study evaluating fenoldopam therapy. At 48 hours, RCN incidence was 19.9% versus 15.9% with fenoldopam and placebo, respectively. At 96 hours, incidence was 33.6% versus 30.1%, respectively. The investigators recruited slightly greater than 300 subjects to accommodate potential subject discontinuation. Based upon the results of this clinical trial, the incidence of RCN was actually higher with fenoldopam than placebo. By conducting a study with a larger sample size, the treatment effect of fenoldopam was more accurately measured compared to the study of only 51 subjects.

Statistical Analysis

Within controlled clinical trials, the use of statistics is a means to analyze sample data and apply it to the population. Many statistical tests are available and readers should be familiar with and have a basic understanding of the most common tests used in clinical trials. Some statistical analysis can be easily conducted using simple computer programs, while others require specialized training and extensive skill. Typically, a biostatistician is consulted as one of the trial investigators to perform the statistical analysis of the trial results.[140,141] However, even with biostatisticians evaluating the data, study results may be biased by using incorrect statistical analyses.[141]

The purpose of statistical analysis of the study data is to collect sufficient evidence to reject the **null hypothesis (H$_0$)** in favor of accepting the **research hypothesis (H$_1$)** (new terminology may refer to this as failure to accept the null hypothesis).[142,143] Prior to the start of the study, the appropriate tests are selected based upon the type of data that will be collected and analyzed. Since the selection of statistical tests is dependent on the type of data, an overview of the types of data is presented here. There are four types of data (Table 4-5)[144]: **nominal, ordinal, interval**, and **ratio** (the latter two are usually referred collectively as continuous). Nominal data are categorical without any sense of order; these data only can be categorized into one of the possible groups (e.g., either

TABLE 4–5. TYPES OF DATA

Type of Data	Definition	Examples
Nominal	Categorical data Data placed in one category, but not more than one category	Yes/No; alive/dead; colors of cars in a parking lot into five categories of either red, white, blue, black, or other
Ordinal	Ranking, ordered	Likert scale; visual analog scale
Interval	Data with measurable equal distances between points, but no absolute zero	Temperature in degrees Fahrenheit
Ratio	Data with measurable equal distances between points and an absolute zero	Temperature in degrees Kelvin, blood pressure, cholesterol levels, white blood count

dead or alive, but not both), hence mutually exclusive. Ordinal data (i.e., ranking) are categorical data with an intrinsic order, but do not have equal intervals between units. Pain severity (or other type of subjective data) measured by a scale is a typical example of ordinal data. For example, a five-point pain scale with a score of zero indicates no pain, while a score of five indicates severe pain. A one-point change in pain intensity on this five-point pain scale is not necessarily the same from one-to-two as from four-to-five on the scale. Interval and ratio data both have measurable equal intervals between data points, but interval data have no absolute zero (e.g., Fahrenheit temperature) while an absolute zero point (e.g., white blood cell count) is a characteristic for ratio data. Readers need to differentiate between the types of data to ensure correct statistical tests were selected in addition to the study being designed appropriately with correct data collection methods.

The type of data collected also dictates the use of inferential or descriptive statistical methods. **Inferential statistics** (e.g., Student's t-test, chi square test) are used to draw conclusions, based upon the sample, for the application of the trial results to the population.[145,146] In other words, data are analyzed to make a conclusion of the study results from the sample that is then inferred to the population. **Descriptive statistics** describe the characteristics of the sample (e.g., average subject age, baseline endpoint values, number of subjects with another disease present) and the results in some studies (e.g., X% had an adverse effect). Descriptive data are typically presented as measures of central tendency (e.g., mean [average], median, mode) and/or measure of variability (e.g., range, standard deviation, variance) (Table 4-6).[147] Refer to Chapter 6 for further information on descriptive and inferential statistics.

The terms in Table 4-6 can be best explained via an example of a trial in which the change in LDL-C was measured. A total of 200 subjects were enrolled in a clinical study designed to measure the reduction in LDL-C with simvastatin versus placebo. The LDL-C is measured in all subjects at the beginning of the trial. The values are then plotted using a histogram (Figure 4-1). For each subject with a specific LDL-C value, a mark is placed

TABLE 4–6. DATA PRESENTATION METHODS

Type of Data	Mode	Median	Mean	Range	Interquartile Range	Standard Deviation
Nominal	X					
Ordinal	X	X		X	X	
Interval and Ratio	X	X	X	X	X	X

Note: Mode: most frequently occurring data point; median: midpoint of the data (point at which 50% of the data lie above and the other 50% below); mean: average of the data points; range: officially the difference between the smallest and largest data point in the data set, although usually described by listing the smallest and largest data points (e.g., "The range is from 5 to 9"); interquartile range: difference between the scores at the 75th and 25th percentile; standard deviation: degree in which individual data points deviate from the mean value of the data set.

Figure 4–1. Histogram of LDL-C with standard deviation ±15 mg/dL.

on the graph for that value. As each subject with the same LDL-C value is plotted on the graph, an upward column for that LDL-C value forms. If the sample of subjects was randomly taken from the population, all the plotted LDL-C values would form a bell-shaped curve (also known as a normally distributed data set). After all LDL-C values are obtained, the values for the terms in Table 4-6 can be calculated. As seen from the graph, the mode (most commonly occurring LDL-C value), median (point at which 50% of the LDL-C values lie above and below), and mean (average) LDL-C are the same. In this data set, an LDL-C of 145 mg/dL represents these three measures of central tendencies. In addition, the range for the LDL-C values can be determined by identifying the lowest and highest LDL-C value. The data also can be organized into quartiles, four groups containing 25% of the data points. The data are arranged from the lowest to highest value; afterwards, the

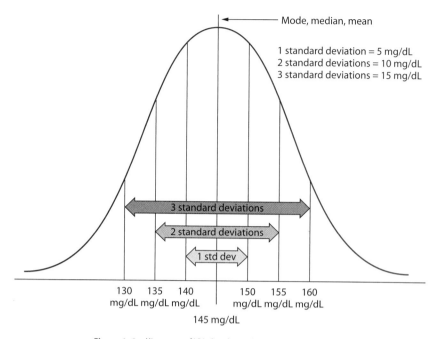

Figure 4–2. Histogram of LDL-C with standard deviation ±5 mg/dL.

data points are divided into four groups: 25th, 50th, 75th, and 100th percentile. Therefore, an LDL-C mg/dL value that corresponds to the 75th percentile would be in the upper limit of this third quartile of the distribution. In addition, the upper limit of the 50th quartile would equal the median value for the data set. The interquartile range is the difference between the scores at the 75th and the 25th percentile.[146]

Since many trials present the results as an average (mean), a more detailed discussion of this measure of central tendency is warranted. Using the LDL-C example, an average LDL-C value is calculated using all the measured values. However, presenting only the sample average does not inform the reader of the diversity in the set of values. Thus, a standard deviation (SD) is calculated using all of the LDL-C values. The SD is presented with the mean value of the sample (e.g., 145 ± 15 mg/dL, where the first number is the mean and the latter number is the SD). The SD is important since the average LDL-C from two distinct samples may be the same, but the dispersion of the LDL-C values may be considerably different. Figure 4-2 displays another set of LDL-C values taken from a different sample of subjects. The average LDL-C value is the same as presented in Figure 4-1, but the spread of the values is not very dispersed away from the average.

The presentation of the mean ± SD allows the readers to calculate the percentage of LDL-C values within portions of the graph. Figure 4-3 illustrates the distribution of LDL-C within one, two, and three SDs from the mean in a data set that has normal distribution

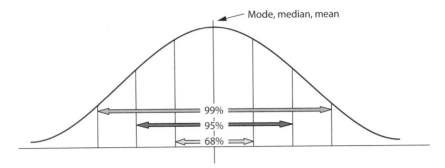

Figure 4–3. Histogram of normal distribution with standard deviations.

of the values. As a rule, ~68% of the LDL-C values would be in ±1 SD, ~95% in ±2 SDs, and ~99% in ±3 SDs. Using Figure 4-1, the average LDL-C is 145 ± 15 mg/dL. Based upon these numbers, 68% of the LDL-C values are in the range of 130 to 160 mg/dL, 95% between 115 and 175 mg/dL, and 99% between 100 and 190 mg/dL. In Figure 4-2, the mean ± SD is 145 ± 5 mg/dL with corresponding values of 140 to 150 mg/dL, 135 to 155 mg/dL, and 130 to 160 mg/dL, respectively. Notice that even though the average of both body weight data sets is the same, 95% of the LDL-C values are in the range of 115 to 175 mg/dL in Figure 4-1, but between 135 and 155 mg/dL in Figure 4-2. The SD allows for the readers to assess more than just the mean for a set of data.

Although SD is commonly used, some investigators may present the standard error of the mean (SEM), which is calculated as the SD divided by the square root of the sample size (SD/$\sqrt{n}$).[145,146,148,149] As seen by this formula, the SEM is smaller than the SD, which implies a smaller dispersion of the data points away from the average. Presenting SEM instead of SD may occur when the investigators want the reader to interpret a small dispersion of the data from the mean value instead of a large variance from the mean if the SD was presented. While SD measures the deviation of the individual values from the mean of the sample, SEM measures the deviation of the individual sample means from the mean of the population.[142] The SEM identifies the variability in the population; 95% of the time, the true mean of the population lies within two SEM of the sample mean.[148] At times SEM is used appropriately (more than one clinical trial) while at most times SEM is incorrectly presented.[148] Readers should be aware of these distinctions and interpret the data accordingly.

Inferential statistics are used to determine if a statistical difference is present between the intervention and control groups. A **p-value** is calculated based upon trial results and statistical tests; afterwards, the p-value is compared to the alpha (α) value established prior to the beginning of the trial (see statistical significance versus clinical difference later in this chapter for further discussion).[144,145] The selection of the statistical test depends on the data being parametric (i.e., normal distribution) versus nonparametric.

Typically, continuous data are assessed via parametric statistics; common tests are Student's t-test, analysis of variance (ANOVA), and analysis of covariance (ANCOVA). Nonparametric tests are used for nominal and ordinal data; examples are chi square (χ^2) and Mann-Whitney U test.[144] A multitude of other statistical analytical procedures are available. An analysis of all research articles in six common pharmacy journals published during 2001 identified that chi square (χ^2), Student's t-test, and ANOVA were the three most common statistical tests used.[150] Chapter 6 of this textbook is devoted to a more in-depth discussion of statistical analyses.

Other statistical terms encountered while reading clinical trials are independent versus paired and one-tailed versus two-tailed statistical analysis. A paired analysis involves the same subject compared to themselves or to a similar matched subject.[142,151] For example, measuring the mean change in LDL-C from baseline to 12 weeks within the same subject receiving simvastatin would be a paired analysis. Analyzing the mean difference in the LDL-C reduction after 12 weeks between two independent groups, one being treated with simvastatin and the other with atorvastatin, would be considered an independent group test. Two-tailed (also known as two-sided) statistical tests are used for trials in which investigators are not sure in which direction the primary endpoint will be affected by the intervention. These tests analyze the results in both directions, for positive or negative effects in comparison to the control.[136] Two-tailed tests are more common because the direction of change (and the degree) is not known.[35,136] For example, a two-tailed test is used for an investigational drug compared to placebo to treat elevated LDL-C. The investigators do not know the effect of the intervention on the LDL-C levels (i.e., the levels can increase or decrease relative to the placebo). A one-tailed test is primarily used in a study in which the direction of the effect of the intervention and active control (e.g., another medication, but not placebo, such as a non-inferiority study) are known or can only go in one direction. The intent of this study type is to measure more precisely the difference in effect between the two groups. Some investigators have used a one-tailed test to determine differences in LDL-C changes in patients receiving statins. Prior research has documented the LDL-C lowering effects of atorvastatin and simvastatin compared to other medications or placebo. Since these research results are available, a one-tailed test could be used to increase the statistical accuracy of detecting a difference in effect between the two statins in lowering LDL-C.

Type I and II Errors/Power Analysis

A clinical trial is conducted to test a research hypothesis that a difference in effect exists between the intervention and control treatments. Before the trial begins, the investigators develop a null hypothesis (H_0; no difference between the groups) and research hypothesis (H_1; a difference is present between the groups). The trial is conducted and the investigators measure the difference in effect between the groups (if any). If a difference is present, this could actually be due to the intervention or happen by random chance (error).[141,142] Hypothesis testing is conducted to examine how likely any observed difference between the intervention and control would be due to chance if the H_0 were true. As the trial results diverge farther and farther from the finding of no difference, the H_0 is rejected (i.e., failure to accept the H_0) between the intervention and control groups.[142]

Two types of errors are possible in hypothesis testing (Table 4-7). A Type I error can occur when the H_0 is falsely rejected and the H_1 is falsely accepted. Thus, the investigators are stating a difference in effect was measured even though there really is no difference between the intervention and control groups (also known as a false-positive finding).[114,133,136,146] On the other hand, a Type II error can occur when H_0 is falsely accepted and the H_1 is falsely rejected. In this case, the investigators are stating no difference in effect is present between the intervention and control even though there really is a difference between the groups (also known as a false-negative finding).[88,136,146,152]

Investigators attempt to control Type I and II error occurrence by setting limits on the probability of these occurring. The only reason that a Type I error can occur is by chance. Since no research is error-proof, methods usually are developed to allow up to a X% (typically 5%) probability that chance was the reason a difference in effect was measured between the intervention and control. The process of setting the probability of a Type I error (false-positive result) to occur no greater than 5% of the time is termed as establishing the alpha (α) value.[133,136,146] This is also referred to setting the statistical significance to 0.05, but can also be phrased as setting the alpha rate at 0.05. Another phrase commonly used to state the α value is p-values <0.05 are considered to be statistically significant. Most clinical trial use an alpha rate of 0.05; however, a few trials may use a more conservative α of 0.01. This latter rate indicates the investigators are more stringent by reducing the possibility of a Type I error to 1%. However, setting $\alpha = 0.1$ is too relaxed and

TABLE 4–7. TYPE I AND II ERRORS POSSIBILITIES

Error Type	Action/Decision	Interpretation
Type I	Statistical difference found even though it is not really present; reject H_0	H_0 is really true, but was rejected, which leads to a false-positive result. The probability equals the α error rate. There is one reason for a Type I error: chance.
Type II	No statistical difference calculated, even though there is one Fail-to-reject ("accept") H_0	H_0 is really false, should be rejected but was accepted, which leads to a false-negative result. The probability equals the β error rate. There are two reasons for a Type II error: chance or small sample size.

permits the Type I error possibility to be very high (at 10%). The alpha rate is a measure of how willing the researchers are to accept the chance of making a Type I error.[141] With the alpha rate at 0.05, this is indicating that in 1 of 20 trials, a difference in effect being measured between the groups can be due to chance.[88,133] An alpha rate of 0.002 indicates that in 2 out of 1,000 trials, a difference in the measured effect between groups can be due to chance. When researchers are interpreting the results of the study, they will compare the probability of making an error (p-value) to the acceptable rate of error (alpha). Thus, the smaller the p-values, the less likely that chance (error) was the reason for finding the differences. Also, the p-value can be expressed as the probability of rejecting a true H_0.[144] This last statement will be explained in the statistical significance section later.

The probability of making a Type II error is referred to as beta (β).[88,136,151] Although investigators want to avoid a Type II error, appropriately designed clinical trials allow this error (false-negative) to occur no greater than 20% of the time.[88,151] Even though investigators want to avoid making both a Type I and Type II error, they are more willing to make a Type II error than Type I error for a few reasons. A Type II error may be easier to determine than a Type I error (specifically in studies with no power analysis and/or too small of a sample size).[141] Also, Type I errors have the potential of being more dangerous in terms of the possible direct effects on patients (see next paragraph). Therefore, this is why the alpha rate is set lower than the beta rate. Investigators, in designing the clinical trial, aim to balance the possibility of a Type I and Type II error knowing that decreasing the probability of one error may increase the probability of the other error occurring.

Making a Type I error means a difference in effect was measured by chance but really no difference in effect exists between the two groups. The danger of using a therapy no different than the control is more serious when the control is a placebo versus an active therapy. A Type II error indicates no difference was measured between the two groups. If the control group is another therapy, then the intervention is shown to be no different. If the control is a placebo, then the intervention may not be considered as a therapy to treat patients. Although the false-negative result is a concern (i.e., a useful therapy may be not used), this is less severe than a false-positive results (i.e., using a therapy that really is no different in effect than the placebo control but was found to be different by chance).

A Type II error can occur by either chance or small sample size in which the latter is usually the reason if the error occurs.[136] The ultimate goal of each clinical trial is to ensure the difference in effect size is properly measured between the intervention and control groups, which require a sufficient sample size.[88] One method for the investigators to ensure a sufficient number of subjects are enrolled in the trial is by conducting a power analysis. The power of a study is defined as the ability to detect a difference in the outcome between the intervention and control if a difference truly exists. Power is calculated from the β-error rate (power = $1 - \beta$).[134,151] As seen from this formula, the lower the β-error rate, the higher the power. Increasing the sample size then reduces the β-error rate, increases study power, and reduces the chance of a false-negative result.[134] In addition, the magnitude of difference in the effect that can be detected between the intervention and control groups is related to the sample size; smaller differences in the effect between the intervention and control can be detected with larger sample sizes.[24,134]

Estimating the absolute difference (δ) in the effect between intervention and control is essential to ensure that the clinical trial has the power to detect differences.[29] This value is not as easily determined as the two other rates; the δ is usually based upon prior preliminary research results or even consensus discussion among the researchers (i.e., educated guess).[134] As an example, IMPROVE-IT investigators used prior research results to assume that the difference between the primary endpoints between the groups was 9.375%.[68]

The sample size needed is influenced by the α-, β-, and δ-values. The purpose of the sample size calculation is to provide sufficient power to be able to reject the H_0 established for the clinical trial's primary endpoint if it is false and should be rejected.[88] Hopefully, a clinical trial with an appropriate sample size will not lead to erroneously detecting a difference in effect when there is no real difference (Type I error), but also have a degree of certainty that the true difference in effects was not missed (Type II error).[133] In theory, a trial having an appropriate sample size increases the precision of estimating the difference in effect (effect size) of the intervention compared to the control.[19] The total number of subjects completing the trial should be similar to the actual sample size calculation for the study to have appropriate power.[134] Normally, the investigators will increase the sample size by some factor above the number calculated to be necessary (previous research can be helpful in determining that number) to account for subject attrition and therapy nonadherence. In addition, investigators can use the study results and conduct an after-the-study calculation to confirm that an appropriate sample size was included.

RESULTS

After the methods section, the results of the clinical trial are presented. This section contains **primary** and **secondary endpoint** results and other useful information, which includes patient demographics, dropout information, and safety information. This section is to be critically appraised to verify if the study objective was met, based upon the data, but also to evaluate the other types of outcomes that may have occurred. Often, data are tabulated or arranged in histogram or line graph format to provide readers a visual interpretation of the study results that may be minimally discussed within the text of the manuscript. The results of a controlled clinical trial should be extrapolated to the patient type enrolled in the study and readers should be aware of the limitations of **surrogate endpoints** and subgroup analysis results.

Subject Demographics

The first type of information provided in the results section describes the subjects actually enrolled and randomized in the clinical trial.[27] A general overview of the average subject is described, and is usually presented in a table of demographic information.[153] Typical information in the table includes average age, gender ratio and disease states, and/or drug therapy use among the study participants at the time of enrollment that could affect the interpretation of the primary endpoint. In addition, any additional lifestyle factors that can affect the endpoint(s) or trial outcome(s) may be described, such as the number of subjects who smoke, amount of caffeine intake, etc.

The patient baseline demographic data need to be compared between treatment groups to ensure the groups are as similar as possible. The groups should not have any significant differences if proper randomization techniques are incorporated by the study investigators; but a few differences can still occur due to chance.[19] Significant dissimilarities between the groups that could contribute to differences in the outcome between the groups need to be closely scrutinized. If the patient baseline differences are substantial, a confounding variable is present and the study investigators must analyze the results to determine if these differences have affected the outcome of the study. Otherwise, the resulting interpretation of results and their subsequent application to practice may be flawed.[136]

An example of baseline subject demographics is illustrated by select patient information from IMPROVE-IT. The simvastatin monotherapy and simvastatin-ezetimibe groups both had a similar number of males (75.9% and 75.5%, respectively) and subjects with hypertension as a diagnosis (61.3% and 61.6%, respectively). Average age, ethnicity, and region of origin also were evenly matched.[68] The disproportion of females and Whites enrolled in the study may be concerning to the beginning reader. However, the similar number of subjects between the two groups is more important in this study, so no differences exist between the two groups. Sometimes the disproportion of gender enrollment in a trial reflects the true prevalence in the population at large (e.g., more males with cardiovascular disease). Nevertheless, for trials that involve disease states in which gender is not a prespecified risk factor, each group should consist of similar number of subjects and not be skewed in one direction for any risk factor, as this sample-based anomaly could affect interpretation and application of study results.

Subject Dropouts/Adherence

After the baseline subject information, data regarding the follow-up (i.e., subject dropout or attrition) and adherence should be presented. Not all subjects randomized in a clinical trial will complete the entire duration, at which time they are then termed a study dropout or lost to follow-up.[113] Reasons vary for discontinuing study participation and include lack of desire to continue, subject relocation (e.g., moving to another city), difficulty finding transportation to clinic visits, subject protocol violation, side effects, and death. Also, not all subjects will be compliant with the therapy. Not accounting for the number of dropouts and nonadherence can have an effect on interpreting the trial results.[113,154,155] As a result, the investigators need to report the number of subjects and major reasons for discontinuing the study, adherence rates, and the techniques of assessing the data for the readers to draw appropriate conclusions about the intervention under study and subsequent trial results. All too often clinicians and industry personnel focus on the efficacy of a medication, but practitioners in particular should clearly analyze the costs of improved efficacy in terms of patient safety. Dropout data can be very revealing about the overall tolerability of a medication, which can illuminate important safety risks associated with emerging therapies compared to conventional therapies. However, readers should be cautioned when evaluating safety data within a study that it may not be adequately powered to draw conclusions about overall adverse effects.

The impact of attrition on the overall study results is dependent on the magnitude of subject discontinuations. A few subjects dropping out of the study may not cause a substantial difference in the results, whereas a sizable percentage of attrition may alter the study results significantly. No threshold of dropout/attrition rates has been established that deems the trial results to be of no clinical value. Similar to demographic information, attrition rates should be analyzed to ensure similarity between treatment arms. Attrition rates of 60% among both groups of a clinical trial, although not ideal, is much less concerning than a study where attrition rates are 10% in one group and 50% in another. Disproportionate attrition rates can be an indicator of significant medication safety considerations for the clinician and should generate further investigation, particularly if safety endpoints were not a primary endpoint of the study.

Frequently, the study results will be analyzed using data collected from all randomized subjects, regardless of whether they completed the entire study duration (i.e., results from dropouts are not discarded, but are considered to be treatment failures). This technique is referred to as the **intention-to-treat** (ITT) principle (see Chapters 5 and 6 for more on ITT and **per-protocol** [PP]). Even in cases where the subject may not have taken even one dose of the medication under investigation, these results are still included in the ITT analysis (i.e., once randomized, always analyzed). The advantage of the ITT analysis is that this analysis better mimics real-life application of an intervention into practice because, similar to real-life, all subjects in a clinical trial may not complete therapy as prescribed.[153] However, a concern with the ITT analysis is that data from subjects discontinuing a trial early may bias the analysis. This is of considerable importance for an endpoint measurement that worsens over time (e.g., cognitive function in subjects with dementia). The last score obtained in a subject discontinuing the trial early may suggest a better response than the last score obtained if this subject discontinued later in the trial.[156]

At times, the study results are analyzed via both ITT and the PP procedure. The latter term refers to analyzing data only from subjects completing the trial per the protocol. The advantage of this technique is for determining the effects of the intervention in subjects that followed the study protocol and completed the entire course of therapy. The ITT and PP analytical methods are simply models under which the study results are analyzed. The ITT analysis can be thought of as a worst-case scenario model, whereas the PP analysis can be thought of as a best-case scenario model. The ITT analysis is typically favored by clinicians or readers of studies when analyzing results due to the desire to determine whether statistically and clinically significant differences are present between the two groups under worst-case scenario conditions. Such results are much stronger than demonstrating statistical or clinical significance under best-case scenario conditions as patients in the greater population are not completely adherent to prescriber instructions. Optimally, study investigators will present both ITT and PP results; the desire is to see no significant differences between the ITT and PP results. If a significant difference exists, this can be an indirect indicator of differences in attrition rates between treatment arms that are represented in the ITT analysis. Furthermore, clinical trials including only the PP results are to be scrutinized more because results from all subjects are not assessed that could result in an overestimation of treatment effects in favor of a treatment arm with high attrition rates.

    An example of analyzing study data according to ITT and PP methods follows. The effect of caffeine therapy on the Epworth Sleepiness Scale (ESS) score in patients with Parkinson disease was assessed.[155] This scoring scheme is based upon questionnaire responses to eight items and the perceived propensity of patients to fall asleep based upon theoretical situations (0 = no chance of sleeping, 3 = high chance of sleeping; total score range: 0 to 24). The primary ITT analysis indicated that caffeine dosed at 200 mg twice daily (n = 30) had no significant effect on ESS scores compared to placebo (n = 31) at 6 weeks (difference of −1.71 points; 95% CI, −3.57, 0.13). However, statistical significance was determined upon PP analysis for the same endpoint and treatment (difference of −1.97 points; 95% CI, −3.87, −0.05), leading the investigators to conclude that caffeine therapy produces marginal but insignificant improvement in daytime sleepiness in patients with Parkinson disease. The difference in results between the ITT and PP populations are tied to the exclusion of four subjects who violated study protocol (two in each group). This example exemplifies that even very small and equal subject attrition or exclusion can significantly affect the interpretation of study results, particularly in studies with small sample sizes, and underscores the importance of analyzing both ITT and PP study results to make the most measured conclusions regarding treatment effect.[157]

Endpoints/Safety

A critical component of the results section is the primary endpoint results. These results can be displayed as tables, graphs, or other illustrations. The information should be presented clearly and completely, using transparent and unbiased methods. In addition, the investigators need to explain the results and present probability values (i.e., p-values). Results of secondary endpoints should follow and are presented in a fashion similar to the primary endpoints; however, endpoints other than the primary endpoint may not be adequately powered to detect differences between the intervention and control. Therefore, if statistically significant results occur with secondary endpoints, the results may be due to chance. Endpoints other than the primary endpoints should be adequately powered to draw meaningful conclusions regarding use in practice and are generally considered hypothesis generating.[27]

One issue to consider in evaluating the results in some clinical trials is whether medication dosing titration is allowed in the methods. The final medication dose of one group may be maximized while the other group did not require maximum doses leading the investigators to make a conclusion based upon misleading information. Readers of a clinical trial should analyze the final doses in each group at the end of the trial. Ideally, both groups should have similar dose titrations at the end of the study instead of one group receiving near the maximum daily dose versus the other group not requiring much of a dose increase. Safety assessments or tolerability of all therapies should be included in the results section.[27] Investigators need to implement valid methods of defining, collecting, and analyzing these results. As with the secondary endpoints, the study may not be powered sufficiently to definitively quantify the safety/tolerability of the intervention. In addition, the frequency and severity of these results may be dissimilar to those observed in clinical practice. Investigators need to monitor the subjects closely and collect these data.[55] Other factors to be considered include the equipotency of doses of medications being studied, clinical trial duration, sample size, and exclusion of selected subjects from being enrolled into the trial, particularly exclusion of persons who are otherwise qualified to be part of the study according to the inclusion and exclusion criteria.

Surrogate Endpoints

Investigators of some clinical trials select a primary endpoint that can be classified as a surrogate endpoint,[158] which is described as "a measure of the efficacy of a treatment can be defined as laboratory values (e.g., HDL-C/LDL-C), symptoms (e.g., pain), or clinical parameters (e.g., blood pressure) that are employed as a substitute for a clinical endpoint (e.g., morbidity, mortality)." Here it is assumed that changes in the **surrogate endpoint** can be directly translated into changes in the definitive clinical endpoint."[159] The primary reason that surrogate endpoints are selected for clinical trials is to quickly measure an effect at a lower overall cost.[158] The established efficacy and other data collected from trials measuring surrogate endpoint provide the rationale for larger trials with clinical endpoints (e.g., MI, stroke, death), which typically are more costly and time-consuming.[30] In certain circumstances, conducting a study using surrogate endpoints versus clinical endpoints maybe more ethical, particularly if a placebo is being used as the control therapy.

The following conditions should be fulfilled before a surrogate endpoint is considered as a valid substitute for a clinical endpoint: convenience (easily and readily assessible); well-established relationship between the surrogate and clinical outcomes (e.g., hemoglobin A_{1C} and risk/severity of diabetes); and determination of clinical benefit as a result of changes in the surrogate endpoint.[158]

The primary limitation of surrogate endpoints is illustrated by the following example. Investigators of the ILLUMINATE trial reported a significant increase in mean HDL-C with adding the investigational agent torcetrapib to atorvastatin versus atorvastatin alone (+72% versus +2%, respectively) along with change in mean LDL-C (−25% versus +3%, respectively) after 12 months of therapy. One would expect these two changes in cholesterol levels to reduce the risk of cardiovascular events (e.g., nonfatal MI, stroke). However, the incidence of a major cardiovascular event was significantly higher in patients treated with torcetrapib than atorvastatin alone (6.2% versus 5%, respectively).[160] This example illustrates that beneficial surrogate endpoint results do not always translate into positive clinical outcomes.

Subgroup Analysis

Investigators often analyze the results of subsets of the study subjects, as divided into various groups that often include gender, age, and presence of diseases or other complicating factors (e.g., diabetes versus no diabetes).[161] Reasons to analyze the results in these subgroups vary but usually relate to providing additional information in these specific patient types as opposed to the overall trial results from all randomized subjects. For example, trial investigators may analyze the results according to various demographics that included age (i.e., ≤65 years and >65 years), race/ethnicity, or gender.

Although the investigators may be able to obtain more information from a trial by using subgroup analysis, limitations and other issues need to be recognized.[27,104,123,160,162] A few prerequisites should be present before subgroup analyses are conducted: (1) the clinical trial should be well-designed with sound study methods, (2) a subgroup analysis should be defined prior to the initiation of the trial and have documented justification (e.g., past studies suggest a benefit in that patient group), and (3) subgroup analyses should come from trials with well-defined study methods and that are internally valid (e.g., ITT, randomization, blinding)—for results from studies that are sufficiently flawed, there is no reason to perform subgroup analysis. Additionally, data analysis should only be conducted from those studies in which the primary endpoint was statistically significant; otherwise, investigators may be perceived to be on a fishing expedition, searching for statistically significant results.[160]

Furthermore, the investigator may have conducted a multitude of subgroup analyses and only reported the statistically significant results. As the number of statistical evaluations on a data set increases, the likelihood of finding a statistical difference by chance alone increases.[160] Therefore, multiple subgroup analyses on the same data set should be avoided, unless authors can demonstrate that they have powered the endpoint for the multiple analyses *a priori* and/or have adjusted error rates statistically to control for multiple comparisons. Also, the power of the subgroup analysis is reduced with subgroup analyses, since results from a smaller number of subjects are analyzed as compared to the entire trial sample; this reduced power could lead to false-positive conclusions (i.e., Type I error).[160,161] Additionally, to avoid making invalid conclusions based on subgroup analyses, the ITT data set of the trial should be utilized to ensure that all dropouts are included for all treatment arms.[160] Subgroup analyses can be helpful in determining future research targets, but, unless powered appropriately, should not be used as a basis for therapeutic decision making.

Readers of clinical trials need to be aware of subgroup analyses being conducted and the potential misleading claims reported by the trial authors. For instance, an evaluation was conducted on clinical trials published during 2007 in which 41% of these trials reported claimed subgroup effects. However, the credibility of the claims was low. The results of this study are not to discourage conducting subgroup analyses, but authors need to be more informative and descriptive of the methods and interpretations of subgroup analyses.[163]

Overinterpretation of subgroup results can occur.[157] Reducing the sample size via a subgroup analysis can lead to a positive result that may have occurred by chance.[97,153,160,161] An illustration of this effect was documented by the African-American Antiplatelet Stroke Prevention Study (AAASPS),[164] which was conducted in response to the subgroup analysis of Ticlopidine Aspirin Stroke Study (TASS).[165] The TASS investigators documented a lower incidence of nonfatal stroke or death from any cause in subjects with recent transient or mild persistent focal cerebral or retinal ischemia taking ticlopidine compared to aspirin (17% versus 19%; p = 0.048). In addition to this overall study result, the investigators reported fewer cases of stroke and death with ticlopidine compared to aspirin in a subgroup analysis of African-Americans enrolled in this trial. The AAASPS results documented a slightly higher incidence of the composite endpoint (recurrent stroke, MI, or vascular death) in patients taking ticlopidine compared to aspirin (14.8% versus 12.4%; p = 0.12). Although the study designs of these two studies were not identical, the AAASPS results serve as an example to the limitations of selecting therapy based upon subgroup analysis. Thus, practitioners should be aware that, although subgroup analysis may document greater benefits in selected individuals, the differences in effect may be due to chance or other factors.

Ancillary versus Adjunctive Therapies

Clinical trials are designed to have almost identical groups with the only difference between the groups being the assignment to the intervention or control. At times, the study design may allow **ancillary therapy** to be included, in which subjects can take another therapy that can distort or confound interpretation of the results.[87] The effect of the ancillary therapy on the study results needs to be assessed and included in the study evaluation. However, readers should not confuse ancillary therapy with **adjunctive therapy**. Some studies may include in the methods an adjunctive therapy, which all participants receive as treatment, while ancillary therapy may not be equally distributed between the intervention and control groups. Thus, any significant difference in effect between the outcomes measured between the groups should be due to the therapies under investigation. For example, a clinical trial investigated the effect of cinnamon extract on glycemic markers in patients with diabetes.[166] Study subjects received either cinnamon extract or placebo; all subjects were taking an adjunctive sulfonylurea agent each day. Although sulfonylureas can lower blood glucose levels, all subjects in the trial received this therapy. Since therapy to control blood glucose should not be withheld in patients with diabetes, the use of a sulfonylurea in this trial was appropriate and use was similar between the two groups. However, ancillary therapy would occur if patients were allowed to take any other agent that could alter blood glucose levels at their own discretion resulting in a difference between the two groups. This would create a situation where the two groups were not similar, besides one group taking the intervention and the other taking the control (i.e., would violate the principles of a controlled clinical trial).

● DISCUSSION/CONCLUSION

The primary purpose of the discussion/conclusion is to evaluate and/or interpret the results of the clinical trial. Investigators should begin with a summary of the key findings of the study. Potential explanations of the study results should be addressed, in addition to discussing internal and external validity of outcomes.[27] The investigators should also interpret the trial results in comparison with results of other similarly designed studies. Also, the trial may be discussed in comparison to other trials assessing the intervention or the disease state under investigation. This is also where clinical trial limitations are identified and discussed.[27] Even though all clinical trials have limitations, these may vary from minor to those that seriously hinder the usefulness of the results, including completely invalidating the study. The discussion section should also address the clinical importance of the clinical trial results and how these results should be used in practice. All of this information should allow the reader to understand the application of the clinical trial results in practice. However, this section needs to be read just as carefully as the other sections, because it can contain biased wording. No new information from the clinical study should be presented in this section that has not been presented before reading it in the discussion section. In addition, authors may only discuss selected items in relationship to the clinical trial.[97]

The investigators should ensure that strategies are included within the study design to minimize biases that may occur. Some of the strategies can include blinding, randomization, and appropriate inclusion/exclusion criteria. In addition, investigators should not be biased in interpreting the results of the trial. Readers should determine the degree that the study results compare with patients encountered in practice. One of the most commonly cited criticisms of clinical trials by clinicians is the lack of external validity of the trials and may be one explanation for the underuse of reportedly favorable treatment options in clinical trials by clinicians.[167] Although some investigators may report beneficial results of an intervention under investigation, the patient population in the clinical trial may be so dissimilar to patients encountered in practice that clinicians are not convinced that the favorable results may be beneficial in their patient population. Several issues may potentially affect the external validity of the clinical trial and should be evaluated to assess the effects of the results in practice. These include the setting of the trial, selection of patients, characteristics of randomized patients, differences between the trial protocol and routine practice, outcome measures, follow-up, and adverse effects of treatment.[166] If the characteristics of the patients and setting are very different from those encountered in practice, the clinical usefulness of the reported information may be questionable.

Potential limitations may include small sample size, short duration of the study, endpoint assessment techniques, or other factors that hinder the clinical usefulness of the study. The investigators should also address methods to circumvent trial limitations in subsequent clinical studies. There is no minimum or maximum number of limitations that investigators should address; a thorough discussion of the limitations should be provided so that readers can determine the applicability of the trial results to their patient population.

Comparison of the current study to previous studies should be conducted. According to the results of one study, discussion sections of trial reports were lacking complete analysis of previous clinical trial results.[168] A total of 33 randomized trials were identified in 19 issues of leading medical journals (e.g., Annals of Internal Medicine, JAMA). The authors of four reports claimed that their study was a first-of-a-kind study; however, reports of similar trials were located for one of these studies. In three of the reports, systematic reviews of earlier trials were mentioned; however, no attempts to incorporate the results of the new trial with the existing results were identified in the remaining 27 reports. The results of other trials should be included to allow the reader to assess the results of the current trial in context to previous trial results. The readers can determine if the study is a first-of-a-kind study that adds substantial information to a topic or is a me-too study that adds no new information to existing knowledge. The discussion section should also address future concerns and unanswered questions.

The conclusion section should provide an overall research recommendation to the readers. The investigators' conclusion should focus on the primary endpoint results, especially if no statistically significant differences between the intervention and control groups were observed, rather than favorable, secondary endpoint results. Conclusions should be limited to only that information discussed in previous sections of the trial; no new information should be discussed in this section. Also, the conclusions should be aligned with the results of the trial. Investigators should not make erroneous conclusions that are not supported by the results of the trial.

Clinical Trial Result Interpretation

Statistical Significance versus Clinical Difference

❽ *Correctly interpreting the p-values is crucial in evaluating a controlled clinical trial; not all statistically significant p-values are clinically important. The magnitude of difference in effect between the intervention and control cannot be determined solely with the p-value.* Once the clinical trial is completed, the investigators calculate a p-value for the endpoints using the collected study results and statistical tests. The p-value is an abbreviation for probability value and is compared to the alpha (α) value established prior to the beginning of the clinical trial (*a priori*) that serves as the benchmark to which p-values are compared to determine if statistical significance is present. Also, since the entire population is not included, the investigators have to estimate the difference in effect from the sample.[141,142,169] Without statistical analysis, the likelihood of chance being the reason for any measured difference in effect is not known.[136] A p-value for the primary endpoint that is less than the **alpha value** indicates the H_0 is rejected and a statistically significant difference is declared between the intervention and control groups. This also indicates chance alone was not likely the reason that a difference in effect was measured. The H_0 is accepted (failed to be rejected) with a p-value equal to or greater than the alpha value and no statistically significant difference is declared.[142,168]

Statistical significance does not automatically mean a clinical difference in the effect between the intervention and control groups.[170] (See next section regarding the assessment of clinical difference.) The reader needs to make a decision in determining if the intervention is worth using instead of the control therapy, which can be dependent on the judgment and experiences of the reader (i.e., assessing both internal and external validity). Not all statistically significant studies have clinically different results (Figure 4-4). A p-value less than the alpha value only represents the probability that a true H_0 has been rejected. In other words, the p-value can be translated into what is the probability of the difference in the effect between the intervention and control due to chance?[141] Lower p-values indicate a lower probability that chance alone could be the reason a difference in effect was measured between the intervention and control. Alternatively stated, what is the chance of observing this difference if there really was no difference between the two groups?[136] Recall that a Type I error is possible after rejecting the H_0; the results may be statistically significant due to chance alone.

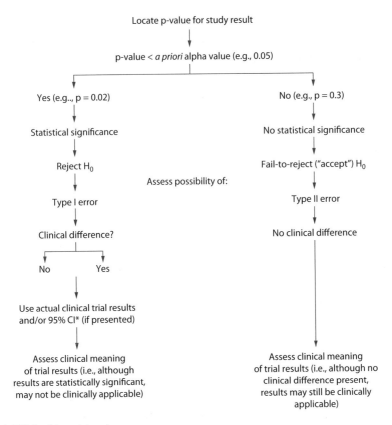

Figure 4–4. Determining statistical significance, clinical difference, and clinical meaningfulness.

Another paramount issue in understanding clinical trials is that the p-value does not express the magnitude of difference in the effect between the intervention and control.[142] Statistically significant results simply signify that the alternative hypothesis (H_1) is accepted. The H_1 states a difference in the effect is present between the intervention and control. From this information, the reader cannot determine complex quantitative differences in effect (i.e., clinical difference between intervention and control groups).[136,144]

In addition, specific p-values should be stated in the text of the article (i.e., p = 0.0012 instead of p < 0.05) to be more informative and helpful to the reader.[136,142] Also, all p-values should be presented in conjunction with associated endpoint results (i.e., investigators concluded that drug A lowered mean DBP more than placebo, −12 versus −3 mmHg, respectively [p = 0.001] as opposed to investigators concluded that drug A lowered mean DBP more than placebo [p = 0.001]). Readers should scrutinize study data that present p-values without endpoint results (naked p-values). Such a situation should prompt the reader to ask if endpoint results were not presented with the p-value because the actual difference in the effect was minimal. Without the endpoint results being presented, statistical significance alone can be concluded with the p-value; however, clinical differences cannot be assessed without accompanying endpoint results. See next sections for further discussion of this issue.

Assessing Clinical Difference

Two critical items needed to assess clinical difference between the intervention and control groups of a clinical trial are the p-value and actual study results used to calculate the p-value. A fundamental first step of determining clinical difference in a given trial begins with determining if statistical significance exists (i.e., p < *a priori* alpha value) (see Figure 4-4). The reader must keep in mind that clinical difference is predicated on statistical significance. In other words, clinical difference between the intervention and control cannot exist with study outcome data if the results are not statistically significant. The second step in assessing clinical differences is evaluating the results used to calculate the p-value. The reader must analyze the magnitude of endpoint difference between the intervention and control results.[136,169] Once a reader determines that statistical significance is present with given study data, no magical formula is available to conclude whether clinical difference exists between the intervention and control.[142] The remainder of the process is based upon clinical knowledge and experience, and may be relative in the reader's opinion to whether clinical difference is present or not. For example, an antihypertensive therapy lowers mean DBP by 14 mmHg versus 3 mmHg with placebo in subjects with a mean baseline DBP of 98 mmHg. In this case, the results are clinically different due to 11 mmHg average difference and subjects are achieving goal DBP values from baseline (<85 mmHg). However, atorvastatin lowering mean LDL-C by 1.7% greater than simvastatin (37.1% versus 35.4%; p = 0.0097[89]) cannot be considered clinically different in subjects with a mean baseline LDL-C of 181 mg/dL. The mean LDL-C was reduced by <2% with atorvastatin compared to simvastatin, a difference that most likely is not associated with producing clinical differences in effect. In addition, the actual mean LDL-C lowering was almost identical (66 mg/dL) and the mean LDL-C level at study end was <116 mg/dL in both groups.

Some readers may consider the trial results to be clinically different while others may not. In fact, two people may have different conclusions after reading the same clinical trial. This situation is very common when interpreting clinical trials in health care practice. In response, readers must justify their own conclusion regarding their decision of clinical difference. A few suggestions and examples are provided to assist in determining clinical difference.

Understanding the instrument that was used in measuring the endpoint is important in assessing clinically significant differences in trials. For example, ordinal data typically use scales or ranking (e.g., pain, depression scales).[143] Thus, the definitions of the minimum and maximum numbers of these scales need to be known. As an example, investigators of a hypothetical clinical trial concluded that glucosamine sulfate (500 mg three times a day) reduced pain greater than placebo in men with osteoarthritis (OA) of the knee. Pain intensity difference at rest was assessed by a 10-point visual analog scale (0 = no pain; 10 = severe pain). The median scores were 3.6 with placebo versus 3.3 with glucosamine (p = 0.03) at the end of the trial. Although results are statistically significant between glucosamine and placebo, the difference in scores between these two groups is minimal, only 0.3 points on a 10-point scale. Stating a clinical difference between glucosamine and placebo would be considered incorrect.

Another issue to consider is that clinical trials with too large of a sample size (i.e., overpowered) lead to smaller p-values versus those with smaller sample sizes.[134,142] The magnitude of the p-value is dependent on sample size; small differences in effect can be statistically significant with large sample size.[136] Thus, statistically significant results can occur even though a small absolute difference in effect is present. An example of this issue is a clinical trial that compared esomeprazole (n = 2,624) versus lansoprazole (n = 2,617). The primary endpoint, incidence of erosive esophagitis healing, was statistically significant in favor of esomeprazole (92.6% versus 88.8%; p = 0.0001).[171] The investigators (and marketing advertisements) concluded esomeprazole to be superior to lansoprazole, although the absolute difference in healing was only 4% between these two drugs. In addition, a significant number of subjects in each group (>88%) experienced erosive esophagitis healing. Even when those results were statistically different, readers can debate whether the difference in effect is clinically different.

A data assessment technique that can be misleading is converting a continuous endpoint measure into a dichotomous value. For instance, in a study measuring blood pressure (continuous value) after an intervention (rofecoxib—later withdrawn from the market) and control (celecoxib) were administered, the subjects with a blood pressure above a predefined cut-off point were classified as being hypertensive (nominal data because subject has a blood pressure value below or above this cut-off point). Significantly more subjects taking rofecoxib versus celecoxib were diagnosed with systolic hypertension (17% versus 11%, respectively; p = 0.032). However, the change in the mean for SBP values was +2.6 versus −0.5 mmHg, respectively (p = 0.007).[172] These two data sets assessed together indicate that rofecoxib may not negatively affect SBP compared to celecoxib. The actual SBP in the subjects taking rofecoxib may have just exceeded the cut-off hypertensive value (increase >20 mmHg with absolute value >140 mmHg) while it was just below this value for the celecoxib (i.e., 141 versus 139 mmHg, respectively). The absolute difference between these two blood pressure values was minimal (2 mmHg), but the number of subjects counted as hypertensive was different (6%). The change in SBP between these two medications did not appear to be clinically different. Even though the measured endpoints between subjects randomized to the intervention were numerically close to the control, the subjects were categorized differently based upon cut-off blood pressure values. This example illustrates the potential biases of this form of data analysis and presentation.

The foundation in determining clinical difference between an intervention and control is the p-value and actual study results. Other items can assist the reader in this endeavor and include 95% **confidence intervals** and calculating measures of association; both of these are described below. However, readers must remember that not all clinical trials may have these latter two items. Thus, the importance of analyzing and interpreting p-values and the magnitude of difference between the intervention and control cannot be overemphasized.

Confidence Intervals

Many clinical trials include 95% confidence intervals (CIs) with the study results, which can assist in assessing clinical difference between the intervention and control. ❾ *The use of 95% confidence intervals can assist the reader in assessing the magnitude of difference in effect between the intervention and control to apply to the population.* CIs provide data that address the size of effect (e.g., mean reduction in DBP) of the intervention under investigation in a clinical trial by presenting a range that likely covers the true but unknown value.[173,174] Although the basis of accepting or rejecting the H_0 is based upon the p-value, a limitation of the p-value is that the magnitude of difference in effect between the intervention and control groups of a clinical trial is not known, since it is not able to be determined based upon a statistical calculation.[142,169] Because of this, the use of a CI can assist in judging the clinical usefulness of the study result.[136] Clinical trials report the effect of an intervention as a point estimate, a single value that can be considered to represent the true effect (e.g., mean reduction in DBP; incidence of MI). For instance, an angiotensin-converting enzyme (ACE) inhibitor lowered mean DBP by 8 mmHg; this value would be termed the point estimate. If the study was repeated, a similar, but not exact, reduction in mean DBP may occur (e.g., −10 mmHg, −12 mmHg). The presentation of the results only as a point estimate provides the reader with limited information. Clinical trials presenting 95% CI in conjunction with the point estimate enables the readers to further critique the study results and determine the usefulness for practice.

A CI provides an indication of the outcome within the population and is interpreted as a range of values in which the true value is included. The 95% CI for an average is calculated using the SEM from the trial sample. Recalling the formula for SEM, the SD is divided by the square root of the sample size $(SD/\sqrt{n})$. A 95% CI is equivalent to approximately two SEM from the sample mean, with an exact formula of CI = mean $\pm$1.96 $\times$ SEM. The SEM is used as opposed to the SD since SEM is more reflective of the population variance, while SD is indicative of the dispersion within the sample.[142,173] A 95% CI is not the only CI reported in the literature and readers of clinical trials need to recognize the changes in the interpretation. A 99% CI indicates more confidence that the true, but unknown, endpoint value is in this range than does a 95% CI. Thus, the 99% CI range is wider in value than a 95% CI, whereas a 90% CI range is narrower (i.e., less confident).[173,175]

A 95% CI for a point estimate is a common method of data presentation. Investigators of a clinical trial reported that the mean reduction in DBP with an ACE inhibitor was -11.3 mmHg (95% CI, -8.2 to -14.4 mmHg) in subjects with a mean baseline DBP of 99 mmHg. This indicates that the investigators are 95% confident that the mean DBP reduction in the population is between -8.2 and -14.4 mmHg. An important issue to recognize in interpreting a 95% CI is a lower probability for the mean reduction in DBP at the upper and lower end of the 95% CI range compared to numbers near the point estimate value.[145] The further away a value lays from the point estimate within the 95% CI range, the lower the probability that this value is representative of the given population. A low probability exists that the ACE inhibitor lowers mean DBP in the population by only 8.2 mmHg compared to a higher probability that mean DBP reduction is closer to the point estimate of 11.3 mmHg (the same is true with the upper end of the 95% CI).

Within this trial, the ACE inhibitor was compared to hydrochlorothiazide (HCTZ) and the mean DBP reduction with HCTZ was -9.9 mmHg (95% CI, -7.5 to -13.3 mmHg). The same principles are used to interpret this 95% CI as with the ACE inhibitor 95% CI; the investigators are 95% confident that the mean reduction of DBP in the population with HCTZ is between 7.5 and 13.3 mmHg. In addition, these two 95% CI ranges can be compared to determine any difference in effect between these two agents. Since both 95% CI ranges overlap considerably, no difference in effect is concluded.[136,142,174] However, if no overlap of the 95% CI for the two groups is present, a clinical difference can be concluded.

Another common method of data presentation is calculating a 95% CI for the difference of the point estimates between two groups. In the above trial example, the point estimate of mean DBP lowering with the ACE inhibitor was -11.3 mmHg while -9.9 mmHg for HCTZ. The difference in mean DBP between these two equals -1.4 mmHg (-11.3 minus $-9.9 = -1.4$). The 95% CI for the difference in the point estimates is calculated to be -3.9 to $+1.1$ mmHg. This is interpreted as being 95% confident that the difference in mean DBP reduction can be 1.1 mmHg greater with HCTZ (i.e., -13.1 mmHg for HCTZ versus -12 mmHg for ACE inhibitor) or 3.9 mmHg greater with the ACE inhibitor (i.e., -16.9 mmHg for ACE inhibitor versus -13 mmHg for HCTZ). Notice the upper end of the 95% CI of the difference in point estimates is a positive number ($+1.1$ mmHg). This does not indicate the mean DBP was increased, only that the difference in mean DBP lowering was 1.1 mmHg greater with HCTZ compared to ACE inhibitor (i.e., −12 minus −13.1 mmHg for ACE inhibitor and HCTZ, respectively). Also, in this 95% CI is the number zero (value of equality); this indicates with 95% confidence that there is no difference in mean DBP between these two groups (i.e., −13.2 minus −13.2 mmHg for both agents equals zero). If no zero is in the 95% CI of the difference between the two point estimates, then a clinical difference in effect between the intervention and control could be concluded.

The interpretation of clinical difference using 95% CI is dependent on clinical experience and appropriate assessment. A 95% CI without a zero in the range does not always indicate a clinical difference between the intervention and control. For example, a 95% CI for mean DBP lowering in a trial comparing an ACE inhibitor and HCTZ was −1.9 to −0.5 mmHg. Even though this 95% CI range does not contain a zero, a mean difference of only 0.5 to 1.9 mmHg greater DBP-lowering effect with one agent would not be considered clinically different.

Interpreting Risks and Number Needed to Treat

Case Study 4–3

ENGAGE AF-TIMI 48 was a randomized double-blinded, double-dummy study that compared two once-daily regimens (60 mg and 30 mg) of edoxaban to warfarin. The target population for the study included atrial fibrillation subjects with moderate-to-high stroke risk, with the primary endpoint of stroke or systemic embolization. The study design analyzed for noninferiority, as well as, superiority between treatments in the context of the primary endpoint.

In total, there were 7,036, 7,035, and 7,034 subjects randomized to the warfarin, 60 mg edoxaban, and 30 mg edoxaban treatment arms, respectively. The annualized rates of primary endpoint occurrence were higher for the warfarin (1.5%) versus high-dose edoxaban group (1.18%), with low-dose edoxaban generating higher rates of primary endpoint occurrence (1.61%) compared to warfarin. In the ITT analysis of the primary endpoint, high-dose edoxaban outperformed warfarin numerically, but not statistically (HR, 0.87; 97.5% CI, 0.73 to 1.04), whereas low dose edoxaban did not perform well versus warfarin in either respect (HR, 1.13; 97.5% CI, 0.96 to 1.34). Major bleeding rates favored both dosing groups of edoxaban: high dose = 2.75%, low dose = 1.61%, warfarin = 3.43% ($p < 0.001$ for high- and low-dose edoxaban versus warfarin). Annualized rates of death from cardiovascular causes were statistically significant in favor of both high- and low-dose edoxaban (2.74% and 2.71%, respectively) versus warfarin (3.17%).

1. This study employed double-dummy blinding. What is double-dummy blinding and was its use necessary?
2. Calculate the RR for the primary endpoint for the high-dose edoxaban group versus warfarin and interpret the value.
3. Calculate RRR for the primary endpoint for the high-dose edoxaban group versus warfarin and interpret the value.
4. Calculate the ARR for the primary endpoint for the high-dose edoxaban group versus warfarin and interpret the value.
5. Calculate the NNT for the primary endpoint for the high-dose edoxaban group versus warfarin and interpret the value.
6. Interpret the confidence interval for the primary endpoint result comparison between low-dose edoxaban and warfarin: HR, 1.13; 97.5% CI, 0.96 to 1.34.

Another technique to critique and interpret clinical trial results is to calculate the measures of association: relative risk (RR), relative risk reduction (RRR), absolute risk reduction (ARR), and number needed to treat (NNT). ● *Calculating measures of association (RR, ARR, RRR, NNT) for nominal data provides further information to evaluate the meaning of controlled clinical trial results.* However, these calculations can only be performed with clinical trials designed to determine if there is a reduction in an outcome that occurs with modification of a risk factor when comparing the intervention to the control. Examples of outcomes could include the incidence of MI, stroke, hospitalization, or death. Since the endpoint is dichotomous (i.e., occurred or did not occur), the results can be set
● up in a table, as illustrated in Table 4-8. As seen from Table 4-8, the subjects randomized to the intervention are represented by either A (number of subjects experiencing the outcome) or B (those without the outcome). Subjects assigned to the control group and experiencing the outcome are designated by C while those without the outcome by D.[174,176]

Table 4-9 displays the formulas to calculate the four measure of association values and provides a description of these measures.[174,175] A description of interpreting these values follows. The RR is calculated as the proportion of the intervention group experiencing the outcome divided by the proportion of the control group with the event. The

TABLE 4-8. PRESENTING NOMINAL DATA STUDY RESULTS

Group	Adverse Event	
	Yes	No
Intervention	A	B
Control	C	D

RR equaled to 1 indicates no difference between the intervention and control (i.e., the incidence of the outcome was not increased or decreased with the intervention compared to control). Anytime a numerator divided by a denominator calculates to 1, these two variables are equal. The RR < 1 signifies the intervention lowered the risk of the outcome compared to the control (i.e., protective effect); a lower proportion of the intervention group compared to the control experienced the outcome. The RR > 1 indicates the

TABLE 4–9. MEASURES OF ASSOCIATION DESCRIPTION AND FORMULAS[a,179]

Measure of Association	Description	Formula
RR	The ratio of risk of an event occurring in one group compared to another group.	[A/(A + B)]/[C/(C + D)] In other words, (% of intervention group with primary endpoint)/(% of control group with primary endpoint)
RRR	Percent of baseline risk removed. The difference in event rates between two groups, expressed as a proportion of the event rate in the untreated group.	1 − RR
ARR	Percentage of subjects treated with the intervention spared the adverse outcome compared with the control.	[C/(C + D)] − [A/(A + B)] In other words, (% of control group with primary endpoint) − (% of intervention group with primary endpoint)
ARI	Percentage of subjects treated with the intervention who experienced the adverse outcome compared with the control.	[C/(C + D)] − [A/(A + B)] In other words, (% of control group with primary endpoint) − (% of intervention group with primary endpoint). The resulting calculation is typically a negative number.
NNT	Number of subjects needed to be treated to prevent one adverse event. A time course is included that represents the average (or median) duration of follow-up during the trial.	1/(ARR)
NNH	Number of subjects needed to be treated to prevent for one adverse event to occur. A time course is included that represents the average (or median) duration of follow-up during the trial. The value is referred to as NNH when the ARR is calculated as a negative number.	1/(ARR)

[a]Barratt A, Wyer PC, Hatala R, McGinn T, Dans AL, Keitz S, Moyer V, for GG; Evidence-Based Medicine Teaching Tips Working Group. Tips for learners of evidence-based medicine: 1. Relative risk reduction, absolute risk reduction and number needed to treat. CMAJ. 2004 Aug 17;171(4):353-8.

intervention increased the risk of the outcome; a greater proportion of the intervention group had the outcome compared to control. As an example, a RR of death equal to 0.70 was reported in a clinical trial in which subjects were randomized to either simvastatin (n = 2,221) or placebo (n = 2,223).[93] The RR was calculated by dividing the proportion of the subjects who died taking simvastatin (n = 182) by the proportion of those who died taking placebo (n = 256). The calculation of RR for this trial is (182/2,221)/(256/2,223). The RR is <1, which indicates simvastatin lowered the risk of death by almost one-third of the baseline risk compared to placebo. RRR indicates the relative change in the outcome rate between the intervention and control groups. The RRR was calculated as 30% ((1 − 0.70) × 100). The risk of experiencing death was 30% lower by treating these subjects with simvastatin instead of placebo. ARR refers to the difference in the outcome rate between the intervention and control groups. A higher proportion of subjects taking placebo died (n = 256 of 2,223 or 11.5%) compared to those taking simvastatin (182 of 2,221 or 8.2%). The ARR for death associated with simvastatin in this trial equals 3.3% (ARR = 11.5% − 8.2%); thus, 3.3% of the subjects receiving simvastatin were spared death compared to placebo. The NNT of this study equals 30 (NNT = 1/0.033), meaning 30 subjects need to be treated for a median of 5.4 years with simvastatin instead of placebo to prevent one case of death. The trial had a median follow-up time period of 5.4 years.

Many clinical trials present an endpoint as a relative change, which can be a misleading value. For instance, the RRR of stroke associated with atorvastatin was 48% compared to placebo in this study. Although this value appears very beneficial to subjects at risk for stroke, the ARR needs to be evaluated besides just the RRR value. The actual incidence of stroke was 1.5% (21 of 1,428 subjects treated with atorvastatin) versus 2.8% (39 of 1,409 subjects treated with placebo), which calculates to an absolute difference of 1.3% (ARR). Even though almost 50% less subjects (a relative difference) experienced a stroke with atorvastatin, this represents only a difference of 18 in a group of just over 2,800 subjects.[177]

All four measures of association can be calculated for clinical trials measuring nominal data and assessed together for the reader to determine the clinical difference in effect between the intervention and control. As seen by the simvastatin example earlier (in addition to Table 4-9), the same study result (e.g., death) can be presented using four different methods with different meanings. However, readers should not be misled by clinical trials that only present and discuss one of these values, which usually is the most appealing value (i.e., the one that seems to show the greatest difference). In fact, studies have documented that practitioners are more inclined to select a therapy presented as RRR more often than if the same study result was presented as all four values (i.e., ARR, RR, RRR, NNT).[178] Thus, investigators may be biased and selectively present the most appealing of these four values to mislead the reader into concluding a greater difference in effect among the intervention and control, even though the difference may be minimal.

CIs can also be calculated for nominal endpoints presented as RR or hazard ratio (HR). The latter is used to describe risks associated with adverse events and/or mortality data. The same formula for RR is used to calculate HR, which refers to whether the hazard of the adverse event (e.g., MI, hospitalization) is lowered or increased with the intervention compared to the control.[179] According to the formula for RR (and HR), a calculated value of 1 signifies that the incidence of the adverse event is equal between the intervention and control (i.e., numerator and denominator are equal and therefore no difference).[136,174] As previously mentioned, a RR < 1 signifies the intervention lowered the risk and a RR > 1 is interpreted as the intervention increasing the risk of the adverse event compared to the control. Therefore, investigators of a clinical trial presenting a RR (or HR) with a 95% CI that lies entirely on one side of 1 (i.e., up to 0.99 or 1.01 and upwards) indicates a difference in effect between the intervention and control. The 95% CI range for death in the simvastatin study was entirely below 1 (0.58 to 0.85),[93] which is interpreted as the investigators are 95% confident that the RR associated with simvastatin is between 0.58 and 0.85 for the population. Since 1 is not in this range, the investigators are 95% confident that the RR of experiencing the adverse event is reduced with simvastatin (i.e., difference in effect). Using another example, the calculated HR for the primary endpoint of CHD was 1.82 with a 95% CI of 1.49 to 2.01. This information indicates the investigators are 95% confident that the risk of CHD is increased with the intervention versus placebo in the population since the HR is >1. Also, the investigators were 95% confident that the intervention increased CHD risk in the population since the 95% CI for this endpoint did not include 1. However, a 95% CI containing the value of 1 indicates that the intervention may have neither lowered nor increased the risk (or hazard) of the adverse event. For instance, an HR for death due to other causes was calculated as 0.92 (95% CI, 0.74 to 1.14). The 95% CI range lies on both sides of 1 and indicates the risk of death could be lowered to 0.74 or increased to 1.14 with the intervention. Thus, the investigator (or reader) would conclude that the intervention is no different than placebo in decreasing or increasing the risk of death.

No Difference Does Not Indicate Equivalency

Using the above items (e.g., 95% CI, measures of association) assists the reader in determining the clinical significance of study results with p-values less than alpha. Remember, study results are not automatically clinically different (or significant) with p-values less than alpha. However, clinical studies reporting p-values greater than the alpha value translate into no statistical significance; thus, no clinical difference in effect is declared between the intervention and control groups. The H_0 is accepted (fail to be rejected) and the H_1 is rejected; in response, the statement of no difference is accepted.[141,168] The H_0 is not written to state that the intervention and control are the same, but stated as no difference in the effect (i.e., endpoint measurement) between the intervention and control. ⓫ *Nonstatistically significant results do not equate to the intervention and control being the same or equal.* Studies accepting the H_0 have the possibility of a Type II error. A difference in effect between the intervention and control groups may be present but either by chance or by a small trial sample size, the difference in effect was not detected. In this latter instance, the clinical trial may not have been powered sufficiently to detect the difference. Usually (but not all of the time) clinical trials in which the H_0 is accepted have too small of a sample size.[136] In fact, some studies may even be designed with an insufficient sample size so the investigators may claim equivalence between the intervention and active control after rejecting the H_0 even though a trial with an appropriate sample size could detect a difference. For instance, a study comparing the blood pressure-lowering effects of a new ACE inhibitor to a highly prescribed ACE inhibitor may use a small sample size to obtain study results that are not statistically different. Unfortunately, the trial results may be incorrectly interpreted by some readers as both ACE inhibitors being the same and/or the new ACE inhibitor being promoted as being equal as the comparative ACE inhibitor. This situation can occur in biased articles and/or presentations. However, the correct interpretation should be no difference detected. As one author stated, "absence of evidence is not evidence of absence."[134]

Assessing the Clinical Relevance of the Results

⓬ *All controlled clinical trial results need to be assessed to determine the clinical relevance (i.e., meaningfulness) of the intervention versus control.*[36,144,169] In other words, what do these results mean to practice? Small treatment effects and/or differences may be statistically different, but really not mean much clinically.[76,97,136] For example, an antihypertensive medication lowered mean DBP by 5 mmHg versus 2 mmHg for placebo ($p = 0.04$). The H_0 was rejected due to statistical difference. However, mean baseline DBP was 98 mmHg and this antihypertensive medication only lowered mean DBP to 93 mmHg, which is still classified as hypertensive.[180] Thus, practitioners would consider these results to be not clinically meaningful. In other words, these results are not useful in treating patients with hypertension.

On the other hand, a small difference in effect that is statistically different may be of clinical importance, depending on the perspective of the reader. A long-term care practitioner who specializes in geriatrics may consider a trial reporting a reduced number of incontinence episodes, on average, by two in a 24-hour period with a new anticholinergic agent compared to placebo to be clinically meaningful compared to an infectious disease practitioner. The new drug may reduce nursing time and improve the overall quality of life in patients with incontinence.

Not all clinical trials reporting nonstatistically significant results are completely devoid of clinical importance. The overall effect of the intervention and control need to be assessed. For example, a study compared lansoprazole (30 mg; n = 421) to omeprazole (20 mg; n = 431); each group received once-daily therapy for a duration of 8 weeks. The healing rates of erosive reflux esophagitis was 87.2% versus 87%, respectively, via ITT analysis (p = nonsignificant [NS]).[181] No clinical difference is concluded from this study, but these results would be considered to be clinically meaningful (i.e., clinically relevant) since >85% of patients were healed with either therapy.

As previously mentioned, clinical trial results of the intervention may be statistically significant and clinically different than the control, but may be not clinically practical. The clinical trial methods need to be reviewed for the ability to replicate these into every day patient care. A clinical trial may be designed that consists of technologies and/or include personnel that may not be readily accessible in patient care areas. In addition, patients may not be able to afford the new intervention. Another issue to consider is the demand on the actual patient. At times investigators offer incentives (e.g., monetary compensation, free medical care) for the subjects to strictly follow the study protocol (i.e., more motivated to be compliant). But in practice, real patients may not be as eager to follow an intricate schedule. For example, bismuth subsalicylate can be taken as a prophylaxis against traveler's diarrhea.[182] Although a clinical trial reported the suspension of subsalicylate bismuth 60 mL four times daily reduced the incidence of this unfortunate experience during travel,[183] some individuals may not be willing to adhere to this dosing schedule. Another issue to consider before applying the clinical trial results into practice is the normal care for patients with the disease/condition under study. Endpoint results of an intervention may be statistically significant and clinically different than the active control, but the control is not normally prescribed for patients with the disease/condition.[97]

BIBLIOGRAPHY

References are a very important part of the manuscript. The reference or bibliography section is at the end of the manuscript and provides documentation to support the information provided in the manuscript or acknowledgment for the work of other authors.[57] Any material that the author uses in the manuscript should be appropriately cited. References included in the manuscript should be recent (e.g., outdated articles should not be used unless the results of the article are pertinent to the manuscript) and complete. Readers should scan the references listed in the bibliography to determine if the authors used material from reputable sources. In addition, authors should refrain from extensively citing only their own work.[184] References should be used only once and typically are listed in numerical order (e.g., Arabic numerals) in which these appear in the manuscript; however, several referencing styles exist and are journal dependent (refer to Appendix 12-3 for further information about referencing). At minimum, the information in the reference section should be sufficient to lead the reader to locating the same arti-cle. With electronic publication, reference numbers throughout the text will appear as hyperlinks to the references. For this reason, many publishers will request that web-links and/or the direct-object identifier (DOI) be included at the end of the citation. In addition, publishers of biomedical information may also request a PubMed identification number (PubMed ID). Weblinks to the reference should be provided following the page number. The information should be listed in the following order: the phrase "Available from" followed by a colon, a space, and then the URL. A period should follow the URL only if it ends with a slash; otherwise, no punctuation is used. In the event that the full content is not freely available (e.g., subscription only), the most accurate URL to lead the person to the content should be used. If the URL length is disrupting to the formatting, the URL may be separated by placing a space after a hyphen or slash in the address.[185] Readers use the references to verify the cited information as well as to locate additional references on a topic.[57]

● ACKNOWLEDGMENTS

Individuals contributing to the clinical trial, but who do not meet the requirements for authorship, can be recognized in this section (see Chapter 12 for more information); how-ever, many journals have a prespecified amount of space for the acknowledgment section that must be adhered to by authors. Examples of persons identified are those providing manuscript preparation, technical assistance, or donors of equipment or supplies. Medical writers or editors also may be listed if their contributions significantly strengthened the clarity of the content. A collaboration or group may receive recognition in the acknowl-edgment section. Authors must obtain written permission from persons acknowledged before listing in this section, so the readers do not infer endorsements of the data and conclusions from these contributors.[41,57]

Other types of information may be included in this section. Such items are financial support (see below for further information) and conflicts of interest, which can help the reader identify or reconcile sources of bias. Indicators that the manuscript underwent peer review, signified by a series of dates and titled received/revised/accepted, may also be included in the acknowledgments. Typically, at least 4 to 8 weeks are between these stages since it is necessary to allow time for the reviewers to comment, the authors to revise, and receive another review of the manuscript. Some journals only present the manuscript acceptance date, which allows readers to determine the lag time between the article being accepted in final form for publication. A minimal time period between the acceptance and publication date is beneficial since this increases content currency.

FUNDING

⓭ *Controlled clinical trial investigators and authors should disclose any funding sources and potential conflicts of interest.* Due to the enormous expense often required to conduct a clinical trial, investigators may seek financial assistance to conduct the research. Various funding sources are available that include pharmaceutical companies, government agencies (e.g., National Institutes of Health [NIH]), national organizations (e.g., American Heart Association), university grants (e.g., faculty development grants), and private donations. Although financial disclosure by industry and investigators is recommended, this may not occur. In 2010, the Patient Protection and Affordable Care Act (also known as The Sunshine Act) "required that pharmaceutical and medical industry manufacturers disclose their financial relationship with physicians."[186] Reporting of payments by pharmaceutical companies to physicians has been assessed in numerous studies. In general, reporting is difficult to evaluate because pharmaceutical companies and journals may have different financial-disclosure thresholds (for what is considered a significant monetary payment); there can be variability in required reporting timeframes (distinct versus unspecified); disclosures may differ depending on whether the requirement is a listing of *all* financial relationships versus those that are related to the research topic being evaluated; and there are inconsistencies in the categories of relationships (e.g., speaking, consulting, research, travel, expert witness) and how to report other nonmonetary support (e.g., meals, continuing education, gifts).[185] Nevertheless, studies have found significant disagreement in reporting of financial relationships. One study that evaluated physician payments >$100,000 from the Dollars for Docs database during years 2009 to 2010 found that 69% of the 103 publications did not contain disclosure of physician payments.[186] Another study that evaluated the agreement between pharmaceutical disclosure and author self-disclosures for payments >$10,000 found that authors and industry only disclosed 19% and 12% of payments, respectively.[185]

During 2015, an estimated $58.8 billion was spent by the pharmaceutical companies for research and development (which includes clinical drug trials). Current estimates indicate that the cost is $2.6 billion to develop a new medication and only 12% of medications that make it into phase I clinical trials are deemed safe and effective enough to be approved by the FDA.[187] The pharmaceutical industry is responsible for a significant amount of the clinical research conducted worldwide and new medications have resulted in a reduction in morbidity and mortality plus improved quality of life for various disease states. Thus, readers of industry-sponsored research should not automatically disregard a clinical trial solely based upon a pharmaceutical company sponsoring the research. However, readers should be cognizant of possible **conflicts of interest**, defined as "a set of conditions in which professional judgment concerning a primary interest (such as a patient's welfare) tends to be unduly influenced by a secondary interest (such as financial gain)"[188] that may result in potential bias. Conflicts of interest arise because the industry may be prompted to publish articles as a means of making their product appear better for a disease state in relation to the standard of care. This research may result in methods bias, premature termination of trials for nonscientific/unethical reasons, or reporting/publication bias.[189] To counter this, investigators are encouraged to promote objectivity by designing studies that have clear methodology with outcomes measures that are transparently reported so that interpretation differences are reduced.[190] Many journals now include a funding and conflicts of interest section in the methodology of the manuscript. The role of the funding source in the design of the study, collection and analysis of data, and the interpretation of study results should be included. Further, this section should state whether the investigators made the decision about publication of the data and the role the investigators had in writing, editing, and approving the manuscript. The ICMJE has adopted a disclosure form for all their member journals to obtain financial associations of the authors submitting manuscripts. The form is posted on the ICMJE website (http://www.icmje.org/coi_disclosure.pdf).[191]

The study design, result presentation, data interpretations, and study conclusions should be assessed appropriately to determine if the funding source had any influences on the overall clinical trial. Pharmaceutical companies need to determine the clinical usefulness of newly developed medications. These companies are expecting to profit from the new medication being approved by the FDA and marketed to prescribers. Many organizations (e.g., government, not for profit) are not prime candidates to offer funding for these studies, which leaves the pharmaceutical company to sponsor the study. Thus, readers are going to encounter pharmaceutical companies sponsoring research and the reader is responsible to determine the quality of the research.

Not all investigator–pharmaceutical industry relationships have the potential to cause a conflict of interest, but readers should decide if a publication is biased. In fact, many well-designed, clinically important studies documenting improved patient health have been sponsored by the pharmaceutical industry and these have changed the standards of practice in treating patients.

However, there have been reports in the literature of selected pharmaceutical companies terminating studies for various reasons unrelated to efficacy and safety,[192] employing inappropriate comparators,[193] using inappropriate study samples,[194] and suppressing the results of negative studies.[195] Also, it can be assumed that a pharmaceutical company would design studies that are most likely to show superiority of their drug in some aspect or another. Furthermore, reports have been published that indicate a favorable conclusion of studies financially supported by the pharmaceutical industry, which can be referred to as **publication bias**. This type of sponsored research usually yields larger treatment effects than not-for-profit funded studies.[97]

Research has documented that the conclusions of some trials funded by for-profit organizations were significantly in favor of the experimental drug as the treatment of choice.

Not all pharmaceutical industry-sponsored research is biased; many study results are clinically meaningful. Readers need to be aware that the pharmaceutical company has a lot at stake for an investigational drug to be approved by the FDA. In response, the pharmaceutical company attempts to design a clinical trial to meet the FDA-approval standards. However, the methods of presenting (i.e., results section), interpreting (i.e., introduction and/or discussion sections), and summarizing the data and results (i.e., conclusion) can be biased and are not governed by the regulations of the FDA. Consequently, readers need to evaluate the trial data critically to assess the appropriateness and validity of the reported conclusions based upon the trial results.[196]

Furthermore, trial registration with an official governmental entity is another method for the reader to discern if publication bias exists in favor of a particular interventional therapy. Specifically, the national clinical trials registry (http://www.clinicaltrials.gov),[197] which is hosted by the NIH, is a very useful resource for the reader of biomedical literature to determine if potentially negative study results are being excluded from discussion in clinical trials or promotional materials. The Food and Drug Administration Amendments Act of 2007 (also known as FDAAA 801) mandates registration and reporting of results from clinical trials utilizing certain drugs, biologics, and devices, regardless of study outcome.[198]

ClinicalTrials.gov indexes more than 224,186 federally and privately funded clinical trials conducted in the United States and more than 192 countries. Furthermore, this resource provides the user details about a trial's purpose, guidelines for participation, study locations, and contact information for more details. The information contained within the national trial registry should be strictly viewed as supplementary to complement care from a health care professional. This website can be searched by a variety of functions, including investigational agent or disease state. With this in mind, the national clinical trials registry is also a very useful tool for the practitioners who may need to identify treatment options for a patient who cannot afford conventional intervention or who has a rare or terminal disease state and is seeking additional treatment options.[197]

COMMENTARIES/CLINICAL TRIAL CRITIQUES

Every journal should provide its readership the opportunity for correspondence to exchange ideas about a topic or relay new information about articles published in the journal.[41,57] ⓮ *Editorials, letters to the editor, and commentary publications can assist in interpreting controlled clinical trial results.* Commentaries can be essential in assisting readers in interpreting and/or critiquing articles published within the journals, by providing strengths and limitations of the original research, an update to published information, or questions to the authors of the original research manuscript.

Editorials, defined as "a written expression of opinion that may reflect the official position of the publication,"[57] are short essays from the editor or other experts in a particular field and are written to convey additional opinions about an article, typically, in the same issue of a journal. Not all editorials reflect the ideas/thoughts of the journal because these are opinions of the editorial author. Although editorials may contain some bias, this literature should always be considered when evaluating a clinical trial by providing additional insight of the results and aid in the comprehension of the clinical application of the trial results. For instance, an editorial in response to IMPROVE-IT was published in the same journal issue.[199] The editorial authors discussed many issues ranging from the large discontinuation rate (42%) in the groups, despite the fact that therapy for hyperlipidemia is long term, to the addition of other agents to lower LDL levels in combination with statins, potentially producing the same effect.[198]

Several issues should be considered during the preparation or evaluation of editorials. Quality editorials are original; those editorials with non-original ideas need to include a clear justification of repeating these ideas. The editorial objective should be clearly presented and reflect a complete message. The content should be significant to merit publication, along with being applicable to practice, accurate, and thorough. The editorial points should be timely with respect to the publication in which the author is responding. Finally, the editorial author should mention the facts clearly and the material should be applicable to the readership of the publication.[200]

Not all original research reports are accompanied by an editorial. Persons seeking an editorial associated with a clinical trial can use a few methods to locate the publication. First, the journal issue that contains the clinical trial will list the editorial title in the journal issue's table of contents. Another way, not always present in all clinical trials, is a notation printed on the first page of the clinical trial referring the reader to another page (i.e., "For comment, see page ..."; "Commentary, page ..."). Readers not having access to the actual clinical trial or journal issue's table of contents can locate the trial citation in PubMed® (using the Single Citation Matcher at http://www.pubmed.gov). Those clinical trials with an accompanying editorial will contain a notation of Comment in and an abbreviated journal citation (i.e., journal name, date, plus volume, issue, and page numbers). Another method is to search the clinical trial topic (i.e., via Medical Subject Heading [MeSH] term in PubMed®) and limit the search to the publication type of editorial.

Some journals/websites are published for the primary purpose of providing editorials/commentaries addressing a clinical trial. These resources are known as secondary journals and are independent of the journals that directly publish the clinical trials.[43,97,201] Secondary journals are publications that assist the busy practitioners in a few vital methods, keeping them current regarding important and relevant studies, plus presenting key study information in a concise format. Clinical trials are presented, usually in a structured abstract style, but not just copying and pasting the exact abstract prepared by the trial investigators. These prepared abstracts may present additional and/or more precise information. In addition, a commentary addressing the study strengths, limitations, and application into practice is authored by a leading practitioner in the field of study. Readers should use these resources while critiquing the biomedical/pharmacy literature.

Examples of secondary journal websites include http://www.theheart.org and http://www.medscape.com. Typically, these publications provide an overview of the study followed by a commentary. Medscape is particularly useful for practitioners since pharmacy-specific topics are addressed in a section of this website. ACP Journal Club is an online resource (included in Annals of Internal Medicine journal issues) in which biomedical literature (i.e., original research, systematic reviews) is selected, based on predefined criteria, and summarized by an expert in the field in the form of structured abstracts followed by a commentary. More than 130 journals are reviewed and are selected due to their potential impact on clinical practice.[202]

Another example is the New England Journal of Medicine (NEJM) Journal Watch, an online resource that is published at least monthly in print[203] and daily on the Internet. Updated information for over 10 specialty areas of medical practice obtained from over 250 medical journals and other vital medical news sources is provided by physicians along with a commentary to help clinicians determine the impact or the research results on their practice.[203] Several specialty editions of Journal Watch are available including Journal Watch Cardiology, Journal Watch Emergency Medicine, Journal Watch Gastroenterology, and Journal Watch Infectious Diseases.[203]

Letters to the Editor

Letters to the editor can provide valuable insight into original research and can include various types of contributions. These may be in the form of comments, addenda, or updates from previously published articles, alerts regarding potential problems in practice, observations/comments on trends in medication use, opinions on trends or controversies in therapy or research, or original research. Authors of letters to the editor must adhere to strict guidelines from the journals regarding the length, number of authors, tables, and references, and format of the publication.[204] The primary content of letters to the editor is feedback from the journal readers regarding the published materials in the journal. In addition, most journals restrict use or reference to unpublished data. Typically, these letters are published within 3 to 6 months of the original publication. The primary content of letters to the editor is feedback from the journal readers regarding the published materials in the journal. The letters may disagree with the design, result interpretation, and/or conclusions of the publication. Also, the letters may ask for additional information that can be used to interpret, clarify, comprehend, and/or critique the information within the publication. Afterwards, the authors of the original publication may provide a response to these published letters. The letters to the editor serve as another source of valuable information for those using and critiquing the biomedical literature.

Conclusion

Practitioners are characterized by having the skills, ability, and knowledge to problem solve, critically think, and formulate recommendations based upon the literature. All practitioners need the skill of efficiently locating, critically evaluating, and effectively formulating and communicating an evidence-based recommendation, regardless of the practice setting. As the role of the practitioners in direct patient care continues to increase, incorporating these skills in daily practice is essential. A multitude of literature is published each year and the quality varies significantly. Readers of the literature should not immediately accept the authors' conclusions; they should be able to assess the strengths and limitations of the source. The information within this chapter identifies and discusses many issues to consider while reading and analyzing controlled clinical trials. Although every clinical trial has limitations, those trials with appropriate design and well-presented results are still important to apply into clinical practice. Using the proper techniques in evaluating clinical trials can allow practitioners to contribute as key stakeholders in an ever-increasing interdisciplinary health care arena.

Self-Assessment Questions

Read the excerpt of the following clinical trial summary and answer the questions that follow.[205]

The STOPAH trial was a multicenter, double-blind, randomized controlled clinical trial that assessed the effectiveness of prednisolone versus pentoxifylline in reducing short-term (28-day) mortality in subjects with alcoholic hepatitis and severe disease. Subjects who met inclusion criteria were randomized in a 2:2 fashion to one of four treatment groups: pentoxifylline placebo and prednisolone placebo, prednisolone and pentoxifylline placebo, pentoxifylline and prednisolone placebo, or prednisolone plus pentoxifylline. Secondary endpoints were 90-day mortality and liver transplantation at 90 and 365 days. Study investigators determined that 1,026 subjects were needed for the total study sample in order to detect 30% and 21% reduction in 28-day mortality between subjects receiving each active therapy or placebo, respectively. Results from all subjects were included in the final analyses and a p-value less than 0.05 was considered significant.

After randomization, data from 1,053 subjects were available for the primary endpoint analysis. Subjects were distributed evenly across all treatment groups based upon predefined characteristics. Incidence of 28-day mortality occurred in 14% (73/526) of subjects receiving prednisolone-based therapy, 18% (95/527) of those not receiving prednisolone,

16% (85/518) of those receiving pentoxifylline, and 16% of those not receiving pentoxifylline (32/535). The resulting ratio for 28-day mortality in individuals receiving pentoxifylline versus no pentoxifylline was 1.07 (95% CI, 0.77 to 1.49; p = 0.69) and with prednisolone versus no prednisolone was 0.72 (95% CI, 0.52 to 1.01; p = 0.06). There was no difference in primary outcome occurrence between prednisolone and pentoxifylline at 28 days as significant overlap between the CI ranges for the individual therapies was present (p = 0.41). Nor was difference between therapies present at prespecified 90-day and 365-day checkpoints. Incidence of serious infections was more common in individuals receiving prednisolone (13%) versus those who did not receive prednisolone (7%) (p = 0.002).

USE THE STUDY NARRATIVE TO ANSWER QUESTIONS 1 TO 9

1. What type of blinding was used in this study?
   a. No blinding
   b. Single-blinding
   c. Open-label
   d. Double-blinding
   e. Triple-blinding

2. Which of the following represents the type of data collected and evaluated for the primary endpoint in this study?
   a. Nominal
   b. Ordinal
   c. Continuous
   d. Interval
   e. Ratio

3. Which of the following statements defines the measures of central tendency that can be performed on the type of data represented by the primary endpoint?
   a. Average numerical value in a data set
   b. Absolute middle value in a data set
   c. Most frequently occurring value in a data set
   d. Measurement of the variability of data around the average
   e. Inclusion of all study subjects in analysis regardless of completion

4. The study narrative states, "There was no difference in primary outcome occurrence between prednisolone and pentoxifylline at 28 days (p = 0.41)." Interpret the meaning of the p-value.
   a. The p-value is less than alpha.
   b. The p-value is due to small sample size.

   c. The probability of a Type II error is 0.41%.
   d. The probability of a Type I error is 59%.
   e. The probability of a Type I error is 41%.

5. Which of the following is included in this study?
   a. Per-protocol analysis since results from subjects who completed the complete study were included in the final analysis.
   b. Run-in phase since baseline demographics were similar between the two groups.
   c. Intention-to-treat since results from all subjects were included in the final analysis.
   d. Subgroup analysis since medication adherence was high.
   e. A subjective primary endpoint that utilized surrogate markers.

6. Which of the following is correct regarding the power of the study?
   a. Since at least 80% of the subjects completed the study, the power is 80%.
   b. Included to estimate a sample size and control for Type II error.
   c. Included to estimate the statistical significance of study endpoints.
   d. Power was not met for this study because not enough subjects were analyzed.
   e. Since results of all subjects are utilized, no power analysis is needed.

7. The study narrative states, "The resulting ratio for 28-day mortality in individuals receiving pentoxifylline versus no pentoxifylline was 1.07 (95% CI, 0.77 to 1.49; $p = 0.69$)." Select the appropriate interpretation of the point estimate and range from the selections below.
   a. The risk of 28-day mortality is lowered by receiving pentoxifylline by 69% because the point estimate is greater than 1.
   b. The risk of 28-day mortality is unchanged by receiving pentoxifylline compared to not receiving pentoxifylline and the investigators are 95% confident that the risk of mortality is 77% to 149% higher in subjects taking pentoxifylline than in those not taking pentoxifylline.
   c. The risk of 28-day mortality is slightly elevated by receiving pentoxifylline in the study sample and the investigators are 95% confident that the risk ranges from 23% reduction of baseline risk to 49% elevation of baseline risk in the general population compared to not receiving pentoxifylline.
   d. The risk of 28-day mortality is increased by 69% by receiving pentoxifylline versus not receiving pentoxifylline.
   e. The risk of 28-day mortality is improved by receiving pentoxifylline compared to prednisolone.

8. The study narrative states, "The resulting ratio for 28-day mortality in individuals receiving . . . prednisolone versus no prednisolone was 0.72 (95% CI, 0.52 to 1.01; p = 0.06)." Select the appropriate interpretation of this information from the selections below.
   a. A clinical difference can be present because the value of equality (one) is in confidence interval range.
   b. The investigators are 95% confident that 5% of the subjects will not experience the primary endpoint by receiving prednisolone.
   c. No clinical difference can be present because this result lacks statistical significance.
   d. Even though statistical significance is not present, the reader can still look at study characteristics to determine if clinical significance is present.
   e. Even though 72% of subjects receiving prednisolone experienced the primary endpoint, the investigators are 95% confident that the real rate of endpoint occurrence in the general population will range from 52% to 101%.

9. Which of the following is correct for the safety endpoint of serious infections?
   a. Not statistically significant and not clinically different
   b. Statistically significant and accept (fail to reject) H_0
   c. Not statistically significant and reject H_0
   d. Not statistically significant but clinically significant
   e. Statistically significant and reject H_0

END OF CASE

10. Which of the following characteristics is associated with controlled clinical trials?
    a. Retrospective
    b. Short duration
    c. Low level of evidence
    d. No IRB approval required
    e. Comparative

11. Which of the following information would be expected to be included in the introduction section of a controlled clinical trial?
    a. Investigator opinions about study results
    b. Statement of primary endpoint
    c. Statistical tests used in the study
    d. Characteristics of subjects enrolled
    e. Inclusion and exclusion criteria

12. Which term below accurately describes characteristics of a study or outside influences that may affect the true study results?
    a. Confounding variable
    b. Statistical significance
    c. Blinding
    d. Randomization
    e. Type I error

13. Which of the following is true regarding data distribution?
    a. A normal distribution occurs when mean, median, and mode are numerically equal.
    b. 68% of data points are included within 2 standard deviations from the mean.
    c. 99% of data points are included within 1 standard deviation from the mean.
    d. 95% of data points are included within 3 standard deviations from the mean.
    e. Standard deviation and standard error of the mean are the same value.

14. Which of the following is true regarding Type I and Type II errors?
    a. Type II errors can occur when the H_0 is rejected.
    b. Type I errors can occur when the H_0 is accepted (fail to reject).
    c. Type I errors are associated with sample size.
    d. Type II errors are associated with statistically significant results.
    e. Type II errors can occur when the H_0 is accepted (fail to reject).

15. Which of the following is an example of a surrogate marker or endpoint?
    a. Death
    b. Hip fracture
    c. Infection
    d. Hospital discharge
    e. Blood pressure

REFERENCES

1. Ware M, Mabe M. The STM report. An overview of scientific and scholarly journal publishing. 34th ed. Published November 2012. Available from: http://www.stm-assoc.org/2012_12_11_STM_Report_2012.pdf. Accessed August 3, 2016.
2. Food and Drug Administration [Internet]. Silver Spring, MD. Novel drug approvals for 2016. [cited 2017 Mar 13]. Available from: https://www.fda.gov/Drugs/DevelopmentApprovalProcess/DrugInnovation/ucm483775.htm
3. Food and Drug Administration [Internet]. 2016 biological license application approvals. [cited 2017 Mar 13]. Available from: https://www.fda.gov/BiologicsBloodVaccines/DevelopmentApprovalProcess/BiologicalApprovalsbyYear/ucm482397.htm

4. PubMed homepage [Internet]. Bethesda, MD: National Library of Medicine. [cited 2017 Mar 13]. Available from: http://www.ncbi.nlm.nih.gov/pubmed/

5. Gallup, Inc. Honesty/Ethics in professions [Internet]. Washington, DC: Gallup, Inc. [cited 2016 Oct 20]. Available from: http://www.gallup.com/poll/1654/honesty-ethics-professions.aspx

6. Sheridan SL, Pignone M. Numeracy and medical student's ability to interpret data. Eff Clin Pract. 2002;5:35-40. Available from: http://ecp.acponline.org/janfeb02/sheridan.pdf. Accessed August 3, 2016.

7. Calis KA, Hutchison LC, Elliott ME, Ives TJ, Zillich AJ Poirier T, Townsend KA, Woodall B, Feldman S, Raebel MA, American College of Clinical Pharmacy. Health People 2010: challenges, opportunities, and a call to action for America's practitioners. Pharmacotherapy. 2004 Sept;24(9):1241-94. PMID: 15460187. doi:10.1592/phco.24.13.1241.38082.

8. Santschi V, Chiolero A, Colosimo AL, Platt RW, Taffé P, Burnier M, Burnand B, Paradis G. Improving blood pressure control through practitioners interventions: a meta-analysis of randomized controlled trials. J Am Heart Assoc. 2014 Apr 10;3(2):e000718. Review. PubMed PMID: 24721801; PubMed Central PMCID: PMC4187511. doi:10.1161/JAHA.113.000718.

9. Hadi MA, Alldred DP, Briggs M, Munyombwe T, Closs SJ. Effectiveness of practitioners-led medication review in chronic pain management: systematic review and meta-analysis. Clin J Pain. 2014 Nov;30(11):1006-14. Review. PubMed PMID: 24480911. doi:10.1097/AJP.0000000000000063.

10. Tan EC, Stewart K, Elliott RA, George J. Practitioners services provided in general practice clinics: a systematic review and meta-analysis. Res Social Adm Pharm. 2014 Jul-Aug;10(4):608-22. Epub 2013 Oct 23. Review. PubMed PMID: 24161491. doi:10.1016/j.sapharm.2013.08.006.

11. Cutler TW. The pharmacy profession and health care reform: opportunities and challenges during the next decade. J Am Pharm Assoc. 2011 Jul-Aug;51(4):477-81.

12. Walker KA, Scarpaci L, McPherson ML. Fifty reasons to love your palliative care practitioners. Am J Hosp Palliat Care. 2010 Dec;27(8):511-3. Epub 2010 May 27. PubMed PMID: 20508241. doi:10.1177/1049909110371096.

13. Nathan JP. Drug information—the systematic approach: continuing education article. J Pharm Prac. 2013;26:78-84. doi:10.1177/0897190012474229.

14. U.S. National Library of Medicine [Internet]. Bethesda, MD: PubMed tutorial. Building the search. [cited 2016 Aug 3]. Available from: https://www.nlm.nih.gov/bsd/disted/pubmedtutorial/020_010.html

15. Nelson SJ, Schulman JL. Orthopaedic literature and MeSH. Clin Orthop Relat Res. 2010 Oct;468(10):2621-26. PMID: 20623263. PMCID: PMC3049625. doi:10.1007/s11999-010-1387-4.

16. Bhandari M, Giannoudis PV. Evidence-based medicine: what it is and what it is not. Injury. 2006 Apr;37(4):302-6. PMID: 16487527. doi:10.1016/j.injury.2006.01.034.

17. Hershenberg R, Drabick DA, Vivian D. An opportunity to bridge the gap between clinical research and clinical practice: implications for clinical training. Psychotherapy. 2012 Jun;49(2):123-34. PMID: 22642520. PMCID: PMC3786339. doi:10.1037/a0027648.

18. Steen RG, Dager SR. Evaluating the evidence for evidence-based medicine: are randomized clinical trials less flawed than other forms of peer-reviewed medical research. FASEB J. 2013;27:3430-6. doi:10.1096/fj.13-230714.

19. Pihlstrom BL, Curran AE, Voelker HT, Kingman A. Randomized controlled trials: what are they and who needs them? Periodontol 2000. 2012 Jun;59(1):14-31.

20. Umscheid CA, Margolis DJ, Grossman CE. Key concepts of clinical trials: a narrative review. Postgrad Med. 2011 Sep;123(5):194-204.

21. U.S. Food and Drug Administration. How drugs are developed and approved [Internet]. Rockville, MD: U.S. Food and Drug Administration; [updated 2015 Aug 18; cited 2016 Aug 3]. Available from: http://www.fda.gov/drugs/developmentapprovalprocess/how-drugsaredevelopedandapproved/default.htm

22. Stanley K. Evaluation of randomized controlled trials. Circulation. 2007;115:1819-22. doi:10.1161/CIRCULATIONAHA.106.618603.

23. Gehlbach S. Interpreting the medical literature. 5th ed. New York, NY: McGraw-Hill Company; 2006.

24. Doll R. Controlled trials: the 1948 watershed. BMJ. 1998 Oct 31;317(7167):1217-20. PMID: 9794864. PMCID: PMC1114161. doi:http://dx.doi.org/10.1136/bmj.317.7167.1217.

25. Kunz R, Oxman AD. The unpredictability paradox: review of empirical comparisons of randomised and non-randomised clinical trials. BMJ. 1998 Oct 31;317(7167):1185-90. PMID: 9794851. PMCID: PMC28700. doi:http://dx.doi.org/10.1136/bmj.317.7167.1185.

26. Kendrach MG, Anderson HG. Fundamentals of controlled clinical trials. J Pharm Pract. 1998 Jun;XI(3):163-80. doi:10.1177/089719009801100308.

27. Schulz KF, Altman DG, Moher D; CONSORT Group. CONSORT 2010 Statement: updated guidelines for reporting parallel group randomised trials. Ann Int Med. 2010;152(11):726-32. doi:10.7326/0003-4819-152-11-201006010-00232.

28. STROBE statement. Strengthening the reporting of observational studies in epidemiology. Version 4. Available from: http://www.strobe-statement.org/fileadmin/Strobe/uploads/checklists/STROBE_checklist_v4_combined.pdf. Accessed August 3, 2016.

29. Friedman L, Furberg C, DeMets D. Fundamentals of clinical trials. 4th ed. New York, NY: Springer; 2010.

30. Lader EW, Cannon CP, Ohman EM, Newby LK, Sulmasy DP, Barst RJ, Fair JM, Flather M, Freedman JE, Frye RL, Hand MM, Jesse RL, Van de Werf F, Costa F, American Heart Association. The clinician as investigator: participating in clinical trials in the practice setting: Appendix 1: fundamentals of study design. Circulation. 2004 Jun 1;109(21):e302-4. PMID: 15173052. doi:10.1161/01.CIR.0000128807.57602.61.

31. Song F, Loke Y, Hooper L. Why are medical and health-related studies not being published? A systematic review of reasons given by investigators. Wicherts JM, editor. PLoS ONE. 2014;9(10):e110418. doi:10.1371/journal.pone.0110418.

32. Mathieu S, Boutron I, Moher D, Altman DG, Ravaud P. Comparison of registered and published primary outcomes in randomized controlled trials. JAMA. 2009 Sep 2;302(9):977-84. PMID: 19724045. doi:10.1001/jama.2009.1242.

33. Krzyzanowska MK, Pintilie M, Tannock IF. Factors associated with failure to publish large randomized trials presented at an oncology meeting. JAMA. 2003 Jul 24;290(3):495-501. PMID: 12876092. doi:10.1001/jama.290.4.495.

34. Irwin RS. The role of conflict of interest in reporting of scientific information. Chest. 2009 Jul;136(1):253-9. PMID: 19584207. doi:10.1378/chest.09-0890.

35. Hayes A, Hunter J. Why is publication of negative clinical trial data important? Br J Pharmacol. 2012 Dec;167(7):1395-7.

36. Sridharan L, Greenland P. Editorial policies and publication bias: the importance of negative studies. Arch Intern Med. 2009 Jun 8;169(11):1022-3.

37. Jones CW, Handler L, Crowell KE, KEil LG, Weaver MA, Platts-Mills TF. Non-publication of large randomized clinical trials: cross sectional analysis. BMJ. 2013;346:f6104. doi:http://dx.doi.org/10.1136/bmj.f6104.

38. Stone GW, Pocock SJ. Randomized trials, statistics, and clinical inference. J Am Coll Cardiol. 2010 Feb 2;55(5):428-31. PMID: 20117455. doi:10.1016/j.jacc.2009.06.066.

39. Cook DA. Randomized controlled trials and meta-analysis in medical education: what role do they play? Med Teach. 2012;34(6):468-73. PMID: 22489980. doi:10.3109/0142159X.2012.671978.

40. Journal of Negative Results in BioMedicine. About the journal. [cited 2016 Aug 3]. Available from: https://jnrbm.biomedcentral.com/about

41. International Committee of Medical Journal Editors. Recommendations for the conduct, reporting, editing and publication of scholarly work in medical journals [Internet]. [place unknown]: International Committee of Medical Journal Editors. [cited 2013 Oct 4]. Available from: http://www.icmje.org/icmje-recommendations.pdf. Accessed September 14, 2016.

42. Armstrong PW, Newby LK, Granger CB, Lee KL, Simes RJ, Van de Werf F, White HD, Califf RM, Virtual Coordinating Centre for Global Collaborative Cardiovascular Research (VIGOUR) Group. Lessons learned from a clinical trial. Circulation. 2004 Dec 7;110(23):3610-4.

43. Augustyn N, Welch SJ, Irwin RS. Managing information overload: the evolution of CHEST. Chest. 2012 Jul;142(1):1-5. PMID: 22796829. doi:10.1378/chest.12-1364.

44. Blumenthal D. Doctors and drug companies. N Engl J Med. 2004 Oct 28;351(18):1885-90. PMID: 15509823. doi:10.1056/NEJMhpr042734.

45. Mintzes B, Lexchin J, Sutherland JM, Beaulieu MD, Wilkes MS, Durrieu G, Reynolds E. Pharmaceutical sales representatives and patient safety: a comparative prospective study of information quality in Canada, France and the United States. J Gen Intern Med. 2013 Oct;28(10):1368-75. Epub 2013 Apr 5. PubMed PMID: 23558775; PubMed Central PMCID: PMC3785667. doi:10.1007/s11606-013-2411-7.

46. Spurling GK, Mansfield PR, Montgomery BD, Lexchin J, Doust J, Othman N, Vitry AI. Information from pharmaceutical companies and the quality, quantity, and cost of physicians' prescribing: a systematic review. PLoS Med. 2010 Oct 19;7(10):e1000352. Review. PubMed PMID: 20976098; PubMed Central PMCID: PMC2957394. doi:10.1371/journal.pmed.1000352.

47. Campbell B. "Throw-away journals": tactics for dealing with office waste. CMAJ. 1990 Jan 15;142(2):100. PMID: 2295024. PMCID: PMC1451725.

48. Wood BD, Ludwig RL. The difference between peer review and nonpeer review. Radiol Technol. 2012 Sep-Oct;84(1):90-2. PMID: 22988268.

49. Harden RM, Lilley P. A fresh approach to publishing and reviewing papers in health professions education. Med Teach. 2013;35(1):1-3.

50. Shahriari N, Grant-Kels JM, Payette MJ. Predatory journals: How to recognize and avoid the threat of involvement with these unethical "publishers". J Am Acad Dermatol. 2016 Sep;75(3):658-9. PMID: 27543229. doi:10.1016/j.jaad.2016.04.056.

51. Rochon PA, Bero LA, Bay AM, Gold JL, Dergal JM, Binns MA, Streiner DL, Gurwitz JH. Comparison of review articles published in peer-reviewed and throwaway journals. JAMA. 2002 Jun 5;287(21):2853-6.

52. Rochon PA, Gurwitz JH, Cheung CM, Hayes JA, Chalmers TC. Evaluating the quality of articles published in journal supplements compared with the quality of those published in the parent journal. JAMA. 1994 Jul 13;272(2):108-13.

53. Schriger DL, Raffetto B, Drolen C, Cooper RJ. The effect of peer review on the quality of data graphs in Annals of Emergency Medicine. Ann Emerg Med. 2016 Sep 7. pii: S0196-0644(16)30366-3. doi:10.1016/j.annemergmed.2016.06.046. [Epub ahead of print]. PMID: 27614587.

54. Wagner E, Middleton P. Effects of technical editing in biomedical journals: a systemic review. JAMA. 2002;287:2821-4.

55. Guyatt GH, Akl EA, Crowther M, Gutterman DD, Schuünemann HJ, American College of Chest Physicians Antithrombotic Therapy and Prevention of Thrombosis Panel. Executive summary: Antithrombotic therapy and prevention of thrombosis, 9th ed: American College of Chest Physicians Evidence-Based Clinical Practice Guidelines. Chest. 2012 Feb;141(2 Suppl):7S-47S. MID: 22315257. PMCID: PMC3278060. doi:10.1378/chest.1412S3.

56. Health on the Net. HON code. What is it? [cited 2016 Sep 14]. Available from: http://www.hon.ch/HONcode/Patients/Visitor/visitor.html

57. Lader EW, Cannon CP, Ohman EM, Newby LK, Sulmasy DP, Barst RJ, Fair JM, Flather M, Freedman JE, Frye RL, Hand MM, Jesse RL, Van de Werf F, Costa F, American College of Cardiology Foundation. The clinician as investigator: participating in clinical trials in the practice setting. Circulation. 2004 Jun 1;109(21):2672-9. PMID: 15173050. doi:10.1161/01.CIR.0000128702.16441.75.

58. Studdert DM, Mello MM, Brennan TA. Financial conflicts of interest in physicians' relationships with the pharmaceutical industry—self-regulation in the shadow of federal prosecution. N Engl J Med. 2004 Oct 28;351(18):1891-900. PMID: 15509824. doi:10.1056/NEJMlim042229.

59. Iverson C, Christiansen S, editors. American Medical Association manual of style. A guide for authors and editors. 10th ed. New York, NY: Oxford University Press; 2007.

60. Nelson HS, Bensch G, Pleskow WW, DiSantostefano R, DeGraw S, Reasner DS, Rollins TE, Rubin PD. Improved bronchodilation with levalbuterol compared with racemic albuterol

in patients with asthma. J Allergy Clin Immunol. 1998 Dec;102(6 Pt 1):943-52. PMID: 9847435. doi:http://dx.doi.org/10.1016/S0091-6749(98)70332-X.

61. Peat J, Elliott E, Baur L, Keena V. Scientific writing: easy when you know how. London: BMJ Books; 2002.

62. Hopewell S, Clarke M, Moher D, Wager E, Middleton P, Altman DG, Schulz KF; CONSORT Group. CONSORT for reporting randomized controlled trials in journal and conference abstracts: explanation and elaboration. PLoS Med. 2008;5(1):e20. PMID: 18215107. PMCID: PMC2211558. doi:10.1371/journal.pmed.0050020.

63. Guimarães CA. Structured abstracts: narrative review. Acta Cir Bras. 2006 Jul-Aug;21(4):263-8. PMID: 16862349. doi:http://dx.doi.org/10.1590/S0102-86502006000400014.

64. Hartley J. Current findings from research on structured abstracts. J Med Libr Assoc. 2004 Jul-Aug;92(3):368-71. PMID: 15243644. PMCID: PMC442180.

65. Harris AH, Standard S, Brunning JL, Casey SL, Goldberg JH, Oliver L, Ito K, Marshall JM. The accuracy of abstracts in psychology journals. J Psychol. 2002 Mar;136(2):141-8. PMID: 12081089. doi:10.1080/00223980209604145.

66. Pitkin RM, Branagan MA, Burmeister LF. Accuracy of data in abstracts of published research articles. JAMA. 1999 Mar 24-31;281(12):1110-1. PMID: 10188662. doi:10.1001/jama.281.12.1110.

67. Ward LG, Kendrach MG, Price SO. Accuracy of abstracts for original research articles in pharmacy journals. Ann Pharmacother. 2004 Jul-Aug;38(7-8):1173-7. PMID: 15150375. doi:10.1345/aph.1D416.

68. Prasad S, Lee DJ, Yuan JC, Barao VA, Shyamsunder N, Sukotjo C. Discrepancies between abstracts presented at International Association for Dental Research annual sessions from 2004 to 2005 and full-text publication. Int J Dent. 2012;2012:859561. Epub 2012 Feb 22. PMID: 22505912. PMCID: PMC3296196. doi:10.1155/2012/859561.

69. Cuddy PG, Elenbaas RM, Elenbaas JK. Evaluating the medical literature. Part I: abstract, introduction, methods. Ann Emerg Med. 1983 Sept;12(9):549-55. PMID: 6614609. doi:10.1016/S0196-0644(83)80296-0.

70. Cannon CP, Blazing MA, Giugliano RP, McCagg A, White JA, Theroux P, Darius H, Lewis BS, Ophuis TO, Jukema JW, De Ferrari GM, Ruzyllo W, De Lucca P, Im K, Bohula EA, Reist C, Wiviott SD, Tershakovec AM, Musliner TA, Braunwald E, Califf RM; IMPROVE-IT Investigators. Ezetimibe added to statin therapy after acute coronary syndromes. N Engl J Med. 2015 Jun 18;372(25):2387-97. Epub 2015 Jun 3. PMID: 26039521. doi:10.1056/NEJMoa1410489.

71. Veith FJ. How randomized controlled trials (RCTs) can be misleading: introduction. Semin Vasc Surg. 2011 Sep;24(3):143-5. PMID: 22153022. doi:10.1053/j.semvascsurg.2011.10.001.

72. Hulley SB, Cummings SR, Browner WS, Grady DG, Newman TB. Designing clinical research. 4th ed. Philadelphia, PA: Lippincott Williams & Wilkins; 2013.

73. Goldberg RJ, McManus DD, Allison J. Greater knowledge and appreciation of commonly-used research study designs. Am J Med. 2013 Feb;126(2):169.e1-8.

74. Kastelein JJ, Akdim F, Stroes ES, Zwinderman AH, Bots ML, Stalenhoef AF, Visseren FL, Sijbrands EJ, Trip MD, Stein EA, Gaudet D, Duivenvoorden R, Veltri EP, Marais AD, de Groot E; ENHANCE Investigators. Simvastatin with or without ezetimibe in familial hypercholesterolemia. N Engl J Med. 2008 Apr 3;358(14):1431-43. doi:10.1056/NEJMoa0800742.

75. Karalis DG, Ross AM, Vacari RM, Zarren H, Scott R. Comparison of efficacy and safety of atorvastatin and simvastatin in patients with dyslipidemia with and without coronary heart disease. Am J Cardiol. 2002 Mar 15;89(6):667-71.

76. Sessler DI, Imrey PB. Clinical research methodology 3: randomized controlled trials. Anesth Analg. 2015 Oct;121(4):1052-64. doi:10.1213/ANE.0000000000000862.

77. Tripepi G, Jager KJ, Dekker FW, Zoccali C. Selection bias and information bias in clinical research. Nephron Clin Pract. 2010;115(2):c94-9.

78. Naylor CD, Guyatt GH, Bass E, Gerstein H, Heyland D, Holbrook A, Moyer V, Newman T, Oxman A, Richardson WS, Tugwell P, Williams J. Users' guides to the medical literature. X. How to use an article reporting variations in the outcomes of health services. The Evidence-Based Medicine Working Group. JAMA. 1996 Feb 21;275(7):554-8. PMID: 8606478. doi:10.1001/jama.1996.03530310060034.

79. Berger VW, Rezvani A, Makarewicz VA. Direct effect on validity of response run-in selection in clinical trials. Control Clin Trials. 2003 Apr;24(2):156-66. PMID: 12689737. doi:10.1016/S0197-2456(02)00316-1.

80. Siddiqi AE, Sikorskii A, Given CW, Given B. Early participant attrition from clinical trials: role of trial design and logistics. Clin Trials. 2008;5(4):328-35. PMID: 18697847. PMCID: PMC2723836. doi:10.1177/1740774508094406.

81. Chan FK, Ching JY, Hung LC, Wong VW, Leung VK, Kung NN, Hui AJ, Wu JC, Leung WK, Lee VW, Lee KK, Lee YT, Lau JY, To KF, Chan HL, Chung SC, Sung JJ. Clopidogrel versus aspirin and esomeprazole to prevent recurrent ulcer bleeding. N Engl J Med. 2005 Jan 20;352(3):238-44. PMID: 15659723. doi:10.1056/NEJMoa042087.

82. Department of Health and Human Services. Recruiting human subjects. Pressures in industry-sponsored clinical research [Internet]. Washington, DC: Department of Health and Human Services; [updated 2000 Jun; cited 2013 Jun 24]. Available from: http://oig.hhs.gov/oei/reports/oei-01-97-00195.pdf

83. Hebert R. Newspaper advertising could distort research results. Nicotine Tob Res. 2000 Nov;2(4):317-8. PMID: 11197310. doi:10.1080/713688156.

84. Sankaré IC, Bross R, Brown AF, Del Pino HE, Jones LF, Morris DM, Porter C, Lucas-Wright A, Vargas R, Forge N, Norris KC, Kahn KL. Strategies to build trust and recruit African American and Latino community residents for health research: a cohort study. Clin Transl Sci. 2015 Oct;8(5):412-20. doi:10.1111/cts.12273.

85. Wei SJ, Metz JM, Coyle C, Hampshire M, Jones HA, Markowitz S, Rustqi AK. Recruitment of patients into an Internet-based clinical trials database: the experience of OncoLink and the National Colorectal Cancer Research Alliance. J Clin Oncol. 2004 Dec 1;22(23):4730-6. PMID: 15570073. doi:10.1200/JCO.2004.07.103.

86. Refolo P, Sacchini D, Minacori R, Daloiso V, Spagnolo AG. E-recruitment based clinical research: notes for Research Ethics Committees/Institutional Review Boards. Eur Rev Med Pharmacol Sci. 2015;19(5):800-4.

87. Maiti R. Clinical trials in India. Pharmacol Res. 2007 Jul;56(1):1-10. PMID: 17391981. doi:10.1016/j.phrs.2007.02.004.

88. Nicholas J. Outsourcing clinical trials. J Natl Cancer Inst. 2012 Jul 18;104(14):1043-5. PMID: 22781429. doi:10.1093/jnci/djs323.

89. Guyatt GH, Sackett DL, Cook DJ. Users' guides to the medical literature. II. How to use an article about therapy or prevention. A. Are the results of the study valid? Evidence-Based Medicine Working Group. JAMA. 1993 Dec 1;270(21):2598-601. PMID: 8230645. doi:10.1001/jama.1993.03510210084032.

90. Julious SA. Sample sizes for clinical trials with normal data. Stat Med. 2004 Jun 30;23(12):1921-86. PMID: 15195324. doi:10.1002/sim.1783.

91. Vickers AJ, de Craen AJ. Why use placebos in clinical trials? A narrative review of the methodological literature. J Clin Epidemiol. 2000 Feb;53(2):157-61. PMID: 10729687. doi:http://dx.doi.org/10.1016/S0895-4356(99)00139-0.

92. Yeh SS, DeGuzman B, Kramer T; M012 Study Group. Reversal of COPD-associated weight loss using the anabolic agent oxandrolone. Chest. 2002 Aug;122(2):421-8. PMID: 12171812. doi:http://dx.doi.org/10.1378/chest.122.2.421.

93. Baker SG, Lindeman KS. Rethinking historical controls. Biostatistics. 2001 Dec;2(4):383-96. PMID: 12933631. doi:10.1093/biostatistics/2.4.383.

94. Brodie MJ. Novel trial designs for monotherapy. Epileptic Disord. 2012 Jun;14(2):132-7. PMID: 22977899. doi:10.1684/epd.2012.0513.

95. Randomised trial of cholesterol lowering in 4444 patients with coronary heart disease: the Scandinavian Simvastatin Survival Study (4S). Lancet. 1994 Nov 19;344(8934):1383-9. PMID: 7968073. doi:10.1016/S0140-6736(94)90566-5.

96. Simons LA, Nestel PJ, Calvert GD, Jennings GL. Effects of MK-733 on plasma lipid and lipoprotein levels in subjects with hypercholesterolaemia. Med J Aust. 1987 Jul 20;147(2):65-8. PMID: 3299016.

97. Avenell A, Grant AM, McGee M, McPherson G, Campbell MK, McGee MA; RECORD Trial Management Group. The effects of an open design on trial participant recruitment, adherence, and retention—a randomized controlled trial comparison with a blinded, placebo-controlled design. Clin Trials. 2004;1(6):490-8. PMID: 16279289. doi:10.1191/1740774504cn053oa.

98. Tramer MR, Reynolds DJ, Moore RA, McQuay HJ. When placebo controlled trials are essential and equivalence trials are inadequate. BMJ. 1998 Sep 26;317(7162):875-80. PMID: 9748192. PMCID: PMC1113953. doi:http://dx.doi.org/10.1136/bmj.317.7162.875.

99. Montori VM, Jaeschke R, Schunemann HJ, Bhandari M, Brozek JL, Devereaux PJ, Guyatt GH. Users' guide to detecting misleading claims in clinical research reports. BMJ. 2004 Nov 6;329(7474):1093-6. PMID: 15528623. PMCID: PMC526126. doi:10.1136/bmj.329.7474.1093.

100. Gluud LL. Bias in clinical intervention research. Am J Epidemiol. 2006 Mar 15;163(6):493-50. PMID: 16443796. doi:10.1093/aje/kwj069.

101. Davidson M, Ma P, Stein EA, Gotto AM Jr, Raza A, Chitra R, Hutchinson H. Comparison of effects on low-density lipoprotein cholesterol and high-density lipoprotein cholesterol

with rosuvastatin versus atorvastatin in patients with Type IIa or IIb hypercholester-olemia. Am J Cardiol. 2002 Feb 1;89(3):268-75. PMID: 11809427. doi:http://dx.doi.org/10.1016/S0002-9149(01)02226-3.

102. Kendrach MG, Kelly-Freeman M. Approximate equivalent rosuvastatin doses for tem-porary statin interchange programs. Ann Pharmacother. 2004 Jul-Aug;38(7-8):1286-92. PMID: 15187217. doi:10.1345/aph.1D391.

103. Schwenzer KJ. Practical tips for working effectively with your Institutional Review Board. Respir Care. 2008 Oct;53(10):1354-61. PMID: 18812000.

104. Enfield KB, Truwit JD. The purpose, composition, and function of an Institutional Review Board: balancing priorities. Respir Care. 2008 Oct;53(10):1330-6. PMID: 18811996.

105. Schwenzer KJ. Protecting vulnerable subjects in clinical research: children, pregnant women, prisoners, and employees. Respir Care. 2008 Oct;53(10):1342-9. PMID: 18811998.

106. Montori A, Onorato M. Why there is a need of an ethics committee in scientific medical societies. Dig Dis. 2008;26(1):32-5. PMID: 18600012. doi:10.1159/000109383.

107. Lema VM, Mbondo M, Kamau EM. Informed consent for clinical trials: a review. East Afr Med J. 2009 Mar;86(3):133-42. PMID: 19702101. doi:http://dx.doi.org/10.4314/eamj.v86i3.54968.

108. Freeman SR, Lundahl K, Schilling LM, Jensen JD, Dellavalle RP. Human research review committee requirements in medical journals. Clin Invest Med. 2008;31(1):E49-54. PMID: 18312748.

109. Byerly WG. Working with the Institutional Review Board. Am J Health Syst Pharm. 2009 Jan 15;66(2):176-84. PMID: 19139484. doi:10.2146/ajhp070066.

110. Mertl SL. The fundamentals of Institutional Review Board operations. J Pharm Pract. 1996;IX:437-43. doi:10.1177/089719009600900060.

111. Macklin R. The ethical problems with sham surgery in clinical research. N Engl J Med. 1999 Sep 23;341(13):992-6. PMID: 10498498. doi:10.1056/NEJM199909233411312.

112. Horng S, Miller FG. Is placebo surgery unethical? N Engl J Med. 2002 Jul 11;347(2):137-9. PMID: 12110744. doi:10.1056/NEJMsb021025.

113. Dumville JC, Hahn S, Miles JN, Torgerson DJ. The use of unequal randomisation ratios in clinical trials: a review. Contemp Clin Trials. 2006 Feb;27(1):1-12. Epub 2005 Oct 19. Review. PMID: 16236557.

114. Egbewale BE. Random allocation in controlled clinical trials: a review. J Pharm Pharm Sci. 2014;17(2):248-53.

115. Guyatt G, Rennie D, Meade MO, Cook DJ. User's guide to the medical literature. A manual for evidence-based clinical practice. 2nd ed. Columbus, OH: McGraw-Hill; 2008.

116. Collins R, MacMahon S. Reliable assessment of the effects of treatment on mortality and major morbidity, I: clinical trials. Lancet. 2001 Feb 3;357(9253):373-80. PMID: 11211013. doi:10.1016/S0140-6736(00)03651-5.

117. Roberts C, Torgerson D. Randomisation methods in controlled trials. BMJ. 1998 Nov 7;317(7168):1301. PMID: 9804722. PMCID: PMC1114206.

118. Kim J, Shin W. How to do random allocation (randomization). Clin Orthop Surg. 2014;6(1):103-9. doi:10.4055/cios.2014.6.1.103.

119. Dibao-Dina C, Caille A, Sautenet B, Chazelle E, Giraudeau B. Rationale for unequal randomization in clinical trials is rarely reported: a systematic review. J Clin Epidemiol. 2014 Oct;67(10):1070-5. doi:10.1016/j.jclinepi.2014.05.015.

120. Dumville JC, Hahn S, Miles JN, Torgerson DJ. The use of unequal randomisation ratios in clinical trials: a review. Contemp Clin Trials. 2006 Feb;27(1):1-12.

121. Slobogean GP, Sprague S, Bhandari M. The tactics of large randomized trials. J Bone Joint Surg Am. 2012 Jul 18;94(Suppl 1):19-23.

122. Pitt B, Segal R, Martinez FA, Meurers G, Cowley AJ, Thomas I, Deedwania PC, Ney DE, Snavely DB, Change PI. Randomised trial of losartan versus captopril in patients over 65 with heart failure (Evaluation of Losartan in the Elderly Study, ELITE). Lancet. 1997 Mar 15;349(9054):747-52.

123. Freemantle N, Calvert M, Wood J, Eastaugh J, Griffin C. Composite outcomes in randomized trials: greater precision but with greater uncertainty? JAMA. 2003 May 21;289(19):2554-9.

124. Lubsen J, Kirwan BA. Combined endpoints: can we use them? Stat Med. 2002 Oct 15;21(19):2959-70. PMID: 12325112. doi:10.1002/sim.1300.

125. Bakal JA, Westerhout CM, Armstrong PW. Impact of weighted composite compared to traditional composite endpoints for the design of randomized controlled trials. Stat Methods Med Res. 2012 Jan 24. [Epub ahead of print]. 2015 Dec;24(6):980-8. PMID: 22275378. doi:10.1177/0962280211436004.

126. Kaul S, Diamond GA. Trial and error: how to avoid commonly encountered limitations of published clinical trials. J Am Coll Cardiol. 2010;55(5):415-27. PMID: 20117454. doi:10.1016/j.jacc.2009.06.065.

127. Cohen M, Demers C, Gurfinkel EP, Turpie AG, Fromell GJ, Goodman S, Langer A, Califf RM, Fox KA, Premmereur J, Bigonzi F. A comparison of low-molecular-weight heparin with unfractionated heparin for unstable coronary artery disease. Efficacy and safety of subcutaneous enoxaparin in Non-Q-Wave Coronary Events Study Group. N Engl J Med. 1997 Aug 14;337(7):447-52. PMID: 9250846. doi:10.1056/NEJM199708143370702.

128. Armstrong PW. Heparin in acute coronary disease—requiem for a heavyweight? N Engl J Med. 1997 Aug 14;337(7):492-4. PMID: 9250854. doi:10.1056/NEJM199708143370710.

129. Ohman EM. Enoxaparin reduced combined coronary events in unstable angina and non-Q-wave MI at 14 and 30 days [Comment]. ACP J Club. 1998;128:34. doi:10.7326/ACPJC-1998-128-2-034.

130. U.S. Department of Health and Human Services. Guidance for clinical trial sponsors. [cited 2017 Mar 13]. Available from: https://www.fda.gov/downloads/RegulatoryInformation/Guidances/ucm127073.pdf

131. Expert panel on detection, evaluation, and treatment of high blood cholesterol in adults. Executive summary of the third report of the National Cholesterol Education Program (NCEP) expert panel on detection, evaluation, and treatment of high blood cholesterol in adults (Adult Treatment Panel III). JAMA. 2001 May 16;285(19):2486-97. PMID: 11368702. doi:10.1001/jama.285.19.2486.

132. Frandsen CS, Dejgaard TF, Holst JJ, Andersen HU, Thorsteinsson B, Madsbad S. Twelve-week treatment with liraglutide as add-on to insulin in normal-weight patients with poorly

controlled type 1 diabetes: a randomized, placebo-controlled, double-blind parallel study. Diabetes Care. 2015 Dec;38(12):2250-7. Epub 2015 Oct 20. PMID: 26486191. doi:10.2337/dc15-1037.

133. American Diabetes Association. Standards of medical care in diabetes—2017. Diabetes Care. 2017;40(1):S1.

134. Lader EW, Cannon CP, Ohman EM, Newby LK, Sulmasy DP, Barst RJ, Fair JM, Flather M, Freedman JE, Frye RL, Hand MM, Jesse RL, Van de Werf F, Costa F; American Heart Association. The clinician as investigator: participating in clinical trials in the practice setting: Appendix 2: statistical concepts in study design and analysis. Circulation. 2004 Jun;109:2672-9. PMID: 15173053. doi:http://dx.doi.org/10.1161/01.CIR.0000128702.16441.75.

135. Whitley E, Ball J. Statistics review 4: sample size calculations. Crit Care. 2002 Aug;6(4):335-41. PMID: 12225610. PMCID: PMC137461.

136. Cannon CP, Blazing MA, Giugliano RP, McCagg A, White JA, Theroux P, Darius H, Lewis BS, Ophuis TO, Jukema JW, De Ferrari GM, Ruzyllo W, De Lucca P, Im K, Bohula EA, Reist C, Wiviott SD, Tershakovec AM, Musliner TA, Braunwald E, Califf RM; IMPROVE-IT Investigators. Ezetimibe added to statin therapy after acute coronary syndromes. N Engl J Med. 2015;372:2387-97. doi:10.1056/NEJMoa1410489.

137. Guller U, DeLong ER. Interpreting statistics in medical literature: a vade mecum for surgeons. J Am Coll Surg. 2004 Mar;198(3):441-58. PMID: 14992748. doi:10.1016/j.jamcollsurg.2003.09.017.

138. Tumlin JA, Wang A, Murray PT, Mathur VS. Fenoldopam mesylate blocks reductions in renal plasma flow after radiocontrast dye infusion: a pilot trial in the prevention of contrast nephropathy. Am Heart J. 2002 May;143(5):894-903. PMID: 12040355. doi:http://dx.doi.org/10.1067/mhj.2002.122118.

139. Stone GW, McCullough PA, Tumlin JA, Lepor NE, Madyoon H, Murray P, Wang A, Chu AA, Schaer GL, Stevens M, Wilensky RL, O'Neill WW; CONTRAST Investigators. Fenoldopam mesylate for the prevention of contrast-induced nephropathy: a randomized controlled trial. JAMA. 2003 Nov 5;290(17):2284-91. PMID: 14600187. doi:10.1001/jama.290.17.2284.

140. Altman DG, Goodman SN, Schroter S. How statistical expertise is used in medical research. JAMA. 2002 Jun 5;287(21):2817-20. PMID: 12038922. doi:10.1001/jama.287.21.2817.

141. Chan AW, Tetzlaff JM, Gøtzsche PC, Altman DG, Mann H, Berlin JA, Dickersin K, Hróbjartsson A, Schulz KF, Parulekar WR, Krleza-Jeric K, Laupacis A, Moher D. SPIRIT 2013 explanation and elaboration: guidance for protocols of clinical trials. BMJ. 2013 Jan 8;346:e7586. PMID: 23303884. PMCID: PMC3541470. doi:10.1136/bmj.e7586.

142. Guyatt G, Jaeschke R, Heddle N, Cook D, Shannon H, Walter S. Basic statistics for clinicians: 1. Hypothesis testing. CMAJ. 1995 Jan 1;152(1):27-32. PMID: 7804919. PMCID: PMC1337490.

143. Whitley E, Ball J. Statistics review 3: hypothesis testing and P values. Crit Care. 2002 Jun;6(3):222-5. PMC137449. doi:10.1186/cc1493.

144. DeMuth JE. Overview of biostatistics used in clinical research. Am J Health Syst Pharm. 2009 Jan 1;66(1):70-81. PMID: 19106347. doi:10.2146/ajhp070006.

145. Salkind NJ. Statistics for people who (think they) hate statistics. Thousand Oaks, CA: Sage; 2000.

146. Whitley E, Ball J. Statistics review 2: samples and populations. Crit Care. 2002 Apr;6(2):143-8. PMCID: PMC137296. doi:10.1186/cc1473.

147. Tu YK, Gilthorpe MS. Key statistical and analytical issues for evaluating treatment effects in periodontal research. Periodontol 2000. 2012 Jun;59(1):75-88. PMID: 22507061. doi:10.1111/j.1600-0757.2011.00431.x.

148. Evans RB, O'Connor A. Statistics and evidence-based veterinary medicine: answers to 21 common statistical questions that arise from reading scientific manuscripts. Vet Clin North Am Small Anim Pract. 2007 May;37(3):477-86. PMID: 17466751. doi:10.1016/j.cvsm.2007.01.006.

149. Glantz SA. Primer of biostatistics. 5th ed. New York, NY: McGraw-Hill; 2002.

150. Lee CM, Soin HK, Einarson TR. Statistics in the pharmacy literature. Ann Pharmacother. 2004 Sep;38(9):1412-8. PMID: 15199191. doi:10.1345/aph.1D493.

151. Swinscow TDV. Statistics at square one. London: British Medical Association; 1983.

152. Kirby A, Gebski V, Keech AC. Determining the sample size in a clinical trial. Med J Aust. 2002 Sep 2;177(5):256-7. PMID: 12197821. doi:10.1.1.156.8676.

153. Elenbaas JK, Cuddy PG, Elenbaas RM. Evaluating the medical literature, Part III: results and discussion. Ann Emerg Med. 1983 Nov;12(11):679-86. PMID: 6356998. doi:10.1016/S0196-0644(83)80416-8.

154. DeMets DL. Statistical issues in interpreting clinical trials. J Intern Med. 2004 May;255(5):529-37. PMID: 15078496. doi:10.1111/j.1365-2796.2004.01320.x.

155. White IR, Carpenter J, Horton NJ. Including all individuals is not enough: lessons for intention-to-treat analysis. Clin Trials. 2012 Aug;9(4):396-407. PMID: 22752633. PMCID: PMC3428470. doi:10.1177/1740774512450098.

156. Le Bars PL, Katz MM, Berman N, Itil TM, Freedman AM, Schatzberg AF. A placebo-controlled, double-blind, randomized trial of an extract of *Ginkgo biloba* for dementia. North American EGb Study Group. JAMA. 1997 Oct 22-29;278(16):1327-32. PMID: 9343463. doi:10.1001/jama.1997.03550160047037.

157. Postuma RB, Lang AE, Munhoz RP, Charland K, Pelletier A, Moscovich M, Filla L, Zanatta D, Rios Romenets S, Altman R, Chuang R, Shah B. Caffeine for treatment of Parkinson disease: a randomized controlled trial. Neurology. 2012 Aug 14;79(7):651-8. PMID: 22855866. PMCID: PMC3414662. doi:10.1212/WNL.0b013e318263570d.

158. Bucher HC, Guyatt GH, Cook DJ, Holbrook A, McAlister FA. Users' guides to the medical literature: XIX. Applying clinical trial results. A. How to use an article measuring the effect of an intervention on surrogate end points. Evidence-Based Medicine Working Group. JAMA. 1999 Aug 25;282(8):771-8. PMID: 10463714. doi:10.1001/jama.282.8.771.

159. Weihrauch TR, Demol P. Value of surrogate endpoints for evaluation of therapeutic efficacy. Drug Inf J. 1998;32(3):737-43. doi:10.1177/009286159803200313.

160. Barter PJ, Caulfield M, Eriksson M, Grundy SM, Kastelein JJ, Komajda M, Lopez-Sendon J, Mosca L, Tardif JC, Waters DD, Shear CL, Revkin JH, Buhr KA, Fisher MR, Tall AR,

Brewer B, for the ILLUMINATE Investigators. Effects of torcetrapib in patients at high risk for coronary events. N Engl J Med. 2007 Nov 22;357(21):2109-22. PMID: 17984165. doi:10.1056/NEJMoa0706628.

161. Cook DI, Gebski VJ, Keech AC. Subgroup analysis in clinical trials. Med J Aust. 2004 Mar 15;180(6):289-91. PMID: 15012568.

162. Ghert M, Petrisor B. Subgroup analyses: when should we believe them? J Bone Joint Surg Am. 2012 Jul 18;94(Suppl 1):61-4. PMID: 22810450. doi:10.2106/JBJS.L.00272.

163. Sun X, Briel M, Busse JW, You JJ, Akl EA, Mejza F, Bala MM, Bassler D, Metz D, Diaz-Granados N, Vandvik PO, Malaga G, Srinathan SK, Dahm P, Johnston BC, Alonso-Coello P, Hassouneh B, Walter SD Heels-Ansdell D, Bhatnagar N, Altman DG, Guyatt GH. Credibility of claims of subgroup effects in randomised controlled trials: systematic review. BMJ. 2012 Mar 15;344:e1553. PMID: 22422832. doi:http://dx.doi.org/10.1136/bmj.e1553.

164. Gorelick PB, Richardson D, Kelly M, Ruland S, Hung E, Harris Y, Kittner S, Leurgans S; African American Antiplatelet Stroke Prevention Study Investigators. Aspirin and ticlopidine for prevention of recurrent stroke in black patients: a randomized trial. JAMA. 2003 Jun 11;289(22):2947-57. PMID: 12799402. doi:10.1001/jama.289.22.2947.

165. Hass WK, Easton JD, Adams HP Jr, Pryse-Phillips W, Molony BA, Anderson S, Kamm B. A randomized trial comparing ticlopidine hydrochloride with aspirin for the prevention of stroke in high-risk patients. Ticlopidine Aspirin Stroke Study Group. N Engl J Med. 1989 Aug 24;321(8):501-7. PMID: 2761587. doi:10.1056/NEJM198908243210804.

166. Lu T, Sheng H, Wu J, Cheng Y, Zhu J, Chen Y. Cinnamon extract improves fasting blood glucose and glycosylated hemoglobin level in Chinese patients with type 2 diabetes. Nutr Res. 2012 Jun;32(6):408-12. PMID: 22749176. doi:10.1016/j.nutres.2012.05.003.

167. Rothwell PM. External validity of randomised controlled trials: "to whom do the results of this trial apply?" Lancet. 2005 Jan 1-7;365(9453):82-93. PMID: 15639683. doi:10.1016/S0140-6736(04)17670-8.

168. Clarke M, Alderson P, Chalmers I. Discussion sections in reports of controlled trials published in general medical journals. JAMA. 2002 Jun 5;287(21):2799-801. PMID: 12038916. doi:10.1001/jama.287.21.2799.

169. Anderson G, Kendrach MG, Trice S. Basic biostatistics and hypothesis testing. J Pharm Pract. 1998 Jun;XI(3):181-95. doi:10.1177/089719009801100309.

170. Pocock SJ, Ware JH. Translating statistical findings into plain English. Lancet. 2009 Jun 6;373(9679):1926-8. PMID: 19375158. doi:10.1016/S0140-6736(09)60499-2.

171. Castell DO, Kahrilas PJ, Richter JE, Vakil NB, Johnson DA, Zuckerman S, Skammer W, Levine JG. Esomeprazole (40 mg) compared with lansoprazole (30 mg) in the treatment of erosive esophagitis. Am J Gastroenterol. 2002 Mar;97(3):575-83. PMID: 11922549. doi:10.1111/j.1572-0241.2002.05532.x.

172. Whelton A, Fort JG, Puma JA, Normandin D, Bello AE, Verburg KM. Cyclooxygenase-2-specific inhibitors and cardiorenal function: a randomized, controlled trial of celecoxib and rofecoxib in older hypertensive osteoarthritis patients. Am J Ther. 2001 Mar-Apr;8(2):85-95. PMID: 11304662.

173. Ranstam J. Why the P-value culture is bad and confidence intervals a better alternative. Osteoarthr Cartil. 2012 Aug;20(8):805-8. PMID: 22503814. doi:10.1016/j.joca.2012.04.001.
174. Guyatt G, Jaeschke R, Heddle N, Cook D, Shannon H, Walter S. Basic statistics for clinicians: 2. Interpreting study results: confidence intervals. CMAJ. 1995 Jan 15;152(2):169-73. PMID: 7820798. PMCID: PMC1337571.
175. Guyatt GH, Sackett DL, Cook DJ. Users' guides to the medical literature. II. How to use an article about therapy or prevention. B. What were the results and will they help me in caring for my patients? Evidence-Based Medicine Working Group. JAMA. 1994 Jan 5;271(1):59-63. PMID: 8258890. doi:10.1001/jama.1994.03510250075039.
176. Jaeschke R, Guyatt G, Shannon H, Walter S, Cook D, Heddle N. Basic statistics for clinicians: 3. Assessing the effects of treatment: measures of association. CMAJ. 1995 Feb 1;152(3):351-57. PMID: 7828099. PMCID: PMC1337533.
177. Colhoun HM, Betteridge DJ, Durrington PN, Hitman GA, Neil HA, Livingstone SJ, Thomason MJ, Mackness MI, Charlton-Menys V, Fuller JH, on behalf of the CARDS investigators. Primary prevention of cardiovascular disease with atorvastatin in type 2 diabetes in the Collaborative Atorvastatin Diabetes Study (CARDS): multicentre randomised placebo-controlled trial. Lancet. 2004 Aug 21-27;364(9435):685-96. PMID: 15325833. doi:10.1016/S0140-6736(04)16895-5.
178. Kendrach MG, Covington TR, McCarthy MW, Harris CM. Calculating risks and number-needed-to-treat: a method of data interpretation. J Managed Care Pharm. 1997 Mar/Apr;3(2):179-83. doi:http://dx.doi.org/10.18553/jmcp.1997.3.2.179.
179. Feinstein AR. Principles of medical statistics. Boca Raton, FL: Chapman & Hall/CRC Press; 2002.
180. Chobanian AV, Bakris GL, Black HR, Cushman WC, Green LA, Izzo JL Jr, Jones DW, Materson BJ, Oparil S, Wright JT Jr, Roccella EJ; National Heart, Lung, and Blood Institute Joint National Committee on Prevention, Detection, Evaluation, and Treatment of High Blood Pressure; National High Blood Pressure Education Program Coordinating Committee. The seventh report of the Joint National Committee on Prevention, Detection, Evaluation, and Treatment of High Blood Pressure: the JNC 7 report. JAMA. 2003 May 21;289(19):2560-72. PMID: 12748199. doi:10.1001/jama.289.19.2560.
181. Castell DO, Richter JE, Robinson M, Sontag SJ, Haber MM. Efficacy and safety of lansoprazole in the treatment of erosive reflux esophagitis. The Lansoprazole Group. Am J Gastroenterol. 1996 Sep;91(9):1749-57. PMID: 8792693.
182. Advice for travelers. Treat Guidel Med Lett. 2012 Jun;10(118):45-56. PMID: 22777212.
183. DuPont HL, Sullivan P, Evans DG, Pickering LK, Evans DJ Jr, Vollet JJ, Ericsson CD, Ackerman PB, Tjoa WS. Prevention of traveler's diarrhea (emporiatric enteritis). Prophylactic administration of subsalicylate bismuth. JAMA. 1980 Jan 18;243(3):237-41. PMID: 6985681. doi:10.1001/jama.1980.03300290019013.
184. Mosdell KW. Chapter 6: Literature evaluation I: controlled clinical trials. In: Malone PM, Mosdell KW, Kier KL, Stanovich JE, editors. Drug information: a guide for practitioners. 2nd ed. New York, NY: McGraw-Hill; 2001:160.

185. Patrias K. Chapter 22: Books and other individual titles on the Internet. In: Wendling DL, technical editor. Citing medicine: the NLM style guide for authors, editors, and publishers [Internet]. 2nd ed. Bethesda, MD: National Library of Medicine; 2007 [updated 2011 Aug 11; cited 2016 Jul 20]. Available from: http://nlm.nih.gov/citingmedicine

186. Alhamoud HA, Dudum R, Young HA, Choi BG. Author self-disclosure compared with pharmaceutical company reporting of physician payments. Am J Med. 2016;129:59-63. Available from: http://dx.doi.org/10.1016/j.amjmed.2015.06.028

187. Pharmaceutical Research and Manufacturers of America. 2016 Biopharmaceutical Research Pharmaceutical Industry Profile 2016 [Internet]. Washington, DC: Pharmaceutical Research and Manufacturers of America; [updated July2016; cited 2016 Sept 1]. Available from: http://phrma.org/sites/default/files/pdf/biopharmaceutical-industry-profile.pdf

188. Thompson DF. Understanding financial conflicts of interest. N Engl J Med. 1993 Aug 19;329(8):573-6. PMID: 8336759. doi:10.1056/NEJM199308193290812.

189. Wynia M, Boren D. Better regulation of industry-sponsored clinical trials is long overdue. J Law Med Ethics. 2009 Fall;37(3):410-9, 395. PMID: 19723252. doi:10.1111/j.1748-720X.2009.00402.x.

190. National Institutes of Health. Responsibility of applicants for promoting objectivity in research for which PHS funding is sought. Available from: http://grants.nih.gov/grants/policy/coi/coi_faqs.htm. Accessed November 2, 2016.

191. International Committee of Medical Journal Editors. ICMJE form for disclosure of potential conflicts of interest resource page. [cited 2013 Mar 7]. Available from: http://www.icmje.org/coi_disclosure.pdf. Accessed September 1, 2016.

192. Lievre M, Menard J, Bruckert E, Cogneau J, Delahaye F, Giral P, Leitersdorf E, Luc G, Masana L, Moulin P, Passa P, Pouchain D, Siest G. Premature discontinuation of clinical trial for reasons not related to efficacy, safety, or feasibility. BMJ. 2001 Mar 10;322(7286):603-5. PMID: 11238162. PMCID: PMC1119794. doi:http://dx.doi.org/10.1136/bmj.322.7286.603.

193. Gotzsche PC, Johansen HK. Meta-analysis of prophylactic or empirical antifungal treatment versus placebo or no treatment in patients with cancer complicated by neutropenia. BMJ. 1997 Apr 26;314(7089):1238-44. PMID: 9154027. PMCID: PMC2126615. doi:http://dx.doi.org/10.1136/bmj.314.7089.1238.

194. Rochon PA, Berger PB, Gordon M. The evolution of clinical trials: inclusion and representation. CMAJ. 1998 Dec 1;159(11):1373-4. PMID: 9861206. PMCID: PMC1229855.

195. Blumenthal D, Campbell EG, Anderson MS, Causino N, Louis KS. Withholding research results in academic life science. Evidence from a national survey of faculty. JAMA. 1997 Apr 16;277(15):1224-8. PMID: 9103347. doi:10.1001/jama.1997.03540390054035.

196. Als-Nielsen B, Chen W, Gluud C, Kjaergard LL. Association of funding and conclusions in randomized drug trials: a reflection of treatment effect or adverse events? JAMA. 2003 Aug 20;290(7):921-8. PMID: 12928469. doi:10.1001/jama.290.7.921.

197. U.S. National Institutes of Health [Internet]. Washington, DC: ClinicalTrials.gov website page. [cited 2013 Jun 27]. Available from: http://www.clinicaltrials.gov/. Accessed September 1, 2016.

198. U.S. National Institutes of Health [Internet]. Washington, DC: FDAAA 801 Requirements Web page [Internet] [reviewed 2012 Dec; cited 2013 Jun 27]. Available from: http://www.clinicaltrials.gov/ct2/manage-recs/fdaaa. Accessed October 26, 2016.

199. Jarcho JA, Keaney JF Jr. Proof that lower is better-LDL cholesterol and IMPROVE-IT. N Engl J Med. 2015;372:2448-50.

200. Sage Publications. Thousands Oak, CA. Annals of Pharmacotherapy journal website. Manuscript Guidelines Web page. [cited 2013 Oct 4]. Available from: http://www.sage-pub.com/journals/Journal202238/title#tabview=manuscriptSubmission.www.theannals.com/site/misc/Guidelines_Com.pdf. Accessed October 27, 2016.

201. Devereaux PJ, Manns BJ, Ghali WA, Quan H, Guyatt GH. Reviewing the reviewers: the quality of reporting in three secondary journals. CMAJ. 2001 May 29;164(11):1573-6. PMID: 11402795. PMCID: PMC81111.

202. ACP Journal Club. ACP Journal Club [Internet]. [cited 2013 Oct 4]. Available from: http://annals.org/aim/pages/acpjc-purpose-and-procedure. Accessed October 26, 2016.

203. NEJM Journal Watch subscription Web page [Internet]. [cited 2016 Oct 26]. Subscribe to Journal Watch Newsletters. Available from: https://secure.jwatch.org/subscribem?cpc=SMAAALLV0513A&promo=OJFLSB21&prc=OJFLSB21&step=0. Accessed October 26, 2016.

204. American Journal of Health-System Pharmacy website. Columns of AJHP [Internet]. [cited 2013 Oct 4]. Available from: http://www.ajhp.org/sites/default/files/assets/AJHP%20PDF%20FILES/AJHP_Sections_Columns.pdf. Accessed October 26, 2016.

205. Thursz MR, Richardson P, Allison M, Austin A, Bowers M, Day CP, Downs N, Gleeson D, MacGilchrist A, Grant A, Hood S, Masson S, McCune A, Mellor J, O'Grady J, Patch D, Ratcliffe I, Roderick P, Stanton L, Vergis N, Wright M, Ryder S, Forrest EH; STOPAH Trial. Prednisolone or pentoxifylline for alcoholic hepatitis. N Engl J Med. 2015 Apr 23;372(17):1619-28. doi:10.1056/NEJMoa1412278.

SUGGESTED READINGS

1. Schulz KF, Altman DG, Moher D; CONSORT Group. CONSORT 2010 statement: updated guidelines for reporting parallel group randomised trials. Ann Intern Med. 2010;152(11):726-32. doi:10.7326/0003-4819-152-11-201006010-00232.

2. Stone GW, Pocock SJ. Randomized trials, statistics, and clinical inference. J Am Coll Cardiol. 2010 Feb 2;55(5):428-31. doi:10.1016/j.acc.2009.06.066.

3. Guyatt G, Rennie D, Meade MO, Cook DJ. User's guide to the medical literature. A manual for evidence-based clinical practice. 2nd ed. Columbus, OH: McGraw-Hill; 2008.

4. Kaul S, Diamond GA. Trial and error: how to avoid commonly encountered limitations of published clinical trials. J Am Coll Cardiol. 2010 Feb 2;55(5):415-27. doi:10.1016/j.jacc.2009.06.065.

5. Guller U, DeLong ER. Interpreting statistics in medical literature: a *vade mecum* for surgeons. J Am Coll Surg. 2004 Mar;198(3):441-58.

6. Pihlstrom BL, Curran AE, Voelker HT, Kingman A. Randomized controlled trials: what are they and who needs them? Periodontol 2000. 2012;59(1):14-31. doi:10.1111/j.1600-0757.2011.00439.x.

7. Tu YK, Gilthorpe MS. Key statistical and analytical issues for evaluating treatment effects in periodontal research. Periodontol 2000. 2012;59(1):75-88. doi:10.1111/j.1600-0757.2011.00431.x.

8. DeMuth JE. Overview of biostatistics used in clinical research. Am J Health Syst Pharm. 2009 Jan 1;66(1):70-81. doi:10.2146/sjhp070006.

9. Whitley E, Ball J. Statistics review 3: hypothesis testing and P values. Crit Care. 2002 Jun;6(3):222-5.

10. Kendrach MG, Covington TR, McCarthy MW, Harris CM. Calculating risks and number-needed-to-treat: a method of data interpretation. J Managed Care Pharm. 1997 Mar/Apr;3(2):179-83.

Chapter Five

Literature Evaluation II: Beyond the Basics

Patrick J. Bryant • Cydney E. McQueen

Learning Objectives

After completing this chapter, the reader will be able to

- Describe other study designs besides the basic controlled clinical trial.
- Discuss the potential utility, limitations, and questions to ask when evaluating other study designs.
- Identify various observational trial designs based on differing characteristics.
- Differentiate between the three types of literature reviews: narrative (nonsystematic) review, systematic review, and meta-analysis.
- Describe common quality-of-life (QOL) measures used in health outcomes research and discuss the appropriate use of these measures in the medical literature.
- Identify issues encountered in dietary supplement (botanical and non-botanical) medical literature.
- Efficiently and effectively begin to evaluate the available evidence associated with a clinical question and categorize the quality of that evidence to develop a recommendation/clinical decision.

Key Concepts

❶ Although the randomized controlled trial is the most frequently used study design for clinical research, several other designs are used in specific situations, such as investigating rare outcome incidences, studying equivalency/non-inferiority between drugs, or minimizing patient exposure to new drugs with inadequate efficacy.

❷ Observational study designs offer an alternative to interventional trials and are used in specific situations, such as when large populations must be followed over extended periods of time. Results from these trials only allow associations to be formed rather than true cause-and-effect relationships.

❸ Case studies, case reports, and case series are observational or interventional reports describing patient or patient group exposure to a drug or technology and can be valuable to record preliminary findings that lead to further study. A key characteristic to these reports is the lack of a control or comparison group.

❹ Survey research is information gathered from an identified group with conclusions drawn and applied to a larger population. This gathered information is considered either descriptive (such as opinions and attitudes) or explanatory (such as explaining a cause and effect) in nature and the validity of the results depends on quality of the study's internal rigor.

❺ Meta-analyses are the only type of review providing new quantitative data derived from combining the results of each study in the meta-analysis and performing a statistical analysis on that data set. The overall reliability of a meta-analysis is ultimately dependent on the quality of the individual studies, homogeneity between these studies, and the appropriateness of the analysis.

❻ The value assigned to the duration of a patient's life when altered by various impairments, functional states, perceptions, and social opportunities that have been modified by disease, injury, treatment, and social policy is termed health-related quality of life (HR-QOL or HRQOL).

❼ The principles and criteria used to analyze the quality of drug literature are used to analyze dietary supplement (DS) literature; however, unique additional points such as standardization and purity must be considered.

❽ An understanding of strength and limitations inherent with each study design is essential to determine the overall quality of the evidence produced. Those trial designs with a high level of quality provide the most reliable evidence and that translates into the strongest recommendation/clinical decision.

Introduction

❶ *Although the randomized controlled trial is the most frequently used study design for clinical research, several other designs are used in specific situations, such as investigating rare outcome incidences, studying equivalency/non-inferiority between drugs, or minimizing patient exposure to new drugs with inadequate efficacy.* Principles that apply to randomized controlled trials (see Chapter 4) also apply to other types of study designs. There are situations where other research designs are more effective in answering specific questions or providing the only data available to answer the questions. For example, there has been a tremendous increase in the use of non-inferiority study design to establish a drug's position in therapy.[1] Typically, a superiority trial design is used in this instance. The issue arises when no statistically significant difference in efficacy between the new drug and control or reference drug (often considered to be standard treatment) is shown. The only conclusion to be made at that time is that the new drug is not superior to the reference drug. When non-inferiority trial design is used AND the results confirm that the new drug is non-inferior to the reference drug, a conclusion can be made that the new drug is "no worse" than the reference drug IN REGARD TO efficacy. If non-inferiority is established, the same data can be analyzed for superiority of the new drug over the reference drug, with a clear superiority margin, or a point of superiority. If no statistically significant difference in efficacy is shown from this analysis and, therefore, no superiority is established, the researcher at least knows the new drug is still no worse than the reference drug. As another example, **adaptive clinical trial** design has become more common in assisting to establish efficacy for a particular drug. Adapting the number of patients, eligibility criteria, drug dose, or randomization allocation can significantly improve the efficiency of drug development and provide a more realistic clinical environment to test a new drug. Table 5-1 lists commonly encountered trial designs in the biomedical literature.

To effectively determine the quality of these trials, the practitioner must first evaluate major considerations that apply to the design. One approach uses a list of essential study components referred to as the **Ten Major Considerations** Checklist.[2] The Ten Major Considerations include:

1. Power of the study set/met (to estimate adequate sample size that will identify a difference between groups if one truly exists)?
2. Dosage/treatment regimen appropriate?
3. Length of study appropriate to show effect?
4. Inclusion criteria adequate to identify target study population?
5. Exclusion criteria adequate to exclude patients who may be harmed or cause confounding results in study?
6. Blinding present?
7. Randomization resulted in similar groups?
8. Biostatistical tests appropriate for type of data analyzed?
9. Measurement(s) standard/accepted?
10. Author's conclusions are supported by the results?

Once this is completed, additional considerations unique to a specific study design discussed in this chapter must be evaluated. For example, how did the investigators

TABLE 5–1. COMMONLY ENCOUNTERED BIOMEDICAL LITERATURE

Study Design	Study Purpose
Clinical study	Determine cause and effect relationships
Non-inferiority study	Identify if one drug is therapeutically no worse than another drug, usually the accepted reference control drug
N-of-1 study	Compare effects of drug to control during multiple observation periods in a single patient
Adaptive clinical trial	Provides flexibility in design to incorporate continuously emerging knowledge generated as the trial progresses
Stability study	Evaluate stability of drugs in various preparations (e.g., ophthalmologic, intravenous, topical, and oral)
Bioequivalence study	Assess the bioequivalency of two or more products
Programmatic research	Determine the impact and/or economic value of clinical services
Cohort (follow-up) study	Determine association between various factors and disease state development
Case-control (trohoc) study	Determine association between disease states and exposure to various risk factors
Cross-sectional study	Identify prevalence of characteristics of diseases in populations
Case study, case report, or case series	Report observations in a single patient or series of patients
Survey research	Study the incidence, distribution, and relationships of sociologic and psychologic variables through use of questionnaires applied to various populations
Postmarketing surveillance study	Evaluate use and adverse effects associated with newly approved drug therapies
Narrative review	Nonsystematic, qualitative, subjective summary of data from multiple studies
Systematic review	Systematic, qualitative, and objective summary of data from multiple studies
Meta-analysis	Combine, statistically evaluate, and create new data from combining multiple studies in a quantitative manner
Outcomes studies (pharmacoeconomic and health-related quality-of-life measures)	Compare outcomes (QOL) and costs (pharmacoeconomics) of drug therapies or services

determine the non-inferiority margin since this is a variable that can be manipulated to provide desired results?

The purpose of this chapter is to familiarize the health care practitioner with these unique study designs. Specific considerations unique to each design, in addition to the Ten Major Considerations, are provided for the practitioner to use when evaluating these types of studies (see Appendix 5-1). Finally, a process is provided to bring all the results of trials focused on a particular clinical question together and develop a recommendation/ clinical decision based on this evidence. For these reasons, this chapter can be extremely valuable and useful to anyone who depends on the medical literature to provide answers to their daily clinical challenges.

This chapter covers the variations on randomized clinical trial design (non-inferiority, **N-of-1 trials**, and adaptive clinical trials), observational trial design (cohort, case-control, and cross-sectional), and uncontrolled study designs (case studies, case series, and case reports). Specific types of studies such as bioequivalency, postmarketing surveillance, and programmatic research are discussed. Differences between narrative (qualitative), systematic (qualitative), and **meta-analysis** (quantitative) reviews are addressed. A discussion of the specialized area of health outcomes research is included to introduce concepts directly related to patient QOL trials. A section on evaluation of dietary supplement (DS) medical literature, including issues specific to these trials and common methodological flaws, is provided.

Good literature evaluation skills and application of a systematic evidence-based medicine (EBM) process provide the foundation that allows clinicians to make the best recommendations and decisions.[3] In light of rapidly emerging evidence and busy practitioner schedules, an understanding of inherent strengths and limitations associated with various types of clinical trial design provides a powerful clinical tool. In general, those trials with a greater number of identified strengths than limitations, especially if those limitations have a minimal effect on the study results, provide a high level of reliability. Using these high-quality trials that represent the best evidence, a stronger recommendation/clinical decision can be made. This in turn ensures the highest level of patient care, whether for one specific patient or large patient populations.

Beyond the Basic Controlled Trial

NON-INFERIORITY TRIALS

Description

Randomized, controlled clinical trials are utilized to determine one of three different outcomes between comparative drugs: superiority, equivalency, or **non-inferiority (NI)**.[4] All three trial designs involve a new test drug compared to the accepted active control or standard of care drug. With superiority trials, the aim is to determine that one drug is superior to the other.[5] In contrast, equivalency trials are designed to determine whether the new drug is therapeutically similar to the control drug. This trial design is used primarily to determine bioequivalence between two drugs. Non-inferiority trials seek to show that any other difference between two treatments is small enough to conclude the test drug has "an effect that is not too much smaller than the active control,"[6] also referred to as the reference drug or standard treatment.[1,6-9] This section will focus on description, interpretation, and evaluation of NI trials.

There has been a dramatic increase in rate of published NI studies since 1999.[1] Along with this increase has come an understanding of several potential study design issues including choice of reference drug, point at which the test drug's treatment effect will be considered inferior to the reference drug, and optimal analytical approaches, therefore, requiring rigor in design and conduct of these trials.[10-12] A NI study design is often considered when superiority of a test drug over a reference drug is not anticipated.[13] In this case, the objective is showing the test drug to be statistically and clinically not inferior to the reference drug based on efficacy, yet the test drug could offer other potential advantages related to safety, tolerability, convenience, or cost.[7,8] These ancillary benefits can justify use of the test drug to replace standard treatment. NI trials are also considered when the use of a superiority trial would be unethical.[6] For example, it is unethical to use a placebo when there is available effective treatment that possesses an important benefit, such as preventing death or irreversible injury to the patient. For this reason, NI trials may provide an alternative method to using superiority trials for meeting U.S. Food and Drug Administration (FDA) marketing approval requirements.[6] Between 2002 and 2009, 14% of the new drug applications (NDAs) approved contained evidence from pivotal NI trials.[14] Rather than going through the process of showing a new drug is therapeutically superior to the reference drug treatment or a placebo, pharmaceutical companies are choosing to use an NI design. This is a developmental strategy to confirm that the new drug has a valid therapeutic effect and that the drug's effect is not worse than the reference drug.[15,16] Often the anticipated key differentiating factor for the test drug in this situation is improved safety profile. For example, a new drug for cardiac arrhythmias is anticipated to have similar efficacy but less serious side effects than the standard treatment. It should be noted that NI design is not recommended when the reference drug treatment effect is not consistently superior to placebo (both statistically and clinically).[17]

Establishing the NI Margin

The NI margin is an important component of an NI trial and is a prespecified value used to show the test drug's treatment effect is not worse than the reference drug by more than this specific degree.[15,18] A combination of statistical reasoning and clinical judgment is required to best determine the NI margin.[7,8,12,19-22] In other words, the NI margin is the extent to which the test drug's effect can be worse than the reference drug, but still be considered no worse.[23] For instance, if the reference drug's minimal treatment effect is determined to be a 5 mmHg drop in diastolic blood pressure compared to placebo, then the test drug could not be worse than this 5 mmHg change to be considered non-inferior to the reference drug. If the results from the NI trial showed the test drug's treatment effect to be 4 mmHg, then the test drug would be considered potentially inferior to the reference drug. The FDA draft guideline document defines the NI margin as the largest clinically acceptable difference (degree of inferiority) of the test drug compared to the reference drug.[6] Methods to determine the NI margin have been proposed; however, concern exists with the subjectivity and potential bias associated with any method that relies on an indirect comparison of historical data rather than a true placebo arm built into the NI study.[24-27]

A simple method to determine the NI margin is to look at the confidence interval (CI) for the reference drug treatment effect (reference drug – placebo = treatment effect). This treatment effect is best determined from examining the historical reference drug versus placebo-controlled trials. A meta-analysis of these historical placebo-controlled trials is preferred over separate evaluation of individual studies to obtain the most accurate overall treatment effect when several studies are involved.[8] The CI around the mean reference drug treatment effect is used to establish the NI margin (see Chapter 6 for further understanding of CIs). The lower bound of that CI represents the smallest expected reference drug treatment effect. For example, if the CI around the mean reference drug treatment effect is 3 to 14 mmHg diastolic blood pressure, then the lower bound of that CI would be 3 mmHg. This lower bound can be used to set the NI margin; however, a 5 mmHg change in diastolic blood pressure could be considered the smallest clinically significant change. Given this information, the NI margin can be set at 5 mmHg.

Interpretation of Results

The NI design focuses on the mean treatment difference between the test drug and the reference drug (Figure 5-1).[15] To determine NI, the CI around the mean treatment difference between the test drug and the reference drug is compared against the NI margin. If the CI around the mean treatment difference includes (or crosses) the NI margin, then the possibility of the test drug being inferior to the reference drug exists (inconclusive), and thus, the test drug fails to exhibit non-inferiority (see Scenario A in Figure 5-1). The test drug would be determined inferior if the entire CI around the mean treatment difference was located on the inferior side of the NI margin (see Scenario B in Figure 5-1). However, if the CI around the mean treatment difference does not include or cross the NI margin, then a conclusion can be made that the test drug is non-inferior to the reference drug (see Scenarios C and D in Figure 5-1).

For example, an NI study of a new antihypertensive agent (test drug) compared to reference drug is published in the literature. The overall treatment effect of the reference drug compared to previous placebo-controlled studies is a reduction of 12 mmHg (CI 6 to 15 mmHg) for a sitting diastolic blood pressure. The lower bound of that CI 6 mmHg, or some percentage of that lower bound based on consideration of the clinical significance, can be used to help set the NI margin. In this case, the lower bound of the CI 6 mmHg treatment effect can be considered a clinically significant difference or change in sitting diastolic blood pressure. Given this, the NI margin is established as 6 mmHg sitting diastolic blood pressure. In other words, when the NI trial is completed, the test drug's lower bound of the CI associated with the mean treatment difference cannot include or cross the set NI margin of 6 mmHg on the graph (Figure 5-2). If the test drug's lower

Figure 5–1. Non-inferiority trial design concept.

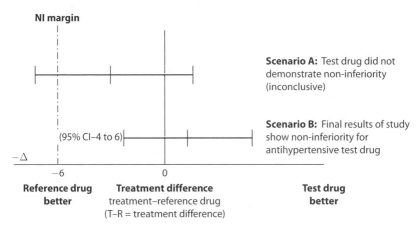

Figure 5–2. Non-inferiority trial design example.

bound of the CI includes (or crosses) the NI margin, this would suggest that the test drug failed to exhibit non-inferiority to the reference drug (see Scenario A in Figure 5-2). This situation would be considered an inconclusive result unless the entire CI for the mean treatment difference is located on the inferiority side of the NI margin of 6 mmHg, confirming inferiority. Upon completion of the example antihypertensive NI study, the actual results confirm non-inferiority of the new antihypertensive agent based on the lower bound of the CI interval for the test drug treatment effect not including (or crossing) the NI margin (see Scenario B in Figure 5-2). In the case where non-inferiority is determined, three assumptions are made: (1) test drug exhibits non-inferiority to the reference drug, (2) test drug performs better than placebo if placebo was included as a comparator group,

TABLE 5–2. DIFFERENCES IN DEFINING PARAMETERS FOR NULL AND ALTERNATIVE HYPOTHESES

Type of Trial	$P \geq 0.05$ (Alpha $= 0.05$) (Not Statistically Sig.) Fail to Reject the H_0	$P \geq 0.05$ (Alpha $= 0.05$) (Statistically Sig.) Reject the H_0 in Favor of H_A
Superiority trial	H_O = No difference	H_A = Difference
Non-inferiority trial	H_O = Inconclusive	H_A = Non-inferior

H_O—Null hypothesis.
H_A—Alternative hypothesis.

and (3) test drug may offer ancillary benefits and these could include safety, tolerability, convenience, or cost.[7]

If an NI margin and/or CI are not provided, then non-inferiority can still be determined if an alpha and p-value have been given. To use p-values for this purpose, there must be an understanding that statistical rationale for NI trials differs from that used with superiority trials.[28,29] Specifically, defining parameters for the null and alternative hypotheses (see Chapters 4 and 6) are different from those used with superiority trials.[15] In fact, the definitions for the two hypotheses are essentially switched or reversed and relabeled compared to superiority trial hypotheses[7,8] (Table 5-2). The null hypothesis for a superiority trial postulates that there is no statistically significant difference between treatment groups, and the alternative hypothesis states there is a statistically significant difference between the treatment groups. With NI trials, the null hypothesis states the test drug fails to exhibit non-inferiority to the reference drug or at the very least the results are inconclusive for non-inferiority versus inferiority.[13,15] The alternative hypothesis states that the test drug is non-inferior to the reference drug (not significantly worse). With NI trials, the null hypotheses must be rejected in favor of the alternative hypothesis to conclude non-inferiority for the test drug. This requires a p-value less than the set alpha value. For example, with an established alpha of 0.05 indicating the significance level, a p-value <0.05 would indicate non-inferiority for the test drug. If the null hypothesis is not rejected, then the test drug fails to exhibit non-inferiority. In this case the p-value would be equal to or greater than the set alpha value. Non-inferiority can be determined when a p-value is provided instead of an NI margin and/or CI around the mean treatment difference.

Some controversy exists whether an NI trial alone can show superiority of the test drug over the reference drug.[5,28,30] One reason for this is that a one-sided statistical test is used for determining non-inferiority, but a two-sided statistical test is needed for establishing superiority.[16] Once NI is established, superiority can be tested using the results for the primary outcome measure(s).[7,8] According to guidance from the FDA, an NI study can be designed to first test for non-inferiority with a predetermined NI margin, and, if successful at proving non-inferiority, the data can be analyzed for potential superiority of the test drug. Note the importance of the sequential process of first proving non-inferiority, then analyzing for superiority. For instance, if the new antihypertensive NI trial discussed earlier provided results that showed the test drug to be non-inferior, then an analysis of superiority would be appropriate and acceptable. This should be stated in the original non-inferiority trial protocol. Superiority can be tested prior to NI, even with a prespecified interim analysis, but the NI margin must be stated *a priori* to avoid potential manipulation of the margin.[31] Adjusting the NI margin to avoid the CI from crossing over would give a false NI result and is unacceptable. In addition, seeking the conclusion of NI from a failed superiority trial (one that shows no statistically significant difference between treatment groups) is not acceptable.[6,32] The only conclusion that can be made from this scenario is that the test drug is not superior to the reference drug. If a non-inferiority conclusion is anticipated, an NI study design should be the initial choice.

Evaluation

Specific study design characteristics must be considered when evaluating the quality of an NI trial.[2,5,33] Of significant importance is how the NI margin used to determine non-inferiority is defined.[28,34] Correctly determining this margin is considered the greatest challenge in the design and interpretation of NI trials.[6] If non-inferiority is established for the test drug, concluding the test drug is efficacious can only be made if the reference drug's efficacy has been confirmed with high-quality clinical trials against placebo. This is referred to as assay sensitivity.[6,26,32] The NI margin is set using historical studies to determine the actual effect of the reference drug. Two approaches to determine the NI margin are most frequently referenced: the fixed margin approach and the synthesis approach. Both these approaches use historical data. The fixed-margin approach is preferred by the FDA since that approach is more conservative than the synthesis approach.[35]

In a non-inferiority trial, it is key that the reference drug used should be superior to placebo. When past trials have been appropriately designed and conducted to confirm the superiority of the reference drug over placebo, the phrase historical evidence of sensitivity to drug effects (HESDE) is used. Meta-analytic methods can be used to develop more precise estimates of reference drug effect when several studies are available. When multiple studies exist, all studies should be considered to avoid overestimating the reference drug's effect.[6] Only after a determination is made that these past studies are similar in design and conduct compared to the NI trial, regarding features that could alter the effect size, can the HESDE be used to select the NI margin. In other words, the historical studies and new NI study should be as identical as possible regarding important characteristics. This is called the **constancy assumption**.[13,26] Note that establishing efficacy for the test drug using an NI trial design is seriously complicated by assay sensitivity and constancy assumptions that cannot be completely verified, leading to potentially inflated Type I error rate (see Chapters 4 and 6).[35] The concern is that approval of an ineffective therapy can result with inflated Type I error rates, since the test drug is falsely determined to be non-inferior to the reference drug.

Another concern called **biocreep** or **placebo creep** can exist that complicates using an active control to confirm efficacy, as is done with an NI trial.[13,26] Biocreep is the phenomenon where a somewhat inferior test drug is chosen as the reference drug for a future generation of NI trials. When this occurs with generation after generation of NI trials, the future reference drug becomes no better than placebo.

As mentioned earlier but important enough to reiterate, setting the NI margin *post hoc* can be interpreted as potential investigator manipulation to show desired results. For this reason, it is critical that the NI margin be set prospectively before the beginning of the trial. This is considered acceptable practice. For all of these reasons, the investigators should provide a detailed description of how the NI margin was determined.

The type of analysis used should also be determined prospectively. For the purposes of NI study analysis, a per-protocol (PP) analysis, where only the patients that completed the study are included in the analysis, is preferred over an intention-to-treat (ITT) analysis (see Chapters 4 and 6).[5,28] The ITT analysis includes all patients that were randomized to treatment regardless of whether they completed the study duration. With the ITT analysis, smaller observed treatment effects can result since patients may not have stayed in the study long enough to see the maximum effect of the test drug. Using an ITT analysis with an NI trial can significantly increase the risk of falsely claiming non-inferiority due to the potential of smaller observed treatment effects.[8,32] For this reason, when an ITT analysis is used, a PP analysis is also used to cross-validate the ITT analysis.[8,36] Note that the PP analysis can be invalidated based on significant variation in dropout rates between treatment groups.[36] For example, a non-inferiority study is completed, but there is an excessively large dropout rate due to safety and lack of return to the clinic visits. This provides a much smaller PP population to be analyzed. If that PP population is less than the required number of patients to meet the set power, then questions arise if no statistical significance ($p \geq 0.05$ if alpha set at 0.05) is shown. This lack of statistical significance shown could be real and the test drug would fail to exhibit non-inferiority (fail to reject the null hypothesis). Since power was not met, the result could represent a Type II error (no statistical significance is shown when there really is one and, therefore, the test drug is non-inferior to the reference drug) that invalidates the PP analysis (see Chapters 4 and 8 for explanation of Type II errors). The FDA and others suggest conducting and reporting both a PP and an ITT analysis.[6,9,36] Any differences in results between these two separate analyses should be examined closely by the reader (Case Study 5-1).

Case Study 5–1: Non-Inferiority Trial Design

A 12-week randomized double-blind double-dummy non-inferiority (NI) trial was conducted to compare the effectiveness and safety of transdermal buprenorphine with sustained-release tramadol for moderate to severe musculoskeletal pain. The primary outcome measure was the difference in mean visual analog scale (VAS) pain scores from baseline to end of study. It was determined, based on the FDA's Guidance for industry non-inferiority clinical trials (draft guidelines) that the NI margin would be −1.5 cm on the VAS. In other words, the mean difference in changes in pain from baseline to end of study between the two study drugs (treatment effect = transdermal buprenorphine – sustained release tramadol) with corresponding 95% CI was used for non-inferiority test. The lower limit of the CI was within −1.5 cm and therefore did not cross this NI margin. Intent-to-treat and per protocol analyses were used. Safety was assessed by the number of reported adverse drug reactions for each drug.

- *Identify the null hypothesis and alternative hypothesis for this non-inferiority study.*
  - ○ *Null hypothesis:*
  - ○ *Alternative hypothesis:*
- *When setting the NI margin, what specific factors did the investigators need to take into consideration?*
- *Did the investigators use the appropriate analysis type for an NI study?*
- *What is your conclusion if the 95% CI around the mean treatment difference for VAS, a measurement of pain between transdermal buprenorphine and sustained release tramadol, does not include or cross over the established NI margin?*
- *If the 95% CI around the mean treatment difference for VAS includes or crosses over the established NI margin, what is your conclusion?*
- *After showing non-inferiority for the two drugs, the investigators performed a superiority analysis on the data. What is your reaction to this second analysis?*

NI trials have a larger sample size compared to superiority trials since the NI margin is frequently smaller than the treatment difference anticipated with superiority trials.[16,32,37] Sample size determination before the study is started can be difficult since variance of the estimated treatment effect and event rate can be unknown for the test drug at this point. When this issue is present for superiority studies, an independent data monitoring group/committee is formed to examine the blinded information during the trial (interim analysis).

This committee is looking for the occurrence of an unexpectedly low event rate so an upward adjustment in sample size can be proposed. This same approach to sample size reassessment and adjustment is applied to NI trials.[38,39] A clear explanation of how the blinded information was handled and how the independent data monitoring committee (IDMC) was conducted should be provided in the article for evaluation.

One simple method that has been proposed to assist in remembering to evaluate some of the above characteristics uses the mnemonic "FACTS."[33] These five steps include:

1. Formulate a null hypothesis.
2. Assess the non-inferiority margin.
3. Compare the ITT and PP analyses.
4. Translate CIs graphically.
5. Summarize the clinical relevance of the results.

Although FACTS is helpful, this method does not cover all characteristics discussed in this section that should be evaluated to determine the quality of an NI trial.

Reporting NI trials in the literature is still not consistent and this can often be the biggest issue when evaluating and interpreting trial results for quality.[12,40,41] The Consolidated Standards of Reporting Trials (CONSORT) statement was first published in 1996 and then updated in 2010 to improve randomized controlled trial reporting in the medical literature.[42,43] Extensions to the CONSORT statement that specifically address reporting of NI trials have been proposed.[5,8,44] Specifically, these points include:

- Rationale for conducting trial
- Research objective(s)
- Clearly defined primary and secondary outcome measures
- Statistical methods used to evaluate objective(s)
- Methods used for sample size determination
- Inclusion/exclusion criteria comparable to previous trials using the active comparator (reference drug/devise/procedure)
- Description accounting for patients that are screened, randomly allocated, violated protocol, and completed study
- Explanation of how NI margin was determined
- Rationale for choosing comparator with historical study results confirming efficacy of this comparator
- Explanation of interim analysis and study discontinuation rules
- Interpretation of the real and estimated treatment exposures
- Explanation of the impact that withdrawals or crossovers could have had on the length of exposure to treatment assigned

- Summary of results for each primary and secondary outcome measures providing estimated effect size and precision (e.g., 95% CI)
- Interpretation of results considering the NI hypothesis, potential biases, and concerns with any multiple analysis

As mentioned previously, an attempt to rescue a failed superiority study by concluding that the results demonstrated NI should not be accepted.[28] Unfortunately, this situation is more common than would be expected.[45] The plan to determine NI of a test drug compared to the reference drug must be established prospectively utilizing the proper study design to test for NI. In other words, lack of superiority in a superiority trial design does not equal NI.

Appendix 5-1 contains a list of additional questions specific to NI studies. These specific questions are in addition to the standard questions used to evaluate other randomized clinical trials noted in Chapter 4; using basic tools such as the Ten Major Considerations Checklist discussed in the Introduction section; and using the pneumonic "FACTS" which has been proposed to help remember five steps associated with evaluation of NI studies.[33]

N-of-1 Trials

DESCRIPTION

The N-of-1 in clinical medicine is simply a crossover trial design that is repeated multiple times in a single patient to determine the relative effectiveness of two different therapies specifically for that one patient.[46,47,48] Multiple sequential treatment periods are involved where the active treatment is paired with a matched intervention (alternative treatment or placebo). The benefit of the crossover design between treatments minimizes the **patient-by-treatment interaction** (i.e., variation in response to therapy due to the heterogeneity of multiple patients' individual characteristics) seen with parallel group trials. In addition, the repeated use of treatment over time increases measurement precision and controls for **treatment-by-time interaction** (chance that the effects associated with each treatment might vary over time).[46,47]

To strengthen the trial design, randomization of treatment by period can be added to reduce **treatment order effects** (the order in which patients receive the treatments in the trial affects the results). Blinding of physician and patient is also added to reduce placebo effects (therapeutic activity provided by administering a placebo) and observer bias (person collecting data from the trial knows or has some idea which intervention each patient is receiving and, therefore, this may have some effect on the results reported).[46] In addition, washout/run-in periods between treatment periods to make sure that there is no carryover effect from the previous treatment period can be used to strengthen the design of the trial. Characteristics which have been identified as essential for the conduct of these trials include a disease that is chronic and stable over time, a relatively short half-life of the therapies being used, a rapid onset of action and offset of therapeutic activity, objective outcome measures that are meaningful to both physician and patient and considered acceptable practice or validated, and therapies that do not alter the underlying cause of the disease state.[46,47]

The N-of-1 trial is useful for individual patient-centered care and comparative effectiveness research.[47,49] Using this design, a clinician can compare effects of different treatments in the same patient.[48] Typically, the clinician performs an informal trial of therapy where the patient may try various treatments and in a subjective manner chooses the drug that seems to be working the best. As an alternative method, the N-of-1 trial provides scientific rigor to this process and improved individualized patient care based on objective comparative evidence.[50] For this approach to be successful, the clinician must institute multiple procedures including explaining the process to their patients, identifying outcomes mutually beneficial and appropriate for both patient and clinician, monitoring the patient on a regular basis, continually evaluating the results and explaining them to the patient, and collaborating with the patient to determine the best therapeutic approach for them based on these results.[46] From this collaborative approach to the N-of-1 study, the patient has a greater awareness and grasp of their disease state, and they feel more in control of decisions regarding their health care.

Observing across multiple N-of-1 studies using the same methods and types of patients could provide investigators the ability to draw conclusions regarding the effectiveness of an intervention in subsets of the population.[48] For instance, this approach could work well in individual patients with rare disease states unable to recruit a large enough study population to conduct classical clinical trials. Using this same reasoning, a series of N-of-1 trials could help identify characteristics that differentiate responders from nonresponders. In addition, trials of multiple doses could identify the most effective dose and the clinical endpoints most influenced by the drug. However, there are some situations where N-of-1 studies would be considered inappropriate or unfeasible.[48] For instance, public health studies involving population-wide intervention would require large numbers of patients to study the outcome of adding fluoride to the drinking water.

Currently, N-of-1 studies face several barriers to being implemented as a common place solution to individualized patient-centered care.[46-48] There is hesitancy by regulatory agencies, researchers, and clinicians to abandon classic clinical studies for generating objective findings. In addition, this study design is time consuming and expensive for the individual clinician, especially those in the primary care area. However, as clinicians recognize that an individual patient's response may not be represented by a mean effect from a large classical clinical trial, using N-of-1 trials could be useful to implement patient-centered care. With patient-centered care and comparative effectiveness at the forefront of contemporary medicine, N-of-1 trials should receive increased attention by health research and clinical care communities.[46,49,51-53]

EVALUATION

General evaluation requirements have been recommended for N-of-1 trials.[46,47] Readers should determine whether the treatment target (or measure of effectiveness) was evaluated during each treatment period. This target should be a symptom or diagnostic test result but must be directly relevant to the patient's well-being (e.g., the visual analog scale for pain). Two other critical characteristics of the N-of-1 trial are that the symptom under investigation shows a rapid improvement when effective treatment is begun and that this improvement regresses quickly (but not permanently) when effective treatment is discontinued. The longer it takes to see a therapeutic effect provided by a drug, the longer the testing period of the trial. This also holds true for how long it takes for the therapeutic effect to disappear after stopping the drug; a longer washout period results in an overall increase in trial duration. The length of the treatment period is important to know. For those diseases that remain constant, this treatment period is easy to establish. When dealing with a disease that is not constant, such as multiple sclerosis, the treatment period must be long enough to observe an exacerbation of the condition. A general rule is that if an event occurs an average of once every X days, then a clinician needs to observe three times X days to be 95% confident of observing at least one event. One should ask if a clinically relevant treatment target is used and can it be accurately measured? It is advisable to measure symptoms or the patient's QOL directly, with patients rating each symptom at least twice during each study period.

If statistical tests are used to analyze the data, the paired t-test is recommended for normally distributed data.[54] It is important to determine if sensible criteria for stopping the trial is established. Specification of the number of treatment pairs in advance strengthens the statistical analysis of the results and it has been advised that at least two pairs of treatment periods are conducted before the study is unblinded.

N-of-1 trials provide more objective information than case reports or case studies because there is a control group, and are useful for providing definitive information for drug prescribing in individual patients. See Table 5-3 for a comparison of N-of-1 trials and case studies.

Appendix 5-1 contains a list of additional questions specific to N-of-1 studies. These specific questions are in addition to the standard questions used to evaluate other randomized clinical trials noted in Chapter 4 and using basic tools such as the Ten Major Considerations Checklist discussed in the Introduction section.

TABLE 5–3. COMPARISON OF N-OF-1 TRIALS AND CASE STUDIES

	N-of-1 Trial	Case Study
Design	Prospective	Retrospective (most often)
Predefined methods	Yes	No
Clearly defined outcome measures	Yes	No
Randomization	Yes	No
Blinding	Yes	No
Multiple treatment periods	Yes	Not usually

Source: Adapted from Spilker.[122]

Adaptive Clinical Trials

DESCRIPTION

Adaptive clinical trial (ACT) design, also known as group sequential design, continues to be a topic of great interest by both the pharmaceutical industry and the FDA.[55,56] The FDA defines ACT as "a study that includes a prospectively planned opportunity for modification of one or more specified aspects of the study design and hypotheses based on analysis of data (usually interim data) from subjects in the study."[57] Note that these revisions are made based on information obtained entirely from inside the specific study itself and not from outside derived information. In simplest form, the ACT could be a well-designed randomized clinical trial with an interim analysis halfway through the study to identify if the original sample size determination is going to be adequate to meet the set power.[58] If this interim analysis shows the original sample size to be inadequate based on treatment effect, the response-adaptation of increasing the number of patients to be entered into the study will assure power is met by the end of the trial.[59,60]

Classical clinical trial design is rigidly structured to investigate a set number of variables and prevent additional variables from being introduced that will confound the results. However, the disadvantage of such rigidity is the inability to make adjustments to the study as it progresses and new information comes from those patients who have completed the trial. For example, if the investigators discover there is a specific patient group that responds to the treatment during the trial, adjustments to include only that patient population are not allowed. For that reason, a significant number of patients who are anticipated to not respond are exposed to a treatment that may cause severe side effects. ACT design provides enough flexibility to incorporate continuously emerging knowledge generated as a trial is carried out, such as limiting inclusion to only that specific patient population that responds.[61]

The ACT study design is attractive because of the potential savings of time and resources along with minimizing the exposure of subjects to possible dangerous therapies.[62] Stopping a trial because of recognition of the inability of that study to achieve its objectives is called **futility**.[63,64] Additional benefits include a more efficient developmental pathway for the drug, that patients benefit from effective therapies earlier, and that prescribers have more information on patients most likely to benefit from the drug.[65,66] The FDA is interested in the advantages offered by ACT design; however, it is remaining cautious in its acceptance due to possible introduction of various biases and confounding factors that could result in false conclusions.[55,57]

A review of ACT studies published between 2000 and 2014 revealed several interesting insights.[67] Results of this review confirmed that ACT studies are increasing in numbers. In addition, the ACT design is used most often in phase II clinical trials and in the area of oncology. Phase III ACT studies most often used a group sequential design where the sample size is not determined before starting the study, but rather once a statistically significant difference is noted at the interim analyses of prespecified adaptation options, such as sample size, change of study endpoints, and modification of dose and/or treatment duration.[55,67] A smaller number of pivotal, efficacy confirming studies have used the ACT design due to company concerns about FDA's skepticism based on the design's potential for bias and increased false-positive (Type I) error rates.[65]

EVALUATION

Studies based on the ACT design are evaluated similarly to other randomized clinical trials; however, there are some questions that are specific for assessing the ACT component:

- Was an IDMC, separate from the study personnel conducting the trial stationed in a different location, formed to follow the information coming out of the ACT over the time of the study?[57,68] This group would also be responsible to identify potential adaptations necessary to be implemented real time by the study personnel. The IDMC should not be included in the analysis and interpretation of the results following completion of the ACT. When appropriate, the IDMC would also use a termination rule for recommending discontinuation of the study after futility or efficacy was established prior to the scheduled end of the ACT.
- How were logistical issues identified by the IDMC communicated to the study personnel? For instance, patient response information can be transferred to a central location and then sent on to the study personnel from the central location. This maintains blinding between the two groups.
- How were adaptive changes determined by the IDMC? All proposed adaptive changes should be based on evidence being created by the continuous flow of

information from the study along with clinical judgment. In some cases, computer-generated adaptations using algorithms already developed prior to the study may be used. Termination rules should already exist with specific criteria to take into consideration.

- Did extensive adaptations to the protocol occur during the ACT? When extensive adaptations are implemented, the primary hypothesis can become unclear and the study's integrity diminished. This is especially important for efficacy-confirming studies.

- Are there any obvious indications that bias entered the study and had effects on the results? Bias is a term used to describe a preference toward a particular result when this preference interferes with the ability to be impartial or objective. Several types of bias have been identified that can have major effects on the results of a study. See Table 5-4 for a list of biases from different causes that should be ruled out as having significant effects on the results of an ACT.[69]

- If an interim analysis was conducted, exactly who had access to the information created from the interim analysis and how could this have affected any of the results? The formation of an IDMC to conduct interim analyses on the patient information received from the ongoing study can alleviate the need for interactions with the company sponsoring the trial.

- If the ACT was stopped early based on an interim analysis, did this have any effect on the results that would prevent the development of strong conclusions? If the discontinuation significantly shortens the period of treatment, evidence may be lacking and therefore it is impossible to make any conclusions. For instance, if the study was discontinued because no efficacy difference was seen between the two agents being studied, the early stopping results in not having enough patients studied to meet power, thus no final conclusion can be made at that time.

The benefits of ACT design are obvious and this encourages continued exploration for appropriate application to clinical programs.[70–77] Adaptations to study eligibility criteria, total sample size, randomization procedure, drug dose, schedule, treatment duration, concomitant treatments, patient evaluations for data collection, primary endpoint, secondary endpoints, and analytical methods to evaluate these endpoints can significantly improve the efficiency of drug development and overall patient care. See Chapter 6 for further discussion of ACT.

Appendix 5-1 contains a list of additional questions specific to ACTs. These specific questions are in addition to the standard questions used to evaluate other randomized clinical trials noted in Chapter 4 and use basic tools such as the Ten Major Considerations Checklist discussed in the Introduction section.

TABLE 5–4. TYPES OF BIAS

Category of Bias	Name of Bias	Description	Methods of Control	Cohort	Case-Control	Cross-Sectional
Selection bias	Admission rate (Berkson) bias	Admission rates of exposed and unexposed cases and controls differ, resulting in a distortion of odds of exposure in hospital-based studies	A priori define inclusion and exclusion criteria		X	
			All groups of subjects should have undergone identical diagnostic testing and there should be no difference in how exposure or disease status is determined			
	Nonresponse bias	Nonrespondents may exhibit exposures or outcomes that differ from respondents, resulting in overestimation or underestimation of odds or risk	Match or adjust for confounding variables	X	X	X
			Use more than one control group			
	Prevalence-incidence (Neyman) bias	Timing of exposure identification causes some cases to be missed		X	X	
	Unmasking bias	An innocent exposure causes a sign or symptom that precipitates search for a disease, but does not itself cause the disease		X	X	±
Information bias	Family history bias	Family members tend to share more information with family members who have similar diseases or exposures	Establish a priori explicit criteria for data collection methods on exposures and outcomes	X	N/A	X
		Those family members without the disease or exposure may be unaware	Blinded interviewer and subject to the hypotheses investigated			
		Family historical information may vary widely depending on whether the person is a case or a control	Standardize data collection procedure, i.e., train observers, develop and refine survey questions and methods of recording answers			

	Difference in how data collection occurs exists between cases and controls, or the exposed and unexposed, resulting in an abnormally high rate of recall of exposure or outcome in one group	Maintain aggressive contact with subjects to limit attrition (cohort designs) For surveys, obtain response rates ≥80%	X	N/A	X
Recall bias		Assess for effects of potential confounders			
Exposure suspicion bias	Knowledge of a subject's disease status may influence both intensity and outcome of a search for exposure		X	N/A	±
Data analysis bias					
Post hoc significance bias	When decisions regarding level of significance are selected *a posteriori*, conclusion may be biased	Establish *a priori* the statistical methods to be used to evaluate data Report how missing data are handled	X	X	X
Data dredging bias	When data are reviewed for all possible associations without prior hypotheses, results are only suitable for hypothesis-forming activities	Assess associations between confounders and exposures and outcomes	X	X	X
Significance bias	Confusing statistical significance with clinical significance		X	X	X
Correlation bias	Correlation does not equate with causation, concluding that correlation equates with causation can lead to serious errors		X	X	X

± = Potentially.
N/A = Not applicable.
Source: Adapted from Fletcher et al.[69]

Stability Studies/*In Vitro* Studies

DESCRIPTION

Stability of a pharmaceutical product is defined by the United States Pharmacopeia (USP) as "extent to which a product retains, within specific limits and throughout its period of storage and use (that is, its shelf-life), the same properties and characteristics that it possessed at the time of its manufacture."[78] To determine the stability of various preparations (e.g., ophthalmologic, intravenous, topical, oral), specific studies are performed under various conditions such as heat, freezing, refrigeration, transport, and room temperature.[79,80] Generally, stability studies are not published but remain unpublished data on file with the pharmaceutical company or compounding pharmacy and, in some cases, not available to the public since they reveal secret manufacturing equipment or techniques used to maintain stability, also known as trade secrets. Although the actual written study is not readily available for evaluation, these studies are extremely important to the practice of pharmacy. For example, pharmacists who prepare intravenous solutions for use by patients at home often want to know how long a drug admixture in a particular solution is stable. Another stability question could be whether the length of time to maintain stability would be increased with freezing the admixture. This information helps determine how many intravenous admixtures may be dispensed at a time. It is also important for pharmacists involved with extemporaneous compounding to know the length of time that a particular preparation remains stable.

EVALUATION

Stability study requirements and expiration dating are presented in the Current Good Manufacturing Practices (cGMPs),[81] the USP,[82] and the FDA and International Council for Harmonization-Quality. The listings for FDA guidelines associated with various stability testing can be located at http://www.fda.gov/RegulatoryInformation/Guidances/default.htm. The International Council for Harmonization (ICH) guidelines on quality web page is located at http://www.ich.org/products/guidelines/quality/article/quality-guidelines.html. The cGMPs require a written testing program designed to assess the stability characteristics of drug products.[81] The USP contains detailed stability and expiration dating information in addition to stability considerations in dispensing practices.[82] Design of stability studies to acquire expiry and product storage, in addition to directions for submission of this information, is found in the FDA guidance documents. The ICH guidelines provide common approaches used by the pharmaceutical industry for assessing stability of drug products.

Appendix 5-1 contains a list of additional questions specific to stability studies. These specific questions are in addition to the standard questions used to evaluate other randomized clinical trials noted in Chapter 4 and using basic tools such as the Ten Major Considerations Checklist discussed in the Introduction section, when appropriate.

Bioequivalence Trials

DESCRIPTION

An ever-increasing number of generic products are becoming available in the marketplace and there is a need to establish that the quality, safety, and efficacy of these generic drugs are the same as the brand name product, which is the purpose of this type of trial.[83] The health care practitioner is often placed in the position of having to select one from among several apparently equivalent products for individual patients or for use on formularies of health care organizations. The more skilled the health care practitioner is at interpreting the data, the more comfortable he or she will be in selecting the appropriate product for the specific patient or organization.

According to the director of the FDA Office for Generic Drugs, "The standards for quality are the same for brand name and generic products."[84] Current FDA regulations require bioequivalence between each new generic product and the brand name product be demonstrated, but do not require that bioequivalence among generic copies of the same brand name drug be demonstrated. This is based on the fact that if each generic copy must show bioequivalence to the brand name product, then the copies should be within the same range of bioequivalency.

A company is required to demonstrate that, in addition to several other things, its drug product is bioequivalent to the reference listed drug (RLD).[83] According to the Federal Food, Drug and Cosmetic Act (FD&C Act), a generic drug is considered bioequivalent to the RLD if "the rate and extent of absorption of the drug do not show a significant difference from the rate and extent of absorption of the listed drug when administered at the same molar dose of the therapeutic ingredient under similar experimental conditions in either a single dose or multiple doses." Bioequivalent studies can be one of several designs in descending order of preference by the FDA: pharmacokinetic, pharmacodynamics, clinical, and *in vitro* studies. For pharmacokinetic studies, the FDA recommends a two-period, two-sequence, two-treatment, single-dose, crossover study design, a single-dose parallel study design, or a replicate study design for bioequivalence studies. The area under the blood concentration time curve (AUC), the peak height concentration (C_{max}), and the time of the peak concentration (T_{max}) are the primary pharmacokinetic parameters used to assess the rate and extent of drug absorption.

EVALUATION

When evaluating bioequivalence trials for application in clinical practice, it is important to focus on the methods of the study. The following are specific components to look for in the methods section[85]:

- Acceptable age and weight range for the subjects are defined.
- Clinical parameters used to characterize a normal, healthy adult (e.g., physical exam observations, hematological evaluations) are described.
- Subjects should be free of all drugs, including caffeine, nicotine, alcohol, and other recreational drugs for at least 2 weeks prior to testing because these factors can affect pharmacokinetic parameters.
- Subjects should be free of all dietary supplements (botanical and non-botanical), as many of these products can interact with products under bioequivalence review.
- All subjects should receive the drug under the same conditions and all blood levels should be taken at the same intervals, which should be based on the half-life of the drug.
- The assay used to determine the blood levels should be validated.
- The same assay should be used for the test and reference drugs. Multiple assays are available to measure serum levels for some products. Results from the same assay for two drugs may demonstrate equivalence. However, if one assay type is used for the reference drug and another assay type is used for the test drug, the results may not demonstrate equivalence because the sensitivity and specificity of assays may be different.
- Bioequivalence testing may be performed in both fasting and fed states to assess the impact of food on bioavailability; however, food intake should be closely monitored and controlled.

One of the most common errors in the use of bioavailability data is comparing two products based on data obtained from separate studies.[85] Different subject populations, study conditions, and assay methodologies are reasons why comparisons of data from different studies are dangerous and can lead to false conclusions.[85] For example, a pharmacy and therapeutics committee may identify two generic products that each have individually shown bioequivalence to the brand product in two separate studies. A false conclusion can be made that both generic products are bioequivalent to each other. Additional information, scientific and medical evaluations by the FDA, is available on the FDA website at http://www.accessdata.fda.gov/scripts/cder/ob/default.cfm.

Appendix 5-1 contains a list of additional questions specific to bioequivalence studies. These specific questions are in addition to the standard questions used to evaluate other randomized clinical trials noted in Chapter 4 and use basic tools such as the Ten Major Considerations Checklist discussed in the Introduction section.

Programmatic Research

DESCRIPTION

Programmatic research, another type of research important to overall health care, is focused on the impact and economic value of programs and services provided by practitioners in community and institutional settings.[85–88] This research is particularly important because limited resources and budget constraints demand that only those services that improve patient care in a cost-effective manner be implemented.[89–91] As an example, the body of evidence in support of the economic benefit of pharmacists providing clinical pharmacy services has grown over the past decade and is diverse.[92–94] The evidence includes contemporary practice sites and services. The study design and methodology has improved, in addition to economic, clinical, and humanistic outcomes assessed in many practice environments. Pharmacists, working in interprofessional settings with physicians and other health care providers, have demonstrated that they can improve drug therapy effectiveness and safety.[95] This study also showed that pharmacists enhanced the efficient delivery of health care in collaboration as part of an interprofessional team, applying their specific drug therapy knowledge, skills, and abilities to complement the other types of care provided by the collaborating professionals. The American College of Clinical Pharmacy (ACCP) has published a succession of position statements that review published literature regarding the value of clinical pharmacy services.[95] These position papers discuss strengths and limitations of existing literature, and include recommendations for further studies in order to facilitate continued documentation of value provided by pharmacists in progressive roles and settings, while utilizing methodology that ensures a high **level of evidence**-based rigor. Note that programmatic research is also used to determine if interventions made to pharmacy school curriculums have the intended benefits on student learning and goals.[96,97]

In general, programmatic research articles consist of a wide array of different study designs that create descriptive information and sometimes analytical data. Some of these designs include survey, pharmacoeconomic, or randomized controlled trial designs. To accurately assess these trials, the specific section in this chapter that relates to the trial design of the study being assessed should be consulted. Appendix 5-1 contains a list of additional questions specific to programmatic research studies. These specific questions are in addition to the standard questions used to evaluate other randomized clinical trials noted in Chapter 4 and use basic tools such as the Ten Major Considerations Checklist discussed in the Introduction section.

Observational Study Design

● ❷ *Observational study designs offer an alternative to interventional trials and are used in specific situations, such as when large populations of patients must be followed over extended periods of time. Results from these trials only allow associations to be formed rather than true cause-and-effect relationships.* They can be prospective, retrospective, or a single snapshot (or slice) in time. Observational study designs involve subject groups that are based on presence or absence of a disease or exposure, with observations being made and recorded regarding patient characteristics. The observational study design seeks to evaluate questions based on less rigidly controlled practice conditions than those used in experimental study designs. Research questions are addressed by comparing outcomes or experiences of patients arising from naturally occurring assignment to different treatments, subject characteristics, or exposures.[98] For instance, if an agent is particularly toxic and of no therapeutic value, it would be unethical to ask subjects to voluntarily expose themselves to the agent, thus an observational study would be used. An example of this type of situation is the evaluation of risk factors for diseases such as cancer. An investigator wishing to evaluate the toxicity of environmental or industrial hazards or the teratogenicity of drugs administered during pregnancy would have to employ specific observational studies that will be discussed in this section to study these problems. These research techniques allow associations rather than cause-and-effect relationships ● to be determined. Thus, when evaluating overall results of any observational study (e.g., cohort, case-control, cross-sectional, case study), it is important to remember that a correlation or an association between exposure and outcome does not prove causation.[99] Other factors possibly related to both the exposure and outcome must be considered.

The following discussion will present observational study designs commonly encountered within health care literature: the cohort, case-control, and cross-sectional designs. Differences between these study designs will be discussed and specific uses identified ● for each design (Table 5-5). In addition, evaluation techniques for each will be discussed.

TABLE 5–5. CHARACTERISTICS OF OBSERVATIONAL STUDY DESIGN

Observational Study Design	Prospective Data Collection	Retrospective Data Collection	Exposure Known at Beginning of Study	Outcome Known at Beginning of Study	Study Determines Exposure Status	Study Determines Outcome Occurrence
Cohort	X	X	X			X
Case-control (trohoc)		X		X	X	
Cross-sectional	X				X	X

See Table 5-5 for differentiating factors between observational trial designs: cohort, case-control, and cross-sectional. In addition, see Table 5-4 for specific types of bias associated especially with observational studies. Note the suggested methods to control for bias, and which types of observational studies are at the highest risk for each bias is discussed.

COHORT STUDIES

Description

The term cohort is derived from the Latin word *cohors*, which means a group of soldiers.[100] In ancient Roman times, soldiers were assigned into 1 of 10 divisions of a legion where they remained over the duration of their service or died. This term is used today to describe a group of individuals with a common characteristic or experience.[101] That experience is often a specific exposure to a particular agent such as a vaccine, medication, procedure, or environmental toxin. Participants in a **cohort study** are grouped by their exposure and followed over time to determine the incidence of symptoms, disease, or death.[101] Two groups are usually compared. Generally, these two groups are made up of those participants exposed and those nonexposed. Other terms for cohort studies are follow-up, incidence, and longitudinal studies. See Figure 5-3 for a schematic representation of this study design.

The study hypothesis for a cohort study attempts to establish a relationship between an exposure or risk factor and a subsequent outcome.[102] A measurement, such as relative risk, is frequently used to determine the extent of this relationship. Relative risk is the risk of developing a disease or adverse event in those participants exposed to a specific variable compared to those not exposed to that variable.[2,103]

The relative risk values can be greater than, less than, or equal to 1. For instance, if the relative risk calculated for a relationship between a specific drug exposure and cervical cancer is 5, this means that participants are five times more likely to develop cervical cancer when given the drug compared to those not being exposed to the drug. Other measurements such as attributable risk, number needed to treat, and life table methods can be used to analyze the data from cohort studies.[102]

Relative risk gives an idea of the magnitude of an effect but does not provide information about precision or statistical significance of the result.[104] Alternatively, calculation of CIs (usually at a level of 95%) is utilized for evaluation of statistical significance of results. The CI provides a range in which the true value for the population lies. The concept is that the wider the CI, the greater the variability and, therefore, range that contains the true value. Because a relative risk of 1 indicates no difference exists between groups, the CI cannot include 1 and still maintain statistical significance. See Chapters 4 and 6 for further discussion on relative risk.

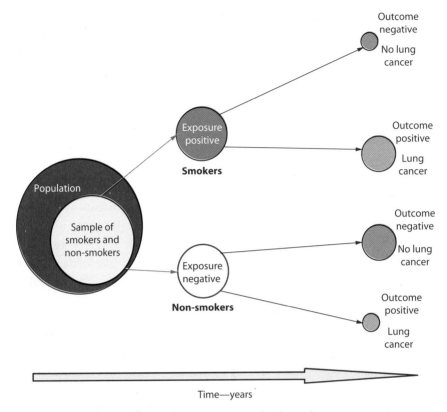

Figure 5–3. Schematic diagram of a cohort study.

Categories of Cohort Studies

There are three basic categories of cohort studies used based on timing of the events: prospective (looking forward in time), retrospective (looking backward in time), and ambidirectional (looking both forward and backward in time).[101] The prospective cohort study, also known as concurrent because participants are monitored over time, groups the participants based on current or past exposure and then follows these groups over time observing the various predetermined outcomes. In the prospective cohort design, outcomes have yet to develop and investigators are required to wait for their occurrence. For example, observing the long-term effects of lead exposure on cognitive function as children grow to be adults.

Retrospective or historical cohort studies, also referred to as nonconcurrent since both the exposure and the outcome are already recorded in a database, use computerized data on patients that have been recorded over the natural course of their health care.[102,105] Information regarding the treatment received by individuals in 2000 is obtained from a database in 2010. In addition, the assessment of outcomes due to this treatment is known and recorded in this database by 2010. For instance, a computer database is searched for all patients who received medication or surgical treatment for a disease in 2000. Once identified, the investigators observe the assignment to study or control groups. The database is then searched to determine the outcomes occurring for each group from 2000 to 2010.

Finally, the ambidirectional cohort study involves both prospective and retrospective components.[101] An example of this type of cohort is the Air Force Health Study looking at men involved in aerial spraying of herbicides, including Agent Orange, during the Vietnam War.[106] The retrospective portion of the study observed the incidence of cancer and mortality from time of exposure in the war through the 1980s,[107,108] while the prospective component involves observing these men well into the future.[109]

Other terms describing cohort studies are based on the characteristics of the population that makes up the cohort, changes or no changes in the exposure over time, and existence of losses to follow-up.[101] Cohort studies where the participants may enter or leave based on changing characteristics, such as smoking, alcohol consumption, occupation, and specific geographical location, are referred to as open or dynamic. For instance, a participant is a member of an open cohort group of Kansas City residents as long as he or she continues to live in Kansas City. A fixed cohort is identified by an unchangeable event such as having undergone a surgical procedure or been exposed to a potential toxin, such as Agent Orange, at a specific time, like the 1960s, and place, such as Vietnam. For this reason, exposures do not change or are considered fixed in this type of cohort. A third type of cohort is referred to as closed. Similar to the fixed cohort, a closed cohort involves an unchangeable event. A closed cohort also has a specific starting and ending point that involves follow-up. For example, a closed cohort may be conducted with participants attending a high school football game to determine if the nachos and spicy cheese consumed at the game provided them discomfort, such as gastritis, throughout the remainder of the evening until morning.

Uses of Cohort Studies

Cohort study designs are primarily used to explore the possible causes or risk factors, but not confirm the cause of a disease or the benefits and safety risks of both medication and procedures.[102] For instance, important information on the risk of cancer in individuals undergoing radiation therapy for noncancerous disease states has been identified. The cohort study is the simplest approach for studying disease incidence.[110] Key characteristics of each participant are determined prior to the study initiation and monitored during the follow-up period. From this information, important risk factors relating to the disease incidence are identified. In this way, risk factors are measured prospectively before the disease occurs. For example, cohort studies have been responsible for identifying the risk factors associated with cardiovascular disease such as high blood pressure, high cholesterol, physical inactivity, obesity, and smoking.

The primary disadvantages of cohort studies are expense and time consumption.[104] For example, with rare outcomes, such as the occurrence of aplastic anemia with use of clozapine, a prospective investigation may require extremely large numbers of patients, need decades of data collection, and accrue large project costs to acquire answers. It takes many years for adequate assessment of disease development or to establish disease-free status.[100] Such research questions are investigated more efficiently with the retrospective case-control design.

Evaluation of Cohort Studies

When critically evaluating a cohort study, the practitioner should be concerned with several points.[99] With a cohort study, there is no randomization process used to ensure that each participant has an equal opportunity to be in either the exposed or nonexposed group. The investigator selects the group each participant is relegated for the duration of the study. Certainly, those who have been, are currently, or will be exposed are assigned to that group, in addition to those who never have or never will be exposed assigned to the nonexposed group. Unlike a randomized controlled trial where patients are similar in their demographic characteristics between groups due to the randomization, a cohort study has no assurance of this similarity. For this reason, two concerns arise: selection bias and confounders.[111,112]

Selection Bias

Selection bias is a potential whenever the investigator is allowed to decide who is brought into the study and who is not selected to participate. This can result in differences within and/or between the groups that can have an impact on the final study results. For instance, an investigator either knowingly or unknowingly selects from the general population only the healthiest individuals to be assigned to the non-exposure group while at the same time a mixture of healthy and unhealthy participants are selected for the exposure group. With this scenario, there is an imbalance between groups that could set the exposed group up for an exaggerated negative effect to the exposure. When compared to the nonexposed group who were extremely healthy from the start of the study, this selection bias can produce an amplified difference that would not have been observed if both groups were balanced in regard to the initial healthiness of the participants. Simply stated, when a study starts out with dissimilar groups, the observed results at the study completion may be due to the exposure or due to the fact that the groups were different from the start.

Confounding Factor

A confounding factor, or confounder, is a variable related to one or more variables defined in the study.[113] These confounding factors can be known or unknown depending on whether they have been discovered. Confounding factors are common in cohort studies since they are the product of not using a randomization schedule that evenly distributes the confounding factors between the exposure and non-exposure groups. For instance, in a cohort trial that is studying the effects of sleep deprivation on pharmacy students during their schooling, sleep deprivation is a defined variable (exposure) and various outcomes associated with sleep deprivation, such as grades, interaction during lectures, and volunteer time provided to student organizations, are other defined variables. An example of a confounder would be age. If there were a greater number of older students in the exposure group, the outcomes could be poorer since older students have established lives with families and possibly other activities competing for their time. These confounding factors could certainly have an effect on the outcome measures, but have nothing to do with sleep deprivation. Confounding factors can mask actual associations or falsely demonstrate an apparent association that actually does not exist between variables in a study.[111] In the example of sleep-deprived pharmacy students, time taken away from studying and volunteer work that results in a negative effect on grades and volunteer time for organizations could be due to other competing activities related to older age (confounding factor) of participants. With age as a confounding factor in this example, it is possible to see how this confounder falsely demonstrates an apparent association between sleep deprivation and negative outcomes. In other words, an association between sleep deprivation and poorer grades or less volunteer time can be made when in reality the difference in age between groups is the real cause of the negative outcomes. Whether the investigators have used a systematic process to identify known confounders should be identified. In addition, careful consideration can sometimes identify confounders not mentioned by the authors. This would be considered a limitation and should raise caution with regard to reliability of the results.

There are methods and techniques that can be used to assess, correct, control, or adjust for confounding variables.[112,113] One method is putting restrictions on the selection criteria.[112] If the investigators had recognized age as a potential confounding factor prior to initiating the pharmacy student sleep deprivation study described earlier, an age range restriction such as 20 to 25 years of age could have been incorporated into the selection criteria. By restricting the age to no greater than 25 years, the confounding factor of older age and the potential effects on the results are removed from the scenario. Other analytical strategies can be used on the data to increase confidence that confounding factors had no or minimal effects on the results.[114] One analytical technique is regression that uses the data to determine if confounders are related to the outcomes. If regression analysis determines confounders have affected the results, an adjusted estimate of the actual exposure effect of interest on the outcomes is provided. For example, if age was shown by regression analysis to have affected the outcomes in the pharmacy student study, an adjusted estimate of actual sleep deprivation without the confounder effect on the outcomes would be provided. Stratification is another analytical technique that creates subgroups that are more balanced regarding baseline participant characteristics than the entire study population. Confounders such as age are balanced between subgroups.

For example, applying a stratification analysis to the sleep deprivation study would result in age being more balanced between subgroups. The overall effect of sleep deprivation is calculated from the difference in average outcomes between the exposure and non-exposure groups within each stratum. The result of stratification is that less confounder effect is seen on the results of the association between sleep deprivation and measured outcomes of pharmacy student grades, lecture interaction, and volunteer time. Whether the investigators have used any of these techniques should be identified. Use of the technique can determine if confounding factors played a significant role in the final results based on what these analysis strategies reveal.

Outcome Measurement

Accurate measurement of the outcome is essential.[104] Surveillance bias is a potential problem when one group, generally the exposed group, is more intensely monitored for changes in the outcome measure than the comparison group. Blinding the investigator responsible for performing the outcome measurement is one potential way of minimizing the chances for surveillance bias. Sources for acquiring the outcome data can vary. When this happens, the different sources can affect the results since one source can be more sensitive than others. For example, the details provided regarding follow-up can be significantly different when looking at medical chart versus nursing notes versus the actual interpretation of the radiology report by an expert. Making sure that the same source is used to obtain all measurements for both groups is crucial. Furthermore, information bias can occur if the same efforts to measure outcomes are not made for both the exposed and nonexposed groups.[110,118]

Follow-Up

Adequate follow-up is important.[101] The practitioner must ensure that the length of follow-up was adequate for the outcome being measured. For instance, a 3-month cohort study to determine risk factors associated with long-term cardiovascular events such as myocardial infarction is inadequate. Also, dropouts should be accounted for by the authors and assessed to determine if there were factors that caused a greater number in one group compared to the other. For instance, participants who are sicker in one group might drop out of the study due to death that is not associated with the risk factor being studied, but rather because they were more prone to death due to some other cause. Studies where loss to follow-up exceeds 20% in either the exposed or nonexposed cohort should be interpreted with caution.[100]

Appendix 5-1 contains a list of additional questions specific to cohort studies. These specific questions are in addition to the standard questions used to evaluate randomized clinical trials noted in Chapter 4 and using basic tools such as the Ten Major Considerations Checklist discussed in the Introduction section (Case Study 5-2).

Case Study 5–2: Cohort Study Design

A cohort study is published in Cancer Epidemiology, Biomarkers, and Prevention. The study is a prospective observation on the relation between coffee consumption and risk of endometrial cancer. Coffee consumption was prospectively assessed in relation to endometrial cancer risk in the Nurses' Health Study with 67,470 females aged 34 to 59. The questionnaires collected the cumulative average coffee intake over a specific time period. Cox regression models calculated incidence rate ratios. The results showed that consumption of fewer than four cups of coffee per day were not related to endometrial cancer risk. Women who consumed four or more cups of coffee had a 25% lower risk of endometrial cancer than those who consumed less than one cup of coffee per day (multivariable RR = 0.75, 95% CI = 0.57 to 0.97; p[trend] = 0.02). Decaffeinated coffee consumption suggested an inverse relationship. The authors concluded that these observations suggest four or more cups of coffee per day are associated with a lower risk of endometrial cancer in women.

- *What would indicate that there is some potential for selection bias in this study?*
- *What would be some of the potential confounding factors associated with this study?*
- *What are some of the other characteristics of a cohort study that should be evaluated?*
- *What cause-effect relationship can be established with this study?*

CASE-CONTROL STUDIES

Description

Case-control studies (also termed case-referent, case history, or retrospective studies) are a type of observational study that offers an epidemiologic research alternative to cohort studies.[99] The latter requires a large number of subjects, and is often expensive and time consuming. Case-control studies seek to retrospectively identify potential risk factors of diseases or outcomes. In a case-control study, subjects (cases) with a particular characteristic or outcome of interest (e.g., disease) are recruited, matched with, and compared to a similar group of subjects (controls) who have not experienced the characteristic or outcome. Data regarding the history of exposures are collected via patient interviews or by reviewing subject data records, and the two groups are compared to identify possible risk factors or contributors for development of the disease or outcome of interest. Note both the exposure and the outcome are known for all subjects at the beginning of the case-control study. This is a key differentiating factor for case-control versus cohort study design. See Figure 5-4 for a schematic of the case-control study design.

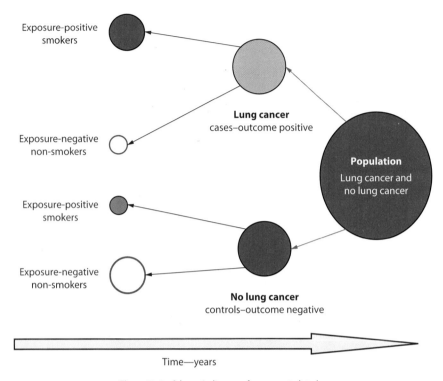

Figure 5–4. Schematic diagram of a case-control study.

Case-control studies can be more useful than cohort studies when diseases have a rare prevalence or when many years of exposure to the risk factor is required.[95,99,100] Case-control studies are always conducted in a retrospective design compared to randomized clinical trials and cohort studies, which are usually performed in a prospective manner and that is why case-control studies are sometimes called trohoc studies (i.e., cohort spelled in reverse).

Exposure of study subjects to the risk factor should reflect what occurs in the general population. If subjects with higher or lower exposure rates to the risk factor are excluded from the study, determination of possible associations between the exposure and a particular disease may be biased and inaccurate. For example, case-controls often use subjects drawn from hospitalized populations, whose risk factor exposure may differ from individuals in the community, a problem termed Berkson's bias.[115] Table 5-4 presents this and other types of bias that may be found within observational study designs, along with methods that provide control of potential biasing factors.

Matching is often used to ensure that cases and controls are similar.[99] Predisposition to the disease of interest should be similar in both cases and controls, except for exposure to the risk factor under investigation; however, this is extremely difficult to ensure. With matching, each case has a comparable control or controls in terms of demographic and exposure characteristics. At the beginning of the study in Figure 5-4, patients with lung cancer and those without have matching demographics and exposure characteristics. Often it is difficult to determine which variables should be used to match cases to controls (e.g., sex, age, and date of admission). Such matching allows assessment of only the risk factor under investigation such as smoking. No other variables that may have contributed to the disease are taken into consideration. Matching may even result in a negative impact on the interpretation of study results if cases and controls are matched for a factor that is itself related to the exposure.[100] Using the example, this type of situation could exist if the patients were required to have a family background of smokers. This exposure to second-hand smoke may confound the results regarding effects of direct smoking on the case group since the non-smokers have been exposed to a factor that is itself related to the exposure. The result is both groups being exposed to indirect smoking in the past, which may contribute to the development of lung cancer.

Cases and controls should undergo the same diagnostic evaluation to determine the presence or absence of the disease under investigation (e.g., chest x-ray and bronchoscopy for definitive diagnosis of lung cancer), because detection of a disease is more likely to be found in individuals who undergo extensive diagnostic testing.[112] In addition, individuals administering the tests should be blinded to the presence or absence of the risk factor to eliminate diagnostic review bias.[110,112] This blinding can be achieved if the x-rays and bronchoscopies are reviewed and interpreted by an independent non-investigator who is unaware of the study protocol details. A problem is that many diagnostic tests can only be performed in individuals suspected of having a particular disease state due to risks associated with their use. This would be the situation with bronchoscopies due to the invasiveness of the test. In this situation, the independent non-investigator is left with only a chest x-ray and the physician's subjective final diagnosis in the medical records.

Case-control study designs have both advantages and disadvantages.[99] These studies are relatively inexpensive and can be completed in a shorter timeframe than cohorts. Both of these advantages are related to how subjects are recruited and data are acquired. When rare events are studied prospectively in a cohort design, recruitment of large numbers of patients is required due to the uncertainty of events occurring during the study period and the resulting need to ensure study power. In contrast, case-control studies reduce the need for large sample sizes, as subjects are recruited based on *a priori* knowledge of occurrence of outcomes as stated in the medical records.

Evaluation

Several points should be considered when evaluating these types of trials.[99] Most limitations inherent to case-control studies are due to the retrospective design. Overall, the two

major methodological issues include appropriate selection of controls and accurate determination of the level of exposure.[111] Historical data used in case-control studies, which
are obtained from medical records, may be inaccurate or incomplete. When patients are
interviewed regarding historical events, equal distribution of patients' ability to recall
events that have happened in the past between the two groups may not be ensured. For
example, patients with lung cancer may be more likely to recall events preceding development of the disease than patients who are healthy. Patients with disease have probably contemplated factors that they believe may have contributed to disease development
(recall bias). For this reason, there should be some explanation in the study addressing
the issue of recall bias. Unblinded investigators who collect data may also question individuals exposed to the disease more intensely than control subjects. To reduce variation
in data obtained from cases and controls, trained data collectors should be blinded to the
status of the subjects as cases or controls (lung cancer to no lung cancer).

Another prominent disadvantage is that information about the exposure and outcome is collected simultaneously, so it is difficult to sort out the temporal relationship
between the two.[111] For instance, it is often difficult to determine if the outcome preceded
the exposure, a situation termed protopathic bias, where the disease may lead to risk
factor exposure rather than vice versa.[111] Consider the following illustration. Abnormal
vaginal bleeding may be an early sign of uterine cancer. Vaginal bleeding, however, may
lead to prescribing hormonal therapies such as progesterone. An investigator may later
erroneously conclude that use of progesterone was associated with development of uterine cancer, when in fact the cancer preceded use of the progesterone in this case.[112]

Some experts have suggested use of several control groups selected on the basis of
different criteria in an attempt to reduce some of the biases discussed above.[99] A well-
designed case-control study may have multiple controls for each case. If results of comparing cases to the various control groups are in agreement with one another, bias in the
control groups is less likely to be present.

Odds ratios are used to help interpret the results from case-control studies. The odds
ratio is an estimate of relative risk.[116]

$$\text{Odds Ratio} = \frac{\#\text{ cases with disease \& exposure} \div \#\text{ cases with disease \& no exposure}}{\#\text{ cases without disease \& exposure} \div \#\text{ cases without disease \& no exposure}}$$

Although relative risk is preferred for prospective trials, the odds ratio is the approximate measure for retrospective studies. Consider the situation presented in Table 5-6,
where industrial exposure to formaldehyde in patients with and without respiratory illness
is assessed. Odds of exposure to formaldehyde is 20/180 (0.11) in cases with respiratory
illness and 5/195 (0.03) in the controls. The odds ratio is calculated as 0.11/0.03 = 3.7.
Interpretation is the same as with relative risk; greater than 1 denotes increased risk,

TABLE 5−6. CASE-CONTROL STUDY—DETERMINATION OF ODDS RATIO IN INDUSTRIAL FORMALDEHYDE EXPOSURE IN PATIENTS WITH RESPIRATORY ILLNESS

Risk Factor	Respiratory Illness	No Respiratory Illness	Total
Formaldehyde exposure	20	5	25
No industrial exposure to formaldehyde	180	195	375
Total	200	200	400

equal to 1 indicates no effect, and less than 1 indicates a protective effect. As with cohort studies, 95% CIs should be calculated. CIs are preferred because they provide some indication of precision and variability of the individual participant's outcome. A narrow CI suggests precision and less variability of the individual outcome measures. The wider the CI, the more variability observed between outcome measurements that make up the mean.

A 22-item checklist has been compiled by a group of international epidemiologists, methodologists, statisticians, researchers, and journal editors who are involved in the conduct and dissemination of observational studies.[117] This group is a collaborative initiative entitled STROBE, which stands for their general purpose of **ST**rengthening the **R**eporting of **OB**servational studies in **E**pidemiology. The purpose of the checklist is to assist with the reporting of observational trials and has been endorsed by a large number of biomedical journals. The checklist was developed to be used for reporting of cohort, case-control, and cross-sectional studies and can be found online at www.strobe-statement.org. This checklist can also be used by clinicians as a guide to assist in determining the quality of an observational trial.

Appendix 5-1 contains a list of additional questions specific to case-control studies. These specific questions are in addition to the standard questions used to evaluate randomized clinical trials noted in Chapter 4 and using basic tools such as the Ten Major Considerations Checklist discussed in the Introduction section.

CROSS-SECTIONAL STUDIES

Description

● Cross-sectional studies or prevalence surveys can be thought of as a snapshot (or slice) of time because data are collected only once on members of the study population over a period of time and evaluated as a single point in time.[118] Members of the study population do not need to all be studied at once, but each member can be studied at a different time. The key is that data are only collected once on each member. These studies differ from longitudinal studies that make a series of observations more than once on each member of the study population over a period of time. The cross-sectional study design is hypothesis generating as opposed to hypothesis testing, and is not suited for testing the effectiveness of interventions.[111] Only an association can be drawn from the results, not a cause-effect relationship. Typical examples of cross-sectional studies are surveys that evaluate opinions or situations at a fixed point in time. For a hypothetical situation concerning a drug, a cross-sectional study design could be developed to look into a large insurance database and determine how many people died suddenly within 5 years of receiving that drug. Cross-sectional studies are relatively quick and easy to perform and may be useful for measuring current health status or setting priorities for disease control.[111]

As mentioned earlier, a study is classified as cross-sectional because measurements are taken at a single point in time, even though observations may cover a period of several months or years. For example, a survey of smokers is cross-sectional when the questionnaire is administered once, even though the questions contained in the survey may focus on smoking habits over the past 10 years.

As in other observational trial designs, the research question and the relevant inclusion and exclusion criteria must be clearly and unambiguously stated.[111] Also, selection of cases must be clearly described.[100]

Evaluation

Problems that may occur during cross-sectional studies include errors in data collection and transient effects that may influence observations. Because measurements occur at only one point in time, inaccuracies in data collection may go unnoticed because there are no prior data for comparison. In studies where multiple observations occur, data collection errors, seen as outlier data, may be more easily recognized. For instance, the prevalence of a disease state may be recorded as 15% of the U.S. population in 2007. However, if looking at the same statistics for 2006, 2008, and 2009, it is possible to see the prevalence was 2.1%, 2.2%, and 2.0%, respectively. Obviously, the 2007 prevalence of 15% is quite different than the prevalence 1 year before and the next 2 years after this observation. The 2007 observation would be considered a data outlier that probably represents a data collection error. The problem is, taken as a single observation without the other years, the 2007 prevalence would appear accurate and not recognized as an error in data collection. Transient effects are temporary occurrences that are found at the time when a cross-sectional study is conducted, but are not identified if the study were repeated. A good example of transient effects is student evaluations of university professors. If a professor chooses to have students evaluate a course after a particularly grueling examination, chances are the evaluations would be poor based on students' response to the examination just taken. However, if the evaluations were administered after a curve had been applied for final grades, students may reflect on the course positively based on overall knowledge they received from the instructor, rather than a single negative experience. Transient effects are difficult to identify by a study evaluator. They may only be uncovered through retrospective evaluation of the study by the investigator. The investigator must perform a thorough assessment of all factors that may have impacted the results of the trial.

Appendix 5-1 contains a list of additional questions specific to cross-sectional studies. These specific questions are in addition to the standard questions used to evaluate other randomized clinical trials noted in Chapter 4 and using basic tools such as the Ten Major Considerations Checklist discussed in the Introduction section.

Reports Without Control Group

CASE STUDIES, CASE REPORTS, AND CASE SERIES

❸ *Case studies, case reports, and case series are observational or interventional reports describing patient or patient group exposure to a drug or technology and can be valuable to record preliminary findings that lead to further study. A key characteristic to these reports is the lack of a control or comparison group.*

Each one is different as described below[119–121]:

- Case study is a record of descriptive research that documents a practitioner's experiences, thoughts, or observations related to the care of a single patient.
- Case report is a descriptive record of a single individual in which the possibility of an association between an observed effect and a specific intervention or exposure, such as an adverse drug reaction, exists.
- Case series is a group of records (case studies) that documents a practitioner's experiences, thoughts, or observations related to the care of multiple patients with similar medical situations.

Because these reports lack comparison to a control group, they do not take into consideration other influencing factors that may also have played a role in observed outcomes.[119,120] In contrast to N-of-1 trials, a case study (either interventional or observational) does not apply clinical trial principles such as randomization and blinding to individual patients. The case study can be prospective or retrospective, whereas the N-of-1 trial design is prospective. The case study usually does not involve multiple treatment periods like that seen with N-of-1 trials. Comparisons of single patient clinical trials (N-of-1) and case studies are presented in Table 5-3.[122]

Design and methods describing conduct of a case study are not well defined, and that can make interpretation of case study results difficult.[120] For example, beneficial effects attributed to a drug or treatment under investigation may actually be a function of spontaneous remission of signs and symptoms of the disease, a placebo effect, and/or related to physicians' attitudes that may influence patient outcome.

Case studies, however, are an integral part of the biomedical literature. They have played an important role in identifying treatments for rare disorders where large subject pools cannot be identified.[118,123] Case studies, reports, or series may also be useful for early recognition of drug toxicities and teratogenicity. A newly recognized value of case reports is utilization for understanding potential toxicities of DS products (botanical and non-botanical). Because the FDA does not regulate these products and adverse event reporting is scarce, often safety information is not well defined for these products. Thus, published case reports may play a somewhat larger role for dietary supplements in suggesting potential safety problems than for traditional drug products.

When possible, results of case studies, reports, or series should be confirmed with randomized controlled clinical trials.[119,120] Case studies, reports, and series serve as an important initial step in the formulation of hypotheses. When case studies, reports, or series show a beneficial effect of a drug or treatment in diseases whose outcomes are consistently grim, or when all other treatments have failed, the results can be applied to patients in clinical practice.

Appendix 5-1 contains a list of additional questions specific to case studies, reports, and series. These specific questions are in addition to the standard questions used to evaluate other randomized clinical trials noted in Chapter 4 and use basic tools such as the Ten Major Considerations Checklist discussed in the Introduction section.

Survey Research

❹ *Survey research is information gathered from an identified group with conclusions drawn and applied to a larger population. This gathered information is considered either descriptive (such as opinions and attitudes) or explanatory (such as explaining a cause and effect) in nature and the validity of the results depends on the quality of the study's internal rigor.* Survey research is used to study the incidence, distribution, and relationships of sociologic and psychological variables.[124] It is used to collect information from a sample and generalize the findings to a larger population. Data obtained from survey research have been used for many purposes including helping investigators identify, assess, and compare respondents' ideas, feelings, plans, beliefs, and demographics.[125] Surveys may be used to determine how health care programs should be implemented by utilizing the opinions of experts with experience in a particular area, to study effectiveness of a program by surveying individuals who have used its services, or to understand attitudes and behaviors of patients or members of the profession the program affects. For example, directors of pharmacy may survey other hospitals to determine salary ranges in order to decide whether salary increases are needed to remain competitive in the job market. Patient surveys are prepared and sent to postsurgical patients to document the care and satisfaction perceptions so changes can be made in the process for improvement. The ability to critically evaluate such literature has become a necessity for the practitioner due to an increased emphasis on this type of research in the medical literature.

TYPES OF SURVEYS

There are two basic types of surveys published in the biomedical literature. Descriptive surveys attempt to identify psychosocial variables such as attitudes, opinions, knowledge, and behaviors in a population, while explanatory surveys attempt to explain causal relationships between variables.[125] The dependent variables, such as knowledge and behavior, are often compared to independent variables such as age, sex, or education.

SURVEY SAMPLES

A key characteristic of survey samples is that they represent the population of interest.[124] Since it is next to impossible to gather data from an entire population, a subset of that population known as a sample (**sample frame**) is utilized. For example, instead of trying to gather data from every person with heart failure in the United States, a sample of patients with heart failure receiving a specific therapy is identified. The larger the sample size, the more likely this subset will accurately reflect the whole population of interest.[124] There are no specific rules that help the investigator determine the exact size of the sample frame; however, a larger number is expected if a difference in specific characteristics by subgroups within the population are to be tested rather than simply describing a population's characteristics.[126] In addition, to more closely represent the entire population of interest, the sample should possess similar characteristics. Any significant differences should be identified and justified by the investigators.

DATA COLLECTION METHODS

The two most common methods of collecting survey data are questionnaires and interviews.[124] Questionnaires can take several forms including paper mailed to participants, electronic format via e-mail, or Internet-based programs, for example, SurveyMonkey®. In some cases, a combination of both paper and electronic formats are used to provide different options for the participant to choose their preferred method. This combination of methods can improve sample coverage in the case that some participants may not have access to a computer. Response rates have been increased by using various techniques such as improving the visual appeal and graphics, using appropriate font size for the sample frame, logically ordering items, and arranging those items in a clear fashion on each page. Needless to say, careful attention to detail is necessary while creating the questionnaire, also referred to as the **survey instrument**.

Interviewing participants by phone, computer, or in person is also used to collect survey data.[124] Key advantages of interviewing in person include visually identifying nonverbal responses or body language and being able to clarify the survey question. Interviewing, in general, allows the interviewer to use follow-up probing questions to gain more information and request clarification of unclear responses. Even though the interview has these additional benefits compared to a questionnaire, increased cost and extensive time requirements make interviewing impractical in some cases such as large sample sizes.

ERRORS AFFECTING PRECISION AND ACCURACY

Four sources of error have been described that can threaten the reliability of survey results and must be evaluated by readers.[125] Each source will be described and how to evaluate a survey article for these errors will be discussed in the Evaluation of Survey section.

Coverage Error

The first type of error, **coverage error**, is a bias in a statistic that occurs when the target population you want to survey does not coincide with the sample population that is actually surveyed. This type of error can compromise the ability to generalize study results.[125] Coverage error can be due to an inadequate sample frame or flaws in execution of the data collection. For example, people without telephones or those with unlisted numbers would be excluded from a sample frame of names from a telephone directory. In the case of a web-based survey of a target population that includes urban and rural areas, those persons without a computer or e-mail address would be excluded from the list of e-mail addresses provided for the survey.

Sampling Error

Sampling error refers to the difference between the estimate derived from a sample survey and the true value that would result if a census of the entire target population were taken under the same conditions. As mentioned earlier, surveying an entire target population is not feasible; however, identifying a sample of the target population is more doable but brings with it the potential for a sampling error. This error occurs when the researcher surveys a subset that does not represent all possible subjects within the population of interest.[125] The use of random sampling procedures and larger sample sizes can be used to minimize sampling error. Sample error is reported usually as the mean + **standard error of the mean (SEM)** (see Chapter 6 for more information).

Measurement Error

Measurement error occurs when the collection of data is influenced by the interviewer or when the survey item itself is unclear from the respondent's point of view. When measurement error occurs, a subject's response cannot be compared to other responses.[125] The survey method used to collect the data may be one source of measurement error. Face-to-face interviewers may influence the responses of the person being surveyed. The survey instrument itself may be ambiguous and open to interpretation. Bias can be introduced into a survey by the cover letter or sponsoring body; either may lead the respondent to one desired response rather than measuring the true response.

Lastly, measurement error can occur when a respondent replies with a preferred or more socially acceptable answer rather than the real answer. A well-designed survey instrument can minimize the chances of this type of error occurring. The well-designed survey instrument takes into account the abilities and motivation of the respondent to respond correctly (i.e., written at an appropriate educational level). **Parallel forms** (usually consisting of alternatively worded items placed throughout the survey) of either specific survey items or the entire survey instrument have been used to increase reliability of survey research. The use of such forms requires the calculation of correlation coefficients (see Chapter 6) between the parallel items and survey instruments.

Accurate assessment of measurement error relies on the availability of the questionnaire or tool used to collect data so that readers may analyze wording. Unfortunately, many articles relating results of survey research do not include the actual questionnaire used in the survey due to space and ownership issues. Lengthy questionnaires take up valuable journal space and the publisher may decide not to include them. Some authors do not want to give away the intellectual work that they invested in developing a good questionnaire and decide not to publish it. These factors make it impossible for the reader to evaluate the wording and, thus, the objectivity of questions or quality of the survey instrument. Readers need to look for author information provided on the reliability and validity of their survey instrument to ensure that quality measures were evaluated.

Nonresponse Error

Finally, **nonresponse error** occurs when a significant number of subjects in a sample do not respond to the survey. A type of bias called **nonresponse bias** can result in surveys, where the answers of respondents differ from the potential answers of those who did not answer (see Table 5-4). If the responders' demographics, characteristics, or responses differ significantly from the nonresponders in a way that influences the results, then nonresponse error would be suspect.[125] Unfortunately, this bias is difficult to assess since the nonresponders' answers are never known. One way researchers attempt to minimize the chances of this error is to strive for high response rates in the 80% to 90% range. However, research into nonresponse error has created results that find no correlation between nonresponse rate and nonresponse bias, suggesting that low response rates are not responsible for causing nonresponse bias.[127–129] Other researches have proposed that nonresponse bias can be determined examining high-quality para-data (data regarding the survey operations) that include call histories, contact histories, the mode used to complete the survey, any incentives provided, and acceptance of any proxy interviews.[130] This information would provide the ability to conduct a nonresponse bias analysis. In addition, transparency should be evaluated along with referencing a publicly available quality profile that includes a nonresponse bias analysis performed by the survey research team. Including comparative demographics and other important variables between the target population and sample frame would also assist in determining how closely the two groups' characteristics match.[131]

EVALUATION OF SURVEY

In order to accurately assess the survey's validity (i.e., robustness) and evaluate these potential sources of error and bias, the methods section should be heavily scrutinized. Foremost, a description of study methodology with enough detail to replicate the study should be provided. The standards for rigor in survey design, conduct, and reporting should be no lower than the standards for other forms of clinical research.[126]

Factual Data and Internal Validity

Attempts to assess validity and reliability of the survey and efforts made to validate factual data should be described. For example, demographics of individual hospitals can be verified using American Hospital Association data. Asking more than one question about a concept can increase the **internal validity** of a survey.[125] For example, a respondent who answers yes to a positively worded statement would be expected to answer no to the same concept when worded in a negative fashion. A correlation analysis such as the Cronbach alpha or similar statistical test that measures correlation between items should be calculated and the coefficient factor(s) reported in the article.[125] The coefficient alpha is interpreted in the same fashion that coefficients of reliability are interpreted (i.e., 0 indicates no consistency between responses while increasing consistency is seen as you approach 0.8 to 1).

Sample Size

Additionally, the reader should evaluate the comprehensiveness, probability of selection, and efficiency of the sample frame.[124,126] A sample frame describes the population that will actually be drawn from to make up the survey sample. A sample is comprehensive if all members of a population had a chance to be chosen and no one was systematically excluded. For example, to survey elderly people, it is appropriate to survey all households that make up the sample frame to determine if elderly individuals live there. In addition to providing information about the sampling frame, the methods section should provide a description of interviewers (age, sex, ethnicity, and so forth) and the effect interviewers may have had on the data.

Sampling Strategy and Response Rates

Sampling strategy and response rates should also be stated. The methods section should supply the reader with enough information to ensure that nonresponse error was assessed and measures were taken to control the error.[130,131] Repeated attempts to obtain completed questionnaires from initial nonrespondents will yield higher response rates and more accurate results than if no follow-ups are performed. For example, attempts at other times of the day should be made for phone surveys and a second reminder postcard should be sent for mailed surveys. For web-based surveys, e-mail reminders serve as follow-ups. Additionally, one way to minimize the problem of poor response rates is to sample (by phone) a small group of nonresponders to determine if their responses differ substantially from responders, although this may not be possible. If results do not differ, the survey remains valid. Furthermore, authors should relate as much information about nonresponders as possible. Although survey result information has not been gathered, authors may have demographic and geographic data based on addresses and other information originally obtained.

Survey Instrument Reliability

The methods section should also describe techniques used to assess the reliability (i.e., can the results of the survey be repeated by another investigator) of the survey instrument and present the results of reliability estimates.[125] As discussed earlier under internal validity, a statistical test that measures correlation between items should be used as a reliability estimate. In general, the higher the reliability estimate (correlation coefficient), the more confidence the reader may place in the results published. A more complete review of correlation analysis is presented later (see Chapter 6). Additionally, any relevant elements of the survey research administration process (i.e., whether a pretest or pilot test was used) should be described. A pretest or pilot test is an assessment of a questionnaire made before full-scale implementation to identify and correct problems such as faulty questions, flawed response options, or interviewer training deficiencies.[126] Subjects administered the pretest not only answer the survey questions, but also answer questions about the clarity, length, and ease of understanding the actual instrument and may contribute other questions that should be included.

Other Considerations

Internet or e-mail-based surveys have increased in popularity due to lower expense and improved efficiency.[126] Even though there is a perception of easier data collection with this method, the researcher should not abandon the good principles used for traditional mail surveys. Web-based surveys have the potential to be forwarded on to inappropriate or unintended subjects. In addition, undeliverable e-mails, due to incorrect e-mail addresses, can affect the response rate and overall most appropriate denominator for calculating response rate and, therefore, nonresponse rate. The researchers should describe the method of dissemination such as e-mail with a link to the survey and what web-based survey program was used.

Surveys are a commonly used research tool and are capable of providing a wealth of information on many aspects of a given target population. Ensuring validity of information gained through survey research, however, relies on critical evaluation of results through a thorough assessment of the study's internal rigor.[124-126] The ability to evaluate such research results is highly dependent on the amount and quality of information presented in the methods section.

Appendix 5-1 contains a list of additional questions specific to survey research studies. These specific questions are in addition to the standard questions used to evaluate other randomized clinical trials noted in Chapter 4 and use basic tools such as the Ten Major Considerations Checklist discussed in the Introduction section.

Postmarketing Surveillance Studies

Prior to approval by the FDA, drugs undergo testing in a relatively limited number of patients.[132] Once approved, experience in patients escalates and previously unrecognized rare adverse events may be identified. The drug may also be found to be useful for conditions not described in the product labeling.

Postmarketing surveillance studies are phase IV studies that follow drug use after market approval. See Chapter 21 for further explanation of the phases of the drug development process. The phase IV studies are useful in identifying new, potentially serious effects of drugs.[133] A number of drugs have been removed from the market after approval following identification of such problems (e.g., fenfluramine, rofecoxib [Vioxx™], valdecoxib [Bextra®], propoxyphene [Darvon®], and hydromorphone hydrochloride extended release capsules [Palladone™ Extended-Release]). Postmarketing surveillance studies also allow assessment of drug use outside of product labeling and may identify areas for further research.

Many types of study designs are used in phase IV studies, including cross-sectional, case-control, cohort, and randomized controlled clinical trials; however, the inclusion and exclusion criteria are not as stringent as clinical trials performed for regulatory market approval.[132] These studies can answer questions about drug interactions, identify potential new indications for the product, and gather information about the consequences of an overdose. In addition, the studies can provide efficacy in a larger and broader population—patients with different disease states and demographics that may not have been fully evaluated in the original clinical trials.

Perhaps one of the most important functions of postmarketing surveillance is in the area of adverse event reporting. The Institute of Medicine has recommended that the FDA look at the risk-benefit profile and make publicly available a Benefit and Risk Management Plan of approved drugs at specific predetermined times after initially entering the market.[134] Currently, most of the information on postmarketing safety of the product comes from spontaneous adverse reaction reports. Reporting of events associated with a product by the health care practitioner to a regulatory agency or organization (FDA MedWatch Program, the Adverse Event Reporting System [AERS or FAERS], the Vaccine Adverse Event Reporting System [VAERS], World Health Organization for International Drug Monitoring [VigiBase™], European Medicines Agency or EMA [EudraVigilance], or the pharmaceutical company that markets the product) is the primary means for gathering this information.[135-137] Pharmaceutical companies are required to maintain a database of these spontaneous reports. This database is monitored for increases in frequency of certain events or the appearance of serious unexpected events. If it is determined there is a causal relationship between the drug and the event, the product labeling may be changed to reflect either new events or events with increasing frequency. For more information about this topic, see Chapter 17.

There are several limitations to this type of data collection.[136] The information is taken from the reporter who must make a diagnosis and assessment of causality. Data may be underreported because it is a voluntary system and this may bias the estimation of incidence. Reports may vary in quality or thoroughness and the database may not be suitable for detecting adverse reactions with high background rates in the population. See Chapter 17 for additional information.

The principles of literature evaluation described in previous sections are also applicable to these studies. The method used to evaluate the study is dependent on the type of information collected. Note that when the purpose of these trials is focused on safety, they may be only powered for efficacy and not safety, which may not be sufficient to identify a statistically significant difference in safety, if one really exists. In this case, there is a possibility of a Type II error with resulting confusion when the results show "no statistically significant difference" between the drug and the comparator for various side effects. The reader is directed to the specific section of this chapter or book for the exact method to evaluate the study.

Appendix 5-1 contains a list of additional questions specific to postmarketing surveillance studies. These specific questions are in addition to the standard questions used to evaluate other randomized clinical trials noted in Chapter 4 and use basic tools such as the Ten Major Considerations Checklist discussed in the Introduction section.

Review Articles

Review articles consist of three very different entities—the narrative review (nonsystematic and qualitative review), the systematic review (qualitative review), and the meta-analysis (quantitative review.) ❺ *Meta-analyses are the only type of review providing new quantitative data derived from combining the results of each study in the meta-analysis and performing a statistical analysis on that data set. The overall reliability of a meta-analysis is ultimately dependent on the quality of the individual studies,* **homogeneity** *between these studies, and appropriateness of the analysis.* Reviews are becoming more common in the literature and are relied on as an efficient method for keeping up with the large amount of information presented to the health care professional every day. Once a reader understands differences between individual study designs and characteristics for evaluating strengths and weaknesses within individual studies, it will become easier to analyze differences between publications that attempt to combine results from multiple studies.

Review articles, with the exception of meta-analysis, that essentially consist of analysis and interpretation of previously conducted research studies are classified as tertiary literature (see Chapter 3), although they are often used as secondary sources because they can lead readers to primary literature references. Meta-analyses are classified as primary literature since they create new data. Review articles discussing treatment of disease states or clinical aspects of drug therapy enable practitioners to gain insight into a topic or question of interest and may provide more current information than textbooks.

Although the purpose of review articles is to present the truth found among conflicting and variable primary literature, this does not always occur. Reviews may be subject to author biases or inaccuracies in the literature search.[138] Narrative (nonsystematic) literature reviews generally do not apply systematic methods, such as formal criteria for selection of studies, and they address broad rather than focused clinical questions. In addition, they provide qualitative rather than quantitative information. They often educate readers about the authors' interpretations of selected evidence rather than using a systematic approach to evidence evaluation. Frequently, authors are experts on the topic and know the conclusions prior to conducting the review.

In contrast, systematic reviews do use formal criteria for trial selection and interpretation of study results and authors determine the conclusions based on the data reviewed. These reviews provide qualitative information that is of a higher quality than narrative reviews based on the fact that a systematic approach was utilized. Meta-analyses (sometimes referred to as quantitative systematic reviews) differ from both narrative and systematic reviews in that they provide new data that are quantitative in nature. Due to increased emphasis on evidence-based practice, narrative reviews have largely been replaced by both systematic reviews and meta-analyses as a source of authoritative, summative information.

It is important to note that it is not uncommon to find conclusions of general overviews, systematic reviews, or meta-analyses conflict with one another.[138] Differences in research methodology may explain conflicting conclusions noted in selected published studies. Other explanations for conflicting conclusions include differences in study populations, type of intervention, or study endpoint, as well as chance or confounding issues.[139] In some cases, the amount of high-quality data may not be sufficient to come to a valid conclusion; in others, clinical judgment of authors may place more weight on certain findings over other results. Readers of review articles need to determine whether studies included in the review are broad enough to apply to their clinical situation. Table 5-7 illustrates the primary differences between narrative reviews—qualitative, systematic reviews—qualitative, and meta-analyses—quantitative reviews.

NARRATIVE (NONSYSTEMATIC) REVIEW—QUALITATIVE

A narrative (nonsystematic) review is a summary of research that lacks a description of systematic methods.[139,140] Narrative reviews are considered tertiary literature because they provide information in much the same manner as found in textbooks, but are sometimes used like secondary references because they also contain extensive and up-to-date bibliographies. Narrative reviews may pertain to one specific clinical question or disease state, or to topics related to pharmacy administration (e.g., pharmacy and therapeutics

TABLE 5-7. COMPARISON OF DIFFERENT TYPES OF REVIEWS

Feature	Narrative Review	Systematic Review	Meta-Analysis
Clinical question	Often broadly defined	Clearly defined and focused	Clearly defined and focused
Literature search	Methods not usually explicitly described	Predefined strategy, explicit and comprehensive	Predefined strategy, explicit and comprehensive
Studies included	Inclusion methods not usually described	Predefined inclusion and exclusion criteria	Predefined inclusion and exclusion criteria
Unpublished literature included	Not usually	Possibly	Possibly
Blinding of reviewers	No	Yes	Yes
Analysis of data—results of that analysis	Variable and subjective—no new data produced	Rigorous and objective—no new data produced	Rigorous and objective—new data produced
Results statistically evaluated	No	No	Yes
Type of results	Qualitative	Qualitative	Quantitative

Source: Reprinted with permission from Bryant PJ, Pace HA. The pharmacist's guide to evidence-based medicine for clinical decision making. Bethesda, MD: American Society of Health-System Pharmacists. ©2009. p. 123.

committees). To ensure the quality of narrative reviews, the reader should determine the level of trustworthiness and narrative truth associated with the review.[141]

It should be noted that a relatively newer method of review has been showing up in the literature called a meta-narrative review.[142] The meta-narrative review examines the historical progress of a research tradition (a series of linked studies that build on each other) over time. The methods for developing the meta-narrative review vary greatly and for this reason they are difficult to evaluate; however, the same evaluative principles used for narrative reviews can be applied to meta-narrative reviews.

In general, narrative reviews are useful educational articles by gathering dispersed information about a topic together into a single readable document. These documents' bibliographies can provide additional articles on a subject that are not identified in a literature search.

Appendix 5-1 contains a list of questions specific to narrative reviews that can be used to evaluate the quality of these reviews. These specific questions are in addition to the standard questions used to evaluate randomized clinical trials noted in Chapter 4 and use basic tools such as the Ten Major Considerations Checklist discussed in the Introduction section.

SYSTEMATIC REVIEW—QUALITATIVE

- A systematic review is defined as a research summary conducted in an organized and reproducible manner that addresses a clinical question.[143,144] Systematic reviews are qualitative in nature and for this reason they should be developed in a responsible manner with the highest level of integrity.[145] A meta-analysis is where selected studies have been statistically pooled or aggregated and analyzed resulting in a single estimated effect.
- Meta-analyses can be thought of as a specific methodological and statistical technique (or tool) for combining quantitative data that generates new data. Meta-analyses will be discussed in greater detail later in this chapter.
- Systematic overviews that summarize scientific evidence (in contrast to nonsystematic narrative reviews that mix opinions and evidence) are becoming increasingly prevalent. These overviews address questions of treatment, causation, diagnosis, or prognosis and are considered superior to nonsystematic (narrative) reviews of any given topic.[146]

Systematic reviews require a set of specific criteria be identified up-front regarding article selection and the process used to evaluate those selected articles.[143,144,146] Systematic reviews should concentrate on a clearly defined issue that is of importance to practice. Specific criteria should be used to select articles from the primary literature to be included in the review.[147] For valid conclusions to be derived from systematic reviews, authors must clearly define the study population or topic of interest and include only those studies using valid research methods. Authors of systematic reviews use a variety of resources to identify studies for the systematic review. Use of a single database is not likely to capture all relevant studies and results in reference bias. A combination of databases (such as MEDLINE®, PubMed®, International Pharmaceutical Abstracts, and Embase® for literature published outside the United States, study bibliographies, and experts in the field) should be used to identify studies for evaluation. For valid conclusions to be derived from systematic reviews, authors must clearly define the study population or topic of interest and include only those studies using valid research methods. For example, authors would have the choice of assessing women who are either pre- or postmenopausal in a systematic review focused on the utility of chemotherapy in improving survival following mastectomy in breast cancer patients. Conclusions of this systematic review are likely to be very different depending on which subsets of breast cancer patients are selected. In addition, the authors' initial literature search would probably reveal a collection of studies that use a wide variety of research techniques. Only those studies meeting strict criteria for validity as discussed in Chapter 4 should be included in the review. Poorly controlled, nonrandomized, unblinded studies should be excluded to produce the most reliable results.

The risk of biases associated with publication selection for the systematic review can exist.[143,148] Consideration should be given to inclusion of unpublished data (e.g., data on file at the manufacturer or personal communication with investigators) in addition to published studies, because it has been determined that published studies are more often of a positive nature than unpublished studies, a situation termed **publication bias.**[149] Researchers are now required to register their individual studies and provide data to an FDA website (http://www.clinicaltrials.gov), and this is a good site to find unpublished studies ongoing or completed. Unfortunately, this website only provides summative information, so the quality of the evidence often cannot be determined. The benefit of using unpublished studies is to include more data from which to draw a conclusion. A drawback is that unpublished studies have likely not undergone a peer review and revision process; errors and unclearly stated conclusions may be present. Language bias, in which only articles published in the author's primary language are used, may also affect results. In order to reduce selection bias, review authors choosing articles should be blinded to (1) names of the study authors (to avoid political or personal issues), (2) institution of publication, and (3) results of the studies. For the initial choice of study inclusion, only the methods section should be reviewed. In addition, because of the subjective nature of some aspects of analysis, two or more authors should critique each study under consideration and all evaluators should concur on which studies will be included in the systematic review.

A systematic review article should provide a table that summarizes the results from each study included in the review.[143,146,148] Outcomes described in the systematic review article should be meaningful and, if the trial is a clinical trial, clinically relevant. For example, improved survival rate is a more desirable endpoint than reduction in total cholesterol for the hydroxymethylglutaryl-Coenzyme A (HMG-CoA) reductase inhibitors literature. Authors should also assess benefits versus risks associated with the therapy under review.

Multiple publications exist that describe the steps and required processes to construct or evaluate a systematic review; however, the Preferred Reporting Items for Systematic reviews and Meta-Analyses (PRISMA) guidelines are considered the gold standard at this point in time.[148] This guideline evolved from the QUality Of Reporting Of Meta-analyses (QUOROM) guidance document developed by an international group in 1996. Of significance with the PRISMA statement is an included 27-point checklist that streamlines the evaluation process.

Appendix 5-1 contains a list of additional questions specific to systematic reviews. These specific questions are in addition to the standard questions used to evaluate other randomized clinical trials noted in Chapter 4 and use basic tools such as the Ten Major Considerations Checklist discussed in the Introduction section.

META-ANALYSIS—QUANTITATIVE

Meta-analysis is an analytical technique designed to statistically combine and weigh the data from multiple studies to provide a quantitative and objective assessment.[150–153] This analysis is widely used to provide supporting evidence for clinical decision making. The use of meta-analyses to generate information has grown to an overwhelming amount over the last 25 plus years.[152]

Types of Meta-Analyses

There are two general approaches being used to conduct a meta-analysis: **pair-wise analysis** and **network analysis**.[154] The pair-wise approach is the traditional method to compile a meta-analysis by synthesizing the results of different trials to obtain an overall estimate of the treatment effect of one intervention relative to the control. The other approach is termed network analysis, also known as multiple treatment comparison or mixed treatment meta-analysis. A network meta-analysis simultaneously compares and ranks a "network" of treatments in which subsets have been compared in individual studies.[154,155]

Pair-wise meta-analyses use one of two statistical models: fixed-effects or random-effects models.[156] Put simply, the fixed-effect model is used when the intention is to apply the results only to the included studies, and the random-effects model is used when the intent is to generalize the results beyond the included studies. The actual decision to select one model or the other is complex and involves specific criteria. Table 5-8 provides a comparison between fixed-effect and random-effects models.

Common statistical tests used to combine the data from multiple studies when developing a pair-wise meta-analysis are the Mantel-Haenszel method and the Inverse Variance method.[151] The Mantel-Haenszel method is used when the primary outcome measure is categorical data. When the primary outcome measure is continuous data, the Inverse Variance method is used to combine the data.

TABLE 5–8. FIXED-EFFECTS COMPARED TO RANDOM-EFFECTS MODEL FOR META-ANALYSIS

Criteria to Consider	Fixed-Effects Model	Random Effects Model
Goal of Statistical Inference	One fixed parameter	No common fixed parameter
	All studies estimate same common fixed parameter	Studies estimate different parameters
Number of Studies Included	Small number – approximately 5 studies	Large number – large enough to make generalization inferences
Statistical Heterogeneity	Use when assume homogeneity between studies	Use when cannot assume homogeneity between studies
Probability of a Common Effect Size	Assume one common effect	Assume each study estimates a different underlying true effect

As mentioned earlier, the network analysis is used when multiple treatments from several studies need to be analyzed simultaneously.[154,157–159] The network meta-analysis is being used more frequently since the mid-2000s, along with a number of publications addressing the methodology used in this approach. The approach has been criticized for its complexity, assumptions involved, and outputs that are not well understood or interpreted by clinicians.[160] These reports have raised concerns about the conduct and reporting of network meta-analyses and put into question whether they are at a sufficiently strong level to be used for clinical decision making.[154]

Uses for Meta-Analyses

Meta-analyses are designed to provide greater insight into clinical dilemmas than individual clinical trials. They are especially useful when previous studies have been inconclusive or contradictory, or in situations where sample size may have been too small to detect a statistically significant difference between treatment and control groups (i.e., power not met with required sample size). Meta-analyses assist in (1) supporting or refuting lesser quality evidence, (2) overcoming reduced statistical power of small studies, (3) assessing occurrence of rare events, (4) providing guidance with limited/conflicting data, (5) displaying sample sizes and treatment effects graphically, (6) assessing heterogeneity between studies and publication bias, (7) evaluating the natural history of disease, (8) improving estimates of effect size, and (9) answering new questions not posed at the start of individual trials.[151] Meta-analyses can be used to look at both clinical trials and epidemiologic research, such as cohort and case-control studies, and are particularly useful when definitive trials cannot be conducted, results of available trials are inconclusive, or while awaiting the results of definitive trials.[151] The meta-analysis study design has been used to address important clinical questions, such as whether aspirin reduces the risk of pregnancy-induced hypertension, cholesterol lowering decreases mortality, fluoxetine increases suicidal ideations, or estrogen replacement therapy increases the risk of breast cancer.[151] The thought process involved in identifying the need for this type of analysis can be presented with a hypothetical situation regarding a drug used for the treatment of myocardial infarction. Suppose this drug is shown to be related to increases in sudden death through proarrhythmic effects based on results from a number of small trials. A meta-analysis could be performed to statistically combine the results of these small trials and increase the power of the finding that there is an association or lack of association with increased sudden death for this drug.

Issues with Meta-Analyses

Meta-analysis is a controversial tool because of the involvement of several critical conditions that, when even slightly violated, can lead to conclusions that are misleading.[152] These small violations usually occur with decisions in the designing and performing stages that require personal judgment and expertise. These stages include study identification, study selection and inclusion, availability of information, data extraction, data analysis and synthesis, and data interpretation and reporting. This can lead to creating personal biases or expectations that potentially influence the results of the meta-analysis.

Study identification and selection can be a very subjective activity.[151,152] A quality meta-analysis must clearly define the clinical question addressed by the analysis and state the hypothesis to be tested. The extensiveness of the search strategy determines the comprehensiveness of the meta-analysis. Controls such as a prospective analysis protocol should be put into place prior to the meta-analysis initiation. A prospective analysis protocol can assist in minimizing the risk of bias such as selective outcomes reporting when *post hoc* decisions are being developed. The PRISMA guidelines mentioned earlier recommend that these prospective analysis protocols be registered through the International Prospective Register of Systematic Reviews (PROSPERO—http://www.crd.york.ac.uk/Prospero/) prior to the initiation of the meta-analysis work.[161] Transparency, resulting in less conscious bias, is an important objective of this registration process. As with systematic reviews, details of literature searches that were conducted to locate primary research articles must be given and criteria for inclusion of studies in the meta-analysis must be determined prior to conducting the analysis.[151] Because computerized searches may not locate all of the relevant articles, other resources such as textbooks, experts in the field, and reference lists from clinical studies should also be consulted.

Publication bias is a form of selection bias where publication of studies is based on the magnitude, direction, or statistical significance of the results.[162] It has been documented that researchers are more likely to publish studies that demonstrate positive effects of drugs. Therefore, studies that show lack of efficacy are less likely to be located in medical literature searches than those that demonstrate beneficial effects of a drug. **Funnel plots** are used to identify the potential existence of publication bias.[151,155,163] A funnel plot is a scatterplot of treatment effect versus sample size of the studies included in the meta-analysis.[164] The treatment effect estimates should cluster around a constant value with variability in this treatment effect decreasing as size of the trial increases with

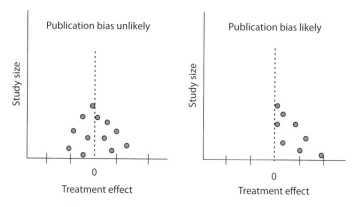

Figure 5–5. Symmetrical versus asymmetrical funnel plots.

a resultant funnel shape.[163] If the funnel plot shows an inverted symmetrical funnel shape, publication bias is probably not present (Figure 5-5). However, if an asymmetrical funnel is noted, this suggests a relationship between treatment effect and study size. An asymmetrical funnel plot indicates the possibility that publication bias is present.

The quality of the meta-analysis depends on the quality of the individual studies used to develop the meta-analysis.[151,152,154,155,165] As mentioned earlier, the actual selection of information found can also be a subjective process.[151] For instance, data from sources such as conference abstracts, unpublished reports, or other documents not distributed or indexed by commercial publishers are known as "**gray literature**." Inclusion of this type of literature can potentially reduce biases; however, these types of documents often have not undergone the rigors of peer review and publisher editing, thereby increasing the chance of bias influencing the meta-analysis. There are risks using data from gray literature, including inaccurate information (not completely correct information), misinformation (incorrect information), and disinformation (false information deliberately provided in order to influence opinions), that can confound the meta-analysis results. To minimize this type of bias, the decision to include or exclude specific studies in the analysis is usually based on some criteria such as study design quality, language, date of publication, and duplicate data or data published multiple times such as interim analysis, final analysis, and analyses of various subgroups all from the same study patient population.[151] Specifically, study quality can be determined via a rating system that takes into consideration important characteristics of a well-done randomized clinical trial. There are several rating systems available; however, one of the more well-known systems is the Jadad Scoring system.[166] Another more recent scoring system that takes into consideration several more study characteristics to determine quality is the Ten Major Considerations Checklist.[2]

One of the main problems with meta-analyses is that the studies included are different, which results in heterogeneity.[151] Some degree of heterogeneity will always exist between the individual studies that go into a meta-analysis. The key is to investigate and determine if the studies can be combined reliably. The Chi-squared test is used to identify if the spread of results between the studies is statistically significant or just due to chance (heterogeneity is present). Once identified, the degree of inconsistency across studies is determined using the I-squared test (value >40% is considered significant inconsistency). The higher the percentage, the greater the heterogeneity. Even heterogeneity brought into the meta-analysis by smaller-sized studies should be determined.[167] Caution should be used when pooling results of heterogeneous studies.

Sensitivity analysis is performed once the data have been extracted from the chosen studies and analysis complete.[151] The sensitivity analysis helps to determine if the results of the meta-analysis are robust. Studies that meet specific criteria are removed, such as those with poor quality, that are less similar to the others, conference abstracts, or unpublished data. The sensitivity analysis is rerun without each of these identified studies to determine the effect that an individual study has on the overall results. Generally, studies that have a significant effect on the results of the meta-analysis are removed from the analysis. Those individual studies with lesser effects are still combined in the meta-analysis; however, they should be reported in the article by the investigators.

The preferred method to present results obtained from meta-analyses is the **forest plot** (Figure 5-6).[151] The forest plot illustrated in Figure 5-6 describes the results of a meta-analysis of a new antiemetic versus standard of care for preventing chemotherapy-induced nausea and vomiting. The mean odds ratio for the new antiemetic compared

Figure 5–6. Forest plot.

to the standard of care (including the 95% CI) is plotted for each study. The odds ratio represents a ratio between two values, for instance nausea and vomiting rates from highly emetic chemotherapy between two interventions such as this new antiemetic and standard of care therapy. The odds ratio is the preferred measurement, rather than relative risk, to be calculated for retrospective analyses. The null hypothesis value defined as no difference between treatment groups for the odds ratio (new antiemetic versus standard of care therapy) is one. Because of this, a statistically significant difference in favor of the new antiemetic would be illustrated as a mean odds ratio and 95% CI greater than 1 (e.g., mean = 2.64 with 95% CI, 1.56 to 3.89), as noted by the #4 study in the forest plot. A statistically significant difference in favor of standard of care over the new antiemetic would be represented as a mean odds ratio less than 1 (0.30 with 95% CI, 0.19 to 0.54). Note there were no studies in this meta-analysis that favored standard of care over the new antiemetic. At the bottom of the forest plot is the pooled odds ratio from all the individually plotted studies included in the meta-analysis. For this meta-analysis, the overall mean odds ratio was 1.80 with a 95% CI of 0.97 to 2.26. These values represent a statistically significant difference in odds ratios favoring the new antiemetic compound compared to standard of care. The advantage of illustrating the meta-analysis results using a forest plot is that each study's results are presented in a visual display. Note: The size of the individual parallelograms represents the relative size of that study's patient population. With this visual display, the practitioner can quickly interpret the overall results of the meta-analysis at the same time, being able to see the contributions made to the overall result by each included study.

Evaluation of Meta-Analyses

Several points should be considered when evaluating meta-analyses.[168] Specific standards have been developed and accepted to help authors improve the reporting of meta-analyses in the literature.[161,169,170] These standards that consist of a 27-item checklist are referred to as the PRISMA statement mentioned earlier. More recently, a 17-item checklist has been proposed to serve as a guideline to assist authors in preparing protocols for planned meta-analyses.[171] The checklist is considered the minimum set of items to be included in the protocol.

Overall, meta-analyses should be interpreted with caution, remembering that conclusions depend on the quality and similarity of the studies included. Meta-analysis can be a powerful way to summarize combined data from clinical trials thereby increasing the sample size in an attempt to present more valid results.[152] Like all types of research evidence, meta-analyses require careful evaluation to determine their validity and applicability in practice.[162]

Appendix 5-1 contains a list of questions specific to meta-analyses.[161] These specific questions are in addition to the standard questions used to evaluate other randomized clinical trials noted in Chapter 4 and use basic tools such as the Ten Major Considerations Checklist discussed in the Introduction section (Case Study 5-3).

Case Study 5–3: Meta-Analysis

A meta-analysis was conducted to determine if there was an increased risk of developing diabetes in patients taking statins for lipid-lowering effects. MEDLINE®, Embase®, and the Cochrane Central Resister of Controlled Trials from 2000 to 2015 were used to identify randomized controlled trials of statins. Only trials with greater than 1,200 patients with identical follow-up for both groups and duration of greater than 1 year were included. Studies in patients with organ transplants or the need for hemodialysis were excluded. Heterogeneity was measured between trials. A calculated risk estimate for the incident of diabetes was used in conjunction with a random-effects meta-analysis approach. Thirteen statin trials with 88,132 participants were identified. Of these 88,132 participants, 4,142 (2,065 were assigned statins and 2,077 control treatment) developed diabetes during a mean 5 years. From the results, statin therapy was associated with an 8% increased risk for incident diabetes (odds ratio [OR] 1.08; 95% CI, 1.01 to 1.16). There was very little heterogeneity between trials (10%). A meta-regression exhibited that the risk of development of diabetes with statins was highest with older participants. The level of significance was set at alpha = 0.05. Begg's funnel plots of trials included in the meta-analysis were performed and showed very little publication bias. Forest plots were utilized to display the results of the meta-analysis. All 13 trials assessed $HbA1_c$ as the primary outcome measure as an indicator of diabetes. In addition, participant attrition was less than 20% in all trials. All 13 trials used a parallel group design and similar lengths of treatment period. The authors concluded that statin therapy is associated with a slightly increased risk of development of diabetes. Patients with moderate to high cardiovascular risk or existing cardiovascular disease should not have their statin therapy discontinued.

- *The quality of this meta-analysis depends on the quality of what component of the meta-analysis?*
- *One concern with meta-analyses is publication bias. What is publication bias and what specifically has this meta-analysis performed to correctly analyze and determine the likelihood of this bias being present?*
- *The studies included in a meta-analysis should be similar. What factors associated with these studies suggest that there is a lack of or minimal heterogeneity between the studies in this meta-analysis?*
- *The results of this meta-analysis are provided in the text of the article. What method did the authors use to provide the results and why is this method preferred?*

Practice Guidelines

The Institute of Medicine defines clinical practice guidelines as "statements that include recommendations intended to optimize patient care, that are informed by a systematic review of evidence and an assessment of the benefits and harms of alternative care options."[172]

Three types of practice guidelines are published at the present time: evidence-based, formal consensus-based, and a mixture of EBM and consensus-based. These various types are differentiated by the source of information used to develop the practice guideline as well as the rigor of the process for evaluating that information. EBM practice guidelines utilize a rigorous systematic process involving review and critical evaluation of the medical literature to develop final recommendations. Formal consensus-based practice guidelines utilize experience of experts in their practice area to draw conclusions and develop recommendations. This is useful when the evidence does not exist, is not complete, or not conclusive enough to allow the development of a final recommendation. In these situations, experts are used to assist completion of practice guidelines using their expertise in those deficient areas. The mixed EBM and consensus-based practice guideline uses evidence to construct the guideline and supplements those steps without evidence with experience of the experts.

Appendix 5-1 contains a list of questions to consider when evaluating a clinical practice guideline in addition to information presented in Chapter 8. Another approach to evaluating a clinical practice guideline is to use the questions noted earlier in Chapter 4 along with the basic tools such as the Ten Major Considerations Checklist discussed in the Introduction section to evaluate key clinical trials included in the guideline. Clinical practice guidelines may not always include recent modifications made in a particular practice area. A medical literature search for quality research articles to fill the gap is sometimes needed along with using the above questions to determine the quality of that evidence when updating a clinical practice guideline for immediate use.

Health Outcomes Research

Health outcomes research encompasses literature pertaining to discussion of pharmacoeconomic, therapeutic, and nontherapeutic outcomes (such as number of visits to the emergency room and number of hospital admissions), along with QOL outcomes. Readers are referred to Chapter 7 for information on evaluating pharmacoeconomic outcome studies. This section will focus on evaluating literature that includes QOL outcome measures.

QUALITY-OF-LIFE MEASURES

Clinical trials have traditionally focused on health outcomes related to physical or laboratory measurements of response.[173] How the patient feels and functions relative to daily activities are not always captured by these measurements. A patient's perception of well-being can be the most important outcome in specific disease states. Investigators make assumptions that changes in therapy improve the patient's QOL. These assumptions require testing. For this reason, additional health outcome measurements have been developed to address a patient's QOL.

As defined by the Centers for Disease Control and Prevention (CDC), QOL is a multidimensional concept that includes subjective evaluations of positive and negative characteristics of an individual's life.[174] There are several different domains associated with the QOL including health, jobs, housing, schools, and neighborhoods, in addition to aspects of culture, values, and spirituality. In this chapter we will focus on the health domain of QOL.

❻ *The value assigned to the duration of a patient's life when altered by various impairments, functional states, perceptions, and social opportunities that have been modified by disease, injury, treatment, and social policy is termed* **health-related quality of life (HR-QOL or HRQL).**[175] HR-QOL focuses on factors that can be influenced by health care providers and systems.[176]

Three reasons exist as to why researchers and clinicians are incorporating HR-QOL into their activities.[175,177] The first reason is the fact that HR-QOL provides the patient's perception regarding their disease state and how the health care team and system is treating that disease state. Second, HR-QOL clarifies a patient's process of adjustment to their disease and the treatment being utilized. Third, HR-QOL provides important patient-specific information that helps to determine treatment regimens, plan for alterations in the current treatment regimen, and evaluate the change in interventions made by the practitioner. It should be pointed out that when utilized to capture information in clinical trials, HR-QOL can clarify the trade-offs between treatments with major benefits and health-related outcome costs.

The classification of HR-QOL measures is based on the types of patients being questioned and the desired outcome to be measured.[175,176] Two general types of HR-QOL measurements exist: generic measures and specific measures. Generic measures cover physical and mental health and are applicable to adult populations of patients. Examples include Short-Form Health Survey (SF-36 [a 36-item questionnaire], SF-12, and SF-8), CDC HRQOL—14 "Healthy Days Measure" (a questionnaire containing 4 basic questions with 10 optional questions), WHO-Quality of Life-BREF (WHOQOL-BREF) which is validated in several countries, and the EQ-5D (a simple QOL questionnaire). Specific measures cover a particular disease state and are applicable to only patients with that disease state. Examples of specific measure instruments include Asthma Quality of Life Questionnaire (33 items giving scores to activity limitations, symptoms, emotional function, and environmental exposure) and the Child Health and Illness Profile/CHIP (with five domains of satisfaction, comfort, resilience, risk avoidance, and achievement).

Although the examples provided are commonly used instruments to measure HR-QOL, there are also many others out there to consider. For this reason, the clinician will need to understand the measurement properties of an appropriate questionnaire for determining HR-QOL. Three categories of measurement are used to determine if the instrument used to collect individual patient HR-QOL is appropriate.[175] The first category is *reliability*. The questionnaire must produce consistent and reproducible measurements on an intra- and inter-observer basis. The second category is *validity* and refers to the extent the items in the questionnaire are sensible. In addition, the measure must agree with a gold standard criterion and have the ability to perform as expected. The third category is *responsiveness*. Responsiveness is the ability of the measure to accurately change over time within a patient.

Often HR-QOL is designated as a secondary endpoint with study power set and sample size calculated to detect differences only in the study's primary outcome measurements. Note that as subgroups are analyzed, the sample size of those subgroups will most likely not be powered to determine a difference; therefore, if no statistically significant difference is observed one must be cautious not to draw conclusions because of the potential for a Type II error. Additional information regarding power can be found in Figure 5-7 in this chapter and in Chapter 6.

Two statistical anomalies that have been reported more commonly in HR-QOL trials and should be watched for when evaluating these studies are the "ceiling effect" and the "floor effect." The ceiling effect is noted when patients starting out at a much higher QOL than average do not have a lot of room for improvement when treated by the intervention

Figure 5–7. Power algorithm.
SOURCE: Reprinted with permission from Bryant PJ, Pace HA. The pharmacist's guide to evidence-based medicine for clinical decision making. Bethesda, MD: American Society of Health-System Pharmacists. ©2009. p. 66.

being evaluated. The opposite is true with the floor effect. In this case, patients starting with a lower QOL than average have much more room for improvement. The potential outcome of either of these effects is skewed end results and the possibility of falsely concluding the treatment's effectiveness positively or negatively.

When evaluating a longitudinal HR-QOL study, the reviewer should be watching for response-shift bias.[178] Response-shift bias can occur when a patient's views, values, or expectations change over the time of the study. This can result in creating another factor of change on the HR-QOL measures over the study duration. For example, a patient may start out with a certain set of values and expectations when first being diagnosed with a potentially treatable form of cancer. Upon several difficult rounds of chemotherapy and the change in prognosis due to the failure of the treatment to eradicate the tumor, those original values and expectations may have changed significantly, providing the possibility of a response-shift bias.

When reviewing a study containing HR-QOL measurements, the practitioner is referred to a list of suggested questions for assistance. Appendix 5-1 contains this list of questions. These specific questions are in addition to the standard questions used to evaluate other randomized clinical trials noted in Chapter 4 and use basic tools such as the Ten Major Considerations Checklist discussed in the Introduction section.

Dietary Supplement Medical Literature

❼ *The principles and criteria used to analyze the quality of drug literature are used to analyze dietary supplement (DS) literature; however, unique additional points such as standardization and purity must be considered.* Dietary supplement (botanical and non-botanical) information is a large and growing body of medical literature that all health practitioners must delve into more frequently as patients continue to use supplements. As with standard drug literature, the ability to discern robust clinical evidence from weak clinical evidence is an essential skill that enables practitioners to make solid recommendations to patients and to other health care professionals.

Provision of DS information is similar to provision of standard drug information. Evidence is described and ranked according to the quality of the literature supporting or refuting DS product claims. The same evidence-based criteria utilized for drug literature analysis applies to DS literature. Thus large, well-designed, randomized, controlled clinical trials or well-done meta-analyses lend stronger support versus retrospective data, case series, observational data, and experiential testimonials. However, it is not unusual to have only poorly designed published trial data to support or refute a DS product's claims. This means that, for some products, the only data available concerning theoretical actions, interactions, and side effects are animal and/or *in vitro* data.

To further compound misinformation and/or misunderstandings, often trials touted as supporting efficacy of a botanical DS have actually been conducted using chemical extracts or single chemical agents. Even if trials are of good quality, it is inappropriate to apply those results to the supplement. For example, if a trial of a concentrated echinacea extract from the whole plant of *Echinacea purpurea* shows positive results for shortening duration and severity of cold symptoms, that trial cannot be used to support efficacy of a product consisting of capsules of ground *Echinacea angustifolia* root. The same concerns apply to different salt forms of non-botanical supplements.

While many evidence-based principles are easily applied to DS literature, what follows are a few issues unique to DS trials as well as the most commonly encountered methodological flaws. In addition to standard literature evaluation criteria, specifics to consider include:

- Location of literature—international literature inclusion
- Standardization of chemical components
- Adequate trial duration and sample size
- Quality and purity of product formulations
- Limited availability of high-quality evidence-based literature

INTERNATIONAL TRIALS AND INFORMATION RETRIEVAL

A majority of DS trials are conducted in Europe and Asia. Just as with prescription drug trials, practitioners must consider the appropriateness of generalizing those trial results to their own patient population. This may be of even greater concern for DS, as many "supplements" are often used as food products as well, either in the United States or in other parts of the world.

Most health professionals are familiar with the MEDLINE® database, whether searched through PubMed® or another platform. Unfortunately, studies of supplements published in foreign language journals may be overlooked when doing a literature search with only one database. Embase® (http://www.embase.com) is another large, commonly used database that indexes abstracts from a wider variety of international journals. Citations and full-text articles are also available more quickly than in MEDLINE®. These journals are often published in English or have English abstracts. While abstracts are useful to estimate the amount of potential supportive data, they do not contain enough information to properly analyze a trial's quality. Therefore, original studies must be reviewed.

No matter which databases are searched, use of adequate keywords or indexing terms is important. This is especially true for botanical supplements—plants have multiple common names and different spellings (e.g., ginkgo, gingko, ginko), different plants share common names, and official taxonomy changes frustratingly frequently. A database search should include multiple search terms in order to ensure thoroughness. Additionally, searching the references of obtained articles (i.e., bibliographic searches) is useful to identify citations of trials.

With the increased use of general online searching to identify scientific literature, the use of misleading or outright fraudulent "publications" by DS manufacturers is on the increase as well. These will often be PDF documents that appear to be full-text from scientific journals, but investigation will reveal that the journal does not actually exist. Any studies located by a general Internet search must be verified as authentic before use.

STANDARDIZATION

One important characteristic to look for in a botanical DS study is standardization of the chemical components. Plant-derived products contain many different chemical entities that fluctuate with the growing and harvesting conditions, the plant's age, and which part of the plant is used. One or more chemical entities could be considered active constituents, that is, responsible for desired pharmacologic action, which may or may not be accurately identified. Other components may be marker compounds, compounds that allow estimation of levels of other, less easily assayed, chemicals. Supplements are standardized by controlling the amount of one chemical entity, either an active constituent (if known) or a marker compound. Using a standardized chemical concentration allows for comparisons between study products and marketed products as well as between various brands of one product. For trial evaluation, it is important to assess standardization methods used by investigators. Trial investigators should discuss and document the plant or chemical substance(s) as well as the strength or salt form utilized. This is an essential element to consider for grouping trials appropriately to make "apples-to-apples" comparisons for decision making.

Plant parts are also important to consider. If a trial evaluated use of an herb's root, but the product about which a practitioner is searching for information contains the herb's leaves and flowers, the results cannot be extrapolated. The "apples-to-apples" concept also applies to non-botanical products, generally in terms of differences in salt forms. For example, glucosamine sulfate monotherapy has more evidence of benefit in osteoarthritis patients, while glucosamine hydrochloride monotherapy has little supportive evidence.

Chemical constituents of botanicals, or products derived from them, can be volatile; possible degradation must be considered in interpreting results of a trial.[179] Researchers should take active steps to verify that products used in studies are stable throughout the duration of a clinical trial.

TRIAL DURATION

As with drug clinical trials, duration of therapy is important for accurate assessment of efficacy and safety. Inadequate duration is a common flaw in DS trials. Dependent on the mechanism of action, some supplements may take several weeks to months before patients experience full benefit. Dietary supplements may appear less efficacious than they actually are if study duration is too short. If benefits are only small to moderate, a short trial may tend to overestimate responses as patients will often exhibit greater responses in the beginning of clinical trials, perhaps because of contributing placebo effect. That response may attenuate as the trial proceeds. And, just as with drug clinical trials, shorter study periods cannot predict outcomes or safety issues associated with long-term use.

TRIAL SIZE

Small subject population is a very common flaw in DS trials. Small-sized groups may not have adequate statistical power to detect a potential difference between a DS and a placebo. Adverse reactions or drug interactions can be overlooked in smaller groups versus a larger one. In addition, a small subject population can decrease trial generalizability to broader patient populations.

BLINDING

Many botanical dietary supplements have very distinctive odors and/or tastes. These characteristics complicate the process of adequately blinding study groups to ensure that participants are not able to determine whether they are taking an active ingredient or a placebo. Therefore, it is essential that researchers take extra steps to ensure that blinding is performed appropriately, and that it is effective, by comparing the percentages of subjects in each study group who are able to correctly guess to which treatment group they were assigned.

QUALITY AND PURITY

Dietary supplements can be adulterated with heavy metals, synthesis byproducts, or prescription medications. Although DS manufacturers of all sizes are now legally required to follow Dietary Supplement Good Manufacturing Practices (GMPs), the reality is that many small companies do not, and many poor quality supplements are on the market. Some manufacturers voluntarily participate in the USP Dietary Supplement Verification Program (USP DSVP, http://www.uspverified.org/), and products must meet USP monograph standards. Approved manufacturers are permitted to display a seal of approval on product labels and are listed on the USP DSVP website.

For companies that do not participate in USP's quality seal program, patients and health care practitioners can use third-party laboratories. ConsumerLab (http://www.consumerlab.com) is an example of an organization that independently evaluates specific DS brands for content purity and accurate labeling, and publishes the results online. When a product meets the quality standard, the company may, for a fee, use a seal of approval on DS labels.

MINIMAL EVIDENCE

For most supplements, few large, controlled, methodologically sound clinical trials exist. Without a body of human data, practitioners must often make counseling decisions or recommendations based on safety and efficacy data that are theoretical, from case reports or flawed trials, or from animal and/or *in vitro* studies. This can be appropriate, especially when the safety profile of the supplement is judged to be good, but decisions to use must include a very patient-specific risk-benefit analysis, that is, weighing risks of occurrence of an interaction or side effect against possible benefits of the supplement. The health literacy level of the patient is an important factor, as it is essential for the patient to be able to accurately self-monitor for adverse effects according to instructions.

OTHER SPECIAL CONSIDERATIONS

Unlike prescription drugs, dietary supplements are not legally required to be reviewed and approved by the FDA for safety and efficacy prior to marketing. The FDA has authority to take action if problems are discovered with safety or efficacy once a product is available to consumers. Patients and health care practitioners must keep in mind that the bottle a consumer purchases in the health store or supermarket cannot be guaranteed to be dosed appropriately. Unless the manufacturer is participating in a quality program such as USP, the supplement cannot be guaranteed to be labeled correctly or appropriately. Therefore, even when clinical evidence clearly supports use of an herb or supplement, the patient may not experience a benefit because the product being used is mislabeled, dosed sub-therapeutically, or incorrectly standardized.

DS use continues to be prevalent despite fluctuations in ages or ethnicities choosing to use supplements, and changes in the popularity of specific products.[180] Pharmacists must serve as reliable and approachable information resources for DS information just as they do for other medications. In community settings, supplements are often placed with over-the-counter products near the pharmacy, making pharmacists easily accessible for consumer questions and counseling. The ability to effectively evaluate DS literature is essential to making informed recommendations and appropriately counseling patients who have DS questions.

As previously mentioned, all DS clinical trials should be evaluated for quality with the same criteria as used for FDA-approved medications, but with the addition of questions that become especially important when considering both internal and external validity of DS trials:

Botanicals
- What plant species was used? Which plant part?
- Was a standardized extract used and was it appropriate?

- Was the study product stability ensured?
- Was the dose appropriate?
- Was blinding ensured and evaluated?
- Was the trial length appropriate to perceive treatment effects or differences?
- Was sample size sufficient to detect a difference between groups if one exists?

Non-botanicals
- Was a specific salt form used and was it appropriate?
- Was the dose appropriate?
- Was the trial length appropriate to perceive treatment effects or differences?
- Was sample size sufficient to detect a difference between groups if one exists?

Appendix 5-1 contains a list of questions specific to evaluation of DS studies. These are in addition to the standard questions used for evaluation of randomized clinical trials noted in Chapter 4 and use basic tools such as the Ten Major Considerations Checklist discussed in the Introduction section (Case Study 5-4).

Case Study 5–4: Trials Testing Natural Products

You are evaluating a trial comparing a natural product called *Pelargonium sidoides* (pelargonium) to placebo for treating acute bronchitis in adults. Pelargonium has been shown to stimulate the immune system and possess some minor bacteriostatic effect. The trial utilized a flavored syrup containing a standardized proprietary dose of pelargonium. The randomized double-blind placebo-controlled trial was conducted in multiple centers throughout Europe. Four hundred adult patients with acute bronchitis were randomized to receive either two teaspoons full of pelargonium syrup or an identical appearing placebo syrup three times daily for 7 days. The primary outcome measure to determine efficacy was a change in intensity of five typical bronchitis symptoms (the Integrative Medicine Outcome Scale [IMOS]). These symptoms include coughing, wheezing/whistling on expiration, expectoration, pain in the chest during coughing, and dyspnea. The IMOS is a five-point scale (from not present to extremely pronounced) and added to produce a total score with a maximum of 20 points. The data were evaluated using an ITT and a PP analysis.

Power was set at 0.80 and met based on the PP analysis. The results of the study showed a statistically and clinically significant reduction in the intensity of the symptoms as measured by the IMOS data ($p = 0.001$; alpha set at 0.05). No side effects that could be attributed to the treatment were noted. The investigators concluded that pelargonium was effective in treating bronchitis in adult patients.

- *You are evaluating this trial because you would like to have pelargonium as an option to include in the overall therapy of acute bronchitis in your patients. You have noticed several different over-the-counter products containing various amounts of pelargonium. How could this proprietary formulation of the product used in this study be a problem to extrapolating the results of this study to your patients?*
- *Like this trial, many natural product trials are conducted outside the United States. Why should you take this into consideration?*
- *Is there any concern with the duration of pelargonium therapy in this trial?*
- *What is your opinion regarding the patient numbers for this trial?*

Getting to a Clinical Decision

❽ *An understanding of strengths and limitations inherent with each design is essential to determine the overall quality of the evidence produced. Those trial designs with a high level of quality provide the most reliable evidence and that translates into the strongest recommendation/ clinical decision.*

Once the study is evaluated, the overall quality of that trial must be determined. Categorizing the quality of the trial is the bridge from literature evaluation to developing a defensible conclusion/recommendation/clinical decision. In general, trial designs can be categorized by quality. This categorization ranks each study design from very low to high in quality. These categories of different quality are referred to as levels of evidence.[2]

Several different scales that rank the quality of evidence have been developed.[181,182] Although many of these levels of evidence scales follow a similar continuum of quality, labeling of each level is highly variable. For instance, one scale may use an alphabetical system (A = highest quality and D = lowest quality of evidence) while another scale uses a numerical system (1 to 5). There are even scales that combine the two systems (e.g., 1a, 1b, 1c, 2a, 2b) to rank the study design from highest to lowest quality within each level. In addition, several of these levels of evidence scales use ambiguous descriptors such as "poorly designed" or "high-quality" study. This complicates the use of the scale and adds subjectivity, which leads to variability between scales. In other words, reproducing the same ratings between scales is difficult.

A standard level of evidence scale developed by combining the best attributes from several individual scales that are currently available has been proposed.[2] Figure 5-8 illustrates this proposed level of evidence scale. Using the level of evidence scale illustrated,

Figure 5–8. Levels of evidence.
SOURCE: Reprinted with permission from Bryant PJ, Pace HA. The pharmacist's guide to evidence-based medicine for clinical decision making. Bethesda, MD: American Society of Health-System Pharmacists. ©2009. p. 98.

the level of quality can be assigned to a trial based on the specific study design characteristics. For example, a randomized, double-blind, controlled, N-of-1 trial used to test the efficacy and safety of a new antihypertensive would be assigned either a Level 1 or Level 2 ranking. On further examination of the study's method section, the practitioner identifies that power was set; however, an inadequate number of patients were entered into the trial to meet the set power. In this case, there is a high risk of a Type II error being present or, in other words, no difference is noted when, in fact, a true difference may actually exist. It is unknown whether adding the additional patients needed to meet power would have resulted in actually observing the true difference between treatment groups. Using the diagram, the practitioner can identify that this study design is ranked as a Level 2 for quality of evidence. Note the one difference between the Level 1 and Level 2 categories is power being set and met. (See Figure 5-8 for a better understanding of how power can affect the quality of a study design.) As mentioned in the Introduction section, additional study characteristics are also considered to further evaluate the strengths and limitations, and how these attributes impact the results of the trial. The greater the number of individual strengths identified, the greater is the quality and reliability of the evidence produced by that trial. From the assigned level of evidence based on the study design and attributes, the practitioner has an understanding of the overall quality of the trial. This understanding allows the practitioner to develop a clinical decision that can be easily defended based on the evidence.

Three inputs have been identified that are involved with developing an EBM recommendation/clinical decision[2]: quality of evidence, logical reasoning, and clinical judgment. Organizing the trials by the highest level of evidence, outcome of the trial, and associated limitations allows the practitioner to formulate an initial recommendation/clinical decision statement. Identifying key points associated with efficacy, safety, cost, and special considerations/special populations can help the practitioner justify and defend his or her recommendation/clinical decision. Note that a conservative approach is taken with population-based decisions such as drug additions to a hospital formulary. These types of decisions require a more conservative approach since a whole population is affected and little detail exists about each patient in that group. This is in contrast to an individual patient therapeutic decision where a great amount of detail from the medical chart is known about that single patient, and for this reason the decision requires a less conservative approach.

Putting it all together in an EBM manner is critically important to clinical decision making. No matter what study design is used, a thorough evaluation and categorization of the quality of that evidence are necessary. Practitioners need high-quality and reliable evidence to make firm clinical recommendations/decisions. Caution should be exhibited making these decisions when lower quality or no evidence is available. In this situation the practitioner must rely on the other two components mentioned: logical reasoning and clinical judgment. Unfortunately, clinical decisions made in this manner tend to overestimate the efficacy of the intervention and underestimate the safety risk to patients.[183] For this reason, clinical decisions and recommendations should be made using the highest quality of evidence available to ensure the best patient care.

Conclusion

Although the randomized controlled trial is the most frequently used study design for clinical research, several other designs are used in specific situations. The design is chosen based on the specific clinical questions needing to be answered. In some cases, a design is used because it represents the only way a particular data set can be obtained ethically. This chapter has provided an overview of those additional types of designs. There are general questions that should be answered when evaluating any study design type. This chapter provides additional questions/points to consider that are unique for each specific design. Many clinical decisions depend on knowledge provided in the medical literature. To ensure the highest quality of care for patients, the practitioner needs to be able to determine, through efficient and effective evaluation practices, the quality and reliability of that knowledge gained from the medical literature.

Self-Assessment Questions

For each of the following questions, please select the *best* answer.

1. All of the following are design characteristics of a N-of-1 trial, except:
   a. Randomized and controlled
   b. Parallel groups
   c. Single patient
   d. Crossover component

2. A patient experiences an adverse drug reaction that is not listed in the package insert. The patient's practitioner realizes this should be shared with other practitioners so she writes and publishes this observation in the medical literature. This type of study is termed:
   a. Case series
   b. Case report
   c. Postmarketing study
   d. N-of-1 design

3. A study design that provides information that helps a practitioner decide if various levothyroxine products made by different companies are interchangeable is a:
   a. Non-inferiority study
   b. Stability study
   c. Bioequivalence study
   d. Case series

4. If the 95% CI crosses the non-inferiority margin in a non-inferiority study, this is the conclusion that can be made:
   a. Inconclusive results
   b. Non-inferiority findings
   c. Inferiority results
   d. Superiority results

5. Which of the following statements does not describe the basic adaptive clinical trial (ACT) design?
   a. Allows adaptation of various components of the design
   b. Assists in deciding adaptations based on interim analysis
   c. Uses adaptive-response strategies
   d. Provides rigor and minimal confounding factors

Trial #1: The investigators have identified and will observe 1,000 patients with coronary artery syndrome and another 1,000 patients similar to the first group but without coronary artery syndrome over a 5-year period. The primary objective of this study is to see what medical complications develop in those patients with coronary artery syndrome.

Trial #2: Investigators developed a protocol to follow as they reviewed medical charts looking for those patients with coronary artery syndrome. They then matched those charts with additional charts of patients very similar to the first group; however, this second group of patients did not have coronary artery syndrome. The investigators extracted information from both groups' charts regarding complications secondary to coronary artery disease.

Trial #3: Seventy-three patients with coronary artery syndrome were followed over a 4-year period to identify any complications that occurred secondary to the coronary artery syndrome. After the 4-year period there were approximately 50% of the patients that developed a secondary complication.

6. From the trial(s) information provided above, determine the study design for each trial in the correct order.
   a. Cohort, case series, case-control
   b. Cohort, case-control, case series
   c. Case-control, case series, cohort
   d. Cohort, cross-sectional, case series

7. Choose the answer below that represents a ranking of trial designs in order of increasing rigor.
   a. Case report < Powered randomized controlled trial < Case series
   b. Case-control < Case report < Case series
   c. Powered randomized controlled trial < Case series < Non-powered randomized controlled trial
   d. Case series < Cohort < Powered randomized controlled trial

8. Choose the correct study design category below for a prospective randomized controlled crossover trial.
   a. N-of-1
   b. Randomized controlled trial—parallel groups
   c. Case-control
   d. Cohort

9. Choose the correct study design category for a prospective observational study design without control group.
   a. Case-control

   b. N-of-1 study

   c. Cohort

   d. Case series

10. All of the following are characteristics of a meta-analysis, except:

   a. Analytical technique

   b. Provides quantitative assessment

   c. Statistically combines studies

   d. Prospective randomized

11. Quality-of-life measures in a study should be:

   a. Validated

   b. Culturally relevant

   c. Minimal potential for investigator bias

   d. All of the above

12. One important characteristic to identify in a dietary supplement study is:

   a. Food and Drug Administration (FDA) approved since plant-derived products are regulated by the FDA

   b. Trial duration because these studies are often long

   c. Standardization since plant-derived products often contain many different chemical entities

   d. a and c

13. A reputable evidence-based medicine process:

   a. Ranks the quality of evidence

   b. Avoids complexity

   c. Systematically evaluates studies

   d. All of the above

14. All of the following components are important for an evidence-based medicine process, except:

   a. Method to determine the quality of the evidence

   b. Method to develop a defendable clinical decision

   c. Method to develop a meta-analysis

   d. a and b

15. The quality of evidence equation includes:

   a. Only trials of highest quality

   b. Key study attributes and study design characteristics

   c. Risk to patients greater than acceptable

   d. All unpublished studies and clinical research reports

Abbreviations

ACCP – American College of Clinical Pharmacists
ACT – adaptive clinical trial
AERS/FAERS – Adverse Event Reporting System/Formal Adverse Event Reporting System
AUC – area under the curve
CDC – Centers for Disease Control and Prevention
cGMPs – current Good Manufacturing Practices
CI – confidence interval
C_{max} – peak maximum concentration
CONSORT – Consolidated Standards of Reporting Trials
DS – dietary supplements
EBM – evidence-based medicine
EMA – European Medicines Agency
FD&C Act – Federal Food, Drug and Cosmetic Act
FDA – Food and Drug Administration
HESDE – historical evidence of sensitivity to drug effects
HMG-CoA – hydroxymethylglutaryl-Coenzyme A (HMG-CoA)
HR-QOL or HRQOL – health-related quality of life
ICH – International Council for Harmonization
IDMC – independent data monitoring committee
IMOS – Integrative Medicine Outcome Scale
ITT – intention/intent to treat
NDA – New Drug Application
NI – non-inferiority
N-of-1 – crossover trial design involving 1 patient
PDF – Portable Document Format
PP – per protocol
PRISMA – Preferred Reporting Items for Systematic reviews and Meta-Analyses
PROSPERO – International Prospective Register of Systematic Reviews
QOL – quality of life
QUOROM – **QU**ality **Of R**eporting **Of M**eta-analyses
RLD – reference listed drug
SEM – standard error of the mean
STROBE – **ST**rengthening the **R**eporting of **OB**servational studies in **E**pidemiology
T_{max} – time of peak maximum concentration
USP – United States Pharmacopeia

USP DSVP – Dietary Supplement Verification Program
VAERS – Vaccine Adverse Event Reporting System
WHO – World Health Organization

Acknowledgments

The authors wish to gratefully acknowledge Kerry Cain at the University of Missouri-Kansas City School of Pharmacy Drug Information Center for retyping, editing, formatting, proofreading, manuscript problem-solving, and taking the lead with citation assistance. Also from the Drug Information Center, the authors wish to thank and acknowledge Denise Woolf, M.Ed., B.S. for her assistance with new diagram development and general manuscript problem-solving, along with Andrea Potter, PharmD, for her assistance with the citations.

REFERENCES

1. Suda KJ, Jurley AM, McKibbin T, Motl Moroney SE. Publication of non-inferiority clinical trials: changes over a 20-year interval. Pharmacotherapy. 2011;31(9):833-9.
2. Bryant PJ, Pace HA, eds. The pharmacist's guide to evidence based medicine for clinical decision making. Bethesda, MD: American Society of Health-System Pharmacists; 2009:198.
3. Fairman KA, Curtiss FR. Rethinking the "whodunit" approach to assessing the quality of health care research—a call to focus on the evidence in evidence-based practice. JMCP. 2008;14(7):661-74.
4. De Muth JE. Basic statistics and pharmaceutical applications. 2nd ed. Boca Raton, FL: Chapman & Hall/CRC; 2006:714.
5. Piaggio G, Elbourne DR, Altman DG, Pocock SJ, Evans SJ. Reporting of non-inferiority and equivalence randomized trials: an extension of the CONSORT statement. JAMA. 2006;295:1152-60.
6. U.S. Department of Health and Human Services, Food and Drug Administration, Center for Drug Evaluation and Research, and Center for Biologics Evaluation and Research. Guidance for industry non-inferiority clinical trials [Internet]. Silver Springs, MD; 2016 Nov [cited 2017 Mar 5]: [63 pp.]. Available from: https://www.fda.gov/downloads/Drugs/Guidances/UCM202140.pdf
7. Kaul S, Diamond GA. Good enough: a primer on the analysis and interpretation of non-inferiority trials. Ann Intern Med. 2006; 145:62-9.
8. Dasgupta A, Lawson KA, Wilson JP. Evaluating equivalence and non-inferiority trials. Am J Health Syst Pharm. 2010;67:1337-43.

9. Head SJ, Kaul S, Bogers AJ, Kappetein AP. Non-inferiority study design: lessons to be learned from cardiovascular trials. Eur Heart J. 2012;33:1318-24.

10. Durkalski V, Silbergleit R, Lowenstein D. Challenges in the design and analysis of non-inferiority trials: a case study. Clin Trials. 2011;8:601-8.

11. Schumi J, Wittes J. Through the looking glass: understanding non-inferiority. Trials. 2011;12:106.

12. Wangge G, Klungel OH, Roes KCB, de Boer A, Hoes AW, Knol MJ. Room for improvement in conducting and reporting non-inferiority randomized controlled trials on drugs: a systematic review. PLoS ONE. 2010;5(10):e13550. doi:10.1371/journal.pone.0013550.

13. D'Agostino RB Sr, Massaro JM, Sullivan LM. Non-inferiority trials: design concepts and issues—the encounters of academic consultants in statistics. Statist Med. 2003;22:169-86.

14. New drug approval: FDA's consideration of evidence from certain clinical trials—Report to Congressional Requesters. Washington, DC: United States Government Accountability Office; 2010 July, 33 pp. Report No.: GAO-10-798.

15. Turner JR, Durham TA. Must new drugs be superior to those already available? The role of noninferiority clinical trials. J Clin Hypertens. 2015;17(4):319-21.

16. Kaji AH, Lewis RJ. Noninferiority trials: is a new treatment almost as effective as another? JAMA. 2015;313(23):2371-2.

17. Gotzsche PC. Lesson from and cautions about non-inferiority and equivalence randomized trials. JAMA. 2006;295(10):1172-4.

18. Guidelines on the choice of non-inferiority margin. London: European Medicines Agency (EMA); 2006.

19. Fleming TR, Odem-Davis K, Rothmann MD, Shen YL. Some essential considerations in the design and conduct of non-inferiority trials. Clin Trials. 2011;8:432-9.

20. Hung JH, Wang SJ, Tsong Y, Lawrence J, O'Neil RT. Some fundamental issues with non-inferiority testing inactive controlled trials. Statist Med. 2003;22:213-25.

21. Wang Y, Harigaya Y, Cavaille-Coll M, Colangelo P, Reynolds KS. Justification of noninferiority margin: methodology considerations in an exposure-response analysis. Clin Pharmacol Therapeut. 2015;97(4):405-10.

22. Fleming TR, Powers JH. Issues in noninferiority trials: the evidence in community-acquired pneumonia. CAP Noninferiority Trials. CID. 2008;47(Suppl 3):S108-20.

23. Musch DC, Gillespie BW. The state of being non-inferior. Ophthalmology. 2006;113(1):1-2.

24. Hung JH, Wang SJ, Tsong Y, Lawrence J, O'Neil RT. Challenges and regulatory experiences with non-inferiority trial design without placebo arm. Biometrical J. 2009;2: 324-34.

25. Huitfeldt B, Hummel J. The draft FDA guideline on non-inferiority clinical trials: a critical review from European pharmaceutical industry statisticians. Pharmaceut Statist. 2011;10:414-9.

26. Julious SA. The ABC of non-inferiority margin setting from indirect comparisons. Pharmaceut Statist. 2011;10:448-53.

27. Wang SJ, Blume JD. An evidential approach to non-inferiority clinical trials. Pharmaceut Statist. 2011;10:440-7.

28. Norman GR, Streiner DL, eds. Biostatistics: the bare essentials. Shelton, CT: People's Medical Publishing House; 2008:393.

29. Chiquette E, Posey LM, eds. Evidence-based pharmacotherapy. Washington, DC: American Pharmaceutical Association; 2007:211.

30. Pater C. Equivalence and non-inferiority trials—are they viable alternatives for registration of new drugs? (III). Current controlled trials in cardiovascular medicine [Internet]. 2004 Aug 17 [cited 2017 Mar 5]; 5(8): [7 pp.] Available from: http://trialsjournal.biomedcentral.com/articles/10.1186/1468-6708-5-8

31. Chen YHJ, Chen C. Testing superiority at interim analyses in a non-inferiority trial. Statist Med. 2012;31:1531-42.

32. Snapinn SM. Non-inferiority trials. Curr Control Trials Cardiovasc Med. 2000;1:19-21.

33. Thornby K-A, Johnson A, Ferrill MJ. Simplifying and interpreting the facts of noninferiority trials: a stepwise approach. Am J Health Syst Pharm. 2014;71:1926-31.

34. Hung JH, Wang SJ, O'Neill R. A regulatory perspective on choice of margin and statistical inference issue in non-inferiority trials. Biometrical J. 2005;47:28-36.

35. Snapinn S, Jiang Q. Controlling the type 1 error rate in non-inferiority trials. Statist Med. 2008;27:371-81.

36. Scott IA. Non-inferiority trials: determining whether alternative treatments are good enough. MJA. 2009;190:326-30.

37. Kaul S, Diamond G. Making sense of non-inferiority: a clinical and statistical perspective on its application to cardiovascular clinical trials. Prog Cardiovasc Dis. 2007;49(4):284-99.

38. Friede T, Kiser M. Blinded sample size reassessment in non-inferiority and equivalence trials. Statist Med. 2003;22:995-1007.

39. Brown D, Volkers P, Day S. An introductory note to CHMP guidelines: choice of the non-inferiority margin and data monitoring committees. Statist Med. 2006;25:1623-7.

40. Henanff AL, Giraudeau B, Baron G, Ravaud P. Quality of reporting of non-inferiority and equivalence randomized trials. JAMA. 2006;295(10):1147-51.

41. Gopal AD, Desai NR, Tse T, Ross JS. Reporting of noninferiority trials in clinical trials.gov and corresponding publications. JAMA. 2015;313(11):1163-5.

42. Mohr D, Hopewell S, Schulz KF, Montori V, Gotzsche PC, Devereaux PH, et al. CONSORT 2010 explanation and elaboration: updated guidelines for reporting parallel group randomized trials. BMJ. 2010;340:c869.

43. Schulz KF, Altman DG, Moher D. CONSORT 2010 statement: updated guidelines for reporting parallel group randomized trials. Int J Surg. 2011;9:672-7.

44. Gomberg-Maitland M, Frison L, Halperin JL. Active-control clinical trials to establish equivalence or non-inferiority: methodological and statistical concepts linked to quality. Am Heart J. 2003;146(3):398-403.

45. Green WL, Concato J, Feinstein AR. Claims of equivalence in medical research: are they supported by the evidence? Ann Int Med. 2000;132:715-22.

46. Kravitz RL, Duan N, eds, and the DEcIDE Methods Center N-of-1 Guidance Panel. Design and implementation of N-of-1 trials: a user's guide. Chap 1. Intro to N-of-1 trials: indications and barriers. AHRQ Pub No. 13(14)-EHC122-EF. Rockbille, MD: Agency

for Healthcare Research and Quality. 2014 Feb [cited 2017 Mar 5]. Available from: www
.effectivehealthcare.ahrq.gov/N-1-Trials.cfm

47. Velengtas P, Mohr P, Messner DA, eds. Making informed decisions: assessing the
    strengths and weaknesses of study designs and analytic methods for comparative effec-
    tiveness research. Center for Medical Technology stakeholders report. 2012 Feb.

48. Schork NJ. Time for one-person trials. Nature. 2015 Apr 30;520:609-11.

49. Duan N, Kravita RL, Schmid CH. Single-patient (n-of-1) trials: a pragmatic clinical decision
    methodology for patient-centered comparative effectiveness research. J Clin Epidemiol.
    2013;66:S21-8.

50. Vohra S, Punja S. N-of-1 trials: individualized medication effectiveness tests. Virtual
    Mentor. AMA J Ethics. 2013;15(1)42-5.

51. Lillie EO, Patay B, Diamant J, Issell B, Topol EJ, Schork NJ. The n-of-1 clinical trial:
    the ultimate strategy for individualizing medicine? NIH PA Author Manuscript. Per Med.
    2011;8(2):161-73. doi:10.2217/pme.11.7.

52. Gabler NB, Duan N, Vohra S, Kravitz RL. N-of-1 trials in the medical literature: a system-
    atic review. Med Care. 2011;49(8):761-8. doi:10.1097/MLR.0b013e318215d90d.

53. Hui D, Zhukovsky DS, Burera E. Which treatment is better? Ascertaining patient prefer-
    ences with crossover randomized controlled trials. American Academy of Hospice and
    Palliative Medicine. J Pain Symptom Manage. 2015;49:625-31.

54. Chen X, Chen P. A comparison of four methods for the analysis of N-of-1 trials. PLoS ONE.
    2014;9(2):e87752. doi:10.1371/journal.pone.0087752.

55. Chow S. Adaptive clinical trial design. Annu Rev Med. 2014;65:405-15.

56. Meurer WJ, Lewis RJ, Table D, Fetters MD, Legocki L, Berry S, Connor J, Durkalski V,
    Elm J, Zhao W, Frederiksen S, Silbergleit R, Palesch Y, Berry DA, Barson WG. An over-
    view of the adaptive designs accelerating promising trials into treatments (ADAPT-IT)
    project. Ann Emerg Med. 2012;60:451-7.

57. Guidance for industry. Adaptive design clinical trials for drugs and biologics. U.S.
    Department of Health and Human Services. Food and Drug Administration. 2010 Feb.

58. Mehta CR. Adaptive clinical trial designs with pre-specified rules for modifying the sam-
    ple size: a different perspective. Statist Med. 2013;32:1276-9.

59. Gottlieb S. Adaptive trial design. Paper presented at: Conference on Adaptive Trial
    Design. 2006 Jul 10; Washington, DC.

60. Levin GP, Emerson SC, Emerson SS. An evaluation of inferential procedures for adaptive
    clinical trial designs with pre-specified rules for modifying the sample size. Biometrics.
    2014;70:556-67.

61. Scher HI, Nasso SF, Rubin EH, Simon R. Adaptive clinical trial designs for simulta-
    neous testing of matched diagnostics and therapeutics. Clin Cancer Res. 2011 Nov
    1;17(21):6634-40.

62. Cook T, DeMets DL. Review of draft FDA adaptive design guidance. [Review]. J Biopharm
    Stat. 2010 Nov;20(7):1132-42.

63. Snapinn S, Chen M-G, Jian Q, Koutsoukos T. Assessment of futility in clinical trials.
    Pharmaceut Statist. 2006;5:273-81.

64. Yi J, Fang L, Su Z. Hybridization of conditional and predictive power for futility assessment in sequential clinical trials with time-to-event outcomes: a resampling approach. Contem Clin Trials. 2012;33:138-42.

65. Adaptive designs in the real world by Deborah Borfitz [Internet]. WHERE: BioITWorld. com. Despite potential advantages, pharma is taking a cautious approach to adaptive designs, resulting in a slow but sure restyling of the research enterprise; 2008 Jun 10 [cited 2013 Apr 2]: [6 pp.]. Available from: http://www.bioitworld.com/issues/2008/june/cover-story-adaptive-trial-designs.html?terms=tessella

66. Chow S, Corey R. Benefits, challenges and obstacles of adaptive clinical trial designs. [Review]. Orphanet J Rare Dis. 2011;6:79.

67. Hatfield I, Allison A, Flight L, Julious S, Dimairo M. Adaptive designs undertaken in clinical research: a review of registered clinical trials. [Review]. Trials. 2016;17:150.

68. Porcher R, Lecocq B, Vray M, participants of Round Table Ndegree 2 de Giens XXVI. Adaptive methods: when and how should they be used in clinical trials? Therapie. 2011 Jul-Aug;66(4)319-26, 309-17.

69. Fletcher RH, Fletcher SW, Wagner EH. Risk. In: Fletcher RH, Fletcher SW, Wagner EH, eds. Clinical epidemiology: the essentials. 3rd ed. Baltimore, MD: Williams & Wilkins; 1996:94-110.

70. Parke T. ISCTM: implementing phase 2 dose finding adaptive clinical trials. [Review]. Eur Neuropsychopharmacol. 2011;21:167-74.

71. Barrett KM, Brott TG, Brown RD Jr, Carter RE, Geske JR, Graff-Radford NR, McNeil RB, Meschia JF, and Mayo Acute Stroke Trial for Enhancing Recovery (MASTER) Study Group. Enhancing recovery after acute ischemic stroke with donepezil as an adjuvant therapy to standard medical care: results of a phase IIA clinical trial. J Stroke Cerebrovasc Dis. 2011;20(3):177-82.

72. Anonymous. Adaptive clinical trial designs proposed to accelerate development of HIV vaccines. Expert Rev Vaccines. 2011;10(6):717.

73. Beckman RA, Chen C. New evidence-based adaptive clinical trial methods for optimally integrating predictive biomarkers into oncology clinical development programs. Chin J Cancer. 2013;32(5)233-41.

74. Kesselheim AS, Gagne JJ. Strategies for postmarketing surveillance of drugs for rare diseases. [Review]. Clin Pharmacol Ther. 2014;95(3):265-8.

75. Meurer WJ, Barsan WG. Spinal cord injury neuroprotection and the promise of flexible adaptive clinical trials. World Neurosurg. 2014;82(3/4):e541-6.

76. Gomeni R. Use of predictive models in CNS diseases. Curr Opin Pharmacol. 2014;14:23-9.

77. Davies GR, Phillips PPJ, Jaki T. Adaptive clinical trials in tuberculosis: applications, challenges and solutions. Int J Tuberc Lung Dis. 2015;19(6):626-34.

78. Bokser AD, O'Donnell PB. Stability of pharmaceutical products. In: Lawson LA, Adejare A, Desselle SP, Felton LA, Moffat AC, et al., eds. Remington: the science and practice of pharmacy. 22nd ed. Philadelphia, PA: Pharmaceutical Press; 2013:335-47.

79. Ammann C. Stability studies needed to define the handling and transport conditions of sensitive pharmaceutical or biotechnological products. AAPS Pharm Sci Tech. 2011;12(4):1264-75.

80. Bajaj S, Singla D, Sakhuja N. Stability testing of pharmaceutical products. J Appl Pharmaceut Sci. 2012;02(03):129-38.

81. Current good manufacturing practice for finished pharmaceuticals [Internet]. U.S. Department of Health and Human Services, Food and Drug Administration. 2016 June 24 [cited 2017 Jan 3]. Available from: https://www.accessdata.fda.gov/scripts/cdrh/cfdocs/cfcfr/CFRSearch.cfm?CFRPart=211

82. United States Pharmacopeia, Inc. U.S. Pharmacopeia 40—National Formulary 35. Rockville, MD: U.S. Pharmacopeia Convention, Inc.; 2017.

83. Guidance for industry: bioequivalence studies with pharmacokinetic endpoints for drugs submitted under an ANDA. Draft guidance [Internet]. U.S. Department of Health and Human Services. FDA. CDER. Biopharmaceutics. 2013 Dec [cited 2017 Jan 3]. Available from: http://www.fda.gov/ucm/groups/fdagov-public/@fdagov-drugs-gen/documents/document/ucm377465.pdf

84. FDA ensures equivalence of generic drugs [Internet]. U.S. Food and Drug Administration. 2002 Aug 1 [cited 2013 Aug 10]. Available from: http://www.fda.gov/drugs/EmergencyPreparedness/BioterrorismandDrugPreparedness

85. Johnson SB. Bioavailability and bioequivalency testing. In: Lawson LA, Adejare A, Desselle P, Felton LA, Moffat AC, Perrie Y, Popovich NG, Shermock KM, Wall DS, eds. Remington: the science and practice of pharmacy. 22nd ed. Philadelphia, PA: Pharmaceutical Press; 2013:349-59.

86. Emden C, Borbasi S. Programmatic research: a desirable (or despotic?) nursing strategy for the future. Collegian. 2000;7(1):32-7.

87. McQueen L, Mittman BS, Demakis JG. Overview of the Veterans Health Administration (VHA) Quality Enhancement Research Initiative (QUERI). J Am Med Inform Assoc. 2004;11(5):339-43.

88. Stetler CB, Mittman BS, Francis J. Overview of the VA Quality Enhancement Research Initiative (QUERI) and QUERI theme articles: QUERI Series. Implement Sci. 2008;3:8.

89. Collignon U, Oborne CA, Kostrzewski A. Pharmacy services to UK emergency departments: a descriptive study. Pharm World Sci. 2010;32:90-6.

90. Whitty JA, Kendall E, Sav A, Kelly F, McMillan SS, King MA, Wheeler AJ. Preferences for the delivery of community pharmacy services to help manage chronic conditions. Res Social Adm Pharm. 2015;11:197-215.

91. Hommel KA, Gray WN, Hente E, Loreaux K, Ittenbach RF, Maddux M, Baldassano R, Sylvester F, Crandall W, Doarn C, Heyman MB, Keljo D, Denson LA. The Telehealth Enhancement of Adherence to Medication (TEAM) in pediatric IBD trial: design and methodology. Contemp Clin Trials. 2015;43:105-13.

92. Willett MS, Bertch KE, Rich DS, Eveshehefsky L. Prospectus on the economic value of clinical pharmacy services. A position statement of the American College of Clinical Pharmacy. Pharmacotherapy. 1989;9:45-56.

93. Giberson SF. Million Hearts™: pharmacist-delivered care to improve cardiovascular health. Pub Health Rep. 2013;128:2.

94. Giberson S, Yoder S, Lee MP. Improving patient and health system outcomes through advanced pharmacy practice. A report to the U.S. Surgeon General. Office of the Chief Pharmacist, U.S. Public Health Service; 2011.

95. Hammond RW, Schwartz AM, Campbell MJ, Remington TL, Chuck S, Blair MM, Vassey AM, Rospond RM, Herner SJ, Webb CE. Collaborative drug therapy management by pharmacists: 2003. Pharmacotherapy. 2003;23(9):1210-25.

96. Overholser BR, Foster DR, Henry JR, Plake KS, Sowinski KM. Instructional design and assessment: the influence of an elective introductory clinical research course on pharmacy student interest in pursuing research-based careers. Am J Pharm Educ. 2010;74(9): Article 165.

97. Ansong MA, James K. Using systematic reviews and cost-justification models to emphasize concepts in a research design course. Pharmacy Practice Faculty Publications. 2012;272. Available from: http://digitalcommons.cedarville.edu/pharmacy_practice_publications/272

98. Mann CJ. Observational research methods. Research design II: cohort, cross sectional, and case-control studies. Emerg Med J. 2003;20:54-60.

99. Song JW, Chung KC. Observational studies: cohort and case-control studies. Plast Reconstr Surg. 2010;126(6):2234-42.

100. Aschengran A, Seage GR, eds. Essentials of epidemiology in public health. 2nd ed. Sudbury, MA: Jones and Bartlett; 2008:516.

101. Greenhalgh T. How to read a paper. 3rd ed. Malden, MA: Blackwell Publishing; 2006: 229.

102. Slaughter RL, Edwards DJ, eds. Evaluating drug literature: a statistical approach. New York, NY: McGraw-Hill; 2001:369.

103. Matthews DE, Farewll VT, eds. Using and understanding medical statistics. 4th ed. Basel, Switzerland: Karger; 2007:322.

104. Gabay M, ed. The clinical practice of drug information. Burlington, MA: Jones and Bartlett Learning; 2016:178.

105. Riegelman R. Studying a study and testing a test. 5th ed. Philadelphia, PA: Lippincott Williams & Wilkins; 2005:356.

106. Lanthrop GD, Wolfe WH, Albanese RA, Moynahan PM. An epidemiologic investigation of health effects in Air Force personnel following exposure to herbicides. Baseline morbidity results. Washington, DC: U.S. Air Force; 1994.

107. Wolfe WH, Michalek JE, Miner JC, Rahe A, Silva J, Thomas WF, Grubbs WD, Lustik MB, Karrison TG, Roegner RH. Health status of Air Force veterans occupationally exposed to herbicides in Vietnam I. Physical health. JAMA. 1990;264:1824-31.

108. Michalek JE, Wolfe WH, Miner JC. Health status of Air Force veterans occupationally exposed to herbicides in Vietnam II. Mortality. JAMA. 1990;264:1832-6.

109. Ketchum NS, Michalek JE. Postservice mortality in Air Force veterans occupationally exposed to herbicides during the Vietnam War: 20 year follow-up results. Mil Med. 2005;1780:406-13.

110. Matthews DE, Farewell VT, eds. Using and understanding medical statistics. 4th ed. Basel, Switzerland: Karger; 2007:322.

111. Rochon PA, Gurwitz JH, Sykora K, Mamdani M, Streiner DL, Gafinkel S, Normand SL, Anderson GM. Reader's guide to critical appraisal of cohort studies: 1. Role and design. BMJ. 2005 Apr 16;330:895-7.

112. Mamdani M, Sykora K, Li P, Normand ST, Austin PC, Rochon PA, Anderson GM. Reader's guide to critical appraisal of cohort studies: 2. Assessing potential for confounding. BMJ. 2005 Apr 23;330:960-2.

113. Normand ST, Sykora K, Li P, Mamdani M, Rochon PA, Anderson GM. Reader's guide to critical appraisal of cohort studies: 3. Analytical strategies to reduce confounding. BMJ. 2005 Apr 30;330:1021-3.

114. Hayden GF, Kramer MS, Horwitz RI. The case-control study. A practical review for the clinician. JAMA. 1982;247:326-31.

115. Westreich D. Berkson's bias, selection bias, and missing data. Epidemiology. 2012;23(1):159-64.

116. Kier KL. Biostatistical applications in epidemiology. Pharmacotherapy. 2011;31(1):9-22.

117. Vandenbroucke JP. STREGA, STROBE, STARD, SQUIRE, MOOSE, PRISMA, GNOSIS, TREND, ORION, COREQ, QUOROM, REMARK ... and CONSORT: for whom does the guideline toll? J Clin Epidemiol. 2009;62:594-6.

118. Grimes DA, Schulz KF. Cohort studies: marching towards outcomes. Lancet. 2002;359:341-5.

119. Baxter P, Jack S. Qualitative case study methodology: study design and implementation for novice researchers. Qual Rep. 2008;13(4):544-59.

120. Nissen T, Wynn R. The clinical case report: a review of its merits and limitations. BMC Res Notes. 2014;7:264.

121. Abu-Zidan FM, Abbas AK, Hefny AF. Clinical "case series": a concept analysis. Afr Health Sci. 2012;12(4)557-62.

122. Spilker B. Single patient clinical trials. Guide to clinical trials. New York, NY: Lippincott-Raven; 1996:277-82.

123. Vandenbroucke JP. In defense of case reports and case series. Ann Intern Med. 2001;134(4):330-4.

124. Ponto J. Understanding and evaluating survey research. J Adv Pract Oncol. 2015;6:168-71.

125. Shi L. Health services research methods. 2nd ed. Clinton Park, NY: International Thomson Publishing; 2008:481.

126. Draugalis JR, Coons SJ, Plaza CM. Best practices for survey research reports: a synopsis for authors and reviewers. Am J Pharm Educ. 2008. Available from: http://www.ajpe.org/view.asp?art=aj720111

127. Groves RM. Nonresponse rates and nonresponse bias in household surveys. Public Opin Q. 2006;70:5:646-75.

128. Davern M, McAlpine D, Beebe TJ, Ziegenfuss J, Rockwood T, Call KT. Are lower response rates hazardous to your health survey? An analysis of three state telephone health surveys. Health Serv Res. 2010 Oct;45:5, Part 1.

129. Lim S, Immerwahr S, Lee S, Harris TG. Estimating nonresponse bias in a telephone-based health surveillance survey in New York City. Am J Epidemiol. 2013;178(8):1337-41.
130. Davern M. Nonresponse rates are a problematic indicator of nonresponse bias in survey research. Health Serv Res. 2013;48(3):905-12.
131. Halbesleben JRB, Whitman MV. Evaluating survey quality in health services research: a decision framework for assessing nonresponse bias. Health Serv Res. 2013 Jun;48(3):913-30.
132. Suvarna V. Phase IV of drug development. Perspect Clin Res. 2010;1(2):57-60.
133. Selvan AT, Mohan CJ, Sundari SKK, Suthakaran R. Study on role of postmarketing surveillance in new drug development. Asian J Manage. 2013;4(1):12-5.
134. Roehr B. FDA should tighten post-marketing surveillance of prescription drugs, says Institute of Medicine. BMJ. 2012;344:e3104. Doi:10.1136/bmj.e3104.
135. FDA postmarketing surveillance programs. 2014 Aug 19 [cited 2017 Jan 3]:[1 screen]. Available from:http://www.fda.gov/Drugs/GuidanceComplianceRegulatoryinformation/Surveillance/ucm090385.htm
136. Sharrar RG, Dieck GS. Monitoring product safety in the postmarketing environment. Ther Adv Drug Saf. 2013;4(5):211-9.
137. FDA Adverse Events Reporting System (FAERS) Electronic Submissions. 2016 Jun 22 [cited 2017 Jan 3]:[1 screen]. Available from: http://www.fda.gov/Drugs/GuidanceComplianceRegulatoryInformation/Surveillance/AdverseDrugEffects/ucm115894.htm
138. Gough D, Thomas J, Oliver S. Clarifying differences between review designs and methods. Syst Rev. 2012;1:28.
139. Green BN, Johnson CD, Adams A. Writing narrative literature reviews for peer-reviewed journals: secrets of the trade. J Chiropr Med. 2006;3(5):101-17.
140. Bae JM. Narrative reviews. Epidemiol Health. 2014;36:e2014018.
141. Loh J. Inquiry into issues of trustworthiness and quality in narrative studies: a perspective. Qual Rep. 2013;18(65):1-15.
142. Greenhalgh T, Wong G. Training materials for meta-narrative reviews. National Institute for Health Research Health Services and Delivery Research Programme (NIHR HS&DR). Project no. 10/1008/07. 2013.
143. Murad MH, Montori VM, Ioannidis JPA, Jaeschke R, Devereaux PJ, Prasad K, Neumann I, Darrasco-Labra A, Agoritsas T, Hatala R, Meade MO, Wyer P, Cook DJ, Guyatt G. How to read a systematic review and meta-analysis and apply the results to patient care. JAMA. 2014;312(2):171-9.
144. Simunovic N, Sprague S, Bhandari M. Methodological issues in systematic reviews and meta-analyses of observational studies in orthopaedic research. J Bone Joint Surg Am. 2009;91(Suppl 3):87-94.
145. Wager E, Wiffen PJ. Ethical issues in preparing and publishing systematic reviews. J Evid Based Med. 2011;4:130-4.
146. Montori VM, Swiontkowski MF, Cook DJ. Methodologic issues in systematic reviews and meta-analyses. Clin Orthop Relat Res. 2003;413:43-54.

147. Hausner E, Guddat C, Hermanns T, Lampert U, Waffenschmidt S. Development of search strategies for systematic reviews: validation showed the noninferiority of the objective approach. J Clin Epidemiol. 2015;68:191-9.

148. Moher D, Liberati A, Tetzlaff J, Altman DG, PRISMA Group. Preferred Reporting Items for Systematic reviews and Meta-Analyses: the PRISMA Statement. Ann Intern Med. 2009;151:264-69.

149. Turlik M. Evaluating the results of a systematic review/meta-analysis. FAOJ. 2009;2(7):5 pp.

150. Walker E, Hernandez AV, Kattan MW. Meta-analysis: its strengths and limitations. Cleve Clin J Med. 2008;75(6):431-9.

151. Crowther M, Lim W, Crowther MA. Systematic review and meta-analysis methodology. Blood. 2010;116(17):3140-6.

152. Greco T, Zangrillo A, Biondi-Zoccai G, Landoni G. Meta-analysis: pitfalls and hints. Heart Lung Vessel. 2013;5:219-25.

153. Pucino F. Use of meta-analysis to support clinical decision making. Paper presented at: Meta-analysis: Principles and Practice Session. Proceedings of the 43rd American Society of Health-System Pharmacists Midyear Clinical Meeting; 2008 Dec 7-11; Orlando, FL.

154. Hutton B, Salanti G, Chaimani A, Caldwell DM, Schmid C, Thorland K, Mills E, Catala-Lopez F, Turner L, Altman DG, Moher D. The quality of reporting methods and results in network meta-analyses: an overview of reviews and suggestions for improvement. PLoS ONE. 2014 Mar;9(3):e92508.

155. Salanti G, Del Giovane C, Chaimani A, Caldwell DM, Higgins JPT. Evaluating the quality of evidence from a network meta-analysis. PLoS ONE. 2014 Jul;9(7):e99682.

156. Tufanaru C, Munn Z, Stephenson M, Aromataris E. Fixed or random effects meta-analysis? Common methodological issues in systematic reviews of effectiveness. Int J Evid Based Healthc. 2015;13:196-207.

157. Li T, Puhan MA, Vedula SS, Singh S, Dickersin K. Network meta-analysis-highly attractive but more methodological research is needed. BMC Med. 2011;9:79.

158. Cipriani A, Higgins JPT, Geddes JR, Salanti G. Conceptual and technical challenges in network meta-analysis. Ann Intern Med. 2013;159:130-7.

159. Neupane B, Richer D, Bonner AJ, Kibret T, Beyene J. Network meta-analysis using R: a review of currently available automated packages. PLoS ONE. 2014 Dec;9(12):e115065.

160. Chaimani A, Higgins JPT, Mavridis D, Spyridonos P, Salanti G. Graphical tools for network-meta-analysis in STATA. PLoS ONE. 2013 Oct;8(10):e76654.

161. Liberati A, Altman DG, Tetzlaff J, Mulrow C, Gotzsche PC, Ioannidis JP, Clarke M, Devereaux PJ, Kleijnen J, Moher D. The PRISMA statement for reporting systematic reviews and meta-analyses of studies that evaluate healthcare interventions: explanation and elaboration. PLoS Med. 2009;6(7):e1000100. doi:10.1371/journal.pmed.1000100.

162. Guyatt G, Rennie D, Meade M, Cook DJ, eds. User's guides to the medical literature: a manual for evidence-based clinical practice. 3rd ed. Chicago, IL: AMA Press; 2015:706.

163. Mavridis D, Giannatsi M, Cipriani A, Salanti G. A primer on network meta-analysis with emphasis on mental health. Evid Based Mental Health. 2015;18:40-6. doi:10.1136/eb-2015-102088.

164. Armitage P, Berry G, Matthews JN, eds. Statistical methods in medical research. 4th ed. Malden, MA: Blackwell Science; 2005:817.

165. LeLorier J, Gregoire G, Benhaddad A, Lapierre J, Derderian F. Discrepancies between meta-analyses and subsequent large randomized, controlled trials. N Engl J Med. 1997;337:536-42.

166. Jadad AR, Moore RA, Carroll D, Jenkinson C, Reynolds DJM, Gavaghan DJ, McQuay HJ. Assessing the quality of reports of randomized clinical trials: is blinding necessary? Control Clin Trials. 1996;17:1-12.

167. Moreno SG, Sutton AJ, Thompson JR, Ades AE, Abrams KR, Cooper NJ. A generalized weighting regression-derived meta-analysis estimator robust to small-study effects and heterogeneity. Statist Med. 2012;31:1407-17.

168. Stroup DF, Berlin JA, Morton SC, Olkin I, Williamson GD, Rennie D, et al. Meta-analysis of observational studies in epidemiology: a proposal for reporting. JAMA. 2000;283(15):2008-2012.

169. Moher D, Cook DJ, Eastwood S, Olkin I, Rennie D, Stroup DF. Improving the quality of reports of meta-analyses of randomized controlled trials: the QUOROM statement. Lancet. 1999;354:1896-900.

170. Moher D, Liberati A, Tetzlaff J, Altman DG, PRISMA Group. Preferred Reporting Items for Systematic reviews and Meta-Analyses: the PRISMA statement. PLoS Med. 2009;6(7):e1000097. doi:10.1371/journal.pmed.1000097.

171. Moher D, Shamseer L, Clarke M, Ghersi D, Liberati A, Petticrew M, Shekelle P, Stewart L, and PRISMA-P Group. Preferred reporting items for systematic review and meta-analysis protocols (PRISMA-P) 2015 statement. Syst Rev. 2015;4:1.

172. About systematic evidence reviews and clinical practice guidelines. National Heart, Lung, and Blood Institute. National Institutes of Health website. [cited 2017 Jan 3]: [1 screen]. Available from: https://www.nhlbi.nih.gov/health-pro/guidelines/about

173. Fairclough DL. Design and analysis of quality of life studies in clinical trials. Boca Raton, FL: Chapman & Hall; 2002:328.

174. Health-related quality of life. Available from: https://www.cdc.gov/hrqol/concept.htm. Viewed 12/12/16.

175. Agency for Healthcare Research and Quality, U.S. Department of Health and Human Services White Paper. A primer for systematic reviewers on the measurement of functional status and health-related quality of life in older adults. 2013; p. 5.

176. HealthKnowledge. Measures of health status, quality of life and health care report [Internet]. England and Wales; 2009 [cited 2017 Mar 21]. Available from: http://www.healthknowledge .org.uk/public-health-textbook/research-methods/1c-health-care-evaluation-hcalth-care-assessment/measures-health-status

177. Lin XJ, Lin IM, Fan SY. Methodological issues in measuring health-related quality of life. Tzu Chi Medical J. 2013;25:8-12.

178. Rapkin BD, Schwartz CE. Toward a theoretical model of quality-of-life appraisal: implications of findings from studies of response shift. Health Qual Life Outcomes. 2004;2(1):1-14.

179. Stoney CM, Coates P, Briggs JP. Integrity of active components of botanical products used in complementary and alternative medicine. JAMA. 2008;300(17):1995.

180. Dickinson A, Blatman J, El-Dash N, Franco JC. Consumer usage and reasons for using dietary supplements: report of a series of surveys. J Am Coll Nutr. 2014;33(2):176-82.

181. Croom M, Bryant PJ, Pace HA, Schnabel L. A comparative analysis of identified hierarchical categorizations of evidence. Paper presented at: Innovations in Drug Information Session. Proceeding of the 42nd American Society of Health-System Pharmacists Midyear Clinical Meeting; 2007 Dec 3; Las Vegas, NV.

182. OCEBM Levels of Evidence Working Group.* "The Oxford 2011 Levels of Evidence." Oxford Centre for Evidence-Based Medicine. Available from: http://www.cebm.net/index.aspx?o=5653. *OCEBM Levels of Evidence Working Group = Jeremy Howick, Iain Chalmers (James Lind Library), Paul Glasziou, Trish Greenhalgh, Carl Heneghan, Alessandro Liberati, Ivan Moschetti, Bob Phillips, Hazel Thornton, Olive Goddard, and Mary Hodgkinson.

183. Cook DJ, Guyatt GH, Laupacis A, Sackett DL. Rules of evidence and clinical recommendations on the use of antithrombotic agents. Chest. 1992;102(Suppl 4):305S-11S.

SUGGESTED READINGS

1. Bryant PJ, Pace HA, eds. The pharmacist's guide to evidence-based medicine for clinical decision making. Bethesda, MD: American Society of Health-System Pharmacists; 2009.

2. Chiquette E, Posey LM, eds. Evidence-based pharmacotherapy. Washington, DC: American Pharmaceutical Association; 2007.

3. Walter RW. The application of statistical analysis in the biomedical sciences. In: Malone PM, Malone MJ, Park SK, eds. Drug information: a guide for pharmacists. 6th ed. New York, NY: McGraw-Hill Medical; 2018.

6

Chapter Six

The Application of Statistical Analysis in the Biomedical Sciences

Ryan W. Walters

Learning Objectives

After completing this chapter, the reader will be able to

- Define the population being studied and describe the method most appropriate to sample a given population.
- Identify and describe the dependent and independent variables and indicate whether any covariates were included in analysis.
- Identify and define the four scales of variable measurement.
- Describe the difference between descriptive and inferential statistics.
- Describe the mean, median, variance, and standard deviation and why they are important to statistical analysis.
- Describe the properties of the normal distribution and when an alternative distribution should be, or should have been, used.
- Describe several common epidemiological statistics.
- Identify and describe the difference between parametric and nonparametric statistical tests and when their use is most appropriate.
- Determine whether the appropriate statistical test has been performed when evaluating a study.

Key Concepts

1 There are four scales of variable measurement consisting of nominal, ordinal, interval, and ratio scales that are critically important to consider when determining the appropriateness of a statistical test.

2 Measures of central tendency are useful to quantify the distribution of a variable's data numerically. The most common measures of central tendency are the mean, median, and mode, with the most appropriate measure of central tendency dictated by the variable's scale of measurement.

3 Variance is a key element inherent in all statistical analyses, but standard deviation is presented more often. Variance and standard deviation are related mathematically.

4 The key benefit to using the standard normal distribution is that converting the original data to z-scores allows researchers to compare different variables regardless of the original scale.

5 The last observation carried forward (LOCF) technique used often with the data from clinical trials introduces significant bias into the results of statistical tests.

6 The central limit theorem states when equally sized samples are drawn from a non-normal distribution, the plotted mean values from each sample will approximate a normal distribution as long as the non-normality was not due to outliers.

7 There are numerous misconceptions about p-values and it is important to know how to interpret them correctly.

8 Clinical significance is far more important than statistical significance. Clinical significance can be quantified by using various measures of effect size.

9 The selection of the appropriate statistical test is based on several factors including the specific research question, the measurement scale of the dependent variable (DV), distributional assumptions, the number of DV measurements as well as the number and measurement scale of independent variables (IVs) and covariates, among others.

Introduction

Knowledge of statistics and statistical analyses is essential to constructively evaluate literature in the biomedical sciences. This chapter provides a general overview of both descriptive and inferential statistics that will enhance the ability of the student or practitioner to interpret results of empirical literature within the biomedical sciences by evaluating the appropriateness of statistical tests employed, the conclusions drawn by the authors, and the overall quality of the study.

Alongside Chapters 4 and 5, diligent study of the material presented in this chapter is an important first step to critically analyze the often avoided methods or results sections of published biomedical literature. Be aware, however, that this chapter cannot substitute for more formal didactic training in statistics, as the material presented here is not exhaustive with regards to either statistical concepts or available statistical tests. Thus, when reading a journal article, if doubt emerges about whether a method or statistical test was used and interpreted appropriately, do not hesitate to consult appropriate references or an individual who has more formal statistical training. This is especially true if the empirical evidence is being considered for implementation in practice. Asking questions is the key to obtaining knowledge!

For didactic purposes, this chapter can be divided into two sections. The first section presents a general overview of the processes underlying most statistical tests used in the biomedical sciences. It is recommended that all readers take the time required to thoroughly study these concepts. The second section, beginning with the Statistical Tests section, presents descriptions, assumptions, examples, and results of numerous statistical tests commonly used in the biomedical sciences. This section does not present the mathematical underpinnings, calculation, or programming of any specific statistical test. It is recommended that this section serve as a reference to be used concurrently alongside a given journal article to determine the appropriateness of a statistical test or to gain further insight into why a specific statistical test was employed.

Populations and Sampling

When investigating a particular research question or hypothesis, researchers must first define the population to be studied. A population refers to any set of objects in the universe, while a sample is a fraction of the population chosen to be representative of the specific population of interest. Thus, samples are chosen to make specific generalizations about the population of interest. Researchers typically do not attempt to study the entire population because data cannot be collected for everyone within a population. This is why a sample should ideally be chosen at random. That is, each member of the population must have an equal probability of being included in the sample.

For example, consider a study to evaluate the effect a calcium channel blocker (CCB) has on blood glucose levels in Type 1 diabetes mellitus (DM) patients. In this case, all Type 1 DM patients would constitute the study population; however, because data could never be collected from all Type 1 DM patients, a sample that is representative of the Type 1 DM population would be selected. There are numerous sampling strategies, many beyond the scope of this text. Although only a few are discussed here, interested readers are urged to consult the list of suggested readings at the end of this chapter for further information.

A random sample does not imply that the sample is drawn haphazardly or in an unplanned fashion, and there are several approaches to selecting a random sample. The most common method employs a random number table. A random number table theoretically contains all integers between one and infinity that have been selected without any trends or patterns. For example, consider the hypothetical process of selecting a random sample of Type 1 DM patients from the population. First, each patient in the population is assigned a number; say 1 to N, where N is the total number of Type 1 DM patients in the population. From this population, a sample of 200 patients is requested. The random number table would randomly select 200 patients from the population of size N. There are numerous free random number tables and generators available online; simply search for "random number table" or "random number generator" in any search engine.

Depending on the study design, a random sample may not be most appropriate when selecting a representative sample. On occasion, it may be necessary to separate the population into mutually exclusive groups called strata, where a specific factor (e.g., race, gender) will create separate strata to aid in analysis. In this case, the random sample is drawn within each stratum individually. This process is termed stratified random sampling. For example, consider a situation where the race of the patient was an important variable in the Type 1 DM study. To ensure the proportion of each race in the population is represented accurately, the researcher stratifies by race and randomly selects patients within each stratum to achieve a representative study sample.

Another method of randomly sampling a population is known as cluster sampling. Cluster sampling is appropriate when there are natural groupings within the population of interest. For example, consider a researcher interested in the patient counseling practices of pharmacists across the United States. It would be impossible to collect data from all pharmacists across the United States. However, the researcher has read literature suggesting regional differences within various pharmacy practices, not necessarily including counseling practices. Thus, he or she may decide to randomly sample within the four regions of the United States defined by the U.S. Census Bureau (i.e., West, Midwest, South, and Northeast) to assess for differences in patient counseling practices across regions.[1]

Another sampling method is known as systematic sampling. This method is used when information about the population is provided in list format, such as in the telephone book, election records, class lists, or licensure records, among others. Systematic sampling uses an equal-probability method where one individual is selected initially at random and every nth individual is then selected thereafter. For example, the researchers may decide to take every 10th individual listed after the first individual is chosen.

Finally, researchers often use convenience sampling to select participants based on the convenience of the researcher. That is, no attempt is made to ensure the sample is representative of the population. However, within the convenience sample, participants may be selected randomly. This type of sampling is often used in educational research. For example, consider a researcher evaluating a new classroom instructional method to increase exam scores. This type of study will use the convenience sample of the students in their own class or university. Obviously, significant weaknesses are apparent when using this type of sampling, most notably, limited generalization.

Variables and the Measurement of Data

A variable is the characteristic that is being observed or measured. Data are the measured values assigned to the variable for each individual member of the population. For example, a variable would be the participant's biological sex, while the data are whether the participant is male or female.

In statistics, there are three types of variables: dependent (DV), independent (IV), and confounding or nuisance. The DV is the response or outcome variable for a study, while an IV is a variable that is manipulated. A confounding variable (often referred to as covariate) is any variable that has an effect on the DV over and above the effect of the IV, but is not of specific research interest. Putting these definitions together, consider a study to evaluate the effect a new oral hypoglycemic medication has on glycosylated hemoglobin (HbA1c) compared to placebo. Here, the DV consists of the HbA1c data for each participant, and the IV is treatment group with two levels (i.e., treatment versus placebo). Initially, results may suggest the medication is very effective across the entire sample; however, previous literature has suggested participant race may affect the effectiveness of this type of medication. Thus, participant race is a confounding variable and would need to be included in the statistical analysis. After statistically controlling for participant race, the results may indicate that the medication was significantly more effective in the treatment group.

SCALES OF MEASUREMENT

❶ *There are four scales of variable measurement consisting of nominal, ordinal, interval, and ratio scales that are critically important to consider when determining the appropriateness of a statistical test.*[2] Think of these four scales as relatively fluid; that is, as the data progress from nominal to ratio, the information about each variable being measured is increased. The scale of measurement of DVs, IVs, and confounding variables is an important consideration when determining whether the appropriate statistical test was used to answer the research question and hypothesis.

A **nominal scale** consists of categories that have no implied rank or order. Examples of nominal variables include gender (e.g., male versus female), race (e.g., Caucasian versus African American versus Hispanic), or disease state (e.g., absence versus presence). It is important to note that, with nominal data, the participant is categorized into one, and only one, category. That is, the categories are mutually exclusive.

An **ordinal scale** has all of the characteristics of a nominal variable with the addition of rank ordering. It is important to note the distance between rank ordered categories cannot be considered equal; that is, the data points can be ranked but the distance between them may differ greatly. For example, in medicine a commonly used pain scale is the Wong-Baker Faces Pain Rating Scale.[3] Here, the participant ranks pain on a 0 to 10 scale; however, while it is known that a rating of 8 indicates the participant is in more pain than a rating of 4, there is no indication that a rating of 8 hurts twice as much as a rating of 4.

An **interval scale** has all of the characteristics of an ordinal scale with the addition that the distance between two values is now constant and meaningful. However, it is important to note that interval scales do not have an absolute zero point. For example, temperature on a Celsius scale is measured on an interval scale (i.e., the difference between $10°C$ and $5°C$ is equivalent to the difference between $20°C$ and $15°C$). However, $20°C/10°C$ cannot be quantified as twice as hot because there is no absolute zero (i.e., the Celsius scale does not have an index of "no temperature").

Finally, a **ratio scale** has all of the characteristics of an interval scale, but ratio scales have an absolute zero point. The classic example of a ratio scale is temperature measured on the Kelvin scale, where zero Kelvin represents the absence of molecular motion. Theoretically, researchers should not confuse absolute and arbitrary zero points. However, the difference between interval and ratio scales is generally trivial as these data are analyzed by identical statistical procedures and are both numerical.

CONTINUOUS VERSUS CATEGORICAL VARIABLES

Continuous variables generally consist of data measured on interval or ratio scales. However, if the number of ordinal categories is large (e.g., seven or more), they may be considered continuous.[4] Be aware that continuous variables may also be referred to as quantitative in the literature. Examples of continuous variables include age, body mass index (BMI), or uncategorized systolic or diastolic blood pressure values.

Categorical variables consist of data measured on nominal or ordinal scales because these scales of measurement have naturally distinct categories. Examples of categorical variables include gender, race, or blood pressure status (e.g., hypotensive, normotensive, prehypertensive, hypertensive). In the literature, categorical variables are often termed discrete or if a variable is measured on a nominal scale with only two distinct categories it may be termed binary or **dichotomous**.

Note that it is common in the biomedical literature for researchers to categorize continuous variables. Although not wholly incorrect, categorizing a continuous variable will always result in loss of information about the variable. For example, consider the role that participant age has on the probability of experiencing a cardiac event. Although age is a continuous variable, younger individuals typically have much a lower probability compared to older individuals. Thus, the research may divide age into four discrete categories: <30, 31 to 50, 51 to 70, and 70+. Note that assigning category cutoffs is generally an arbitrary process. In this example, information is lost by categorizing age because after categorization, the exact age of the participant is unknown. That is, an individual's age is defined only by their age category. For example, a 50-year-old individual is considered identical to a 31-year-old individual because they are in the same age category and qualitatively different from a 51-year-old individual given they are in different categories.

Descriptive Statistics

There are two types of statistics—descriptive and inferential. Descriptive statistics present, organize, and summarize a variable's data by providing information regarding the appearance of the data and distributional characteristics. Examples of descriptive statistics include measures of central tendency, variability, shape, histograms, boxplots, and scatterplots. These descriptive measures are the focus of this section.

Inferential statistics indicate whether a difference exists between groups of participants or whether an association exists between variables. Inferential statistics are used to determine whether the difference or association is real or whether it is due to some random process. Examples of inferential statistics are the statistics produced by each statistical test described later in the chapter. For example, the t statistic produced by a t-test.

MEASURES OF CENTRAL TENDENCY

❷ *Measures of central tendency are useful to quantify the distribution of a variable's data numerically. The most common measures of central tendency are the mean, median, and mode, with the most appropriate measure of central tendency dictated by the variable's scale of measurement.*

The **mean** (indicated as M in the literature) is the most common and appropriate measure of central tendency for normally distributed data (see the Common Probability Distributions section later in this chapter) measured on an interval or ratio scale. The mean is the arithmetic average of a variable's data. Thus, the mean is calculated by summing a variable's data and dividing by the total number of participants with data for the specific variable. It is important to note that data points that are severely disconnected from the other data points can significantly influence the mean. These extreme data points are termed outliers.

The **median** (indicated as Mdn in the literature) is most appropriate measure of central tendency for data measured on an ordinal scale. The median is the absolute middle value in the data; therefore, exactly half of the data is above the median and exactly half of the data is below the median. The median is also known as the 50th percentile. Note that the median can also be presented for continuous variables with skewed distributions (see the Measures of Distribution Shape section later in chapter) and for continuous variables with outliers. A direct comparison of a variable's mean and median can give insight into how much influence outliers had on the mean.

Finally, the **mode** is the most appropriate measure of central tendency for nominal data. The mode is a variable's most frequently occurring data point or category. Note that it is possible for a variable to have multiple modes; a variable with two or three modes is referred to as bimodal and trimodal, respectively.

MEASURES OF VARIABILITY

Measures of variability are useful in indicating the spread of a variable's data. The most common measures of variability are the range, interquartile range, variance, and standard deviation. These measures are also useful when considered with appropriate measures of central tendency to assess how the data are scattered around the mean or median. For example, consider the two histograms in Figure 6-1. Both histograms present data for 100 participants that have identical mean body weight of 185 pounds. However, notice the variability (or dispersion) of the data is much greater for Group 2. If the means for both groups were simply taken at face value, the participants in these two groups would be considered similar; however, assessing the variability or spread of data within each group illustrates an entirely different picture. This concept is critically important to the application of any inferential statistical test because the test results are heavily influenced by the amount of variability.

The simplest measure of variability is the range, which can be used to describe data measured on an ordinal, interval, or ratio scale. The range is a crude measure of variability calculated by subtracting a variable's minimum data point from its maximum data point. For example, in Figure 6-1 the range for Group 1 is 30 (i.e., 200 – 170), whereas the range from Group 2 is 95 (i.e., 235 – 140).

The interquartile range (indicated as IQR in the literature) is another measure of dispersion used to describe data measured on ordinal scale; as such, the IQR is usually presented alongside the median. The IQR is the difference between the 75th and 25th percentile. Therefore, because the median represents the 50th percentile, the IQR presents the middle 50% of the data and always includes the median.

Figure 6–1. Differences in variability between two groups with identical means.

The final two measures of variability described are the variance and standard deviation. These measures are appropriate for normally distributed continuous variables measured on interval or ratio scales. ❸ *Variance is a key element inherent in all statistical analyses, but standard deviation is presented more often. Variance and standard deviation are related mathematically.* Variance is the average squared deviation from the mean for all data points within a specific variable. For example, consider Figure 6-1 where the mean for both Group 1 and Group 2 was 185 pounds. Say a specific participant in Group 1 had a body weight of 190 pounds. The squared deviation from the mean for this participant would be equal to 25 pounds. That is, $190 - 185 = 5$ and $5^2 = 25$. To calculate variance, the squared deviations are calculated for all data points. These square deviations are then summed across participants and then divided by the total number of data points (i.e., N) to obtain the average squared deviation. Some readers may be asking why the deviations from the mean are squared. This is a great question! The reason is that summing unsquared deviations across participants would equal zero. That is, deviations resulting from values above and below the mean would cancel each other out. While the calculation of variance may seem esoteric, conceptually all that is required to understand variance is that larger variance values indicate greater variability. For example, the variances of Group 1 and Group 2 in Figure 6-1 were 25 and 225, respectively. While the histograms did not present these numbers explicitly, the greater variability in Group 2 can be observed clearly. The importance of variance cannot be overstated. It is the primary parameter used in all parametric statistical analyses, and this is why it was presented in such detail here. With that said, variance is rarely presented as a descriptive statistic in the literature. Instead, variance is converted into a standard deviation as described in the next paragraph.

As a descriptive statistic, the standard deviation (indicated as SD in the literature) is often preferred over variance because it indicates the average deviation from the mean presented on the same scale as the original variable. Variance presented the average deviation in squared units. It is important to note that the standard deviation and variance are directly related mathematically, with standard deviation equal to the square root of the variance (i.e., $SD = \sqrt{\text{variance}}$). Thus, if the standard deviation is known, the variance can be calculated directly, and vice versa. When comparing variability between groups of participants, the standard deviation can provide insight into the dispersion of scores around the mean, and, similar to variance, larger standard deviations indicate greater variability in the data. For example, from Figure 6-1, Group 1 had a standard deviation of 5 (i.e., $\sqrt{25}$) and Group 2 had a standard deviation of 15 (i.e., $\sqrt{225}$). Again, the greater variability within Group 2 is evident.

MEASURES OF DISTRIBUTION SHAPE

Skewness and kurtosis are appropriate measures of shape for variables measured on interval or ratio scales, and indicate asymmetry and peakedness of a distribution, respectively. They are typically used by researchers to evaluate the distributional assumptions of a parametric statistical analysis.

Skewness indicates the asymmetry of distribution of data points and can be either positive or negative. Positive (or right) skewness occurs when the mode and median are less than the mean, whereas negative (or left) skewness occurs when mode and median are greater than the mean. As stated previously, the mean is sensitive to extremely

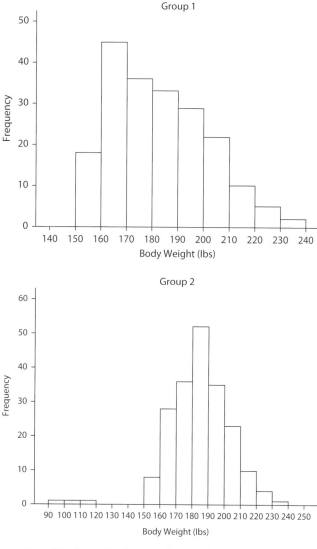

Figure 6–2. True positive skewness and negative skewness due to outliers.

disconnected data points termed outliers; thus, it is important to know the difference between true skewness and skewness due to outliers. True skewness is indicated by a steady decrease in data points toward the tails (i.e., ends) of the distribution. Skewness due to outliers is indicated when the mean is heavily influenced by data points that are extremely disconnected from the rest of the distribution. For example, consider the histogram in Figure 6-2. The data for Group 1 provides an example of true positive skewness, whereas the data for Group 2 provides an example of negative skewness due to outliers.

Kurtosis indicates the peakedness of the distribution of data points and can be either positive or negative. Plotted data with a narrow, peaked distribution and a positive kurtosis value is termed leptokurtic. A leptokurtic distribution has small range, variance, and standard deviation with the majority of data points near the mean. In contrast, plotted data with a wide, flat distribution and a negative kurtosis value is referred to as platykurtic. A platykurtic distribution is an indicator of great variability, with large range, variance, and standard deviation. Examples of leptokurtic and platykurtic data distributions are presented for Group 1 and Group 2, respectively, in Figure 6-2.

GRAPHICAL REPRESENTATIONS OF DATA

Graphical representations of data are incredibly useful, especially when sample sizes are large, as they allow researchers to inspect the distribution of individual variables. There are typically three graphical representations presented in the literature—histograms, boxplots, and scatterplots. Note that graphical representations are typically used for continuous variables measured on ordinal, interval, or ratio scales. By contrast, nominal, dichotomous, or categorical variables are best presented as count data, which are typically reported in the literature as frequency and percentage.

A histogram presents data as frequency counts over some interval; that is, the x-axis presents the values of the data points, whether individual data points or intervals, while the y-axis presents the number of times the data point or interval occurs in the variable (i.e., frequency). Figures 6-1 and 6-2 provide examples of histograms. When data are plotted, it is easy to observe skewness, kurtosis, or outlier issues. For example, reconsider the distribution of body weight for Group 2 in Figure 6-2, where each vertical bar represents the number of participants having body weight within 10-unit intervals. The distribution of data has negative skewness due to outliers, with outliers being participants weighing between 90 and 120 pounds.

A boxplot, also known as a box-and-whisker plot, provides the reader with five descriptive statistics.[5] Consider the boxplot in Figure 6-3, which presents the same data as the Group 2 histogram in Figure 6-2. The thin-lined box in a boxplot indicates the IQR, which contains the 25th to 75th percentiles of the data. Within this thin-lined box is a thick, bold line depicting the median, or 50th percentile. From both ends of the thin-lined box extends a tail, or whisker, depicting the minimum and maximum data points up to 1.5 IQRs beyond the median. Beyond the whiskers, outliers and extreme outliers are identified with circles and asterisks, respectively. Note that other symbols may be used to identify outliers depending on the statistical software used. Outliers are defined as data points 1.5 to 3.0 IQRs beyond the median, whereas extreme outliers are defined as data points greater than 3.0 IQRs beyond the median. The boxplot corroborates the information provided by the histogram in Figure 6-2 as participants weighing between 90 and 120 pounds are defined as outliers.

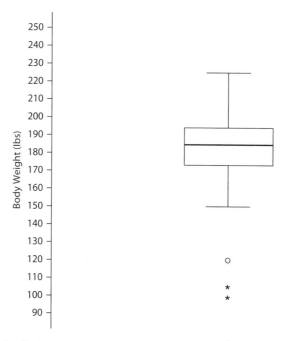

Figure 6–3. Boxplot of body weight with outliers. Circles represent values 1.5 to 3.0 IQRs, asterisks represent values >3.0 IQRs.

Finally, a scatterplot presents data for two variables both measured on a continuous scale. That is, the *x*-axis contains the range of data for one variable, whereas the *y*-axis contains the range of data for a second variable. In general, the axis choice for a given variable is arbitrary. Data are plotted in a similar fashion to plotting data on a coordinate plane during an introductory geometry class. Figure 6-4 presents a scatterplot of height in inches and body weight in pounds. The individual circles in the scatterplot are a participant's height in relation to their weight. Because the plot is bivariate (i.e., there are two variables), participants must have data for both variables in order to be plotted. Scatterplots are useful in visually assessing the association between two variables as well as assessing assumptions of various statistical tests such as linearity and absence of outliers.

Common Probability Distributions

Up to this point, data distributions have been discussed using very general terminology. There are numerous distributions available to researchers; far too many to provide a complete listing, but all that needs to be known about these available distributions is that each

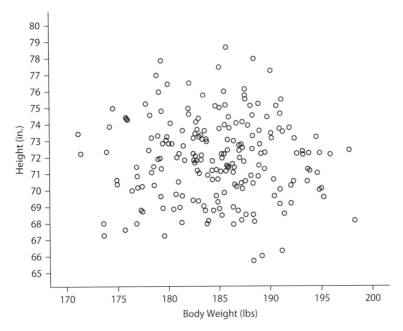

Figure 6–4. Scatterplot of height by weight.

has different characteristics to fit the unique requirements of the data. Globally, these distributions are termed probability distributions, and they are incredibly important to every statistical analysis conducted. Thus, the choice of distribution used in a given statistical analysis is nontrivial as the use of an improper distribution can lead to incorrect statistical inference. Of the distributions available, the normal and binomial distributions are used most frequently in the biomedical literature; therefore, these are discussed in detail. To provide the reader with a broader listing of available distributions, this section also presents brief information about other common distributions used in the biomedical literature and when they are appropriately used in statistical analyses.

THE NORMAL DISTRIBUTION

The normal distribution, also called Gaussian distribution, is the most commonly used distribution in statistics and one that occurs frequently in nature. It is used only for continuous variables measured on interval or ratio scales. The normal distribution has several easily identifiable properties based on the numerical measures of central tendency, variability, and shape. Specifically, this includes the following characteristics:

1. The primary shape is bell-shaped.
2. The mean, median, and mode are equal.

3. The distribution has one mode, is symmetric, and reflects itself perfectly when folded at the mean.
4. The skewness and kurtosis are zero.
5. The area under a normal distribution is, by definition, equal to one.

It should be noted the five properties above are considered the gold standard. In practice, however, each of these properties will be approximated; namely, the curve will be roughly bell-shaped, the mean, median, and mode will be roughly equal, and skewness and kurtosis may be evident but not greatly exaggerated. For example, the distribution of data for Group 2 in Figure 6-1 is approximately normal.

Several additional properties of the normal distribution are important; consider Figure 6-5. First, the distribution is completely defined by the mean and standard deviation. Consequently, there are an infinite number of possible normal distributions because there are an infinite number of mean and standard deviation combinations. In the literature, this property is often stated as the mean and standard deviation being sufficient statistics for describing the normal distribution. Second, the mean can always be identified as the peak (or mode) of the distribution. Third, the standard deviation will always dictate the spread of the distribution. That is, as the standard deviation increases, the distribution becomes wider. Finally, roughly 68% of the data will occur within one standard deviation above and below the mean, roughly 95% within two standard deviations, and roughly 99% within three standard deviations.

THE STANDARD NORMAL DISTRIBUTION

Among the infinite number of potential normal distributions, only the standard normal distribution can be used to compare all normal distributions. Although this may seem confusing on the surface, a clearer understanding of the standard normal distribution is made possible by considering the standard deviation. Initially, when converting a normal distribution to a standard normal distribution, the data must be converted into standardized scores referred to as **z-scores**. A z-score converts the units of the original data into standard deviation units. That is, a z-score indicates how many standard deviations a data point is from the mean. When converted to z-scores, the new standard normal distribution will always have a mean of zero and a standard deviation of one. The standard normal distribution is presented in Figure 6-5.

It is a common misconception that converting data into z-scores creates a standard normal distribution from data that was not normally distributed. This is never true. A standardized distribution will always have the same characteristics of distribution from which it originated. That is, if the original distribution was skewed, the standardized distribution will also be skewed.

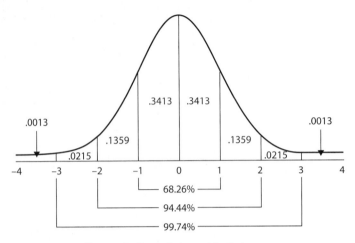

Figure 6–5. The standard normal distribution.

❹ *The key benefit to using the standard normal distribution is that converting the original data to z-scores allows researchers to compare different variables regardless of the original scale.* Remember, a standardized variable will always be expressed in standard deviation units with a mean of zero and standard deviation of one. Therefore, differences between variables may be more easily detected and understood. For example, it is possible to compare standardized variables across studies. It should go without stating that the only requirement is that both variables measure the same construct. After z-score standardization, the age of two groups of participants from two different studies can be compared directly.

THE BINOMIAL DISTRIBUTION

Many discrete variables can be dichotomized into one of two mutually exclusive groups, outcomes, or events (e.g., dead versus alive). Using the binomial distribution, a researcher can calculate the exact probability of experiencing either binary outcome. The binomial distribution can only be used when an experiment assumes the four characteristics listed below:

1. The trial occurs a specified number of times (analogous to sample size, n).
2. Each trial has only two mutually exclusive outcomes (success versus failure in a generic sense, x). Also, be aware that a single trial with only two outcomes is known as a Bernoulli trial, a term that may be encountered in the literature.
3. Each trial is independent, meaning that one outcome has no effect on the other.
4. The probability of success remains constant throughout the trial.

An example may assist with the understanding of these characteristics. The binomial distribution consists of the number of successes and failures during a given study period. When all trials have been run, the probability of achieving exactly x successes (or failures) in n trials can be calculated. Consider flipping a fair coin. The coin is flipped for a set number of trials (i.e., n), there are only two possible outcomes (i.e., heads or tails), each trial is not affected by the outcome of the last, and the probability of flipping heads or tails remains constant throughout the trial (i.e., 0.50).

By definition, the mean for the binomial distribution is equal to the number of successes in a given trial. That is, if a fair coin is flipped 10 times and heads turns up on six flips, the mean is 0.60 (i.e., 6/10). Further, the variance of the binomial distribution is fixed by the mean. While the equation for the variance is not presented, know that the variance is largest at a mean of 0.50, decreases as the mean diverges from 0.50, and is symmetric (e.g., the variance for a mean of 0.10 is equal to the variance for a mean of 0.90). Therefore, because variance is fixed by the mean, the mean is the sufficient statistic for the binomial distribution.

In reality, the probability of experiencing an outcome is rarely 0.50. For example, biomedical studies often use all-cause mortality as an outcome variable, and the probability of dying during the study period is generally lower than staying alive. At the end of the trial, participants can experience only one of the outcomes—dead or alive. Say a study sample consists of 1,000 participants, of which 150 die. The binomial distribution allows for the calculation of the exact probability of having 150 participants die in a sample of 1,000 participants.

OTHER COMMON PROBABILITY DISTRIBUTIONS

As mentioned in the introduction to this section, there are numerous probability distributions available to researchers, with their use determined by the scale of measurement of the DV as well as the shape (e.g., skewness) of the distribution. When reading journal articles, it is important to know whether the appropriate distribution has been used for statistical analysis as inappropriate use of any distribution can lead to inaccurate statistical inference.

Table 6-1 provides a short list of the several commonly used distributions in the biomedical literature. Of note here is that alternative distributions are available when statistically analyzing non-normally distributed continuous data or data that cannot be normalized such as categorical data. The takeaway message here is that non-normal continuous data does not need to be forced to conform to a normal distribution.

The only DV scale presented in Table 6-1 that has not been discussed thus far is count data. An example of count data would be a count of the number of hospitalizations during a 5-year study period. It is clear from the example that count data cannot take on negative values. That is, a participant cannot have a negative number of hospitalizations.

TABLE 6–1. COMMON PROBABILITY DISTRIBUTIONS AND WHEN THEY ARE APPROPRIATE TO USE

Distribution Name	DV Scale	Distribution Characteristics	Comments
Normal	Continuous		
Gamma	Continuous	Positive skew	
Inverse Gaussian	Continuous	Positive skew	
Exponential	Continuous	Positive skew	Data has to be >0
Log-normal[a]	Continuous	Positive skew	Data has to be >0
Weibull	Continuous	Positive or negative skew	
Gompertz	Continuous	Positive or negative skew	
Poisson	Count	Mean $=$ variance	Data ≥ 0
Negative binomial	Count	Mean $\neq$ variance	Data ≥ 0
Bernoulli	Binary		One trial; 2 categories
Binomial	Binary		Repeated Bernoulli trials; 2 categories
Categorical	Categorical		One trial; >2 categories
Multinomial	Categorical		Repeated trials; >2 categories

[a]Log $=$ natural log or ln.

Both the Poisson and negative binomial distributions are used when analyzing count data. The Poisson distribution assumes the mean and the variance of the data are identical. However, in situations where the mean and variance are not equal, the negative binomial distribution allows the variance of the distribution to increase or decrease as needed. As a point of possible confusion, the negative binomial distribution does not allow negative values. The negative in negative binomial is a result of using a negative exponent in its mathematical formula.

TRANSFORMATION OF NON-NORMAL DISTRIBUTIONS

Transformations are usually employed by researchers to force a non-normal distribution into a distribution that is approximately normal. Although on the surface this may appear reasonable, data transformation is an archaic technique. As such, transformation is not recommended for the three reasons provided below.

First, although parametric statistical analyses assume normality, the distribution of the actual DV data is not required to be normally distributed. As stated in the previous section, and highlighted in Table 6-1, if non-normality is observed, alternative distributions exist allowing proper statistical analysis of non-normal data without transformation. For this reason alone, transformation is rarely necessary.

Second, transforming the DV data potentially prevents effects of an IV from being observed. As an overly simplistic example, consider the distribution of body weight data

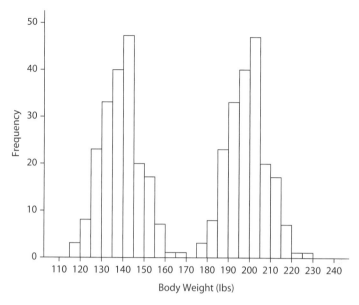

Figure 6–6. Body weight data for a group of men and women.

• presented in Figure 6-6. Say the body weight data were collected from a sample of men and women. Obviously, the data in Figure 6-6 is bimodal and not normally distributed. In this situation, a researcher may attempt to transform the data, but transformation would obscure the effects of an obvious IV—gender. That is, women tend to be lighter compared to men, and this is observed in these data, with women being grouped in the left distribution and men grouped in the right distribution. If transformation were performed successfully, inherent differences between men and women would be erased.

Third, although data transformation will not affect the rank order of the data, it can significantly cloud interpretation of statistical analyses. That is, after transformation all results must be interpreted in the transformed metric, which can become convoluted quickly making it difficult to apply results to the untransformed data used in the real world. Thus, when reading a journal article where the authors employed any transformation, be aware that the results are in the transformed metric and ensure that the authors' interpretations remain consistent with this metric.

Although transformation is not recommended, it can be used appropriately, and it will inevitably be encountered when reading the literature, especially for skewed distributions. Therefore, it is useful to become familiar with several of the techniques used to transform data. Transformations for positive skewness differ from those suggested for negative skewness. Mild positive skewness is typically remedied by a square root transformation. Here, the square root of all data is calculated and this square root data is used in analysis. When positive skewness is severe, a natural log transformation is used. When data are skewed negatively, researchers may choose to reflect their data to make it positively skewed and apply the transformations for positive skewness described above. To reflect data, a 1 is added to the absolute value of the highest data point and all data points are subtracted from this new value. For example, if the highest value in the data is 10, a 1 is added to create 11, and then all data points are subtracted from 11 (e.g., $11 - 10 = 1$, $11 - 1 = 10$). In this manner, the highest values become the lowest and the lowest become the highest. It should be clear that this process considerably convolutes data interpretation!

Epidemiological Statistics

The field of epidemiology investigates how diseases are distributed in the population and the various factors (or exposures) influencing this distribution.[6] Epidemiological statistics are not unique to the field of epidemiology, as much of the literature in the biomedical sciences incorporates some form of these statistics, such as odds ratios. Thus, it is important to have at least a basic level of understanding of these statistics. In this section, the most commonly used epidemiological statistics are discussed briefly including ratios, proportions, rates, incidence and prevalence, relative risk and odds ratios as well as sensitivity, specificity, and predictive values.

RATIOS, PROPORTIONS, AND RATES

Ratios, proportions, and rates are terms used interchangeably in the medical literature without regard for the actual mathematical definitions. Further, there are a considerable number of proportions and rates available to researchers, each providing unique information. Thus, it is important to be aware of how each of these measures are defined and calculated.[7]

- A ratio expresses the relationship between two numbers. For example, consider the ratio of men to women diagnosed with multiple sclerosis (MS). If, in a sample consisting of only MS patients, 100 men and 50 women are diagnosed, the ratio of men to women is 100 to 50, or 100:50, or 2:1. Remember, that the order in which the ratio is presented is vitally important; that is, 100:50 is not the same as 50:100.

- A proportion is a specific type of ratio indicating the probability or percentage of the total sample that experienced an outcome or event without respect to time. Here, the numerator of the proportion, representing patients with the disease, is included in the denominator, representing all individuals at risk. For example, say 850 non-MS patients are added to the sample of 150 MS patients from the example above to create a total sample of 1,000 patients. Thus, the proportion of patients with MS is 0.15 or 15% (i.e., 150/1,000).

A rate is a special form of a proportion that includes a specific study period, typically used to assess the speed at which the event or outcome is developing.[8] A rate is equal to the number of events in a specified time period divided by the length of the time period. For example, say over a 1-year study period, 50 new cases of MS were diagnosed out of the 850 previously undiagnosed individuals. Thus, the rate of new cases of MS within this sample is 50 per year.

INCIDENCE AND PREVALENCE

Incidence quantifies the occurrence of an event or outcome over a specific study period within a specific population of individuals. The incidence rate is calculated by dividing the number of new events by the population at risk, with the population at risk defined as the total number of people who have not experienced the outcome. For example, consider the 50 new cases of MS that developed from the example above from the 850 originally undiagnosed individuals. The incidence rate is approximately 0.06 (i.e., 50/850). Note the denominator did not include the 150 patients already diagnosed with MS because these individuals could longer be in the population at risk.

Prevalence quantifies the number of people who have already experienced the event or outcome at a specific time point. Prevalence is calculated by dividing the total number of people experiencing the event by the total number of individuals in the population. Note that the denominator is everyone in the population, not just individuals in the population at risk. For example, the diagnosed MS cases (i.e., 50 + 150 = 200) would be divided by the population that includes them. That is, the prevalence of MS in this sample is 0.20 (i.e., 200/1,000).

Finally, it is important to consider both incidence and prevalence when describing events or outcomes. This is because prevalence varies directly with incidence and the duration of the sickness or disease. For example, consider influenza where the duration of the sickness is relatively short. Thus, while incidence of new influenza cases may be high, the overall prevalence may be low because most individuals recover quickly. By contrast, consider individuals diagnosed with asthma. Because asthma is incurable, the prevalence of the disease may be high, whereas the incidence may be low depending on the total number of new cases diagnosed throughout the year.

RELATIVE RISK AND ODDS RATIO

Relative risk is defined as the ratio (or probability) of the incidence of an event occurring in individuals exposed to a stimulus compared to the incidence of the event in those not exposed to the stimulus. Relative risk can be calculated directly from the cohort study design (see Chapter 5). Briefly, this design is typically a prospective observational design comparing the incidence of experiencing an event in cohorts of exposed and unexposed individuals over time.

Relative risk is used when comparing the probability of an event occurring to all possible events considered in a study. For example, consider the risk of developing lung cancer in those who are exposed and unexposed to secondhand smoke over a 10-year study period. Upon study conclusion, the 2 × 2 contingency table, shown in Figure 6-7, is created containing frequency counts of events for two groups exposed and unexposed to the secondhand smoke stimulus. This table provides all data necessary to calculate the incidence of the event for both exposed and unexposed individuals. Relative risk is calculated by dividing the proportion of individuals who suffered the event in the exposed group (i.e., A/A+B) by the proportion of individuals who suffered the event in the unexposed group (i.e., C/C+D). Relative risk provides a single number ranging from zero to infinity, and there are three resulting interpretations provided below.[6]

1. If relative risk equals 1, the risk of experiencing the event was equal within the exposed and unexposed groups. Thus, there is no association of being exposed to the stimulus.
2. If relative risk is greater than 1, the exposed group has a greater risk of experiencing the event compared to the unexposed group. Thus, there is a positive association or detrimental effect (risk factor) of being exposed to the stimulus.
3. If relative risk is less than 1, the exposed group has a lower risk of experiencing the event compared to the unexposed group. Thus, there is a negative association or protective effect of being exposed to the stimulus.

When relative risk cannot be calculated, researchers will often present an odds ratio. Odds are calculated by dividing the proportion of people experiencing an event by the proportion of people not experiencing an event. Thus, an odds ratio is a ratio of two odds; one for individuals exposed to the stimulus and the other for those not exposed to the stimulus. Odds ratios range from zero to infinity. They have three interpretations identical to those presented above for relative risk, simply substitute the odds ratio for relative risk. Odds ratios can be calculated for both cohort and case-control designs. A case-control study compares cases that have experienced the event and controls who have not, and

	Event	No Event	
Exposed	A	B	A + B
Unexposed	C	D	C + D
	A + C	B + D	A + B + C + D

Figure 6–7. Example of a 2 × 2 contingency table.

then assesses whether each individual was exposed to a stimulus or not. Thus, a case-control study is retrospective.

Odds ratios are used when comparing events to nonevents with its calculation depending on the study design. For example, consider comparing a group of individuals who developed measles to those who did not and then determining whether they received all recommended vaccinations. In a cohort study, the odds ratio is calculated by dividing the odds of experiencing the event in the exposed group (i.e., A/B) by the odds in the unexposed group who experienced the event (i.e., C/D). In a case-control study, the odds ratio is calculated by dividing the odds that cases were exposed to the risk (i.e., A/C) by the odds that the controls were exposed (i.e., B/D).

Relative risk and odds ratios are comparable in magnitude only when the outcome under study is rare (e.g., some cancers). It is important to consider that odds ratios consistently overestimate risk when the outcome is more common (e.g., hyperlipidemia). As a result, relative risk should be used if possible and caution should be exhibited when interpreting odds ratios.

SENSITIVITY, SPECIFICITY, AND PREDICTIVE VALUES

Sensitivity, specificity, and positive and negative predictive values indicate the ability of a test to identify correctly those experiencing the event and those who did not. For example, consider the ability of a blood glucose screening test to correctly identify individuals with diabetes. Four outcomes result from this test that are required for the calculation of sensitivity, specificity, and the predictive values:

1. True positives (TP) have the disease and have a positive test result.
2. False positives (FP) do not have the disease, but have a positive test result.
3. True negatives (TN) do not have the disease and have a negative test result.
4. False negatives (FN) have the disease, but have a negative test result.

Sensitivity is the probability a diseased individual will have a positive test result and is the true positive rate of the test. It is calculated by dividing true positives by all individuals who actually have the disease (i.e., TP/TP+FN). **Specificity** is the probability that a disease-free individual will have a negative test result and is the true negative rate of the screening test. It is calculated by dividing true negatives by all disease-free individuals (i.e., TN/TN+FP).

Positive and negative predictive values are calculated to measure the accuracy of the screening test. Both predictive values are directly related to disease prevalence; that is, the higher the prevalence, the higher the predictive value.[6] Positive predictive value provides the proportion of individuals who test positive for the disease that actually have the disease. It is calculated by dividing true positives by all individuals with a positive test result (i.e., TP/TP+FP). Negative predictive value provides the proportion of individuals who test negative and who are actually disease-free. It is calculated by dividing true negatives by all individuals with a negative test result (i.e., TN/TN+FN).

It is important to identify the implications all four values have to new and existing research. When designing a study involving a screening test, researchers must indicate a standard cutoff score for their screening. That is, qualify who is to be considered diseased and who will be considered disease-free. This decision clearly reflects the repercussions of classifying individuals as false negatives or false positives. For example, consider a screening tool for early-stage breast cancer, where there are considerable consequences for both false positives and false negatives. On the one hand, a patient with a false positive may be referred for unnecessary testing that is painful and expensive, not to mention emotionally taxing. On the other hand, a false negative has more serious implications, since the patient may not receive any treatment until the disease has progressed.

Types of Study Design

The distinction between experimental, quasi-experimental, and nonexperimental research is important, both from a study design perspective and when evaluating literature. Although experimental designs are considered the gold standard by many, do not discount research conducted using quasi-experimental and nonexperimental designs, as long as the limitations are considered. Each of these types of designs is discussed in this section.

EXPERIMENTAL DESIGNS

In the biomedical sciences, experimental designs are typically referred to as a randomized controlled trial (RCT). A full treatment of experimental design is presented in Chapters 4 and 5, so the discussion provided here will only touch the tip of the iceberg on experimental designs. Interested readers are encouraged to consult the suggested readings provided at the end of this chapter for more information.

First, experimental designs always allow the researcher to manipulate levels of an IV. For example, consider a drug trial assessing the effectiveness of a new cancer medication. For this trial, four groups of participants are randomly assigned to a different dose of a medication. Thus, there are four levels of the IV. The researcher, within ethical and theoretical constraints, can manipulate the size of the dose, if the participants will be measured multiple times, and the length of the study period.

Second, in experimental design, participants are randomly assigned to levels of the IV. Thus, any participant has a chance of being placed in any single group, which theoretically provides initial equivalence of participants across study groups. There are many different methods and theories of randomization and the chance of being in one group versus another does not necessarily have to be equal. For example, consider a study that has two treatment groups and one placebo group where the researcher is interested in the difference between the treatment groups. Because the difference in the DV between the placebo and either treatment group will usually be larger than the difference in the DV between the treatment groups, the researcher may randomize more participants to the treatment groups to increase statistical power to detect the difference between treatments. Note that the concept of statistical power is discussed in the Statistical Inference section as well as in Chapter 4. Often a 2:1 or 3:1 randomization schedule will be used with two or three times as many participants, respectively, being randomized to treatment as opposed to placebo.

Third, causality can be determined with proper experimental control of error. For example, the effectiveness of a cancer drug can be better explained by reducing sources of error due to the participant (e.g., age, health status), setting (e.g., prescriber's office), or diagnostic tests (e.g., measurement accuracy).

Finally, it should be noted RCTs have limitations. The primary limitation is cost, as RCTs are extremely costly requiring many considerations including space, personnel, and participants. RCTs also may have limited external validity and generalizability due to extreme control over experimental conditions (e.g., efficacy study) that do not necessarily translate to real-world situations (e.g., effectiveness study). Third, it is difficult, if not impossible, to study rare events with an RCT due to ethical concerns and the considerable sample size required.

QUASI-EXPERIMENTAL DESIGNS

Quasi-experimental designs are used more often in the social sciences but can be observed in the biomedical literature. On the surface, these types of designs appear to be experimental; however, they lack one key aspect, random assignment.

For example, consider examining the effectiveness of a new dialysis treatment. Most dialysis patients are already in the care of a nephrologist at a specific clinic. Because nephrologists typically see numerous patients, randomizing patients to specific levels of treatment (i.e., the IV) within a group that is under the care of the same nephrologist may be infeasible logistically or may lead to medication errors. Thus, the entire clinic must be randomized. That is, all patients within a specific clinic will receive one treatment.

Advantages of quasi-experimental designs include reduced cost and a quicker timeline compared to RCTs with the addition of possible increases in external validity due to conditions being more consistent with the real world. The disadvantages, however, are considerable. This is most notable with the lack of random assignment. Nonrandom assignment may create dissimilar groups based on any number of characteristics that are potentially related to the success of the treatment. For example, consistent differences in patient demographics (e.g., sickness) may result from a dialysis clinic in the suburbs being compared to a dialysis clinic in a more urban setting. Further, causation cannot be implied and statistical analysis can potentially be rendered uninformative.[9]

NONEXPERIMENTAL DESIGNS

Nonexperimental designs have several advantages over RCTs, primarily lower cost, a quicker timeline to publication, and a broader range of participants.[10] The advantages of nonexperimental studies over RCTs have prompted their widespread use in the biomedical sciences. Overall, these studies tend to be nonrandomized, retrospective, and correlational in nature and are distinct because the researcher cannot manipulate the IV(s).

For example, consider a 5-year retrospective study assessing the effectiveness of statin therapy on preventing cardiac events. The researcher has knowledge of which patients initiated statin therapy, but has no control over the drug, dose, adherence, etc. Although the researcher may assign patients to groups based on different doses, the researcher cannot randomly assign patients to a specific drug nor can they manipulate the dose. In addition, nonexperimental research often fails to indicate causality, which is due to lack of experimental control and randomization as well as inability to identify all confounding variables. Finally, it is important to note that while nonexperimental designs are ubiquitous in the biomedical sciences, treatment effects may be different when compared to RCTs[11] (Case Study 6-1).

Case Study 6–1

In the past, blood loss in patients undergoing total knee replacement had been managed through electro-cauterization and tourniquet. More recently, however, the use of antifibrinolytic medications have become common to further decrease blood loss. Two common antifibrinolytics include tranexamic acid (TXA) and ε-aminocaproic acid (EACA). Given that TXA is much more expensive than EACA, an orthopedic surgeon is interested in whether 14 g of EACA can produce a similar blood-sparing effect to 2 g of TXA (note that TXA is at least seven times more potent than EACA on a molar basis). The surgeon plans to enroll his own patients as well as patients from six other surgeons in his practice. All patients and surgeons will be blinded from the medication used as the medication will be distributed by the hospital's pharmacist in a 250 cc vial of saline. Following consent, patients will be randomized such that an equal number of patients receive either TXA or

EACA; the randomization schedule will stratify patients by biological sex and weight to account for blood volume differences. Blood loss will be estimated using hemoglobin measured at preoperative physical and immediately after surgery; both pre- and postoperative hemoglobin will be treated as continuous variables.

Please answer the following questions:

1. Who is the population of interest?
2. What sampling strategy or strategies were used?
3. Would this study be considered a randomized controlled trial? Why or why not?
4. What is the DV for this study? What is the scale of measurement for the DV? Is the DV repeatedly measured?
5. What is the IV for this study? What is the scale of measurement for the IV? How many levels does the IV have?
6. Based on the study description, should any confounding variables or covariates have been considered for this study? If so, please describe.
7. The researcher is planning on presenting pre- and postoperative hemoglobin as mean and standard deviation. In what situation would this be the correct approach?

The Design and Analysis of Clinical Trials

The U.S. National Institutes of Health (NIH) defines clinical trials into two types: interventional and observational studies.[12] In this chapter, two specific types of interventional clinical trials are discussed—the randomized controlled trial (RCT) and adaptive clinical trial (ACT). The experimental design of RCTs and ACTs are discussed at length in Chapters 4 and 5, so the descriptions provided in this chapter are minimal. Briefly, RCTs and ACTs are both protocol-based, meaning that every step of the study from design to analysis is identified *a priori*. They are prospective studies where participants are followed over time using strict experimental control to indicate reliably the causality between the DV and manipulated IV.

THE DESIGN OF CLINICAL TRIALS

Parallel-Groups Design

The most common RCT is a parallel-groups design where the IV typically involves participants randomized into fixed levels of treatment, also known as treatment arms, with each arm indicating a different treatment or comparison.[13-16] That is, participants are randomly assigned to one, and only one, treatment arm. As stated in the previous section, the sample size within each group does not have to be equal and can vary depending on estimated statistical power to detect treatment effects.

There are two parallel-groups designs frequently used in the biomedical sciences—group comparison and matched pairs.[15] Briefly, a group comparison design simultaneously compares at least two groups of participants after each group is randomized to a different level of the IV. In a matched pairs design, participants are matched based on one or more characteristics (e.g., age, race) and then randomized to levels of the IV.

Crossover Design

The second most common RCT is a crossover design. A crossover design has the primary advantage of each participant serving as his or her own control.[13,15] The primary advantage of a crossover design is that it requires fewer participants in comparison to a parallel-groups design due to the fact that at the end of the study all participants will have been in all treatment arms. A disadvantage is that a crossover design cannot be used in a study where the first drug may cure the participant (e.g., an antibiotic given for an infection), since there would be no reason for the participant to crossover to the other agent.

For example, consider a 1-month study that includes two treatment arms. For a parallel-groups design, say 20 participants are required; that is, 10 participants are randomized to each treatment arm. By contrast, in a crossover design, only 10 subjects are required because each participant receives both treatments—10 participants receive the first treatment and the same 10 participants receive the second treatment. While both designs have two total measurements, in the parallel-groups design, two individual groups of participants provide one measurement each, whereas in the crossover design the same group of participants provides both measurements.

At this point, a common question is whether the effect of the first treatment carries over to influence the effect of the second treatment. This is a considerable concern in crossover designs and is dealt with by including a washout period between treatments. The maximum duration of the washout period is arbitrary. I must be long enough that the effect of the first treatment is absent prior to the beginning of the second treatment, but not be so long that participant attrition becomes a concern.

Adaptive Design

A more recent advancement to the RCT is the adaptive design or ACT. Although an ACT is possibly cheaper and more ethical than an RCT, this design is much more complex to both implement and analyze. Briefly, ACTs implement changes or adaptations in the design of the study based on the results of a predetermined set of interim statistical analyses. Interim analyses can be based on blinded or unblinded data, with the resulting adaptations aimed at establishing a more efficient, safer, and informative trial that is more likely to demonstrate treatment effects.[17]

For example, consider a 3-year study examining the effect of three different large doses of vitamin D on parathyroid hormone. Because implementing large doses of vitamin D is controversial, ethical considerations require this study to be adaptive. Here, the interim analyses would provide important information regarding the effectiveness and safety of the doses. Say, for example, that the ACT has interim analyses scheduled quarterly. Further, say that at the end of the second quarter of the first year the interim analyses indicated that the group receiving the highest dose of vitamin D had twice the risk of developing kidney stones compared to the other two groups. Thus, the group receiving the highest dose of vitamin D could have their dose reduced or the group could be dropped from the study completely. After these adaptations are implemented, the study continues as designed.

THE ANALYSIS OF CLINICAL TRIALS

The analysis of clinical trials typically involves evaluating repeated measures data where participants are followed prospectively over time or conducting an endpoint analysis using only the last observation or measurement. Regardless of the study design, the choice of the appropriate statistical test to analyze these data is based primarily on the scale of measurement of the DV, but other factors should also be considered (see the Selecting the Appropriate Statistical Test section later in the chapter).

Because an endpoint analysis is straightforward conceptually, a brief discussion of repeated measures design and analysis considerations is presented. Using a repeated measures design allows researchers to study the treatment effects over time in a smaller sample of participants due to the increased statistical power. Briefly, a repeated measures design increases statistical power by removing the error variance due to the participant. That is, each participant serves as his or her own control. Removing error variance is important because it results in larger test statistics and an increased probability of achieving statistical significance. However, a repeated measures design has limitations relevant to clinical trials, primarily participant attrition and nonadherence.

Attrition and nonadherence can assume many forms in a clinical trial. For example, participants may drop out of the study, fail to complete all required measurements, receive incorrect treatment or doses, or a myriad of other possible protocol violations. Thus, the first part of this section will discuss how the analysis of clinical trials typically handles missing data due to attrition and nonadherence. The final sections discuss the analysis of parallel-group, crossover, and adaptive designs.

Intent-to-Treat and Per-Protocol Approaches

Two analytical approaches exist for clinical trials—intent-to-treat (ITT) and per-protocol (PP). The ITT approach is often employed in the presence of violations to protocol or patients being lost to follow-up. ITT is the approach most often used in the biomedical literature. ITT requires the analysis to include all participants in the arm to which they were randomized originally. That is, treatment effects are best evaluated by the planned treatment protocol rather than the actual treatment given.[18]

For example, consider a participant randomized to receive treatment A but instead receives treatment B. For analysis, this participant would be considered as receiving treatment A. It should be noted that if a large number of protocol violations of this nature occur, the study would be discontinued; thus, these occurrences are relatively rare. It is important to note that the ITT approach has considerable weaknesses. Most notably, for ITT to be unbiased, attrition and nonadherence are considered to occur completely at random.[14] However, this is an untestable hypothesis. Further, the ITT approach can dilute treatment effects simply by including nonadherent participants by employing the last observation carried forward (LOCF) technique discussed later in this section.

By comparison, the PP approach evaluates only compliant participants with complete data. Although this analysis is straightforward analytically and allows researchers to evaluate a more accurate treatment effect, it has substantial limitations, primarily, reduced statistical power compared to an ITT approach, because participants with incomplete data are not considered in analysis.[18]

Because the ITT approach considers all participants with at least one measurement, an imputation or replacement method is often employed for missing measurements. The LOCF technique is one of the most commonly used imputation methods. This method uses the last recorded measurement for a participant for every missing measurement. For example, consider a study measuring HbA1c on six occasions over a 1-year study period. If a participant had only the first three measurements, the third (i.e., last) measurement would be imputed for measurements four through six. ❺ *From this example, it is clear the LOCF technique not only dilutes treatment effects, but also introduces significant bias into the results of statistical tests.* Therefore, be cautious when evaluating a study that has employed the LOCF technique. As a result of these limitations, better imputation approaches have been suggested including multiple imputation and the use of maximum likelihood estimation. These techniques are beyond the scope of this chapter, but are valid and produce unbiased estimates if data are considered missing at random.[19,20]

Analyzing Parallel-Groups Designs

When analyzing a parallel-groups design, the traditional approach is to conduct an endpoint analysis using only the final measurement. If the DV is continuous, analysis will typically require an independent samples t-test for two groups, one-way analysis of variance (ANOVA) for more than two groups, or analysis of covariance (ANCOVA) for two or more groups, statistically controlling for a baseline DV measurement. If the DV is categorical, an endpoint analysis will typically require a chi square test or logistic regression analysis. Note that these analyses are discussed in detail in the Statistical Tests section later in the chapter.

For example, consider a study designed to assess the effect of lubiprostone compared to placebo in treating chronic constipation associated with Parkinson's disease. Following randomization, this 1-month study will assess constipation symptoms twice—at the end of the second and fourth week. An endpoint analysis would only consider the treatment effect at the end of week 4, ignoring the measurement at the end of week 2. Thus, it is clear that this type of analysis does not consider the repeated measures, and, as a result, does not consider the changes occurring over time. Further, an endpoint analysis does not take full advantage of statistical power increases from a longitudinal design as discussed in The Analysis of Clinical Trials section.

By contrast, to assess for change over time using repeated measures for a continuous DV, researchers often employ a mixed between-within ANOVA or mixed-effects linear regression. Briefly, these analyses assess differences between treatment groups as well as changes over time within treatment groups. The major benefit of these analyses is provided by the interaction effect, which evaluates whether the change over time was different between the two treatment arms (Figure 6-8). To evaluate group differences in change over time for a categorical DV, researchers are required to employ a mixed-effects logistic regression. This analysis allows the researcher to evaluate group differences and interaction effects. In general, mixed-effects analyses are extremely complex and even a brief overview of this analysis is well beyond the scope of this chapter. With that said, when these analyses are most appropriate is provided in the Selecting the Appropriate Statistical Test section. Interested readers are encouraged to consult the suggested readings at the end of the chapter for a treatment of this analysis.

As an example of analyzing a parallel-groups design, reconsider the lubiprostone example. Say the results are presented graphically in Figure 6-8. Notice that two groups experience drastically different change in constipation symptoms between the end of week 2 and the end of week 4. The between-group difference in constipation symptoms over time is the interaction effect. Because a lower number of symptoms are indicative of treatment success, Figure 6-8 shows that the effect of lubiprostone is more effective compared to placebo over the study period.

Following a statistically significant interaction effect, researchers can conduct follow-up or *post hoc* tests to determine where the significant difference occurred. In Figure 6-8, there is likely no statistically significant difference in constipation symptoms between groups at the end of week 2, but there is a likely statistically significant difference at the end of week 4. Therefore, *post hoc* tests can assist researchers in identifying the shortest treatment time or minimum effective dose by indicating where treatment effects diminish (e.g., the slope plateaus) or indicating when differences between doses converge and are no longer statistically significant.

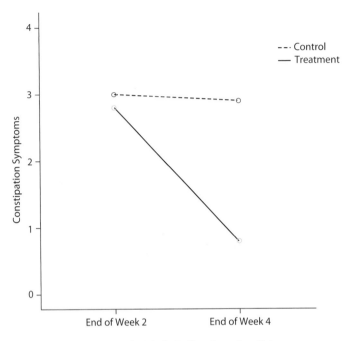

Figure 6–8. Statistically significant interaction effect.

Analyzing Crossover Designs

The purpose of the crossover design is to study treatment effects using the participant as his or her own control. Remember, in a crossover design each participant receives all treatment arms, with an adequate washout period occurring between arms to prevent the carryover of treatment effects. For example, consider the lubiprostone example described in the Analyzing Parallel-Groups Designs section. Instead of having two treatment arms as in a parallel-groups design, the crossover design would randomize participants into a different treatment order. That is, Group A would receive lubiprostone and Group B would receive placebo for the first 2 weeks. At the end of the 2-week study period, constipation symptoms are assessed. Next, all participants are required to have a 3-week washout period purported to effectively eliminate any carryover effects of the lubiprostone. Note that during the washout period the placebo is not given either. After the washout period, Group A would receive placebo and Group B would receive lubiprostone for 2 weeks. At the end of this second 2-week study period, constipation symptoms are assessed again.

Statistically, a crossover design requires an initial test for order effects. If the DV is continuous, order effects are assessed by evaluating the interaction effect between order of treatment and the IV using a mixed between-within ANOVA or a mixed-effects linear

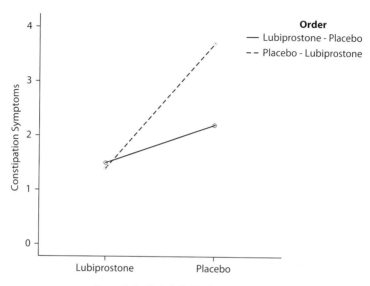

Figure 6–9. Statistically significant order effect.

regression. These analyses are described in detail in the Selecting the Appropriate Statistical Test section later in the chapter, but for now consider both analyses useful when evaluating interaction effects. When testing for order effects, a statistically significant interaction indicates that the order in which the treatments were received influenced the treatment effect. For example, say that receiving lubiprostone prior to placebo had a different treatment effect than receiving placebo prior to lubiprostone. A clear order effect is presented in Figure 6-9. Notice the effect of placebo differs depending on the order in which it was received. The presence of a statistically significant order effect can have multiple explanations. Considering the example and Figure 6-9, it is clear the washout period may not have been long enough, as the effectiveness of lubiprostone carried over to measurement of the placebo. In addition, the groups may have been initially different following randomization. Whenever a statistically significant order effect is identified, no further analysis is conducted as any subsequent analyses are biased by this order effect. However, if the interaction is nonsignificant and the DV is continuous, an endpoint analysis is typically evaluated via paired-samples *t*-test (also explained in detail in the Selecting the Appropriate Statistical Test section later in the chapter). That is, treatment differences between lubiprostone and placebo are assessed without respect to the order in which the treatments were received.

Analyzing Adaptive Designs

The statistical analyses and considerations used when analyzing adaptive designs are similar to parallel-groups and crossover designs. If the DV is continuous, statistical tests used during the interim analyses or on the study endpoint typically include an independent-samples t-test for comparing two groups, one-way ANOVA for comparing more than two groups, or ANCOVA for statistically controlling baseline DV measurement. Note that the DV for the interim analyses is the most recent measurement. If the DV is categorical, an interim analysis will typically require a chi square test or logistic regression analysis. All of the analyses mentioned are discussed in detail in the Statistical Tests section later in the chapter.

Several important considerations are required when analyzing and interpreting the results from adaptive designs.[17] First, all interim and endpoint analyses suffer the potential risk of inflated Type I errors. Briefly, a Type I error can be thought of as a false positive. That is, the statistical test could indicate a statistically significant result when the result is actually not significant. Type I error has been discussed in Chapter 4 and is discussed in the Statistical Inference section later in the chapter. With this definition in mind, as the number of interim analyses increase, the probability of finding a false positive might increase as well. To adjust for this possibility, researchers will often make the criteria for achieving statistical significance more conservative by adjusting alpha (see the Statistical Inference section later in the chapter for a full description of alpha). Note that adjusting alpha is not a ubiquitous practice and there is no universal recommendation for doing so. Just be aware that inflated Type I errors may be an issue in an ACT.

Second, estimates of population parameters may be biased. That is, any adaptation can reduce the generalizability to the original population sampled, produce underestimated or overestimated parameter estimates, and produce misleading confidence intervals. Researchers must carefully document and provide rationale for adaptations resulting from interim analysis. Failure to do so will indicate that results should be viewed with extreme caution.

Finally, when all adaptations are considered, the overall results of the endpoint analyses may actually be invalid, providing inaccurate support for treatment effects. Consumers of research are urged strongly to consider these factors when interpreting and evaluating research using adaptive designs.

Statistical Inference

Inferential statistics provide the probability that a difference or association is actually observed in the population based on the analysis of sample data. Inferential statistics allow researchers to make rational decisions in the presence of random processes and variation. This section presents several requirements that need to be considered prior to conducting and evaluating the result of a statistical test. First, the sampling distribution and application of the **Central Limit Theorem** are discussed, followed by hypothesis testing, as well as

Type I and Type II errors and statistical power. Then, the difference between statistical and clinical significance is presented. Finally, the appropriate uses of parametric and non-parametric statistical tests are provided as well as a brief description of degrees of freedom.

SAMPLING DISTRIBUTIONS AND THE CENTRAL LIMIT THEOREM

Statistical inference uses sampled data to make conclusions about a specific population. Because quality samples are chosen randomly, the means produced from these samples are also random.[21] Given this information, it is important to remember that the mean may not be exactly representative of the population and will vary from sample to sample. However, the law of large numbers states that as the size of the sample increases, the sample mean will move closer to the population mean. Further, as the number of samples increases, the mean of the sample means will begin to approximate the population mean.

❻ *The central limit theorem states when equally sized samples are drawn from a non-normal distribution, the plotted mean values from each sample will approximate a normal distribution as long as the non-normality was not due to outliers.*

A distribution of the sampled means calculated from repeated samples is termed the distribution of sampling means. For example, consider a study to analyze the mean value of blood urea nitrogen (BUN) in the general, healthy population, where the researcher selects 100 random samples of 10 healthy participants. Each sample of 10 will provide a mean BUN value. Although mean BUN will vary from sample to sample, when the 100 sample means are plotted in a histogram, this distribution of sampling means will begin to approximate the actual population distribution.

The Central Limit Theorem states that sufficiently large samples should approximate a normal distribution of sampling means as long as the data do not contain outliers. A sufficiently large sample is generally considered to consist of 30 or more participants or a situation where the degrees of freedom for the statistical test are greater than 20.[22] Note that degrees of freedom are discussed later in this section. In addition, researchers must be careful not to confuse the issue of having a large enough sample to achieve statistical significance and a large enough sample to be representative of the population.

As with any normal distribution, the standard deviation of the distribution of sampling means can be calculated. This is termed the standard error of the mean (SEM). The SEM is equal to the standard deviation divided by the square root of the sample size, and reflects variability within the sample means. Further, standard error is used in the majority of statistical tests. It is important when evaluating the literature to understand the relationship between the standard deviation and the SEM. Researchers often present the SEM to show variability or noise in their data. Note that the SEM will always be smaller than the standard deviation. Thus, the use of SEM will suggest the data is less variable and often more appealing.

HYPOTHESIS TESTING

A hypothesis indicates a theory about the population regarding an outcome the researcher is interested in studying. The statistical analyses discussed in this chapter evaluate two types of hypotheses, the null hypothesis and the alternative or research hypothesis. That is, the analyses discussed employ procedures generally known as null hypothesis significance testing (NHST). The **null hypothesis** (H_0) assumes no difference or association between the different study groups or variables, whereas the **alternative hypothesis** (H_A or H_1) states that there is a difference or association between the different study groups or variables. A representative, ideally random, sample is then drawn from the population of interest to estimate the difference or relationship and test whether this difference or relationship rejects or fails to reject the null hypothesis. It is important to note that failing to reject the null hypothesis does not indicate the null hypothesis is true. This is a common misconception observed frequently in the literature. There are often many other reasons for failing to reject the null hypothesis including inadequate experimental design, inadequate control over extraneous variables, and inadequate sample size to detect the effect of interest, among others.

When testing a specific hypothesis, a researcher is required to determine whether their hypothesis is directional or not. A directional hypothesis requires a **one-tailed** hypothesis test, whereas a nondirectional hypothesis requires a **two-tailed** hypothesis test. For example, consider a hypothesis which states that initiating statin therapy will lower low-density lipoproteins (LDL). Note that use of the term lower implies directionality and requires a one-tailed test. If, however, the researchers were looking for any effect of statin therapy, whether lowering or raising LDL, the hypothesis is nondirectional and would require a two-tailed test. In the literature, it is generally more acceptable to use a two-tailed test, even if the hypothesis is directional because a two-tailed test is more conservative statistically, thereby reducing the probability of a spurious statistical significance.

ERROR AND STATISTICAL POWER

It is essential that researchers establish how much error they are willing to accept before initiating a study. NHST can only result in four possible outcomes, which can be observed in Table 6-2. Type I and Type II errors have been discussed at length in Chapter 4, but briefly, a **Type I error** occurs when a statistical test rejects the null hypothesis by indicating a statistically significant difference when, in fact, the null hypothesis is true (i.e., false positive). A **Type II error** occurs when the researcher fails to reject the null hypothesis by not indicating a statistically significant difference when, in fact, the null hypothesis is false (i.e., false negative). Type I and Type II errors are interconnected; that is, as the probability of one error increases the other decreases. Researchers must consider these

TABLE 6–2. FOUR POSSIBLE OUTCOMES OF NULL HYPOTHESIS SIGNIFICANCE TESTING (NHST)

	Truth	
Decision	**False H_0**	**True H_0**
Reject H_0	Correctly reject H_0	Type I error
Fail to reject H_0	Type II error	Correctly fail to reject H_0

two errors carefully when designing studies, weighing whether a false positive is more or less concerning than a false negative.

Statistical power was developed as a method allowing researchers to calculate the probability of finding a statistically significant result, when, in fact, one actually exists. This topic has been discussed in Chapter 4. Essentially, increasing statistical power reduces the probability of committing a Type II error; however, it can also increase the probability of committing a Type I error as described in the previous paragraph. Statistical power is influenced by four factors: alpha defined as the probability value at which the null hypothesis is rejected, effect size defined as the size of the treatment effect (discussed later), error variance defined as the precision of the measurement instrument, and the sample size. Statistical power can be increased by increasing alpha, effect size, or sample size as well as by decreasing error variance. Note that statistical power of 0.80 has been defined as adequate.[23] However, some researchers use 0.90 or higher in the biomedical sciences, indicating that a false negative is more detrimental than a false positive, such as when evaluating the effectiveness of a novel breast cancer treatment.

STATISTICAL VERSUS CLINICAL SIGNIFICANCE

Alpha and *p*-Values

The next step in the research process is to employ a statistical test to assess whether a difference or relationship is due to random variation. The researcher is interested in determining whether the observed difference or relationship rejects or fails to reject the null hypothesis. **Alpha** (α) is the conventionally designated decision criterion for rejecting the null hypothesis and ranges from 0 to 1. Alpha is defined as the theoretical probability of rejecting the null hypothesis conditional on the null hypothesis being true. Alpha does not represent the exact Type I error rate; instead, alpha is the upper bound of the Type I error rate. Although most studies typically set alpha at 0.05, this value is arbitrary. A more conservative (i.e., $\alpha = 0.01$) or liberal ($\alpha = 0.10$) alpha may be used in an attempt to show greater support for rejecting or retaining the null hypothesis, respectively. As an example, conservative alpha levels are often used to protect against Type I errors, whereas liberal alpha values are often used in drug equivalency trials where researchers are using data to show nonsignificant differences between the drugs.

Conceptually related to alpha is the probability value (i.e., **p-value**). Statistical tests produce p-values that range from 0 to 1. The formal definition of a p-value is the probability of obtaining a test statistic as large as or larger than the one obtained, conditional on the null hypothesis being true. Graphically, a p-value is directly indicative of the area under the probability distribution used by the statistical test. Note that the area under any proper probability distribution is 1. A quick glance at the appendices of any introductory statistics textbook will provide area under the curve values for various distributions. In more general terms, $p = 0.05$ indicates 5% of the distribution's area is to the left or right of the associated test statistic depending on whether it is positive or negative. For example, consider a one-tailed statistical test with a positive test statistic and reconsider Figure 6-5. A z-score of 1.645 leaves approximately 5% of the distribution to the right of this value. This example highlights how a p-value less than 0.05 indicates that less than 5% of the values (or area) lies beyond a specific test statistic value. As an alternative example, consider a two-tailed (i.e., nondirectional) statistical test. A z-score of 1.96 leaves approximately 2.5% of the distribution to the right of this value, whereas a z-score of -1.96 leaves approximately 2.5% of the distribution to the left of this value. Thus, a two-tailed test also leaves 5% of the area under the distribution when the two parts are aggregated. Regardless of whether a one- or two-tailed test was used, in general, if a p-value is less than the specified alpha, the researcher rejects the null hypothesis and the difference or relationship is considered statistically significant. Alternatively, if the p-value is equal to or greater than alpha, the researcher has failed to reject the null hypothesis and the difference or relationship is not considered statistically significant.

    ❼ *There are numerous misconceptions about p-values and it is important to know how to interpret them correctly.* Be aware that there is continuing difficulty when interpreting p-values, even among statisticians.[24] Therefore, it is important to be cognizant of several misconceptions about p-values that are stated commonly in the literature. First, a p-value is not the exact probability of committing a Type I error. Second, the p-value is not the probability that the null hypothesis is true, nor is $1 - p$ the probability that the alternative hypothesis is true. Third, a small p-value is not evidence that the results will replicate, nor can p-values be compared directly across studies. Fourth, a p-value indicates nothing about the magnitude of a difference or relationship. For example, a small p-value (e.g., $p = 0.00001$) does not indicate a larger treatment effect than a larger p-value (e.g., $p = 0.049$). Finally, for better or worse, alpha in NHST is treated like a cliff. For example, if alpha is set at 0.05 and a p-value of 0.051 is obtained, a researcher will often state that a p-value of 0.051 was trending toward significance or that the p-value indicated marginal or moderate significance. These statements are often wholly incorrect! Thinking back to the discussion of one-tailed versus two-tailed significance tests provided in the Hypothesis Testing section, trending can only occur if the hypothesis is directional using a one-tailed test and the result obtained was in the hypothesized direction. Results can never be trending toward significance if the hypothesis was nondirectional using a two-tailed test because the alternative claim that the result was trending away from significance cannot be challenged.

Confidence Intervals

Statistical significance can also be established by calculating a confidence interval around the estimated population parameters (e.g., sample means, slopes) or test statistics (e.g., t). A confidence interval provides a range of scores likely to contain the unknown population parameter, and generally, a confidence interval is reported using a 95% confidence level. The calculation of confidence intervals includes both sample size and variability where smaller confidence intervals indicate less variability in the data. A 95% confidence interval is calculated by multiplying 1.96 by the SEM and adding or subtracting this value from the estimated parameter to find the upper and lower confidence limits, respectively. A 95% confidence interval indicates that if repeated random sampling occurs within the population of interest under consistent conditions (e.g., sample size), the true population parameter would be included in the interval 95% of the time (i.e., the interval is random and the population parameter is fixed).

Confidence intervals can be used to indicate statistical significance without the use of statistical tests. This process varies according to whether the researcher is examining population parameters or test statistics. For example, consider Figures 6-10 to 6-12. In each figure, HbA1c values are being compared for a treatment and placebo group. Further, mean HbA1c for each group is presented as the circle, while the 95% confidence intervals are the whiskers extending above and below the means. The overlap of the confidence intervals between groups is directly related to p-values; that is, less overlap

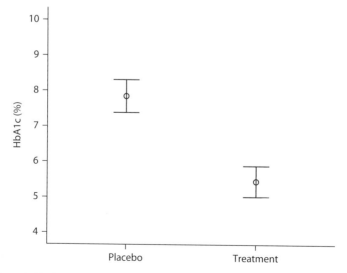

Figure 6–10. Statistically significant result indicated by nonoverlapping 95% confidence intervals.

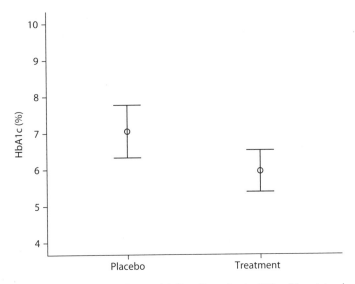

Figure 6–11. Statistically significant result indicated by overlapping 95% confidence intervals.

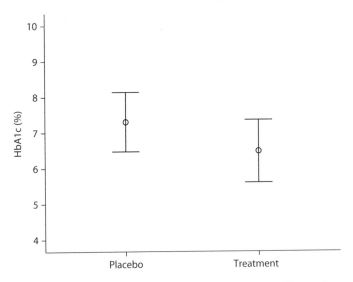

Figure 6–12. Overlapping 95% confidence interval indicating a nonsignificant result.

is indicative of larger differences resulting in smaller p-values. In Figure 6-10, notice that the confidence intervals do not overlap; thus, this difference can be assumed statistically significant at least at $p < 0.05$. Statistical significance can also be indicated when the confidence intervals overlap as long as the overlap is less than approximately 50% of a whisker, as in Figure 6-11.[25] Finally, as shown in Figure 6-12, substantial overlap in confidence intervals indicates a nonstatistically significant difference (i.e., $p > 0.05$).

Determining statistical significance using confidence intervals around test statistics (e.g., t) uses procedures that vary based on the statistical test employed. For most parametric tests of group differences and correlation, a 95% confidence interval around the test statistic containing zero is not considered statistically significant at an alpha of 0.05. That is, statistical significance for these types of analyses are essentially testing that the differences or relationship are different from zero (i.e., $H_0 = 0$). Thus, a 95% confidence interval containing zero essentially indicates that it is plausible the true population difference or relationship could be zero.[26] For example, consider the commonly used independent-samples t-test to evaluate for a difference between two group means (this statistical test is discussed in the Statistical Tests section). Say that the test statistic produced was 2.0, but the confidence interval ranged from -0.50 to 4.50. Based on this sample, the difference would not be considered statistically significant because it is plausible that in 95% of samples of the same size, the true population parameter could in fact be zero.

Alternatively, the 95% confidence interval for test statistics based on ratios (e.g., odds ratios) that contain 1 is not considered statistically significant at an alpha of 0.05. Remember from the Epidemiological Statistics section, that an odds ratio or relative risk of 1 indicates no difference. Thus, a 95% confidence interval for a relative risk or an odds ratio that contains 1 indicates that it is plausible the true population parameter could in fact be an odds ratio or relative risk of 1. For example, say the result of a logistic regression analysis produced an odds ratio of 2.5 (this statistical test is discussed in the Statistical Tests section). This value is greater than 1, indicating an increase in odds of experiencing the event. However, say the 95% confidence interval ranged from 0.50 to 15.0. Because the confidence interval contains 1, the odds ratio of 2.5 is not statistically significant using an alpha of 0.05.

Clinical Significance and Effect Size

8 *Clinical significance is far more important than statistical significance. Clinical significance can be quantified by using various measures of effect size.* When evaluating the significance of the finding, keep in mind that statistical significance (e.g., $p < 0.05$) does not indicate clinical significance. Statistical significance can be manipulated in several ways, most easily by increasing sample size drastically. A sample size increase may artificially reduce error variance, which in turn reduces the standard error on which the test statistic is based. Reducing the standard error increases the value of the test statistic necessarily resulting in a smaller p-value.

As an example, using a sample of 10,000 patients, researchers may find a CCB reduced blood glucose significantly in Type I DM patients. However, on examining the estimated parameters, the statistically significant difference in blood glucose was only 2 mg/dL, a decrease considered clinically insignificant.

This example highlights the importance of identifying and interpreting the clinical significance or effect size of all studies. While a complete discussion of effect size is beyond the scope of this chapter, larger effect size values are always preferred. Briefly, two different types of effect sizes exist. First, standardized difference effect sizes indicate a standardized difference between groups in standard deviation units. Examples commonly seen in the literature include Cohen's **d**, Glass' Δ, and Hedges' **g**. As indicated by their name, standardized difference effect sizes are used when evaluating mean differences between groups. Further, because the effect sizes are standardized, it may be easier to think of them as z-scores. Standardized difference effect sizes range from $-\infty$ to $+\infty$, with larger absolute values indicating larger effects. Second, effect size may also be reported as the proportion of variance explained. That is, how much of the reason a participant had a specific value of the DV is due to the IV. Examples commonly observed in the literature include R^2, ω^2, and η^2. Proportion of variance effect sizes are specific to tests of relationships or association as described in the Statistical Tests section. Their values range from 0 to 1, with higher values indicating larger effects.

Given this information, it is important to remember that the definition of clinical significance varies by substantive area; thus, the definition of clinical significance to a bench researcher may be qualitatively different from an evidence-based practitioner. Finally, not all studies will provide an effect-size estimate, especially in the biomedical sciences. Thus, research must be viewed with warranted skepticism until it can be determined whether the statistically significant difference or relationship is clinically meaningful.

PARAMETRIC VERSUS NONPARAMETRIC STATISTICAL TESTS

The primary difference between parametric and nonparametric statistical tests is that parametric tests make assumptions regarding the descriptive characteristics of the normal distribution (i.e., mean, variance, skewness, and kurtosis). Nonparametric tests make a few or no distributional assumptions. In general, **parametric tests** are used only for interval and ratio scales, whereas **nonparametric tests** can be employed for any scale of measurement. Regardless, if the DV is measured on a continuous scale, the decision of which statistical test to employ typically begins with parametric tests. Because they assume a normal distribution, all parametric tests have several conservative and easily violated assumptions. These assumptions are testable, but vary depending on the statistical test employed. Therefore, in the Statistical Tests section, all assumptions are described for each statistical test. It is important to know that employing a parametric test in the presence of a non-defined distribution will lead to inaccurate, biased, and unreliable parameter estimates. Therefore, when reading a journal article, if the authors neglect to provide information regarding assumption testing, caution should be exercised as it is unknown how much bias exists in their results.

Some assumption violations challenge the robustness of parametric tests greater than others. **Robustness** is defined as the ability of the statistical test to produce correct inferences in the presence of assumption violations. In most situations, any assumption violation requires the researcher to employ a nonparametric test, and most parametric tests have a widely used nonparametric alternative. Most, but not all, nonparametric statistical tests are distribution free, meaning they do not make inferences based on a defined probability distribution. Further, additional strengths of nonparametric tests include the ability to assess small sample sizes and the ability to assess data from several different populations.[27] However, it must be noted if the assumptions of a parametric test are tenable, parametric tests have greater statistical power to detect real effects compared to their nonparametric alternative(s).[28]

DEGREES OF FREEDOM

Degrees of freedom (df) are a vital component of all statistical tests, as most probability distributions, and statistical significance are based on them. Degrees of freedom are provided for all statistical tests and are a useful indicator of adequate sample size in the presence of assumption violations. For example, recall that the Central Limit Theorem states the distribution of sampling means is approximately normal with degrees of freedom greater than 20. Thus, the Central Limit Theorem operates independently of the distribution of the actual raw data. Therefore, if a researcher indicates that degrees of freedom for the statistical test is greater than 20, the results can typically be viewed as robust.

The definition of degrees of freedom is obscure and beyond the scope of this chapter; however, a brief description is provided. Degrees of freedom are conceptually defined as the number of data points that are free to vary. Not all data are free to vary because values may have to be fixed by a specific sample parameter, such as the group mean. For example, consider a group of three participants who have a mean age of 50. Because the mean is 50, two of the participants can be of almost any age greater than zero. The third participant, however, must be of the age that creates the mean of 50. Thus, if participant A is 40 and participant B is 45, participant C must be 65. That is, [40+45+65]/3 = 50. If instead, participant A is 75 and participant B is 40, then participant C must be 35. Therefore, because the age of two of the three participants could be just about any age greater than zero, there are two degrees of freedom (i.e., 2df).

Calculating degrees of freedom become increasingly complex in accordance with the complexity of the statistical test. That is, degrees of freedom for bivariate tests, such as those evaluating the difference between two group means, are easier to calculate and conceptualize than multivariate tests with multiple DVs. For the analyses described in the Statistical Tests section later in the chapter, calculation of degrees of freedom is not explained explicitly, but it is important to note that the distribution, probability, and statistical significance of all statistical tests are based on degrees of freedom. Further, degrees of freedom will usually be subscripted next to the test statistic for all parametric tests as well as for some nonparametric tests, such as the chi square test. Subscripted degrees of freedom should be provided in the brief results section for all statistical tests described.

Selecting the Appropriate Statistical Test

While the information presented in this chapter has outlined the underlying processes of most statistical tests used in the biomedical sciences, the remainder of the chapter uses all previous information as a base to begin to integrate more directly useful information. This section presents decision trees that allow for determination of whether the appropriate statistical test was used in a journal article.

 ❾ *The selection of the appropriate statistical test is based on several factors including the specific research question, the measurement scale of the DV, distributional assumptions, the number of DV measurements as well as the number and measurement scale of IVs and covariates, among others.* Tables 6-3 and 6-4 provide decision trees to identify the most appropriate statistical test based on the unique set of factors for statistical tests of group differences and statistical tests of association, respectively.

FACTOR 1: THE RESEARCH QUESTION

The first factor that needs to be addressed when selecting the most appropriate statistical test is whether the research question is phrased to evaluate differences or associations. In general, the last paragraph of the Introduction to any journal article should explicitly state the research questions, so give close attention to the phrasing of these questions. This may seem mundane, but it is important to note that all parametric tests of group differences are mathematically equivalent to parametric tests of association. Therefore, various parametric statistical tests can often be used interchangeably to answer the same research question. This can be seen in Tables 6-3 and 6-4 where one-way ANOVA can be used in the same situations as simple linear regression analysis. The overall statistical inference would be identical. This can be an overwhelmingly confusing concept for those with more novice statistical backgrounds. However, in general, when a research question is phrased to evaluate group differences (e.g., to determine whether three treatment groups differ on some outcome) follow the decision tree provided in Table 6-3, and when a research question is phrased to evaluate associations between variables (e.g., to determine whether a patient's age is associated with some outcome), follow Table 6-4.

TABLE 6–3. CHOOSING THE MOST APPROPRIATE STATISTICAL TEST OF GROUP DIFFERENCES

	DV Scale	Distributional Assumptions Met	Repeated DV Measurements	Number of DV Measurements	Number of IVs	IV Levels	Covariates Allowed	Appropriate Statistical Test
Differences from known population	Continuous	Yes	No	1	0		No	One-sample z-test
	Continuous	Yes	No	1	0		No	One-sample t-test
	Dichotomous		No	1	0		No	Binomial test
	Continuous		No	1	0		No	Kolmogorov-Smirnov test
Between-group differences	Continuous	Yes	No	1	1	2	No	Independent-samples t-test
	Ordinal or higher	No	No	1	1	2	No	Mann-Whitney test
	Ordinal or higher	No	No	1	1	2	No	Median test
	Continuous	Yes	No	1	1	≥ 2	No	One-way ANOVA
	Ordinal or higher	No	No	1	1	≥ 2	No	Kruskal-Wallis test
	Continuous	Yes	No	1	1	≥ 2	Yes	ANCOVA
	Continuous	Yes	No	1	≥ 2	≥ 2	No	Factorial ANOVA
Within-group differences	Continuous	Yes	Yes	2	0		No	Paired-samples t-test
	Ordinal or higher	No	Yes	2	0		No	Signed-rank test
	Ordinal or higher	No	Yes	2	0		No	Sign test
	Continuous	Yes	Yes	≥ 2	0		No	One-way RM-ANOVA
	Ordinal or higher	No	Yes	≥ 2	0		No	Friedman test
	Continuous	Yes	Yes	≥ 2	1	≥ 2	No	Mixed BW-ANOVA
	Dichotomous		Yes	2	0		No	McNemar test
	Dichotomous		Yes	≥ 2	0		No	Cochran Q test

TABLE 6–4. CHOOSING THE MOST APPROPRIATE STATISTICAL TEST OF ASSOCIATION

	DV Scale	Distributional Assumptions Met	Number of IVs	IV Scale	Covariates Allowed	Appropriate Statistical Test
One sample association	Categorical		1	Categorical	No	Chi square test
	Categorical		1	Categorical	No	Fisher's exact test
	Categorical		1	Categorical	Yes	Mantel–Haenszel test
Correlation and regression	Continuous	Yes	1	Continuous	No	Pearson's correlation
	Continuous	No	1	Continuous	No	Spearman's rank order correlation
	Continuous	Yes	1	Any	No	Simple linear regression
	Continuous	Yes	≥2	Any	Yes	Multivariable linear regression
	Dichotomous		1	Any	No	Simple logistic regression
	Dichotomous		≥2	Any	Yes	Multivariable logistic regression
Within–group regression	Continuous	Yes	≥0	Any	Yes	Mixed-effects linear regression[a]
	Dichotomous		≥0	Any	Yes	Mixed-effects logistic regression[a]
Time-to-event	Continuous	Yes	≥2		Yes	Cox proportional-hazards model
Reliability	Nominal		0		No	Kappa

[a]Mixed-effects linear and logistic regression models are complex analyses beyond the scope of this chapter. Therefore, they are not described in the Statistical Tests section. However, be aware that these analyses are available. Also, note that there is varying terminology used among researchers when describing these types of models; thus, in the literature mixed-effects models may be termed multilevel, hierarchical, nested, random effects, random coefficient, or random parameter models. The actual procedure for conducting the analyses remains identical regardless of the label attached to them.

FACTOR 2: SCALE OF MEASUREMENT

● The second factor to consider is the measurement scale of the DV. This is a much more concrete concept, but requires a thorough understanding of the four scales of variable measurement. Remember, nominal and ordinal scales are roughly classified as discrete or categorical, whereas interval and ratio scales are classified as continuous. Although it is often inappropriate, continuous variables may be also categorized into discrete variables. For example, categorization often occurs in the biomedical sciences with variables such as blood pressure, where exact systolic or diastolic blood pressure values are combined and categorized into low, normal, or high blood pressure.

FACTOR 3: DISTRIBUTIONAL ASSUMPTIONS

● The distributional assumptions of a statistical test involve complex explanations beyond the scope of this chapter. However, there are a few concepts to remember regarding distributions, most of which have been described in the Common Probability Distributions section. First, distributional assumptions are required for all statistical tests using a continuous DV. Remember, the search for the most appropriate statistical test usually begins with parametric options, and all parametric statistical tests require a normal distribution (or application of the Central Limit Theorem). Second, the distribution of the actual DV data is never considered when assessing distributional assumptions. Distributional assumptions are based on residual values, which represent the difference between the outcome predicted by the statistical model and the actual, observed outcome. Residuals are discussed in detail later in the simple linear regression analysis section. Third, if the distributional assumptions are violated, two options are generally available. First, the researcher could use a more appropriate distribution (see Table 6-1) or, second, they could employ a nonparametric statistical test. It is also common to see data transformation to attempt to force a normal distribution, but the considerable downside of this archaic technique was discussed previously in the Transforming Non-Normal Distributions section. It is more common in the biomedical literature to see a nonparametric test used, but be aware more statistically savvy researchers will use alternative distributions if the distributional assumption is violated.

FACTOR 4: REPEATED MEASURES

● The number of DV measurements is critically important to determine whether an appropriate statistical test was used. Note that studies using one DV measurement are known as **cross-sectional**, whereas studies using two or more DV measurements are known as **longitudinal**. If the DV was measured on multiple occasions, there is inherent association or correlation across DV measurements. That is, DV values from the same person inherently have a higher correlation compared to DV values from different people. Therefore, if a statistical test does not account for this correlation, the standard errors will be biased and improper statistical inference will occur.

FACTOR 5: INCLUSION OF COVARIATES

It is also critically important to consider the number of IVs and covariates, their scale of measurement, the number of categorical IV levels, and whether the IVs and/or covariates interact. Note that the distribution of the IV or covariate is never considered in the statistical analysis. With that said, the scale of measurement for each IV and covariate is important when deciding which statistical test to employ. In general, ANOVA will usually be employed for categorical IVs, whereas regression analysis is required for continuous IVs. Note that the wording of the last sentence was chosen specifically. That is, although it was stated earlier that ANOVA and regression are mathematically equivalent, ANOVA cannot be used with continuous IVs. However, regression analysis can be used with any combination of IVs and covariates measured on any scale. This can be a confusing distinction.

Another important concept is the number of levels for each categorical IV. Remember, a level can be thought of as the number of groups being studied and evaluated. When testing group differences, researchers will typically employ a t-test for two levels and ANOVA for three or more groups. Determining the number of levels is important because with three or more groups, the statistical test is an **omnibus test**. That is, an overall test result will be provided indicating a difference between at least two of the groups, but the test will not indicate specifically which groups differ. The concept of an omnibus test is discussed throughout the Statistical Tests section later in the chapter. Finally, whether an IV interacts with another IV or covariate is critically important. It is important to note that ANOVA can handle interactions between categorical IVs. Remember, an interaction indicates that the value of one IV is dependent on the value of another IV. For example, treatment group differences may be smaller in older patients (i.e., a treatment group-by-age interaction). However, if there is an interaction between a categorical IV and a continuous covariate, an ANOVA-type analysis, such as ANCOVA, cannot be used and a form of regression analysis must be used instead. Whether an interaction exists is an empirical question that is testable and described in the ANCOVA section later in the chapter.

FACTOR 6: CLUSTERING

Finally, other factors exist when determining whether the appropriate statistical test was used, but many are beyond the scope of this chapter. One key factor worth considering, however, is based on the concept of clustering (also known as nesting). Classic examples of clustering include children nested within the same classroom or patients nested within the same doctor. Clustering creates statistical issues that are similar to using a cross-sectional analysis on longitudinal data. That is, DV measurements from children nested within the same classroom have greater associations compared to DV measurements from children in different classrooms. Failing to account for clustering will result in biased standard errors and incorrect statistical inference. Although a description of the statistical analysis for clustered data is too complex for this chapter, recognizing when an analysis should account for (or should have accounted for) clustering is relatively easy, and the number of clustering levels can get as complex as the researcher desires. For example, patients could be nested within a doctor, the doctor could be nested within a clinic, the clinic could be nested within a hospital system, the hospital system could be nested within a city, and so on. When reading a journal article, take time to consider whether clustering should have been considered by the researchers. Do not be disheartened by the possibility of seeing an exorbitant number of clustering levels in any journal article. If clustering is considered, most studies in the biomedical sciences will only use two or three clustering units. The takeaway message is that careful thought must be undertaken when evaluating a study, especially when considering clustering. If clustering levels were not considered, but should have been, interpret all results with caution.

As an example of how to use Tables 6-3 and 6-4, say a researcher wanted to examine the effect a new statin medication had on the number of LDLs using a sample of 200 healthy patients. Although LDL has received a bad reputation, research has shown that the size of the LDL particles carrying the cholesterol is more predictive of future cardiovascular problems than the absolute LDL value measured in mg/dL.[29] More specifically, cholesterol carried by large, buoyant LDLs (i.e., Pattern A) has little association with cardiovascular problems, whereas cholesterol carried by small, dense LDLs (i.e., Pattern B) has been associated with a myriad of cardiovascular problems.[30] Therefore, a statin that only targets cholesterol carried by small, dense LDL is needed. Based on lipoprotein particle profile (LPP) testing, patients were placed into one of two groups based on LDL particle size (i.e., the IV: Pattern A versus Pattern B). The outcome for the study was LDL measured in mg/dL. Baseline measurements and demographic data were used as covariates and included categorized age (i.e., 40 to 49, 50 to 59, etc.), race, socioeconomic status indicated by whether the patient's mother graduated from high school, comorbid conditions, concurrent medications, and baseline LDL. The researchers hypothesized that the statin should reduce LDL significantly more in Pattern A patients compared to Pattern B patients. The analysis was completed at the end of a 6-month study period. In the method section, the researchers stated that baseline characteristics and demographic data were compared between the two groups of patients. Due to the presence of outliers, Mann-Whitney tests were used for all continuous variables and chi square tests were used for categorical variables. For the primary analysis, multiple linear regression was used. No assumption violations were indicated.

The example above contains similar information to what is typically provided in the overwhelming majority of published literature. Thus, using the example information above, Tables 6-3 and 6-4 can be used to determine whether the statistical tests employed were appropriate. Note that all three of these tests are described in detail later in the chapter. For the baseline and demographic data, using Table 6-3, the Mann-Whitney test was used because the DV scale was continuous, distributional assumptions were not met due to outliers, the DV was only measured on one occasion, there was one IV with two levels, and no covariates were considered. Further, using Table 6-4, chi square tests were used because both the DV and IV were categorical and no covariates were considered. For the primary analysis, using Table 6-4, multiple linear regression analysis was used because the scale of the DV was continuous, the distributional assumptions were met, there was one IV with two levels, covariates were considered measured on both categorical and continuous scales, and although the DV was measured twice, the baseline measurement was used only as an additional covariate. Based on this information, all three statistical tests were used appropriately (Case Study 6-2).

Case Study 6–2

The questions for Case Study 6-2 use the study described in Case Study 6-1. Briefly, the surgeon planned to enroll his own patients as well as patients from six other surgeons in his practice. Following consent, patients were randomized so that an equal number of patients received either TXA or EACA; patients were stratified by biological sex and weight. All patients and surgeons were blinded to the medication. Blood loss was estimated using hemoglobin measured at the preoperative physical and immediately after surgery; both pre- and postoperative hemoglobin were continuous variables. The primary hypothesis was that EACA will have postoperative blood-sparing effects similar to TXA. In this case, the surgeon defined a "similar blood-sparing effect" was no more than a 10% difference in postoperative hemoglobin. A statistical power analysis indicted that 380 participants (or 190 per group) were required to achieve 80% power. Based on this sample size estimate, the surgeon expected that this study would require about 3 years. Planned interim analyses were conducted at the end of first and second study years.

Please answer the following questions:

1. Is the design parallel-groups, crossover, or adaptive? Why?
2. What does it mean to say that the study achieved 80% power?
3. The surgeon planned to use a two-tailed hypothesis for this study. Is this appropriate? Why or why not?

4. At the end of the first study year, data from 140 patients were collected. For this interim analysis, the distributional assumptions were met and the surgeon initially considered estimating a mixed between-within repeated-measures analysis of variance (ANOVA) model. In terms of hemoglobin in the EACA and TXA groups, what research question would this model answer? Is this model the most appropriate to test the surgeon's hypothesis?

5. At the end of the second study year, data from 250 patients were collected. For this interim analysis, the distributional assumptions were met and the surgeon initially considered estimating a multivariable linear regression model to evaluate postoperative hemoglobin after controlling for preoperative hemoglobin as well as the patient's biological sex and weight. Does it make sense to statistically control for biological sex and weight? Why or why not?

6. The surgeon decides to stop the trial at the end of the second study year because results of a one-way ANCOVA model, in which the mean difference in postoperative hemoglobin was adjusted for preoperative hemoglobin, indicated the difference in postoperative hemoglobin between the EACA and TXA groups was statistically significant with $p < 0.000001$. Does this very small p-value indicate that the difference in postoperative hemoglobin is large and clinically meaningful? Does this p-value indicate that this result is likely to replicate if the study was conducted again? Is a p-value enough justification for stopping a trial? What associated statistical information should the surgeon present to provide the clinical significance of this study?

Introduction to Common Statistical Tests

The remainder of this chapter describes the application and assumptions of numerous parametric and nonparametric statistical tests commonly used in the biomedical sciences. Note that this section only covers statistical tests applicable to study designs with one measured DV. A description and list of assumptions are provided for each statistical test as well as an example with an associated results section as it would likely appear in the literature. It is important to take careful note of the assumptions for each statistical test, as these assumptions are vital in determining whether correct statistical inference can be inferred from the statistical test results. The discussion of statistical tests begins with tests for nominal and categorical data, followed by statistical tests for evaluating group differences and associations. Finally, a brief discussion of a Bayesian framework and its estimation methods is provided.

TESTS FOR NOMINAL AND CATEGORICAL DATA

Nonparametric Tests

Pearson's Chi Square Test

Pearson's chi square test (or simply the chi square test) is one of the most common statistical tests used in the biomedical sciences. It is used to assess for significant differences between two or more mutually exclusive groups for two variables measured on a nominal scale. Note that the data may also be ordinal if the number of rank ordered categories is small; however, the test does not consider rank order. The chi square test assesses for differences between actual or observed frequency counts and the frequency count that would be expected if there actually were no differences in the data.

As an example, consider a study to determine whether a significant difference in gender exists between three treatment groups. In most journal articles, a 2×3 (i.e., gender by treatment group) contingency containing the observed frequency counts within each cell will typically be presented. This table would appear similar to Figure 6-7 but with another row or column. The expected frequencies are rarely presented in the literature. Next, a chi square (χ^2) statistic should be presented with appropriate degrees of freedom subscripted next to the chi square symbol (e.g., χ^2_2 for two degrees of freedom). As stated above, the number of degrees of freedom will vary based on the analysis. If the probability of the difference is below alpha, that is, if the observed frequencies are different from the expected frequencies, the test is considered statistically significant indicating a significant gender difference between the groups. The results of a statistically significant gender difference are presented as follows:

The results of the chi square test indicated a statistically significant gender difference between treatment groups ($\chi^2_2 = 11.59$, $p < 0.05$).

When the chi square test is based on a contingency table larger than 2×2, the test is considered an omnibus test. That is, in the example above for the 2×3 table, the chi square test indicated that a statistically significant gender difference existed between at least two treatment groups, but failed to indicate specifically which treatment groups differed. In these situations, *post hoc* chi square tests (or Fisher's exact tests if expected frequencies are low; see the next section) are used to determine where statistically significant differences occurred. For example, in the 2×3 chi square above, three 2×2 *post hoc* chi square tests are required. Specifically, gender compared between groups A and B, gender compared between groups A and C, and gender compared between groups B and C. A sample results section including the *post hoc* chi square test results is presented below:

Statistically significant gender differences were indicated across the three treatment groups ($\chi^2_2 = 11.59$, $p < 0.05$). Post hoc chi square tests indicated statistically significant gender differences between groups A and B ($\chi^2_1 = 6.54$, $p < 0.05$) and between groups B and C ($\chi^2_1 = 10.26$, $p < 0.05$), with group B including significantly more males compared *to both groups A and C. Further, no statistically significant gender difference was indicated between groups A and C.*

The assumptions of the chi square test include:

1. Data for both variables being compared must be categorical.
   a. Note that continuous data can be categorized; however, information will be lost via categorization.
2. The categories must be mutually exclusive.
   a. That is, each individual can fall into one, and only one, category.
3. The total sample size must be large.
   a. The expected frequencies in each cell must not be too small. For chi square tests with degrees of freedom greater than 1 (i.e., when the number of columns and/or rows are greater than 2), no more than 20% of the cells should have expected frequencies less than 5. Further, no cell should have an expected frequency less than 1.[31] This is a difficult assumption to verify from the literature, outside of calculating the expected frequencies by hand. However, if an article fails to indicate this assumption was tested, view results with caution.

Fisher's Exact Test

Fisher's exact test is ubiquitous in the biomedical literature. The test can only be applied to 2 × 2 contingency tables and is most useful when the sample size is small. It is often used when the third assumption of the chi square test is violated. Conceptually, Fisher's exact test is identical to the chi square test, in that the two variables being compared must be nominal and have mutually exclusive categories.

For example, consider a study assessing for differences in cardiac events in dialysis patients who initiated beta-blocker therapy compared to patients who did not initiate therapy. Note, both variables are dichotomous (i.e., event versus no event; beta blocker versus no beta blocker). Fisher's exact test provides the exact probability of observing this particular set of frequencies within each cell of the contingency table. Results of a statistically significant Fisher's exact test are presented below. Notice only a p-value is provided:

The results of a Fisher's exact test indicated patients initiating beta-blocker therapy had significantly fewer cardiac events compared to patients failing to initiate therapy ($p < 0.05$).

The assumptions of Fisher's exact test include:

1. Data for both variables being compared must be dichotomous.
   a. Note that continuous data can be dichotomized; however, information will be lost via categorization.
2. The dichotomous categories must be mutually exclusive.
   a. That is, each individual can fall into one, and only one, category.

Mantel-Haenszel Chi Square Test

The Mantel-Haenszel chi square test (aka, Cochran-Mantel-Haenszel test or Mantel-Haenszel test) measures the association of three discrete variables, which usually consists of two dichotomous IVs and one categorical confounding variable or covariate used as a stratification variable.

For example, consider a study assessing the presence or absence of lung cancer in smokers and nonsmokers (the IVs) after stratifying for frequent exposure to secondhand smoke (the dichotomous covariate; exposure versus no exposure). A 2×2 contingency table is created at each level of secondhand smoke. That is, a contingency table for exposure and another for no exposure. This test produces a chi square statistic (χ^2_{MH}), with a statistically significant result indicating a significant difference in the presence of lung cancer for smokers and nonsmokers across the levels of the covariate (i.e., exposed versus unexposed). A statistically significant result is presented as follows:

The results of a Mantel-Haenszel chi square test indicated the proportion of nonsmokers developing lung cancer was significantly greater for those exposed to secondhand smoke ($\chi^2_{MH} = 29.67$, 1 df, $p < 0.05$).

The assumptions of the Mantel-Haenszel chi square test include:

1. Data of the IVs must be dichotomous.
   a. Note that continuous data can be dichotomized; however, information will be lost via categorization.
2. The dichotomous categories must be mutually exclusive.
   a. That is, each individual can fall into one, and only one, category.
3. Data of the covariate must be categorical.
   a. Again, note that continuous data can be dichotomized; however, information will be lost via categorization.

The Kappa Statistic

The kappa statistic (aka, Cohen's kappa or κ) is a measure of inter-rater reliability or agreement for a categorical variable measured on a nominal scale. That is, kappa indicates how often individual raters using the same measurement scale indicate identical scores. Kappa provides the proportion of agreement corrected for chance and ranges from 0 indicating no agreement to 1 indicating perfect agreement. Be aware that there are no methodological studies defining a threshold for what could be considered good agreement. The definition of good agreement varies by substantive area. That is, what is considered good agreement in medical literature may not be considered good agreement in psychology, or vice versa. In general, however, a higher kappa is always better.

Because this statistic corrects for chance agreement, it is more appropriate than simply calculating overall percent agreement.[32] In fact, percent agreement should rarely be used and published results using percent agreement should be viewed with caution. Kappa can be applied to a variable with any number of categories, with the understanding that as the number of categories increase, overall agreement will undoubtedly decrease. That is, the more choices two raters have, the less likely they are to agree.

As an example, consider 100 professional school applicants, who each interview with two faculty members. After the interview is complete, each faculty member rates the applicant as accept, deny, or waitlist. Kappa is then used to calculate the agreement between faculty members. Results using the kappa statistic are presented as follows:

Cohen's kappa was employed to measure the agreement between faculty members in determining whether applicants should be accepted, denied, or waitlisted. Results indicated moderate agreement between faculty members ($\kappa = 0.75$).

The assumptions of the kappa statistic include:

1. Each object (e.g., the applicant in the example above) is rated only one time.
2. The outcome variable is nominal with mutually exclusive categories.
    a. That is, each individual can fall into one, and only one, category.
3. There are at least two independent raters.
    a. That is, each rater provides one, and only one, response for each applicant.

TESTING FOR DIFFERENCES FROM THE POPULATION

Parametric Tests

One-Sample z-Test

The one-sample z-test is used to assess for a difference between the mean of the study sample and a known population mean using a continuous DV.

For example, consider data collected from a random sample of 1,000 patients with borderline high cholesterol, for which their mean serum total cholesterol was 210.01 mg/dL. The researcher is interested in determining whether the total cholesterol of this sample is significantly higher than the mean total cholesterol within the general population. The 2007 to 2008 National Health and Nutrition Examination Survey (NHANES) determined the mean serum total cholesterol level for individuals in the United States aged 6 years and older is 186.67 mg/dL with a standard deviation of 42.15.[33] A one-sample z-test provides a z-score indicating how many standard errors the sample mean is from the known population mean and if this difference is large enough to be considered statistically significant based on specific degrees of freedom. Note that degrees of freedom will be subscripted next to the z-score (e.g., z_{999}). Results of a statistically significant one-sample z-test with no assumption violations are provided as follows:

Results of a one-sample z-test indicated a statistically significant difference in total cholesterol between the study sample and population ($z_{999} = 2.10$, $p < 0.05$), with the study *sample having significantly higher total cholesterol compared to the general population (210.01 mg/dL versus 186.67 mg/dL, respectively).*

Assumptions of the one-sample z-test include:

1. The DV is measured on an interval or ratio scale.
2. The sampling distribution of means for the DV is normal.
   a. This can be assured by applying the Central Limit Theorem.
3. The population mean and standard deviation are known.
4. The observations are independent.
   a. That is, each participant provides one, and only one, observation (i.e., data or response).

One-Sample t-Test

Only in rare cases is the population standard deviation known; thus, test statistics often must be based on sample data (i.e., standard deviation and sample size). The one-sample t-test is used in situations where only the population mean is known, or can at least be estimated by very large amounts of data. It is used only for a continuous DV.

For example, consider a study to compare the mean total cholesterol of a random sample of 1,000 adults aged 20 years of age or older with borderline high cholesterol (e.g., 231.26 mg/dL) to the mean total cholesterol of the general population. In 2006, the National Center for Health Statistics determined that the mean serum total cholesterol for adults in the United States aged 20 years and older was 199.00 mg/dL.[34] Notice, no population standard deviation is available; thus, a one-sample t-test is required. Note that this test produces a t-statistic, which can be considered similar to a z-score when samples are large. In general, a t-test will approximate a z-test with a sample size of around 30. The result of a statistically significant one-sample t-test with no assumption violations is presented as follows:

Results of a one-sample t-test indicated a statistically significant difference in total cholesterol between the study sample and population ($t_{999} = 2.23$, $p < 0.05$), with the study sample having significantly higher total cholesterol compared to individuals aged 20 or older in the general population (231.26 mg/dL versus 199.00 mg/dL, respectively).

Assumptions of the one-sample t-test include:

1. The DV is measured on an interval or ratio scale.
2. The sampling distribution of means for the DV is normal.
   a. This can be assured by applying the Central Limit Theorem.
3. The population mean is known.
4. The observations are independent.
   a. That is, each participant provides one, and only one, observation (i.e., data or response).

Nonparametric Tests

Binomial Test

The binomial test is used when the DV is dichotomous and all of the possible data or outcomes fall into one, and only one, of the two categories. The binomial test uses the binomial distribution to test the exact probability of whether the sample proportion differs from the population proportion. Further, the binomial test is often used in the literature when sample sizes are small and violate the assumptions of the chi square test, specifically low expected frequencies.[27]

For example, say a fair coin is flipped 10 times, and lands on heads 6 of the 10 flips. The expected population proportion is 0.50; that is, if the coin is fair, as the number of flips increases the coin should land on heads 50% of the time. Because the coin landed on heads 6 of the 10 flips, the statistical test is whether this proportion (i.e., 6/10 or 0.60) is statistically different from the expected proportion (i.e., 0.50). In this case, the binomial test indicates the difference between these proportions is not significant and results are presented as follows:

Results of the binomial test indicated the probability of flipping six heads in 10 flips was not statistically different from the expected population proportion of 0.50 ($p > 0.05$).

The assumptions of the binomial test include:

1. Data for both variables being compared must be dichotomous.
    a. Note that continuous data can be dichotomized; however, information will be lost via categorization.
2. The dichotomous categories must be mutually exclusive.
    a. That is, each individual can fall into one, and only one, category.
3. The population proportion is known.
4. The observations are independent.
    a. That is, each participant provides one, and only one, observation (i.e., data or response).

Kolmogorov-Smirnov One-Sample Test

The Kolmogorov-Smirnov one-sample test is a goodness-of-fit test used to determine the degree of agreement between the distribution of a researcher's sample data and a theoretical population distribution.[27] That is, it allows researchers to compare the distribution of their sample data against a given probability distribution for a continuous DV (see Table 6-1).

For example, consider a study where HbA1c data were collected for a random sample of 100 patients with diabetes. The researcher is interested in determining whether the HbA1c data were sampled from a population of patients with an underlying normal distribution. That is, the researcher is interested in whether the sample data is normally distributed. A nonsignificant Kolmogorov-Smirnov test indicates the sample distribution and the hypothesized normal distribution are not statistically different; that is, the distribution of sample data can be considered normally distributed. Results of the Kolmogorov-Smirnov test are presented as follows:

Results of the Kolmogorov-Smirnov test indicated HbA1c variable had a nonsignificant departure from normality (p > 0.05); thus, the data are considered to result from a normal distribution.

The assumptions of the Kolmogorov-Smirnov one-sample test include:

1. The DV is measured on an interval or ratio scale.
2. The underlying population distribution is theorized or known.
   a. That is, the researcher must specify the correct probability distribution to test the sample data against. If the distribution is unknown, the test is inappropriate.
3. The observations are independent.
   a. That is, each participant provides one, and only one, observation (i.e., data or response).

TESTING FOR DIFFERENCES BETWEEN GROUPS

Parametric Tests

Independent-Samples t-Test

The independent-samples t-test (aka, student's t-test) is used to assess for a statistically significant difference between the means of two independent, mutually exclusive groups using a continuous DV.

For example, consider testing for a mean difference in a methacholine challenge at the end of an 8-week study period in two groups of asthma patients receiving either rosiglitazone or placebo. Methacholine challenge was measured by a 20% decrease in forced expiratory volume in 1 second (FEV1; PC20). The independent-sample t-test provides the t statistic and probability of obtaining a difference of this size or larger based on specific degrees of freedom, which are usually subscripted (e.g., t_{31}). Results of a statistically significant independent-samples t-test with no assumption violations are presented as follows:

The results of an independent-samples t-test indicated a statistically significant difference between groups (t_{31} = 9.654, p < 0.05), with asthma patients receiving rosiglitazone displaying significantly better lung function compared to placebo (mean PC20 = 10.7 mg/mL versus 3.8 mg/mL, respectively).

The assumptions of the independent-samples t-test include:

1. The DV is measured on an interval or ratio scale.
2. The sampling distribution of means for the DV within each level of the IV (i.e., group) is normal.
   a. This can be assured by applying the central limit theorem.

3. The IV is dichotomous.

   a. Note that continuous data can be dichotomized; however, information will be lost via categorization.

4. The IV categories are mutually exclusive.

   a. That is, each individual can fall into one, and only one, category.

5. Homogeneity of variance is assured.

   a. That is, the variance within each group is similar. A crude indicator of a violation of this assumption (i.e., heterogeneity) is the ratio of the largest variance to smallest variance being greater than 10:1.[22] For example, most studies do not provide the variance for each variable; however, the standard deviation is reported consistently. Remember, variance is simply the standard deviation squared. Thus, consider two variables with standard deviations of 5 and 10. The homogeneity of variance assumption can be tested by squaring the standard deviations (i.e., $5^2 = 25$ and $10^2 = 100$, respectively) and finding their ratio (i.e., $100/25 = 4$). In this case, the ratio is less than 10:1; thus, the assumption is not violated.

6. The observations are independent.

   a. That is, each participant provides one, and only one, observation (i.e., data or response).

One-Way Between-Groups Analysis of Variance

A one-way between-groups analysis of variance (ANOVA) is an extension of the independent-samples t-test to situations where researchers want to assess for mean differences between three or more mutually exclusive groups using a continuous DV.

For example, consider the rosiglitazone example from the Independent-Samples t-Test section, but in addition to the placebo group, include two groups receiving different doses of rosiglitazone (e.g., 4 mg and 8 mg). The use of three independent-samples t-tests to test for mean differences between groups (i.e., 4 mg versus placebo, 8 mg versus placebo, 4 mg versus 8 mg) is inappropriate due to a possible increase in Type I error. Instead, one-way ANOVA is used to partition the variance between and within groups to determine if a statistically significant group difference exists. This partitioning can be observed in the two numbers presented for degrees of freedom (i.e., $F_{2,27}$ indicates 2 between-group degrees of freedom and 27 within-group degrees of freedom). The result of a statistically significant one-way ANOVA with no assumption violations is presented as follows:

Results of a one-way ANOVA indicated a statistically significant difference between groups ($F_{2,27} = 6.89$, $p < 0.05$).

ANOVA provides an omnibus F test, that is, an overall test assessing the statistical significance between the three or more group means. A statistically significant omnibus F test indicates a statistically significant difference between at least two group means. To determine which groups differ specifically, a series of *post hoc* tests are conducted. *Post hoc* tests are simply tests comparing individual groups to one another; thus, *post hoc* tests can be viewed as a series of independent-samples *t*-tests. That is, two-group comparisons. Because *post hoc* tests increase the number of statistical tests used, they often use a more conservative alpha to control for potential Type I errors. With this in mind, the significant one-way ANOVA in the example above would require three adjusted *post hoc* tests. That is, 4 mg versus placebo, 8 mg versus placebo, and 4 mg versus 8 mg. The most commonly used *post hoc* tests in the literature include the Tukey and Scheffé tests. Be aware that the Scheffé test is the most conservative *post hoc* test available and some methodologists argue that the test may be too conservative increasing the probability of committing a Type II error. A suitable alternative is the Tukey test, which is conservative but to a lesser degree. In most cases, the two tests will indicate similar results and both are viewed as acceptable.

The results of a statistically significant one-way ANOVA including *post hoc* tests are presented as follows:

Results of a one-way ANOVA indicated a statistically significant difference between groups ($F_{2,27} = 6.89$, $p < 0.05$). Post hoc Tukey tests indicated statistically significant differences (at $p < 0.05$) between placebo (3.8 mg/mL) and 4 mg dose of rosiglitazone (10.7 mg/mL) as well as between placebo and the 8 mg dose of rosiglitazone (12.2 mg/mL). No statistically significant differences were indicated between the 4 mg and 8 mg doses of rosiglitazone.

The assumptions for one-way ANOVA include:

1. The DV is measured on an interval or ratio scale.
2. The sampling distribution of means for the DV within each level of the IV is normal.
   a. This can be assured by applying the Central Limit Theorem.
3. The levels of the IV are mutually exclusive.
   a. That is, each individual can fall into one, and only one, category.
4. Homogeneity of variance is assured.
   a. That is, the variance within each group is similar. A crude indicator of a violation of this assumption (i.e., heterogeneity) is the ratio of the largest variance to smallest variance being greater than 10:1.[22] For example, most studies do not provide the variance for each variable; however, the standard deviation is reported consistently. Remember, variance is simply the standard deviation squared. Thus, consider two variables with standard deviations of 5 and 10. The homogeneity of variance assumption can be tested by squaring the standard deviations (i.e., $5^2 = 25$ and $10^2 = 100$, respectively) and finding their ratio (i.e., $100/25 = 4$). In this case, the ratio is less than 10:1; thus, the assumption is not violated.
5. The observations are independent.
   a. That is, each participant provides one, and only one, observation (i.e., data or response).

Factorial Between-Groups Analysis of Variance

A factorial between-groups analysis of variance (aka, factorial ANOVA) is an extension of the one-way between-groups ANOVA to a study with more than one IV using a continuous DV.

For example, consider a study to evaluate for differences in heart rate measured by beats per minute (bpm) between men and women following either a 25 mg dose of pseudoephedrine or placebo. In the literature, this may be described as a 2 × 2 factorial design indicating two IVs (i.e., gender and treatment) each with two levels (i.e., male versus female; pseudoephedrine versus placebo). This type of design produces two main effects—one for gender and one for treatment—and an interaction effect between gender and treatment. Thus, three separate F tests are provided, one for each effect, with statistical significance determined separately for each effect.

It is extremely important to note that if the interaction effect is statistically significant, the results of the main effects cannot be interpreted directly, as the IVs are dependent on each other. From the example, a statistically significant interaction effect indicates treatment effects differ depending on the gender of the participant. That is, pseudoephedrine had a different effect for males than it did for females. However, if the interaction effect is not significant, main effects can and should be interpreted. When interpreting the main effect of an IV, the levels of the other IV are averaged or marginalized. That is, interpreting the main effect of gender is done irrespective of whether the participants received pseudoephedrine or placebo. Likewise, interpreting the main effect of treatment is done irrespective of the participant's gender.

Similar to one-way between-groups ANOVA, following a statistically significant main effect or interaction, *post hoc* tests may be required to identify where statistically significant differences occurred. There are a number of *post hoc* tests available depending on whether the interaction or main effects are statistically significant including the Tukey and Scheffé tests.[35] Each *post hoc* test adjusts alpha more or less conservatively to reduce potential Type I errors. *Post hoc* tests for factorial ANOVA used in the literature are often termed simple comparisons, simple contrasts, simple main effects, or interaction contrasts. While each uses a slightly different procedure, they are used to accomplish the same goal—identify group differences.

In the biomedical sciences, the results of a nonsignificant interaction effect for a 2 × 2 factorial between-groups ANOVA with no assumption violations are presented as follows:

Results of a 2 (gender; male versus female) × 2 (treatment; pseudoephedrine versus placebo) factorial between-groups ANOVA indicated a nonsignificant interaction effect between gender and treatment (p > 0.05). However, the main effect for gender was statistically significant ($F_{1,26} = 21.36$, p < 0.05), with males having significantly higher heart rates than females (91.6 bpm versus 84.3 bpm, respectively). Further, the main effect of treatment was also statistically significant ($F_{1,26} = 15.24$, p < 0.05), with pseudoephedrine resulting in a significantly higher heart rate compared to placebo (70.3 bpm versus 65.2 bpm, respectively).

The results of a 2×2 factorial between-groups ANOVA with a statistically significant interaction and no assumption violations are presented as follows:

Results of a 2 (gender; male versus female) × 2 (treatment; pseudoephedrine versus placebo) factorial between-groups ANOVA indicated a statistically significant interaction effect between gender and treatment ($F_{1,26} = 15.42$, $p < 0.05$). Simple main effects were assessed to identify at which treatment level gender differed. Results indicated pseudoephedrine increased heart rate significantly higher for males compared to females (90.5 bpm versus 82.4 bpm, respectively). No statistically significant gender difference in heart rate was indicated for the placebo group.

The assumptions of factorial between-groups ANOVA include:

1. The DV is measured on an interval or ratio scale.
2. The sampling distribution of means for the DV within each level of the IV is normal.
   a. This can be assured by applying the Central Limit Theorem.
3. The levels of the IVs are mutually exclusive.
   a. That is, each individual can fall into one, and only one, category.
4. Homogeneity of variance is assured.
   a. That is, the variance within each group is similar. A crude indicator of a violation of this assumption (i.e., heterogeneity) is the ratio of the largest variance to smallest variance being greater than 10:1.[22] For example, most studies do not provide the variance for each variable; however, the standard deviation is reported consistently. Remember, variance is simply the standard deviation squared. Thus, consider two variables with standard deviations of 5 and 10. The homogeneity of variance assumption can be tested by squaring the standard deviations (i.e., $5^2 = 25$ and $10^2 = 100$, respectively) and finding their ratio (i.e., 100/25 = 4). In this case, the ratio is less than 10:1; thus, the assumption is not violated.
5. The observations are independent.
   a. That is, each participant provides one, and only one, observation (i.e., data or response).

Analysis of Covariance

Analysis of covariance (ANCOVA) is an extension of both one-way between-groups ANOVA and factorial between-groups ANOVA. ANCOVA evaluates main effects and interactions using a continuous DV after statistically adjusting for one or more continuous confounding variables. That is, ANCOVA adjusts all group means to create the situation as if all participants scored identically on the covariate.[22]

For example, consider a study comparing atenolol to placebo (IV) and assessing their effects on systolic blood pressure (DV). The researchers note, however, that previous research has shown systolic blood pressure and BMI to be highly correlated.[36] Thus, the analysis will include BMI as a covariate assessing the effect of atenolol on systolic blood pressure over and above the effect of BMI on systolic blood pressure. If the atenolol group has greater BMI values compared to the placebo group, ANCOVA will adjust the systolic blood pressure within both groups to account for this initial difference in BMI.

In ANCOVA, covariates are continuous, measured before the DV, and correlated with the DV. It should be noted that ANCOVA is closely related to linear regression. Thus, although not completely necessary, it may be useful to revisit this section after reading the sections on Simple Linear Regression and Multivariable Linear Regression presented later in the chapter. In ANCOVA, group means are statistically adjusted by the magnitude of the association (i.e., slope) between the DV and covariate.[39] That is, the greater the association, the more useful the covariate and better the adjustment. Thus, the goal of the covariate is to reduce error variance thereby increasing the statistical power of the test. From the example, mean systolic blood pressure for the atenolol and placebo groups are adjusted by the association between BMI and systolic blood pressure. Because previous research has shown the association between systolic blood pressure and BMI to be considerable, the statistical power of this test will undoubtedly be increased.

When presenting the results of ANCOVA, researchers should provide adjusted means; that is, the mean of the DV at each level of the IV after adjusting for the covariate. Published research that does not present adjusted means should be viewed with caution. Further, the effect of the covariate must also be presented which provides information regarding the effectiveness of the covariate in adjusting group means. Finally, it should be noted that ANCOVA is more suited for experimental design in which participants are randomized to groups, as opposed to nonexperimental designs without randomization. Remember, ANCOVA is used to adjust group means as if all participants had identical covariate values. However, in nonexperimental research, important covariates may have been missed and causality is difficult to infer—a characteristic intrinsic to all nonexperimental work. Thus, the limitations may be significant when applying ANCOVA to nonexperimental designs and results must be viewed cautiously.[9]

In the biomedical sciences, the results of a statistically significant ANCOVA with no assumption violations are presented as follows:

Results of a one-way ANCOVA indicated a statistically significant group differences in systolic blood pressure after adjusting for BMI ($F_{1,17} = 7.98$, $p < 0.05$), with patients receiving atenolol having significantly lower systolic blood pressure compared to placebo (adjusted means = 118 mmHg versus 141 mmHg, respectively). The relationship between systolic blood pressure and BMI was also statistically significant after adjusting for group ($F_{1,17} = 39.85$, $p < 0.05$) with a pooled within-group correlation of 0.61.

The assumptions of ANCOVA include:

1. The DV is measured on an interval or ratio scale.
2. The sampling distribution of means for the DV and covariate(s) within each level of the IV is normal.
   a. This can be assured by applying the Central Limit Theorem.
3. The levels of the IV are mutually exclusive.
   a. That is, each individual can fall into one, and only one, category.
4. Homogeneity of variance is assured.
   a. That is, the variance within each group is similar. A crude indicator of a violation of this assumption (i.e., heterogeneity) is the ratio of the largest variance to smallest variance being greater than 10:1.[22] For example, most studies do not provide the variance for each variable; however, the standard deviation is reported consistently. Remember, variance is simply the standard deviation squared. Thus, consider two variables with standard deviations of 5 and 10. The homogeneity of variance assumption can be tested by squaring the standard deviations (i.e., $5^2 = 25$ and $10^2 = 100$, respectively) and finding their ratio (i.e., $100/25 = 4$). In this case, the ratio is less than 10:1; thus, the assumption is not violated.
5. Homogeneity of regression is assured.
   a. This assumption requires the association between the DV and covariate to be the same within each level of the IV. A violation of this assumption renders ANCOVA inappropriate, and the authors should use linear regression instead. However, violation is difficult to detect from the literature, as most authors fail to provide the appropriate information in the narrative. Thus, when reading a journal article employing ANCOVA, if the author fails to indicate whether this assumption was tested, results must be viewed with caution.
6. The covariate(s) is measured reliably and without error.
7. The observations are independent.
   a. That is, each participant provides one, and only one, observation (i.e., data or response).

Nonparametric Tests

Mann-Whitney Test

The Mann-Whitney test is the nonparametric alternative to the independent-samples t-test and is one of the most powerful nonparametric tests.[27] It is used when the distributional assumptions for the parametric test are violated or when the DV is measured on an ordinal scale. The Mann-Whitney test is based on ranked data. That is, instead of using the actual values of the DV, as an independent-samples t-test does, each participant's DV value is ranked with the highest value receiving the highest rank and the lowest value receiving the lowest rank. The ranks within each group are then summed and the test assesses whether the difference in ranked sums between groups is statistically significant.

For example, consider a performance improvement study assessing gender differences in patient satisfaction of hospital stay following total hip replacement surgery. The measurement instrument uses a Likert-type scale with four possible responses anchored from Strongly Disagree to Strongly Agree. A statistically significant Mann-Whitney test indicates gender differences in patient satisfaction, with the group with the highest ranked sums indicating higher satisfaction. The results of the Mann-Whitney test are presented as follows:

The results of a Mann-Whitney test indicate a statistically significant gender difference in patient satisfaction following total hip replacement surgery ($z = 2.65$, $p < 0.05$), with males indicating higher satisfaction scores compared to females.

The assumptions of the Mann-Whitney test include:

1. The DV is measured on an ordinal, interval, or ratio scale.
2. The IV is dichotomous.
   a. Note that continuous data can be categorized into a dichotomous variable; however, information will be lost.
3. The levels of the IV are mutually exclusive.
   a. That is, each individual can fall into one, and only one category.
4. The observations are independent.
   a. That is, each participant provides one, and only one, observation (i.e., data or response).

Median Test

The median test is used to assess whether two mutually exclusive groups have different medians. There is no parametric alternative to the median test; however, the nonparametric Mann-Whitney test can be used as an adequate alternative. The test calculates the medians within each group and then classifies the data within each group as either above or below the respective group median. Further, because the test is based on the median, it can be used appropriately for skewed distributions or data containing outliers.

For example, consider a study evaluating gender differences in childhood autism as measured by the Childhood Autism Spectrum Test (CAST).[37] The CAST measures difficulties and preferences in social and communication skills using the total score of a 37-item questionnaire, with lower scores indicating fewer symptoms. Because autism is a relatively rare disorder, the distribution of CAST scores is expected to have severe positive skewness due to outliers. That is, most children will score low, while a few autistic children will have high scores. The median test was used to determine whether statistically significant gender differences existed in CAST scores. The results of a statistically significant median test are presented as follows:

The results of the median test indicated gender differences in CAST scores ($p < 0.05$), with boys having a significantly higher median score compared to girls (median = 5 versus median = 4, respectively).

Assumptions of the median test include:

1. The DV is measured on an ordinal, interval, or ratio scale.
2. Samples sizes are sufficiently large.
   a. If sample sizes are small, say less than five in each group, Fisher's exact test should be used instead. From the example, this means using a 2 (group; male versus female) × 2 (median; above versus below) contingency table.
3. The observations are independent.
   a. That is, each participant provides one, and only one, observation (i.e., data or response).

Kruskal-Wallis One-Way ANOVA by Ranks

The Kruskal-Wallis one-way ANOVA by ranks (or simply, the Kruskal-Wallis test) is the nonparametric alternative to the one-way between-groups ANOVA. The test is an extension of the Mann-Whitney test to assess group differences between three or more mutually exclusive groups. The Kruskal-Wallis test is typically used when distributional assumptions are violated or when the DV is measured on an ordinal scale. Further, the Kruskal-Wallis test is based on rank sums similar to the Mann-Whitney test. The DV scores are ranked from highest to lowest, summed, and statistically significant group differences are evaluated based on these rank sums.

For example, consider a study evaluating regional differences in whether volunteer preceptors believe they have adequate time available to dedicate to their experiential pharmacy students.[38] In this study, the DV was measured on an ordinal 4-point Likert-type scale; thus, the Kruskal-Wallis test was used in lieu of one-way between-groups ANOVA. The results of the statistically significant Kruskal-Wallis test are presented as follows:

Results of the Kruskal-Wallis test indicated regional differences regarding whether volunteer preceptors believe they have adequate time to dedicate to experiential students ($\chi_6^2 = 33.07, p < 0.05$).

Similar to a one-way between-groups ANOVA, the Kruskal-Wallis test is an omnibus test. That is, the test will determine whether an overall statistically significant difference exists between groups, but will not indicate specifically which groups differed statistically. Thus, *post hoc* tests are required. In this situation, the Mann-Whitney test is used to compare all two-group combinations. From the example, *post hoc* tests would include West versus Midwest, West versus South, West versus Northeast, and so on for a total of six *post hoc* tests. The results of the Kruskal-Wallis test including Mann-Whitney *post hoc* tests are presented as follows:

Results of the Kruskal-Wallis test indicated regional differences regarding whether volunteer preceptors believe they have adequate time to dedicate to experiential students ($\chi^2_6 = 33.07, p < 0.05$). *Post hoc Mann-Whitney tests indicated preceptors in the West disagreed more compared to preceptors located in the Midwest (p < 0.05) and agreed less with preceptors in the South (p < 0.05). No other statistically significant group differences were indicated.*

The assumptions of the Kruskal-Wallis test include:

1. The DV is measured on an ordinal, interval, or ratio scale.
2. The IV is categorical.
   a. Note that continuous data can be categorized; however, information will be lost.
3. The levels of the IV are mutually exclusive.
   a. That is, each individual can fall into one, and only one category.
4. Each group has approximately the same distribution.
   a. Although the Kruskal-Wallis test does not assume data are distributed normally, if the distribution for one level of the IV is skewed negatively and the other levels are skewed positively, the results produced by the test may be inaccurate.
5. The data do not include a large number of ties.
   a. Tied values are given average ranks. Typically, if less than 25% of the data are ties, the test is unaffected.[27]
6. The observations are independent.
   a. That is, each participant provides one, and only one, observation (i.e., data or response).

TESTING FOR WITHIN-GROUP CHANGE

Parametric Tests

Paired-Samples t-Test

The paired-samples *t*-test (aka, matched *t*-test or nested *t*-test) is used when one group of participants is measured twice or two groups of participants are matched on specific characteristics. In both cases, the assumption of independence, or mutually exclusive groups, is violated. This statistical test is only appropriate using a continuous DV.

When one group of participants is measured twice, it is known as a repeated measures design. Repeatedly measuring participants is a valid method for reducing error and increasing statistical power, which requires fewer participants. The simplest repeated measures design is termed a pretest-posttest design. For example, consider measuring the therapeutic knowledge of 20 fourth-year pharmacy (P4) students prior to clinical rotations (i.e., pretest) and following rotations (i.e., posttest) to assess for increases in therapeutic knowledge. Therapeutic knowledge was measured using a discriminating 20-question test. The paired-samples t-test assesses for a statistically significant change in correct responses from pretest to posttest.

When two groups of participants are matched on specific characteristics, it is called a matched design. For example, when studying the effects of a new statin medication on hyperlipidemia, researchers would identify a group of patients to receive the statin and then identify a matched control group by matching individuals based on age, race, gender, BMI, and years with diagnosis. Note that the matched control group does not receive any medication. Matching participants serves the same purpose as repeated measures—reduce error variance—but is often more difficult because as the number of matching criteria increases, the probability of finding a suitable match decreases.

Results of a statistically significant paired-samples t-test with no assumption violations using the pretest-posttest design example above is presented as follows:

The results of a paired-samples t-test indicated a statistically significant difference in therapeutic knowledge between pretest and posttest scores ($t_{19} = 3.25, p < 0.05$). Therapeutic knowledge increased significantly following clinical rotations (mean = 10.4 correct responses at pretest versus a mean of 16.5 at posttest).

The assumptions of the paired-samples t-test include:

1. The DV is measured on an interval or ratio scale.
2. The two DV measurements are associated.
3. The sampling distribution of means for both DV measurements is normal.
   a. This can be assured by applying the Central Limit Theorem.
4. Homogeneity of variance for both DV measurements is assured.
   a. That is, the variance within each group is similar. A crude indicator of a violation of this assumption (i.e., heterogeneity) is the ratio of the largest variance to smallest variance being greater than 10:1.[22] For example, most studies do not provide the variance for each variable; however, the standard deviation is reported consistently. Remember, variance is simply the standard deviation squared. Thus, consider two variables with standard deviations of 5 and 10. The homogeneity of variance assumption can be tested by squaring the standard deviations (i.e., $5^2 = 25$ and $10^2 = 100$, respectively) and finding their ratio (i.e., $100/25 = 4$). In this case, the ratio is less than 10:1; thus, the assumption is not violated.

One-Way Repeated Measures Analysis of Variance

A one-way repeated measures ANOVA (aka, repeated measures ANOVA) is an extension of the paired-samples t-test to situations where the continuous DV is measured three or more times. Again, this can occur when the same participants are measured repeatedly or when three or more matched groups are measured once. A repeated measures ANOVA is used to indicate whether statistically significant change occurred between the repeated measurements.

For example, reconsider the pretest-posttest design described in the Paired-Samples *t*-Test section early in the chapter. Briefly, a researcher is interested in testing whether therapeutic knowledge of 20 pharmacy students in their last year of college changes before and after clinical rotations. To be applicable to repeated measures ANOVA, students would be tested on a third occasion 6 months after posttest to assess knowledge retention. That is, the design measures therapeutic knowledge at pretest, posttest, and 6-month follow-up. The repeated measures ANOVA is then used to test whether a statistically significant change occurred between the repeated measurements.

It should be noted that some researchers prefer to use repeated measures ANOVA over paired-samples *t*-tests when participants are only measured twice. This is an appropriate use of repeated measures ANOVA as repeated measures ANOVA can be used in any situation when a paired-samples *t*-test is appropriate. The results would be identical. However, the test statistic from the repeated measures ANOVA will be an F value instead of a t value produced by the paired-samples *t*-test. This is a nonissue, though, as the F value in this situation is simply t^2.

In most cases, repeated measures ANOVA has more statistical power than a paired-samples *t*-test. This has been alluded to in The Analysis of Clinical Trials and Paired-Samples *t*-Test sections earlier in the chapter. In general, increasing the number of repeated measures further reduces error, which allows for more precise measurement and decreases the overall probability of committing a Type I error. With that said, increasing the number of repeated measurements has diminishing returns in statistical power. That is, for most studies, statistical power will increase drastically by adding a few additional repeated measurements, but the magnitude of this increase weakens rapidly between four and six measurements, with little to no increases in statistical power beyond the seventh measurement.[39] Finally, if a study has more than 10 repeated measurements, a time series analysis may be more appropriate than repeated measures ANOVA.

In addition, a brief discussion of the key assumption of repeated measures ANOVA is useful as a basic understanding of this assumption will assist in determining whether the test statistics produced from the analysis are correct. This key assumption, known as sphericity, states that the variances of the differences between repeated measurements are equal. For example, consider a study with three repeated measurements. For the sphericity assumption to be satisfied, the variance of the difference between the first and second measurements must be similar to the variance of the difference between the first and third and second and third. This assumption tends to be restrictive, as most differences closer in time tend to have less variability compared to measurements further apart in time. Sphericity is a testable assumption using Mauchly's test, and a violation can severely bias the statistical inference. Therefore, when reading a journal article, if the authors fail to provide information regarding the assurance or violation of the sphericity assumption, results and interpretations must be viewed with caution.

Briefly reconsider the example provided above where 20 pharmacy students in their final year have therapeutic knowledge measured before clinical rotations (i.e., pretest), once immediately after rotations (i.e., posttest), and at a 6-month follow-up. That is, therapeutic knowledge is measured on three separate occasions. A statistically significant repeated measures ANOVA with no assumption violations will be presented as follows:

The results of a one-way repeated measures ANOVA indicated a statistically significant difference in therapeutic knowledge between pretest, posttest, and 6-month follow-up $(F_{2,38} = 9.87, p < 0.05)$.

With more than two repeated measurements the one-way repeated measures ANOVA is an omnibus test. That is, the F test will identify whether a statistically significant difference exists between repeated measures, but will not indicate specifically which repeated measurements differ. Thus, *post hoc* tests, known as pairwise comparisons, are required. Similar to other analysis requiring *post hoc* tests, there are numerous adjusted pairwise comparisons available. Each type of pairwise comparison adjusts alpha differently, with some being more conservative. It may be simpler to think of these comparisons as a series of paired-samples *t*-tests with adjusted alpha values, that is, adjusted paired-samples *t*-tests comparing the first and second repeated measurements, the first and third, the second and third, and so on. The additional information required to present results of a statistically significant one-way repeated measures ANOVA with no assumption violations are presented as follows:

The results of a one-way repeated measures ANOVA indicated a statistically significant difference in therapeutic knowledge between pretest, posttest, and 6-month follow-up $(F_{2,38} = 9.87, p < 0.05)$. Results of the pairwise comparisons indicated a statistically significant increase in therapeutic knowledge from pretest to posttest (mean = 5.50 versus 15.90, respectively, p < 0.05). Further, no statistically significant difference was indicated from posttest to 6-month follow-up (mean = 15.90 versus 15.50, respectively) indicating therapeutic knowledge was retained for 6 months following clinical rotations.

The assumptions of the one-way repeated measures ANOVA include:

1. The DV is measured on an interval or ratio scale.
2. All DV measurements are associated.
3. The sampling distribution of means for all DV measurements is normal.
   a. This can be assured by applying the Central Limit Theorem.
4. Homogeneity of variance for all DV measurements is assured.
   a. That is, the variance within each group is similar. A crude indicator of a violation of this assumption (i.e., heterogeneity) is the ratio of the largest variance to smallest variance being greater than 10:1.[22] For example, most studies do not provide the variance for each variable; however, the standard deviation is reported

consistently. Remember, variance is simply the standard deviation squared. Thus, consider two variables with standard deviations of 5 and 10. The homogeneity of variance assumption can be tested by squaring the standard deviations (i.e., $5^2 = 25$ and $10^2 = 100$, respectively) and finding their ratio (i.e., $100/25 = 4$). In this case, the ratio is less than 10:1; thus, the assumption is not violated.

5. Sphericity is assured for designs with three or more repeated measurements.

    a. This is a complex assumption discussed above. In general, sphericity is violated when the variance of the differences between measurements is not similar.

Mixed Between-Within Analysis of Variance

A mixed between-within analysis of variance (aka, factorial ANOVA with repeated measures or split-plot ANOVA) is a combination of factorial between-groups ANOVA and repeated measures ANOVA. The mixed terminology highlights this combination, and indicates that the design considers two or more levels of the IV when a continuous DV is measured repeatedly. It is important to note that a mixed between-within ANOVA is qualitatively different from a mixed-effects analysis involving random effects (see Table 6-4). The simplest case is a 2×2 pretest-posttest design, using two mutually exclusive treatment groups measured on two separate occasions. The primary advantage of this analysis is that it allows researchers to assess the interaction effect evaluating whether two groups changed differently over time in addition to between-subjects main effect indicating the overall effect irrespective of measurement and within-subjects main effect indicating the overall effect irrespective of group.

As an example, consider a study examining the effectiveness of a relatively new FDA-approved tricyclic antidepressant (TCA) compared to amitriptyline over a 12-week study period. The researcher hypothesizes that the new TCA is more effective than amitriptyline in reducing symptoms of clinical depression. Prior to initiating treatment, 20 patients with diagnosed clinical depression are measured on the Beck Depression Inventory II (BDI-II).[40] Following this pretest or baseline measurement, each patient is randomized to receive one of two treatment options, the new TCA or amitriptyline, with 10 patients in each group. Patients then initiate the prescribed medication therapy and at the end of the 12-week study period BDI-II scores are measured again. A mixed between-within ANOVA provides researchers with a separate F tests for the interaction effect, between-groups main effect, and within-groups main effect each evaluated with specific degrees of freedom. Within this example, the primary effect of interest is the interaction effect, evaluating whether BDI-II scores changed differently within the new TCA group compared to the amitriptyline group from pretest to posttest.

Similar to factorial ANOVA discussed above, only if the interaction effect is nonsignificant can the researcher evaluate the statistical significance of overall group mean difference or between-group main effect and the overall change in BDI-II scores or within-group main effect. That is, a statistically significant interaction effect indicates that the change in BDI-II scores from pretest to posttest changed differently in the group receiving the new TCA group compared to the group receiving amitriptyline or vice versa. Stated another way, the reduction in symptoms from pretest to posttest was dependent on whether the patient received the new TCA or amitriptyline. In this example, the researcher's hypothesis would be supported by a statistically significant interaction effect; that is, the new TCA was more effective at reducing the symptoms associated with clinical depression compared to amitriptyline.

Although the example above was for a 2 (group: new TCA versus amitriptyline) × 2 (measurement: pretest versus posttest) design, a mixed between-within ANOVA can be used for a design with any number of IVs with any number of levels or repeated measures. This is often seen in the literature. For example, consider the pretest-posttest study evaluating the effectiveness of three treatment groups (e.g., new TCA, amitriptyline, and placebo) in reducing symptoms of clinical depression. This would be considered a 3 × 2 design. Or, consider the same study evaluating for additional gender differences within these three treatments. This would be considered a 3 × 2 × 2 design. It must be noted that as the number and levels of the IVs increase so does the complexity of interpreting results. Thus, extreme care must be taken when interpreting results and implementing suggestions supported by these types of designs. Consultation with an individual well versed in research methodology and statistical analysis is advised prior to implementing findings into an evidence-based practice.

Because a mixed between-within ANOVA is an extension of factorial between-groups ANOVA and repeated measures ANOVA, *post hoc* tests or pairwise comparisons may be required for any IV with three or more levels. That is, when there are more than three levels of the between-groups IV (e.g., new TCA, amitriptyline, and placebo), the between-groups main effect is an omnibus test. A statistically significant between-groups main effect indicates that a statistically significant difference in BDI-II scores exists, but does not indicate specifically which groups differ significantly. Further, with three or more repeated measures, a statistically significant within-groups main effect indicates a difference between repeated measures, but fails to indicate specifically which measurements differ significantly. The *post hoc* tests and pairwise comparisons for factorial between-groups ANOVA and repeated measures ANOVA, respectively, are also appropriate for a mixed between-within ANOVA.

The results of a 2 × 2 mixed between-within ANOVA with no assumption violations for a nonsignificant interaction effect and statistically significant between- and within-groups main effects are presented as follows:

The results of a 2 (group: new TCA versus amitriptyline) × 2 (measurements: pretest versus posttest) mixed between-within ANOVA failed to indicate a statistically significant interaction ($F_{1,18} = 1.215$, $p > 0.05$). However, both main effects were statistically significant. Overall, patients receiving the new TCA had lower BDI-II scores compared to patients receiving amitriptyline ($F_{1,18} = 27.97$, $p < 0.05$; mean = 29.41 versus 47.50, respectively).

Further, an overall decrease in depressive symptoms was indicated from pretest to posttest ($F_{1,18}$ = 24.74, p < 0.05; mean = 49.86 versus 35.72, respectively).

With a statistically significant interaction effect, results of the mixed between-within ANOVA with no assumption violations are presented as follows:

The results of a 2 (group: new TCA versus amitriptyline) × 2 (measurements: pretest versus posttest) mixed between-within ANOVA indicated a statistically significant interaction effect ($F_{1,18}$ = 10.37, p < 0.05). Simple main effects were assessed to identify statistically significant treatment differences at pretest and posttest individually. Results indicated no statistically significant difference between the new TCA and amitriptyline at pretest (mean = 48.53 versus 50.23, respectively). However, at posttest, a statistically significant difference was indicated, with the new TCA having significantly lower BDI-II scores compared to amitriptyline (mean = 24.63 versus 47.53, respectively).

The assumptions of a mixed between-within ANOVA include:

1. The DV is measured on an interval or ratio scale.
2. All DV measurements are associated.
3. The sampling distribution of means at each level of the IV(s), collapsed across the repeated DV measurements, is normal.
   a. This can be assured by applying the Central Limit Theorem.
4. Homogeneity of variance for all DV measurements within each level of the IV(s) is assured.
   a. That is, the variance within each group is similar. A crude indicator of a violation of this assumption (i.e., heterogeneity) is the ratio of the largest variance to smallest variance being greater than 10:1.[22] For example, most studies do not provide the variance for each variable; however, the standard deviation is reported consistently. Remember, variance is simply the standard deviation squared. Thus, consider two variables with standard deviations of 5 and 10. The homogeneity of variance assumption can be tested by squaring the standard deviations (i.e., $5^2 = 25$ and $10^2 = 100$, respectively) and finding their ratio (i.e., $100/25 = 4$). In this case, the ratio is less than 10:1; thus, the assumption is not violated.
5. Sphericity is assured for designs with three or more repeated measurements.
   a. This is a complex assumption discussed briefly above for one-way repeated measures ANOVA. In general, sphericity is violated when the variance of the differences between measurements is not similar.

Nonparametric Tests

Wilcoxon Signed-Rank Test

The Wilcoxon signed-rank test (aka, signed-rank test) is the nonparametric alternative to a paired-samples *t*-test. The test is used typically to assess for differences between two repeated measurements or two matched groups when distributional assumptions are violated or when the DV is measured on an ordinal scale. The signed-rank test is based on ranked difference scores (e.g., difference between pretest and posttest), with the highest difference score receiving the highest rank and the lowest difference score receiving the lowest rank.

For example, consider single group pretest-posttest study evaluating the secondary effect of weight loss in pounds while on exenatide therapy in a sample of 20 Type I DM patients. Prior to initiating exenatide therapy, all patients are weighed (i.e., pretest). At the end of a 1-year study period, patients are weighed again (i.e., posttest). For this study, the DV has numerous outliers; thus, the signed-rank test is used in lieu of paired-samples t-test to assess for a change in patient weight from pretest to posttest. The result of a statistically significant signed-rank test is presented as follows:

The results of the signed-rank tests indicated a statistically significant decrease in body weight from pretest to posttest ($z = 2.32$, $p < 0.05$).

The assumptions of the signed-rank test include:

1. The DV measured repeatedly on an ordinal, interval, or ratio scale.
2. The two DV measurements are associated.
3. The two measurements come from populations with the same median.
4. There should not be a large number difference scores equal to zero.
   a. That is, the number of participants having no change (i.e., difference score of zero) should be low.

Friedman Two-Way ANOVA by Ranks

The Friedman two-way ANOVA by ranks test (aka, Friedman's test) is the nonparametric alternative to the one-way repeated measures ANOVA and is an extension of the signed-rank test to a situation with three or more repeated measurements. Similar to the other nonparametric tests, it is most often used when distributional assumptions are violated or the DV is measured on an ordinal scale. The Friedman test is based on ranked data, with higher scores receiving higher ranks, and is used to assess for statistically significant differences between repeated measurements.

For example, reconsider the exenatide example described in the Wilcoxon Signed-Ranks section above. Briefly, the example consisted of a one-time pretest-posttest study evaluating the secondary effect of weight loss in pounds while on exenatide therapy in a sample of 20 Type I DM patients. To extend this design to be applicable to Friedman's test, consider a study where patients are weighed prior to initiating exenatide therapy, 6 months after initiation, and 1 year after initiation. Thus, each patient is weighed on three occasions. Because the distribution of weight has numerous outliers, Friedman's test is employed. The results of a statistically significant Friedman's test are presented as follows:

The results of Friedman's test indicated statistically significant differences in body weight between the three repeated measurements ($\chi_2^2 = 15.21$, $p < 0.05$).

Similar to the one-way repeated measures ANOVA, Friedman's test is an omnibus test. That is, it assesses whether a statistically significant difference exists between the repeated measurements, but does not indicate specifically which measurements differ significantly. Thus, a series of *post hoc* tests are required. For the example above, three signed-ranks tests are required to test for differences between measurements: pretest versus 6 months, pretest versus 1 year, and 6 months versus 1 year. The results of a statistically significant Friedman's test including the additional *post hoc* tests are presented as follows:

The results of Friedman's test indicated statistically significant differences between the three repeated measurements ($\chi_2^2 = 15.21$, $p < 0.05$). Post hoc signed-rank tests indicated a statistically significant decrease in body weight from pretest to 6-month follow-up ($z = 2.65$, $p < 0.05$), with no statistically significant difference between the 6-month and 1-year follow-up ($z = 0.51$, $p > 0.05$). Thus, results suggest weight loss occurred rapidly, within 6 months of initiating exenatide therapy, and was sustained through 1 year of therapy.

The assumptions of the Friedman test include:

1. The DV is measured repeatedly on an ordinal, interval, or ratio scale.
2. All DV measurements are associated.
3. The DV measurements come from populations with the same median.

The Sign Test

The sign test is another nonparametric alternative to the paired-samples *t*-test. Similar to the signed-rank test, the sign test is used typically when distributional assumptions are violated or when the DV is measured on an ordinal scale. The sign test is used to assess for differences between two repeated measurements or two matched groups. It must be noted that the sign test is typically less powerful than the signed-rank test as the signed-rank test uses more information from the data to calculate the test statistic. Nevertheless, the sign test is presented here because it is seen in the literature; however, in most situations, the signed-rank test should have been used.

For example, consider a pretest-posttest study to evaluate change in BMI following a physical activity intervention in a sample of 20 third-grade students. In this study, BMI was measured at the beginning of the school year (i.e., pretest) and again after school year was complete (i.e., posttest). The sign test assesses whether statistically significant change occurred between the two measurements. The results of a statistically significant sign test are presented below. Notice that no test statistic is presented, only a *p*-value.

The results of the sign test indicated a statistically significant decrease in BMI from pretest to posttest ($p < 0.05$).

The assumptions of the sign test include:

1. The DV is measured repeatedly on an ordinal, interval, or ratio scale.
2. The two DV measurements are associated.

The McNemar Test of Change

The McNemar test of change (aka, McNemar's test) is an extension of the chi square and Fisher's exact test when participants are measured on two separate occasions and assesses the statistical significance of observed changes between the two repeated measurements. McNemar's test is only applicable to a DV measured on a nominal scale; however, continuous variables can be artificially dichotomized, with the understanding that information will be lost.[27,41]

McNemar's test is often used for pretest-posttest studies to assess change following an intervention or treatment. For example, consider a study to determine the effectiveness of an influenza vaccination across two consecutive flu seasons. At the beginning of the first flu season, 20 participants are randomized to receive either vaccination or placebo with 10 in each group. At the end of the first flu season, participants are asked whether they were diagnosed with the flu or not (i.e., yes versus no). Then, at the beginning of the second flu season, participants who received the vaccination originally will receive placebo and those who received placebo originally will receive the vaccination. At the end of the second flu season, participants are asked again whether they were diagnosed with flu. McNemar's test is used in this study to statistically test whether the flu vaccination was effective, where participants diagnosed with flu while taking placebo should not have developed flu with the vaccination. That is, the participant's outcome changed depending on the treatment received.

A critically important caveat is that McNemar's test only considers participants who changed between the two repeated measurements, with participants who did not change removed from analysis. Thus, if a researcher believes that change will be rare, the McNemar test may be inappropriate because the statistical power of this test may be extremely reduced due to the sample size decrease from removing participants who did not change.

Based on the example above, the results of a statistically significant McNemar test are presented below. Notice that no test statistic is provided, only the p-value.

The results of a statistically significant McNemar's test indicated a statistically significant change between treatment and placebo ($p < 0.05$), with the vaccination significantly reducing influenza diagnoses compared to placebo.

The assumptions of the McNemar's test include:

1. The DV is measured repeatedly on a dichotomous scale.
2. The two DV measurements are associated.

The Cochran Q Test

The Cochran Q test (aka, Cochran's Q) is an extension of McNemar's test to situations where participants are measured repeatedly on three or more separate occasions.[27] Similar to McNemar's test, the DV must be measured repeatedly on a nominal scale.

In the biomedical literature, Cochran's Q is often used to assess stability of a treatment over time or to compare the effectiveness of several treatments. For example, consider a study evaluating the effectiveness of the combination treatment sildenafil and psychotherapy in reducing symptoms of erectile dysfunction (ED).[42] Eight patients with psychogenic ED attended weekly psychotherapy sessions and ingested 50 mg of sildenafil citrate orally as needed over a 6-month period. Symptoms of ED were assessed at baseline, 6 months (i.e., end of treatment), and at a 3 month posttreatment follow-up. For this study, Cochran's Q was used to evaluate a change in the stage of remission for patients dichotomized into ED versus no ED. A statistically significant finding indicated change from baseline and the possibility of sustaining effects at posttreatment follow-up. That is, all patients were diagnosed with ED at baseline, thus a statistically significant change in patients indicated remission of ED symptoms at some point.

In the literature, the results of the Cochran Q test may be presented with a χ^2 statistic and a p-value; however, in other studies, the results may only present a p-value. Although failing to include the test statistic provides less information, it does not necessarily damage the integrity of results. The result of a statistically significant Cochran's Q for the example above is presented as follows:

The results of Cochran's Q indicated a statistically significant change in psychogenic ED symptoms from baseline (p <0.05) suggesting a combination of psychotherapy and 50 mg sildenafil are effective in reducing ED symptoms.

Because Cochran's Q is used to assess change over three or more repeated measures, it is an omnibus test. That is, the test will determine whether a statistically significant change occurred between the repeated measurements, but will not indicate where the change occurred. Thus, *post hoc* tests are required. For Cochran's Q, a series of McNemar tests comparing each repeated measurement serve as *post hoc* tests. In this example, three separate McNemar tests are required comparing baseline versus 6 months, baseline versus posttreatment follow-up, and 6 months versus posttreatment follow-up. The results of a statistically significant Cochran's Q including results of *post hoc* McNemar tests are presented as follows:

The results of the Cochran Q test indicated a statistically significant change in psychogenic ED symptoms from baseline (p < 0.05). Post hoc McNemar's tests indicated statistically significant changes from baseline at 6 months as well as at posttreatment follow-up (all p < 0.05). These results suggest the combination of psychotherapy and sildenafil are effective in reducing ED symptoms and this effect continued to reduce ED symptoms up to 3 months following treatment completion.

The assumptions of the Cochran test include:

1. The DV measured repeatedly on a dichotomous scale.
2. All DV measurements are associated.

TESTING FOR RELATIONSHIPS OR ASSOCIATIONS

When exploring the association or relationship between two or more variables, two specific types of analyses are employed—correlation or regression. These analyses are applied to determine the magnitude and direction of an association or relationship. Correlation analysis indicates the co-relationship of two variables. That is, correlation described how one variable changes in relation to another. It is critically important to note that correlation cannot imply causation.

For example, consider the positive association between creatinine and BUN. In most cases, as creatinine increases so does BUN, but increasing creatinine does not cause BUN to increase or vice versa. Instead, the cause of the BUN and creatinine increase might be due to renal failure.

Regression analysis is a type of correlational analysis used to predict the value of one variable from the value of another variable. In this type of analysis, researchers attempt to determine the amount of variance in the DV that is explained by the IVs or covariates. Note that regression analysis can also permit multiple IVs and/or covariates measured on any scale. With the inclusion of multiple IVs or covariates this type of analysis is often referred to as multivariable regression analysis. While the definition of an IV and covariate is not always concrete, it is easier to think of an IV as the primary variable of interest and a covariate as a variable correlated with the DV, but not of specific interest.

For example, consider a multivariable analysis assessing the effect statin use (IV) had on all-cause mortality due to heart failure (DV) during a 5-year study period after statistically controlling for age, gender, race, comorbid conditions, and concurrent medications (covariates). The covariates may explain the reason a patient died, but are not of specific research interest.

This section begins by discussing bivariate, or two-variable, techniques followed by multivariable techniques. The discussion in this section will progress in a similar fashion to the statistical tests already presented where parametric tests will be discussed first, followed by the nonparametric alternatives.

Parametric Tests

Pearson's Product-Moment Correlation

Pearson's product-moment correlation (aka, Pearson's correlation or Pearson's r) is one of the most commonly used correlation measures. It measures the direction and strength of a linear relationship between two continuous variables. Pearson's r ranges from -1 and

+1, with r of 0 indicating no relationship. That is, as the correlation is stronger as it approaches -1 or 1. A positive correlation (e.g., 0.30 or 0.99) indicates that as the values of one variable increase so do the values of the other variable, while a negative correlation (e.g., -0.50 or -0.80) indicates that as the values of one variable increase, the values of the other variable decrease. Pearson's r tests whether the correlation of two variables is different from 0 (i.e., no relationship); thus, a statistically significant r indicates the slope of the linear relationship is not horizontal.

For example, research has shown a moderate, but statistically significant, positive correlation ($r = 0.25$) between weight in kilograms and platelet count in men aged 20 to 55.[43] Thus, in men, as weight increases, so does platelet count. However, the magnitude of this increase varies from person to person. That is, for any individual man, a 1-kg increase in body weight may indicate an increase in platelet count that is different from the platelet count increase for another man. It should be noted the value of r is dimensionless because it is based on standardized scores. That is, measuring weight in pounds or kilograms in the example above will not change the value of the correlation. Finally, be aware that r is substantially affected by outliers, so researchers must identify and remove them from analysis or use the nonparametric Spearman's rho discussed below.

The relationship between two variables can be assessed visually by plotting the data on a scatterplot. In fact, this practice is highly recommended.[5] The magnitude of the correlation is directly related to the strength of the linear relationship. Take a moment to consider Figures 6-13 and 6-14. In Figure 6-13, the value of Pearson's r is approximately 1 indicating a near perfect relationship between the two variables. Notice the dots on the scatterplot lay near the best fit line and that the slope of this line is fairly steep. The positive correlation coefficient indicates that as the values of continuous variable 1 increase so do the values of continuous variable 2. In Figure 6-14, Pearson's r is approximately 0. Here, notice the dots are scattered all over the plot with no real direction, and the best fit line is almost perfectly horizontal, which indicates no relationship between the two continuous variables.

To highlight the substantial effect outliers have on Pearson's r, take a moment to draw an outlier on Figure 6-13, say, a value of 45 for continuous variable 1 and a value of 25 for continuous variable 2. Visualize what effect this outlier has on the previously strong positive correlation and how it would pull the best fit line toward horizontal significantly weakening the correlation.

The result of a statistically significant Pearson's product-moment correlation with no assumption violations using the example above is presented as follows:

The results of a Pearson's product-moment correlation indicate a statistically significant moderate relationship between body weight in kilograms and platelet count ($r_{81} = 0.252$, $p < 0.05$) indicating body weight increased in concordance with platelet count.

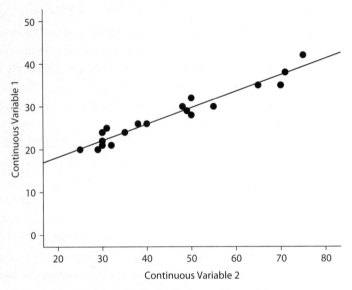

Figure 6–13. Scatterplot showing a positive correlation.

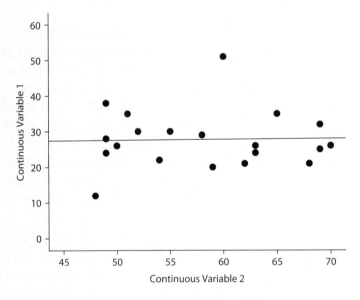

Figure 6–14. Scatterplot showing no correlation.

Assumptions of the Pearson's product-moment correlation include:

1. Both variables are measured on an interval or ratio scale.
2. There are no outliers.
3. The relationship between the variables is linear.

4. **Homoscedasticity** is assured.
   a. The assumption states that the variability around the best fit line of the linear relationship is the same for all data. A violation of this assumption can be seen within a scatterplot. For example, consider a scatterplot where the lower values for a variable fall near the best fit line and higher values for this same variable fall far from the best fit line. In this situation, the variability around the line is not constant. The tenability of this assumption is difficult to ascertain in a journal article; thus, ensure the authors noted that it was tested.
5. The observations are independent.
   a. That is, each participant provides one, and only one, observation (i.e., data or response) for each variable.

Simple Linear Regression

As stated in the previous section, the magnitude or size of the correlation is directly related to the strength of the linear relationship. The pattern of this linear relationship is typically indicated by the regression line, which is another name for the best fit line presented in Figures 6-13 and 6-14. The regression line is a best fit line describing how the continuous DV changes as values of the IV change. Similar to Pearson's r, the statistical test in simple linear regression is whether the slope of the regression line is statistically different from zero, or, stated another way, whether the regression line has no slope or is horizontal. Simple linear regression, however, takes Pearson's r one step further, where the regression line is used to predict values of the DV for a given value of the IV.[21] This is incredibly useful to evidence-based practitioners looking to implement findings into their practice.

The algebraic linear regression equation is: $\hat{y} = a + bx$. Here, a is the intercept of the regression line with the y-axis, b is the slope of the regression line, x is the value of the IV, and $\hat{y}$ (pronounced y-hat) is the predicted value of the DV. The intercept is interpreted as the predicted value of the DV when the value of the IV is zero. The slope is interpreted as the overall change in the DV for a one-unit increase in the IV. Further, it is important to note that the value of Pearson's correlation between the DV and IV is incorporated into the mathematical equation for the slope.

As an example, consider the association between systolic blood pressure measured in millimeters of mercury (mmHg) and height in centimeters for 100 children aged 5 to 7 years.[44] The results of this study indicated a positive Pearson correlation between height and systolic blood pressure of 0.33. Moving beyond basic correlation, the researchers used a simple linear regression analysis to predict a child's systolic blood pressure from their height. Results indicated an intercept value of 46.28 mmHg and a slope of 0.48. Using these values, the linear regression equation would be: $\hat{y} = 46.28 + (0.48 \times \text{height})$. Using the interpretation of the intercept and slope provided above, the intercept value of 46.28 is the predicted systolic blood pressure for a child 0 cm tall, whereas the slope indicates that a 1-cm increase in height increases systolic blood pressure 0.48 mmHg. From this interpretation, it is obvious that a child with a height of 0 cm is impossible. This is a prime example of the awareness readers must have when interpreting the intercept. That is, unless it makes theoretical sense to have a meaningful zero point for the IV, the interpretation of the intercept is never useful. This situation, however, should not suggest the intercept is meaningless to prediction. Instead, the intercept is simply a starting point for predicting the outcome. For example, say we want to predict systolic blood pressure for a child that is 115 cm tall; the linear regression equation becomes: $\hat{y} = 46.28 + (0.48 \times 115)$, which equals 101.48 mmHg.

It is important to note that the predicted values of the DV are rarely identical to the actual observed values. That is, a child 115 cm tall in this sample may actually have a systolic blood pressure of 105 mmHg, but have a predicted value of 101.48 mmHg. The difference between the actual and predicted scores is referred to as a **residual value** or residual error. For the example child above, the residual value is 3.52 mmHg (i.e., 105 − 101.48). Residual values are always calculated for all participants included in the regression analysis, and one of the assumptions of linear regression is that the residual values follow a normal distribution; this is where the assumption of normality originates for all parametric statistical tests. The tenability of this assumption is a key indicator of the reliability of the results. Therefore, if a researcher fails to describe the distribution of residuals alongside their results, the study should be read and interpreted with caution.

In addition, the interpretation of slope used in the above example is only appropriate for IVs measured on a continuous scale. If instead the IV is categorical, interpretation is slightly different. For example, consider replacing height in the example above with the dichotomous IV gender. In this situation, the researcher must specify which level of gender will serve as the reference or comparison category that is coded 0 for analysis. That is, specify which level of the IV the calculated slope represents. Note that every published study should indicate which group served as the reference category, and if the authors fail to provide a reference category, interpretation becomes impossible. Continuing, if females are specified as the reference category, the slope for gender provides the overall difference in predicted systolic blood pressure for males compared to females. Interpretation follows this logic. For example, using an example similar to the above, say a simple linear regression analysis indicated the intercept was 115.54 and the slope for gender was 15.20 with females considered the reference category. The new linear regression equation would be: $\hat{y} = 115.54 + 15.20 \times$ male. Thus, the intercept value of 115.54 now represents the average systolic blood pressure for a women (i.e., when male = 0) and the slope indicates that the predicted value of systolic blood pressure will be 15.20 mmHg higher for a man (i.e., when male = 1) compared to a woman. Admittedly, these interpretations can be confusing, but understanding this concept is critically important to proper interpretation of study results.

The primary test used in simple linear regression is an omnibus between-groups ANOVA. It may seem esoteric, but linear regression and ANOVA are mathematically equivalent. The omnibus ANOVA provides an F test indicating whether the IV explains a statistically significant amount of variance in the DV. Stated another way, the omnibus test determines whether the IV reliably predicts the DV. Only if the ANOVA is statistically significant is the slope of the individual IV interpreted. Most research studies will provide the results of the ANOVA prior to presenting the slope of the IV. Further, the ANOVA results presented in simple linear regression will be presented identically to the one-way between-groups ANOVA examples discussed above. The statistical significance of the IV will most often be presented with the regression slope and potentially an associated t-value. The slope is critical to proper interpretation of any regression analysis; thus, if the slope is not presented in the narrative portion or in a table, complete interpretation of the regression analysis is impossible and the study is essentially useless.

Finally, the amount of variance in the DV explained by the IV must also be considered. That is, how much of the reason why a participant has a particular value on the DV is attributable to his or her IV value. As a side note, the word "explained" should not and does not imply causality, as causality in correlational studies is extremely difficult to determine. The amount of variance explained in simple linear regression is quantified by an effect size estimate termed the coefficient of determination. This coefficient is calculated by squaring the Pearson's r between the IV and DV (i.e., r^2). In the literature, it will often be referred to simply as r^2, or identically as R^2. Note that how this value is referred to in a study is dependent on the researcher, but regardless of whether r^2 or R^2 is reported, their values will be identical and, thus, interpreted identically. The coefficient will often be presented as a proportion, ranging from 0 to 1, with higher values indicating more reliable prediction. From the example above, remember the correlation between a child's height and systolic blood pressure was 0.33. Thus, approximately 0.11 (i.e., 0.33^2) of the child's measured systolic blood pressure can be explained by the child's height. Said another way, approximately 11% of the reason a child has a particular systolic blood pressure value is explained by his or her height.

In the literature, the result of a statistically significant simple linear regression analysis with no assumption violations will be presented as follows:

The results of a simple linear regression analysis indicated a child's height significantly predicts systolic blood pressure ($F_{1,98} = 12.03$, $p < 0.05$, $r^2 = 0.11$), with a 1-cm increase in height resulting in a 0.48 mmHg increase in systolic blood pressure.

The assumptions of simple linear regression include:

1. The DV is measured on an interval or ratio scale.
2. There are no outliers.
3. The relationship between the DV and IV is linear.

4. Homoscedasticity is assured.

   a. The assumption states that the variability around the regression line is the same for all data. A violation of this assumption can be seen within a scatterplot. For example, consider a scatterplot where the lower values for a variable fall near the regression line and higher values for this same variable fall far from the regression line. In this situation, the variability around the regression line is not constant. The tenability of this assumption is difficult to ascertain in a journal article; thus, ensure the authors noted that it was tested.

5. Residuals are distributed normally.

   a. Residuals are the difference between the actual and predicted values. Authors will need to state that they tested this assumption.

6. The observations are independent.

   a. That is, each participant provides one, and only one, observation (i.e., data or response) for each variable.

Multivariable Linear Regression

Multivariable linear regression (aka, multiple linear regression) is an extension of simple linear regression for designs with one continuous DV and multiple IVs or covariates measured on any scale. Remember, an IV is defined as an explanatory variable of specific research interest, while a covariate is a nuisance variable that is significantly associated with the DV, but not of specific research interest. That is, covariates are typically included because they are related to the DV or because previous research has indicated they are important. In multiple linear regression, IVs can be any combination of continuous or discrete variables (e.g., height, gender). Further, this analysis is often a better option than simple linear regression because the inclusion of additional IVs often explains a higher percentage of variance in the DV. That is, multiple linear regression produces higher R^2 values.

For example, previous research has shown a statistically significant negative Pearson's correlation between serum 25-hydroxyvitamin D (25OHD; ng/mL) and serum parathyroid hormone (PTH; pg/mL) of -0.28.[45] Based on this correlation, the percentage of variance in serum PTH explained by serum 25OHD is 8% (i.e., -0.28^2). That is, 8% of the reason a participant has a predicted serum PTH value is due to their serum 25OHD level. In an effort to increase this percentage of variance explained, a new study is designed to determine the effect serum 25OHD has on serum PTH after statistically adjusting for age, BMI, total calcium intake, and serum creatinine. Thus, a multiple linear regression analysis will be used to determine whether there is an effect of serum 25OHD on serum PTH over and above the effect of the covariates. That is, multiple linear regression assesses the unique correlation between 25OHD and serum PTH after removing the effects already accounted for by age, BMI, total calcium intake, and serum creatinine.

The percentage of variance explained in multiple linear regression is always referred to as R^2, where the R indicates the multiple correlation. That is, R is the multivariate extension of Pearson's r and is defined as the combined or total correlation between all IVs and the DV. Similar to Pearson's r, R ranges from -1 to 1, with 0 indicating no relationship. Thus, as R approaches -1 or 1, the association between the IVs and DV becomes stronger. In addition, most studies will also present an adjusted R^2 value, sometimes labeled R^2_{adj} in the literature. Adjusted R^2 is interpreted exactly the same as R^2, but it is adjusted for the sample size used in the study. When reading a study, comparing R^2 and adjusted R^2 is incredibly useful to interpretation, as large differences between the two indicates significant issues with the analysis, such as inadequate sample size, which essentially render the regression model useless and not generalizable to the population. Finally, it should be noted that a multiple linear regression model will never explain 100% of the variance in the DV. However, do not disregard studies reporting low values of R^2 because the definition of what constitutes a large R^2 value varies by research arena. That is, lower R^2 values are expected when using human participants because measurement error is usually high. For example, consider a study using participant self-reported daily calorie intake. Large R^2 values are expected for bench research studies because in well-conducted bench research measurement error is typically not an issue. For example, think about a biomedical research study using analytic chemistry.

In general, the results of a multiple linear regression model are interpreted in an almost identical fashion to simple linear regression. As a result, please reconsider the section on simple linear regression if necessary. Similar to simple linear regression, multiple regression produces a regression equation allowing for prediction of DV values based on the y-intercept and the slope of the regression line for each IV or covariate. Briefly, the intercept is the predicted value of the DV when all values of the IVs and covariates are 0, while the slope quantifies the change in the predicted DV with a one-unit increase in the IV or covariates. Again, the regression equation is incredibly useful to evidence-based practitioners looking to implement findings into their practice. For example, consider the multiple regression example above, where serum PTH was predicted from 25OHD and a set of covariates. Based on the regression equation from this study, the practitioner can provide the patient with empirical evidence regarding which variables (i.e., age, BMI, total calcium intake, serum creatinine, and serum 25OHD) to increase or decrease, if possible, in an effort to optimize serum PTH levels and increase bone production.

The overall test of the multiple linear regression model is an omnibus between-groups ANOVA, which indicates at least one of the IVs or covariates significantly predicts the DV. However, this omnibus test fails to indicate which IVs or covariates significantly predict the DV. Thus, the statistical test for each IV or covariate is considered. Each of the statistical tests for the IVs and covariates can be considered similar to a *post hoc* test; however, unlike the *post hoc* tests discussed for ANOVA-type models above, alpha remains unadjusted. In most studies, the results of the individual IVs or covariates are presented as regression slope or t-values. Note that regardless of which result an author presents, the p-values will be identical. Further, interpretation of the slopes for the individual coefficients is also slightly different compared to simple linear regression. In multiple linear regression, interpretation of a particular IV or covariate is statistically adjusted for all other IVs and covariates in the regression model similar to ANCOVA.

An example may help clarify this information. Consider a situation where the result of a statistically significant multiple linear regression analysis based on the example above indicates 25OHD has a statistically significant slope of -1.5 pg/mL. Because the analysis is multivariable, this slope must be interpreted considering all covariates included in the model. Thus, the slope of -1.5 pg/mL indicates that after adjusting for age, BMI, total calcium intake, and serum creatinine, a 1-ng/mL increase in 25OHD decreases predicted serum PTH 1.5 pg/mL.

Based on the example, the results of a statistically significant multiple linear regression analysis with no assumption violations are presented below. Notice the effects of statistically significant covariates (i.e., BMI and serum creatinine) are also described; however, authors will vary on which covariates, if any, they choose to interpret.

The results of a multivariable linear regression analysis indicated age, BMI, total calcium intake, serum creatinine, and 25OHD significantly predicted serum PTH ($F_{5,472}$ = 21.82, $p < 0.05$, adjusted $R^2 = 0.18$). After adjusting for covariates, 25OHD significantly predicted serum PTH (slope = -1.5, $p < 0.05$). That is, with all else held constant, a 1-ng/mL increase in serum 25OHD resulted in a 1.5-pg/mL decrease in serum PTH. Regarding the individual covariates, after adjustment, increases in BMI and serum creatinine (slope = 0.75 and 2.12, respectively, both $p < 0.05$) resulted in higher serum PTH levels. Finally, after adjustment, age and total calcium intake were not associated with serum PTH.

The assumptions of multiple linear regression include:

1. The DV is measured on an interval or ratio scale.
2. Absence of **multicollinearity** is assured.
   a. That is, no Pearson's r between any IVs and covariates should be greater than 0.90, as correlations this high indicate the variables are redundant. That is, high correlations indicate the variables may be measuring the same construct. Including redundant variables will significantly bias results. Most published studies provide Pearson correlations between the DV, IVs, and covariates; thus, a violation of this assumption is easy to identify.
3. There are no outliers.
4. The relationship between the DV and IVs and between the DV and covariates is linear.
5. Homoscedasticity is assured.
   a. The assumption states that the variability around the regression line is the same for all data. A violation of this assumption can be seen within a scatterplot. For example, consider a scatterplot where the lower values for a variable fall near

the regression line and higher values for this same variable fall far from the regression line. In this situation, the variability around the regression line is not constant. The tenability of this assumption is difficult to ascertain in a journal article; thus, ensure the authors noted that it was tested.

6. Residuals are distributed normally.

   a. Residuals are the difference between the actual and predicted values.

7. The observations are independent.

   a. That is, each participant provides one, and only one, observation (i.e., data or response) for each variable.

Nonparametric Tests

Spearman Rank-Order Correlation Coefficient

The Spearman rank-order correlation coefficient (r_s), also known as Spearman's rho (ρ), is the nonparametric alternative to Pearson's r. This correlation is used when two continuous variables have outliers, when the variables are measured on an ordinal scale, or when the relationship is nonlinear. Similar to the other nonparametric statistical tests discussed previously, this correlation is based on rank-ordered data as opposed to the actual values. The value of r_s ranges between −1 and 1, with 0 indicating no association. Thus, as r_s approaches −1 or 1, the association between the two variables becomes stronger. A statistically significant r_s indicates that the association is significantly different from 0.

As an example, consider a study assessing the association between triglyceride content and lag time in LDL oxidation in a sample of 18 renal transplant patients.[46] Spearman's rank-order correlation was used in this study because outliers were identified in the sample, and because the sample was small, removing outliers was not a viable option. The study found a statistically significant negative r_s of −0.502, suggesting that as triglyceride content increased, LDL oxidation decreased.

Based on the example above, the result of a statistically significant Spearman rank-order correlation coefficient is presented as follows:

The Spearman rank-order correlation analysis was employed in lieu of Pearson's correlation due to the presence of outliers and small sample size. Results indicated a statistically significant negative association between triglyceride content and lag time in LDL oxidation ($r_s = -0.502$, $p < 0.05$), which suggest increases in triglyceride content translate into decreases in LDL oxidation.

The assumptions of the Spearman rank-order correlation coefficient include:

1. The two variables are measured on an ordinal, interval, or ratio scale.
2. The relationship between the two rank-ordered variables is linear.

   a. Although the relationship between the two variables based on their actual values may be nonlinear, the relationship based on rank-ordered data must be linear. This assumption typically cannot be tested by what the authors provide in the narrative. Thus, when authors fail to indicate whether the assumption was tested, results should be viewed with caution.

3. The observations are independent.

    a. That is, each participant provides one, and only one, observation (i.e., data or response) for each variable.

Logistic Regression

The interpretation of a logistic regression analysis is similar to linear regression; thus, a basic understanding of the interpretation of simple and multiple linear regression is extremely useful. Please reconsider reading the sections discussing simple and multivariable linear regression as much of the material discussed here is simply an extension of the material described in detail previously.

Logistic regression is used when the DV is measured on a dichotomous scale and the relationship between the DV and IV is nonlinear. This analysis is ubiquitous in the biomedical sciences. It is important to note that in any logistic regression analysis, the measurement scale of the DV is always considered unordered. That is, the dichotomous DV is always considered to be measured on a nominal scale. While the logistic regression analyses discussed here are only for a dichotomous DV, an extension of logistic regression is available for a categorical DV with three or more categories. This analysis is termed multinomial logistic regression, with the definition of multinomial being multiple nominal categories. Interpretation of results from this analysis is similar to the analyses discussed in this section and interested readers are encouraged to consider the suggested readings at the end of the chapter.

As an example of a design requiring a simple logistic regression analysis, consider a 5-year study designed to assess the effect that the duration of statin use measured as percentage of time on any statin during the study period has on all-cause mortality in a sample of Veterans Administration patients previously experiencing congestive heart failure. Note that the DV is dichotomous (i.e., dead versus alive). Further, a simple logistic regression analysis can always be extended to a multivariable analysis by including additional IVs and covariates in an effort to explain more of the reason why patients experienced the outcome of interest. For example, consider a multivariable extension to the study above where the effect duration of statin use has on all-cause mortality is assessed after controlling for age, race, gender, concurrent medications, and comorbid conditions.

For all logistic regression models, researchers must choose a reference category for the DV. When identified, the reference category is used as a comparison group for the primary outcome of interest. In most situations, the reference category is typically the category determined by the researcher to be of less specific interest. For example, consider all-cause mortality, a dichotomous DV (i.e., dead versus alive). Most studies are interested in the individuals who died; essentially the researcher wants to identify the primary reasons for death. Thus, with patients alive at the end of the study period considered as the reference category, all regression slopes are calculated for patients who died compared to patients who lived. Thus, the first step in properly interpreting the results of logistic regression analysis is to identify the primary outcome of interest and the reference category within the DV. It should be noted that most authors will not explicitly identify the primary outcome of interest or the reference category; however, this information can be obtained easily as all results and interpretations are typically written in relation to the primary outcome of interest.

Similar to linear regression, a logistic regression analysis provides a regression equation that can be used to predict the probability of experiencing primary outcome of interest. Briefly, the regression equation contains a y-intercept and slope values for all IVs included in the analysis. This equation is interpreted slightly different from linear regression because the association between the DV and IV is nonlinear. That is, because probability is bounded between 0 and 1, the slope must essentially shut off at these bounds. However, the usefulness of the equation is the same. That is, the equation can be used to assist evidence-based practitioners in instructing patients regarding what changes need to be made to optimize or prevent a specific outcome.

The primary statistical test in logistic regression determines whether the logistic model including all IVs or covariates better predicts the probability of experiencing the outcome of interest compared to the model with no IVs or covariates. That is, a logistic regression analysis determines whether the IVs significantly predict the primary outcome of interest. Similar to linear regression, this overall test is an omnibus chi square test. If this omnibus chi square test is statistically significant, the statistical significance of each IV or covariate is assessed and interpreted. These tests of individual predictors can be thought of as *post hoc* tests, and typically no adjustment is made to alpha. When interpreting the results for individual predictors, authors typically provide two values, the slope and odds ratio.

The slope is interpreted similar to linear regression; however, slopes in logistic regression indicate changes in the **log-odds** (aka, **logits**) of experiencing the outcome of interest. That is, a one-unit increase in the IV indicates a change in the predicted log-odds of experiencing the primary outcome of interest. While a full description of log-odds or logits is beyond the scope of this chapter, they can be thought of simply as a linear transformation of probability. That is, after transformation, log-odds or logits are linear; thus, their values can be interpreted similarly to slopes in linear regression. For example, reconsider the 5-year study assessing the effect duration of statin use, measured as percentage of time on any statin during the study period, has on all-cause mortality. Say, the slope for statin use is -0.25. With death considered the primary outcome of interest and alive serving as the reference category, this slope suggests that a 1% increase in statin use during the study period resulted in a 0.25 unit decrease in the log-odds of dying. Note this was a decrease because the slope was negative. Based on this interpretation, a common question is, what does a 0.25 unit decrease in log-odds mean? While the slope is integral in producing the regression equation, the interpretation in log-odds can be fairly convoluted. Thus, logistic regression provides an alternative value that some individuals find easier to interpret—the odds ratio.

The odds ratio produced by a logistic regression analysis is calculated and interpreted similarly to the odds ratios discussed in the Epidemiological Statistics section earlier in the chapter. Briefly, odds ratios range from 0 to infinity, with 1 indicating no association. Therefore, an odds ratio above 1 indicates an increase in the odds of experiencing the primary outcome of interest, whereas an odds ratio below 1 indicates a decrease in the odds of experiencing the primary outcome of interest. For example, reconsider the example above with a slope of -0.25. The associated odds ratio for this slope is 0.78. Because the odds ratio is below 1, a 1% increase in statin use is associated with a 22% (i.e., $1 - 0.78$) decrease in the odds of dying during the study period.

It is important to be aware that authors will vary the information they present in journal articles, as one article may only provide slopes as log-odds and another article may provide odds ratios. This is not an issue, however, because there is a direct mathematical relationship between slopes and odds ratios. That is, the slope is the natural log of the odds ratio (i.e., $\ln 0.78 = -0.25$) and the odds ratio is simply the exponentiated slope (i.e., $e^{-0.25} = 0.78$). It should become clear that this mathematical relationship is where the definition of log-odds originates; they are literally the log of the odds. Given this relationship, if an author provides log-odds, the odds ratio can be easily calculated to ease interpretation. Also, note that regardless of which value the authors present, the associated p-value will be identical. That is, a statistically significant slope will have a statistically significant odds ratio, and vice versa.

Finally, similar to linear regression, the primary reason a researcher includes additional IVs and covariates in a multivariable logistic regression model are to increase the amount of variance explained in the primary outcome of interest. That is, multivariable logistic regression models aim to better identify the reason why participants experienced the outcome of interest. However, unlike R^2 in linear regression, there is no accepted measure for quantifying explained variance in logistic regression. While a detailed description regarding why is beyond the scope of this chapter, it has to do with the fixed variance of the logistic distribution used to model the residual values. However, be aware that several pseudo-R^2 values may be presented in the literature, with the most common including the Nagelkerke R^2 and the Cox and Snell R^2. These pseudo-R^2 values are used to approximate R^2 from linear regression and are interpreted in similar fashion. For example, reconsider the 5-year study assessing the effect of statin use on all-cause mortality. Say the Nagelkerke R^2 value from the logistic regression analysis was 18%. This value indicates that 18% of the reason why patients died was due to their statin use. Again, it is important to note that these pseudo-R^2 values will never be near 100%, and the definition of a large or small pseudo-R^2 value is determined by the specific research arena, as discussed in the section on multivariable linear regression.

Based on the example described above, the result of a simple logistic regression analysis is presented as follows:

The results of a simple logistic regression analysis indicated a statistically significant association between duration of statin use and all-cause mortality ($\chi^2_1 = 13.65$, $p < 0.05$) where a 1% increase in duration of statin use resulted in a 22% decrease in the odds of dying during the study period.

An example of a multivariable logistic regression analysis, with the addition of age, race, gender, concurrent medications, and comorbid conditions as covariates, is presented below. Notice in this example, the researcher is not interested in the individual effects of the covariates, as they are not interpreted.

The results of a multivariable logistic regression analysis indicated a statistically significant overall association between the variables as a set and all-cause mortality ($\chi^2_1 = 156.02$, $p < 0.05$). After controlling for age, race, gender, concurrent medications, and comorbid conditions, duration of statin use significantly predicted all-cause mortality (OR = 0.62, $p < 0.05$). Thus, holding all variables constant, a 1% increase in statin use resulted in a 38% decrease in all-cause mortality.

The assumptions of logistic regression include:

1. The DV is discrete with mutually exclusive categories.
2. The sample size is large.
   a. A very rudimentary rule is to have at least 50 participants per variable included in the model. A large sample is required so that the parameters (e.g., slopes, standard errors) are estimated accurately.[47] Using this rule, a model with 10 IVs or covariates requires a minimum of 500 participants (i.e., $10 \times 50 = 500$).
3. Adequacy of expected frequencies is assured.
   a. This assumption applies only to categorical IVs and is the same assumption as the chi square test. That is, no more than 20% of cells can have expected frequencies less than 5. This is a difficult assumption to verify, outside of calculating the expected frequencies by hand. Thus, if an article fails to indicate this assumption was tested, view results with caution. However, most studies using logistic regression will have large sample sizes and this assumption is rarely violated.
4. Linearity in the logit is assured.
   a. Remember, logit and log-odds are synonyms. This is a convoluted assumption, and difficult to explain without getting into mathematical detail. However, the

logit is defined as the linear transformation of probability. This assumption is tested by determining whether the relationship between continuous IVs or covariates and the DV is linear. This is a key assumption, and a violation severely biases results. Thus, if authors do not mention the assumption was assured in the methods or results sections, view results with caution.

5. Absence of multicollinearity assured.

    a. That is, no Pearson's r between any continuous IVs and covariates should be greater than 0.90, as correlations this high indicate the variables are redundant. That is, high correlations indicate the variables may be measuring the same facet. Including redundant variables will significantly bias results.

6. There are no outliers.

7. The observations are independent.

    a. That is, each participant provides one, and only one, observation (i.e., data or response) for each variable.

SURVIVAL ANALYSIS

Survival analysis (or failure analysis) consists of three of the most commonly used statistical techniques in the biomedical sciences—life tables, the Kaplan-Meier method, and Cox proportional-hazards model or Cox regression. Survival analysis is concerned with time-to-event data; that is, the time to experience an outcome of interest. For example, consider a study designed to examine whether a new hormone therapy, in comparison to chemotherapy, prolongs remission in women previously diagnosed with breast cancer over a 20-week study period.

In survival analysis, participants who do not experience the outcome of interest are considered to survive, while those who experience the event are considered to fail. Although this is fairly grim terminology, survival and failure do not necessarily imply living or dying. For example, in the example above failure was defined as breast cancer recurrence, not death. In survival analysis, the outcome will typically be dichotomous, patients do not need to enter the study at the same time because enrollment can be continuous, and patients are followed until the study ends which is known as end of follow-up.

Patients who do not experience the event by the end of follow-up, who are lost to follow-up, or who drop out of the study are termed censored. The key advantage survival analysis has over the analyses presented above, particularly logistic regression, is that it can handle censored data, which is essentially incomplete data. That is, censored data are considered incomplete because the researcher does not know when or if participants experienced the event. Survival analysis can handle censored data because the DV is time, which is a continuous variable allowed to vary for each participant. Thus, as long as a participant has a survival time indicated, he or she is included in analysis. The key point here is that survival time for a censored participant is the time until he or she was censored, whether that is end of follow-up or whether he or she left the study for reasons other than suffering the event. Thus, all participants who entered the study are included in analysis regardless of whether they experienced the event or are censored because the analysis only considers the time they were in the study.

Life Tables

Life tables present time-to-event data in table format. That is, a life table tabulates the time that has elapsed until an event is experienced. Life tables are used to indicate the proportion of individuals surviving or not experiencing the event based on fixed or varying time intervals.

For example, reconsider the example above evaluating the effectiveness of the new hormone therapy in preventing recurrence of breast cancer. A life table allows the researcher to tabulate the cumulative proportion of women who do not have a recurrence of breast cancer at any interval, whether it is 6 months, 1 year, or 3 years.

As stated in the introduction to this section, life tables can be based on fixed or varying time intervals. Life tables based on fixed time intervals have a significant weakness, as they do not consider the exact time within the specified interval when the patient experienced the event. Thus, depending on the length of the time interval, a great amount of information could be lost regarding the exact time the event was experienced. That is, the longer the time interval, the less precise a researcher can be regarding the exact moment the event occurred. Thankfully, better methods have emerged, particularly the Kaplan-Meier method.

The Kaplan-Meier Method

The Kaplan-Meier method is the most widely used estimator of survival time in the biomedical sciences.[48] The Kaplan-Meier method is an extension of the life table using varying time intervals. Using this method, the cumulative proportion surviving is recalculated every time an event occurs.[49]

As an example, instead of assessing the total number of women who have a breast cancer recurrence at fixed intervals of 6 months, the Kaplan-Meier method recalculates the proportion of women surviving every time a woman in the study has a recurrence. In most studies, Kaplan-Meier data are presented as a graph of the cumulative survival over the study period known as a Kaplan-Meier curve. The Kaplan-Meier curve presents either a survival or hazard functions, where the survival function is the cumulative frequency of participants not experiencing the event, whereas the hazard function is the cumulative frequency of participants experiencing the event. A Kaplan-Meier curve is provided in the vast majority of published literature using survival analysis and will appear similar to the survival curve presented in Figure 6-15. Note that for ease of interpretation, the curve in Figure 6-15 only presents data for the sample of women initiating the new hormone

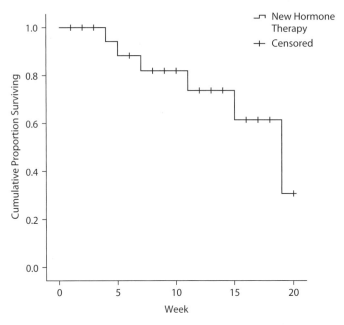

FIGURE 6–15. Kaplan-Meier curve.

therapy and does not include data for women initiating chemotherapy. Notice that the
y-axis indicates the cumulative proportion of women surviving, while the x-axis indicates
the total number of weeks of the study. The solid line represents the survival function.
That is, the cumulative proportion of women not experiencing the event at any given time.
The survival function indicates when a woman experienced the event when the function
steps down. For example, by week 5, two women have experienced the event, indicated
by the two steps in the survival function. Further, notice the vertical dashes throughout
the survival function. These dashes indicate individual women who were censored. That
is, women dropped out of the study for reasons other than experiencing the event such as
side effects or they simply were lost to follow-up by moving out of the area. Few studies
provide explicit information regarding censored participants on the Kaplan-Meier curve
because most survival analyses involve large samples. Thus, the dashes in Figure 6-15 are
usually omitted from the curve; however, frequency counts of censored participants are
always provided within the narrative or in table format.

The Kaplan-Meier curve can also be presented for multiple groups. For example,
consider the overall survival of women initiating the new hormone therapy compared to
women initiating chemotherapy. Figure 6-16 presents a Kaplan-Meier curve where the
survival functions for both treatment groups are presented simultaneously. Interpretation
of these survival functions is identical to the methods described above for Figure 6-15.
However, with two or more treatment groups, a statistical test must be conducted to

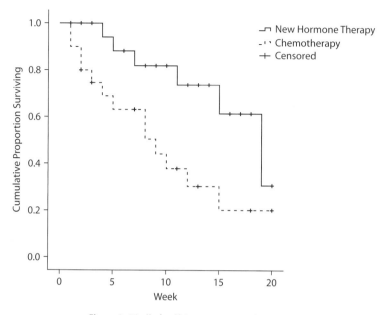

Figure 6–16. Kaplan-Meier curve—comparing groups.

assess for a statistically significant group difference in survival rate. The most common test in the biomedical literature is the log-rank test (aka, the Mantel-Cox test).[49] A statistically significant log-rank test indicates there is a significant difference in survival rate between the groups. However, it is important to note that a Kaplan-Meier curve and associated log-rank test have no way of indicating why the breast cancer recurred beyond the possibility of the therapy being ineffective.

Based on the survival functions presented in Figure 6-16, the results of a statistically significant log-rank test are presented as follows:

Based on Kaplan-Meier curves, the results of the log-rank test indicated a statistically significant difference in duration of breast cancer remission between the new hormone therapy and chemotherapy groups ($\chi^2_1 = 5.68$, $p < 0.05$), with women initiating the new hormone therapy experiencing significantly longer breast cancer remission.

It should be noted that when more than two treatment groups are being compared the log-rank test is an omnibus test. That is, with three or more groups, a statistically significant log-rank test will indicate that a statistically significant difference exists between groups, but will not indicate specifically which groups differ. Thus, *post hoc* log-rank tests are required to determine where a significant difference in survival occurred.

For example, consider the addition of another treatment group to the breast cancer example, say, women who do not want to initiate any therapy. Following a statistically significant omnibus log-rank test, three *post hoc* log-rank tests would be required to determine whether statistically significant differences in survival rate occurred between hormone therapy versus chemotherapy, hormone therapy versus no therapy, and chemotherapy versus no therapy.

The results of statistically significant *post hoc* tests are presented as follows:

Based on Kaplan-Meier curves, the results of the log-rank test indicated a statistically significant difference in breast cancer recurrence between the three treatment groups ($\chi^2_2 = 9.76, p < 0.05$). Post hoc log-rank tests indicated women initiating the new hormone therapy experienced significantly longer breast cancer remission compared to women receiving chemotherapy or women choosing not to receive therapy (both $p < 0.05$). No statistically significant difference was indicated between women initiating chemotherapy and women receiving no therapy.

Cox Proportional-Hazards Model

Although the Kaplan-Meier method is effective in assessing for overall differences in survival, the analysis is unable to identify the association between covariates and survival. That is, the Kaplan-Meier method cannot identify whether the IV significantly predicts survival, and for many studies prediction is a far more important consideration. Thus, a form of regression analysis is required. The Cox proportional-hazards model (aka, Cox regression) is a semiparametric method used to predict the time to experience an event of interest. Note that the DV is time-to-event, the event is usually a dichotomous variable, and the analysis is considered semiparametric because it includes both parametric and nonparametric components. In addition, all predictor variables in a Cox regression are termed covariates. That is, in the literature, authors will not identify a distinction between IVs and covariates. Finally, it should also be noted that most published studies progress from Kaplan-Meier curves and log-rank tests to Cox regression analysis. That is, the Kaplan-Meier curve will first present the survival functions for the covariate of interest as well as associated log-rank tests and then authors will present the results of a Cox regression assessing for the relationship between covariates and the event of interest.

The interpretation of Cox regression can be considered a combination of linear and logistic regression; however, the primary difference is that in Cox regression results are considered time dependent. That is, Cox regression is concerned with the time-dependent risk of experiencing the event instead of the overall occurrence of events as in logistic regression. Remember, the DV is time. For example, consider a study designed to assess the effect duration of statin use, measured as percentage of time in any statin during the study period, has on all-cause mortality in a sample of Veterans Administration patients previously experiencing congestive heart failure. If the researchers were interested in the effect duration of statin use had on prolonging the time until death during the study period a Cox regression analysis is the analysis of choice. Again, the primary consideration in Cox regression is time-to-event, not in the overall probability of the event as in logistic regression.

Similar to linear and logistic regression, Cox regression can be simple or multivariable. For example, in the example above a simple Cox regression analysis was required because only duration of statin use was used to predict the risk of death. However, if the study was extended to statistically control for age, gender, race, comorbid conditions, and concurrent medications, a multivariable Cox regression is appropriate. That is, assess the effects duration of statin use had on the risk of death over and above the effects of the other covariates.

Similar to logistic regression analysis, within the DV the researcher must choose the primary event of interest and the associated reference category. When identified, the reference category is used as a comparison group for the event of interest. In most situations, the reference category is typically the category determined by the researcher to be of less specific interest. For example, consider all-cause mortality, a dichotomous outcome variable, in which most studies are interested in the individuals who died. Thus, patients who lived are usually considered the reference category and all regression slopes are calculated for patients who died compared to patients who lived. Therefore, the first step in properly interpreting the results of a Cox regression analysis is to identify the event and the reference category. If an author does not explicitly state the reference category, this information can be obtained easily as all results and interpretations are typically written in relation to the primary event of interest.

It is critically important to note that in the literature, authors will report using one of two different Cox regression analyses—with or without time-varying covariates. The decision of which model to use is based on whether the proportionality of hazards assumption was violated. This assumption typically applies to all categorical covariates and states that, although events can begin to occur at any time during the study period, when events do begin, the rate at which events occur between levels of a categorical covariate must remain constant over time. That is, when events begin to occur, the survival functions for the groups must be the same or roughly parallel.

For example, reconsider Figure 6-16. Here, the proportionality of hazards assumption is not violated because events occur at approximately the same rate in each group. Notice women initiating the new hormone therapy did not begin experiencing breast cancer recurrence until week 4, as indicated by no steps in the curve until week 4, whereas women in the chemotherapy group began experiencing the recurrence at week 1, steps occurred immediately. However, when events began to occur in either group, they occurred at approximately the same rate. That is, the slopes of the survival functions are roughly parallel. Thus, the proportionality of hazards assumption is not violated and the treatment group covariate is assumed to have constant survival rates over time. More specifically, in this situation a Cox regression without time-varying covariates is appropriate.

By contrast, a violation of the proportionality assumption is provided in Figure 6-17. Notice that in this figure, events began occurring at roughly around weeks 3 and 4 within

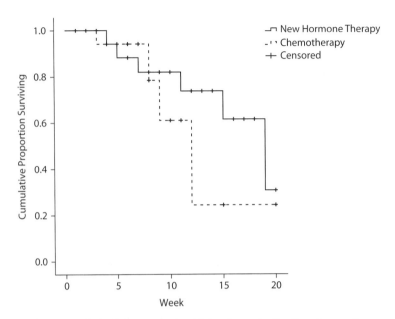

Figure 6–17. Kaplan-Meier curve showing violation of proportionality of hazards assumption.

both treatment groups. However, the survival functions are drastically different, and in fact intersect twice. In general, any time survival functions intersect, the proportionality of hazards assumption can be considered violated, because the rate of survival within each group varies across time. In this situation, Cox regression with time-varying covariates would be required.

In conclusion, when reading a journal article, take careful notice of the Kaplan-Meier curves presented prior to the Cox regression analysis. Clear violation of this assumption is apparent at any time survival functions intersect. If a violation is observed, identify whether the appropriate Cox regression analysis was employed. That is, if a violation is indicated, Cox regression with time-varying covariates must be used. If Cox regression without time-varying covariates was used in the presence of a violation, results and interpretations are extremely misleading.

Similar to the other forms of regression discussed, Cox regression allows researchers to produce a regression equation useful in determining the overall risk score for a patient based on specific characteristics. The primary difference in Cox regression, however, is that there is no y-intercept representing the baseline hazard function. Thus, overall risk is calculated simply by using the slopes for the covariates. Even without the intercept, however, this regression equation remains useful for evidence-based practitioners when consulting their patients on changes required for decreasing the risk of experiencing an unfavorable event.

Identical to logistic regression, the overall statistical test in Cox regression is whether the model including the covariates predicts the time elapsed prior to experiencing the event significantly better than the model with no covariates. That is, a Cox regression analysis determines whether the covariates significantly predict the time elapsed prior to experiencing the primary event of interest. This overall test is an omnibus chi square test. Only if this omnibus chi square test is statistically significant does the researcher evaluate the statistical significance of each covariate. The tests of individual predictors are usually more important and these will be presented in all studies using a Cox regression model. Tests of individual predictors will be presented by regression slopes and/or hazard ratios.

In Cox regression, slopes are interpreted similar to logistic regression. However, for this analysis, a one-unit increase in a covariate results in an increase or decrease in the log-hazard or log-risk of experiencing the event. While a full description of log-risk is beyond the scope of this chapter, they can be thought of simply as a linear transformation of probability of experiencing the event. That is, after transformation, log-risks are linear and their values can be interpreted similarly to slopes in linear regression. For example, say the slope for women initiating the new hormone therapy was -0.65. That is, women initiating chemotherapy served as the reference or comparison group. Thus, the slope represents a 0.65 unit decrease in the log-risk of breast cancer recurrence for the new hormone therapy compared to chemotherapy. A 0.65 unit decrease in log-hazard is difficult to explain and beyond the scope of this chapter; thus, the presentation and interpretation of hazard ratios are often a useful alternative.

The hazard ratio produced by a Cox regression analysis is calculated and interpreted similarly to the relative risk discussed in the Epidemiological Statistics section. However, it is important to note that a hazard ratio is not identical to relative risk. Briefly, hazard ratios range from 0 to infinity, with 1 indicating no association. Therefore, a hazard ratio above 1 indicates an increase in the risk of experiencing the event, whereas a hazard ratio below 1 indicates a decrease in the risk of experiencing the event. For example, reconsider the example above where the slope for the new hormone therapy was -0.65. The associated hazard ratio for this slope is 0.52. Because the hazard ratio is below 1, initiating the new hormone therapy resulted in a 48% (i.e., $1 - 0.52$) decrease in the risk of breast cancer recurrence compared to chemotherapy.

It is important to consider that authors may vary the information they present in journal articles, as one study may only provide slopes and another study may only provide hazard ratios. This is not an issue because there is a direct mathematical relationship between slopes and hazard ratios. That is, the slope is simply the natural log of the hazard ratio (i.e., $\ln 0.52 = -0.65$), whereas the hazard ratio is simply the exponentiated slope (i.e., $e^{-0.65} = 0.52$). It should become clear that this mathematical relationship is where the definition of log-risk originates; they are literally the log of the risk. Thus, if an author only provides slopes, the hazard ratio can be easily calculated to ease interpretation. Also, note that regardless of which value the authors present, the associated *p*-value will be identical. That is, a statistically significant slope will have a statistically significant hazard ratio, and vice versa.

Finally, no pseudo-R^2 exists for Cox regression to indicate proportion of variance explained. Although several have been suggested they are not interpreted as the percentage of variance explained and these values do not indicate how much of the overall reason why a participant experienced the event.[48] Thus, when reading a journal article, do not be discouraged by authors failing to provide this information.

Based on the breast cancer example, a statistically significant multivariable Cox regression analysis is presented below. Note that this Results section will typically be presented in addition to the results of the Kaplan-Meier analysis presented before.

No violation of the proportionality of hazards assumption was indicated; thus, a Cox regression without time-dependent covariates was conducted to assess the effectiveness of a new hormone therapy compared to chemotherapy in preventing breast cancer recurrence after adjusting for age, concurrent medications, and comorbid conditions. Results indicated the covariates, as a set, significantly predicted time to breast cancer recurrence ($\chi^2_8 = 63.12$, $p < 0.05$). Holding age, concurrent medications, and comorbid conditions constant, women initiating the new hormone therapy experienced a 48% decrease in the risk of breast cancer recurrence compared to women initiating chemotherapy.

The assumptions of Cox regression include:

1. Time is measured on an interval or ratio scale.
2. Sample size must be large.
   a. A very rudimentary rule is to have at least 50 participants per variable included in the model. A large sample is required so that the parameters (e.g., slopes, standard errors) are estimated accurately.[47] Using this rule, a model with 10 IVs and covariates requires a minimum of 500 participants (i.e., $10 \times 50 = 500$).
3. Proportionality of hazards is assured.
   a. The survival functions for all categorical covariates must be similar.
4. No differences between withdrawn and remaining cases exist.
   a. Because Cox regression can handle censored data, participants who are lost to follow-up must not differ from those whose outcome is known. That is, participants who dropped out of the study must not be different from those who completed it. For example, women who dropped out of the new hormone group because they are experiencing unbearable side effects that do not occur in the chemotherapy group.

5. Absence of multicollinearity is assured.
    a. That is, no Pearson's r between any continuous covariates should be greater than 0.90, as correlations this high indicate the variables are redundant. High correlations indicate the variables may be measuring the same facet. Including redundant variables will significantly bias results.
6. There are no outliers.
7. Observations are independent.
    a. That is, each participant provides one, and only one, observation (i.e., data or response) for each variable.

Conclusion

A thorough understanding of statistical methods is integral to effectively evaluating medical literature. Being cognizant of the effect study design has on results, interpretation, and generalization is incredibly important to implementing evidence-based practice. Statistical analyses are simply a piece of the puzzle when evaluating literature, since the study design and research question determine the appropriate analyses. It must be noted that simply because a study is published does not define it as a quality study. Further, all research has flaws, some trivial, others significant. A reader's task is to determine whether these flaws prevent the research from being credible.[50] Thus, when reviewing an empirical study, the following steps must be considered carefully:

1. Thoughtfully consider the study design (see Chapters 4 and 5). This includes, but is not limited to, the theory, specific research question(s), randomization, sample characteristics, data collection methods, variables, and outcomes. A poor design will lead to inaccurate or biased estimates, leading to an inferior study.
2. Evaluate the statistical test. Is it appropriate for the research question? Did the author test for assumption violations? If no assumption tests are stated, can violations be determined from the descriptive statistics provided? Was the test interpreted properly? Were effect size (i.e., clinical significance) measures provided?
3. Evaluate the discussion section. Are the results interpreted within the context of the sample and population? Are generalizations accurate? What were the limitations? How does the study lend itself to future research?

Finally, to reiterate, this chapter is by no means exhaustive of all statistical tests, nor does it provide a complete overview of statistical tests. Interested readers are encouraged to consult any of the suggested readings at the end of this chapter for a more thorough treatment of the topics discussed.

Self-Assessment Questions

1. Consider a city with one hospital system consisting of six individual hospitals. Say that a researcher plans to collect data from patients who see a physician at any of these six hospitals. What type of sampling design is this?
   a. Convenience sample
   b. Cluster sample
   c. Stratified random sample
   d. Multistage sample

2. An example of a continuous variable is:
   a. Data measured on an interval or ratio scale
   b. Survey responses ranging from Strongly Disagree to Strongly Agree
   c. Age >75 years
   d. None of the above

3. Say a continuous variable, such as board scores from the North American Pharmacist Licensure Examination (NAPLEX), is categorized into pass versus not pass, where ≥75 is determined to be the cutoff for passing. If this new categorical variable were included in a statistical analysis, pharmacists who passed the NAPLEX with a score of 75 would be considered qualitatively superior from individuals who did not pass with a score of 74.
   a. True
   b. False

4. The most appropriate measure of central tendency for categorical data is:
   a. Mean
   b. Median
   c. Mode
   d. Range

5. Variance is an incredibly important descriptive statistic that is used in all statistical analyses. Although most journal articles will only report the standard deviation, it is easy to translate between variance and standard deviation. For example, say the variance of a continuous variable is reported to be 100. What is the standard deviation?
   a. 100
   b. 1
   c. 10,000
   d. 10

6. What does the length of the whiskers in a boxplot represent?
   a. The interquartile range
   b. The range of data up to 1.5 interquartile ranges from the median
   c. Outliers
   d. Extreme outliers

7. A z-score of -2.75 indicates that a specific data point is what?
   a. The data point is 2.75 standard deviations above variable's mean.
   b. The data point is 2.75 interquartile ranges from the variable's median.
   c. The variable has a range of 2.75.
   d. The data point is 2.75 standard deviations below the variable's mean.

8. An odds ratio of 0.75 indicates:
   a. There is a 25% decrease in the odds of experiencing some outcome.
   b. There is a 75% increase in the odds of experiencing some outcome.
   c. One group is 25% less likely to experience the outcome compared to another group.
   d. There is a 25% increase in the odds of experiencing some outcome.

9. A study in which data are collected from retrospective chart review would be:
   a. Nonexperimental
   b. Experimental
   c. Quasi-experimental
   d. None of the above

10. A 2-year study in which participants receive one, and only one, treatment and planned interim analyses are conducted throughout the study period is an example of what type of study design?
    a. A crossover design
    b. A randomized controlled trial
    c. A parallel-groups design
    d. An adaptive design

11. A statistical test is used to evaluate for differences between two treatment groups. Alpha is set at 0.05. The statistical test indicates $p = 0.0001$, which is statistically significant. This small p-value indicates a clinically significant difference.
    a. True
    b. False

12. A Type I error indicates:
    a. The test result was not statistically significant when in fact the result does exist in the population.

b. An erroneously large effect size.

c. The statistical test result is significant when in fact the result does not exist in the population.

d. The result of the statistical test is true in the population.

13. The 95% confidence interval indicates:

a. There is a 95% probability that the true population parameter is within the interval.

b. If repeated random sampling occurred from the population of interest using identical sample sizes, the true population parameter would be included in the 95% of intervals.

c. There is 95% certainty that the parameter estimate is correct.

d. None of the above.

14. The mean difference between two treatment groups has a Cohen's d of 0.50. This indicates:

a. The treatment group variable explains 50% of the variability in the outcome.

b. Irrelevant. Cohen's d is inappropriate to use when comparing two group means.

c. The statistical test was an independent-samples t-test.

d. The two means are 0.50 standard deviations apart.

15. A drug safety trial is designed to evaluate the proportion of patients who suffered congestive heart failure (i.e., yes versus no) after taking a new drug compared to placebo. Patients were followed for 2 years. The analysis will control for a variety of patient characteristics (e.g., age, biological sex, comorbidities, etc.). Which analysis is appropriate given the research question?

a. A multivariable logistic regression model

b. The multivariable Cox proportional-hazards model

c. Pearson's chi square test

d. Mantel-Haenszel chi square test

REFERENCES

1. United States Census Bureau. Census regions and divisions of the United States. Available from: http://www.census.gov/geo/www/us_regdiv.pdf. Accessed June 24, 2010.

2. Stevens SS. On the theory of scales of measurement. Science. 1946;103(2684):677-80.

3. Hockenberry MJ, Wilson D. Wong's essentials for pediatric nursing. 8th ed. St. Louis, MO: Mosby; 2009.

4. Tabachnick BG, Fidell LS. Using multivariate statistics. 5th ed. Boston, MA: Pearson Education; 2007.

5. Tukey JW. Exploratory data analysis. Reading, MA: Addison-Wesley; 1977.

6. Gordis L. Epidemiology. Philadelphia, PA: Saunders Elsevier; 2009.

7. Hennekens CH, Buring JE. Epidemiology in medicine. Mayrent SL, ed. Philadelphia, PA: Lippincott, Williams, and Wilkins; 1987.

8. Friis RH. Epidemiology 101. Sudbury, MA: Jones and Bartlett Publishers; 2010.

9. Campbell DT, Stanley JC. Experimental and quasi-experimental designs for research. Chicago, IL: Rand McNally & Company; 1963.

10. Feinstein AR. Epidemiologic analyses of causation: the unlearned scientific lessons of randomized trials. J Clin Epidemiol. 1989;42(6):481-9.

11. Ioannidis JP, Haidich AB, Pappa M, Pantazis N, Kokori SI, Tektonidou MG, et al. Comparison of evidence of treatment effects in randomized and nonrandomized studies. JAMA. 2001;286(7):821-30.

12. United States National Institutes of Health. Understanding clinical trials. Available from: http://clinicaltrials.gov/ct2/info/understand#Q18. Accessed June 25, 2010.

13. Hopewell S, Dutton S, Yu L-M, Chan A-W, Altman DG. The quality of reports of randomized trials in 2000 and 2006: comparative study of articles indexed in PubMed. BMJ. 2010;340(c723):1-8.

14. Everitt BS, Pickles A. Statistical aspects of the design and analysis of clinical trials. 2nd ed. River Edge, NJ: Imperial College Press; 2004.

15. Chow S, Liu J. Design and analysis of clinical trials: concepts and methodologies. 2nd ed. Hoboken, NJ: John Wiley & Sons; 2004.

16. International Conference on Harmonisation of Technical Requirements for Registration of Pharmaceuticals for Human Use (ICH). Statistical principles for clinical trials E9. Available from: http://www.ich.org/LOB/media/MEDIA485.pdf. Accessed June 26, 2010.

17. United States Department of Health and Human Services. Guidance for industry: Adaptive designclinicaltrialsfordrugsandbiologics. Availablefrom: http://www.fda.gov/downloads/Drugs/GuidanceComplianceRegulatoryInformation/Guidances/UCM201790.pdf. Accessed June 18, 2010.

18. Lachin JM. Statistical considerations in the intent-to-treat principle. Control Clin Trials. 2000;21(3):167-89.

19. Enders CK. A primer on the use of modern missing-data methods in psychosomatic medicine research. Psychosom Med. 2006;68(3):427-36.

20. Rubin DB. Inference and missing data. Biometrika. 1976;63(3):581-92.

21. Moore DS. The basic practice of statistics. 2nd ed. New York, NY: W. H. Freeman and Company; 2000.

22. Tabachnick BG, Fidell LS. Experimental design using ANOVA. Belmont, CA: Duxbury Press; 2007.

23. Cohen J. Statistical power analysis for the behavioral sciences. 2nd ed. Hillsdale, NJ: Lawrence Erlbaum; 1988.

24. Nickerson RS. Null hypothesis significance testing: a review of an old and continuing controversy. Psychol Methods. 2000;5(2):241-301.

25. Cumming G, Finch S. Inference by eye: confidence intervals and how to read pictures of data. Am Psychol. 2005;60(2):170-80.

26. Cumming G, Finch S. A primer on the understanding, use, and calculation of confidence intervals that are based on central and noncentral distributions. Educ Psychol Meas. 2001;61(4):532-74.

27. Siegel S, Castellan NJ. Nonparametric statistics for the behavioral sciences. 2nd ed. New York, NY: McGraw-Hill; 1988.

28. Sheskin DJ. Handbook of parametric and nonparametric statistical procedures. 3rd ed. Boca Raton, FL: CRC Press; 2000.

29. Krauss RM, Burke DJ. Identification of multiple subclasses of plasma low density lipoproteins in normal humans. J Lipid Res. 1982;23(1):97-104.

30. Austin MA, King MC, Vranizan KM, Krauss RM. Atherogenic lipoprotein phenotype. A proposed genetic marker for coronary heart disease risk. Circulation. 1990;82:495-506.

31. Cochran WG. Some methods for strengthening the common χ^2 tests. Biometrics. 1954;10(4):417-51.

32. Cohen J. A coefficient of agreement for nominal scales. Educ Psychol Meas. 1960;20(1):37–46.

33. United States Centers for Disease Control and Prevention. National Health and Nutrition Examination Survey. Available from: http://www.cdc.gov/nchs/nhanes/. Accessed August 29, 2016.

34. Schober SE, Carroll MD, Lacher DA, Hirsch R. High serum total cholesterol—an indicator for monitoring cholesterol lowering efforts; U.S. adults, 2005–2006. NCHS data brief no. 2. Hyattsville, MD: National Center for Health Statistics; 2007.

35. Keppel G, Wickens TD. Design and analysis: a researcher's handbook. 4th ed. Upper Saddle River, NJ: Prentice Hall; 2004.

36. Hardy R, Kuh D, Langenberg C, Wadsworth ME. Birthweight, childhood social class, and change in adult blood pressure in the 1946 British birth cohort. Lancet. 2003;362(9391):1178-83.

37. Williams JG, Allison C, Scott FJ, Bolton PF, Baron-Cohen S, Matthews FE, et al. The Childhood Autism Spectrum Test (CAST): sex differences. J Autism Dev Disord. 2008;38:1731-9.

38. Skrabal MZ, Jones RM, Walters RW, Nemire RE, Soltis DA, Kahaleh AA, et al. National volunteer preceptor survey of experiential student loads, quality of time issues, and compensation: differences in responses based on region, type of practice setting, and population density. J Pharm Pract. 2010;23(3):265-72.

39. Vickers AJ. How many repeated measures in repeated measure designs? Statistical issues for comparative trials. Br Med Res Methodol. 2003;3(22):1-9.

40. Beck AT, Steer RA, Brown GK. Manual for Beck depression inventory-II. San Antonio, TX: Psychological Corporation; 1996.

41. Jekel JF. Epidemiology, biostatistics, and preventative medicine. 3rd ed. Philadelphia, PA: Saunders Elsevier; 2007.

42. Melnik T, Abdo CHN. Psychogenic erectile dysfunction: comparative study of three therapeutic approaches. J Sex Marital Ther. 2005;31(3);246-55.

43. Siebers RWL, Carter JM, Wakem PJ, Maling TJB. Interrelationship between platelet count, red cell count, white cell count and weight in men. Clin Lab Hematol. 1990;12(3); 257-62.

44. Petrie A, Sabin C. Medical statistics at a glance. 2nd ed. Malden, MA: Blackwell; 2005.

45. Need AG, Horowitz M, Morris HA, Nordin BEC. Vitamin D status: effects of parathyroid hormone and 1,25-dihydroxyvitamin D in post-menopausal women. Am J Clin Nutr. 2000; 71(6):1577-81.

46. Sutherland WH, Walker RJ, Ball MJ, Stapley SA, Robertson MC. Oxidation of low density lipoproteins from patients with renal failure or renal transplants. Kidney Int. 1995; 48(1):227-36.

47. Aldrich JH, Nelson FD. Linear probability, logit, and probit models. Sage University paper series on quantitative applications in the social sciences, series no. 07-045. Newbury Park, CA: Sage; 1984.

48. Allison PD. Survival analysis using the SAS System: a practical guide. 2nd ed. Cary, NC: SAS Institute; 2010.

49. Kleinbaum DG, Klein M. Survival analysis: a self-learning text. 2nd ed. New York; NY: Springer; 2005.

50. Simon SD. Is the randomized clinical trial the gold standard of research? J Androl. 2001;22(6):938-43.

SUGGESTED READINGS

The suggested readings below are for interested readers to gain further insight into some of the topics covered in this chapter. Note that most of the information provided in the first half of this chapter can be obtained in any introductory statistics textbook.

Epidemiological Statistics

Gordis L. Epidemiology. Philadelphia, PA: Saunders Elsevier; 2009.

Clinical Significance and Effect Size

Cohen J. Statistical power analysis for the behavioral sciences. 2nd ed. Hillsdale, NJ: Lawrence Erlbaum; 1988.

Study Design and Randomized Controlled Trials

Campbell DT, Stanley JC. Experimental and quasi-experimental designs for research. Boston, MA: Houghton Mifflin Company; 1966.

Chow S, Liu J. Design and analysis of clinical trials: concepts and methodologies. 2nd ed. Hoboken, NJ: John Wiley & Sons; 2004.

Nonparametric Statistical Tests

Siegel S ,Castellan NJ. Nonparametric statistics for the behavioral sciences. 2nd ed. New York, NY: McGraw-Hill, Inc.; 1988.

ANOVA Designs

Keppel G, Wickens TD. Design and analysis: a researcher's handbook. 4th ed. Upper Saddle River, NJ: Prentice Hall; 2004.

Linear Regression, Logistic Regression, Survival Analysis

Tabachnick BG, Fidell LS. Using multivariate statistics. 5th ed. Boston, MA: Pearson Education; 2007.

Stevens J. Applied multivariate statistics for the social sciences. 4th ed. Mahwah, NJ: Lawrence Erlbaum; 2002.

Cohen P, Cohen J, West SG, Aiken LS. Applied multiple regression/correlation analysis for the behavioral sciences. 3rd ed. Mahwah, NJ: Lawrence Erlbaum; 2003.

Hosmer DW, Lemeshow S. Applied logistic regression. 3rd ed. New York, NY: John Wiley & Sons; 2013.

Kleinbaum DG, Klein M. Survival analysis: a self-learning text. 2nd ed. New York; NY: Springer; 2005.

Clustering and Nesting

Snijders TAB, Bosker RJ. Multilevel analysis: an introduction to basic & advanced multilevel modeling. 2nd ed. Thousand Oaks, CA: Sage; 2011.

Hox J. Multilevel analysis: techniques and applications. 2nd ed. New York, NY: Routledge; 2010.

Raudenbush SW, Bryk AS. Hierarchical linear models: applications and data analysis methods. 2nd ed. Newbury Park, CA: Sage; 2002.

Statistical Analysis in the Bayesian Framework

Gelman A, Hill J. Data analysis using regression and multilevel/hierarchical models. New York, NY: Cambridge University Press; 2007.

Kruschke JK. Doing Bayesian data analysis: a tutorial with R, JAGS, and Stan. 2nd ed. Waltham, MA: Academic Press; 2015.

Gelman A, Carlin JB, Stern HS, Dunson DB, Vehtari A, Rubin DB. Bayesian data analysis. 3rd ed. Boca Raton, FL: CRC Press; 2013.

Chapter Seven

Pharmacoeconomics

James P. Wilson • Karen L. Rascati

Learning Objectives

After completing this chapter, the reader will be able to

- Describe the four types of pharmacoeconomic analysis: cost-minimization analysis (CMA), cost-benefit analysis (CBA), cost-effectiveness analysis (CEA), and cost-utility analysis (CUA).
- Describe the advantages and disadvantages of the different types of pharmacoeconomic analyses.
- List and explain the 10 steps that should be found in a well-conducted pharmacoeconomic study.
- List the six steps in a decision analysis.
- Give examples of the application of the pharmacoeconomic evaluation techniques to the formulary decision process, including decision analysis.
- Apply a systematic approach to the evaluation of the pharmacoeconomic literature.

Key Concepts

1. Pharmacoeconomics has been defined as the description and analysis of the costs of drug therapy to health care systems and society—it identifies, measures, and compares the costs and consequences of pharmaceutical products and services.

2. Pharmacoeconomic studies categorize costs into four types: direct medical, direct nonmedical, indirect, and intangible.

3. Perspective is a pharmacoeconomic term that describes whose costs are relevant based on the purpose of the study.

4. There are four ways to measure outcomes, and each type of outcome measurement is associated with a different type of pharmacoeconomic analysis: cost-minimization analysis (CMA), cost-benefit analysis (CBA), cost-effectiveness analysis (CEA), and cost-utility analysis (CUA).

❺ There are two common methods that economists use to estimate a value for health-related consequences, the human capital approach and the willingness-to-pay approach.

❻ A CUA takes patient preferences, also referred to as utilities, into account when measuring health consequences.

❼ All four types of analyses described (CMA, CBA, CEA, and CUA) should follow 10 general steps.

❽ A sensitivity analysis allows one to determine how the results of an analysis would change when these best guesses or assumptions are varied over a relevant range of values.

❾ Decision analysis is the application of an analytical method for systematically comparing different decision options. Decision analysis graphically displays choices and performs the calculations needed to compare these options.

Introduction

Change continues to be a leading factor in health care deliveries and costs. The continued introduction of new technologies, including many new drugs, has been among these changes. During 2016, 22 novel drugs were approved by the U.S. Food and Drug Administration (FDA).[1] New biotechnology drugs can cost over $10,000 per course of therapy. The increase in the number of new drugs combined with the increase in costs of drugs provides a great challenge for all health care. The new organizations created by the Affordable Care Act to provide access to health care insurance for Americans, in addition to existing managed care organizations (MCOs), all desire to deliver quality care while minimizing costs.[2]

Pharmacy and therapeutics (P&T) committees are responsible for evaluating these new drugs and determining their potential value to organizations (see Chapters 13 and 14). Evaluating drugs for formulary inclusion can often be an overwhelming task. The application of pharmacoeconomic methods to the evaluation process may help streamline formulary decisions.

This chapter presents an overview of the practical application of pharmacoeconomic principles as they apply to the formulary decision process. Students and health professionals are often asked to gather and evaluate literature to support the decision process.

Pharmacoeconomics: What Is It and Why Do It?

❶ *Pharmacoeconomics has been defined as the description and analysis of the costs of drug therapy to health care systems and society—it identifies, measures, and compares the costs and consequences of pharmaceutical products and services.*[3] Decision makers can

Figure 7–1. The pharmacoeconomic equation.

use these methods to evaluate and compare the total costs of treatment options and the outcomes associated with these options. To show this graphically, think of two sides of an equation: (1) the inputs (costs) used to procure and use the drug and (2) the health-related outcomes (see Figure 7-1).

The center of the equation, the drug product, is symbolized by R_x. If only the left-hand side of the equation is measured without regard for outcomes, this is a cost analysis (or a partial economic analysis). If only the right-hand side of the equation is measured without regard to costs, this is a clinical or outcome study (not an economic analysis). In order to be a true pharmacoeconomic analysis, both sides of the equation must be considered and compared.

Relationships of Pharmacoeconomics to Outcomes Research

Outcomes research is defined as an attempt to identify, measure, and evaluate the end results of health care services. It may include not only clinical and economic consequences, but also outcomes, such as patient health status and satisfaction with their health care. Pharmacoeconomics is a type of outcomes research, but not all outcomes research is pharmacoeconomic research.[4]

Models of Pharmacoeconomic Analysis

The four types of pharmacoeconomic analyses all follow the diagram shown in Figure 7-1, they measure costs or inputs in dollars and assess the outcomes associated with these costs. Pharmacoeconomic analyses are categorized by the method used to assess outcomes. If the outcomes are assumed to be equivalent, the study is called a **cost-minimization analysis** (CMA); if the outcomes are measured in dollars, the study is called a **cost-benefit analysis** (CBA); if the costs are measured in natural units (e.g., cures, years of life, blood pressure), the study is called a **cost-effectiveness analysis** (CEA); if the outcomes take into

TABLE 7–1. FOUR TYPES OF PHARMACOECONOMIC ANALYSIS

Methodology	Cost Measurement Unit	Outcome Measurement Unit
Cost-minimization analysis (CMA)	Dollars	Assumed to be equivalent in comparable groups analysis
Cost-benefit analysis (CBA)	Dollars	Dollars
Cost-effectiveness analysis (CEA)	Dollars	Natural units (life years gained, mm Hg blood analysis [CEA] pressure, mmol/L blood glucose)
Cost-utility analysis (CUA)	Dollars	Quality-adjusted life year (QALY) or other utilities

account patient preferences (or utilities), the study is called a **cost-utility analysis** (CUA) (Table 7-1). Each type of analysis includes a measurement of costs in dollars. Assessment of these costs is discussed first, followed by further examples of how outcomes are measured for these four types of studies.

Assessment of Costs

First, the assessment of costs (the left-hand side of the equation) will be discussed. A discussion of the four types of costs and timing adjustments for costs follows.

TYPES OF COSTS

Costs are calculated to estimate the resources (or inputs) that are used in the production of an outcome. ❷ *Pharmacoeconomic studies categorize costs into four types.* **Direct medical costs** are the most obvious costs to measure. These are the medically related inputs used directly in providing the treatment. Examples of direct medical costs would include costs associated with pharmaceutical products, physician visits, emergency room visits, and hospitalizations. **Direct nonmedical costs** are costs directly associated with treatment, but are not medical in nature. Examples include the cost of traveling to and from the physician's office or hospital, babysitting for the children of a patient, and food and lodging required for patients and their families during out-of-town treatment. **Indirect costs** involve costs that result from the loss of productivity due to illness or death. Please note that the accounting term indirect costs, which is used to assign overhead, is different from the economic term, which refers to a loss of productivity of the patient or the patient's family due to illness. **Intangible costs** include the costs of pain, suffering, anxiety, or fatigue that occur because of an illness or the treatment of an illness. It is difficult to measure or assign values to intangible costs.

Treatment of an illness may include all four types of costs. For example, the cost of surgery would include the direct medical costs of the surgery (medication, room charges, laboratory tests, and physician services), direct nonmedical costs (travel and lodging for the preoperative day), indirect costs (cost due to the patient missing work during the surgery and recuperative period), and intangible costs (due to pain and anxiety). Most studies only report the direct medical costs. This may be appropriate depending on the objective of the study or the perspective of the study. For example, if the objective is to measure the costs to the hospital for two surgical procedures that differ in direct medical costs (e.g., using high-dose versus low-dose aprotinin in cardiac bypass surgery), but that are expected to have similar nonmedical, indirect, and intangible costs, measuring all four types of costs may not be warranted.

In order to determine what costs are important to measure, the perspective of the study must be determined. ❸ *Perspective is a pharmacoeconomic term that describes whose costs are relevant based on the purpose of the study.* Economic theory suggests that the most appropriate perspective is that of society. Societal costs would include costs to the insurance company, costs to the patient, and indirect costs due to the loss of productivity. Although this may be the most appropriate perspective according to economic theory, it is rarely seen in the pharmacoeconomic literature. The most common perspectives used in pharmacoeconomic studies are the perspective of the institution or the perspective of the payer. The payer perspective may include the costs to the third-party plan, the patient, or a combination of the patient copay and the third-party plan costs.

TIMING ADJUSTMENTS FOR COSTS

When costs are estimated from information collected for more than a year before the study or for more than a year into the future, adjustment of costs is needed. If retrospective data are used to assess resources used over a number of years, these costs should be adjusted to the present year. For example, if the objective of the study is to estimate the difference in the costs of antibiotic A versus B in the treatment of a specific type of infection, information on the past utilization of these two antibiotics might be collected from a review of medical records. If the retrospective review of these medical records dates back for more than a year, it may be necessary to adjust the cost of both medications by calculating the number of units (doses) used per case and multiplying this number by the current unit cost for each medication.

If costs are estimated based on dollars spent or saved in future years, another type of adjustment, called discounting, is needed. There is a time value associated with money. Most people (and businesses) prefer to receive money today, rather than at a later time. Therefore, a dollar received today is worth more than a dollar received next year—the time value of money. Discount rate, a term from finance, approximates the cost of capital by taking into account the projected inflation rate and the interest rates of borrowed money and then estimates the time value of money. From this parameter, the present value (PV) of future expenditures and savings can be calculated. The discount factor is equal to $1/(1 + r)^n$, where r is the discount rate and n is the year in which the cost or savings occur. For example, if the costs of a new pharmaceutical care program are $5,000 per year for the next 3 years, and the discount rate is 5%, the PV of these costs is $14,297 ($5,000 year 1 + $5,000/1.05 year 2 + $5,000/[1.05]^2$ year 3) (note that discounting does not start until year 2). The most common discount rates currently seen in the literature are 3% to 5%, the approximate cost of borrowing money today.

Assessment of Outcomes

The methods associated with measuring outcomes (the right-hand side of the equation) will be discussed in this section. ❹ *As shown in Table 7-1, there are four ways to measure outcomes: CMA, CBA, CEA, and CUA.* Each type of outcome measurement is associated with a different type of pharmacoeconomic analysis. The advantages and disadvantages of each type of analysis will be discussed in this section.

COST-MINIMIZATION ANALYSIS

● For a CMA, costs are measured in dollars, and outcomes are assumed to be equivalent. One example of a CMA is the measurement and comparison of costs for two therapeutically equivalent products, like glipizide and glyburide.[5] Another example is the measurement and comparison of using prostaglandin E2 on an inpatient versus an outpatient basis.[6] In both cases, all the outcomes (e.g., efficacy, incidence of adverse drug interactions) are expected to be equal, but the costs are not. Some researchers contend that a CMA is not a true pharmacoeconomic study, because costs are measured, but outcomes are not. Others say that the strength of a CMA depends on the evidence that the outcomes are the same. This evidence can be based on previous studies, publications, FDA data, or expert opinion.

● The advantage of this type of study is that it is relatively simple compared to the other types of analyses because outcomes need not be measured. The disadvantage of this type of analysis is that it can only be used when outcomes are assumed to be identical.

Examples

A hospital needs to decide if it should add a new intravenous antibiotic to the formulary, which is therapeutically equivalent to the current antibiotic used in the institution and has the same adverse event profile. The advantage of the new antibiotic is that it only has to be administered once per day versus three times a day for the comparison anti-biotic. Because the outcomes are expected to be nearly identical, and the objective is to assess the costs to the hospital (e.g., the hospital perspective), only direct medical costs need to be estimated and compared. The direct medical costs include the daily costs of each medication, the pharmacy personnel time used in the preparation of each dose, and the nursing personnel time used in the administration of each dose. Even if the cost of the new medication is a little higher than the cost of the current antibiotic, the lower cost of preparing and administering the new drug (once a day versus three times per day) may offset this difference. Direct nonmedical, indirect, and intangible costs are not expected to differ between these two alternatives and they need not be included if the perspective is that of the hospital, so these costs are not included in the comparison.

Mithani and Brown[7] examined once-daily intravenous administration of an aminogly-coside versus the conventional every 8-hour administration (Table 7-2). The drug acquisi-tion cost was in Canadian dollars ($Can) 43.70 for every 8 hours dosing, and $Can 55.39 for the single-dose administration. Not including laboratory drug level measurements, the costs of the intravenous bag ($Can 29.32), preparation ($Can 13.81), and administration ($Can 67.63) were $Can 110.76 for the three-times daily administration versus $Can 42.23 (intravenous bag $Can 10.90, preparation $Can 6.20, and administration $Can 25.13) for the single daily dose. With essentially equivalent clinical outcomes, the once-daily admin-istration of the aminoglycoside minimized hospital costs ($Can 97.62 versus $Can 154.46).

COST-BENEFIT ANALYSIS

A CBA measures both inputs and outcomes in monetary terms. One advantage to using a CBA is that alternatives with different outcomes can be compared, because each outcome is converted to the same unit (dollars). For example, the costs (inputs) of providing a pharmacokinetic service versus a diabetes clinic can be compared with the cost savings (outcomes) associated with each service, even though different types of outcomes are expected for each alternative. Many CBAs are performed to determine how institutions

TABLE 7–2. EXAMPLE OF COST MINIMIZATION

Type of Cost	Every 8 Hours	Once Daily
Drug acquisition cost	$43.70	$55.39
Minibag cost	$29.32	$10.90
Preparation cost	$13.81	$6.20
Administration costs	$67.63	$25.13
Total cost	$154.46	$97.62

Note: Costs are presented in Canadian dollars.

can best spend their resources to produce monetary benefits. For example, a study conducted at Walter Reed Army Medical Center looked at costs and savings associated with the addition of a pharmacist to its medical teams.[8] Discounting of both the costs of the treatment or services and the benefits or cost savings is needed if they extend for more than a year. Comparing costs and benefits (outcomes in monetary terms) is accomplished by using one of two methods. One method divides the estimated benefits by the estimated costs to produce a benefit-to-cost ratio. If this ratio is more than 1, the choice is cost beneficial. The other method is to subtract the costs from the benefits to produce a net benefit calculation. If this difference is positive, the choice is cost beneficial. The example at the end of this section will use both methods for illustrative purposes.

Another more complex use of CBA consists of measuring clinical outcomes (e.g., avoidance of death, reduction of blood pressure, and reduction of pain) and placing a dollar value on these clinical outcomes. This type of CBA is not often seen in the pharmacy literature, but will be discussed here briefly. This use of the method still offers the advantage that alternatives with different types of outcomes can be assessed, but a disadvantage is that it is difficult to put a monetary value on pain, suffering, and human life. ❺ *There are two common methods that economists use to estimate a value for these health-related consequences, the human capital (HC) approach and the willingness-to-pay (WTP) approach.* The HC approach assumes that the values of health benefits are equal to the economic productivity that they permit. The cost of disease is the cost of the lost productivity due to the disease. A person's expected income before taxes and/or an inputted value for nonmarket activities (e.g., housework and child care) is used as an estimate of the value of any health benefits for that person. The HC approach was used when calculating the costs and benefits of administering a meningococcal vaccine to college students. The value of the future productivity of a college student was estimated at $1 million in this study.[9] There are disadvantages to using this method. People's earnings may not reflect their true value to society, and this method lacks a solid literature of research to back this notion. The WTP method estimates the value of health benefits by estimating how much people would pay to reduce their chance of an adverse health outcome. For example, if a group of people is willing to pay, on average, $100 to reduce their chance of dying from 1:1,000 to 1:2,000, theoretically a life would be worth $200,000 [$100/(0.001−0.0005)]. Problems with this method include the issue that what people say they are willing to pay may not correspond to what they actually would pay, and it is debatable if people can meaningfully answer questions about a 0.0005 reduction in outcomes.

Example

An independent pharmacy owner is considering the provision of a new clinical pharmacy service. The objective of the analysis is to estimate the costs and monetary benefits of two possible services over the next 3 years (Table 7-3). Clinical Service A would cost $50,000

TABLE 7–3. CBA EXAMPLE CALCULATIONS

	Year 1 Dollars (No Discounting in Year 1)	Year 2 Dollars (Discounted Dollars)	Year 3 Dollars (Discounted Dollars)	Total Dollars (Discounted Dollars)	Benefit-to-Cost Ratio Dollars (Discounted Dollars)	Net Benefit Dollars (Discounted Dollars)
Costs of A	$50,000	$20,000	$20,000	$90,000	$120,000/$90,000 = 1.33:1	$120,000 − $90,000 = $30,000
	($50,000)	($19,048)	($18,140)	($87,188)	($114,376/87,188 = 1.31:1)	($114,376 − 87,188 = 27,188)
Benefits of A	$40,000	$40,000	$40,000	$120,000		
	($40,000)	($38,095)	($36,281)	($114,376)		
Costs of B	$40,000	$30,000	$30,000	$100,000	$135,000/100,000 = 1.35:1	$135,000 − 100,000 = 35,000
	($40,000)	($28,571)	($27,211)	($95,782)	($128,673/95,782 = 1.34:1)	($128,673 − 95,782 = 32,891)
Benefits of B	$45,000	$45,000	$45,000	$135,000		
	($45,000)	($42,857)	($40,816)	($128,673)		

in start-up and operating costs during the first year, and $20,000 in years 2 and 3. Clinical Service A would provide an added revenue of $40,000 each of the 3 years, Clinical Service B would cost $40,000 in start-up and operating costs the first year and $30,000 for years 2 and 3. Clinical Service B would provide added revenue of $45,000 for each of the 3 years. Table 7-3 illustrates the comparison of both options using the perspective of the independent pharmacy with no discounting and when a discount rate of 5% is used. Although both services are estimated to be cost beneficial, Clinical Service B has both a higher benefit-to-cost ratio and a higher net benefit when compared to Clinical Service A.

COST-EFFECTIVENESS ANALYSIS

This is the most common type of pharmacoeconomic analysis found in the pharmacy literature. A CEA measures costs in dollars and outcomes in natural health units such as cures, lives saved, or blood pressure. An advantage of using a CEA is that health units are common outcomes practitioners can readily understand and these outcomes do not need to be converted to monetary values. On the other hand, the alternatives used in the comparison must have outcomes that are measured in the same units, such as lives saved with each of two treatments. If more than one natural unit outcome is important when conducting the comparison, a cost-effectiveness ratio (CER) should be calculated for each type of outcome. Outcomes cannot be collapsed into one unit measure in CEAs as they can with CBAs (outcome = dollars) or CUAs (outcome = **quality-adjusted life years [QALYs]**). Because CEA is the most common type of pharmacoeconomic study in the pharmacy literature, many examples are available. Bloom and others[10] compared two medical treatments for gastroesophageal reflux disease (GERD), using both healed ulcers confirmed by endoscopy and symptom-free days as the outcomes measured. Law and others[11] assessed two antidiabetic medications by comparing the percentage of patients who achieved good glycemic control as the outcome measure.

A cost-effectiveness grid (Table 7-4) can be used to illustrate the definition of cost-effectiveness. In order to determine if a therapy or service is cost-effective, both the costs and effectiveness must be considered. Think of comparing a new drug with the current standard treatment. If the new treatment is (1) both more effective and less costly

TABLE 7-4. COST-EFFECTIVENESS GRID

Cost-Effectiveness	Lower Cost	Same Cost	Higher Cost
Lower effectiveness	A	B	C
Same effectiveness	D	E	F
Higher effectiveness	G	H	I

(cell G), (2) more effective at the same price (cell H), or (3) has the same effectiveness at a lower price (cell D), the new therapy is considered cost-effective. On the other hand, if the new drug is (1) less effective and more costly (cell C), (2) has the same effectiveness but costs more (cell F), or (3) has lower effectiveness for the same costs (cell B), then the new product is *not* cost-effective. There are three other possibilities: (1) that the new drug is more expensive and more effective (cell I)—a very common finding, (2) less expensive but less effective (cell A), or (3) has the same price and the same effectiveness as the standard product (cell E). For the middle cell E, other factors may be considered to determine which medication might be best. For the other two cells, an incremental cost-effectiveness ratio (ICER) is calculated to determine the extra cost for each extra unit of outcome. It is left up to the readers to determine if they think the new product is cost-effective, based on a value judgment. The underlying subjectivity as to whether the added benefit is worth the added cost is a disadvantage of CEA.

Example

An MCO is trying to decide whether to add a new cholesterol-lowering agent to its preferred formulary. The new product has a greater effect on lowering cholesterol than the current preferred agent, but a daily dose of the new medication is also more expensive. Using the perspective of the MCO (e.g., direct medical costs of the product to the MCO), the results will be presented in three ways in Tables 7-5 to 7-7 to illustrate the various ways that costs and effectiveness are presented in the literature. Table 7-5 presents the simple listing of the costs and benefits of the two alternatives. Sometimes for each alternative,

TABLE 7–5. **LISTING OF COSTS AND OUTCOMES**

Alternative	Costs for 12 Months of Medication	Lowering of LDL in 12 Months (mg/dL)
Current preferred medication	$1,000	25
New medication	$1,500	30

LDL = low-density lipoprotein.

TABLE 7–6. **COST-EFFECTIVENESS RATIOS**

Alternative	Costs for 12 Months of Medication	Lowering of LDL in 12 Months	Average Cost per Reduction in LDL
Current preferred medication	$1,000	25 mg/dL	$40 per mg/dL
New medication	$1,500	30 mg/dL	$50 per mg/dL

LDL = low-density lipoprotein.

TABLE 7–7. INCREMENTAL COST-EFFECTIVENESS RATIO

Alternative	Costs for 12 Months of Medication	Lowering of LDL in 12 Months	Incremental Cost per Marginal Reduction in LDL
Current preferred medication	$1,000	25 mg/dL	($1,500 − $1,000)/(30 mg/dL − 25 mg/dL) = $100 per mg/dL
New medication	$1,500	30 mg/dL	

LDL = low-density lipoprotein.

the costs and various outcomes are listed but no ratios are conducted—this is termed a cost-consequence analysis (CCA).

The second method of presenting results includes calculating the average CER for each alternative. Table 7-6 shows the CER for the two alternatives. The CER is the ratio of resources used per unit of clinical benefit, and implies that this calculation has been made in relation to doing nothing or no treatment. In this case, the current medication costs $40 for every 1 mg/dL decrease in LDL while the new medication under consideration costs $50 for the same decrease. In clinical practice, the question is infrequently "Should we treat the patient or not?" or "What are the costs and outcomes of this intervention versus no intervention?" More often the question is "How does one treatment compare with another treatment in costs and outcomes?" To answer this more common question, an ICER is calculated. The ICER is the ratio of the difference in costs divided by the difference in outcomes. Most economists agree that an ICER (the extra cost for each added unit of benefit) is the more appropriate way to present CEA results. Table 7-7 shows the incremental cost-effectiveness (the extra cost of producing one extra unit) of the new medication compared to the current medication. For the new medication, it costs an additional $100 for every additional decrease in LDL of 1 mg/dL. The formulary committee would need to decide if this increase in cost is worth the increase in benefit (improved clinical outcome). In this example, the costs and benefits of the medications are estimated for only 1 year; discounting is not needed. If incremental calculations produce negative numbers, this indicates that one treatment is both more effective and less expensive, or dominant, compared to the other option. The magnitude of the negative ratio is difficult to interpret, so it is suggested that authors instead indicate which treatment is the dominant one. As mentioned before, when one of the alternatives is both more expensive and more effective than another, the ICER is used to determine the magnitude of added cost for each unit in health improvement (see CEA grid, cell I, Table 7-4).

Clinicians must then wrestle with this type of information—it becomes a clinical call. Many economists will argue that this uncertainty is why cost-effectiveness may not be the preferred method of pharmacoeconomic analysis.

COST-UTILITY ANALYSIS

❻ *A CUA takes patient preferences, also referred to as utilities, into account when measuring health consequences.*[12] The most common unit used in conducting CUAs is QALYs. A QALY is a health utility measure combining quality and quantity of life, as determined by some valuations process. The advantage of using this method is that different types of health outcomes can be compared using one common unit (QALYs) without placing a monetary value on these health outcomes (like CBA). The disadvantage of this method is that it is difficult to determine an accurate QALY value. This is an outcome measure that is not well understood or embraced by many providers and decision makers. Therefore, this method is not commonly seen in the pharmacy literature. One reason researchers are working to establish methods for measuring QALYs is the belief that 1 year of life (a natural unit outcome that can be used in CEAs) in one health state should not be given the same weight as 1 year of life in another health state. For example, if two treatments both add 10 years of life, but one provides an added 10 years of being in a healthy state and the other adds 10 years of being in a disabled health state, the outcomes of the two treatments should not be considered equal.

Adjusting for the quality of those extra years is warranted. When calculating QALYs, 1 year of life in perfect health has a score of 1 QALY. If health-related **quality of life** (HR-QOL) is diminished by disease or treatment, 1 year of life in this state is less than 1 QALY. This unit allows comparisons of morbidity and mortality. By convention, perfect health is assigned 1 per year and death is assigned 0 per year, but how are scores between these two determined? Different techniques for determining scales of measurement for QALY are discussed below.

There are three common methods for determining QALY scores: rating scales (RS), standard gamble (SG), and time trade-off (TTO). A rating scale consists of a line on a page, somewhat like a thermometer, with perfect health at the top (100) and death at bottom (0). Different disease states are described to subjects, and they are asked to place the different disease states somewhere on the scale indicating preferences relative to all diseases described. As an example, if they place a disease state at 70 on the scale, the disease state is given a score of 0.7 QALYs.

The second method for determining patient preference (or utility) scores is the SG method. For this method, each subject is offered two alternatives. Alternative one is treatment with two possible outcomes: either the return to normal health or immediate death. Alternative two is the certain outcome of a chronic disease state for life. The probability (*p*) of dying is varied until the subject is indifferent between alternative one and alternative two. As an example, a person considers two options: a kidney transplant with a 20% probability of dying during the operation (alternative one) or dialysis for the rest of his life (alternative two). If this percent is his or her point of indifference (he or she would

TABLE 7–8. SELECTED QALY ESTIMATES

Disease State	QALY Estimate
Complete health	1.00
Moderate angina	0.83
Breast cancer: removed breast, unconcerned	0.80
Severe angina	0.53
Cancer spread, constant pain, tired, not expected to live long	0.16
Death	0.00

not have the operation if the chances of dying during the operation were any higher than 20%), the QALY is calculated as $1 - p$ or 0.8 QALY.

The third technique for measuring health preferences is the TTO method. Again, the subject is offered two alternatives. Alternative one is a certain disease state for a specific length of time t, the life expectancy for a person with the disease, then death. Alternative two is being healthy for time x, which is less than t. Time x is varied until the respondent is indifferent between the two alternatives. The proportion of the number of years of life a person is willing to give up $(t - x)$ to have his or her remaining years (x) of life in a healthy state is used to assess his or her QALY estimate. For example, a person with a life expectancy of 50 years is given two options: being blind for 50 years or being completely healthy (including being able to see) for 25 years. If the person is indifferent between these two options (he or she would rather be blind than give up any more years of life), the QALY for this disease state (blindness) would be 0.5. Table 7-8 contains examples of disease states and QALY estimates for each disease state listed.

As one might surmise, QALY measurement is not regarded as being as precise or scientific as natural health unit measurements (like blood pressure and cholesterol levels) used in CEAs. Some issues in the measurement of QALYs are debated in the literature. One issue concerns whose viewpoint is the most valid. An advantage of having patients with the disease of interest determine health state scores is that these patients may understand the effects of the disease better than the general population, whereas, some believe these patients would provide a biased view of their disease compared with other diseases they have not experienced. Some contend that health care professionals could provide good estimates because they understand various diseases and others argue that these professionals may not rate discomfort and disability as seriously as patients or the general population.

Another issue that has been addressed regarding patient preference or utility-score measures is the debate over which is the best measure. Utility scores calculated using one method might differ from those using another. Finally, utility measures have been criticized for not being sensitive to small, but clinically meaningful, changes in health status.

Example

An article by Kennedy and associates[13] assessed the costs and utilities associated with two common chemotherapy regimens (vindesine and cisplatin [VP], and cyclophosphamide, doxorubicin, and cisplatin [CAP]) and compared the results with the costs and utilities of using best supportive care (BSC) in patients with non-small cell lung cancer. The perspective was that of the health care system or the payer. Using the TTO method, treatment utility scores were estimated by personnel of the oncology ward. Although the chemotherapy regimens provide a longer survival (VP = 214 days, CAP = 165 days) than BSC (112 days), the quality of life TTO score was higher for BSC (0.61) compared with the chemotherapy regimens (0.34). When survival time is multiplied by the TTO scores, the use of BSC results in an estimated 0.19 QALYs, which is similar to VP (0.19 QALYs), but higher than CAP (0.15 QALY). The costs to the health care system for the three options are about $5,000 for BSC, $10,000 for VF, and $7,000 for CAP (the authors reported median costs instead of average costs due to the abnormality of the cost data). Cost-utility ratios are calculated similarly to cost-effectiveness ratios, except that the outcome unit is QALYs. Therefore, the cost-utility ratio is about $26,000/QALY for BSC and about $44,000 to $52,000/QALY for the chemotherapy regimens. Because BSC is at least as effective, as measured by QALYs, and is less expensive than the other two options, a marginal (or incremental) cost-utility ratio does not need to be calculated. Marginal cost-utility ratios only need to be calculated to estimate the added cost for an added benefit, not when the added benefit comes at a lower cost.

Performing an Economic Analysis

Conducting a pharmacoeconomic analysis can be challenging. Resources (time, expertise, data, and money) are limited. Data used to construct a model may be impossible to obtain due to lack of computer automation. Comparative studies of drug treatments may not be available or poorly designed. Results of clinical trials may not apply at the institution performing the analysis due to lack of resources.

Methods for conducting a pharmacoeconomic analysis have been described. ❼ *All four types of analyses described (CMA, CBA, CEA, and CUA) should follow 10 general steps.* See Table 7-9. A modified practical approach to these steps based on the work developed by Jolicoeur and others[14] will be reviewed.

TABLE 7–9. STEPS IN PERFORMING AN ECONOMIC ANALYSIS

Step 1	Define the problem
Step 2	Determine the study's perspective
Step 3	Determine specific treatment alternatives and outcomes
Step 4	Select the appropriate pharmacoeconomic method or model
Step 5	Measure inputs and outcomes
Step 6	Identify the resources necessary to conduct the analysis
Step 7	Establish the probabilities for the outcomes of the treatment alternatives
Step 8	Construct a decision tree
Step 9	Conduct a sensitivity analysis
Step 10	Present the results

● STEP 1: DEFINE THE PROBLEM

This step is self-explanatory. What is the question or objective that is the focus of the analysis? An example might be, "The objective of the analysis is to determine what medications for the treatment of urinary tract infections (UTIs) should be included on formulary." Perhaps one of the drugs being evaluated is a new drug recently approved by the FDA. Should the new drug be added to the drug formulary? The important thing to remember with this step is to be specific.

● STEP 2: DETERMINE THE STUDY'S PERSPECTIVE

It is important to identify from whose perspective the analysis will be conducted. As mentioned in the Assessment of Costs section, this will determine the costs to be evaluated. Is the analysis being conducted from the perspective of the patient or from that of the health system, clinic, accountable care organization, or society? Depending on the perspective assigned to the analysis, different results and recommendations based on those results may be identified. If deciding on whether to add a new antibiotic to a formulary for treating UTIs, the perspective of the institution or payer would probably be used.

● STEP 3: DETERMINE SPECIFIC TREATMENT ALTERNATIVES AND OUTCOMES

In this step, all treatment alternatives to be compared in the analysis should be identified. This selection should include the best clinical options and/or the options that are used most often in that setting at the time of the study. If a new treatment option is being considered, comparing it with an outdated treatment or a treatment with low efficacy rates is a waste of time and money. This new treatment should be compared with the next best alternative or the alternative it may replace. Keep in mind that alternatives may include drug treatments and nonpharmacologic treatments. For the UTI example, a new antibiotic would probably be compared with fluoroquinolones or sulfa drugs, or even the use of cranberry juice—old or gold standard therapy—but still the usual and most commonly used therapy. Today's expensive new chemical entities are very unlikely to cost less than standard therapy, and because of this, newer drugs are sometimes compared to the most recent, more expensive drugs used as alternative therapy.

The outcomes of those alternatives should include all anticipated positive and negative consequences or events that can be measured. Remember, outcomes may be measured in a variety of ways: lives saved, emergency room visits, hospitalizations, adverse drug reactions, dollars saved, QALYs, and so forth. For the UTI example, cure rates would be the most important outcome.

STEP 4: SELECT THE APPROPRIATE PHARMACOECONOMIC METHOD OR MODEL

The pharmacoeconomic method selected will depend on how the outcomes are measured (see Table 7-1). Costs (inputs) for all four types of analyses are measured in dollars. When all outcomes for each alternative are expected to be the same, a CMA is used. If all outcomes for each alternative considered are measured in monetary units, a CBA is used. When outcomes of each treatment alternative are measured in the same nonmonetary units, a CEA is used. When patient preferences for alternative treatments are being considered, a CUA is used. For the UTI example, cure rates are a natural clinical unit measure, so a CEA would be conducted.

STEP 5: MEASURE INPUTS AND OUTCOMES

All resources consumed by each alternative should be identified and measured in monetary value. The cost for each alternative should be listed and estimated (see Assessment of Costs section). The types of costs that will be measured will depend on the perspective chosen in Step 2. When evaluating alternatives over a long period of time (e.g., greater than 1 year), the concept of discounting should be applied. For the UTI example, if the perspective is an acute care hospital, only inpatient costs of treatment are measured. If the perspective is that of the third-party payer, all direct medical costs for the treatment are included whether they are provided on an inpatient or outpatient basis.

Measuring outcomes can be relatively simple (e.g., cure rates) or relatively difficult (e.g., QALYs). Outcomes may be measured prospectively or retrospectively. Prospective measurements tend to be more accurate and complete, but may take considerably more time and resources than retrospective data retrieval. Prospectively it is possible to define exactly what data to capture, but because it is necessary to wait for the patients to complete therapy, these types of studies may take months to years to complete. A data set on the shelf (computer) can be available now, and may have all the data fields of interest. For the UTI example, cure rates attributed to the new product may be estimated from previous clinical trials, expert opinion, or measured prospectively in the population of interest.

STEP 6: IDENTIFY THE RESOURCES NECESSARY TO CONDUCT THE ANALYSIS

The availability of resources to conduct the study is an important consideration. Lack of access to important data can severely limit the validity of an analysis, as can the accuracy of the data itself. Data may be obtained from a variety of sources, including clinical trials, medical literature, medical records, prescription profiles, or computer databases. Before proceeding with the project, evaluate whether reliable sources of data are accessible or the data can be collected within the timeframe and budget allocated for the project.

STEP 7: ESTABLISH THE PROBABILITIES FOR THE OUTCOMES OF THE TREATMENT ALTERNATIVES

Probabilities for the outcomes identified in Step 3 should be determined. This may include the probability of treatment failures or success, or adverse reactions to a given treatment or alternative. Data for these can be obtained from the medical literature, clinical trials, medical records, expert opinion, prescription databases, as well as institutional databases. For the UTI example, probabilities of a cure rate for the new medication can be found in clinical trials or obtained from the FDA-approved labeling information (see Table 7-10). Probabilities of cure rates for the previous treatments (e.g., sulfas) can also be found in clinical trials or by accessing medical records. If prospective data collection is conducted, the probabilities of all alternatives will be directly measured instead of estimated.

STEP 8: CONSTRUCT A DECISION TREE

Decision analysis can be a very useful tool when conducting a pharmacoeconomic analysis (see the section on Decision Analysis for a step-by-step review). Constructing a

TABLE 7-10. STEPS IN DECISION ANALYSIS

Step 1	Identify the specific decision (therapeutic or medical problem)
Step 2	Specify alternatives
Step 3	Specify possible outcomes and probabilities
Step 4	Draw the decision analysis structure
Step 5	Perform calculations
Step 6	Conduct a sensitivity analysis (vary cost estimates)

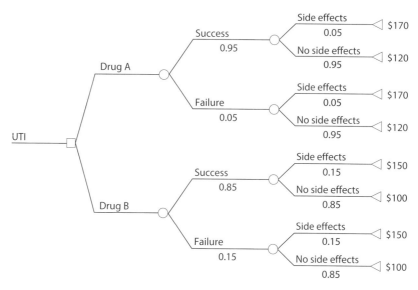

Figure 7–2. Decision tree for UTI example.

decision tree creates a graphic display of the outcomes of each treatment alternative and the probability of their occurrence. Costs associated with each treatment alternative can be determined and the respective cost ratios derived. An example using a decision tree is provided in Figure 7-2.

STEP 9: CONDUCT A SENSITIVITY ANALYSIS

Whenever estimates are used, there is a possibility that these estimates are not precise. These estimates may be referred to as assumptions. For example, if the researcher assumes the discount rate is 5%, or assumes the efficacy rate found in clinical trials will be the same as the effectiveness rate in the general population, this is a best guess used to conduct the calculations. ❽ *A* **sensitivity analysis** *allows one to determine how the results of an analysis would change when these best guesses or assumptions are varied over a relevant range of values.* For example, if the researcher makes the assumption that the appropriate discount rate is 5%, this estimate should be varied from 0% to 10% to determine if the same alternative would still be chosen within this range. In order to vary many assumptions at one time, a probabilistic sensitivity analysis (changing each variable at random and recalculating) can be conducted that simulates many patients randomly being processed through the decision model using a range of estimates chosen for the analysis.[15]

STEP 10: PRESENT THE RESULTS

The results of the analysis should be presented to the appropriate audience, such as P&T committees, medical staff, or third-party payers. The steps outlined in this section should be employed when presenting the results. State the problem, identify the perspective, and so on. It is imperative to acknowledge or clarify any assumptions.

Although none of the models presented above are perfect, their utility may lead to better decision making when faced with the difficult task of evaluating new drugs or technology for health care systems.

What Is Decision Analysis?

Decision analysis is a tool that can help visualize a pharmacoeconomic analysis. ❾ *It is the application of an analytical method for systematically comparing different decision options. Decision analysis graphically displays choices and performs the calculations needed to compare these options.* It assists with selecting the best or most cost-effective alternative. Decision analysis is a tool that has been utilized for years in many fields, but has been applied to medical decision making more frequently in the last 10 years. This method of analysis assists in making decisions when the decision is complex and there is uncertainty about some of the information.

Discussions of the medical uses of decision analysis have been included in collections of pharmacoeconomic bibliographies,[16-20] and in such specific topic areas as CEAs,[21] CUAs,[22] CBAs,[23] CMAs,[24] policies,[25] formulary processes,[26] pharmacy practices,[27] and drug product development.[28]

STEPS IN DECISION ANALYSIS

The steps in the decision process are enumerated in greater detail in several articles,[29-33] and are relatively straightforward, especially with the availability of computer programs that greatly simplify the calculations.[33] Articles reporting a decision analysis should include a picture of the decision tree, including the costs and probabilities utilized. The steps in a decision analysis will be outlined using the UTI example. The six steps involved in performing a decision analysis are provided below, and in Table 7-10.

Step 1: Identify the Specific Decision

Clearly define the specific decision to be evaluated (what is the objective of the study?). Over what period of time will the analysis be conducted (e.g., the episode of care, a year)?

Will the perspective be that of the ill patient, the medical care plan, an institution/organization, or society? Specifying who will be responsible for the costs of the treatment will determine how costs are measured. For the UTI example, the decision was whether to add a new antibiotic to the formulary to treat UTIs. The perspective was that of the institution and the time period is 2 weeks.

Step 2: Specify Alternatives

Ideally, the two most effective treatments or alternatives should be compared. In pharmacotherapy evaluations, makers of innovative new products may compare or measure themselves against a standard (older or well-established) therapy. This is most often the case with new chemical entities. For pharmaceutical products, dosage and duration of therapy should be included. When analyzing costs and outcomes of pharmaceutical services, these services should be described in detail. For the UTI example, the use of the new medication (drug A) will be compared with that of a sulfa drug (drug B).

Step 3: Specify Possible Outcomes and Probabilities

Consequences, and outcomes calculated in dollars, yield a cost per outcome in natural medical units, such as mg/dL, which is a CEA. For each potential outcome, an estimated probability must be determined (e.g., 95% probability of a cure or a 7% incidence of adverse events).

Table 7-11 shows the outcomes and probabilities for the UTI example. The probabilities represent the chances or likelihood of treatment success or adverse events, and the costs associated with them.

Step 4: Draw the Decision Analysis Structure

Lines are drawn to joint decision points (branches or arms of a decision tree), represented either as choice nodes, chance nodes, or final outcomes. Nodes are places in the decision tree where decisions are allowed; a branching becomes possible at this point. There are three types of nodes: (1) a choice node is where a choice is allowed (as between two drugs or two treatments), (2) a chance node is a place where chance (natural occurrence) may influence the decision or outcome expressed as a probability, and (3) a terminal node is

TABLE 7–11. OUTCOMES AND PROBABILITIES, UTI EXAMPLE

	Drug A	Drug B
Effectiveness probability	0.95	0.85
Side effect probability	0.05	0.15
Cost of medication	$120	$100
Cost of side effects	$50	$50

the final outcome of interest for that decision. Probabilities are assigned for each possible outcome, and the sum of the probabilities must add up to one. Most computer-aided software programs utilize a square box to represent a choice node, a circle to represent a chance node, and a triangle for a terminal branch or final outcome. Figure 7-2 illustrates the decision tree for the UTI example.

Step 5: Perform Calculations

The first consideration should be the present value, or cost, of money. If the study is over a period of less than 1 year, actual costs are utilized in the calculations. If the study period is greater than 1 year, then costs should be discounted (converted to PV). For each branch of the tree, costs are totaled and multiplied by the probability of that arm of the tree. These numbers (costs × probabilities) calculated for each arm of the option are added for each alternative. Example calculations are given in Tables 7-12, 7-13, and 7-14. The UTI example would be a cost-effectiveness type of study, so the difference in the cost for each arm would be divided by the difference in effectiveness for each arm to produce a marginal CER (see Table 7-14).

Step 6: Conduct a Sensitivity Analysis (Vary Cost Estimates)

Because these decision trees or models are constructed with best guesses, a sensitivity analysis is conducted. The highest and lowest estimates of costs and probabilities are inserted into the equations to determine the best case and worse case answers. These estimates should be sufficiently varied to reflect all possible true variations in values.

TABLE 7–12. DECISION ANALYSIS CALCULATIONS FOR DRUG A

	Cost	Probability	Probability × Cost ($)
Outcome 1	$120 + $50 = $170	0.95 × 0.05 = 0.0475	8.08
Outcome 2	$120	0.95 × 0.95 = 0.9025	108.30
Outcome 3	$120 + $50 = $170	0.05 × 0.05 = 0.0025	0.42
Outcome 4	$120	0.05 × 0.95 = 0.0475	5.70
Total		1	122.5

TABLE 7–13. DECISION ANALYSIS CALCULATIONS FOR DRUG B

	Cost	Probability	Probability × Cost ($)
Outcome 1	$100 + $50 = $150	0.85 × 0.15 = 0.1275	19.12
Outcome 2	$100	0.85 × 0.85 = 0.7225	72.25
Outcome 3	$100 + $50 = $150	0.15 × 0.15 = 0.0225	3.38
Outcome 4	$100	0.15 × 0.85 = 0.1275	12.75
Total		1	107.50

TABLE 7–14. INCREMENTAL COST-EFFECTIVENESS RATIO

	Alternative Costs of Drug and Treating Side Effects ($)	Effectiveness in Treating UTI (%)	Incremental Cost per Treatment Success
Drug A	$122.50	95	($122.50 − $107.50)/ (0.95 − 0.85) = $150
Drug B	$107.50	85	

For the UTI example, the new drug (drug A) would be added to the formulary if the committee thought the added cost ($150) was worth the added benefit (one more successful treatment) (see Table 7-12). Some might not agree with the probability of the adverse events of drug A; because the therapy is new, they may believe 5% may be an underestimate. If the estimate is increased to a 10% adverse event rate for the new drug and the marginal CER is recalculated, the recalculated ratio would be $175 per added treatment success. Again, the committee would have to decide if the added cost is worth the added benefit.

Decision analysis is being used more commonly in pharmacoeconomic evaluations. The use and availability of computer programs[32] to assist with the multiple calculations make it fairly easy for someone to automate their evaluations. Examples of software available for this purpose include TreeAge Pro (http://www.treeage.com), DPL (http://www.syncopation.com), and DecisionPro® (http://www.decisionpro.biz). The prices for these software packages range from less than $100 for student versions to over $1,000 for professional versions. Decision analyses can also be conducted using Microsoft Excel (http://office.microsoft.com/en-us/excel).

Example

An article by Botteman and others[34] used a decision tree analysis to model the cost-effectiveness of enoxaparin compared to warfarin for the prevention of complications (deep vein thrombosis, venous thromboembolisms, and postthrombotic syndromes) due to hip replacement surgery. Data for this model were obtained through published literature and expert opinion. The model was created to assess both short-term (immediately after surgery) and long-term (followed until death or 100 years old) costs and consequences. The perspective was that of the payer, and a discount rate of 3% was used for the long-term analysis. Results: for the short-term model, therapy with enoxaparin was more expensive (+$133 per patient), but had a better outcome (+0.04 QALY per patient). For the long-term model, therapy with enoxaparin saved money (−$89 per patient) and had a better outcome (+0.16 QALY per patient), and was therefore the dominant (saves money and has a better outcome) choice. Both univariate (one item varied) and probabilistic (multiple items varied) sensitivity analyses were conducted and indicated that the results were robust.

Steps in Reviewing Published Literature

It is more likely that a practicing pharmacist will be asked to evaluate published literature on the topic of pharmacoeconomics, rather than actually conduct a study. When evaluating the pharmacoeconomics literature for making a formulary decision, or selecting a best product for an institution, a systematic approach to evaluating the pharmacoeconomics literature can make the task easier.

Several authors[14,35-40] cite methodology to assist in systematically reviewing the pharmacoeconomic literature. If a study is carefully reviewed to ensure that the author(s) included all meaningful components of an economic evaluation, the likelihood of finding valid and useful results is high. The steps for evaluating studies are similar to the steps for conducting studies, because the readers are determining if the proper steps were followed when the researcher conducted the study. When evaluating a pharmacoeconomic study, at least the following 10 questions should be considered.

1. Was a well-defined question posed in an answerable form? The specific questions and hypotheses should be clearly stated at the beginning of the article.

2. Is the perspective of the study addressed? The perspective should be explicitly stated, not implied.

3. Were the appropriate alternatives considered? Head-to-head comparisons of the best alternatives provide more information than comparing a new product or service with an outdated or ineffective alternative.

4. Was a comprehensive description of the competing alternatives given? If products are compared, dosage and length of therapy should be included. If services are compared, explicit details of the services make the paper more useful. Could another researcher replicate the study based on the information given?

5. What type of analysis was conducted? The paper should address if a CMA, CEA, CBA, or CUA was conducted. Some studies may conduct more than one type of analysis (i.e., a combination of a CEA and a CUA). Some studies, especially older published studies, incorrectly placed the terms benefit or effectiveness analysis in the title of the article, when many were actually CMA studies.

6. Were all the important and relevant costs and outcomes included? Check to see that all pertinent costs and consequences were mentioned. The clinician needs to evaluate his or her situation and compare it to his or her practice situation.

7. Was there justification for any important costs or consequences that were not included? Sometimes, the authors will admit that although certain costs or consequences are important, they were impractical (or impossible) to measure in their study. It is better that the authors state these limitations, than to ignore them.

8. Was discounting appropriate? If so, was it conducted? If the treatment cost or outcomes are extrapolated for more than 1 year, the time value of money must be incorporated into the cost estimates.

9. Are all assumptions stated? Were sensitivity analyses conducted for these assumptions? Many of the values used in pharmacoeconomic studies are based on assumptions. For example, authors may assume the adverse event rate is 5%, or that adherence with a regimen will be 80%. These types of assumptions should be stated explicitly. For important assumptions, was the estimate varied within a reasonable range of values?

10. Was an unbiased summary of the results presented? Sometimes, the conclusions seem to overstate or exaggerate the data presented in the results section. Did the authors use unbiased reasonable estimates when determining the results? In general, are the study results believable? (Case Study 7-1)

Case Study 7-1

Title: Cost-Utility Analysis of Best Supportive Care versus Oncoplatin and Oncotaxel in the Treatment of Recurrent Metastatic Breast Cancer

Background: For patients diagnosed with recurrent metastatic breast cancer, the prognosis is grim. Two agents, Oncoplatin and Oncotaxel, have been used to help prolong the lives of these patients (authors would cite clinical literature here for real pharmaceutical products). As with other chemotherapy treatments, the toxic effects of the medications can be severe and vastly decrease the patient's quality of life. Some would argue that the small increase in life expectancy from these agents might not be worth the trade-off in suffering from the adverse effects of the agents during the treatment period. Instead of chemotherapy, palliative treatments, such as best supportive care (BSC), have been suggested as an option. BSC includes measures to keep the patient comfortable. These may include medications to alleviate pain, antibiotics, or radiotherapy to reduce tumor size. The objective of this study was to compare the costs and utility of two chemotherapy treatments, Oncoplatin and Oncotaxel, with those of BSC in patients with recurrent metastatic breast cancer.

Methods: The practice sites for data collection included three oncology clinics that are part of a multihospital, multiclinic health care system. Utility scores were collected via the **time trade-off** (TTO) method. A panel of experts helped create descriptions of the health states of patients undergoing the different treatment options. Based on these descriptions, utility scores were elicited from two sources: oncology nurses at the three clinics and a random sample of patients from general (non-oncology) clinics associated with the health care system.

Data on treatment and survival time were collected for the past 3 years from a retrospective analysis of charts at three oncology clinics. Medical services and procedures associated with these treatment options were recorded. Treatment data included medications and their administration, as well as laboratory, radiology, and various types of medical visits (physician, clinic, emergency room, and hospital). Charges listed by the health care system in 2013 were used to estimate current costs for each service or procedure.

● **Results:** Table 7-15 lists the costs and survival times found by the review of charts. Using the TTO method, treatment utility scores were estimated by nurses from the oncology clinics and a random sample of patients who did not have cancer. Although the chemotherapy regimens provided a longer survival (Oncoplatin, 200 days; Oncotaxel, 160 days) than BSC (130 days), the utility score was higher for BSC (0.60–0.61) compared with the chemotherapy regimens (0.32–0.35). Oncology nurses gave similar estimates compared with the group of non-oncology patients.

If the difference in quality of life is not incorporated into the analysis, cost-effectiveness calculations based on survival time alone (life years saved [LYS]) indicate that chemotherapy is more effective but at a higher cost (Table 7-16). When survival time is adjusted for the differences in utilities (preferences) for treatment, the use of BSC is dominant over both chemotherapy treatments because of its lower cost and higher QALY estimate.

Sensitivity analyses were conducted by reducing cost estimates using the clinic's cost-to-charge ratio of 0.83:1 and by varying the days of survival by their 95% confidence

TABLE 7–15. COMPOSITE ARTICLE DATA

	BSC	Oncoplatin	Oncotaxel
	(*n* = 29)	(*n* = 36)	(*n* = 35)
Treatment charges			
Mean	$5,000	$10,000	$7,000
(SD)	($1,000)	($2,000)	($2,000)
Survival (days)			
Mean	130 days	200 days	160 days
Range	110–140 days	180–215 days	110–190 days
Utility scores			
Oncology nurses	0.60	0.35	0.35
Utility scores			
Non-oncology patients	0.61	0.32	0.32

TABLE 7–16. COMPOSITE ARTICLE CALCULATIONS

	BSC	Oncoplatin	Oncotaxel
	(*n* = 29)	(*n* = 36)	(*n* = 35)
Cost effectiveness			
Cost per LYS = (cost/days) × 365 days/year	$14,038	$18,250	$15,969
Incremental cost per LYS = [Δcosts/Δdays] × 365 days/year		Oncoplatin vs. BSC = $26,071 per additional LYS	Oncotaxel vs. BSC = $24,333 per additional LYS
Cost utility			
QALY = $\dfrac{\text{days} \times \text{utility}}{365 \text{ days/year}}$	O=0.21 QALY P = 0.22 QALY	O = 0.19 QALY P = 0.17 QALY	O = 0.15 QALY P = 0.14 QALY
Average cost per QALY Cost/QALY	O = $23,809 P = $22,727	O = $52,631 P = $58,823	O = $46,667 P = $50,000
Incremental cost per QALY = [Δcosts/ΔQALYs]	Both Oncoplatin and Oncotaxel dominated by BSC For both O and P estimates	Oncoplatin vs. Oncotaxel O = $75,000 per additional QALY P = $100,000 per additional QALY	

BSC = Best supportive care; LYS = life-years saved; QALY = quality-adjusted life year; O = based on utility scores from oncology nurses; P = based on utility scores from non-oncology patients.

intervals. As with the comparison of oncology nurses versus patient utility estimates, the results were robust.

Conclusion: There are some limitations to this study. The data were collected from a small sample of patients. Although data were collected from three clinics, these clinics were all part of the same health care system. Oncology treatment in other clinics may vary in both costs and outcomes. Although utility scores were collected from health care professionals and general patients, they were not collected from patients with metastatic breast cancer. We believed that administering the instrument to these women might have placed an undue burden on patients with a poor prognosis. Actual cost data were not available, so charge data were used as a proxy, and a sensitivity analysis was conducted on this variable.

As with previous research, using BSC was found to be less expensive than using chemotherapy agents to treat advanced cancer. Although BSC may not be as effective as chemotherapy in traditional measures of effectiveness (e.g., survival time, progression-free survival time), when preferences for a less toxic treatment are factored into the decision, BSC may become the preferred treatment, and it should be considered as an option.

■ CRITIQUE OF CUA ARTICLE

1. Complete title: The title identified the type of study (CUA), the treatments that were being compared (BSC, Oncoplatin, and Oncotaxel), and the disease state (metastatic breast cancer).

2. Clear objective: The objective of this study was "to compare the costs and utility of two chemotherapy treatments, Oncoplatin and Oncotaxel, with those of best supportive care." This was clear.

3. Appropriate alternatives: The three alternatives were BSC, Oncoplatin, and Oncotaxel. A case was made that BSC is sometimes overlooked as a valid option. Based on the clinical literature cited, the readers would determine if the two chemotherapy options were appropriate.

4. Alternatives described: Chemotherapy dosing is very individualized, and data were collected from three clinics; average doses of agents were not included. BSC was defined as keeping the patient comfortable, including providing pain medications, antibiotics, and radiotherapy, if needed.

5. Perspective stated: The perspective of the study was not explicitly stated. Because the researchers only report measuring direct medical costs, the perspective could have been that of the payer or that of the health care system that included the three oncology clinics. Charges were measured, so the perspective is still unclear. If actual costs to the health system were estimated, the perspective could have been the health care system. If reimbursed costs were used, the perspective could have been that of the average third-party payer.

6. Type of study: The study was correctly identified as a CUA because outcomes were valued in QALYs. For comparison purposes, incremental cost-effectiveness ratios were also calculated based on length of survival for the three options, so the answer could be that both a CUA and a CEA were conducted.

7. Relevant costs: Because we are unsure of the perspective of the study, it is difficult to determine if relevant costs were measured. It seems as if all relevant direct medical costs were measured. Patient costs, such as time traveling to and from the clinic, might be different for BSC than for chemotherapy, but these costs were not measured.

8. Relevant outcomes: Outcomes of the treatment were measured by determining the length of life from chart reviews and utilities via two groups, oncology nurses and general patients. The TTO technique was used to elicit utility scores. A description of the health states used in eliciting these responses would have been a helpful addition to the article.

9. Adjustment or discounting: Data were collected from charts that spanned a 3-year period. To adjust for this, units of service were multiplied by current charges for each service. Discounting was not needed because neither costs nor outcomes were extrapolated into the future.

10. Reasonable assumptions: One assumption was that utility scores from the oncology staff would be accurate. To test this assumption, scores were also obtained from another group (a random sample of non-oncology patients). Another assumption was that charges were a valid substitute for actual costs.

11. Sensitivity analyses: Sensitivity analyses were conducted. Utility scores from two groups were compared, and costs and survival time were varied. Although the authors indicated that results were insensitive to these analyses, a table with the numbers based on these new calculations would have been useful.

12. Limitations addressed: The authors did address some of their limitations at the beginning of the conclusion section. One limitation that was not addressed is that patients were not randomized to the three treatment options. It is possible that patients who received BSC were different from those who received chemotherapy. They may have been older or may have been in a more advanced stage of the disease.

13. Generalizations appropriate: Because data on both costs and outcomes were collected from only one health care system (albeit from three clinics within the system), caution should be used when extrapolating to other populations who are treated in other settings.

14. Unbiased conclusions: The authors state that when survival is adjusted for patient preferences, BSC is a valid option for treating patients with recurrent metastatic breast cancer. BSC costs less than chemotherapy treatments and provides a higher QALY score. Sensitivity analyses found the results to be robust (i.e., not sensitive to changes in estimates).

Many articles, several journals, and numerous texts have been devoted to pharmacoeconomics. Research and further development and refinement of the analysis tools are ongoing. It can be expected that the literature on pharmacoeconomics will continue to expand rapidly, not only for use in proving the value of new therapies, but for invalidating the worth of standard therapies. Grutters,[35] Husereau,[36] Duran,[37] Chiou,[38] Ofman,[39] Edwards,[40] among others, cite references to assist readers in understanding and assessing economic analyses of health care as well as providing checklists (with examples and explanations) to evaluate published articles.[41]

TABLE 7–16.   SELECTED WEBSITE REFERENCES

Canadian Agency for Drugs and Technologies in Health	https://www.cadth.ca/
Cochrane Collaboration home page	http://www.cochrane.org
Department of Defense Pharmacy Outcomes Research Team	https://health.mil/pod
Institute of Health Economics	http://www.ihe.ca
International Society for Pharmacoeconomics and Outcomes Research	http://www.ispor.org/links_index.asp

Selected Pharmacoeconomic Websites

Articles that provide an overview of the field of pharmacoeconomics, its changing methodologies, and recent advances can often be found readily at Internet sites devoted to this area of specialization. These sites usually highlight articles that are not necessarily drug or therapy specific, but many present an overview or validation of methodologies. Several pharmacoeconomic websites are included as references. They were selected because they all have multiple links to other pharmacoeconomic-related sites (see Table 7-16).

Educational opportunities in pharmacoeconomics have grown tremendously over the past 15 years, especially in U.S. Colleges of Pharmacy.[42]

Conclusion

Many health care organizations continue to be challenged with managing costs of pharmacotherapy. With the proliferation of health care programs under the Affordable Care Act, each entity will be building pharmacoeconomic models that can be useful tools for evaluating the costs of pharmaceuticals in these plans. The ability to objectively measure and compare costs may also produce better decisions about the choice of pharmaceuticals for a formulary. Decision analysis is one of the many tools finding increased utilization in the field of medicine, and pharmacoeconomics specifically. As the science of pharmacoeconomics becomes more standardized, rigorous comparisons among several papers on the same topic will be possible and necessary. For a more in-depth review of the principles and concepts of pharmacoeconomics, please see textbooks devoted to the topic, such as *Essentials of Pharmacoeconomics*[43] or *Methods for the Economic Evaluation of Health Care Programmes*.[44]

Self-Assessment Questions _____

1. A patient is anxious about waiting 2 weeks for a test result—this can be categorized as what type of cost?
   a. Direct medical cost
   b. Direct nonmedical cost
   c. Indirect cost
   d. Intangible cost

2. A parent staying home from work to care for their sick child is categorized as what type of cost?
   a. Direct medical cost
   b. Direct nonmedical cost
   c. Indirect cost
   d. Intangible cost

3. For which of the following would Alternative A be considered cost-effective when compared to the standard Alternate B.
   a. Alternative A costs less than Alternative B.
   b. Alternative A is more effective than Alternative B.
   c. Alternative A is more effective than Alternative B, and Alternative A costs less than Alternative B.
   d. Alternative A is less effective than Alternative B, but Alternative A costs more than Alternative B.

4. When an article states that the results of an analysis are *insensitive* to a particular variable this means:
   a. The results vary depending on the range of that variable, thereby strengthening your confidence in the study results.
   b. The results vary depending on the range of that variable, thereby weakening your confidence in the study results.
   c. The results do not vary depending on the range of that variable, thereby strengthening your confidence in the study results.
   d. The results do not vary depending on the range of that variable, thereby weakening your confidence in the study results.

5. If Project A costs $30,000 this year, $40,000 in year 2, and $50,000 in year 3, what is the total 3-years cost in present value (PV) terms using a 5% discount rate? Do not begin discounting until year 2. Round to the nearest $1,000.
   a. $100,000
   b. $113,000

    c. $120,000

    d. $127,000

6. If a researcher evaluates cost per quality-adjusted life year saved, what type of study is being conducted?

    a. CEA

    b. CBA

    c. CMA

    d. CUA

7. Most economists agree that the most appropriate way to present cost-effectiveness data is using:

    a. An incremental cost-effectiveness ratio

    b. A simple cost-effectiveness ratio

    c. A net benefit ratio

    d. A benefit-to-cost ratio

8. In order to estimate utilities, researchers use:

    a. Rating scale methods

    b. Time trade-off methods

    c. Standard gamble methods

    d. Any of the above methods may be used

9. A disadvantage of using the human capital method to value health is:

    a. The value estimated depends on a person's earning potential.

    b. People may not pay what they indicate they are willing to pay.

    c. Both of the above.

    d. None of the above.

10. Drug A cost $3,000 and saves $5,000. What is the benefit-to-cost ratio for Drug A?

    a. 0.60:1

    b. 0.80:1

    c. 1.67:1

    d. 2.50:1

11. Drug B cost $5,000 and saves $4,000. What is the benefit-to-cost ratio for Drug B?

    a. 0.75:1

    b. 0.80:1

    c. 1.67:1

    d. 1.33:1

12. Based on these results from questions 10 and 11 which option would you choose?
    a. Drug A is most cost-beneficial option.
    b. Drug B is the most cost-beneficial option.
    c. They are equally cost-beneficial.
    d. Not able to calculate based on information given.

For questions 13 to 15 use the following abstract:

Title: Cost-utility of asthmazolimide (fictitious drug) in the treatment of severe persistent asthma.

Background: Some patients with severe persistent asthma are not controlled with standard treatment (defined in this study as a combination of long-acting beta agonists [LABAs] and inhaled corticosteroids [ICS]). Clinical trials have shown improved outcomes for these patients if asthmazolimide is added to their regimen.

Objective: The objective of this study was to estimate the cost per quality-adjusted life year (QALY) of the addition of asthmazolimide to standard treatment for patients enrolled in a randomized controlled trial. The perspective of the study was the third-party payer.

Methods: Patients with severe persistent asthma in a health plan were enrolled in the study using a pre-post study design. The index date for each patient was his or her date of enrollment. Two years of pre-index utilization and costs of medical services were recorded using retrospective data collection, and patients were followed prospectively for 1 year after their index date. For the first 12 months after enrollment, patients recorded their use of any asthma-related medical services and prescriptions and kept a daily symptom diary. Then patients had asthmazolimide added to their regimen for the next 12-month period and again kept tract of their asthma-related medical services and prescriptions and a diary of daily symptoms. Costs of pre-index services were adjusted to 2008 costs to the health plan. QALYs were calculated using utility weights for various asthma-related symptoms that were estimated from a previous study using the time trade-off (TTO) method.

Results: A total of 216 patients were enrolled in and completed the study. Asthma-related health plan costs increased after the addition of asthmazolimide (mostly from an increase in prescription costs) by an average of $800 per year. Fewer symptoms and less severe symptoms were reported after the addition of the new drug, resulting in an average increase of 0.1 QALY, for an incremental cost per QALY ratio of x (*for calculating the answer, see question 13, below*).

Conclusion: For these 216 patients, the addition of asthmazolimide to their medication regimen resulted in a reduction of symptoms at a reasonable cost to the health plan.

13. What number should be included in the blank in the abstract?
    a. $800
    b. $8,000
    c. $80
    d. $80,000

14. In the abstract, was discounting needed? Was it conducted?
    a. Not needed, not conducted
    b. Needed, not conducted
    c. Needed, conducted
    d. Not needed, conducted

15. In the abstract, was adjustment needed? Was it conducted?
    a. Not needed, not conducted
    b. Needed, not conducted
    c. Needed, conducted
    d. Not needed, conducted

REFERENCES

1. U.S. Food and Drug Administration. Novel drugs summary 2016 [Internet]. [cited 2017 Mar 26]. Available from: https://www.fda.gov/Drugs/DevelopmentApprovalProcess/DrugInnovation/ucm534863.htm
2. Wang Z, Salmon JW, Walton SM. Cost effectiveness analysis and the formulary decision-making process. J Manag Care Pharm. 2004;10(10):48-59.
3. Bootman JL, Townsend RJ, McGhan WF. Introduction to pharmacoeconomics. In: Bootman JL, Townsend RJ, McGhan WF, eds. Principles of pharmacoeconomics. 2nd ed. Cincinnati, OH: Harvey Whitney Books; 1996:5-11.
4. Rascati KL. Essentials of pharmacoeconomics. Philadelphia, PA: Wolters Kluwer/Lippincott Williams & Wilkins; 2009:3.
5. Nadel HL. Formulary conversion from glipizide to glyburide: a cost-minimization analysis. Hosp Pharm. 1995;30(6):467-9, 472-4.
6. Farmer KC, Schwartz WJ, Rayburn WF, Turnball G. A cost-minimization analysis of intra-cervical prostaglandin E2 for cervical ripening in an outpatient versus inpatient setting. Clin Ther. 1996;18(4):747-56.
7. Mithani H, Brown G. The economic impact of once-daily versus conventional administration of gentamicin and tobramycin. PharmacoEconomics. 1996;10(5):494-503.
8. Bjornson DC, Hiner WO, Potyk RP, Nelson BA, Lombardo FA, Morton TA, et al. Effects of pharmacists on health care outcomes in hospitalized patients. Am J Hosp Pharm. 1993;50:1875-84.
9. Jackson LA, Schuchat A, Gorsky RD, Wenger JD. Should college students be vaccinated against meningococcal disease? A cost-benefit analysis. Am J Pub Health. 1995;85(6):843-5.

10. Bloom BS, Hillman AL, LaMont B, Liss C, Schwartz JS, Stever GJ. Omeprazole or ranitidine plus metoclopramide for patients with severe erosive oesophagitis. PharmacoEconomics. 1995;8(4):343-9.

11. Law AV, Pathak DS, Segraves AM, Weinstein CR, Arneson WH. Cost-effectiveness analysis of the conversion of patients with non-insulin-dependent diabetes mellitus from glipizide to glyburide and of the accompanying pharmacy follow-up clinic. Clin Ther. 1995;17(5):977-87.

12. Kaplan RM. Utility assessment for estimating quality-adjusted life years. In: Sloan FA, ed. Valuing health care: costs, benefits, and effectiveness of pharmaceuticals and other medical technologies. Cambridge, NY: Cambridge University Press; 1995.

13. Kennedy W, Reinharz D, Tessier G, Contandriopoulos AP, Trabut I, Champagne F, et al. Cost-utility analysis of chemotherapy and best supportive care in non-small cell lung cancer. PharmacoEconomics. 1995;8(4):316-23.

14. Jolicoeur LM, Jones-Grizzle AJ, Boyer JG. Guidelines for performing a pharmacoeconomic analysis. Am J Hosp Pharm. 1992;49:1741-7.

15. Shaw JW, Zachry WM. Application of probabilistic sensitivity analysis in decision analytic modeling. Formulary. 2002;37:32-4, 37-40.

16. McGhan WF, Lewis NJW. Basic bibliographies: pharmacoeconomics. Hosp Pharm. 1992;27:547-8.

17. Wanke LA, Huber SL. Basic bibliographies: cancer therapy pharmacoeconomics. Hosp Pharm. 1994;29:402.

18. Skaer TL, Williams LM. Basic bibliographies: biotechnology pharmacoeconomics I. Hosp Pharm. 1994;29:1053-4.

19. Skaer TL, Williams LM. Basic bibliographies: biotechnology pharmacoeconomics II. Hosp Pharm. 1994;29:1136.

20. McGhan WF. Basic bibliographies: pharmacoeconomics. Hosp Pharm. 1998;33:1270, 1273.

21. Duggan AE, Tolley K, Hawkey CJ, Logan RF. Varying efficacy of *Helicobacter pylori* eradication regimens: cost effectiveness study using a decision analysis model. BMJ. 1998;316:1648-54.

22. Messori A, Trippoli S, Becagli P, Cincotta M, Labbate MG, Zaccara G. Adjunctive lamotrigine therapy in patients with refractor y seizures: a lifetime cost-utility analysis. Eur J Clin Pharmacol. 1998;53(6):421-7.

23. Ginsberg G, Shani S, Lev B. Cost benefit analysis of risperidone and clozapine in the treatment of schizophrenia in Israel. PharmacoEconomics. 1998 Feb 13;231-41.

24. Sesti AM, Armitstead JA, Hall KN, Jang R, Milne S. Cost-minimization analysis of hand held nebulizer LC vs UC metered dose inhaler protocol for management of acute asthma exacerbations in the emergency department. ASHP Midyear Clinical Meeting; 32: MCS-7; 1997 Dec 8–12; New Orleans, LA.

25. Hinman AR, Koplan JP, Orenstein WA, Brink EW. Decision analysis and polio immunization policy. Am J Pub Health. 1988;78:301-3.

26. Kessler JM. Decision analysis in the formulary process. Am J Health-Syst Pharm. 1997; 54:S5-8.

27. Einarson TR, McGhan WF, Bootman JL. Decision analysis applied to pharmacy practice. Am J Hosp Pharm. 1985;42:364-71.

28. Walking D, Appino JP. Decision analysis in drug product development. Drug Cosmet Ind. 1973;112:39-41.

29. Rascati KL. Decision analysis techniques practical aspects of using personal computers for decision analytic modeling. Drug Benefit Trends. 1998; July:33-6.

30. Richardson WS, Detsky AS. Users' guides to the medical literature. Part 7. How to use a clinical decision analysis. Part A. Are the results of the study valid? JAMA. 1995;273:1292-5.

31. Richardson WS, Detsky AS. Users' guides to the medical literature. Part 7. How to use a clinical decision analysis. Part B. What are the results and will they help me in caring for my patients? JAMA. 1995;273:1610-3.

32. Baskin LE. Practical pharmacoeconomics. Cleveland, OH: Advanstar Communications; 1998.

33. Sacristán JA, Soto J, Galende I. Evaluation of pharmacoeconomic studies: utilization of a checklist. Ann Pharmacother. 1993;27:1126-32.

34. Botteman MF, Caprini J, Stephens JM, Nadipelli V, Bell CF, Pashos CL, et al. Results of an economic model to assess cost-effectiveness of enoxaparin, a low-molecular-weight heparin, versus warfarin for the prophylaxis of DVT and associated long-term complications in total hip replacement surgery in the United States. Clin Ther. 2002:24(11):1960-86.

35. Grutters J, Seferina S, Tjan-Heijnen V, van Kampen R, Goettsch W, Joore M. Bridging trial and decision: a checklist to frame health technology assessments for resource allocation decisions. Value Health [serial online]. 2011 Jul;14(5):777-84.

36. Husereau D, Drummond M, Loder E, et al. Consolidated Health Economic Evaluation Reporting Standards (CHEERS) statement. Value Health [serial online]. 2013 Mar;16(2):e1-5.

37. Doran C. Critique of an economic evaluation using the Drummond checklist. Appl Health Econ Health Policy [serial online]. 2010;8(6):357-9.

38. Chiou C, Hay J, Ofman J, et al. Development and validation of a grading system for the quality of cost-effectiveness studies. Med Care [serial online]. 2003 Jan;41(1):32-44.

39. Ofman J, Sullivan S, Hay J, et al. Examining the value and quality of health economic analyses: implications of utilizing the QHES. J Manag Care Pharm [serial online]. 2003 Jan;9(1):53-61.

40. Edwards R, Charles J, Lloyd-Williams H. Public health economics: a systematic review of guidance for the economic evaluation of public health interventions and discussion of key methodological issues. BMC Public Health [serial online]. 2013 Oct 24;13(1):1001.

41. Mullins CD, Flowers LR. Evaluating economic outcomes literature. In: Grauer DW, et al., eds. Pharmacoeconomics and outcomes: applications for patient care. 2nd ed. Kansas City, MO: American College of Clinical Pharmacy; 2003.

42. Makhinova T, Rascati KL. Pharmacoeconomics education in U.S. colleges and schools of pharmacy. Am J Pharm Educ. 2013;77(7):145.

43. Rascati KL. Essentials of pharmacoeconomics. 2nd ed. Philadelphia, PA: Wolters Kluwer/ Lippincott Williams & Wilkins; 2013.

44. Drummond MF, Sculpher MJ, Torrance GW, O'Brien BJ, Stoddart GL. Methods for the economic evaluation of health care programmes. 3rd ed. Oxford, NY: Oxford University Press; 2005.

SUGGESTED READINGS

1. Bingefors K, Pashos CL, Smith MD, Berger ML, Hedbloom EC, Torrance GW. Health care costs, quality, and outcomes: ISPOR book of terms. Lawrenceville, NJ: International Society for Pharmacoeconomics and Outcomes Research; 2003.

2. Drummond MF, Sculpher MJ, Torrance GW, O'Brien BJ, Stoddart GL. Methods for the economic evaluation of health care programmes. New York, NY: Oxford University Press; 2005.

3. Edwards R, Charles J, Lloyd-Williams H. Public health economics: a systematic review of guidance for the economic evaluation of public health interventions and discussion of key methodological issues. BMC Public Health [serial online]. 2013 Oct 24;13(1):1001.

4. Husereau D, Drummond M, Loder E, et al. Consolidated Health Economic Evaluation Reporting Standards (CHEERS) statement. Value Health [serial online]. 2013 Mar;16(2):e1-5.

5. Rascati KL. Essentials of pharmacoeconomics. 2nd ed. Philadelphia, PA: Wolters Kluwer/ Lippincott Williams & Wilkins; 2013.

8

Chapter Eight

Evidence-Based Clinical Practice Guidelines

Kevin G. Moores • Jeanine P. Abrons

Learning Objectives

● *After completing this chapter, the reader will be able to*

- Define clinical practice guideline.
- Define evidence-based medicine.
- Discuss collaboration and roles of health care professionals and pharmacists in the development and use of evidence-based clinical practice guidelines.
- Describe the methodology for development of evidence-based clinical practice guidelines.
- Discuss appropriate use of the GRADE system for grading the quality of evidence and the strength of recommendations.
- Describe application of the AGREE II instrument for evaluating clinical practice guidelines.
- Identify the key issues involved in the implementation and use of clinical practice guidelines.
- Identify sources of published clinical practice guidelines.

Key Concepts

❶ Clinical practice guidelines are recommendations for providing optimal patient care. These guidelines are developed through a systematic review of available evidence, incorporation of expert knowledge, and assessment of the benefits and harms of health care interventions for a particular topic or disease state.

❷ Evidence-based medicine (EBM) is a practice philosophy or approach to making clinical decisions for patients that involves individualization of patient care decisions based on the best available evidence and clinical experience.

❸ Evaluation of guideline quality, applicability, and appropriateness of use in a given setting depends primarily on an ability to distinguish methods that minimize potential biases in development.

❹ Formulation and articulation of clinical questions to be addressed by a guideline is a pivotal step, which provides direction for subsequent steps in the development of a guideline.

❺ Evaluation of evidence quality, which is the basis for recommendations, is a key aspect for interpretation and use of a practice guideline.

❻ The GRADE (Grading of Recommendations, Assessment, Development, and Evaluation) system presents an advantage that all evidence that is important for making a decision has been judged with explicit criteria. Judgments made are transparent. Evidence profiles and tables summarizing findings have been created. This consequently facilitates the use of best evidence.

❼ Prior to selecting a clinical practice guideline for implementation in any practice setting by a health care professional, it is important that the quality of published guidelines be evaluated. A useful tool for evaluating clinical practice guidelines was created by the Appraisal of Guidelines for Research and Evaluation (AGREE) collaboration.

❽ The most effective methods for implementing guidelines to achieve the desired effects of improved quality of care have not been determined.

❾ The National Guideline Clearinghouse website serves as a repository of clinical practice guidelines. Similar websites and peer-reviewed medical literature from secondary databases may allow for awareness and identification of practice standards.

Introduction

❶ Use of clinical practice guidelines to optimize patient care:

Clinical practice guidelines are recommendations for providing optimal patient care. These guidelines are developed through a systematic review of available evidence, incorporation of expert knowledge, and assessment of the benefits and harms of health care interventions for a particular topic or disease state.[1] Interventions evaluated may include use of medications and other types of therapy, such as radiation, surgery, and physical therapy. Clinical practice guidelines are developed by a variety of groups and organizations including federal and state government, professional associations, managed care organizations, third-party payers, quality assurance organizations, and utilization review groups. The purpose of the guidelines, the methods used in the development of the guidelines, format of the documents, and the strategies suggested for implementation vary widely.

Clinical practice guidelines have the potential to influence thousands to millions of decisions on medical interventions; therefore, it is incumbent for health care professionals to be thoroughly familiar with and evaluate the criteria used to judge the validity of guidelines. These professionals must be trained to develop appropriate skill sets and knowledge to determine appropriate application on a situation- and practice-specific basis.

Development and implementation of clinical practice guidelines require similar skillsets and steps to other areas of patient care and use of drug information. Required skillsets include an ability to clearly articulate or specify clinical questions, aptitude in literature search and evaluation strategies, knowledge of epidemiology and biostatistics, establishment and maintenance of clinical expertise, and development of adequate abilities to write, articulate, edit, format, and communicate knowledge and the basis of recommendations. Health care professionals benefit from the use of clinical practice guidelines as information resources.

Appropriately developed clinical practice guidelines provide concise summaries of the most up-to-date and highest quality evidence to differentiate efficacious and non-efficacious health care interventions. Available information and technologies used in health care rapidly evolve. Without clinical practice guidelines, individual health care providers are forced to locate, synthesize, and evaluate benefits and risks of treatments and technologies themselves. Guidelines are vital to organize and summarize the best evidence and knowledge available. Guidelines assist health care providers in clinical decision making, individualization of patient care, and to facilitate discussion of care options consistent with patient needs and preferences. Guidelines also may enhance interprofessional collaboration among health care professionals and may establish a basis for continuity of care, especially when decisions require involvement of multiple health care professionals and transitions of care between different settings.[2]

A significant time lag occurs in translation and incorporation of research into practice. One goal in the development and implementation of evidence-based clinical practice guidelines is to accelerate common use of evidence in practice. Delay in knowledge of well-studied and efficacious treatments has resulted in underutilization of these interventions and continued use of interventions proven to be ineffective.[3] Development of accurate, complete, and transparent guidelines and the incorporation of these guidelines into evidence-based clinical practice may facilitate more rapid adoption of available and strong evidence into clinical practice.

Clinical practice guidelines can assist with identification of indicators for establishment and assessment of care quality. The key issues in reforming the U.S. health care system are access to care, cost, and quality. Quality and safety were a major focus as evidenced by landmark reports published by the National Academy of Medicine, formerly known as the Institute of Medicine (IOM), regarding quality of care problems in the United States, recommendations to focus on improvements in patient safety, and recommendations to reduce preventable medical errors.[4-7] The central concepts in these reports and recommendations relate to using the best available evidence, providing decision support tools, use of informatics, and participation of patients in health care decisions and responsibilities. The National Academy of Medicine reports dealt specifically with standards for clinical practice guidelines, systematic reviews of comparative effectiveness research, and providing care at a lower cost.[1,8,9] These documents and standards highlighted improvements in technology, information technology, quality of access to electronic records, and greater ability to use the data from processes of care to provide valuable information to learn what works best. These concepts were central to improving the validity and usefulness of clinical practice guidelines.

Methods currently recommended as the most valid for development of clinical practice guidelines emphasize an evidence-based approach, formal quantitative techniques to calculate risks and benefits, and incorporation of the patient's preference. The concepts of an evidence-based approach and use of methods to grade the quality of evidence and strength of recommendations are critical elements that will be reviewed in more detail in this chapter. The evidence-based health care movement and the implementation of continuous quality improvement (CQI) programs stimulated growth in guideline development. Advancements continue to be made for the methods of evaluating and summarizing the best available evidence. Development of information databases of systematic reviews and new informatics resources have facilitated the production of clinical practice guidelines and improved access to this information.

This chapter will present a review of the background of clinical practice guidelines and evidence-based medicine; review evidence-based methods for guideline development, evaluation, and implementation; and provide directions to locate sources of guidelines.

Evidence-Based Medicine and Clinical Practice Guidelines

❷ *Evidence-based medicine (EBM) is a practice philosophy or approach to making clinical decisions for patients that involves individualization of patient care decisions based on the best available evidence and clinical experience.*[10] The practice of EBM integrates individual clinical expertise with the best available published clinical evidence from systematic research. EBM is often mistaken for, or reduced to, one of its several components, critical appraisal of the literature. However, EBM requires both clinical expertise and an intimate knowledge of the individual patient's circumstance, beliefs, priorities, and values to be useful. External evidence must be used to inform, but not replace, individual clinical expertise. It is clinical expertise that determines if the external evidence may be applied to the individual patient and, if so, how it should be used in decision making by the patient and the health care provider. The development and application of clinical practice guidelines are among the tools used in EBM. In fact, the first published use of the term evidence-based was in the context of clinical guidelines.[11] An understanding of EBM is necessary to understand recommended methods for production and implementation of guidelines.

Physicians at McMaster University in Hamilton, Ontario are cited as being the first to use the term evidence-based medicine. These physicians, known as the Evidence-Based Medicine Working Group, published a description of what they considered a new paradigm for medical practice and teaching.[12] The article presented by the group articulated views on changes that were occurring in medical practice relating to the use of medical literature to more effectively guide decision making. They stated that the foundation for the paradigm shift rested in significant advances in clinical research, such as the development of the randomized controlled trial and meta-analysis.

The practice of EBM has been described as focusing on five linked activities: (1) converting the information need into a clearly defined answerable clinical question, (2) conducting a search for the best available evidence for the problem, (3) critically appraising the validity, impact, and applicability of the evidence, (4) incorporating the critical appraisal with clinical expertise and the patient's unique characteristics, and (5) evaluating effectiveness and efficiency in executing the first four activities and identifying ways to improve them.[13] These activities are remarkably similar to the systematic approach to drug information requests as outlined by Watanabe and colleagues in 1975 which are still used today.[14]

Following the original paper on EBM by the Evidence-Based Medicine Working Group,[12] the lead individuals published a description of appropriate training methods on evidence-based care to enable practitioners to locate, evaluate, and apply the best evidence.[15] The description recognized that not all practitioners have the time or an interest to use primary literature. The description noted that sources of appropriately pre-appraised evidence could be used. Examples of pre-appraised evidence include clinical practice guidelines and systematic reviews that have been produced with evidence-based methods. The authors noted that skill in interpreting the medical literature is still necessary to judge the quality of the pre-appraised resources. This skill enables the health care professional to know when recommendations provided by pre-appraised resources are applicable, and to determine when to use the original literature when pre-appraised resources are unavailable.[15]

In a review of the philosophy of EBM, Eddy described an approach that is similar to the Evidence-Based Medicine Working Group.[11] The Evidence-Based Medicine Working Group's original description of the practice was referred to as evidence-based individual decision making. Eddy referred to evidence-based guidelines as a second approach to EBM. This second approach has four important features: (1) small, specially trained groups analyze evidence and develop the guideline, (2) an explicit, rigorous process is used, (3) the guideline is not specific to an individual patient but rather should be applicable to a class or group of patients, and (4) the guideline should indirectly help, guide, or motivate health care providers to deliver certain types of care to people, not directly determine the care for a specific patient.[11] Eddy explained further that the most appropriate definition of EBM was a combination of these two approaches. The combination provides for medical practice that will achieve the most efficient and effective use of evidence.

Health care professionals face the complicated reality of constantly changing and increasing medical knowledge. To practice effective, high-quality medicine, it is not necessary to memorize vast amounts of information; it is necessary to develop skills to acquire and critically assess information that is necessary to make clinical decisions.[16] The philosophy of EBM is consistent with the philosophy of clinical practice guidelines. The decision-making process of EBM is supported by access and use of clinical practice guidelines.

Guideline Development Methods

A thorough understanding of the methodology used for clinical practice guideline development is critical for health care practitioners. Although relatively few practitioners actually participate in guideline development, this understanding will prepare them for involvement in appropriate evaluation and implementation of these guidelines. ❸ *Evaluation of guideline quality, applicability, and appropriateness of use in a given setting depends primarily on the ability to distinguish methods that minimize potential biases in development.* A lack of understanding of the requirements for guideline development could lead to inappropriate interpretation, or acceptance of inappropriate levels of enforcement of biased guideline recommendations. Application of biased guidelines may result in provision of ineffective or harmful therapy. Due to the central importance of guideline development methods, a significant portion of this chapter is devoted to this topic.

Many organizations produce clinical practice guidelines, and although there are currently no uniformly endorsed standards for their development, substantial progress has been made through cooperative efforts. For example, The EQUATOR network, which stands for Enhancing the QUAlity and Transparency Of health Research, serves as an "umbrella organization that brings together researchers, medical journal editors, peer reviewers, developers of reporting guidelines, research funding bodies, and other collaborators with mutual interest in improving the quality of research publications and of research itself." A comprehensive collection of reporting guidelines for main study types is maintained and use of guidelines is actively promoted.[17] Many endorsed standards for research can be located here and should be applied to ensure literature incorporated into clinical practice guidelines is sound. In 2008, the former IOM was charged with developing and promoting standards for systematic reviews of comparative effectiveness research and evidence-based clinical practice guidelines.[1] Two committees were formed: the Committee on Standards for Systematic Reviews of Comparative Effectiveness Research and the Committee on Standards for Developing Trustworthy Clinical Practice Guidelines. In 2011, the committees published proposed standards for systematic reviews of comparative effectiveness research[8] and for developing rigorous, trustworthy clinical practice guidelines.[1]

The IOM proposed eight standards (Table 8-1) for developing evidence-based clinical practice guidelines. The major steps in their proposed standards include[1]

- Establishing transparency
- Management of conflict of interest
- Guideline development group composition
- Clinical practice guideline-systematic review intersection
- Establishing evidence foundations for and rating strength of recommendations
- Articulation of recommendations
- External review
- Updating the guideline

Each of these steps will be discussed separately below.

ESTABLISHING TRANSPARENCY

The standard for this step calls for the processes by which the guideline was developed and funded to be transparent. In other words, how the guideline was developed and funded should be explicitly detailed and the public should have access to this information. Transparency helps users understand how the recommendations were made, who developed them, and what bias was potentially introduced. The clinical experience of the guideline development group's members and potential conflicts of interest (COI) should be stated as well.[1]

MANAGING CONFLICTS OF INTEREST

The standard for this step provides details for managing of potential COI by members of the guideline development group. COI include not only financial COI, but also include intellectual conflicts that may occur as a result of previous research published by the individual, institutional COI, and patient-public activities.[1]

TABLE 8–1. STANDARDS FOR DEVELOPING TRUSTWORTHY CLINICAL PRACTICE GUIDELINES[1]

1. Establishing transparency
   1.1 The processes by which clinical practice guidelines are developed and funded should be detailed explicitly and publicly accessible.
2. Management of conflicts of interest (COI)
   2.1 Prior to selection of the guideline development group (GDG), individuals considered for membership should declare all interests and activities potentially resulting in COI with guideline development, by written disclosure to those convening the GDG:
      - Disclosure should reflect all current and planned commercial (including services from which a clinician derives a substantial proportion of income), noncommercial, intellectual, institutional, and patient-public activities pertinent to the potential scope of the clinical practice guideline.
   2.2 Disclosure of COI within GDG:
      - All COI of each GDG member should be reported and discussed by the prospective development group prior to the onset of his or her work.
      - Each panel member should explain how his or her COI could influence the clinical practice guideline development process or specific recommendations.
   2.3 Divestment
      - Members of the GDG should divest themselves of financial investments in which they or their family members have, and not participate in marketing activities or advisory boards of entities whose interests could be affected by clinical practice guideline recommendations.
   2.4 Exclusions
      - Whenever possible, GDG members should not have COI.
      - In some circumstances, a GDG may not be able to perform its work without members who have COI, such as relevant clinical specialists who receive a substantial portion of their incomes from services pertinent to the clinical practice guideline.
      - Members with COI should represent no more than a minority of the GDG.
      - The chair or cochairs of a guideline should not have COI.
      - Funders should have no role in clinical practice guideline development.
3. Guideline development group composition
   3.1 The GDG should be multidisciplinary and balanced, comprising a variety of methodological experts and clinicians, and populations to be affected by the clinical practice guideline.
   3.2 Patient and public involvement should be facilitated by including (at least at the time of clinical question formulation and draft clinical practice guideline review) a current or former patient, and a patient advocate or patient/consumer organization representative in the GDG.
   3.3 Strategies to increase effective participation of patient and consumer representatives, including training in appraisal of evidence, should be adopted by GDGs.
4. Clinical practice guideline-systematic review intersection
   4.1 Clinical practice guideline developers should use systematic reviews that meet standards set by the Institute of Medicine's Committee on Standards for Systematic Reviews of Comparative Effectiveness Research.
   4.2 When systematic reviews are conducted specifically to inform particular guidelines, the GDG and systematic review team should interact regarding the scope, approach, and output of both processes.
5. Establishing evidence foundations for and rating strength of recommendations
   5.1 For each recommendation, the following should be provided:
      - An explanation of the reasoning underlying the recommendation, including:
         ○ a clear description of potential benefits and harms;

continued

TABLE 8–1. STANDARDS FOR DEVELOPING TRUSTWORTHY CLINICAL PRACTICE GUIDELINES (*CONTINUED*)

- ◦ a summary of relevant available evidence (and evidentiary gaps), description of the quality (including applicability), quantity (including completeness), and consistency of the aggregate available evidence;
- ◦ an explanation of the part played by values, opinion, theory, and clinical experience in deriving the recommendation.
- A rating of the level of confidence in (certainty regarding) the evidence underpinning the recommendation
- A rating of the strength of the recommendation in light of the preceding bullets
- A description and explanation of any differences of opinion regarding the recommendation

6. Articulation of recommendations
   6.1 Recommendations should be articulated in a standardized form detailing precisely what the recommended action is, and under what circumstances it should be performed.
   6.2 Strong recommendations should be worded so that compliance with the recommendation(s) can be evaluated.

7. External review
   7.1 External reviewers should comprise a full spectrum of relevant stakeholders, including scientific and clinical experts, organizations (e.g., health care, specialty societies), agencies (e.g., federal government), patients, and representatives of the public.
   7.2 The authorship of external reviews submitted by individuals and/or organizations should be kept confidential unless that protection has been waived by the reviewer(s).
   7.3 The GDG should consider all external reviewer comments and keep a written record of the rationale for modifying or not modifying a clinical practice guideline in response to reviewers' comments.
   7.4 A draft of the clinical practice guideline at the external review stage or immediately following it (i.e., prior to the final draft) should be made available to the general public for comment. Reasonable notice of impending publication should be provided to interested public stakeholders.

8. Updating guidelines
   8.1 The date of clinical practice guideline publication, date of pertinent systematic evidence review, and proposed date for future clinical practice guideline review should be documented in the clinical practice guideline.
   8.2 Literature should be monitored regularly following clinical practice guideline publication to identify the emergence of new, potentially relevant evidence and to evaluate the continued validity of the clinical practice guideline.
   8.3 Clinical practice guidelines should be updated when new evidence suggests the need for modification of clinically important recommendations. For example, a clinical practice guideline should be updated if new evidence shows that a recommended intervention causes previously unknown substantial harm; that a new intervention is significantly superior to a previously recommended intervention from an efficacy or harms perspective; or that a recommendation can be applied to new populations.

Individuals being considered for membership on a guideline development panel should be asked to declare potential COI. Individuals with a potential conflict of interest may still be considered for participation on a panel depending on the type and degree of conflict, along with appropriate levels of management and disclosure.[18] Rigid adherence to exclusion of any possible conflict could result in guideline panels excluding the majority of individuals with the critical expertise needed. Surveys have shown the need for attention to this issue as guideline authors frequently have some relationship with pharmaceutical manufacturers.[19] Controversies over the sponsorship of guideline development and publication[20] and potential COI by panel members[21] have occurred.

The American College of Chest Physicians is one prominent guideline development group that placed an emphasis on dealing with conflict of interest in their most recent complete edition of their Guideline on Antithrombotic Therapy and Prevention of Thrombosis.[22] The primary leadership and responsibility for authorship of each article was assigned to a methodologist with no COI, who in most cases also was a practicing physician, but not an expert on the topic of thrombosis. Some experts nominated to participate in a panel were not accepted because of the magnitude of financial COI. Panel members who had conflicts, either financial or intellectual, could be limited to some extent in participation in discussions and could not participate in the final process of decisions regarding the direction or strength of a recommendation.[22,23]

ESTABLISHING A MULTIDISCIPLINARY GUIDELINE DEVELOPMENT GROUP

The standard for this step relates to the composition of the group to develop the guideline and includes patient and public involvement in the process. Patient involvement is especially important in helping to formulate and prioritize the questions to be addressed by the guideline. This standard also provides direction for how to obtain input from panel members, reach consensus, and make decisions through the group process.[1]

Clinical practice guideline development should involve a multidisciplinary team. Ideally, all groups that have a stake in the development and implementation of a guideline are represented in the process. Participants should include physicians with special expertise in the condition being considered; primary care providers involved in the treatment of patients with the identified condition; representatives of other health care disciplines involved in providing care for the identified condition (e.g., pharmacy, physical therapy, respiratory therapy, nursing, occupational therapy, social work, dentistry); experts in research methods applicable to the topic; individuals with expertise in conducting a systematic search for evidence; individuals with administrative, health services, economics, and other health care systems expertise; and patient representatives or caregivers. Organizational skills, project management, and editorial ability also are key to successfully developing a guideline (Case Study 8-1).

Case Study 8-1

You have been selected to evaluate clinical practice guidelines to be implemented within your health system. You have been given no required criteria to evaluate the clinical practice guidelines that you review. You know that there is the Institute of Medicine (IOM) process for developing evidence-based clinical practice guidelines. As you think about evaluation of clinical practice guidelines, what are the first four steps that you want to ensure that IOM panel members have taken?

CLINICAL PRACTICE GUIDELINE AND SYSTEMATIC REVIEW INTERSECTION

The standard for this step acknowledges the overlap between clinical practice guidelines and systematic reviews (see Chapter 5 for more information on systematic reviews). It recognizes that systematic reviews are important for preparing a synthesis of evidence for the guideline development group to use in formulating recommendations that will be based on the best and most complete available evidence.[1] This standard recommends that clinical practice guideline developers conduct systematic reviews that meet the standards in the IOM's previously mentioned companion publication for systematic reviews of comparative effectiveness research. A few key steps in the companion publication for systematic reviews of comparative research include the following (these are described in more detail below)[8]:

- Select an appropriate topic for creation of a guideline.
- Define the clinical questions to be addressed.
- Determine the study screening selection criteria.
- Conduct a systematic search for evidence.
- Critically appraise individual studies.
- Synthesize the body of evidence.

Select an Appropriate Topic for Creation of a Guideline

Selecting a topic for guideline development has aspects in common with selecting topics for a medication use evaluation, or in a broader sense for any quality improvement program (see Chapter 16). Guidelines are intended to improve the quality and outcomes of care. Therefore, it is important to consider the potential to achieve this improvement when a topic is chosen. As with any clinical management decision, the potential benefits of development and implementation of a guideline should be assessed. Disease states with the maximum potential for benefit from guideline development and implementation share common characteristics including the following:

- High prevalence
- High frequency and/or severity of associated morbidity or mortality
- Availability of high-quality evidence for the efficacy of treatments that may reduce morbidity or mortality
- Feasibility of implementation of the treatment based on expertise and resources required

- Potential cost-effectiveness
- Evidence that current practice is not optimal
- Evidence of practice variation; that is, patients with similar characteristics are provided different services or a substantially different frequency of services in different locations
- Availability of personnel, expertise, and resources to develop and implement the practice guideline

As an example, the American Heart Association (AHA) identified the following reasons for developing evidence-based guidelines for cardiovascular disease prevention in women[24]:

- Cardiovascular disease is the leading cause of death of women in the United States.
- It is essential that coronary heart disease (CHD) be prevented because it is often fatal, and the majority of women who die suddenly have not had any previous symptoms.
- There was an increased need to review and develop strategies for the prevention of CHD in women following the Women's Health Initiative and the Heart and Estrogen/Progestin Replacement Study.
- The number and percentage of women participating in clinical trials has been increasing, which provides more evidence of efficacy of different treatment strategies.
- Characteristics of patients seen in clinical practice may not be similar to those of clinical trial participants. Therefore, it is necessary to evaluate the ability to apply these data in practice.

Define the Clinical Questions to be Addressed

After the topic has been selected, the next step is to further define the specific issues for which the recommendations will ultimately be provided. The guideline development group will consider what specific decision-making or action steps can be improved with recommendations related to disease surveillance or screening methods for disease detection, confirmation of the diagnosis, or treatment. Decision-making points can be expressed as clinical questions. ❹ *Formulation and articulation of clinical questions to be addressed by a guideline is a pivotal step, which provides direction for subsequent steps in the development of a guideline.* The questions are important to provide direction to the systematic review of the literature, and also provide the outline for the recommendations that the guideline will provide. The importance of this phase cannot be overemphasized. Just as in the systematic approach to a drug information question, it is critical to first clearly define the question to be successful in searching for the necessary evidence, and subsequently be able to provide useful valid conclusions.

A clear description of the questions to be addressed by the guideline also is a good starting point for a practitioner to determine if a guideline could be useful in his or her practice. Depending on the overall goals of a guideline, questions may be about the best diagnostic test, methods of screening, what forms of treatment or prevention are most effective, quantification of the potential harms of treatment, what comorbidities change recommendations, or what costs are associated with different management strategies.

One of the important steps for guideline developers, and perhaps even more important for guideline users, is the careful framing of the clinical questions. Many guideline development groups use the Patients-Interventions-Comparison-Outcomes (PICO) model for framing the questions, which includes the following parts[13]:

- *P*atients: Which patients are being considered for the guideline, how can they be described, and do any subgroups require special consideration? This is similar to inclusion and exclusion criteria in a clinical study, however, usually not as restrictive.
- *I*nterventions: Which intervention or treatment should be considered?
- *C*omparison: What other interventions or treatment should be compared with the intervention being considered?
- *O*utcome: What is most important to the patient (e.g., mortality, morbidity, treatment complications, rates of relapse, physical function, quality of life, costs)?

The clinical questions should define the relevant patient population, the management strategies that will and will not be considered, and the outcomes of care that the guideline intends to achieve. All the questions that are necessary for consideration of patient management in a given clinical scenario are delineated to make sure that the recommendations provided by the guideline will be of sufficient scope to avoid important gaps in decision making. There is no specific standard for the number of questions required for each guideline. However, most guideline development groups state that if the number exceeds 30, or in some cases 40 questions, it may be necessary to break the guideline into subtopics. Subtopics may be determined to construct a guideline for making recommendations for screening or diagnosis in one guideline and recommendations for treatment in another. Other subtopics may be based on differentiation of populations that have different levels of severity of disease, for example, New York Heart Association classes of heart failure, or based on other demographic factors that might call for different recommendations for care of those patients. The American College of Chest Physicians guidelines on antithrombotic therapy created several subtopics such as antithrombotic therapy in pregnancy, in persons with peripheral artery disease, in ischemic stroke, in valvular disease, in atrial fibrillation, and others.

In some instances, a preliminary review of the literature may be necessary to assist with delineation of the focused clinical questions to be considered in the guideline.

Clinical experts in the field as well as patients provide critical input in formulating the clinical questions.

Determine the Study Screening Selection Criteria

It is necessary to define the admissible evidence, that is, the types of published or unpublished research to be considered so that an appropriate literature search may be performed. Key words from the focused clinical questions define the types of patients, interventions, comparators, and outcomes of studies that are considered to provide useful evidence. The guideline panel may decide that it will consider evidence from previous guidelines, meta-analyses or systematic reviews, and randomized controlled trials. The panel also may decide to consider evidence from observational studies, diagnostic studies, economic studies, and qualitative studies. This direction is necessary for the information specialists that will conduct the search for evidence. Detailed criteria also are important in this step. This ensures that evidence will be retrieved and selected for inclusion in the review with a minimum of bias, that the search is reproducible, and that the entire process is as transparent as possible. In most cases, more than one person is involved in searching for evidence and selecting evidence for consideration in the review. Clear criteria must be used so that there is consistency among all individuals involved in this process. Inconsistency in the retrieval of evidence between evaluators would add a potential for bias in the review.

The process to define admissible evidence also may be revisited at a later stage of guideline development depending on the results of the initial search. It is conceivable, and in fact common, that based on the initial review of evidence, the questions may be modified or new questions formed, and a decision may be made to expand the scope of admissible evidence. Documentation of these decisions, and the reasons for any changes, is another indicator of a guideline that has been developed with rigorous methods.

Conduct a Systematic Search for Evidence

Evidence-based guidelines require that all relevant evidence is located and appraised. A thorough literature search must be conducted. Many guideline development groups will first conduct a search to identify previously completed guidelines or systematic reviews of the same or closely related questions. The literature retrieval process should include a search of the available bibliographic resources such as MEDLINE®, Current Contents®, EMBASE, Science Citation Index, The Cochrane Library, International Pharmaceutical Abstracts, and Cumulative Index to Nursing and Allied Health Literature (CINAHL). A number of specialized databases exist and should be considered depending on the subject of the search. Also, evidence may be obtained from citations listed in published bibliographies, textbooks, and any literature that may be identified by researchers and other individuals on the expert list that the panel may create. Specific key words and other search constraints, for example, Medical Subject Headings (MeSH) terms from MEDLINE®, limits by publication year, language, randomized controlled trials or other study types, and so forth should be recorded to allow verification of the process. Each retrieved article should then be judged for its relevance and compliance to criteria for inclusion as predetermined by the panel. A log should be kept of excluded studies and the rationale for their rejection.

A review of all the details regarding search strategies, such as controlled vocabulary searching, text word searching, truncation of terms, use of the vocabulary tree structures to explode select terms, and adjacency of terms are beyond the scope of this chapter. Most guideline development groups use highly trained methodologists and librarians to perform this critical search for evidence. Drug information specialists also are well qualified to complete this task. A carefully planned and executed search is necessary to obtain a result that is very sensitive to avoid missing important evidence and at the same time as specific as possible to avoid the requirement to manually screen many irrelevant citations.

Critically Appraise Individual Studies

There are a variety of methods for evaluating individual studies. The purpose of this process is to identify issues with trial design or biases that would affect internal or external validity. Issues to consider include the basic trial design (i.e., randomized, controlled, clinical trial, cohort study, and case-control study), sample size, statistical power, selection bias, inclusion/exclusion criteria, choice of control group, randomization methods, comparability of groups, definition of exposure or intervention, definition of outcome measures, accuracy and appropriateness of outcome measures, attrition rates, data collection methods, methods of statistical analysis, confounding variables, unique characteristics of the study population, and adequacy of blinding. There are other factors to be considered in the overall body of evidence. For example, whether the results of different trials are consistent with each other or if there is significant heterogeneity. The amount of evidence, or how many individuals are evaluated over what length of time, also is an important consideration. This is particularly important in consideration of the safety of treatments. Potential serious adverse events that occur infrequently will not be identified in databases that do not contain sufficient sample size or in sample populations that are too narrowly defined. See Chapters 4 and 5 for information on literature evaluation. It also may be necessary to review Chapter 7 for information on how to evaluate cost information.

Synthesize the Body of Evidence

Evidence from selected studies should be summarized in a way that allows the panel to begin developing conclusions. Clear formats enable review of characteristics and quality of individual studies, consistency of results between studies, overall size of the evidence database, and size of treatment effects for benefits and harms. If necessary evidence is available, a meta-analysis may be appropriate to present the summary estimate of the treatment effect size (see Chapter 5 for information on meta-analyses) (Case Study 8-2).

Building on Case 8-1, you are asked to evaluate how the clinical questions addressed were defined. You are asked to present and describe the PICO format and how it can be used to frame clinical questions and the potential usefulness in clinical practice guideline development. How would you do this?

ESTABLISHING EVIDENCE FOUNDATIONS FOR AND RATING STRENGTH OF RECOMMENDATIONS

This step focuses on the important process of rating the quality of the evidence and strength of recommendations of the guideline produced. The Grading of Recommendations, Assessment, Development, and Evaluation (GRADE) Working Group has developed the most accepted system for determining strength of recommendations and rating quality of evidence.[25] The **GRADE system**, although not specifically endorsed by the National Academy of Medicine, meets essential qualities of the National Academy of Medicine recommended standards. This also is the system used with minor modification by the American College of Chest Physicians[23] and by many other developers of high-quality guidelines. Greater detail on the GRADE system is provided below because the approach to rating the quality of evidence (or the confidence in the estimates of the effects) and the approach for grading the strength of the recommendations are key characteristics for the clinical use of a guideline.

GRADE System of Grading Quality of Evidence and Strength of Recommendations
The GRADE Working Group began in 2000 as an informal international collaboration of people who recognized shortcomings of the grading systems available at that time and wished to offer recommendations for improvement.

The GRADE Working Group first published standardized grading methods for the quality of the evidence and the strength of recommendations in practice guidelines in 2004.[26] The Working Group believed that consistent judgments about the quality of evidence and strength of recommendations, combined with better communication about those judgments, would be achieved by use of the GRADE system. Ultimately, the Working Group felt that the GRADE system would support better informed choices in health care.[26] A five-part series of updated information on GRADE was published in 2008,[27] and a 22-part series was started in 2011.[25]

❺ *Evaluation of evidence quality, which is the basis for recommendations, is a key aspect for interpretation and use of a practice guideline.* However, before deciding to implement a guideline recommendation, it is also necessary for the user to have information to consider the balance between benefits and harms. It also is necessary to have the ability to translate evidence to specific circumstances (i.e., external validity). A system to communicate the strength of a recommendation should consider all of these factors. The designated strength of a recommendation should convey the level of confidence that adherence to that recommendation will do more good than harm.[26]

The GRADE system uses precise definitions of quality of evidence and strength of recommendation. The quality of evidence indicates the amount of confidence that an estimate of effect is correct. The strength of a recommendation indicates the amount of confidence that following the recommendation will do more good than harm.[25] Use of the GRADE system requires assessment of the validity of results of individual studies for important outcomes and sequential judgments about the following[26]:

- The quality of evidence across studies for each important outcome
- Which outcomes are critical to a decision
- The overall quality of evidence across these critical outcomes
- The balance between benefits and harms
- The strength of the recommendations

The GRADE system starts with clearly defined clinical questions using the PICO model. It considers all outcomes that are important to patients.[28] The GRADE system classifies each outcome as critical, important but not critical, or of limited importance. Guideline developers also may use a 9-point scale with 7 to 9 representing critical outcomes, 4 to 6 representing important outcomes, and 1 to 3 representing outcomes of limited importance. Critical outcomes are given more weight in the final recommendation. Outcomes related to possible harms of therapy also must be considered.[28]

Evidence quality of each outcome should be decided on the basis of a systematic review using explicit criteria. The GRADE system initially considers randomized trials to be high-quality evidence and observational studies to be low-quality evidence.[29] These ratings may then be increased or decreased based on additional factors (Table 8-2). There are five reasons for lowering the level of confidence rating (risk of bias, inconsistency, indirectness, imprecision, publication bias). Three reasons for rating the level of confidence higher are provided (large effect, dose response, all plausible confounding).[29]

Basic study design does not tell the whole story of the quality of evidence. The risk for bias is assessed by the guideline panel based on several factors.[30] Factors include that randomization, when it is used correctly, has tremendous power to reduce the potential bias in the results. However, there are randomized controlled trials in which other aspects of the study design are seriously flawed. There are observational studies (e.g., follow-up, case-control, interrupted time series, controlled before and after) with very strong methods that may produce high-quality evidence. Consideration for the quality of a study method

TABLE 8–2. GRADE SYSTEM TO RATING CONFIDENCE IN EFFECT ESTIMATES[28]

1. Establish Initial Level of Confidence		2. Consider Lowering or Raising Level of Confidence		3. Final Level of Confidence Rating
		Reasons for considering lowering or raising confidence		
Study design	Initial confidence in an estimate of effect	↓ Lower if	↑ Higher if	Confidence in an estimate of effect across those considerations
Randomized trials →	High confidence	Risk of bias −1 Serious −2 Very serious Inconsistency −1 Serious −2 Very serious Indirectness −1 Serious −2 Very serious Imprecision −1 Serious −2 Very serious Publication bias −1 Likely −2 Very likely	Large effect +1 Large +2 Very large Dose response +1 Gradient found All plausible residual confounding and bias +1 Would reduce a demonstrated effect or +1 Would suggest a spurious effect if no effect was observed	High ⊕⊕⊕⊕ Moderate ⊕⊕⊕ Low ⊕⊕ Very low ⊕
Observational studies →	Low confidence			

GRADE = Grading of Recommendations, Assessment, Development, and Evaluation.

must include criteria such as adequacy of allocation concealment, blinding, completeness of follow-up, appropriate and relevant outcome reporting, stopping early for benefit, use of validated outcome measures, and lack of other design or execution errors in the study.[30]

The inconsistency of results between different studies also can reduce confidence that the results are valid. If the point estimates of results vary widely across studies, confidence intervals show overlap, or statistical tests for heterogeneity are significant and the differences are not explained, the quality of evidence will be rated lower.[31]

The directness of the results refers to the extent to which subjects, interventions, and outcomes of a study are similar to the target population for a given treatment recommendation.[32] If study subjects differ from the patients treated in ways that may predict a different response based on identifiable factors, the quality of evidence for the clinician's decision making is not as great. Common examples of these identifiable factors may include age, gender, race, other comorbidities or severity of illness. In addition, studies using **surrogate endpoints**, or intermediate outcomes, are not as reliable for estimation of ultimate treatment benefits. Surrogate endpoints are laboratory values or physical assessments that are markers that predict the actual clinical events, but the time from the presence of the surrogate outcome and the ultimate clinical outcome may be long in some cases. They also may be an imperfect predictor of the important clinical outcome. Surrogate endpoints include measurements such as changes in bone mineral density rather than incidence of fractures, and effects of a medication on pulmonary function rather than on mortality. Another example in which indirect evidence must be used is when there are no studies comparing different interventions directly and the evaluation must be made across different studies. This is a common problem with new drugs that have been studied only in comparison to placebo and not to other effective treatments. With this type of comparison, it is difficult to determine which treatment is more effective, and it is even more difficult to estimate the size of a potential treatment difference.[32] The recent development of new oral anticoagulants provides both a positive and negative example of this issue. All of the new oral anticoagulants were studied in direct comparison with warfarin for various indications. However, none of the four new medications that were evaluated have been directly compared with each other. This fact influenced how the ACCP made recommendations in the update of Antithrombotic Therapy Guidelines.[33]

The measure of imprecision in study results is primarily assessed by examination of the 95% confidence interval (see Chapter 6).[34] If the 95% confidence interval crosses the boundary of benefit versus harm, the treatment would not be considered to be proven effective. For example, with a relative risk of a clinical event measured as 0.8, but a 95% confidence interval of 0.5 to 1.1, the result is not considered to be statistically significant. Such a confidence interval does not exclude the possibility of either a reduction or an increase in risk of the event. Also, if the confidence interval extends into a point in which the size of the clinical benefit no longer would be judged to be greater than the potential adverse effects, burden of treatment, and costs, the level of evidence should be graded down. It also is recommended that the absolute risk difference or number needed to treat (NNT) be the value for consideration of the size of the treatment benefit.[34] Absolute risk differences take into consideration the baseline risk, or the risk of the event with no treatment, and are therefore a more meaningful value to represent the size of the potential treatment benefits for a specific patient.

Publication bias also may be a reason to lower the rating of evidence quality. Risk of publication bias is generally greatest early in the development of a new therapy, when there are relatively few studies published and particularly when the sample size is small.[35] Many factors may contribute to publication bias. Industry sponsors may be reluctant to publish negative results. Authors, journal editors, and peer reviewers all have been implicated in a bias against publication of negative results. Negative results are often slower to be published and are more likely to be published in non-English or limited-circulation journals. One method to assess the potential of publication bias is the funnel plot; however, it is not very sensitive or precise.[35] See Chapter 5 for more information about publication bias and funnel plots.

Increases to the confidence rating of evidence made by the GRADE system may occur for one of three reasons. The most common reason to increase the confidence rating of evidence is for a large treatment effect.[36] Another reason for increasing the level of confidence in an observational study by one level is if it shows at least a twofold increase or decrease in risk (odds ratio or relative risk—see Chapters 4 through 6) and by two levels if the effect is a fivefold difference in risk. The third reason to increase the rating level is if a dose-response relationship has been demonstrated in the treatment effect.[36] A dose-response relationship has been considered a factor in causality assessment since the Bradford Hill criteria[37] were published in 1965. If all plausible confounding factors would predict that an observational study in fact underestimated the size of a beneficial treatment effect, that also would be a reason to increase the level of confidence rating of the evidence.[36] In general, decisions to rate the quality of evidence at a higher level should only be considered in the absence of one or more of the five factors mentioned above that are cause for rating the evidence lower.

Based on consideration of the components described above, the GRADE system arrives at one of the following grades of evidence to express the degree of confidence that the true effect is close to the estimate of the effect[29]:

- High = very confident
- Moderate = moderately confident
- Low = limited confidence
- Very low: very little confidence

Many guideline development groups collapse the low and very low confidence grades into a single grade.

The evidence for harms should be graded using the same system as the evidence for benefits. This creates a challenge when making judgments about the balance of benefits and harms because the evidence quality for harms is rarely on the same level as the evidence for benefits. An example is evidence for harms for rosiglitazone (Avandia®), where obtaining high-quality evidence about harm is a more difficult process. The magnitude of the balance of the benefits compared to the harms, as well as value judgments of the desirability of the benefits and harms, also must be considered for treatment recommendations. In addition, information should be provided to demonstrate how evidence translates into specific circumstances. Assessment of what adjustments may be necessary for individuals with different baseline risks, or who are receiving treatment in different settings should be given. The GRADE Working Group recommends the following definitions to categorize the trade-off between benefits and harms[26]:

- *Net benefits:* The intervention clearly does more good than harm.
- *Trade-offs:* There are important trade-offs between the benefits and harms.
- *Uncertain trade-offs:* It is not clear whether the intervention does more good than harm.
- *No net benefits:* The intervention clearly does not do more good than harm.[26]

Factors that should be considering in arriving at one of these designations include the estimated size and confidence intervals of the effect for the main outcomes, quality of evidence, ability to extrapolate evidence to different patients or care settings, and uncertainty of the baseline risk of disease events in the population of interest.[26]

Finally, the GRADE system assigns one of the following categories for a recommendation for an intervention: strong recommendation for using an intervention, weak recommendation for using an intervention, weak recommendation against an intervention, or a strong recommendation against using an intervention.[25] Factors involved in arriving at one of these four categories include the balance of benefits to risk, the quality rating of the evidence, the variability in the values and preferences that may occur between different patients in different circumstances, and resource use implications. Implications on resource use are often the most difficult to use in making a recommendation for political and scientific reasons and because they can change substantially over time and in different settings.[25]

❻ *The GRADE system presents an advantage that all evidence that is important for making a decision has been judged with explicit criteria. Judgments made are transparent. Evidence profiles and tables summarizing findings have been created. This consequently facilitates the use of best evidence.*

Although the system recommended by the GRADE Working Group may appear complex, it provides a balance of the need for simplicity and a need for full explicit consideration of important issues in clinical decision making. It provides transparency for judgments made to arrive at recommendations. The evidence profile[38] and summary of findings tables[38-40] produced with the GRADE process are useful for documentation of judgments made leading to recommendations and for the clinical use of the guideline. See Appendix 8-1 for an example of an evidence profile.

Articulate Recommendations

This step addresses details of phrasing of guideline recommendations and specifies actions that should be taken and in what settings and circumstances. Standardized language should be used to detail exactly what the recommendation is and when it should be done. When justified by evidence, recommendations should be clear and concise with statements that are actionable and employ active voice. Recommendations should avoid vague and nonspecific language.[1] This section also calls for strong recommendations to be worded so that implications for quality of care monitoring systems can incorporate these recommendations into criteria for care.[1] The specifics of the expected clinical behavior of who should do what, for whom, under what circumstance is necessary to permit the guideline recommendations to be incorporated into computerized clinical decision support tools. Of course, if evidence does not support a specific action, but only different options for consideration, it is important that the guideline recommendation reflect that. That is a feature of the GRADE system as well. After using the GRADE system, a strong recommendation would be introduced by terms such as "We recommend" or "Clinicians should" and a weak recommendation would begin with the terms "We suggest" or "Clinicians might" or "Clinicians may."

The basis of the draft document is provided by the graded recommendations. A formal narrative summary should be provided with all relevant details of decisions made in the development of the guideline. It is highly desirable for the finished guideline to include details of guideline scope including target patient population, population restrictions, interventions considered, specific outcomes or performance measures, intended users of the guideline (e.g., specialty and care setting), and the overall objective of the guideline. A clear description of authorship, sponsorship, and potential COI should be provided. Detailed descriptions of all production and methods including recommendations for considering in applying the guideline in practice (e.g. consideration of patient variables, setting, provider, and estimates of how these factors affect and alter outcomes) are helpful to apply guidelines locally. Comments about ongoing studies, which may affect recommendations, and any plans for updating guidelines should be stated.

It also is desirable for a guideline to be written in different formats and levels of detail for different audiences and purposes. Many guideline developers produce quick reference guides, which give only essential information on the recommendations. These documents are more convenient to use in a patient care setting than a full guideline document. It is important for users of quick reference guides to review the full document before deciding that the guideline is valid for individual use, and to recognize any specific limitations in use of the particular guideline. A guideline summary is another useful format that may be used for patient education purposes.

Reaching clear decisions on recommendations for clinical practices is often difficult because the data are not adequate to clearly label the practice as appropriate or inappropriate. Unfortunately, many practices fall into this gray zone category because of uncertainties about the benefits and harms, variability in patients and responses to treatment, and differences in patient preferences about the desirability of outcomes and aversion to risk. The use of rigid language to produce clear-cut recommendations can be dangerous, particularly when presented as simplistic algorithms that fail to recognize the complexity of medical decision making and the need for individual clinical judgment. This danger can be avoided by describing uncertainty and providing broad boundaries for appropriate practice that allows for legitimate differences of opinion. The development of rigid guidelines, when the data are not conclusive, is worse than having no written guidelines.

It is important to consider the information needs of the guideline's user. Practitioners will want specific, quantitative estimates of the relevant health outcomes if a recommendation is followed, a statement of the strength of the evidence and expert judgment supporting the guidelines, information on patient preferences, projections of cost, details of the reasoning behind the recommendations, and the ability to review the data independently, if they so choose. Guidelines should be written such that they may be perceived as an explanation of the thinking process that is used in evaluating and applying the information. If guidelines are perceived as information only, the recommendations may be rejected out of fear that they will become cookbooks for managing specific conditions/disease states. Such guidelines also would not achieve the educational goals to focus further research efforts on gaps in the current evidence.

Depending on the clinical practice guideline subject, more or less emphasis may be placed on sections of the guideline. In addition, recommendations for future research may be included. The process of developing practice guidelines often calls attention to gaps in scientific information. Direction provided for future research is an important result of the practice guideline development process. Practice guidelines that fail to address research priorities may discourage innovation and negatively influence funding decisions for needed research in the area. For the few examples in which clear answers are already provided by high-quality scientific evidence, waste of research resources may be avoided by stopping generation of data that would not increase understanding of a disease process or treatment.

Conduct an External Review

This step details how the guideline should undergo external review, categories for types of stakeholders and participants to be involved in the review, and calls for a draft to be made available for general public comment.[1] All relevant stakeholders should be involved in the external review. Based on feedback from external review, revisions may be required for the guideline to meet its intended goals. As with many steps in the guideline development, documentation is a key activity in this step. Decisions and actions taken in response to the recommendations from external review should be carefully documented. For critical recommendations that the guideline panel rejects, it is particularly important that the reason for that decision be documented.

Establish a Plan for Updating the Guideline

This step addresses the need to keep guidelines up-to-date with new information when available. It calls for clarity of the publication date, dates of systematic reviews utilized in the guideline, regular review of literature to identify new technology or new evidence that may impact the guideline, and a specific plan for updating or expiration of a guideline.[1]

A review interval to update the guideline should be established. The duration of the interval is dependent on the topic and knowledge of ongoing studies (Case Study 8-3).

Case Study 8-3

You are ready to implement a series of clinical practice guidelines within your health care system. You know that the most effective methods for implementing guidelines have not been determined. You hope to address barriers to guideline implementation that should be considered in an implementation plan. Describe the seven identified barrier categories to guideline implementation.

Guideline Evaluation Tools

❼ *Prior to selecting a clinical practice guideline for implementation in any practice setting by a health care professional, it is important that the quality of published guidelines be evaluated. A useful tool for evaluating clinical practice guidelines was created by the Appraisal of Guidelines for Research and Evaluation (AGREE) collaboration. The AGREE* collaboration is an international group of researchers and policy makers. This collaboration has produced a structured instrument, which can be used for critical appraisal of clinical practice guidelines. The collaboration refined the original instrument, which has resulted in the **AGREE II instrument**.[41,42] The purpose of the AGREE II instrument is to provide a framework to assess guideline quality, provide a methodological strategy for guideline development, and inform what guideline information should be reported.[42] For organizations or individuals who wish to perform an assessment of a guideline, the AGREE II instrument provides a tool that is structured, reliable, and reasonable to use. The AGREE II instrument does not assess clinical content or quality of evidence. Its purpose is to assess the quality of the process of guideline development methods and the reporting quality.

The AGREE II instrument addresses 23 quality items. It is organized in six domains and two global rating items for overall assessment (Table 8-3). Individual items for consideration in the development of the instrument are grouped into six quality domains: (1) scope and purpose, (2) stakeholder involvement, (3) rigor of development, (4) clarity and presentation, (5) applicability, and (6) editorial independence.[40,41] Each of the 23 items and two global rating items are rated on a 7-point scale with 1 representing strongly disagree and 7 representing strongly agree.[41] The user's manual[42] provides more detail for each item, guidance on how to rate each item, and directions on where to look in the guideline for information on the item.

Guideline users may benefit from using this instrument to evaluate the guideline quality before considering adoption of the guideline. Although the primary intent of the AGREE II instrument is to provide a tool for guideline evaluation by users, guideline developers also may use the instrument to ensure that the guideline methodology and documentation provided will meet minimum standards.

Implementation of Clinical Practice Guidelines

❽ *The most effective methods for implementing guidelines to achieve the desired effects of improved quality of care have not been determined.* Institutional, organizational, local practice, political characteristics, and even individual practitioner characteristics should be considered when planning an implementation strategy for a practice guideline. It was previously believed that implementation strategies using multiple methods would be the most likely to succeed. In a systematic review of clinical practice guidelines adoption, the variables that affected the success of implementation included guideline-specific qualities, health care professional characteristics, practice setting characteristics, incentives, regulation, and patient factors.[43] Implementation methods shown to be weak were

TABLE 8–3.   AGREE II DOMAINS AND ITEMS FOR ASSESSMENT[42]

Domain 1. Scope and Purpose

1. The overall objective(s) of the guideline is (are) specifically described.

2. The health question(s) covered by the guideline is (are) specifically described.

3. The population (patients, public, etc.) to whom the guideline is meant to apply is specifically described.

Domain 2. Stakeholder Involvement

4. The guideline development group includes individuals from all the relevant professional groups.

5. The views and preferences of the target population (patients, public, etc.) have been sought.

6. The target users of the guideline are clearly defined.

Domain 3. Rigor of Development

7. Systematic methods were used to search for evidence.

8. The criteria for selecting the evidence are clearly described.

9. The strengths and limitations of the body of evidence are clearly described.

10. The methods for formulating the recommendations are clearly described.

11. The health benefits, side effects, and risks have been considered in formulating the recommendations.

12. There is an explicit link between the recommendations and the supporting evidence.

13. The guideline has been externally reviewed by experts prior to its publication.

14. A procedure for updating the guideline is provided.

Domain 4. Clarity of Presentation

15. The recommendations are specific and unambiguous.

16. The different options for management of the condition or health issue are clearly presented.

17. Key recommendations are easily identifiable.

Domain 5. Applicability

18. The guideline describes facilitators and barriers to its application.

19. The guideline provides advice and/or tools on how the recommendations can be put into practice.

20. The potential resource implications of applying the recommendations have been considered.

21. The guideline presents monitoring and/or auditing criteria.

Domain 6. Editorial Independence

22. The views of the funding body have not influenced the content of the guideline.

23. Competing interests of guideline development group members have been recorded and addressed.

Overall Guideline Assessment

Rate the overall quality of the guideline 1 lowest possible quality—2,3,4,5,6—7 highest possible quality

I would recommend this guideline for use Yes, Yes with modifications, No

AGREE = Appraisal of Guidelines for Research and Evaluation.

traditional continuing medical education (CME) and mailings. Audit and feedback was moderately effective, especially if it was concurrent, targeted to specific providers, and delivered by peers or key opinion leaders. Strong methods were reminder systems, use of multiple intervention systems, and **academic detailing**. Academic detailing is a process by which a health care educator visits physicians to provide a 15- to 20-minute educational intervention on specific topics. Information provided is based on physician prescribing patterns and EBM.[42] See Chapter 23 for more information on academic detailing.

Despite this prior belief that using multiple methods was more effective, a subsequent, extensive review of guideline dissemination and implementation strategies concluded that imperfect evidence exists to support decisions about which guideline dissemination and implementation strategies are best. A study explored whether effects of multiple interventions to disseminate guidelines increased the effects. In the study, Grimshaw and colleagues[44] conducted a systematic review of 235 studies that reported 309 comparisons of strategies for guideline dissemination and implementation. Overall, multifaceted interventions were involved in 73% of comparisons. Eighty-four of the 309 comparisons (27%) were performed on single interventions compared to no intervention or usual care. One hundred thirty-six (44%) of the comparisons were of multifaceted interventions compared to no intervention or a usual care group. Multifaceted interventions were compared to a control intervention. Control interventions were either a single intervention or an alternative multifaceted intervention. Eighty-four of the 309 comparisons (27%) of the comparisons involved a single guideline implementation strategy. Of the single interventions compared to no intervention, the most common strategies used and the percentage of all comparisons in the systematic review were reminders (13%), educational materials (6%), audit and feedback (4%), and patient-directed interventions (3%). The most frequent strategies used in multifaceted interventions were educational materials (48%), educational meetings (41%), reminders (31%), audit and feedback (24%), and patient-directed interventions (18%).[44]

Intervention effect sizes were described in one of four categories based on the absolute difference in the post-intervention measures, which were generally process measures of care. The four categories of effect size were: small—an effect size ≤5%; modest—an effect size >5% and ≤10%; moderate—an effect size >10% and ≤20%; and large—an effect size >20%. Examples of the process of care measures included frequency of prescribing a specific therapy, providing patient education, or ordering laboratory tests in accordance with the guideline. Overall, 86% of interventions tested achieved positive improvements in process of care measures. There was considerable variation in the intervention effect sizes in different studies and in some studies between different interventions. The majority of interventions produced modest to moderate improvements in care. Lack of consistency of differences between and within interventions did not permit any conclusion regarding the most effective strategy for guideline implementation. Multifaceted interventions were not found to be consistently more effective than single intervention strategies, and the number of components in the multifaceted interventions did not appear to be associated with effect size. Authors of this systematic review also noted that the overall quality of methodology and reporting of the included studies were poor.[44] This review also concluded that further research is required to develop and validate systems for estimation of efficacy and efficiency of different strategies to implement patient, health professional, and organizational behavior change. Decision makers will have to evaluate choices of implementation strategies carefully. Local factors, potential facilitators, and barriers to implementation are recommended for prominent consideration in this decision.[44]

As noted above, barriers to guideline implementation should be considered when making plans regarding implementation strategies. Cabana and colleagues[45] conducted a systematic review of the literature regarding barriers to physician adherence to clinical practice guidelines. A barrier was defined as any factor that limits or restricts complete physician adherence to a guideline. Authors identified seven general categories of barriers and provided examples or a description of each (Table 8-4). The relative importance of different barriers will vary depending on characteristics of the specific guideline and on many local health care system characteristics.[44] Paying appropriate attention to these potential barriers in the planning and development of guidelines will facilitate successful implementation.

An observational study of general practice in the Netherlands identified the following characteristics that influenced the use of guidelines: (1) specific attributes of the guidelines determine whether they are used in practice (e.g., changes required; compatibility with current values and routines; resources required), (2) evidence-based recommendations are better followed in practice than those not based on scientific evidence, (3) precise definitions of recommended performance improve use (e.g., specificity of the advice; perceived consequences for providers if used), (4) testing the feasibility and acceptance of clinical guidelines among target groups is important to provide insight into why some guidelines are effective and some are not, and (5) the people setting the guidelines need to understand the attributes of effective evidence-based guidelines (e.g., translating scientific literature into clinical practice feasibility).[46]

CLINICAL DECISION SUPPORT SYSTEMS

A computerized **clinical decision support system** (CDSS) is an information system designed to improve clinical decision making[47] and is one method thought to facilitate guideline implementation. Garg and colleagues[47] conducted a systematic review of controlled trials assessing the effects of CDSSs. Of the 100 trials they reviewed, 88% were randomized; 49% of these were cluster randomized; and 40% used a cluster as the unit of analysis or adjusted for clustering. Twenty-nine studies involved drug dosing or prescribing. For single-drug dosing studies ($n = 24$), 15 (62%) demonstrated improved practitioner performance with guidelines, and 2 of the 18 studies assessing patient outcomes showed positive improvement. Five systems used computer order entry for multidrug prescribing. Four or these systems improved practitioner performance, but none improved patient outcomes. There were 40 studies of systems for disease management of conditions, such

TABLE 8–4. SEVEN CATEGORIES OF BARRIER[45]

Barrier Category	Examples of Barriers Identified or Description of Barrier
Lack of awareness	Did not know the guideline existed
Lack of familiarity	Could not correctly answer questions about guideline content or self-reported lack of familiarity
Lack of agreement	Difference in interpretation of the evidence
	Benefits not worth patient risk, discomfort, or cost
	Not applicable to patient population in their practice
	Credibility of authors questioned
	Oversimplified cookbook
	Reduces autonomy
	Decreases flexibility
	Decreases physician self-respect
	Not practical
	Makes patient-physician relationship impersonal
Lack of self-efficacy	Did not believe that they could actually perform the behavior or activity recommended by the guideline, e.g., nutrition or exercise counseling
Lack of outcome expectancy	Did not believe intended outcome would occur even if the practice was followed, e.g., counseling to stop smoking
Inertia of previous practice	This barrier relates primarily to motivation to change practice, whether the motivation is professional, personal, or social. It was also noted that guidelines that recommend eliminating a behavior are more difficult to implement than guidelines that recommend adding a new behavior
External barriers	Patient resistance/nonadherence
	Patient does not perceive need
	Perceived to be offensive to patient
	Causes patient embarrassment
	Lack of reminder system
	Not easy to use, inconvenient, cumbersome, confusing
	Lack of educational materials
	Cost to patient
	Insufficient staff, consultant support, or other resources
	Lack of time
	Lack of reimbursement
	Increased malpractice liability
	Not compatible with practice setting

as diabetes, cardiovascular disease prevention, urinary incontinence, human immunodeficiency virus infection, and acute respiratory distress. Thirty-seven of these studies evaluated practitioner performance with 23 (62%) demonstrating improvement. Only 5 (18%) of the 27 disease management trials evaluating patient outcomes demonstrated improvement. Of 21 trials of reminder systems for preventive care, 16 (72%) found improvements in practitioner performance according to practice guidelines. Of the 10 trials that evaluated CDSSs for diagnostic systems, only 4 (40%) found improvements in practitioner performance. Of the five trials of diagnostic systems that evaluated patient outcomes, none found improvement, which is a concern that requires further study.[47]

The authors also reported that improved practitioner performance was associated with CDSSs that automatically prompted the practitioner compared to systems that required the practitioner to initiate system use.[47] Improved performance was noted in 73% of trials of automated systems compared to 47% of user-initiated systems ($p = 0.02$). It also was interesting to note that the best predictor of success of CDSSs was a study in which the authors were also the developers of the system. Studies conducted by the developer of the system were more likely to find success (74%), compared to 28% when the authors were not the developers ($p = 0.001$).[47]

It is clear that as with other methods for implementation of guidelines and achieving performance or behavior change, further research is needed on the use of CDSSs to provide clear guidance on predictable success rates. Many individual factors will need to be considered in the decision making for implementation of these systems.[48]

ACADEMIC DETAILING

A randomized, controlled trial of CQI and academic detailing to implement clinical guidelines for the primary care of hypertension and depression produced mixed results.[49] The authors concluded that both academic detailing and CQI interventions involve complex social interactions that produce varied implementation success across the different organizations.

EFFECT OF GUIDELINES

Grimshaw and Russell[50] published one of the first systematic literature reviews and evaluations of the effect of practice guidelines. They conducted an extensive literature search and identified 59 studies considered to have appropriate methods to evaluate the effect of guidelines on either physician behavior or patient outcomes. All but four of the studies showed some benefit from the guidelines; however, the magnitude of the benefit and the patient care significance was not impressive in all cases.

Clinical practice guidelines represent an early application of decision support systems to facilitate quality clinical care. When done well, clinical practice guidelines should contain all necessary elements of routine care for most individuals with a specific condition. They should prompt consideration of what specific characteristics of an individual patient might warrant departures from the guideline. When effectively implemented, such systems save clinicians' time. They should be assisted by computerized systems that, among other functions, can catalog past histories, check orders for medications against measures of hepatic and renal function, and schedule reminders for screening tests or preventive services. They should be part of the continuous improvement of systems of care. Guidelines will not be perfect at the outset; systems that use them must be constructed so that experience can be applied to improve the guidelines, just as the guidelines indicate where care delivery can be improved.[16]

CHALLENGES WITH GUIDELINE IMPLEMENTATION

Even with the many improvements in clinical practice guideline development methods that have been described in this chapter, there remain a number of challenges with implementation, updating, and evaluation of the impact of guidelines.[51] Some of these challenges relate to a lack of high-quality evidence for decision making in specific circumstances. In particular, there is a lack of evidence for implementation of guidelines for patients with multiple concurrent disease conditions. Most guidelines are developed for the management of a single condition. It is possible that harm may result from following recommendations from multiple individual guidelines for patients with multiple medical conditions. Treatments may become overly complex, costly, and interact with each other.[52] Although not yet proven, it might be possible to adapt guidelines to facilitate decisions in the presence of multimorbidity.[53]

Another problem with implementation occurs when guidelines are developed by different groups on the same topic and they arrive at different recommendations. Although written with an admitted degree of satire, Packer[54] describes such a problem with recently developed heart failure guidelines. He reviews areas of differences in these guidelines that were developed by the European Society of Cardiology in comparison with those by the American College of Cardiology/American Heart Association/Heart Failure Society of America. Examples of the differences involved details of the indications for one medication, or class of medication, compared to alternatives, and differences in recommended doses. He also mentioned issues with recommendations of therapy in patients with diabetes in addition to heart failure. The differences in recommendations in the guidelines most likely occurred because of differences in judgement when there are gaps in the evidence, or when evidence suffers from some of the shortcomings mentioned in the section in this chapter on grading including indirectness and imprecision.

FUTURE METHODS

The GRADE Working Group is continuing to evaluate improved methods for presentation of information to make recommendations in guidelines that will be more adaptable and feasible for use by clinicians and also more effective for implementation.[55,56] One focused effort is evaluation of new ways of formatting, and use of explanatory footnotes in evidence tables, to improve understanding of the certainty of evidence judgements.[57–59] Members of the group have published resources to educate health professionals on how to interpret and use recommendations in guidelines developed with the GRADE approach.[60] This work may result in future changes in the GRADE methodology. For pharmacists or other health professionals who are charged with implementation of clinical practice guidelines, further review of these references would be useful.

TOOLS FOR IMPLEMENTATION

Additional tools are publically available for those who are developing and implementing guidelines. Understanding the development details will also support implementation within a health system and even improve individual practitioner's best use of guidelines. A guideline development checklist called the Guideline International Network (GIN)—McMaster Guideline Development Checklist (https://cebgrade.mcmaster .ca/guidecheck.html) is available based on a partnership between GIN and McMaster University. The checklist is intended for use by guideline developers to plan and track the process of guideline development. The Guidelines International Network (G-I-N) (http:// www.g-i-n.net) is an international nonprofit association of international organizations and individuals involved in clinical practice guidelines. McMaster University has also partnered with others to provide GRADEpro, https://cebgrade.mcmaster.ca/gradepro.html, which is a web application that "aims to support the complete process of developing health care guidelines, starting from the team composition and management and subject inception to the generation of the recommendations, authoring of the final recommendation document, and the dissemination of the guidelines." One section of the program is an application to create, manage, and share evidence profiles and summary of findings tables. This section in particular would be useful for education of all health professionals who need to understand this critical aspect of guideline development. Video tutorials regarding multiple aspects of guideline development are available from this organization through the following link: https://gradepro.org/guidelines-development#develop-tuts (Case Study 8-4).

Case Study 8-4

Referring back to Case 8-1, you implemented the clinical practice guidelines within your health care system. Over time, you become recognized as an expert in your field. One of the guidelines needs to be updated based on new evidence and you are asked to sit on the panel formed to update the guideline. Describe the importance of the consideration of updates to clinical practice guidelines in initial guideline formation.

Sources of Clinical Practice Guidelines

❾ *The National Guideline Clearinghouse website serves as a repository of clinical practice guidelines. Similar websites and peer-reviewed medical literature from secondary databases may allow for awareness and identification of practice standards.* Systematic reviews that can be helpful in developing or assessing specific practice guidelines are available from organizations such as the Cochrane Library, in addition to other websites that collect and provide health care-related information designed to support EBM such as the Agency for Healthcare Research and Quality (AHRQ).

There are several mechanisms to locate completed clinical practice guidelines or systematic reviews. The National Guideline Clearinghouse (NGC) (http://www.guideline.gov) is maintained by AHRQ. The mission of the NGC is to provide an accessible mechanism for obtaining objective, detailed information on clinical practice guidelines and to further their dissemination, implementation, and use. Components of the NGC include structured abstracts about the guideline and its development, a utility for comparing attributes of two or more guidelines in a side-by-side comparison, synthesis of guidelines covering similar topics, highlighting areas of similarity and difference, links to full-text guidelines where available and/or ordering information for print copies, and annotated bibliographies on guideline development methodology implementation and use. The NGC has published criteria for guidelines to be considered for inclusion in the Clearinghouse (http://www .guideline.gov/about/inclusion-criteria.aspx) from 1997 (in effect through May 31, 2014) and 2013 (revised, effective since June 1, 2014). These criteria provide useful information for quality consideration for guidelines. There are also links that present very useful commentary for further understanding of definitions of guidelines, guideline characteristics for developers, methods of producing and formatting guidelines, and expectations for documentation of these details. The new criteria reflect the most recent recommendations from the National Academy of Medicine that have been described in this chapter. A limitation can be determining which guideline is most frequently used in clinic practice.

Many guidelines published in the peer-reviewed medical literature can be located in MEDLINE®. A variety of search techniques may be used, but the most efficient may be to search for *practice guideline* in the publication type field of the record, or use the MeSH term *practice guideline* or *clinical guideline* in conjunction with other terms for the specific disease or therapy of interest. Additional publication types that may be searched include the terms consensus development conference, guideline, and meta-analysis. Systematic review articles are also useful in preparation of clinical practice guidelines. Key differences of systematic reviews compared to narrative review articles are that systematic reviews begin with focused clinical questions, involve comprehensive searches for evidence, use criterion-based selection that are uniformly applied to include evidence in the reviews, perform rigorous critical appraisal of studies chosen, and provide a quantitative summary of the evidence (i.e., meta-analysis).[61] Literature search strategies have been published for locating systematic reviews.[62,63]

Of note, the National Library of Medicine provides access to the National Institutes of Health (NIH) consensus statements, the U.S. Preventative Services Task Force (USPSTF) Guide to Clinical Preventive Services and Evidence Syntheses, AHRQ evidence reports and summaries, comparative effectiveness reviews, technical reviews and summaries, publications and reports of the Surgeon General, and other resources available from these websites and collectively at the Health Services/Technology Assessment Texts (HSTAT) website (http://www.ncbi.nlm.nih.gov/books/NBK16710).

The G-I-N Library (http://www.g-i-n.net) provides access to the International Guideline Library, development and training resources, relevant literature, health topic collection, relevant links, and other tools. Some of the resources from this website require membership for access.

Multiple professional organizations, academic centers, independent research centers, and government agencies are involved in development of clinical practice guideline activities. Updated information may be obtained by contacting these organizations directly and many have provided access to guidelines on their websites. Finally, the Cochrane Collaboration has a list of databases offering online access to medical evidence (http://www.cochrane.org/about-us/evidence-based-health-care/webliography/databases).

Conclusion

Clinical practice guidelines have become a significant tool in health care with the focus on evidence-based practice. Guidelines have the potential to assist medical decision making and ultimately improve quality of care and patient outcomes, and make more efficient use of resources. Significant advances have been made in guideline methodology to enhance the validity. Information technology and understanding of optimal methods for implementation of guidelines will maximize improvements to quality of care. Practitioners' active involvement in preparation and implementation of evidence-based clinical practice guidelines is vital. A thorough understanding of evidence-based methodology will prepare health care providers to participate in this process. Training in drug information is ideal in the preparation and implementation of evidence-based clinical practice guidelines.

Self-Assessment Questions

1. Which of the following groups or types of organizations have been involved in development of clinical practice guidelines?
   a. Federal and state government
   b. Professional societies and associations
   c. Managed care organizations
   d. Third-party payers
   e. All of the above

2. Which of the following is a common characteristic of practice guideline development and drug information practices?
   a. Decision making and recommendations based on individual experience
   b. Assurance of cost savings
   c. Clear specific definition of clinical questions
   d. Lack of interdisciplinary participation
   e. All of the above

3. Clinical practice guidelines are important to getting research information into practice because:
   a. Well-studied new treatments proven effective are substantially underutilized
   b. Interventions proven ineffective or harmful continue to be provided
   c. Research information is not readily available for implementation into practice
   d. a and b only are important
   e. b and c only are important

4. Recommendations for optimizing patient care that are developed by systematically reviewing the evidence and assessing the benefits and harms of health care interventions is the definition for:
   a. Strengths of recommendations
   b. Evidence-based medicine
   c. Conflicts of interest
   d. Clinical practice guidelines
   e. Systematic reviews

5. Which of the following are among the five core competencies for health professionals as recommended in a landmark Institute of Medicine report?
   a. Deliver patient-centered care
   b. Participate in interdisciplinary teams
   c. Emphasize evidence-based practice

    d. Utilize informatics

    e. All of the above

6. The first step in the Institute of Medicine's proposed standards for developing evidence-based clinical practice guidelines is:

    a. Conduct a systematic review for qualifying evidence

    b. Establish a multidisciplinary guideline development group

    c. Establish transparency

    d. Manage conflict of interest

    e. Conduct an external review

7. Development of a clinical practice guideline should:

    a. Include a hospital administrator

    b. Be a multidisciplinary process

    c. Be made up of panel members without any conflicts of interest

    d. Have a pharmacist leading the effort

    e. All of the above

8. Which of the following characteristics associated with a disease would suggest that it would be a good topic for development and implementation of a practice guideline?

    a. Low prevalence

    b. Evidence that current practice is optimal

    c. Evidence of little variation in current practice

    d. Availability of high-quality evidence for the efficacy of treatments that reduce morbidity or mortality

    e. Low frequency and/or severity of morbidity or mortality

9. In the PICO model for framing clinical questions, the C represents:

    a. Collaboration

    b. Comparison

    c. Clinical

    d. Control

    e. Cohort

10. When using the GRADE system, which of the following information should be incorporated with guideline recommendations?

    a. Quality of evidence across studies for each important outcome

    b. Strength of the recommendations

    c. Balance between benefits and harms

    d. a and b only

    e. a, b, and c

11. When using the GRADE system, all of the following are reasons for lowering the level of confidence rating *except*:
    a. Risk of bias
    b. Publication bias
    c. Imprecision
    d. Indirectness
    e. Consistency

12. When using the GRADE system, which of the following is/are reason(s) for rating the level of confidence higher?
    a. Dose response
    b. Large effect
    c. All plausible confounding
    d. b and c only
    e. a, b, and c

13. All of the following are true regarding the AGREE II instrument for guideline evaluation *except*:
    a. Created by an international group of researchers and policy makers
    b. Provides a framework to assess the quality of guidelines
    c. Assesses the quality of the clinical content
    d. Intended for use by organizations and individuals
    e. Provides a methodological strategy for the development of guidelines

14. External barriers to clinical practice guideline implementation include all of the following *except*:
    a. Lack of familiarity with the guideline
    b. Cost to patient
    c. Increased malpractice liability
    d. Insufficient staff, consultant support, or other resources
    e. Lack of reimbursement

15. All of the following statements about clinical practice guidelines are true *except*:
    a. Clinical practice guidelines *should* contain all necessary elements of routine care for most individuals with a specific condition.
    b. Clinical practice guidelines *should not* prompt consideration of what specific characteristics of an individual patient might warrant departures from the guideline.
    c. Clinical practice guidelines represent an early application of decision support systems to facilitate providing quality clinical care.
    d. Clinical practice guidelines will not be perfect at the outset.
    e. Clinical practice guidelines should be part of the continuous improvement of systems of care.

REFERENCES

1. Institute of Medicine, Committee on Standards for Developing Trustworthy Clinical Practice Guidelines. Clinical practice guidelines we can trust. In: Graham R, Mancher M, Wolman DM, Greenfield S, Steinberg E, eds. Washington, DC: National Academies Press; 2011. [cited 2016 Sept]. Available from: http://nationalacademies.org/HMD/Reports/2011/Clinical-Practice-Guidelines-We-Can-Trust.aspx

2. Jones RH, Ritchie JL, Fleming BB, Hammermeister KE, Leape LL. 28th Bethesda Conference. Task Force 1: Clinical practice guideline development, dissemination and computerization. J Am Coll Cardiol. 1997;29:1133-41.

3. President's Advisory Commission on Consumer Protection and Quality in the Health Care Industry. Quality first: better health care for all Americans. [cited 2012 Dec 14]. Available from: http://archive.ahrq.gov/hcqual/final/

4. Institute of Medicine, Committee on Quality Health Care in America. Crossing the quality chasm: a new health system for the 21st century. Washington, DC: National Academy Press; 2001. [cited 2016 Sept]. Available from: https://www.nap.edu/catalog/10027/crossing-the-quality-chasm-a-new-health-system-for-the

5. Institute of Medicine, Committee on Data Standards for Patient Safety. Patient safety: achieving a new standard for care. In: Aspden P, Corrigan JM, Wolcott J, Erikson SM, eds. Washington, DC: National Academies Press; 2004. [cited 2016 Sept]. Available from: https://www.nap.edu/read/10863/chapter/1

6. Institute of Medicine, Committee on Quality of Health Care in America. To err is human: building a safer health system. In: Kohn LT, Corrigan JM, Donaldson MS, eds. Washington, DC: National Academy Press; 2000. [cited 2016 Sept]. Available from: https://www.nap.edu/read/9728/chapter/1#ix

7. Institute of Medicine, Committee on Identifying and Preventing Medication Errors. Preventing medication errors. In: Aspden P, Wolcott J, Bootman JL, Cronenwett LR, eds. Washington, DC: National Academies Press; 2007. [cited 2016 Sept]. Available from: https://www.nap.edu/read/11623/chapter/1

8. Institute of Medicine, Committee on Standards for Systematic Reviews of Comparative Effectiveness Research. Finding what works in health care: standards for systematic reviews. In: Eden J, Levit L, Berg A, Morton S, eds. Washington, DC: National Academies Press; 2011. [cited 2016 Sept]. Available from: https://www.nap.edu/catalog/13059/finding-what-works-in-health-care-standards-for-systematic-reviews

9. Institute of Medicine, Committee on the Learning Health Care System in America. Best care at lower cost: the path to continuously learning health care in America. In: Smith M, Saunders R, Stuckhardt L, McGinnis JM, eds. Washington, DC: National Academies Press; 2012. [cited 2016 Sept]. Available from: http://www.nationalacademies.org/hmd/Reports/2012/Best-Care-at-Lower-Cost-The-Path-to-Continuously-Learning-Health-Care-in-America.aspx

10. Sackett DL, Rosenberg WM, Gray JA, Haynes RB, Richardson WS. Evidence based medicine: what it is and what it isn't. BMJ. 1996;312:71-2.

11. Eddy DM. Evidence-based medicine: a unified approach. Health Aff. 2005;24:9-17.

12. Evidence-Based Medicine Working Group. Evidence-based medicine. A new approach to teaching the practice of medicine. JAMA. 1992;268:2420-5.

13. Straus SE, Glasziou P, Richardson WS, Haynes RB. Evidence-based medicine: how to practice & teach it. 4th ed. New York, NY: Churchill Livingstone; 2011.

14. Watanabe AS, McCart G, Shimomura S, Kayser S. Systematic approach to drug information requests. Am J Hosp Pharm. 1975;32:1282-5.

15. Guyatt GH, Meade MO, Jaeschke RZ, Cook DJ, Haynes RB. Practitioners of evidence based care. Not all clinicians need to appraise evidence from scratch but all need some skills. BMJ. 2000;320:954-5.

16. Chassin MR. Is health care ready for Six Sigma quality? Milbank Q. 1998;76:565-91, 510.

17. Enhancing the QUAlity and Transparency Of health Research—The EQUATOR network. [cited 2016 Oct]. Available from: http://www.equator-network.org/about-us/equator-network-what-we-do-and-how-we-are-organised/

18. Fye WB. The power of clinical trials and guidelines, and the challenge of conflicts of interest. J Am Coll Cardiol. 2003;41:1237-42.

19. Choudhry NK, Stelfox HT, Detsky AS. Relationships between authors of clinical practice guidelines and the pharmaceutical industry. JAMA. 2002;287:612-7.

20. Curtiss FR. Consensus panel, national guidelines, and other potentially misleading terms. J Manag Care Pharm. 2003;9:574-5.

21. Van der Weyden MB. Clinical practice guidelines: time to move the debate from the how to the who. Med J Aust. 2002;176:304-5.

22. Guyatt GH, Akl EA, Crowther M, Schunemann HJ, Gutterman DD, Zelman LS. Introduction to the ninth edition: antithrombotic therapy and prevention of thrombosis, 9th ed: American College of Chest Physicians evidence-based clinical practice guidelines. Chest. 2012;141:48S-52S.

23. Guyatt GH, Norris SL, Schulman S, Hirsh J, Eckman MH, Akl EA, et al. Methodology for the development of antithrombotic therapy and prevention of thrombosis guidelines: antithrombotic therapy and prevention of thrombosis, 9th ed: American College of Chest Physicians evidence-based clinical practice guidelines. Chest. 2012;141:53S-70S.

24. Mosca L, Appel LJ, Benjamin EJ, Berra K, Chandra-Strobos N, Fabunmi RP, et al. Evidence-based guidelines for cardiovascular disease prevention in women. J Am Coll Cardiol. 2004;43:900-21.

25. Guyatt GH, Oxman AD, Schunemann HJ, Tugwell P, Knottnerus A. GRADE guidelines: a new series of articles in the Journal of Clinical Epidemiology. J Clin Epidemiol. 2011;64:380-2.

26. Atkins D, Best D, Briss PA, Eccles M, Falck-Ytter Y, Flottorp S, et al. Grading quality of evidence and strength of recommendations. BMJ. 2004;328:1490.

27. Guyatt GH, Oxman AD, Vist GE, Kunz R, Falck-Ytter Y, Alfonso-Coello P, et al. GRADE: an emerging consensus on rating quality of evidence and strength of recommendations. BMJ. 2008;336:924-6.

28. Guyatt GH, Oxman AD, Kunz R, Atkins D, Brozek J, Vist G, et al. GRADE guidelines: 2. Framing the question and deciding on important outcomes. J Clin Epidemiol. 2011;64:395-400.

29. Balshem H, Helfand M, Schunemann HJ, Oxman AD, Kunz R, Brozek J, et al. GRADE guidelines: 3. Rating the quality of evidence. J Clin Epidemiol. 2011;64:401-6.

30. Guyatt GH, Oxman AD, Vist G, Kunz R, Brozek J, Alfonso-Coello P, et al. GRADE guidelines: 4. Rating the quality of evidence—study limitations (risk of bias). J Clin Epidemiol. 2011;64:407-15.

31. Guyatt GH, Oxman AD, Kunz R, Woodcock J, Brozek J, Helfand M, et al. GRADE guidelines: 7. Rating the quality of evidence—inconsistency. J Clin Epidemiol. 2011;64:1294-302.

32. Guyatt GH, Oxman AD, Kunz R, Woodcock J, Brozek J, Helfand M, et al. GRADE guidelines: 8. Rating the quality of evidence—indirectness. J Clin Epidemiol. 2011;64:1303-10.

33. Kearon C, Akl EA, Ornelas J, Blaivas A, Jimenez D, Bounameaux H, et al. Antithrombotic therapy for VTE disease: CHEST guideline and expert panel report. Chest. 2016;149:315-52.

34. Guyatt GH, Oxman AD, Kunz R, Brozek J, Alfonso-Coello P, Rind D, et al. GRADE guidelines 6. Rating the quality of evidence—imprecision. J Clin Epidemiol. 2011;64:1283-93.

35. Guyatt GH, Oxman AD, Montori V, Vist G, Kunz R, Brozek J, et al. GRADE guidelines: 5. Rating the quality of evidence—publication bias. J Clin Epidemiol. 2011;64:1277-82.

36. Guyatt GH, Oxman AD, Sultan S, Glasziou P, Akl EA, Alfonso-Coello P, et al. GRADE guidelines: 9. Rating up the quality of evidence. J Clin Epidemiol. 2011;64:1311-6.

37. Hill AB. The environment and disease: association or causation? Proc R Soc Med. 1965;58:295-300.

38. Guyatt G, Oxman AD, Akl EA, Kunz R, Vist G, Brozek J, et al. GRADE guidelines: 1. Introduction—GRADE evidence profiles and summary of findings tables. J Clin Epidemiol. 2011;64:383-94.

39. Guyatt GH, Oxman AD, Santesso N, Helfand M, Vist G, Kunz R, et al. GRADE guidelines: 12. Preparing summary of findings tables—binary outcomes. J Clin Epidemiol. 2013;66:158-72.

40. Guyatt GH, Thorlund K, Oxman AD, Walter SD, Patrick D, Furukawa TA, et al. GRADE guidelines: 13. Preparing summary of findings tables and evidence profiles—continuous outcomes. J Clin Epidemiol. 2013;66:173-83.

41. Brouwers MC, Kho ME, Browman GP, Burgers JS, Cluzeau F, Feder G, et al. AGREE II: advancing guideline development, reporting and evaluation in health care. CMAJ. 2010;182:E839-42.

42. AGREE Next Steps Consortium. Appraisal of Guidelines for Research & Evaluation (AGREE) II Instrument. [cited 2016 Sept]. Available from: http://www.agreetrust.org/wp-content/uploads/2013/10/AGREE-II-Users-Manual-and-23-item-Instrument_2009_UPDATE_2013.pdf

43. Davis DA, Taylor-Vaisey A. Translating guidelines into practice. A systematic review of theoretic concepts, practical experience and research evidence in the adoption of clinical practice guidelines. CMAJ. 1997;157:408-16.

44. Grimshaw JM, Thomas RE, MacLennan G, Fraser C, Ramsay CR, Vale L, et al. Effectiveness and efficiency of guideline dissemination and implementation strategies. Health Technol Assess. 2004;8:iii-72.

45. Cabana MD, Rand CS, Powe NR, Wu AW, Wilson MH, Abboud PA, et al. Why don't physicians follow clinical practice guidelines? A framework for improvement. JAMA. 1999;282:1458-65.

46. Grol R, Dalhuijsen J, Thomas S, Veld C, Rutten G, Mokkink H. Attributes of clinical guidelines that influence use of guidelines in general practice: observational study. BMJ. 1998;317:858-61.
47. Garg AX, Adhikari NK, McDonald H, Rosas-Arellano MP, Devereaux PJ, Beyene J, et al. Effects of computerized clinical decision support systems on practitioner performance and patient outcomes: a systematic review. JAMA. 2005;293:1223-38.
48. Wears RL, Berg M. Computer technology and clinical work: still waiting for Godot. JAMA. 2005;293:1261-3.
49. Horowitz CR, Goldberg HI, Martin DP, Wagner EH, Fihn SD, Christensen DB, et al. Conducting a randomized controlled trial of CQI and academic detailing to implement clinical guidelines. Jt Comm J Qual Improv. 1996;22:734-50.
50. Grimshaw JM, Russell IT. Effect of clinical guidelines on medical practice: a systematic review of rigorous evaluations. Lancet. 1993;342:1317-22.
51. Kredo T, Bernhardsson S, Machingaidze S, Young T, Louw Q, Ochodo E, et al. Guide to clinical practice guidelines: the current state of play. Int J Qual Health Care. 2016; 28:122-8.
52. Boyd CM, Darer J, Boult C, Fried LP, Boult L, Wu AW. Clinical practice guidelines and quality of care for older patients with multiple comorbid diseases: implications for pay for performance. JAMA. 2005;294:716-24.
53. Guthrie B, Payne K, Alderson P, McMurdo ME, Mercer SW. Adapting clinical guidelines to take account of multimorbidity. BMJ. 2012;345:e6341.
54. Packer M. The room where it happens: a skeptic's analysis of the new heart failure guidelines. J Card Fail. 2016;22:726-30.
55. Alonso-Coello P, Schünemann HJ, Moberg J, Brignardello-Petersen R, Akl EA, Davoli M, et al.; GRADE Working Group. GRADE Evidence to Decision (EtD) frameworks: a systematic and transparent approach to making well informed healthcare choices. 1: Introduction. BMJ. 2016;353:i2016.
56. Alonso-Coello P, Oxman AD, Moberg J, Brignardello-Petersen R, Akl EA, Davoli M, et al.; GRADE Working Group. GRADE Evidence to Decision (EtD) frameworks: a systematic and transparent approach to making well informed healthcare choices. 2: Clinical practice guidelines. BMJ. 2016;353:i2089.
57. Carrasco-Labra A, Brignardello-Petersen R, Santesso N, Neumann I, Mustafa RA, Mbuagbaw L, et al. Improving GRADE evidence tables part 1: a randomized trial shows improved understanding of content in summary of findings tables with a new format. J Clin Epidemiol. 2016;74:7-18.
58. Langendam M, Carrasco-Labra A, Santesso N, Mustafa RA, Brignardello-Petersen R, Ventresca M, et al. Improving GRADE evidence tables part 2: a systematic survey of explanatory notes shows more guidance is needed. J Clin Epidemiol. 2016;74:19-27.
59. Santesso N, Carrasco-Labra A, Langendam M, Brignardello-Petersen R, Mustafa RA, Heus P, et al. Improving GRADE evidence tables part 3: detailed guidance for explanatory footnotes supports creating and understanding GRADE certainty in the evidence judgments. J Clin Epidemiol. 2016;74:28-39.

60. Neumann I, Santesso N, Akl EA, Rind DM, Vandvik PO, Alonso-Coello P, et al. A guide for health professionals to interpret and use recommendations in guidelines developed with the GRADE approach. J Clin Epidemiol. 2016;72:45-55.

61. Cook DJ, Mulrow CD, Haynes RB. Systematic reviews: synthesis of best evidence for clinical decisions. Ann Intern Med. 1997;126:376-80.

62. Hunt DL, McKibbon KA. Locating and appraising systematic reviews. Ann Intern Med. 1997;126:532-8.

63. Montori VM, Wilczynski NL, Morgan D, Haynes RB. Optimal search strategies for retrieving systematic reviews from Medline: analytical survey. BMJ. 2005;330:68.

SUGGESTED READINGS

1. AGREE Next Steps Consortium. Appraisal of Guidelines for Research & Evaluation (AGREE) II Instrument. Available from: http://www.agreetrust.org/wp-content/uploads/2013/10/AGREE-II-Users-Manual-and-23-item-Instrument_2009_UPDATE_2013.pdf

2. Guyatt GH, Oxman AD, Schunemann HJ, Tugwell P, Knottnerus A. GRADE guidelines: a new series of articles in the Journal of Clinical Epidemiology. J Clin Epidemiol. 2011; 64:380-2.

3. Institute of Medicine Committee on Standards for Developing Trustworthy Clinical Practice Guidelines. Clinical practice guidelines we can trust. In: Graham R, Mancher M, Wolman DM, Greenfield S, Steinberg E, eds. Washington, DC: National Academies Press; 2011. [cited 2016 Sept]. Available from: http://nationalacademies.org/HMD/Reports/2011/Clinical-Practice-Guidelines-We-Can-Trust.aspx

4. Institute of Medicine Committee on Standards for Systematic Reviews of Comparative Effectiveness Research. Finding what works in health care: standards for systematic reviews. In: Eden J, Levit L, Berg A, Morton S, eds. Washington, DC: National Academies Press; 2011. [cited 2016 Sept]. Available from: https://www.nap.edu/catalog/13059/finding-what-works-in-health-care-standards-for-systematic-reviews

Chapter Nine

Journal Clubs

Benjamin A. Witt

Learning Objectives

● *After completing this chapter, the reader will be able to*

- Describe the process of developing a journal club presentation.
- Discuss the benefits of journal club participation.
- Apply the concepts of literature evaluation to a journal club presentation.
- Describe effective strategies to increase interest and participation in journal clubs.
- Describe methods to add clinical relevance to journal club presentations.

Key Concepts

❶ There is no standard method of implementing a journal club. Journal clubs are flexible in design and execution to meet the needs of the participants.

❷ A journal club can often target articles specific to their area of practice, and practitioners use the journal club as a way to stay current with new developments and clinical evidence in one's specialty area.

❸ Case reports, letters, and nonsystematic reviews should not be the focus of a journal club discussion.

❹ Journal club presenters should draw their own conclusions related to the findings of the study that they are presenting. Evidence to support this critique should be shared with the group.

❺ Discussion among journal club participants can serve as an outlet of providing interesting clinical cases and differing clinical insight and perspectives.

Introduction

Journal clubs have become a staple in the professional development and continuing professional education of health care practitioners across many disciplines. ❶ *However, there is no standard method for implementing a journal club. Journal clubs are flexible in design and execution to meet the needs of the participants.* The purpose of this chapter is to provide general guidance and suggestions that can be used to design a successful journal club that will meet the needs of the reader.

Journal clubs are groups of individuals who meet on a regular basis to discuss and critically evaluate the biomedical literature.[1,2] Documentation of journal clubs dates back to the 1800s, at which time they served the purpose of sharing educational resources to keep current with new findings published in the medical literature.[1,2] As postgraduate education and training of health care practitioners continues to evolve, so does the journal club. Presently, journal clubs are widely used by health care professionals of many disciplines.

Due to the sheer volume of the present-day literature, it is impractical to expect to be able to read every piece of original research that is published. Journal clubs are one solution to help keep current with literature in one's area of practice. Members of a particular journal club often have similar professional interests and practice areas. ❷ *Thus, a journal club can often target articles specific to an area of practice, and practitioners use the journal club as a way to stay current with new developments and clinical evidence in one's specialty area.* Additional aims of journal clubs include teaching and practicing **critical appraisal** skills, improving understanding of statistical methods and research design, and fostering the development of evidence-based practice.[2-4] Journal club participation can also help presenters hone their public speaking and meeting facilitation skills, improve professionalism and ethics, and serve as an outlet for socialization among peers.[5] Due to these benefits, it is clear why journal club presentations have become a mainstay of literature-evaluation education in the training of health care professionals in the United States, and are a primary active-learning method used when teaching literature-evaluation skills.[6] Journal clubs are also used in practice to help answer clinical questions, with the intent of applying the knowledge gained to a current or anticipated treatment decision. Journal clubs can also choose to focus on nonclinical topics, such as management and leadership, depending on the need of the participants.[7,8] No matter the intent, journal clubs are a great way to learn about new drug therapies, apply literature-evaluation techniques, and apply clinical reasoning skills.

Conducting the Journal Club

There are numerous considerations when implementing a journal club, and there is no one correct design for proper execution. The method of delivery and setting can vary considerably to meet the needs of the participants and achieve the intended purpose. The main factor to achieve a successful journal club is to clearly define the expectations of participants and presenters. See Table 9-1 for common considerations when starting a journal club.

EXPECTATIONS OF PARTICIPANTS

Journal clubs should have a facilitator who is commonly a practitioner or academician.[9] The facilitator is responsible for the logistics of the journal club, including designating the presenter or presenters for each session, inviting participants, securing the meeting space, and communicating the logistics of the journal club to all the participants in a timely manner.[9] The facilitator may also select the journal article to be evaluated; however, the presenter(s) may take more ownership if they are allowed to select their own article.[10] If not selected by the facilitator, articles should still be screened and approved by the facilitator to assure relevance to practice and suitability for presentation. Once selected, the article should be announced to or shared with all the participants before the presentation date, via an agreed method, so that they may be prepared for a meaningful discussion at the journal club.

A journal club will have a designated presenter (or presenters) who is responsible for providing an overview of the selected article, along with their critique. The presenter is also responsible for engaging other participants by steering the conversation with carefully constructed and thought-provoking questions. Either the facilitator or presenter

TABLE 9–1. CONSIDERATIONS WHEN PREPARING A JOURNAL CLUB

Who will be invited to attend?	How often will the journal club meet?
Who will facilitate the meetings?	How long will each session last?
How will articles be selected?	What format will be used for presentation?
Is a handout or slide set required?	Will food be provided or permitted?
Will attendance be mandatory?	What technology or resources will need to be obtained?
Where is the presentation held?	
When will the group meet?	

should assume the role of keeping the discussion on track and focused, making sure that the discussion starts and ends on time, and that each participant is meaningfully contributing to the discussion.

Ideally, a content expert will be present to participate in the discussion. In clinical practice, a content expert is typically a practitioner with expertise in the area that is the focus of discussion. Having a content expert present in the discussion helps provide practical insight into how the intervention being discussed applies to real practice. Additionally, inclusion of a drug information specialist or clinician with advanced training in clinical investigation can help add depth to discussion of research methods, study design, and biostatistics.

JOURNAL CLUB SETTING

Journal clubs can take place in many settings and may depend on the structure. Journal clubs that are integrated into coursework will typically take place in the classroom setting, a familiar space often rich in technology that can help aid in discussion. Commonly, this setting is more structured than a practice setting and follows a format designed by the faculty. However, journal clubs can take place in more informal settings, such as in a home or in a public place; such a setting may make newer participants more comfortable and likely to engage in discussion. Journal clubs that take place at work may also be held on patient units or in an office setting. While the content of the discussion should not change, knowing the setting will help the presenter best prepare based on knowledge of available resources. For example, if presenting a journal club formally, by using a set of PowerPoint® slides, it is important for the facilitator or the presenter to ensure that the setting includes a working computer and a projector. Keeping a recurring schedule and meeting place may help increase attendance.[9] Additionally, providing food has been shown to increase journal club turnout when attendance is not mandatory.[11] No matter the setting, it is important for a presenter to be aware of the given setting and prepared to maximize the learning opportunities of a journal club.

JOURNAL CLUB FORMAT

There are several journal club formats that can be used. First is a presentation-based journal club, in which the presenter will present an overview of a study, along with their critique (as discussed in Chapters 4 to 6). This format is commonly used for student presenters, as it is the easiest to evaluate and assess their personal critique and evaluation of the article. This format is often integrated into health sciences curricula as a method to develop, apply, and assess the principles of literature evaluation and biostatistics, in addition to development of public-speaking skills. This format will often be accompanied by the creation of a slide set or a handout, and should allow time for questions and discussion.

The second style of journal club is a discussion-based journal club, which is often the more prevalent style of journal club outside of the classroom setting. In this format, all attendees are expected to have read and critiqued the selected article in advance, and are expected to participate. In this capacity, the presenter may be expected to provide enough background to set the stage for the article, including any relevant treatment guidelines, related therapies, and more information about the disease state in question. The presenter should also be prepared to keep the discussion focused and on track with the use of guiding questions. Typically, this format of journal club is used to evaluate current literature for new and emerging therapies but is also a great time to practice the critical evaluation skills that were presented in Chapters 4 through 6. Slide sets and handouts are less common in this setting, but may be used if determined by the facilitator. Suggestions of questions and other items for discussion are provided in Appendices 4-1 and 5-1.

Lastly, this age of ever-expanding technologies has paved the way for the online journal club. Using video-conferencing software, clinicians from various locations can meet together to help increase access and attendance to the journal club. This format is particularly attractive for multisite health systems in which a commute may be a deterrent to participation, and may also be used among nonaffiliated sites wishing to hold interactive journal clubs focused on specialty topics.[12,13] In this format, the journal club may also serve a purpose of socializing and professional networking by increasing communication among practitioners of similar interest and training, such as among postgraduate residents and fellows within specialty tracks. Asynchronous online journal clubs are also an option and may increase participation due to increased convenience (Case Study 9-1).[14]

Case Study 9–1

A pharmacist in a hospital with a newly started residency program is looking at starting a journal club. The pharmacist is hoping to get the club going by making the discussion a required part of rotation for pharmacy students and residents at the site. However, after a few months of the new program, interest from pharmacy staff appears low and turnout has been less than anticipated.

- *What measures can be taken to increase participation from staff members?*

Preparing the Presentation

SELECTING THE ARTICLE

Articles can be selected in a variety of fashions. Typically, high-quality articles from reputable journals and landmark trials are selected for student presentations in the classroom. One way to gauge the prominence of a journal is by its **impact factor**. Alternately, an instructor may pick articles that appear in popular news sources (e.g., television, newspaper, electronic media), which allows students to understand the significant limitations of what may be learned from such sources. For practicing clinicians, the focus is typically on reviewing a new article to keep abreast of literature, evaluating a piece of original research to help answer a clinical question, or for teaching purposes related to a recent patient case or clinical scenario encountered during the course of clinical practice. One way for clinicians to keep abreast of new literature is to identify a few key journals relevant to one's practice and monitor the table of contents of each new issue for articles that appear useful to one's practice. Articles surrounding clinical controversies are particularly well-suited for journal clubs because participants may have different insight and evidence to provide to the discussion. Ideas may also be solicited from participants in advance of the meeting in order to gather ideas for therapies or disease states target as the topic of discussion. This gives participants the opportunity to offer suggestions of topics that they believe to be timely or clinically relevant, and may help to spur interest and subsequent turnout and participation. Note that articles do not need to produce positive results to be the topic of discussion; an article which does not demonstrate the benefit of a therapy, including therapies already in use, may still have the potential to affect practice and can certainly be the focus of a journal club. Certainly, drotrecogin alfa (activated; Xigris®) was the topic of countless journal clubs following publication of the PROWESS-SHOCK trial.[15] While the randomized controlled trial is a mainstay of the journal club, it is important to review other study designs that were discussed in Chapters 4 and 5; this is an opportune time to review other study designs such as cohort studies, non-inferiority studies, and meta-analyses. ❸ *Case reports, letters, and nonsystematic reviews should not be the focus of a journal club discussion.*

CONSIDERATIONS FOR PREPARATION

When evaluating the article, the reader should collect enough background information to obtain an adequate perspective. The onus of providing enough background to set the stage for discussion is typically on the presenter, who should address any pertinent treatment guidelines, comparable therapies and the place in therapy of the agent being studied, and any disease state specific information such as epidemiological information. The reader should always review any supplements or appendices to selected articles when these are available. Each participant should be supplied with the article for discussion well in advance, to allow time for thoughtful critique. As described above, handouts may or may not be used. If the decision to use a handout is made, it should be brief; remember that each participant should have already read the article. Slide sets are often not necessary for discussion-based journal clubs and may inadvertently distract from the discussion. As previously described, the presenter should come prepared with questions aimed at generating discussion. Questions should be open-ended to gather as many opinions as possible and to allow participants to expand upon their ideas. Participants may also be provided with questions to answer or a checklist to complete prior to attending the journal club, if desired. This may help new participants feel more prepared and likely to actively participate during the discussion.

DELIVERING THE PRESENTATION

Presenters should always set the stage for the discussion by first communicating the reason for choosing the selected article and providing any pertinent background for the study. The amount of detail provided will depend on the audience, how well the background was described within the article, and the nature of the article. For instance, if the research being discussed is the **pivotal trial** for a new medication with a novel mechanism of action, it is worth dedicating extra time to discussing the pharmacology of the new therapy. Pertinent background pertaining to related articles (e.g., a letter to the editor, commentaries) and previous trials with the same therapy should be included.

After setting the stage and stating the purpose of the study, the study methods should be discussed. How were patients recruited? Were the selected outcome variables appropriate for what was being studied? Was the trial of adequate length? This is also a great time to incorporate statistics into the discussion. Were statistical methods described? If so, were they appropriate or adequate? If the presenter disagrees with the methods, this is the perfect time to state what should ideally have been done. If the presenter had to review the statistical tests or concepts used, it is likely that others can benefit from this knowledge as well. As a general rule, if it was necessary to look it up, consider including it in the discussion! These are just a few of the most common items discussed from the methods section; see Appendices 4-1 and 5-1 for more comprehensive examples that can also be used to prepare a check sheet for presenters to consider.

Next, the results and conclusions of the study are discussed. Are the results well described? Are results presented for each specified endpoint? How many patients were lost to follow-up? It is important to address the strengths and limitations of the study during discussion, keeping in mind the internal and external validities of the results. Keep in mind that there may be more strengths and limitations to add than those included in the article. The authors' conclusions should be clearly stated. ❹ *However, journal club presenters should draw their own conclusions related to the findings of the study that they are presenting. Evidence to support this critique should be shared with the group* (Case Study 9-2).

Case Study 9–2

The pharmacist in Case 9-1 has been able to increase turnout to their monthly journal club discussion. However, there is often debate on whether or not certain aspects of the study are valid. This often leads to disagreement among members.

- *What is a reasonable approach to help address these issues?*

ADDING CLINICAL RELEVANCE

After presenting and critiquing the article in its entirety, it is time to put the findings of the article into perspective. How should this new information be used in practice? If the study is investigating a new medication, how should it be recommended or used? If the presenter would use or recommend it, in what specific patient population or clinical scenario would the therapy be most appropriate? This is an opportune time to present a case vignette of how this therapy might be used in a real-life scenario. ❺ *Discussion among journal club participants can serve as an outlet of providing interesting clinical cases and differing clinical insight and perspectives.*

Other key items to consider when presenting a journal club include practical issues and external validity, which may not be thoroughly discussed by the study's investigators. For instance, is the new agent significantly more expensive than the comparator or standard of care? Is the medication available only via a restricted access, such as a Risk Evaluation Mitigation Strategy (REMS)? Is there significant dose burden or complex dosage regimen which may be a barrier to adherence? Answering these questions can help tie the results of the study to clinical practice. Keep in mind that the external validity of the study's results cannot exist if the internal validity of the study (i.e., how well the study was conducted) was not established.

After critical appraisal and journal club discussion of a recently published article, participants may choose to write a **letter to the editor** to describe their analysis of the study.[4,16] Authoring a letter to the editor for publication has been shown to be an enjoyable learning method for reinforcing critical appraisal skills, and many participants will find the group format less intimidating than pursuing this scholarly activity alone. Well-constructed and thoughtful letters should be considered for submission to the journal in which the article was published.[16] Many journals outline their requirements for submission of a letter. The possibility of a potential publication may serve as an outlet for stimulating interest in journal club attendance and participation (Case Study 9-3).

Case Study 9–3

The pharmacist from Cases 9-1 and 9-2 has seen great success with the implementation of their journal club program, and their third-shift pharmacy staff is hoping to find a way to participate.

- *What option could you suggest?*

Conclusion

The focus and execution of journal clubs can vary greatly, and should be tailored to meet the specific need of the group. Careful and critical analysis of study design and statistical methods should be included when discussing original research. Use of a checklist or template will help guide participants through the literature-evaluation process. Presenters should aim to maximize practical information and clinical relevance in their presentation to increase the benefit to other participants.

Self-Assessment Questions

1. Which one of the following is *NOT* a primary goal of journal club participation?
   a. Practice critical appraisal skills
   b. Become a content expert in a therapeutic discipline
   c. Keep current with newly published literature
   d. Improve understanding of statistical methods and research design

2. Which one of the following is *NOT* a function of the journal club facilitator?
   a. Secure a meeting space
   b. Invite guests
   c. Approve articles to be discussed
   d. Provide an overview of the study

3. Critical appraisal is the process of systematically and critically evaluating a scientific study for relevance and value within a specific context.
   a. True
   b. False

4. Discussion of a clinical controversy should be avoided during a journal club discussion.
   a. True
   b. False

5. Which of the following is most suitable for a journal club presentation?
   a. A case series
   b. A letter to the editor
   c. A nonsystematic review
   d. A meta-analysis

6. Which of the following is least likely to help promote participation in discussion?
   a. Use of a presentation-style format and slide set
   b. Use of open-ended questions
   c. Sending participants a literature review checklist
   d. Sending participants the selected article in advance

7. Journal clubs are the most frequently used active learning strategy when teaching medical literature evaluation.
   a. True
   b. False

8. Which of the following should be the *first* item discussed during a journal club presentation?
   a. Critique of overall study design
   b. Critique of statistical methods
   c. Whether your conclusions match the author's
   d. Rationale for selecting the study

9. Only trials with positive results are suitable for journal club discussion.
   a. True
   b. False

10. Which of the following is **LEAST** likely to promote attendance at journal club?
    a. Using an online format
    b. Having each session at a different time of day
    c. Meeting in a casual setting
    d. Writing a letter to the editor after each session

11. An impact factor is an objective way to gauge the relative prestige of a scientific journal.
    a. True
    b. False

12. If you disagree with the findings of a study, the best option is to:
    a. Avoid using this article for a journal club discussion
    b. Contact the authors of the study
    c. Write a letter to the editor
    d. Change your opinion to agree with the authors

13. Monitoring the table of contents of several journals can help you identify articles related to your practice.
    a. True
    b. False

14. Journal clubs were started in the 1800s as a means to share resources.
    a. True
    b. False

15. Information about directions for use and cost of a medication should be avoided during a journal club discussion.
    a. True
    b. False

REFERENCES

1. Linzer M. The journal club and medical education: over one hundred years of unrecorded history. Postgrad Med J. 1987;63(740):475-8.
2. Lizarondo LM, Grimmer-Somers K, Kumar S. Exploring the perspectives of allied health practitioners toward the use of journal clubs as a medium for promoting evidence-based practice: a qualitative study. BMC Med Educ. 2011;11:66.
3. Matthews DC. Journal clubs most effective if tailored to learner needs. Evid Based Dent. 2011;12(3):92-3.
4. Stallings A, Borja-Hart N, Fass J. New Practitioners Forum: strategies for reinventing journal club. Am J Health Syst Pharm. 2011;68(1):14-6.
5. Cave MT, Clandinin DJ. Revisiting the journal club. Med Teach. 2007;29(4):365-70.
6. O'Sullivan TA, Phillips J, Demaris K. Medical literature evaluation education at US schools of pharmacy. Am J Pharm Educ. 2016;80(1):5.
7. Flarey DL. Journal club: a tool for health care management and development. Health Care Superv. 1993;11(3):53-8.
8. Wombwell E, Murray C, Davis SJ, Palmer K, Nayar M, Konkol J. Leadership journal club. Am J Health Syst Pharm. 2011;68(21):2026-7.
9. Hattoy SL, Childress B, Jett A, Motney J. Enhancing experiential education: implementing and improving the journal club experience. Curr Pharm Teach Learn. 2015;7:389-94.
10. Al Achkar M. Redesigning journal club in residency. Adv Med Educ Pract. 2016;7:317-20.
11. Lee AG, Boldt HC, Golnik KC, Arnold AC, Oetting TA, Beaver HA, Olson RJ, Carter K. Using the journal club to teach and assess competence in practice-based learning

and improvement: a literature review and recommendation for implementation. Surv Ophthalmol. 2005;50(6):542-8.

12. Miller Quidley A, LeClaire A, Glick Frasiolas J, Berger K, Gonzales JP, Oyen L. Implementation of a national, web-based critical care pharmacy journal club. Am J Health Syst Pharm. 2015;72(15):1260, 1262.

13. Devabhakthuni S, Reed BN, Watson K. Interactive web-based regional journal club for postgraduate year 2 pharmacy residents in cardiology. Am J Health Syst Pharm. 2016;73(17):1300.

14. Lizarondo L, Kumar S, Grimmer-Somers K. Online journal clubs: an innovative approach to achieving evidence-based practice. J Allied Health. 2010;39(1):e17-22.

15. Ranieri VM, Thompson BT, Barie PS, Dhainaut JF, Douglas IS, Finfer S, Gardlund B, Marshall JC, Rhodes A, Artigas A, Payen D, Tenhunen J, Al-Khalidi HR, Thompson V, Janes J, Macias WL, Vangerow B, Williams MD, PROWESS-SHOCK Study Group. Drotrecogin alfa (activated) in adults with septic shock. N Engl J Med. 2012;366(22):2055-64.

16. Green BN, Johnson CD. Use of a modified journal club and letters to editors to teach critical appraisal skills. J Allied Health. 2007;36(1):47-51.

SUGGESTED READINGS

1. Green BN, Johnson CD. Use of a modified journal club and letters to editors to teach critical appraisal skills. J Allied Health. 2007;36(1):47-51.

2. Guyatt G, Rennie D, Meade MO, Cook DJ. Users' guides to the medical literature: a manual for evidence-based clinical practice. 3rd ed. New York, NY: McGraw-Hill; 2015.

3. Lizarondo L, Kumar S, Grimmer-Somers K. Online journal clubs: an innovative approach to achieving evidence-based practice. J Allied Health. 2010;39(1):e17-22.

4. McLeod P, Steinert Y, Boudreau D, Snell L, Wiseman J. Twelve tips for conducting a medical education journal club. Med Teach. 2010;32(5):368-70.

5. Miller Quidley A, LeClaire A, Glick Frasiolas J, Berger K, Gonzales JP, Oyen L. Implementation of a national, web-based critical care pharmacy journal club. Am J Health Syst Pharm. 2015;72(15):1260, 1262.

6. Stallings A, Borja-Hart N, Fass J. New Practitioners Forum: strategies for reinventing journal club. Am J Health Syst Pharm. 2011;68(1):14-6.

7. Stapleton JJ. The successful journal club. Clin Podiatr Med Surg. 2007;24(1):51-5.

Chapter Ten

Legal Aspects of Drug Information Practice

Martha M. Rumore

Learning Objectives

After completing this chapter, the reader will be able to

- Describe the legal issues related to the provision of drug information (DI).
- Apply various legal theories that impose liability on pharmacists providing DI.
- Describe how pharmacists can help protect themselves from malpractice claims resulting from the provision of DI.
- Explain the Doctrine of Drug Overpromotion as it pertains to the 1997 Food and Drug Administration (FDA) Modernization Act (FDAMA).
- Identify the liability concerns inherent with off-label drug use and informed consent.
- Describe U.S. copyright law as it pertains to the provision of DI.
- Identify copyright, liability, and privacy issues arising from the Internet and social media.
- Describe the legal and ethical challenges emerging in telemedicine and cybermedicine.
- Describe the DI plan that addresses the Health Insurance Portability and Accountability Act (HIPAA) of 1996.
- Explain the legal issues involved with industry support for pharmaceutical educational activities.

Key Concepts

❶ Currently, most litigation concerning pharmacists involves negligence.

❷ There are a number of ways in which tort liability can relate to the provision of DI: incomplete information, inappropriate quality information, outdated information, inappropriate analysis, or dissemination of information.

❸ There are at least three key areas of labeling and advertising liability: the learned intermediary rule, which is a defense to failure to warn actions; the doctrine of overpromotion, under which adequate warning is alleged to have been diluted by communications failing to adequately convey the full impact of the warning; and promotion of off-label use or FDA unapproved indications.

❹ DI is currently being obtained from a number of Internet/social media and mobile apps and there is the possibility of DI liability for information obtained from these sources.

❺ Pharmacists providing DI must have a working knowledge of copyright law both to avoid liability and to protect their own literary works.

❻ The Health Insurance Portability and Accountability Act of 1996 (HIPAA) Privacy Rule is not intended to disrupt or discourage adverse event reporting or drug information in any way.

❼ The FDA, the American Council for Continuing Medical Education (ACCME), and the Pharmaceutical Research and Manufacturers of America (PhRMA) have established educational policies, guidelines, or guidances which allow communication between industry and the continuing medical education (CME) providers.

Introduction

An understanding of the legal aspects of drug information (DI) can help a practitioner in day-to-day practice, as well as provide some possible ways to protect himself or herself in the legal system. This chapter is intended to examine legal issues and should not be considered legal advice.

There are a myriad of legal issues confronting the various facets of DI. These legal issues cross over a number of traditional legal specialties, including computer law, advertising law, privacy law, intellectual property law, telecommunications law, and tort law. This chapter provides an overview and discussion of the key legal issues involving intellectual property rights, torts, privacy, and advertising and promotion that may arise in the provision of DI.

Decades after the genesis of DI services, the legal duties of pharmacists providing DI are still evolving. Today, most pharmacy curriculums, board certifications, and postgraduate year one (PGY-1) residencies include DI, realizing that whether a student specializes in DI or not, it is an integral part of pharmacist-supervised patient care. Pharmacists can and will be held liable for their conduct relating to DI. This chapter begins with an examination of the expanded liability of the DI specialist, which is defined as those pharmacists who either work in DI centers or who spend the majority of their working day providing DI (e.g., clinical managers, DI specialists, and PGY-1 and postgraduate year two [PGY-2] residents). The liability inherent in the provisions of DI to patients as an integral component of pharmacist-supervised patient care will be covered as will recommendations for prevention and mitigation of liability. The chapter then explores copyright, privacy, legal issues pertaining to Internet/social media, direct-to-consumer-advertising, off-label use, as well as industry support for educational activities.

Tort Law

- Pharmacists' functions such as online searching, monitoring or recommending drug therapy, preparing drug alerts and pharmacy bulletins, participating in pharmacy and therapeutics (P&T) committees, conducting medication use evaluations (MUE), writing and revising medication policies, training residents, pharmacy students, and pharmacy staff, and identifying adverse drug events entail legal obligations of proper performance.

  Minimal practice standards for clinicians have been put forth to delineate functions and activities that may be considered essential to the provision of DI services. Position papers and standards of the American Society of Health-System Pharmacists (ASHP) and The Joint Commission (TJC), as well as Accreditation Council for Pharmacy Education (ACPE) curriculum standards, and literature regarding appropriate management of DI requests remove any doubt about the level of expertise needed.[1-3] Minimal standards of performance and a consistent level of competence must be assured by clinicians pro-
- moting or offering DI regardless of the practice site. Although there are no standards to accredit DI centers, professional standards of performance may be used by courts as an objective measuring tool for the standard of care.

  The pharmacy profession is assuming an increased legal responsibility to provide DI in accordance with the Pharmacist's Patient Care Process adopted by the Joint Commission of Pharmacy Practitioners.[4] The physician has been considered the learned intermediary, responsible for communicating the manufacturer's warnings to the patient. However, cases in which pharmacists failed to counsel or warn patients
- are showing a trend in pharmacist liability.[5] Although most cases still maintain that the pharmacist has no duty to warn, a minority of cases in various jurisdictions demonstrate that the pharmacist's duty to warn of foreseeable complications of drug therapy is becoming a recognized part of the expanded legal responsibility of pharmacists.

Courts have been more willing to apply a duty to warn where the pharmacist voluntarily assumes the duty, or has special knowledge about a patient, or the prescription is dangerous as written.[6]

Where the patient is at higher risk than the general population, the courts have uniformly found liability. Today pharmacists providing DI are more likely to be held to the same standards as physicians when determining standard of care.

❶ *Currently, most litigation concerning pharmacists involves negligence.* Traditionally, physicians remain responsible for their patients and must exert **due care**; that is, a physician who knows or should have known that the information provided was improper may be held liable for negligence. Therefore, it is safe to assume that a legal cause of action pertaining to the provision of DI will be founded on the theory of negligence as the direct or **proximate cause** of personal injury or death. Malpractice liability based on negligence refers to failure to exercise the degree of care that a prudent (reasonable) person would exercise under the same circumstances. Elements of negligence include the four Ds: (1) duty breached, (2) damages, (3) direct causation, and (4) defenses absent. To establish a negligent failure, actual conduct must be compared with what is considered standard professional conduct. Typically, this is accomplished by introducing evidence of the relevant professional standards or testimony from expert witnesses such as college of pharmacy faculty or other DI practitioners. Once the duty of care is established, the plaintiff would need a preponderance of evidence to prove that (1) the information provided was materially deficient, (2) the deficient information was a proximate cause of injury suffered (or at least a substantial contributing factor), (3) the recipient reasonably relied on the information provided, (4) the information deficiency was due to failure to exercise reasonable care, and (5) the pharmacist knew or should have known that the safety or health of another may have depended on the accuracy of the information provided.

Expanding on the first element of negligence, duty breached, it is important to be aware of the fact that the duty must be a legal duty, not a moral or ethical duty. Although there are many ethical dilemmas pertaining to the provision of DI by pharmacists and they can sometimes give rise to a cause of action, an ethical breach is not necessarily a legal breach. Similarly, conduct that is considered unprofessional in the broad sense (e.g., rudeness) is distinct from legal duty.

In a study of DI requests, those from consumers rather than health professionals raised more ethical issues.[7] For example, should a pharmacist respond to a drug identification request for someone else's medication? Is the situation different if the medication is a drug of abuse and the inquiry is from a parent, relative, teacher, or police officer? Current law provides little guidance for disclosure of DI for questionable purposes; therefore, pharmacists must exercise independent professional judgment and assume legal responsibility for that judgment when exercised.

Case Study 10–1

The anticoagulation pharmacist receives an order for enoxaparin in a patient who is receiving warfarin. The patient's current INR is 5.2. The anticoagulation pharmacist is a board certified ambulatory care pharmacist (BCACP). The pharmacist dispenses the enoxaparin and the patient is harmed.

- *What factors favor finding the pharmacist liable for negligence?*
- *Is the prescription dangerous as written?*
- *Is the specialist more liable than the generalist?*
- *Who may be liable in this situation—the pharmacist, the physician, or the clinic?*

Suppose a patient develops a reaction that is believed to be caused by a drug, and the pharmacist is consulted to find any case reports of this drug causing the reaction. If the case is available online, but not in print, and the pharmacist had access to online databases, but did not consult them, was the pharmacist required to do so? Did the pharmacist exert reasonable care? Reasonable care (i.e., that which is considered acceptable and responsible) is the standard applied for negligence. What if the pharmacist searched MEDLINE® but not Embase® databases, or vice versa, and thereby failed to retrieve the case? Should the pharmacist have searched both? There are no clear answers here. Who can say what a reasonable search might have been on a given day? However, using outdated references would more likely constitute an inadequate search. In a German case, a court held a business and patent information service to be responsible for not having used updated materials.[8]

In a highly publicized case involving a clinical trial being conducted at Johns Hopkins University, a researcher conduced an incomplete PubMed search only back to 1966 regarding lung damage from hexamethonium.[9] Although articles published in the 1950s and other sources such as TOXLINE® and Micromedex® warned of such dangers, the researcher had not consulted these references resulting in a patient's death.

Cases against pharmacists have held that pharmacists who gain information about the unique susceptibility of a patient are liable for failure to warn of the risks. In *Dooley v. Everett*, the court held the pharmacist liable for failing to warn a patient of the interaction of theophylline with erythromycin that produced seizures and consequent brain damage.[10] Similarly, in *Hand v. Krakowski*, the pharmacist failed to alert either the patient or physician of the drug interaction between the patient's psychotropic drug and alcohol.[11] The fact that the medication profile indicated that the patient was an alcoholic created a foreseeable risk of injury and, therefore, a duty to warn on the part of the pharmacist.

Case Study 10–2

The health system pharmacist receives a prescription order for metformin 500 mg twice daily for a 55-year-old male patient who has severe renal impairment. The pharmacist dispenses the drug without checking the patient's renal function in the computer. The pharmacy department medication use manual policy for metformin requires the pharmacist to check and document the patient's creatinine clearance prior to dispensing metformin.

- *If the patient is harmed, did the pharmacist fall below the standard of care? Could the pharmacist be judged negligent?*

Recently, this liability applied to DI advice the pharmacist provided on a nonprescription (over the counter [OTC]) product. Pharmacists can be sued for malpractice and negligence for inaccurate advice (requires affirmative misrepresentations) regarding OTC drugs that harms the patient. In *Whiting v Rite Aid Pharmacy*,[12] the decedents' estate sued the pharmacist for a recommendation that the patient could safety take phenylpropanolamine and pseudoephedrine. The plaintiff contended that she informed the pharmacist of the decedents' prostate problems. The pharmacist denied the conversation occurred. The plaintiff asserted that the use of the drug exacerbated the patient's prostate condition, resulting in several surgeries, and ultimately, his death several years later. The pharmacy contended that **learned intermediary doctrine** protects pharmacists from such liability and the pharmacists' duty of care does not require giving adequate advice about OTC drugs. The court ruled the learned intermediary doctrine only applies to prescription drugs. Additionally, the court was clear in stating:

> "Pharmacists in Utah clearly have duties regarding nonprescription drugs. If a pharmacist answers a customer's question and offers advice about nonprescription drugs, the pharmacist must advise and act in a non-negligent manner consistent with a reasonably prudent pharmacist's response to a customer's question about the safety of a nonprescription drug."

In *Baker v. Arbor Drugs, Inc.*, the court ruled that by advertising its drug interaction software, the defendant pharmacy voluntarily assumed a duty to use its computer technology with due care. The pharmacy technician had overridden the drug interaction between tranylcypromine (Parnate®) and clemastine fumarate/phenylpropanolamine hydrochloride (Tavist-D®) that the system detected from the patient's medication profile. The patient committed suicide after suffering a stroke from the combination.[13] In another case, the pharmacist chose to override the computer alert regarding an interaction between tramadol and methadone, resulting in the patient's death. A $6 million verdict was returned against the pharmacy for failure to warn.[14]

❷ *There are a number of ways in which* **tort liability** *can relate to the provision of DI: incomplete information, inappropriate quality information, outdated information, inappropriate analysis, or dissemination of information.*

INCOMPLETE DRUG INFORMATION

Is the pharmacist liable when the DI provided is incomplete? Should the pharmacist provide all the medication information via a DI sheet or patient package insert (PPI)? There have been several cases against pharmacists for failure to dispense mandatory PPIs for certain drugs that later caused harm. In *Parkas v. Saary*, the court addressed the issue of whether the pharmacist's failure to dispense the FDA mandated PPI for progesterone was the proximate cause of a congenital eye defect that occurred.[15] Because congenital defects, but not eye deformities, were specified in the PPI, failure to provide the PPI could not be proven to be the proximate cause. Therefore, judgment was in favor of the pharmacy. In *Frye v. Medicare-Glaser Corporation*, the pharmacist counseled the patient regarding drowsiness with Fiorinal® (aspirin, butalbital, caffeine), but failed to provide a warning not to consume alcohol. The patient died presumably as a result of combining the drug with beer. Here, the DI provided was incomplete. The trial court did not find the pharmacist had a duty to warn.[16] Although this case was decided before Omnibus Budget Reconciliation Act of 1990 (i.e., OBRA '90), with its mandatory patient counseling provisions in effect, its outcome would probably not have changed as a result.

In a number of cases where the plaintiffs asserted that the pharmacist breached a duty to warn as required under OBRA '90, the courts have held that OBRA does not create an independent or private cause of action.[17–19]

Other cases are finding pharmacists have a responsibility for patient counseling and drug therapy monitoring.[20] In *Sanderson v. Eckerd Corporation*, where the pharmacy advertised that its computer system would detect drug interactions or warn patients about adverse drug reactions, pharmacists were held liable when they failed to detect and warn the patient of a potential adverse reaction.[21] In *Horner v. Spalitto*, the court imposed a duty on a pharmacist to alert the prescriber when the dose prescribed is outside the therapeutic range.[22] In *Happel v. Wal-Mart Stores*, the pharmacy's computer system was overridden, and the pharmacist failed to warn a patient allergic to aspirin and ibuprofen of the potential for cross-allergenicity with ketorolac.[23] The court found a duty to warn when a contraindicated drug is prescribed. In *Morgan v. Wal-Mart Stores*, where the plaintiffs alleged that the pharmacist's failure to properly warn of the known dangers of desipramine was the proximate cause of the patient's death, the court held pharmacists have a duty beyond accurately filling a prescription "based on known contraindications, which would alert a reasonably prudent pharmacist to a potential problem."[24] However, the court did not find for the plaintiff opining that pharmacists do not have knowledge that desipramine may cause hypereosinophilic syndrome. Liability could also attach where there is a Risk Evaluation and Mitigation Strategy (REMS) requirement where either a pharmacist is required to provide a MedGuide or where patient consent is required for failure to adhere to some other component of the REMS program, such as patient or provider enrollment.

Clearly, these cases demonstrate an expansion of pharmacist's duties from the non-discretionary standard of technical accuracy to a discretionary standard that requires pharmacists to perform professional functions—that is, from a technical model to a pharmacist-supervised patient care model. Knowledge of, or access to, DI is becoming an important factor that courts consider in determination of the pharmacist's duty to warn.

In a case of first impression, a court decided whether a hospital pharmacist contacting a physician regarding a colchicine dosage had a duty of care to the physician to provide complete DI.[25] While the pharmacist advised regarding a correct oral dosage, he did not advise of the correct dose in a renally impaired patient. The plaintiff alleged that the hospital pharmacy's voluntary undertaking to provide DI, and the pharmacist's voluntary intervening between the patient and physician created a duty on the part of the pharmacist to the physician. This is different from other duty to warn cases where plaintiff alleges the pharmacist has a duty to warn the patient. In this case, the plaintiff alleged the hospital's pharmacy voluntarily undertook to be a DI resource and the hospital pharmacist voluntarily intervened between the patient and physician, thereby creating a duty to the physician. The court, however, rejected the argument that a voluntary undertaking of a duty to a physician was created based on a pharmacist's interaction with the patient's physician. The court further held that the learned intermediary doctrine forecloses any duty of care on the part of the pharmacist to the patient, based on the pharmacist's statements to the physician. Significantly, the court commented that even if such a duty were placed on the pharmacist, the duty was not breached inasmuch as the pharmacist correctly followed the hospital's intervention policy.

While pharmacists are in a position to provide DI, providing the patient with all information may have a detrimental effect. In fact, it is the FDA's position that the information contained in professional labeling can be safely used only under the supervision of the licensed prescriber. It has, therefore, been the practice not to provide the patient with the professional labeling unless the patient specifically requests it. With regard to the duty to disclose to the patient low percentage risks, court rulings are inconsistent. One court allowed **strict liability** against a pharmacy. In *Heredia v. Johnson*, the pharmacist dispensed an otic solution without warning of the risk of tympanic membrane rupture and the need to discontinue the drug if certain symptoms appeared. The plaintiff claimed that because of the lack of warning he suffered from severe and permanent injury including brain damage.[26] However, in *Marchione v. State*, a prison inmate alleged lack of informed consent based on failure of the prison physician to inform him about adverse effects of prazosin (Minipress®), which caused permanent impotence. The physician argued his duty was only to warn of severe or frequent adverse effects. The *Marchione* court concluded the physician need not disclose a laundry list of 31 remote adverse effects. The adverse effect had a reported incidence of only two or three cases out of several million prescriptions and was, therefore, rare. The plaintiff also did not have any unique risk factors that would increase the likelihood of the reaction occurring.[27] The courts seem to look at risk factors unique to the patient in deciding whether the health professional is required to indicate the likelihood of occurrence of the risks.

Hall and Honey[28] divided the risks associated with a particular drug into two groups, inherent or noninherent. Inherent risks are unavoidable unique to the drug and usually identified in the package insert (PI), but do not include probable or common adverse effects. However well a drug is researched, manufactured, and prescribed, it still may have the ability to produce certain adverse effects. Examples of inherent drug risks are stroke from oral contraceptives or teeth discoloration from tetracyclines. Noninherent risks are created by the particular drug in combination with some extrinsic factor about which the pharmacist should reasonably know, and include maximum safe dosages, interactions, patient characteristics influencing pharmacokinetics, and probable or common adverse effects. Examples of noninherent risks would be nephrotoxicity from aminoglycosides in patients with renal impairment. The responsibility of the pharmacist to provide DI about noninherent risks is expanding.

What liability does the pharmacist incur for DI outside of the PI? Physicians may prescribe drugs as they see fit, without adhering to the specific therapeutic indications or dosing guidelines within the labeling. The FDA regulates the manufacture and promotion of drugs, not the practice of medicine. However, it has been held that a physician's deviation from the PI was ***prima facie*** (i.e., not requiring further support to establish validity, on its face value) evidence of negligence if the patient's injury resulted from the failure to adhere to the recommendations.[29] However, the states appear to be split on whether recommendations in a PI are *prima facie* evidence of the standard of care. It would be prudent for clinicians to consult the PI when responding to DI inquiries and include such information in the response, especially if the response contradicts what is in the PI.

A disciplinary action by a state pharmacy board highlights the importance of checking the PI or literature concerning the proposed use of a product. In *re Michael A. Gabert*,[30] a pharmacist received a prescription for 5% silver nitrate for bladder instillation. The pharmacist contacted a DI center and was told there was no literature supporting the proposed use. The pharmacist then requested evidence from the prescriber for such use and was referred to a published Mayo Clinic newsletter. The pharmacist did not seek or obtain a copy of the publication for the pharmacy records. Significant patient harm resulted when the solution was instilled into the patient's bladder. The Mayo Clinic newsletter pertained to silver argyrol, not silver nitrate.

INAPPROPRIATE QUALITY DRUG INFORMATION

It has long been recognized by law that false information provided to another could result in harm to the recipient if the recipient acted relying on the false information. Although **negligent misrepresentation** has not been applied to DI, there is no guarantee that it will not in the future.[31] The relevant law is the *Restatement (Second) of Torts, §311, Negligent Misrepresentation Involving Risk of Physical Harm*, which states:

> "One who negligently gives false information to another is subject to liability for physical harm caused by action taken by the other in reasonable reliance upon such information[...] Such negligence may consist of failure to exercise reasonable care in ascertaining accuracy of the information, or in the manner in which it is communicated."[32]

Thus, the DI itself may be faulty for one or more reasons: it may be dated; it may simply be wrong; it may be incomplete and, therefore, misleading; or none may have been provided because of an incomplete search or incompetent searcher. Information negligence may occur because of (1) **parameter negligence** (failure to consult the correct source) or (2) **omission negligence** (consulting the correct source, but failure to locate the correct answer[s]). A study evaluated the accuracy of a drug identification response by 56 DI centers. Approximately 30% correctly identified the investigational drug product; 67% could not make the identification; most importantly, 3.6% (two DI centers) made an incorrect identification. The study found inconsistencies in responses of DI centers.[33] Another study evaluated the quality of DI responses provided by 116 DI centers to multiple queries. The correct response rates varied from 5% for a question pertaining to erythromycin for diabetic gastroparesis to 90% for a drug interaction question pertaining to didanosine-dapsone. For each of three patient-specific questions, the percentages of centers eliciting vital patient data were 5%, 27%, and 86%. The findings suggest that many DI centers continue to fail to elicit patient-specific information necessary for informed responses and focus instead on procedural and technical matters.[34] As an example, despite the peer-review process, the structure of bilirubin was found to be incorrect in an article and the three leading biochemistry textbooks in the United States.[35]

DI of inappropriate quality is not limited to the print media. Several studies have evaluated the use of mobile device apps, such as Epocrates®, Medscape, Lexicomp, Skyscape®, and MIMS for providing DI.[36] A recent quality assessment study of the top

100 apps in medical categories revealed deficiencies in appropriateness, reliability, usability, and privacy. For DI apps, most did not allow for product identification and did not provide supporting references for the DI. Apps with a drug interaction checker had only ~67% overall quality rating, which the authors of the studies conclude may be providing unreliable DI to clinicians. Additionally, differences in functionality were found when using different platforms, such as Apple or Android versions.[37] Another quality study of 270 drug summaries in five online compendia found a median of 782 errors with the greatest number occurring with dosage and administration, patient education, and warnings and precautions. A majority were classified as incomplete, followed by inaccurate and omitted.[38]

Mobile device apps do not undergo any quality assessment and DI apps are no exception. FDA only regulates medical apps that are defined as medical devices where functionality could pose a risk to patient safety if they do not function as intended (e.g., smartphone app to evaluate electrocardiogram data).[39] The FDA has explicitly stated that it will exercise enforcement discretion for all other mobile apps including DI apps.

Inappropriate quality information may be the result of ghostwriting or publication marketing. Ghostwriting occurs when a pharmaceutical company develops the concept for an article to counteract criticism of a drug or embellish its benefits, hires a professional writing company to draft the article, retains a health professional to sign off as the author, and finds a publisher to unwittingly publish the work. In a recent product liability case, the court ordered the pharmaceutical company to disclose its documents pertaining to its ghostwriting practices.[40] In some instances, posters and meeting abstracts may actually be generated by pharmaceutical industry or incomplete and lacking in peer review. For example, the reader has no way of knowing whether the abstract results are reflective of the entire study population or merely a small subset.

Can pharmacists providing DI be held responsible for retrieving information that is itself inaccurate? What responsibility does the information producer incur for errors in information sources? An unskilled searcher or one with insufficient searching knowledge may not find correct or complete information, which can lead to the wrong answer. The fault can lie anywhere in the information dissemination chain, publication, collection, storage, retrieval, dissemination, or utilization. Errors are often encountered in DI databases.[41] DI pharmacists are constantly finding errors and reporting the errors to the vendor or publisher. For example, when completing a class review of potential probiotic agents for the drug formulary, it was noted that only capsules were listed for one product, although the product was available as a liquid and granules. Although very few cases have been brought before courts concerning the liability of print or online information sources, there is some case law to guide under the theory of strict liability.

Strict liability applies where a defective product proximately causes physical harm. Where the service rendered is deemed to be a professional service, the courts exhibit a reluctance to impose strict liability. With exceptions, persons physically injured because of their reliance on defective and unreasonably dangerous information have only negligence as a cause of action, and only against the author, not the publisher;[42] only if the publisher is negligent or offers intentionally misleading information, could it be held liable. This was tested in *Jones v. J.B. Lippincott Co.*, where a nursing student was injured after consulting and relying on a nursing textbook that recommended hydrogen peroxide enemas for the treatment of constipation. The courts rejected the plaintiff's claim that strict liability should be applied to the publisher.[43] Similarly, in a German case, a misprint in a medical textbook resulted in the injection of 25% rather than 2.5% sodium chloride solution, injuring a patient. Again, the court rejected strict liability for the publisher on the basis that any medically educated person should have noticed the misprint.[44] In *Roman v. City of New York*, the plaintiff sued for an alleged misstatement in a booklet distributed by a Planned Parenthood organization that resulted in a "wrongful conception." The court found that "a publisher cannot assume liability for all misstatements, said or unsaid, to a potentially unlimited public for a potentially unlimited period."[45] In *Winter v. G.R Putnam's Sons*, two people required liver transplants after collecting and eating poisonous wild mushrooms. They relied on an *Encyclopedia of Wild Mushrooms* in choosing to eat the mushrooms that caused this severe harm.[46] The court refused to hold the publisher liable and found a publisher has no duty to investigate the accuracy of information it publishes.

In *Delmuth Development Corp. v. Merck & Co.*, the plaintiff claimed lost sales because of publication of erroneous information in the *Merck Index*. The court considered the duty of a publisher to a reader to publish accurate information in a compendium.[47] The court noted a publisher's right to publish without fear of liability is guaranteed by the First Amendment and societal interest. It further held that even if it had a duty to publish with care, the plaintiff could not claim suffered damages because of reliance on this information.

Recently, an Austrian DI company, Diagnosia Enterprise, was sued by the global pharmaceutical company Sanofi for the way its product and its side effect profile were classified in a drug decision support software app. While the court did not grant Sanofi an **injunction**, the litigation and claim for injurious falsehood remain ongoing.[48] Inasmuch as Diagnosia has refused to change the information regarding the drug, the case does have implications for other DI companies.

What liability is incurred by an author or publisher for publication of product comparisons? Recently, a pharmacy journal publisher and author were sued for defamation by a device manufacturer where the publication compared and opined on the performance of devices for compounding sterile products.[49] The court granted the defendants motion to dismiss stating lack of actual malice (a necessary element of defamation). In this ruling, the court protected the First Amendment rights of scientists to report product comparisons and the rights of publishers regarding the peer-review process and publication of such comparisons.[50]

In *Libertelli v. Hoffman La Roche, Inc. & Medical Economics Co.*, the plaintiff became addicted to diazepam (Valium®) and sued the publisher of the *Physician's Desk Reference* (PDR).[51] The claim was based on the absence of warnings in the PDR regarding the addictive nature of the drug. The court dismissed the case against the publisher. Under a long line of cases, a publisher is not liable for matters of public interest if it has no knowledge of its falsity. Although some effort should be made to verify search results, the pharmacist cannot be held responsible for knowing and verifying the contents of all sources, whether in print or online. However, checking a second reference to verify information is prudent.

In a recent case, the patient developed Stevens-Johnson syndrome from lamotrigine and sued the prescriber, pharmacy chain, publisher, and software company for providing an abbreviated monograph sheet.[52] The software company had switched from a five-page monograph (with no sections for "Before Using This Medication," "Overdose," and "Additional Information") to a full eight-page monograph. To save printing costs, the pharmacy chain requested software customization so that it could continue to use the truncated monograph. The plaintiff claimed that she would not have taken the medication had she seen the redacted information. The publisher won on the basis of California law that it owed no duty to the plaintiff as it is neither a drug manufacturer nor a seller. The software company maintained that the DI monographs were protected by the First Amendment and it could not be held liable for omitting information. The court disagreed and this case is one of the first to hold a software vendor liable where it did not sell the plaintiff anything, did not write the monograph, and gave the pharmacy access to an abbreviated monograph meeting specifications set by the pharmacy itself. Evidence was, however, presented showing that the software company had requested and received a release of liability and an indemnity agreement from the pharmacy chain. Duty was found under the Good Samaritan liability, which holds that a person who undertakes to render services necessary to protect another is subject to liability resulting from failure to exercise reasonable care.[53]

Strict liability would appear applicable to software that is licensed without significant modification as a standard packaged system, as has been found with defective medical computer programs.[54] Clinicians providing DI should be aware of computer-related lawsuits that have arisen involving defects (or bugs) in software that caused erroneous results. These cases result in greater damage awards based on **consequential damages** (i.e., special as opposed to actual) suffered. An example of consequential damages would be damage to a firm's reputation. Perhaps the most widely cited software-related accidents involve malfunctioning computerized radiation machines where overdosages have caused patient deaths.[55] Radiation overdosages from faulty software continue to occur today; grim reminders of the problems faced by reliance on software.[56] In one particularly relevant case, the court held that the National Weather Service was liable for the deaths of four fishermen off Cape Cod, Massachusetts. The Weather Service had forecasted calm weather because of faulty software. Although the verdict was overturned on technical grounds, the U.S. District Court let stand the precedent holding an entity liable for information it provides.[57]

In another case, Jeppesen, an information provider, was held liable for an airplane crash caused by faulty data from the Federal Aviation Administration on flight patterns. A pilot used one of the faulty charts and crashed into a mountain, killing the crew and destroying the plane. The company paid $12 million in damages.[58] The court held the information provider strictly liable because the charts were considered a product. In *Jeppesen*, the mass production and mass marketing of the charts rendered them a product. Similarly, in *Greenmoss Builders v. Dun & Bradstreet*, the issue involved the erroneous listing of Greenmoss Builders as a company in bankruptcy in Dun & Bradstreet Business Information Report database. A jury awarded $350,000, including $300,000 in punitive damages. The case was appealed all the way to the Supreme Court, where Dun & Bradstreet lost the case.[59]

In *Daniel v. Dow Jones & Co., Inc.*, where a subscriber brought action against a provider of a computerized database alleging that he relied on a false news report in making investments, the court found that the subscriber did not have a special relationship with the database provider necessary to impose liability for negligent misstatements. First Amendment guarantees of freedom of the press also protected the provider from liability.[60]

As mentioned previously, DI provided may be inaccurate because it is dated, incomplete, or wrong. For example, inappropriate quality information may occur because references are updated differently. Even electronic references are updated differently— some monthly, others weekly. Most DI services require documentation of an answer in at least two different sources. The double-check procedure is common practice when preparing chemotherapy and avoiding drug administration errors. In many of the cases described above, liability could have been prevented by checking the information in more than one reference or source. Thus, checking a DI response in several references is the standard of practice.

INAPPROPRIATE ANALYSIS/DISSEMINATION OF DRUG INFORMATION

Is liability for providing DI a rhetorical supposition or a real possibility? The responsibility of pharmacists providing DI goes beyond that of mere information intermediary, the person between the information producer and the user. Published studies for DI centers have reported that 41% to 83% of requested information is patient specific or judgmental in nature.[61] In addition to liability for the negligent information retrieval and dissemination, the pharmacist's role involves information interpretation, evaluation, and giving advice.

This role falls into a consultative model and differs greatly from that of librarians. Librarians are not equipped to give advice. The pharmacist's role as evaluator and interpreter of the information creates a duty sufficient to sustain liability.

The paucity of case law in the area does not negate liability. The issue deserves consideration because of the potential for harm caused by DI provided by pharmacists. There have only been three cases, two cases involving poison information centers, one of which also was a DI center and a third involving the omission to provide DI while on rounds with the medical team. In *Reben v. Ely*, the plaintiffs filed suit against the DI center for injuries sustained by inadvertent administration of cocaine solution instead of acetaminophen to a 10-year-old patient. The local pharmacy had colored the 10% cocaine solution red and labeled it red solution to thwart abuse. When the nurse realized the mistake, she contacted the Arizona Poison and DI Center. The DI pharmacist described the symptomatology of cocaine overdose, but did not go far enough in recommending that the patient seek emergency care. The patient developed seizures and cardiopulmonary arrest with brain damage that required lifetime nursing care. At the trial, the expert witness testified that the DI center operated below the standard of care. The issue was not erroneous information, but whether the center went far enough in its responsibility in handling the call. The plaintiff was awarded $6.5 million; the DI center was held liable for $3.6 million.[62]

In another case, a lawsuit named a poison information center that was called for assistance when a student died after swallowing a toxic substance during a laboratory experiment. The poison center was named in the $2.5 million suit because it refused to release proof of its claim that the person who called had given the wrong name for the solution that the student drank.[63]

In a recent case, the court denied the motion to dismiss a case where the pharmacist rounding with a medical team "should have known that the patient was receiving the wrong drug for his condition" and failed to make a recommendation.[64] How this case is decided may expand liability for incomplete DI where the pharmacist has proximity to the patient (i.e., rounds).

From a liability standpoint, there are disadvantages to the formal combination of poison control and DI centers. For example, poison inquiries usually require immediate answers in critical situations without written documentation and sometimes without supporting references.[65,66] The outcomes of poisonings (e.g., overdoses, suicide attempts) are more likely to result in patient morbidity and mortality and require medical backup for acute treatment decisions. Some states (e.g., Arkansas, Oregon, Washington, Arizona, New Jersey) have statutory provisions for joint poison control and DI centers. In several of these states, such as Arkansas, immunity from personal liability in judgment (in contrast to carelessness or inadvertence) would not be actionable as malpractice unless a lack of due care can be shown. However, not all DI centers are protected from liability. Additionally, there have been other lawsuits involving poison control centers but these have mostly involved medical toxicologists serving as poison control center consultants, not DI pharmacists.[67]

Defenses to Negligence and Malpractice Protection

Even if the plaintiff can establish all the necessary elements of negligence, legal defenses can avoid or reduce liability. Some defenses might include a statute of limitations, comparative or contributory negligence, informed consent, or governmental immunity. It is important to keep in mind that there may be differences in both types of defenses to negligence and insurance coverage for individuals and employers. Further information on defenses will be described in the following sections.

DEFENSES FOR INDIVIDUALS

Assumption of the risk via informed consent and comparative or contributory negligence are defenses to negligence. Under informed consent, the defendant could assert that the patient knowingly assumed the risk for a new or experimental therapy or regimen. However, the risks the patient assumes does not include negligence on the part of the physician or pharmacist. There is no assumption of the risk for negligent behavior.

Comparative negligence is the allocation of responsibility for damages incurred between the plaintiff and defendant, based on the relative negligence of the two. **Concurrent negligence** is the wrongful acts or omissions of two or more persons acting independently, but causing the same injury. Under comparative or concurrent negligence, the pharmacist may also be held liable, either alone or together with the information requestor (e.g., physician and nurse), for inaccurate information or information that does not ensure maximal protection for the patient.

In the landmark case *Harbeson v. Parke Davis*, a federal court ruled that the doctrine of informed consent required a physician to furnish a patient contemplating pregnancy with information concerning the teratogenicity of the phenytoin she was taking. The physician had a duty to provide information reasonably available in the medical literature, but failed to do so. Even though the physician was not aware of the potential effects of phenytoin, studies were reported in the medical literature.[68] This case represents the only case in which a lack of a literature search resulted in liability.

Cases of **vicarious liability** are not new to medical malpractice. Vicarious liability is the attribution of liability upon one person for the actions of another. Through the doctrine of vicarious liability, a pharmacist could become associated with professional liability actions as part of a case against a hospital or a physician. Physicians have been found negligent for the negligence of nurses, therapists, and others working under their supervision. Significantly, no cases were found where physicians were found negligent from the negligence of pharmacists working under them. If a physician requests DI, he or she would also be held liable if a patient suffers because the search was deficient or the information incorrect. For example, in the *Harbeson* case, if the physician had requested the pharmacist to search for information about the teratogenicity of phenytoin and no references were found because of a faulty search, the pharmacist would share in the negligence together with the physician. The institution would probably also be named as a party in such legal action.

Delegation of authority does not mean abdication of responsibility. Under vicarious liability, a pharmacist who has not been personally negligent could be held responsible for the negligence of others. Supervision and adequate training of subordinates (e.g., interns, pharmacy technicians, other employees) are essential. Incompetence and substandard training of these individuals can lead to liability. An example might include a breach of confidentiality (e.g., revealing someone has a loathsome disease) by an employee.

From a legal standpoint, does charging a fee increase liability for the DI provider? Fee-based providers would appear to be at greater malpractice risk, especially if the relationship is a contractual one. If any of the contractual expectations are not met, the client has a contractual cause of action against the DI center. The courts will look to the terms of the agreement and the reasonable expectations of the parties. However, where bodily injury results, tort law may impose liability even where the defective information is given gratuitously and the DI provider derives no benefit from giving it.

A decision to comment on a physician's therapeutic recommendations, even if factually correct and in the patient's best interest, may result in a legal liability. Prescribers have brought defamation claims against pharmacies where the pharmacist made statements about the patient's physician who wrote the prescription. When the pharmacist wrote the words "pill mill" on the back of the prescription (libel), the defamation case was dismissed as only the defamed person can bring such a lawsuit.[69] In *LeFrock v. Walgreen Co.*, the court held, however, that the pharmacist did not commit slander (oral defamation) against the physician as the necessary element of malice was missing.[70] In addition, the pharmacist's comments during the consultation were privileged. However, in another case, the judge denied the chain pharmacy's allegation that the pharmacist's comments about the patient's physician were protected by a privilege.[71] Pharmacists have a legal and professional responsibility to detect and resolve problems with drug therapy and screen prescriptions for controlled substances. Meeting that responsibility may involve strong language when consulting with patients. Without removing the fear of civil liability as to anything said during patient counseling, pharmacists can be placed in an untenable position. At least a qualified privilege should apply where the alleged defamatory statements bear some connection to the ordinary course and scope of the pharmacist's practice.

DEFENSES FOR EMPLOYERS

Is the provider the hospital, university, or pharmacy where the DI is provided, or the practitioner providing the DI? The employer-employee relationship is a significant factor under either common law *respondeat superior* doctrine or, alternatively, a theory of negligent hire or supervision. Respondeat superior refers to the proposition that the employer is responsible for the negligent acts of its agents or employees. The injured party may also sue the employer for its negligence in hiring or supervising the employee. Under a negligent hire theory, it must be shown that the employee was unfit for the position and that a reasonable, preemployment interview or postemployment supervision would have discovered this fact.[72]

Although the person who provides the information is liable for the harm caused by it, the employer may also be held liable in the absence of sovereign or charitable immunity. For pharmacists providing DI employed by the government (e.g., Veteran's Administration [VA] or Public Health Service [PHS]), there are statutes providing governmental immunity, also called sovereign immunity, from **civil liability**. Such immunity, however, will not protect an intentionally or grossly negligent person.

Even if the lawsuit is nonmeritorious, DI providers affiliated with hospitals or universities represent a deep pocket for contribution to the settlement. With exceptions, suing the practitioner alone would fail to provide a windfall settlement for plaintiffs. The board of directors/trustees of the hospital or university where the DI is provided would be jointly liable. Joint and several liability refers to the sharing of liabilities among a group of people collectively and also individually. If the defendants are jointly and severally liable, it means that the injured party may sue some or all of the defendants together, or each one separately, and may collect equal amounts or unequal amounts from each. In states where joint and several liability applies, the pharmacist provides additional assurance that there will be sufficient assets to recover. The DI provider will be held responsible for the standard of care in the response to DI inquiries and may be found negligent.

PROTECTING AGAINST MALPRACTICE

Methods to protect against lawsuits include contracts covering financial arrangements, adequate documentation, disclaimers, and insurance.[73] For example, a disclaimer can be placed on results of online searches stating that the data being provided are from a source believed to be reliable and factually correct.[74] The best way to avoid omission negligence is to learn from experience, anticipate mistakes that may appear in electronic sources, and keep abreast of changes in DI sources. Even if the delivery of false information is the result of inaccurate information itself, the pharmacist would likely be named as a defendant if the database producer were sued.

Adequate documentation may spell the difference between refuting or not refuting an unfounded claim of malpractice. Such documentation includes responses to inquiries, as well as a record of steps taken in a search. Designing and following procedures to document the research process can help avoid negligence. In *Fidelity Leasing Corp. v. Dun & Bradstreet, Inc.*, the court looked at the operation procedures and adherence to them in the particular instance to determine liability for providing false information.[74]

The key to provision of quality DI is the availability of current, objective information. Procedures should be in place to ensure that data is continually reviewed and updated. Quality assurance (QA) standards for the timeliness, thoroughness, and accuracy of information could also insulate against liability.

Problem areas common to DI regardless of practice site include files not updated and incomplete documentation of responses to requests. With regard to inquiries about adverse reactions, details of the adverse event should be taken and reported to the FDA reporting program. Cases may be clinically urgent and the physician or nurse may have a patient waiting. Response via e-mail, even with alerts attached, is not prudent in such situations as there is no guarantee that the caller is at their desk to receive such e-mails. All statements made should be traceable to the literature. Additionally, information should be confirmed with other references to ensure consistency between various resources. DI centers should address at least some of the items in Table 10-1.

Insistence on a good educational background for entry-level positions including PGY-1 and, ideally PGY-2 residencies in DI, followed by the continuing education of DI professionals, certification in online training courses, and good interpersonal communication skills, may also protect against malpractice. Several studies have shown that physicians who were sued frequently had poor interpersonal skills, that is, patients did not like them.[75] It is also important to keep abreast of changes in sources of DI via regular advanced training, conferences, and reading. All courses in DI should teach situations in ethical conflict that will assist in the decision making and value judgments encountered in the provision of DI.

Under the tort law doctrine of *respondeat superior*, both the practitioner providing DI and the employer are jointly and severally liable for the damages. This enables the plaintiff to have access to the practitioner's personal assets where the employer's assets are not sufficient to cover an adverse judgment. Professional liability insurance provides protection to cover exactly this kind of liability. Consideration should be given to obtaining professional indemnity insurance for the DI practitioner.

Most policies now provide coverage on either an occurrence or claims-made basis. Occurrence means any incident that occurs during the policy period, no matter when the claim is filed, within the applicable statute of limitations. Claims-made policies cover only claims that are filed while the policy is active. To cover claims that are filed after a claims-made policy is terminated, the DI practitioner can purchase tail coverage from the insurer.

TABLE 10–1. QUALITY ASSURANCE AS A LIABILITY REDUCING FACTOR

- Identify scope of activities and personnel requirements.
- Develop and follow policies and procedures or formal call triaging protocols.
- Keep standard operating procedure manual available for consultation.
- Avoid violations of statutes and regulations.
- Unapproved uses or doses should be well documented and if a use or dose differs from the labeling, the requestor must be so notified.
- Do not recommend a use or dose of a drug based solely on foreign literature or animal studies or questionable resources or references that are not peer reviewed.
- Never extrapolate pediatric or geriatric dosages from usual adult dosages.
- Maintain knowledge of the current literature, new drug applications and supplemental approvals, labeling changes, and new warnings.
- Do not present inadequate data or ignore contrary data.
- Avoid overly enthusiastic or exaggerated efficacy and safety claims.
- Do not attempt to diagnose or treat acute poisoning—direct such inquiries to a poison control center or an emergency room.
- Know the circumstances of the case and appropriate background information (e.g., knowledge of causality assessment scales [e.g., Naranjo Algorithm—see Chapter 17]), laboratory findings, concurrent drugs necessary for adverse drug reaction inquiries.
- Exert special care for drug identification questions in view of the growth of counterfeit drugs.
- Responses of new employees, students, residents should be checked—document, document, document. Maintain reasonable response time; if necessary, prioritize requests.
- Obtain peer concurrence or outside professional consultation, if necessary.
- Develop a quality assurance (QA) mechanism to ensure that service is maintained at a high level of quality (e.g., periodic audits or surveys).
- Maintain up-to-date files and reference texts (e.g., paper files should be randomly checked to be sure that they contain articles at least as recent as 2 years old).
- For Internet-specific data, check currency, authorship, publisher, length of time site has existed, site reviews, links to/from other sites, biases/objectiveness, intended audience, quality of the writing, references provided (information without references should receive little weight in clinical decision making), who maintains the site (owner/sponsor or whether the site has an expert advisory board), affiliations (commercial, organization "org," governmental "gov"), and seal of approval from organizations that review health care sites. (See Chapter 3 for further information regarding evaluating Internet websites.)

Tail coverage insures for an incident that occurred while the insurance was in effect but was not filed by the time the insurer-policyholder relationship terminated. It is important to be aware of the limitations and exclusions in these policies, such as some policies no longer covering intravenous compounding. Many do not require the carrier to obtain the consent of the insured before settling a claim. In these policies, the right to protect one's reputation may conflict with the economic interest of the insurer to dispose of the claim as inexpensively as possible. Therefore, it is imperative that individuals obtain insurance coverage policies separate from those of their employers. Most common exclusions are coverage for dishonest, fraudulent, criminal, or malicious acts; property damage; and personal injury coverage. In these cases, the practitioner faces such liability alone, and in certain situations can be ruined financially.

Finally, limiting language in subscriber contracts (i.e., **exculpatory clauses**) may serve to restrict monetary awards in certain circumstances. Such clauses could be included in either contracts for subscribers or signed on acceptance of responses to inquiries. A provision could be included that specifically disclaims any responsibility to a third party who might rely on the information. Written information (e.g., a bulletin) should carry a disclaimer specifying that the DI provided is issued on the understanding that it is the best available from the resources available to the service at a particular time.

An attorney could draft a standard agreement providing that the application of the research by the recipient would not be subject to any implied warranty of fitness for that purpose. However, certain jurisdictions have held that contracts that purport to exculpate a party from negligence will be subjected to strict judicial scrutiny. Courts in certain jurisdictions have declared contracts that attempt to exempt a party's willful or grossly negligent conduct to be void. Further, no exculpatory clause will protect a pharmacist who is grossly or intentionally negligent.

Labeling and Advertising

The FDA defines labeling as written, oral, or electronic information used to supplement or explain a product regardless of whether the information accompanies the product. As such, even literature, textbooks, reprints of articles, scientific seminars may constitute labeling. Labeling requires full disclosure. Advertisements, on the other hand, require a fair balance, meaning there must be a discussion of both benefits and risks, so as not to be misleading, and substantial evidence from clinical trials must be included for comparative claims.[76] The FDA has issued a number of recent guidance documents pertaining to advertising with regard to Internet/social media platforms (e.g., messages on Twitter® [i.e., tweets], individual product pages on social networking sites such as Facebook®, blogs, microblogs, online communities, YouTube™, live podcasts, and online web banners).[77–79]

❸ *There are at least three key areas of labeling and advertising liability: the learned intermediary doctrine, which is a defense to failure to warn actions; the doctrine of overpromotion, under which adequate warning is alleged to have been diluted by communications failing to adequately convey the full impact of the warning; and promotion of off-label use or FDA unapproved indications.*

Direct-to-Consumer (DTC) Drug Information

In 1997, the FDA relaxed the standards for direct-to-consumer advertising (DTCA).[80] DTCA involves magazine, television, website, cell phone, and text advertisements, suggesting the use of various prescription drugs for medical conditions the viewer might experience and also suggesting the viewer ask their physician if the medication would be appropriate for them.

Today, prescription drug advertising is a multibillion-dollar industry. Prescription drug advertising is governed by the Food, Drug, and Cosmetic Act (FDCA) and 21 U.S.C. §331, which prohibits the misbranding of a prescription drug.[81] The primary regulation aimed at pharmaceutical product advertising is found at 21 C.F.R. § 202.1 that pertains to all "advertisements in published journals, magazines, other periodicals, newspapers, and other advertisements broadcast through media such as radio, television, and telephone communication systems." These implementing regulations specify that prescription drug advertisements cannot omit material facts, and must present a fair balance between effectiveness and risk information. Further, for print advertisements, the regulations specify that every risk addressed in the product's approved labeling must also be disclosed in the advertisements. The regulations further require that the advertisement contain a summary of "all necessary information related to adverse effects and contraindications" or "provide convenient access to the product's FDA-approved labeling and the risk information it contains." DTCA of off-label uses of prescription drugs is prohibited.[82]

There is evidence that DTCA is becoming more aggressive.[83] The FDA has cited unsubstantiated safety claims and minimization of risk, including "websites that omit or bury important safety information," as areas of particular concern.[84] In some cases, the advertising does not focus on a product but rather on patient education. One company has developed a campaign to bring mental health educational forums to college campuses featuring free screenings for depression. In another case, a 24-hour television network directed to a captive audience (i.e., hospitalized patients) was launched. As federal regulations require patient education, this programming may be used by hospitals for patient education. Other manufacturers offer monetary rewards or gifts (e.g., free exercise video) to patients who visit their physician regarding the product or offer a rebate or sweepstakes opportunity if the patient completes a questionnaire. Manufacturers are also sending out video press releases about drugs that are often aired as news stories. Many advertisements provide an 800 number to encourage consumers to seek additional information about the products; others offer free videotapes, brochures, and information packets discussing the product.[85] There also exist DI search tools and apps for use directly by consumers (e.g., PDR.net, http://www.pdr.net).[86]

Another popular DTCA vehicle is blog posts. For example, YouTube™ videos about products from patients are being posted on pharmaceutical company websites without review. Often these patient testimonials go well beyond what a company is permitted to advertise about the product. In general, patient testimonials minimize product risks and adverse events and are unbalanced. In August 2015, FDA issued a guidance pertaining to risk information in DTCA via print.[87] In January 2014, FDA issued a draft guidance on interactive promotional media such as firm-sponsored microblogs (e.g., Twitter®), social networking sites (e.g., Facebook®), and firm blogs.[78] In March 2012, the FDA issued a draft guidance on DTCA via television, but has not issued a final guidance. Nor has the FDA issued formal guidelines regarding online DTCA.

While DTCA bypasses the advice of the physician, only a few cases have created an exception to the learned intermediary doctrine on the ground that foundational tenets of the doctrine are no longer applicable in the context of DTCA. In *Perez v. Wyeth Laboratories Inc.*,[88] the New Jersey Supreme Court created an exception for Norplant®, an implantable contraceptive that provided contraception for up to 5 years, but was removable. The plaintiffs alleged personal injury and failure to warn of the contraceptive's adverse effects, including removal complications, which resulted in pain, and scarring. The plaintiffs asserted that based on the mass advertising campaign to women that the pharmaceutical manufacturer had a duty to warn patients directly. According to the majority in *Perez*, the learned intermediary doctrine has four theoretical premises: (1) a reluctance to undermine the physician-patient relationship, (2) an absence for the need for the patient's informed consent, (3) the inability of drug manufacturers to communicate with patients, and (4) the complexity of the subject matter. The court asserted that each of these bases, except the fourth, is obviated in DTCA of prescription drugs. According to *Perez*, when direct advertising influences a patient to request a particular drug, and the physician does not adequately consult with the patient, "neither the physician nor the manufacturer should be entirely relieved of their respective duties to warn."[89]

Despite the ruling in *Perez*, a decade and a half later, plaintiffs have not been able to convince any other jurisdiction to recognize the DTCA exception to the Learned Intermediary Rule. In fact, no court other than *Perez* has allowed a DTCA exception for prescription drugs. Therefore, the duty to warn runs to the prescriber, not the patient.

Increasingly, the courts are holding that the pharmacist has a duty to warn patients and intervene on their behalf. In 1991, Pharmacists Mutual reported no claims involving drug utilization review. In 1999, drug review claims accounted for 9% of all pharmacist liability claims. A 2002 study by the same firm found that drug review claims were continuing in a straight-line increase.[90] In 2010, drug review claims at 7.9% represented the largest category of intellectual errors (as opposed to mechanical or dispensing errors). Counseling claims account for 1.6% of all claims.[91]

In any event, pharmacists must remain vigilant to ensure that DTCA does not promote false expectations. Clearly, DTCA achieves its goals of encouraging consumerism, whereby patients go to seek prescription information from health professionals. DTCA increasingly lead patients to seek information that will confirm or refute the manufacturer's claims that differentiate a product from its competitors. When confronted with the influences of such advertising, pharmacists are on the front lines educating patients regarding these products, including the cost effectiveness of prescription drug options. Pharmacists have a responsibility to provide objective information, to educate the patient, and to serve as a DI resource.[92] Refer to Chapter 23 for additional information.

DOCTRINE OF DRUG OVERPROMOTION

The doctrine of overpromotion is based on liability where an adequate warning is alleged to have been diluted by communications that do not adequately convey the full impact of the warning and are so overpromoting of a drug that members of the medical profession prescribe when it was not warranted. In other instances, overpromotion involves promoting a drug to a group for an off-label use. Recent examples include promoting an opioid indicated for cancer pain to non-oncologists; promoting a birth control pill to treat premenstrual syndrome and/or acne; promoting an antipsychotic approved for bipolar disorder and schizophrenia for anxiety, obsessive compulsive disorder, dementia, and autism.

On August 9, 2003, Prescription Access Litigation Project filed the first class action lawsuit against a pharmaceutical company in connection with DTCA. The class action was brought for allegedly deceptive advertising and overpricing of Claritin®.[93] Plaintiffs alleged that the company's DTCA overstated the limited efficacy of its product and that the company deliberately left out any information about the drug's efficacy.

In yet other cases, the overpromotion failed to warn of the potential for serious adverse effects. While product liability laws vary by jurisdiction, counts of fraud/intentional misrepresentation, negligent misrepresentation, and breach of warranty are often found in the lawsuit pleadings. Another DTCA lawsuit involves Paxil®, one of the top selling drugs in the world.[94] Plaintiffs allege the drug causes withdrawal symptoms, such as severe nausea and other psychological problems, and that the company failed to tell plaintiffs, their physicians, or the public of this adverse effect.[94] If the adverse reaction is not listed in the labeling, the health care provider is exonerated, leaving the pharmaceutical company liable. Recent cases have involved tendon rupture from fluoroquinolone antibiotics, amputation from inadvertent promethazine intravenous extravasation,[95] and neuropathy and polyneuropathy from 3-hydroxy-3-methylglutaryl-coenzyme A (HMG CoA) reductase inhibitors.[96]

Off-Label Use and Informed Consent

Off-label use involves use for indications not specifically approved by the FDA. It is an accepted principle that once FDA approves a drug for marketing, a physician's discretionary use of that product is not restricted to the uses indicated on FDA-regulated labeling. This is particularly important in the areas of oncology and acquired immunodeficiency syndrome (AIDS), where a significant portion of drug use is off-label. While patients and medical innovation, in general, benefit from having their physicians informed about off-label uses, off-label use information from manufacturers has been restricted. In fact, manufacturer promotion of off-label use constitutes misbranding under the FDCA.[97]

Under the 1997 FDAMA, specifically Section 401, the FDA attempted to strengthen regulation of information pertaining to off-label uses.[98] One requirement under FDAMA was FDA review of material to be disseminated to ensure that it does not pose a significant risk to public health and is not false and misleading.[99] However, the authority of the FDA under the FDAMA to regulate the promotion of off-label uses was successfully challenged and Section 401 ceased to be effective on September 30, 2006.[100] In favoring the commercial free speech doctrine, the court ruled that the FDA had to permit drug company-sponsored advertisements for off-label use, as long as they were directed at physicians and not consumers.[101] In 2009, FDA released a guideline allowing for distribution of reprints about off-label uses from peer-reviewed publications.[102] In February 2014, the FDA issued a new draft guidance regarding off-label use, updating the 2009 guidance. Major provisions of both guidelines, which refer to what is considered "Good Reprint Practices" and clarifying FDA's position on manufacturer dissemination of scientific journal articles, scientific or medical reference texts, and clinical practice guidelines are found in Table 10-2.[103] The FDA agrees that off-label uses by unbiased researchers in bona fide published literature should be discussed.

Moreover, medical science liaisons are permitted to provide off-label information in response to unsolicited medical inquiries. The types of nonpromotional information that can be provided include general education, report of a clinical trial, follow-up to a question originally posed to a sales representative, and advice for formularies. Insurers and government plaintiffs have increasingly attempted to claim a "formulary influence" theory of liability, alleging that manufacturers engaged in off-label promotion or kickbacks that caused states to wrongfully include a medication on their Medicaid formularies or gave medications preferred tier status. In one such case, however, *United States ex rel. v. Solvay S.A.*, the product information sent to the P&T committees was requested and the court held that any temporal relationship between sale representative visits to P&T committee members was too tenuous.[104]

TABLE 10–2.   MAJOR PROVISIONS OF THE 2009 AND 2014 FDA GUIDANCES FOR INDUSTRY—GOOD REPRINT PRACTICES FOR THE DISTRIBUTION OF MEDICAL JOURNAL ARTICLES AND MEDICAL OR SCIENTIFIC REFERENCE PUBLICATIONS, REFERENCE TEXTS, AND CLINICAL PRACTICE GUIDELINES ON UNAPPROVED NEW USES OF APPROVED DRUGS

Journal articles
- Article(s) should:
  - Be published by an organization with an editorial board.
  - Be peer reviewed.
  - Be an unabridged reprint, copy of an article, or reference publication.
  - Be accompanied by the approved labeling and, when such information exists, a comprehensive bibliography of well-controlled clinical studies.
  - Be disseminated with a representative publication which reaches contrary or different conclusions.
  - Contain information that describes/addresses well-controlled clinical investigations.
- Article(s) should not:
  - Be a special supplement or funded by a manufacturer of the product that is the subject of the article.
  - Be primarily distributed by a manufacturer but should be generally available via other distribution channels.
  - Be written, edited, excerpted, or published specifically at the request of a manufacturer or edited or influenced by someone having a significant financial relationship with the manufacturer.
  - Be false or misleading or discuss a clinical trial that the FDA has indicated is not adequate and well controlled.
  - Pose a significant risk to public health, if relied upon.
  - Be marked, highlighted, summarized, or characterized by the manufacturer.
- Not consistent with Good Reprint Practices are:
  - Letters to the editor
  - Abstracts of a publication
  - Reports of Phase I trials in healthy subjects
  - Reference publications with little or no substantive discussion of relevant investigation or data
- Articles should be distributed separately from information that is promotional:
  - They may not distribute in exhibit halls or during promotional speakers' programs.
  - Articles should not be attached to specific product information.
- Articles should be accompanied by a prominently displayed and affixed statement disclosing:
  - That the uses are off-label.
  - The manufacturer's interest in the subject drug of the article.
  - Any person known to the manufacturer as having a financial interest and the nature of that interest.
  - All significant risks/safety concerns known to the manufacturer.
  - Any author who has received financial compensation from the manufacturer and the nature and amount of same.

Scientific or Medical Texts and Clinical Practice Guidelines*
- Should:
  - Be based on a systematic review of existing evidence.
  - Be published by an independent publisher.
  - Be the most current version.
  - Be authored, edited, and/or contributed to by experts.
  - Be peer reviewed by experts.
  - Be sold through the usual and customary independent distribution channels.
  - Be delivered separately from promotional material.

continued

TABLE 10-2.   MAJOR PROVISIONS OF THE 2009 AND 2014 FDA GUIDANCES FOR INDUSTRY—GOOD REPRINT PRACTICES FOR THE DISTRIBUTION OF MEDICAL JOURNAL ARTICLES AND MEDICAL OR SCIENTIFIC REFERENCE PUBLICATIONS, REFERENCE TEXTS, AND CLINICAL PRACTICE GUIDELINES ON UNAPPROVED NEW USES OF APPROVED DRUGS (*CONTINUED*)

- ○ Contain a prominently displayed affixed statement identifying both.
  the distributing manufacturer and that some of the uses are off-label.
- ○ Be disseminated with the approved product labeling.
- Should not:
- ○ Be false or misleading.
- ○ Contain information that makes the product dangerous to health when used in the manner suggested.
- ○ Be primarily distributed by a manufacturer.
- ○ Be edited or significantly influenced by a manufacturer or any individuals having a financial relationship.
- ○ Be written or published at the request of a manufacturer.
- ○ Be abridged or excerpted in any manner.
- ○ Be attached to any product information other than approved labeling.

*There are additional requirements for dissemination of chapters.

   Problematic are responses to inquiries that are not really unsolicited or formulary advice that borders on preapproval promotion (known as new product seeding).[105] Additionally, pharmaceutical companies may freely distribute to health professionals copies of articles from peer-reviewed professional journals or reference textbooks containing discussions of off-label product usage. However, sales representatives are not permitted to use this information to promote the company's products. In December 2011, the FDA issued a draft guidance for industry entitled "Responding to Unsolicited Requests for Off-Label Information About Prescription Drugs and Medical Devices."[106] An entire section of this document is devoted to unsolicited requests for off-label information through emerging electronic media. The FDA is recommending that the public DI response to off-label information be limited to providing the firm's contact information and should not include any off-label information. This will ensure that the communication occurs solely between the firm and the individual who made the request and circumvents both broad distribution and issues regarding the enduring nature of online responses.

   Researchers continually conduct studies to determine new uses for already marketed drugs and effective combinations of drugs for new indications with the results being published in the literature. Additionally, with up to 40% of all prescriptions being for off-label use, off-label use comprises a large component of providing DI, especially for queries that involve pediatrics.[107] These queries are often from physicians seeking evidence to support a particular off-label use. Problems arise when the off-label use is not really off-label, but rather, crosses the line and is experimental (in which case an Investigational New Drug Application and/or Institutional Review Board [IRB] approval for study is required).[125] Refer to the Investigational Drugs chapter (Chapter 21) for more detailed information.

Unfortunately, once an off-label use becomes rampant, the market drives it and there remains little incentive for the pharmaceutical company to provide more data or conduct further research regarding that off-label use. This disincentive arises not only because of the expense involved in conducting clinical trials but also because trial results could actually have an adverse effect on sales by showing lack of efficacy or safety. For example, it was a study of rofecoxib (Vioxx®) for an off-label use that first uncovered the cardiovascular risks that eventually led to market withdrawal.[108]

Medicare Parts B and D are required to cover off-label uses of drugs in cancer treatment when the use is supported by a citation in at least one of the following references: *AHFS Drug Information (AHFS-DI), The National Comprehensive Cancer Network's Drugs and Biologics Compendium (NCCN), DRUGDEX® by Truven Health Analytics, Inc.,* or *Clinical Pharmacology by Elsevier/Gold Standard,* or the use is supported by clinical research in peer-reviewed articles published in respected medical journals.[109] Medicaid utilized only *AHFS Drug Information*® and *DRUGDEX*®.[110] When providing DI, it should be realized that not all compendia include revision dates for the monographs. Moreover, a recent study revealed that update policies were not followed, certain off-label indications were excluded without rationale, and for common off-label cancer treatments, outdated literature and incomplete or inconsistent evidence was found in the compendia.[111] Under the Medicare Improvements for Patients and Providers Act of 2008 (MIPPA), the criteria for medically accepted off-label uses are now the same for both Medicare Part B and Part D.[112] For non-cancer Part B and Part D drugs, the off-label coverage is limited to uses in *DRUGDEX*®, *Clinical Pharmacology,* or *AHFS Drug Information,* but only if the FDA has approved the drug for some other use. There is a divergence between Parts B and D for the use of peer-reviewed literature to support off-label use of non-cancer drugs. Peer-reviewed literature (excluding abstracts, meeting abstracts, and in-house publications) can be used to support Part B but not Part D. There is much litigation in this area and the question as to whether CMS reliance on proprietary compendia, not accessible to the public for Part D off-label approval raises serious due process issues.

Following these guidelines for DI queries pertaining to an off-label use would appear to be a prudent practice. Similarly, in providing responses to DI requests pertaining to off-label uses (including usages of off-label dosages), it is prudent to provide complete information, so that a decision may be made whether the information is enough to warrant a particular off-label use. For example, letters to the editor or abstracts would not be complete information. When there is another drug on the market with an approved-label use for the same indication that the off-label product is being considered, the response to the DI request should mention that labeled alternative.[113] Moreover, it is also important to be cognizant of the implications of disseminating off-label information in the context of patient safety and liability. Responding to consumer requests for information about off-label uses is not advised, simply because, unlike health professionals, most often they are not in a position to evaluate the literature and extrapolate to a particular situation.

Off-label use of pharmaceuticals has resulted in liability. For example, physicians have been the target of lawsuits involving gabapentin (Neurontin®), an antiepileptic drug prescribed for numerous off-label uses. The drug has been linked to suicide. Another example is bevacizumab (Avastin®), an oncology drug, used off-label to treat macular degeneration, which caused blindness in some patients.

While there is no question that patients should be advised if a proposed treatment is truly investigational or experimental, off-label use is not necessarily experimental or investigational, thus, informed consent is not necessary whenever an off-label use is proposed.[114] Federal informed consent regulations governing investigational drugs do not apply to off-label use.[115] State informed consent laws vary but usually require discussion of the nature, risks, benefits, and alternative modes of treatment. For example, the New York statute states:

> "Lack of informed consent means the failure of the person providing the professional treatment or diagnosis to disclose to the patient such alternatives thereto and the reasonably foreseeable risks and benefits involved as a reasonable medical...practitioner under similar circumstances would have disclosed, in a manner permitting the patient to make a knowledgeable evaluation."[116]

Actions for informed consent are, therefore, limited to the nondisclosure of medical information. However, failure to disclose FDA status does not raise a **material issue of fact** as to informed consent. That is, it would not result in a summary judgment in a lawsuit.

Liability Concerns for Internet/Social Media Information

❹ *DI is currently being obtained from a number of Internet/social media and mobile apps, and there is a possibility of DI liability for information obtained from these sources.* Google Scholar, Wikipedia, RxWiki, PubDrug, and web citations in general are increasingly being accessed for handling DI queries. It has been reported that half of U.S. physicians use Wikipedia for medical information.[117] The percentage of those who use Wikipedia for DI is unknown. Recently, Internet/social media DI sources have appeared as references in publications.[118] More than 25% of the Internet's content involves health care and medical information.[119] The browser of Internet information resources can now expect to find full prescribing information for most heavily marketed drugs. The situation is complicated by links to investigational products or investigational uses and vice versa. The question is whether this is promotion of off-label uses.[120] Refer to Chapter 23 for further information on this topic.

Liability concerns arise in the area of whether a manufacturer's website content is considered labeling or advertising. It appears to be necessary to distinguish between Internet promotion directed to health professionals and consumers. DTCA on the Internet is considered labeling, rather than advertising and, as such, the FDA has principal authority to regulate it.[121]

On February 2004, the FDA issued new industry guidelines, entitled "Help-Seeking and Other Disease Awareness Communications by or on Behalf of Drug and Device Firms and Brief Summary: Disclosing Risk Information in Consumer-Directed Print Advertisements." While these guidelines are intended to improve the brief summaries of adverse effects that must be included in DTCA, they do not address Internet advertisements.

QUALITY OF INTERNET DRUG INFORMATION

Not all websites are reputable and currently there is no way to distinguish which sites providing DI are authoritative and which are not. Problems have arisen such as **hyperlink** obsolescence, defunct websites, broken links, altered content, and an inability to determine currency.[113] Moreover, it is common for websites to change or move.

Entries in Wikipedia, an encyclopedia project, recently ranked as one of the top 10 sites visited, can be the subject of erroneous entries, fraud, conflict of interest, or even criminal mischief.[122] For example, pharmaceutical companies may edit or delete their product information as the site is user edited. Thus, sites such as Wikipedia are not authoritative and can only be supplementary to, rather than the sole source of DI.[123] In a recent study of the accuracy and completeness of DI in Wikipedia versus Micromedex using PIs as a standard comparator, Wikipedia was found to lack the accuracy and completeness of the clinical reference, Micromedex. Lower completeness, and importantly, accuracy scores for Wikipedia compared with Micromedex (mean composite scores 18.55 versus 38.4, respectively; $p < 0.01$), led to the conclusion that Wikipedia is inappropriate for clinical decision making.[124]

Google Scholar includes both published and unpublished (hence not peer reviewed) information and, unlike PubMed, it may not contain the latest literature. However, as the number of Internet-only journals not indexed in PubMed increases, there will be increased reliance on Google Scholar as an easy to use source for locating primary literature. In fact, in a recent comparison with PubMed, no significant differences were found regarding the number of primary literature articles, although PubMed did retrieve more specific articles.[125]

What about liability for DI obtained from the Internet and electronic journals or apps (such as Epocrates®)? Is there a possibility of pharmacist liability occurring via cyberspace?

As mentioned above, the Internet contains a growing hodgepodge of sources with little organization and uneven credibility. In fact, material on the Internet may contain innocent mistakes and/or deliberate fraud, as well as outdated material. Several situations may result in search results that are not comprehensive. Examples include faulty search strategies and failing to search for historical information. Many databases including PubMed do not contain material prior to the 1940s. Searchers may not even be aware that pre-Internet or old nonelectronic material exists. Old MEDLINE® articles from 1949 through 1965 may not be updated with MeSH terms and may not contain searchable abstracts.[126] For e-books (e.g., online textbooks) with their own built-in search engine (e.g., Merck Manual), there is a possibility of patient harm occurring when the computer malfunctions. Currently, there are no laws pertaining to, and no means for, ensuring the accuracy of DI posed on the Internet. It is possible for information on the Internet to be false, misleading, corrupted by an outside source, or otherwise harmful to the reader to apply it to their specific situation. There is a potential for misinformation to be disseminated, while the reader unknowingly assumes the DI to be accurate and true via the Internet and related technologies.

The Health Summit Working Group, which consists of professional societies including ASHP, and the Health on the Net Foundation (HON) are currently working to improve the quality of DI on the Internet. HON has developed a code (HONcode) for quality and reliability which, if displayed, increases the likelihood that the information is reliable. A seal of approval may also be given from other organizations that approve health care sites such as Internet Healthcare Coalition, Verified Internet Pharmacy Practice Sites (VIPPS®), and Medical Matrix. Unfortunately, these instruments may be difficult to use and their actual validity is unclear. Additionally, a seal of approval should in no way replace critical clinical judgment of the content. Also, the application of the National Information Infrastructure to consumer health information is one of the priorities of the federal government. Examples of website QA criteria are included in Table 10-1 and are found in Chapter 16.

Another venue where the quality of DI may be suspect is social media and/or e-mail communication. Both the American Medical Association and the American Medical Informatics Association have issued guidelines for physicians using e-mail to communicate with patients.[127] These guidelines encourage physicians to be cautious when using e-mail because of the possibility of liability due to misunderstanding and privacy concerns.[128] Perhaps in the near future, health insurers will cover calls made to online pharmacists providing DI, much the same way as Medicare now covers teleconferencing.

The Internet is at the forefront of practice, where pharmacists will consult with each other, thereby learning from one another and benefiting their DI clients and patients.[129] Web applications facilitate interactive information sharing, such as Wikis, blogs, hosted-services, and networking sites. Specific examples include the University Health System Consortium, WebMD, and Google Scholar. In the fast-paced practice of

DI, Internet information may provide a quick starting point for an answer to a query. However, other non-web-based references should also be consulted. DI professionals should never rely solely on a search retrieved from Google Scholar to respond to a DI query. Additionally, when using web citations, it is recommended to include the date accessed to provide readers with some indication of how current the information is (refer to Appendix 12-3).

TELEMEDICINE AND CYBERMEDICINE

Legal issues are emerging from e-health technologies, such as telemedicine and cyber-medicine programs. **Telemedicine** is defined as the use of telecommunications and interactive video technology to provide health care services to patients who are at a distance. **Cybermedicine** is a broader concept that includes the marketing, relationship creation, advice, prescribing, and selling pharmaceuticals and devices in cyberspace. Therefore, telepharmacy is a subset of telemedicine and the terms are used interchangeably here. As telemedicine and cybermedicine expand, questions regarding liability for pharmacists providing DI on the Internet will need to be addressed. For example, health professionals, such as pharmacists, are licensed by states. Which state law applies when the pharmacist is located in New York, the patient is in Florida, and the website is maintained by a company in California? Who is liable for technical problems that make it impossible for the information to be received in a timely manner or for breaches of confidentiality caused by those who would invade private files? Already some sites offer fee-based live physician offices and nurse-triage services (e.g., OptumHealth Care NurseLine) for self-diagnosis and health screening. Additionally, some DI providers provide information over the Internet.

Although the courts have yet to test liability for medical malpractice involving the practice of pharmacy or medicine on the Internet, such a case is bound to surface soon. The most important determination of whether there is such malpractice is whether or not a health care provider-patient relationship has been created by the consultation in the absence of physical contact. Hard copy printouts of Internet discussions would be discoverable before trial and could be uncovered in the defendant's computer files by a plaintiff's attorney. It is likely that where a physician consults with a pharmacist for DI via telemedicine, the pharmacist will not be deemed to have established a pharmacist-patient relationship. Telephone consultations between physicians are most analogous and have not been held to create a physician-patient relationship.[130] Similarly, as previously mentioned, no pharmacist-physician relationship has been found based on a provision of DI to the physician.[28] This is largely because of the public policy interest of promoting consultations, professional association, and education, as well as the assumed limited information conveyed to the consulting physician. However, in view of advancing technology where the patient's entire medical history and test results are available on the computer, this situation may change, especially where a consultation fee is involved. Also, where a pharmacist posts a website and is paid to provide DI, the courts will surely find such cybermedical consultation to create a pharmacist-patient relationship.

Although there have been several lawsuits for false information on online bulletin boards (e.g., Usenet News, CompuServe®), the basis of these lawsuits has been defamation, not malpractice.[131,132] The offering of general medical advice and judgments online (e.g., chat rooms) does not appear to be creating a formal physician-patient relationship. Nor does it appear that the giving of generic advice will generate liability for either the provider or the publisher. If, however, the information is fraudulent or quackery, then courts do have authority under both state and federal computer statutes to stop the activity. Similarly, Internet (or telephone) medical call centers, or triage services used by some health care plans can expect to be held liable when misdiagnosis occurs. On the other hand, liability is lessened where Internet discussions resemble an academic conference between health care providers, rather than a formal consultancy. Similarly, the issuance of a disclaimer in writing with the original subscription and with each message written may help insulate from any liability.

Some websites now carry disclaimers to protect the authors from liability. The limitation of the remedies available should be displayed prominently. A cap equal to the price of the service sold may be included. The following is an example:

> "Please read this agreement entirely and carefully before assessing this website. By accessing the site, you agree to be bound by the terms and conditions below. If you do not wish to be bound by these terms and conditions, you may not access or use this site. Our maximum liability to you under all circumstances will be equal to the purchase price you paid for any goods, services, or information."

This statement is then followed by disclaimers pertaining to accuracy, currency, copyright, no medical advice, no warranties, a disclaimer of endorsement, disclaimer regarding liability for third-party content, and a general disclaimer of liability including negligence with a statement that the user assumes all responsibility and risk for use.[133] It may also be desirable to include a provision that any dispute will be brought in the city of the site owner's principal place of business.

SOCIAL MEDIA

There is a growing use of social media that allows health professionals to share information with their colleagues and, more often recently, their patients. Social media allows for large groups of individuals to share information, expand contact, and serve as a means for professional news and a tool for discussion of pharmacy-related issues. Examples include Facebook®, LinkedIn®, Amazon.com®, Twitter®, YouTube, Pinterest®, blogs, and forums. In fact, most state pharmacy organizations have a Twitter® presence. A number of legal issues for DI pharmacists who use social media warrant consideration—ranging from patient privacy under HIPAA and state privacy torts, creation of a pharmacist-patient relationship to anti-kickback issues. Privacy controls vary by site and change frequently, but patient information must never be disclosed on such sites. Breaches can occur easily such as inquiring about how a patient's diabetes is on Facebook® or discussing celebrities getting medications in pharmacies. Posting of comments and breaches of patient confidentiality, especially by students, are common.[134] Even text messaging with patients can present legal issues that health professionals may not have considered. In addition to the text messaged PHI not being accorded the necessary privacy and security protection, the health professional must always be certain that any information they send and receive must be added to the patient's medical and/or pharmacy profile and retained for the required period of time. While many health care professionals simply delete texts they have read, they may be violating the law. From a liability standpoint, not having a copy of texts a clinician has sent to or received from a patient who is suing him or her for malpractice is a precarious position and may amount to spoliation of evidence. Best practice is to retain posts and texts to and from patients and colleagues. There has been a recent increase in lawsuits brought under invasion of privacy. For discovery purposes, opposing counsel may review any public social network of a witness or party to discover social media posts.

While there are no legal rules on this, friending patients is not a good idea. ASHP has developed a statement on use of social media by pharmacy professionals.[135] However, there is still no clear picture of issues such as the duty to warn in social media.[136] While the Joint Commission originally opined against physicians or other health care providers texting orders to hospitals and other health care settings, it has since stated, "Licensed independent practitioners....may text orders as long as a secure text messaging platform is used and the required components of an order are included."[137]

Questions have also been raised whether providing DI over social media is tantamount to unlicensed practice in a state where the pharmacist is not licensed. Moreover, harmful patient-specific advice may lead to malpractice. Some pharmacists have placed a disclaimer on their blog to indicate "Reading this blog should not be construed to mean that you and I have a pharmacist-patient relationship." Besides privacy and negligence issues other liability may follow for defamation, copyright infringement, discrimination, or harassment.

Some pharmaceutical manufacturers have developed patient blogs and other social media websites especially for patients with chronic illnesses such as diabetes. In some cases, testimonials by what appear to be patients are actually being made by people paid or allied with the pharmaceutical company. While the effect of social media on patient care is currently unclear, the FDA is currently drafting guidelines to cover drug companies' social media presence.

Fraud and Abuse

Another consideration pertains to fraud and abuse laws, such as the anti-kickback laws.[138] The Anti-Kickback Statute prohibits physicians participating in the Medicaid and Medicare programs from submitting any false remuneration, including any kickback, bribe, or rebate to induce referrals of patients.[139] Certain aspects of e-health promotional and marketing tools, such as per-click payment arrangements, are particularly susceptible to violation of the Anti-Kickback Statute. The violation occurs because the health care provider is receiving remuneration based on the referral rate provided by the fee charged per click. Likewise, promotional banners on a health care organization or pharmacist's website that link to a pharmacy or other type of patient care items are most likely in violation because the referring provider is receiving a benefit (i.e., per-click arrangements involve the payment of a fee based on the clicking on a particular link on a website) in exchange for referrals.[140] Similarly, the provision of free e-mail services, online publications, computer equipment, or other types of computer ventures are in violation of the Anti-Kickback Statute when these companies sell items or services reimbursable under Medicaid or Medicare programs.

Another area of uncertainty pertains to the handling of links between web pages. A link is any component of a web page that connects to another web page. The issue of whether pharmaceutical manufacturers will be liable for material posted on sites they have not sponsored, but have merely linked to their own, is yet to be decided in the courts.

At least according to cases over the past few years, mere hyperlinking does not constitute copyright or trademark infringement.[141] Copyright law does not require that permission be obtained for linking, but if there is copyrighted graphic material, people will be reproducing and displaying copyrighted material they do not own. The copyright owner's permission needs to be obtained to use the graphic image, unless fair use is utilized (fair use is discussed further under the section for copyright law). Where the information being linked to is violating the copyright law, it is also possible that a website owner who links to a site containing infringing material may be liable for contributory copyright infringement. Contributory copyright infringement is established when a defendant, with knowledge of another's infringing activity, causes or materially contributes to the infringing conduct.

Moreover, whether deep linking (i.e., bypassing the home page and linking to an internal page of the linked site) is copyright infringement is currently unclear.[142] However, if a web page specifically states to ask permission before linking, it is possible that linking to the site without the owner's permission may be trespass or breach of contract where there are terms of use to which were agreed.[143]

Additionally, certain businesses, who do not want their valuable content associated with or connected to certain sites, have brought legal action under theories of trademark, defamation, disparagement, unfair competition, false advertising, invasion of privacy, and other laws. In *Playboy Enterprises, Inc. v. Universal Tel-A-Talk, Inc.*, an X-rated website linked to the Playboy website.[144] Playboy sued and proved that users of the site may be confused as to whether Playboy sponsored or endorsed the adult site. Playboy also proved that its trademark bunny logo would be blurred or tarnished by the association with the adult site. Also, in *Coca-Cola Co. v. Purdy*, the Court entered judgment for several well-known trademark owners on their infringement claims where an antiabortionist used a host of domain names incorporating their famous marks.[145] The antiabortionist linked the domain names (e.g., *mycoca-cola.com*) with a website associated with *abortion-ismurder.com*. According to the decision, the "quick and effortless nature of 'surfing' the Internet makes it unlikely that consumers can avoid confusion through the exercise of due care."[146]

The practice of using framing to incorporate third-party content into a website is also an area of unsettled law. The framing site can surround the framed pages with its own advertising, logos, or promotions. Framing may trigger a dispute under copyright and trademark law theories because a framed site arguably alters the appearance of the content and creates the impression that its owner endorses or voluntarily chooses to associate with the framer.[147] However, liability for framing has not been fully or clearly resolved by the courts.[148]

Advances in technology may render this dilemma moot. Technology now exists to keep undesired links or frames off a website. In any event, it is advisable not to link to or frame another website without the express (i.e., explicit, written) permission of that site. However, if a website owner is concerned about liability for links or frames, a prominently placed disclaimer may be added. Additionally, if a webmaster wants to obtain permission before someone links to their site, a "request permission" notice needs to be posted and require users to agree to the terms by clicking "I agree" on the home page.

The Internet raises a variety of legal issues, most of which are unresolved but evolving. Future goals should be for pharmaceutical manufacturers to promote their products to consumers more responsibly, for the FDA to regulate DTCA more effectively, and for the medical and pharmacy communities to educate the public about prescription drugs more constructively.

Intellectual Property Rights

COPYRIGHT

The current copyright law is codified at 17 U.S.C.A. § 101 *et seq.* A copyright is a property right in an original work of authorship that is fixed in tangible form.[149] It is a statutory requirement that literary, dramatic, and musical works, for example, must have been recorded or produced in some physical object (or fixed) before copyright can subsist. A copyright holder in a work is granted certain exclusive rights to control use of the work created. A work of authorship must be original in order to qualify for copyright protection. This requirement has two facets. First, the author must have engaged in some intellectual endeavor of his or her own, and not just have copied from a preexisting source. Second, the work must exhibit a minimal amount of creativity. Copyright protection covers both published and unpublished works. Also, the fact that the previously published work is out of print does not affect its copyright. Works of authorship under copyright and items not entitled to copyright are found in Table 10-3.

❺ *Pharmacists providing DI must have a working knowledge of copyright law both to avoid liability and to protect their own literary works.* Under the 1976 Copyright Act, an author is protected as soon as a work is recorded in some concrete way. The process of registering for a copyright involves depositing material with the Copyright Office to be reviewed by an examiner, followed by publication with a copyright notice, usually the symbol ©. Under the Copyright Term Extension Act (CTEA) of 1998, such work is

TABLE 10–3. COPYRIGHT PROTECTION

Works of authorship entitled to copyright protection include the following:
- Literary works
- Musical works, including any accompanying words
- Dramatic works, including any accompanying music
- Pantomimes and choreographic works
- Pictorial, graphic, and sculptural works
- Motion pictures and other audiovisual works
- Sound recordings
- Architectural works

Not entitled to copyright protection:
- Ideas, concepts, principles, or discovery
- Procedures, processes, systems, methods of operation
- Mere compilations of facts

protected until 70 years after the death of the author or for 95 years for corporate copyright holders. In effect, the CTEA retroactively extended copyright terms by 20 years.[150] The constitutionality of CTFA has been challenged and upheld by the Supreme Court. The author or copyright owner has the exclusive right to make copies of the work, control derivative works or adaptations, and sue for damages and injunctive relief (an injunction is a judicial remedy issued in order to prohibit a party from doing or continuing to do a certain activity) against infringers. Public domain works may be copied and distributed without copyright permission. Works of the U.S. government (e.g., General Accounting Office [GAO] reports, Congressional Record, FDA releases) are considered part of the public domain.

Ownership of copyright usually rests with the author at the time when the work is created. The exception is a work made for hire (i.e., "a work prepared by an employee within the scope of the employment relationship, or a work specially ordered or commissioned for use as a contribution to a collective work, as part of a motion picture or other audiovisual work, as a translation, as a supplementary work, as a compilation, as an instructional text, as a test, as an answer material for a test, or as an atlas, if the parties expressly agree in a written instrument signed by them that the work shall be a work made for hire" [Copyright Law of the United States, 17 U.S.C. Sec 106]).[151] Another exception is the first-sale doctrine, which in effect, permits interlibrary loan of materials. Under the first-sale doctrine, a person who legitimately owns a copy of a work is one who purchased the work or otherwise acquired ownership of the work with the permission of the copyright owner, and has full authority to "sell or otherwise dispose of the possession of that copy."[152]

Since the Berne Convention in 1989, the copyright formalities of registration and notice have lost almost all their legal significance. Registration, although not mandatory, affords the copyright claimant certain advantages. For example, it prevents an infringer from pleading innocent infringement. Similarly, the only substantive legal effect of copyright registration is that attorney fees and statutory damages are only recoverable for postregistration infringements. That is, U.S. authors must register before bringing suit. However, for works prior to 1989 and the Berne Convention, copyright can be lost if notice was omitted and that omission was not cured within 5 years of publication by registration and affixation of notice to the remaining copies.

Under the fair use provision of the 1976 Copyright Act, if a use is fair, permission of the copyright owner need not be received, nor royalties paid. Fair use is determined by a four-pronged test: (1) nature and character of use, (2) nature of the work, (3) the proportional amount copied, and, most importantly, (4) the effect on the market for the copied work.[153]

The first factor in the fair use analysis is the nature and character of the use. Uses for research, teaching, scholarship, and news reporting are more likely to be considered fair than strictly commercial uses. In addition, there is a narrow special exemption for educators. The mere fact that the use is educational and not for profit does not insulate the use from a finding of infringement.

The second factor in the fair use analysis is the nature of the work. This factor centers on whether a copyrighted work is creative or informational, and whether it is published or unpublished. The scope of fair use is greater when the copyrighted work is informational. This is because it is generally recognized that there is a greater need to disseminate factual material than works of fiction or fantasy.[154] An unpublished work is given greater copyright protection than a published work and is, therefore, less likely to be subjected to a valid assertion of fair use.[155] In *Harper & Row Publishers, Inc. v. Nation Enterprises*, *Nation* obtained an unauthorized manuscript of former President Ford's memoirs before they were published in a book form under a contract with Harper & Row. The fact that President Ford's memoirs had not yet been published by the time *Nation* published them was a deciding factor.[156] That is, in looking at the nature of the work, an unpublished work seems to be entitled to greater protection than a published work.

The third factor is the amount copied. There does not appear to be a minimal amount or threshold quantity (e.g., five sentences) standard where fair use will be presumed. Many copyrighted works are accessed through a campus license that overrides copyright. Libraries vigorously negotiate licenses for such materials. Although the statute itself does not set the maximum standards for educational fair use, classroom guidelines have been agreed upon by educational, author, and publisher organizations.[157] Multiple copies for classroom use, but not to exceed in any event more than one copy per pupil in a course, are permissible, provided each copy bears a copyright notice and meets the test of (1) brevity, (2) spontaneity, and (3) cumulative effect. For example, to meet the test of brevity the classroom guidelines prohibit multiple copying of complete articles longer than 2,500 words. They prohibit copying excerpts longer than 1,000 words or 10% of the work, whichever is shorter. For motion media, up to 10% or 3 minutes, whichever is less, in the aggregate of a copyrighted motion media work may be reproduced or otherwise incorporated as part of an educational multimedia project. To meet the test of spontaneity, the copying must be at the instance and inspiration of the individual teacher, where the teacher's decision to use the work in class does not allow for a timely reply to request for permission. To meet the cumulative effect requirement, the copying must be for only one course in the school, and except for current news periodicals, newspapers, and current news sections of periodicals, only one article or two excerpts therefrom, may be copied from the same author, or three excerpts from the same collective work or periodical volume. Additionally, the copying must be for only one class term; and no more than nine instances of such multiple copying for one course during one class term. In other words, the copied material may only be used for one semester and permission for longer use must be obtained. Further, students may not be charged for the copy beyond the actual cost of photocopying.

Case Study 10–3

You are publishing a guide regarding "do not crush" drugs for which you will receive compensation. You are merely listing all drugs that should not be crushed. However, the material for this publication is derived from a number of published references, all of which are copyright protected. You adopt an entire table from one of the articles without permission. You also take several direct sentences without providing any source reference. One of the references you are using is out of print.

- *Which of these acts would constitute a violation of the copyright law? What steps should have been taken to avoid copyright violation?*

In *Association of American Publishers v. New York University*, the issue was the production and distribution of custom-made anthologies sold to students. Although the classroom guidelines allow students to make single copies for personal use, the court found infringement when anthologies were sold for profit.[158] The action was settled with the adoption of certain procedures by New York University.

The fourth factor in a fair use analysis is the impact the infringing work will have on the market or potential market of the copyrighted work. The Supreme Court has decided that all four factors of the fair use test should be given equal weight.[159] Under the Copyright Act of 1976, these four fair use factors provide a broad and flexible defense against copyright infringement.

Fair use is an equitable defense to copyright infringement, determined by the courts on a case-by-case basis. Unfortunately, in court decisions on educational photocopying to date, the ruling in almost every case has been against fair use. Copying by nonprofit medical libraries has been held to be a fair use where the photocopying of medical journals by federal nonprofit institutions was made solely for the purpose of medical research. In *Williams & Wilkins Co. v. United States*, the library was copying a single copy for each request and the court found that "medical science would be seriously hurt if such library photocopying were stopped."[160] In *Williams & Wilkins*, the copying of medical journals was by two governmental libraries, that is, the National Institutes of Health and the National Medical library, a repository of much of the world's medical literature.[161] The public benefits of fair use apparently held considerably more weight than any commercial considerations presented before the courts. However, where the photocopying of medical journals by scientists occurred in a large for-profit company, the court decided the making of unauthorized copies of copyrighted articles published in scientific journals for use by research scientists was not fair use. The court determined that the publishers had created through the Copyright Clearance Center, Inc., a viable market for institutional users to obtain licenses to allow photocopying of individual articles. However, in *Princeton University Press v. Michigan Document Services, Inc.*, the court held that a copy shop selling coursepacks, which are compilations of various copyrighted and uncopyrighted materials such as journal articles, sample test questions, course notes, and book excerpts, infringed the copyrights of several publishers.[162] In deciding this was not a fair use, the court noted that the copying was substantial and commercial. Similarly, in *Basic Books v. Kinko's Graphic Corp.*, the court held that a copy shop's reproduction and sale of coursepacks to students was not a fair use of the copyrighted material.[163]

Course management systems and digital course packs, which post copyrighted articles, book excerpts, and research data, are used today by 90% of U.S. colleges and universities. Simply because the material is online does not mean it is free from copyright protection. Unless fair use or some other exemption applies, permission is required before posting.[164] When fair use does not apply, the institution must obtain permission from the rightsholder, who may charge a fee for such permission based on the amount of content and the number of people, usually students, who will view the content. Additionally, reporting of the same material for use in a subsequent semester requires a new permission. Moreover, it violates the intent and spirit of copyright law to use course management systems as a substitute for the purchase of books, subscriptions, or other materials when substantial portions of the material are required for educational purposes. When scanning in paper materials (such as textbooks) to create electronic copies, be sure that legally obtained copies of the work are used, either purchased or owned by the institution. All posted materials in a course management system should contain both the copyright notice from, and complete citation to, the original material, as well as a caution against further electronic distribution.[154] Instant permission may be obtained at http://www.copyright.com through the Copyright Clearance Center for use in course management systems, coursepacks, e-reserves, classroom handouts, and other formats.

The court has also ruled that there is only a limited copyright protection available to a compilation of works written by another author. In *Silverstein v. Penguin Putnam*, the plaintiff had compiled a collection of 122 unpublished Dorothy Parker poems.[165] He presented the compilation to Penguin, which rejected it and subsequently inserted the poems into a new edition of Parker's work published by Penguin. The court held that Silverstein would not be entitled to injunctive relief as he did not hold the copyright on the poems. Thus, his efforts to gather the poems were not protectable in copyright. Additionally, the court looked at Silverstein's arrangement of the poems and found that Penguin did not copy his arrangement.

In 2008, in *Warner Bros. Entm't Inc. v. RDR Books*, a lexicon of terms from the *Harry Potter* series of books, initially posted on a free Internet website and then scheduled for publication, was held as copyright infringement.[166] The legal issues involved were whether there is a distinction in the law between digital and printed copyright and what is a third-party's right to create a new reference book designed to help others better understand the original work (i.e., a study guide). The court held that the print version of the lexicon was not a derivative work, especially in view of the number of places where copying was deemed excessive. However, the court explicitly stated that authors do not have the right to stop the publication of reference guides and companion works.

Copyright infringement requires a showing of copying, which can be proven circumstantially by demonstrating that the defendant had access to the copyrighted work and that the defendant's work is substantially similar to that work. Copyright infringement for purposes of commercial advantage or private financial gain is punishable under 18 U.S.C. §2319. Although the act allows for damages of as much as $100,000 per infringement, innocent infringers (e.g., educators and universities) may be entitled to a remission of statutory damages. They are only liable for actual damages, such as profits earned by the infringer or profits denied to the copyright holder. This provision lowers the incentive for the publishing industry to sue. Recently, publishers have resorted to unsavory tactics in their attempts to control educational copying, such as sending letters threatening to sue copy shops for infringement unless they agree to pay royalties.

Newsletter copying is strictly prohibited and violators risk not only the statutory damages ($100,000), but can be subject to criminal penalties. These newsletters require a fee to be paid to the Copyright Clearance Center even for internal or personal copying and offer rewards to those who report violations. Washington Business Information, Inc. has won major payments in infringement actions against pharmaceutical manufacturers for photocopying its *Food & Drug Letter.*

Section 201(c) of the Copyright Act has produced electronic copyright issues for freelance articles and photography in electronic databases. Specifically, a series of cases involves whether or not permission is required from authors to place their articles on commercial databases or in the electronic public domain (e.g., MEDLINE®). In *New York Times v. Tasini*, the U.S. Supreme Court ruled that publishers cannot republish printed works electronically without obtaining permission from authors.[167] *Tasini* should not have much impact on new work as most publisher agreements now address electronic publication rights. Problematic, however, are older works published without a written agreement. The publishers argued unsuccessfully that the use of the articles in a database was no different from issuing a microfilm or microfiche copy of a newspaper. However, permissibility of electronic republication of an entire issue of a newspaper, magazine, newsletter without further payment to authors, remains unresolved.[168] Rather than attempt to contact freelancers and offer compensation for articles, some database producers have already begun to purge their databases of freelance contributions.

Photocopies fall within the territory of the Copyright Act. When sending copies of original articles, a statement to the effect that the copies are only for personal or private use must be made. The most effective way for any DI facility to protect itself against copy infringement lawsuits is to copy the page with the copyright notice and stamp the first page of the copies with a statement that the enclosed document is protected by copyright, thus putting the burden of responsibility on the recipient of the one copy. Such a notice might state, "This material is subject to the United States Copyright Law (17 U.S. Code): unauthorized copying may be prohibited by law."

The Computer Software Act of 1980 amended the Copyright Act to extend protection to computer software. However, copyright laws do not provide sufficient protection for information transmitted over the Internet and other information networks. Although copyright protection applies when copyrighted material is converted into a digital form, the havoc that cyberspace can wreak on copyright owner's rights cannot be overestimated. A debate is currently raging over whether existing copyright law can successfully adapt to the Internet.

Google recently settled two class action lawsuits regarding application of copyright protection to the indexing of scanned documents.[169,170] The lawsuits involve the Google Library Project where in 2004, the company announced that it has entered into agreement with several libraries to digitalize books and other documents from those libraries collections. The books and documents were also to be indexed for search purposes. Thus, the legal question of whether indexing for search purposes is fair use. Google was sued by publishers and authors when attempting to create an unprecedented extensive digitalized library of books. The authors and publishers claimed the scanning and indexing was not fair use but commercial in nature.[171] The case was settled and not decided by a court. However, on March 22, 2011, the court denied the final settlement approval. The parties are currently considering their next steps. Until then, the question of the legal fair defense of unauthorized copying of the works remains unresolved. Meanwhile Google continues to scan books although some of the digitalization efforts have shifted to European collections perhaps because of the litigation.[172] By April 2013, the Google database encompassed 30 million scanned books.[173]

On October 3, 2002, Congress enacted the Technology, Education, and Copyright Harmonization (TEACH) Act, fully revising §110(2) of the U.S. Copyright Act governing the lawful uses of existing copyright materials in distance education. The TEACH Act defines the conditions and circumstances on which educators may clip pieces of text, images, sound, and other works and include them in distance education. Table 10-4 outlines the key provisions of the TEACH Act. If a particular use does not fit these conditions, one may still consider whether the use is a fair use.[174]

Access to works on the Internet or those publicly available does not automatically mean that these can be reproduced and reused without permission or royalty payment

TABLE 10-4. MAJOR PROVISIONS OF THE TEACH ACT

- Expanded range of allowed works (e.g., nondramatic literary works; nondramatic musical works; audiovisual works).
- Expanded receiving locations. Educational institutions may now reach students through distance education at any location.
- Storage of transmitted content. Allows retention of the content and student access for a brief period of time especially with regard to digital transmission systems.
- Allows for digitalizing of analog works but only if the work is not already available in digital form.
- Educational institutions must now institute policies regarding copyright although the details of content of those policies are not provided.
- Transmission of content must be made solely to students officially enrolled in a course for which the transmission is made. Technological restrictions on access are required.

and, furthermore, some copyrighted works may have been posted on the Internet without authorization of the copyright holder. Publicly available is not to be confused with the legal concept of public domain, which comprises all works that are either no longer protected by copyright or never were. With the ease of retrieval of material electronically, copyright holders are likely to uncover those who are violating their copyright. Publishers who did not previously press for royalty payments of small segments of works can now trace the borrowing of snippets of text and create systems of payment and collection. Research downloading, with deletion of material after use, appears to be a fair use of the material. However, downloading to create a personal database and avoid payment of connect fees and higher user fees is illegal unless covered under special agreements between the database owner and subscriber. Also, linking to a work is always an option. Copyright law does not preclude anyone from linking to a copyright work on a website. However, it is important to remember that if the link contains copyrighted graphic material, it cannot be used without permission of the copyright holder. Further, although the Berne Convention is the principal copyright treaty, there is no such thing as an international copyright. The treaty obligates signatory countries to extend the protection of their copyright law to foreigners whose works are infringed within their borders.[175]

Current copyright law denies protection to compilations of facts unless such facts are arranged or organized with some minimal element of originality. Even then, it is the creative aspect of such arrangements or organization that may be protected and not the underlying facts themselves. Legislation has been repeatedly introduced, advocated primarily by large database companies, aimed at codifying into law a new unique form of intellectual property protection for databases. The situation is different in Europe where the European Union (EU) 1996 Database Directive grants copyright protection for the selection and arrangement of information in a European database, and calls downloading and hyperlinking unfair extraction of information.

Related to copyright infringement is plagiarism and fictitious reporting. Plagiarism is a legal offense or crime. The owner of a copyright (i.e., author) could sue the plagiarist in federal court for violation of the copyright. Fictitious reporting may simply constitute poor journalism or it may rise to the level of fraud or libel. Plagiarism involves not citing material while factitious reporting involves citing things that do not exist.

The definition of plagiarism is subjective and vague. History, facts, and ideas are not copyrighted, although they may be plagiarized. The addition of original material by the plagiarist in no way excuses the act of plagiarism. In fact, trivial changes in copied text, in an attempt to avoid copyright infringement, is specifically prohibited by the copyright law. Additionally, there is no fixed number or percentage of words that can be used without exposure to charges of plagiarism.[176] Verbatim quotes are permitted, provided it falls within the fair use protection. Software and web-based technologies (e.g., Turnitin®) now exist that can scan millions of documents almost instantly to compare what has been written before to what is being written today. Further information on plagiarism is contained in Chapter 12.

Privacy

HEALTH INSURANCE PORTABILITY AND ACCOUNTABILITY ACT OF 1996

Information security concerns are at the forefront of legal issues involved in electronic communications, specifically, questions of authenticity of medical or pharmacy records and confidentiality or privacy of the contents of medical and personal information of patients. Today, an individual's health information is often used for payment, QA, research, peer review, accreditation, and a multitude of other purposes. Further, communicating with patients using mobile devices such as iPhones, iPads, or Android phones is an increasing trend among health care providers.

Congress enacted the Health Insurance Portability and Accountability Act of 1996 (HIPAA).[177] While security and privacy under HIPAA are inextricably linked, there are distinctions. HIPAA *Privacy* Rule protects the privacy of individually identified health information. HIPAA *Security* Rule sets standards for the security of *electronic* protected health information (ePHI). The security rule standards define the administrative, physical, and technical safeguards (e.g., encryption) to protect the confidentiality, integrity, and availability of ePHI.

HIPAA's security standards are intended to protect the security of the environment in which health care information is maintained and transmitted. The privacy rule, by contrast, sets standards for how PHI should be controlled by setting forth what uses and disclosures are authorized or required and what rights patients have with respect to their health information. The privacy rule applies to information in any form, whereas the security rule only applies to ePHI.

Increased use of personal mobile devices such as tablets and smartphones by health care providers and professionals to access and exchange ePHI triggers the HIPAA security rule. In addition to the security risks inherent in the way these devices store data and/or lack of encryption software features, mobile devices are particularly vulnerable to loss and theft. The Office of the National Coordinator for Health Information Technology has outlined best practice steps organizations should take to manage mobile devices used by health care professionals.[178]

For pharmacies, the security standards are applicable only to ePHI, not paper, facsimile, nor telephone transmissions. HIPAA's privacy standards govern the use and disclosure of protected health information. Many aspects of HIPAA fall outside the scope of this chapter. In any event, reasonable steps should always be taken to ensure that fax, text, or e-mail transmissions are sent to and received by the intended recipient. Examples of such steps for faxes include confirming with the intended recipient that the receiving fax machine is located in a secure area or the intended recipient is waiting by the fax machine; preprogramming and testing fax numbers for frequent recipients of DI faxes to avoid errors associated with misdialing; double checking the recipient's fax number prior to transmission; using a fax cover sheet with an erroneous transmission statement and advising to notify the sender immediately and arrange for return or destruction of the fax; promptly checking all fax confirmation sheets to determine that faxed material was received at the intended fax number.

Individual PHI is information, including demographic data, that relates to the individual's past, present, or future physical or mental health or condition; the provision of health care to the individual, or the past, present, or future payment for the provision of health care to the individual, and that identifies the individual or for which there is a reasonable basis to believe it can be used to identify the individual.[179] Individually identifiable health information includes many common identifiers such as name, address, birth date, and social security number.

However, there are no restrictions on the use or disclosure of de-identified health information.[180] De-identified health information neither identifies nor provides a reasonable basis to identify an individual. There are two methods for de-identifying protected health information: the statistical method and the safe-harbor method via removal of certain identifiers.[181] De-identified data sets, which separate individuals' identities from their protected health information, are becoming increasingly available through the Centers for Medicare and Medicaid Services and the National Institutes of Health.[182] This data is proving useful for outcomes and medical error research not associated with the original data collection protocol.

Under HIPAA, a covered entity may engage in research activities in four ways: (1) by using or disclosing only de-identified information, (2) by obtaining a waiver or an authorization from the individual to use and disclose the information for research purposes, (3) by obtaining a waiver of an authorization from an IRB, or (4) by representing that the use or disclosure is solely of the protected health information of a deceased individual. Clinical investigators are most likely to choose option three.[183]

HIPAA specifically permits covered entities such as health care professionals or hospitals to report adverse events and other information related to the quality, effectiveness, and safety of FDA-regulated products to both the manufacturers and directly to FDA. Under this exception, a pharmacist need not obtain an authorization from a patient before notifying a pharmaceutical company and the FDA that the patient had an adverse reaction to a drug manufactured by the drug company.[184] ❻ *It is important to keep in mind that the HIPAA Privacy Rule is not intended to disrupt or discourage adverse event reporting or DI in any way.*

In responding to DI questions, it is of utmost importance to obtain specific patient identification information including, but not limited to, patient name, age, height, weight, or medical record number. Nothing in HIPAA would diminish or affect that responsibility. In the DI arena, HIPAA allows disclosure of patient information for treatment, payment, and health care operations. Examples of health care operations include quality management, QA, outcomes evaluation, development of clinical guidelines, peer review, and credentialing. While not specifically mentioned, DI would appear to fall under both treatment and health care operations. In most instances, HIPAA should not affect DI requests from health care providers as patient identity is usually not required or is provided via medical record number only. However, when patient identifying information is communicated, protection of information within the DI center (or pharmacy) is an important HIPAA requirement. Policies and procedures governing use and disclosure of confidential information should be in place. These policies should include guidance on training and strategies for mitigating risks during all stages of the DI request processing (receipt, triage, and response). For example, procedures should be in place to verify the identity of the requestor of information. Patient information security safeguards should be in place, for example, requiring personal identifiers to be removed as soon as feasible, physical controls, software controls, and formal oversight.[185]

Case Study 10–4

A drug information question involves a patient who has a socially stigmatic disease. In responding to the question, the pharmacist needs to share the patient's PHI with the laboratory and pharmacokinetic services. However, in sharing this information the pharmacist discusses it as well as the diagnosis in an area where it was easily overheard by others not entitled to know. Additionally, the patient's personal information is faxed by the pharmacist to a fax machine in an unsecured area where many people have access to the fax machine.

- *Does HIPAA prohibit any of the pharmacist's actions?*
- *What safeguards should be taken when discussing the patient and his/her information?*
- *What reasonable steps are necessary to ensure that fax transmissions are sent and recorded by the intended recipient?*

There are several other situations in pharmacy practice where HIPAA compliance issues may be triggered. For example, in clinical case reports, whether for publication or teaching purposes, the patient should only be referred to via his or her initials, age, or sex (e.g., RM, a 35-year-old female). When writing a case report or article for publication, always remove any patient identifiers. In some cases, the patient consent may be required to publish the report.

HIPAA permits a pharmacist to counsel individuals other than the patient (e.g., a friend, family member, or neighbor picking up the patient's prescription) even though some of the patient's protected health information may be revealed in such a situation. However, the regulation is clear that such disclosures must be limited and should only be made when the provider believes it is in the patient's best interest. For example, there can be no doubt that disclosing that the medication picked up is for treatment of HIV infection would not be necessary. Under HIPAA, personnel representatives, defined as individuals legally authorized, under state or other applicable law, to make health care decisions on behalf of a patient, are to be treated in the same way as a patient. However, in some cases the personal representative's authority is limited to a specific matter, such as treatment for a life-threatening illness. In these cases, the personal representative may only access protected health information directly related to that illness. Additionally, many states have enacted laws that protect persons with illnesses that are seen as particularly stigmatizing, such as HIV, mental illness, and drug addiction. The Public Health Service Act and implementing regulations govern the confidentiality of substance abuse records maintained by federally assisted drug and alcohol abuse programs.[186]

Similarly, parents are considered the personal representative of a minor child and can access the minor's health records. Exceptions exist when the minor consents to health care and consent of the parent is not required under state or other law, or when the minor obtains health care at the direction of a court, or when the minor is emancipated. Other exceptions exist if a provider believes that a patient or minor is subject to abuse, neglect, or domestic violence by their personal representative.[187] Many states specifically authorize minors to consent to contraceptive services, testing and treatment for HIV and other sexually transmitted diseases, prenatal care and delivery services, treatment for alcohol and drug abuse, and outpatient mental health care.

HIPAA also requires that pharmacies make a good faith effort to obtain a patient's acknowledgment that they have received a copy of the Notice of Privacy Practices. The notice describes how the pharmacy uses and discloses protected health information to carry out treatment, payment or health care operations, and the patient's rights. The notice is to be distributed to patients on or before the first treatment encounter. Where the prescription is being picked up by someone other than the patient, the pharmacy must attempt to deliver the notice to the patient. Examples of a good faith effort include providing the notice in the prescription bag or mailing the notice to the patient together with some type of return receipt means. However, the pharmacy is not in violation if the return receipt is not returned. The pharmacy needs to only document its efforts.[188]

Under HIPAA, pharmacists will be held accountable for handling confidential information properly. Civil and criminal penalties for violating patient confidentiality exist. A patient cannot use a HIPAA violation as a basis of a private lawsuit as there is no "right of private action." However, if the HIPAA violation amounts to negligence or malpractice then such cases may be brought under state laws. Plaintiffs use evidence of a HIPAA violation as proof of a breach of duty in negligence or state law invasion of privacy cases. Increasingly, HIPAA is being used as the basis of negligence claims.

COMMUNICATION PRIVACY

The Telephone Consumer Protection Act (TCPA) sets rules prohibiting unsolicited commercial faxes and text messages. A Federal Communication Commission (FCC) regulation implementing the act requires businesses and nonprofit groups to get signed written permission from clients or members before faxing unsolicited materials containing advertisements. Litigation under the TCPA is increasing, particularly in the area of junk fax class actions and insurance coverage for TCPA damages. There have also been a number of recent cases against pharmacies for sending robo-texts to patients regarding pharmacy services or automated refill reminders without patients' consent.[189,190] The statute provides statutory damages of ~$16,000 for each violation, which are paid to the consumer.

Privacy is also an issue on the Internet (e.g., e-health sites) where the dominant privacy issue arises from the growing practice of data collection. Some websites are interactive; that is, they may require the patient to complete a survey or will send visitors a prescription refill reminder. These sites then link to privacy policies that address any concerns prospective patients may have about filling out an online survey. Disclosure of an online privacy policy together with an opt-out feature can provide assurances about the protection of consumer privacy and personal information. The policy should also address passive disclosure of information, for example, from cookies (a feature which allows web servers to recognize a specific user or computer to access the website) or web server logs. Unfortunately, e-health sites were not included under HIPAA. Some of these e-health Internet sites violate their own privacy policies and transfer patient-identifiable information to third parties.[191]

E-mail use in health care has developed without encryption and HIPAA does not directly address e-mail in any of its standards. However, because e-mail may involve protected health information in electronic form, both HIPAA's privacy and security rules apply. The security of unencrypted e-mail is low. Passwords, firewalls, and other conventional network security should exist to secure electronic DI communications.[192]

There has also been litigation in this area. In *re Pharmatrak Inc. v. Privacy Litigation*, the plaintiffs alleged that numerous pharmaceutical companies secretly intercepted and accessed their personal information through the use of computer cookies and other devices,[193] in violation of state and federal laws such as the Electronic Communications Privacy Act.[194]

Industry Support for Educational Activities

Many pharmacists attend conferences, sometimes funded by pharmaceutical companies to further their professional education. Dialogue between health professionals and the pharmaceutical industry is an opportunity to pass along scientific and educational information, and product risks and benefits. Such dialogue encourages and supports medical research, while providing the health professional with an opportunity to address questions, discuss issues, and offer expertise.

GUIDELINES AND GUIDANCE

❼ *The FDA, the American Council for Continuing Medical Education (ACCME), and the Pharmaceutical Research and Manufacturers of America (PhRMA)*[195] *have established educational policies, guidelines, or guidances which allow communication between industry and the continuing medical education (CME) providers* with the proviso that the final decisions and control rest with the accredited provider. The Office of Inspector General (OIG) issued a guidance that prohibits the pharmaceutical industry from direct communication with CME providers and calls for an intermediary organization to develop CME programs.[196] The following factors are provided in the OIG Guidance: Does the arrangement skew clinical decision making? Is the information complete, accurate, and non-misleading? Does the arrangement have the potential to be a disguised discount or result in inappropriate over- or underutilization? Does the arrangement raise patient safety, quality, or care concerns? Importantly, for pharmacists providing DI as industry clinical education consultants or medical liaisons, the ACPE no longer accredits pharmaceutical and biomedical manufacturers.[197] However, not all states actually require all of a pharmacist's continuing education activities to be accredited by the ACPE.[198]

The PhRMA Code, which became effective in July 2002, and updated in January 2009, is the most specific and stringent and deals with various interactions between industry and health care professionals, such as informational presentations, professional meetings, consultant activities, scholarships and educational funds, and educational and practice-related items.[199] Scholarships for pharmacists, students, and residents to attend selected educational conferences may be provided. Salient features of the latest PhRMA Code are found in Table 10-5 and at http://www.phrma.org/sites/default/files/pdf/phrma_marketing_code_2008.pdf.

The FDA Guidance seeks to draw a distinction between educational activities that the FDA considers non-promotional and those it considers promotional. The distinction is important, especially with regard to off-label uses, which can be an important component of educational activities. The FDA's Factors to Determine Independence of the Educational Activity are found in Table 10-6.[200]

Some health care institutions have established their own best practices approach to developing ethical guidelines for pharmaceutical industry support. The practice involves a process similar to weighing the risks and benefits of a particular medication or therapeutic intervention, whereby each proposal for support can be viewed as having potential value, which may or may not outweigh any potential drawbacks inherent in the involvement of funding from a for-profit company. Often a committee assesses proposals based on the apparent balance between these factors and a set of guidelines developed by the institution.[201]

In general, most policies and procedures prohibit acceptance of commercial support of educational activities if such acceptance would appear to (1) create an atmosphere limiting academic freedom and the free exchange of ideas and information, (2) introduce bias or otherwise threaten objectivity, (3) create a conflict of interest, or (4) be in conflict with the mission and profit status of the health care organization.[202]

RELATIONSHIP TO THE ANTI-KICKBACK STATUTE

Particular arrangements between pharmacists and the pharmaceutical industry pose potential risks under the Anti-Kickback Statute. The Anti-Kickback Statute makes it a criminal offense to knowingly and willfully offer, pay, solicit, or receive any remuneration (in cash or in kind) to induce (or in exchange for) the purchasing, ordering, or

TABLE 10–5. PhRMA CODE ON INTERACTIONS WITH HEALTH CARE PROFESSIONALS

- Gifts
  - Generally prohibited
  - Exceptions—$100 or less that benefits patients or educate health care professionals; e.g., medical textbooks or anatomical models permitted, but not stethoscopes that are primarily used for treating patients
  - Pens, pads, etc. no longer permitted
  - Product samples allowed
- Meals
  - Modest meals accompanying informational presentations
  - Can only be offered occasionally
  - Can only be **directly** provided in office or at hospital (no restaurants or resorts)
- Entertainment
  - Prohibited
  - May sponsor meals or reception at conferences
- Spouses
  - Never appropriate for lodging, travel, meals, entertainment
- Consultants
  - Must be *bona fide* via written contract, appropriate venue, and selection criteria related to purpose of service, must exclude spouses
  - Special disclosure requirements for health care professionals that set up formularies or develop clinical practice guidelines—disclosure requirements extend two years beyond the terms of any speaker or consultant arrangements
  - Legitimate need identified in advance of entering into agreement required
  - Number of consultants cannot be greater than number reasonably needed to achieve purpose
- Financial sponsorship of educational conferences
  - Support should be provided to CPE sponsor, not individual speaker/author
  - Sponsor should control selection of content, faculty, educational materials, and venue
  - Faculty, but not attendees or spouses, may be paid/reimbursed for time, travel, and lodging
  - Exception—companies may pay for travel/lodging for students to attend educational conferences; educational institutional must select individual students
- Informational presentations
  - Should be modest by local standards
  - Should occur in a venue and manner conducive to informational communication
  - Should provide scientific or educational value
  - Can recommend to continuing education providers topics of interest that manufacturer would sponsor

recommending of any good or service reimbursable by any federal health care program.[203] Funding that is conditioned, in whole or in part, on the purchase of product implicates the statute, even if the educational or research purpose is legitimate. Several cases hold that intent is improper if one purpose, not the sole or even primary purpose, is to induce the purchase or recommendation of a company's goods or services.[204,205] When a grant is provided to a customer or potential customer, it may violate the Anti-Kickback Statute if one purpose is to induce the customer to buy the company's product.

TABLE 10–6. FACTORS USED BY THE FDA TO DETERMINE INDEPENDENCE OF AN EDUCATIONAL ACTIVITY

- Control of content and selection of faculty: Is there scripting or other actions designed to influence the content by the supporting company?
- Disclosures: Does it include company funding the program, relationship between provider(s) and presenters to the supporting company, and off-label discussion?
- The focus of the program: Does the title accurately represent the presentation? Is there fair-balanced educational discussion?
- Relationship between provider and supporting company: Is there a legal, business, or other relationship between the parties?
- Provider involved in sales or marketing: Are provider employees also doing marketing or promotional programs?
- Provider's demonstrated failure to meet standards: Does the provider have a history of biased programs?
- Multiple presentations: Do they serve public health interests?
- Audience selection: Is the audience generated by sales or marketing departments to influence marketing goals?
- Opportunities for discussion: Is there an opportunity for meaningful discussion?
- Dissemination: Is the supporting company distributing additional information after the activity; unless requested by participant and then through an independent provider?
- Ancillary promotional activities: Are promotional activities taking place in the educational meeting room?
- Complaints: Are provider(s), faculty, or others complaining about the supporting company?

Educational grants, for example, were at the heart of the $161 million Caremark, LLC settlement[206] and research grants were at the heart of the $450,000 Hoffman-La Roche, Inc. settlement.[207] Furthermore, to the extent the manufacturer has any influence over the substance of an educational program or the presenter, there is a risk that the educational program may be used for inappropriate marketing purposes.

In the area of DI, specific practices that may be problematic under the Anti-Kickback Statute include gifts, use of pharmacists who are customers as consultants or members of speaker's bureaus, and questionable research grants. Problems under the Anti-Kickback Statute could arise where the DI pharmacist participates in any of these activities and also advises on formulary choices or is a member of a formulary committee or subcommittee or is involved with purchasing decisions. If a product or service is recommended and the recommender stands to make financial gain from it, and that service is paid for in part or in whole by the federal government, that person may be violating the Anti-Kickback Statute. Similarly, no gifts should be accepted if there are strings attached.

Educational activities or speakers can be funded by the pharmaceutical industry, whereas promotional marketing activities that purport to be of an educational purpose but serve no direct patient benefit are prohibited. Hiring DI pharmacists under the guise of a consultant or advisor, or focus group participant or advisory board member, or even as a speaker at a meeting, could be considered payments for referrals. Similarly, compensating DI pharmacists as consultants, when all they do is attend conferences primarily in a passive capacity, is suspect. Other suspect activities include compensation for speaking, researching, listening to marketing pitches, or providing preceptor, shadowing or ghostwriting services. However, where the pharmacist is compensated for actual, reasonable, and necessary services, the activities may be considered legitimate.

The Anti-Kickback Statute prohibits involvement with research contracts that come through a pharmaceutical company's marketing department, research not reviewed by the manufacturer's scientific or medical department, research that is unnecessarily duplicative or not needed for any purpose other than the generation of business, and post-marketing research used as a pretense for product promotion.[208] Manufacturers should use Chinese walls (i.e., ethical barriers prohibiting exchange of confidential information between different departments of an organization) for marketing and grant-funding activities to demonstrate that grants are bona fide and not improperly influenced by marketing considerations. The Anti-Kickback Statute requires that grants be given in exchange for fair market value research consideration. This is often difficult to accomplish, since the precise costs and schedules of research activities are not knowable in advance and sometimes not conducive to being reduced to written agreements.

Conclusion

By now, the reader has undoubtedly discovered that the liability aspects of DI include more than just negligence. Liability for off-label uses, consumer advertising, copyright infringement, liability issues unique to the Internet, privacy concerns, and industry support for educational activities are all connected to DI practice. The DI practitioner and pharmacists in general must at least have a working awareness of these areas. DI services provide a foundation for the provision of pharmacist supervised patient care. To date, pharmacists providing DI have only speculated about and not actually faced malpractice lawsuits. Hopefully, this chapter has shed some light on how courts would react to malpractice suits against pharmacists for negligent provision of DI. However, legal precedents cannot be relied upon to predict the future. There is no way to predict how a court will rule in a particular case. What can be done to avoid malpractice and other causes of action? First, always strive for excellence. Second, have good relations with requestors and make sure they are aware of alterations or modifications in information systems and sources. Third, make no outrageous claims about the accuracy and thoroughness of the information provided. Finally, pharmacists should carry their own malpractice insurance policy.

The future of pharmacists as DI providers clearly lies in their ability to provide consultative DI services. While in the past, most of the reported appellate decisions against pharmacists have involved routine dispensing errors, not mistakes in DI or other expanded practice areas, in the future this situation may change. Pharmacists should not be preoccupied with the risk of incurring liability, but should take the necessary steps to limit exposure and develop an appreciation of modern legal philosophy. Definitive guidelines need not emerge only through court decisions. It remains most important that DI be recognized as a liability-reducing factor for the institution and personnel who provide health care to patients.

Self-Assessment Questions

1. All of the following would result in holding the pharmacist providing drug information to a higher standard **except**:
   a. The drug information query pertains to pediatrics and the pharmacist is a Board Certified Pediatric Pharmacist (BCPP).
   b. The pharmacist knows the patient is an alcoholic and Nyquil® elixir is prescribed.
   c. The pharmacist graduated at the top of her class from one of the best pharmacy schools in the country.
   d. The pharmacist runs a drug information center.
   e. The pharmacist is aware that the patient is opioid naïve and fentanyl patch is prescribed.

2. In which of the following scenarios would tort liability attach to the provision of drug information if harm occurs:
   a. Upon recommendation to the P&T Committee by the Drug Information coordinator, the hospital's formulary preferred statin is now simvastatin. Via a therapeutic interchange protocol, the patient was placed on simvastatin. Myopathy developed.
   b. The pharmacy is contacted by a nurse and asked the following drug information question: Can ceftriaxone be administered in the same IV line with calcium gluconate? The pharmacist says they are compatible but does not consult either Trissel's or King's Guide, both of which identify the combination as incompatible. The patient is harmed when crystals form in the IV line.
   c. A pharmacist correctly recommends the right medication for a specific patient at the correct dose and regimen. The patient develops an iatrogenic reaction to the drug.
   d. a and b
   e. a, b, and c

3. Which of the following drug information scenarios may result in vicarious liability?
   a. The pharmacist undertakes to warn the patient about the adverse effects from ciprofloxacin, but fails to warn of tendonitis.
   b. The pharmacist is too busy to counsel the patient on the warning against sunbathing while on doxycycline. She instructs the pharmacy technician to counsel the patient instead. The technician instructs the patient not to take a bath while taking the drug. The patient goes to the beach and harm results.
   c. The pharmacist receives a drug information query from a prescriber asking what the common adverse effects of metformin are. The pharmacist provides the correct response; the prescriber counsels the patient incorrectly.
   d. b and c
   e. a and c

4. For which of the following scenarios would the "learned intermediary" doctrine **NOT** apply:
   a. The pharmaceutical manufacturer advertises its product direct-to-consumers on television.
   b. The prescriber writes a prescription for the medication because the patient has requested that specific medication.
   c. The prescriber is a nurse practitioner.
   d. The pharmacist recommends a nonprescription product.
   e. The "learned intermediary" doctrine applies to each of these scenarios.

5. Which of the following statements is/are false:
   a. The drug information consultation between the pharmacist and patient has been determined by courts to be privileged.
   b. Since the drug information provided is oral and not written, no liability can attach.
   c. A malpractice case is brought against the pharmacist who failed to warn the patient about driving while taking the medication. The pharmacist is not protected via his professional liability insurance policy if the lawsuits brought after the policy expired, even if the event occurred while the policy was effective.
   d. b and c are false.
   e. a, b, and c are false.

6. A violation of the Anti-Kickback Statute would occur when:
   a. The pharmacist contacts the patient's physician to recommend the patient be switched to a particular drug within a therapeutic class. For each patient, the pharmacist is able to obtain a switch, he/she receives a fee from the pharmaceutical company.

b. A hospital pharmacist is preparing the monograph for P&T and making the recommendation whether the hospital should add the medication to formulary or not. The pharmacist's spouse is employed by the pharmaceutical company that manufactures the medication.

c. Compensation is provided to a drug information pharmacist by a pharmaceutical editor to ghost write a review article about their new product. The pharmaceutical company makes the final decision regarding the article content.

d. b and c

e. a, b, and c

7. Which of the following is correct with regard to off-label use of medication?

a. An investigational new drug application (IND) is needed before a medication may be prescribed for an off-label use.

b. Patient informed consent is necessary before a pharmacist should recommend an off-label use to a prescriber.

c. Off-label use of a medication is common in certain patient groups such as pediatric patients.

d. Off-label refers to the fact that the use is not listed in any drug information reference.

e. None of the above.

8. Problems using the Internet for responding to drug information queries include:

a. Information may contain innocent or deliberate mistakes.

b. There are no laws for assuring the accuracy of information on the Internet.

c. May include unpublished (not peer reviewed) information.

d. The information may be outdated or not evidence-based.

e. All of the above.

9. DM is a new pharmacist at XYZ Hospital. During his first week, he identifies a great case report for publication. He takes a photo of the patient's mole on the patient's face and talks about his patient case in the elevator. He leaves his computer with patient information open unattended while he grabs lunch. At lunch, he sees Dr. Jones so they sit alone together and discuss the mutual patient. When DM presents his case, he invites Dr. Jones to the presentation. The first slide reveals the patient's MR#. When he publishes the case report, he includes a patient identifier. How many separate violations of HIPAA has pharmacist DM committed?

a. Three

b. Four

c. Five

    d. Six

    e. Eight

10. Which of the following would constitute fair use under the copyright law?

    a. Obtaining a copyright to prohibit use of a list of medications that cause seizures.

    b. Scanning and distributing to all drug information colleagues an entire chapter from *Drug Information: A Guide For Pharmacists*.

    c. You, Professor Lee, photocopy an excerpt from an article which is about 3% of the work. You will only be using the excerpt for one lecture of a course for one semester only.

    d. You, Professor Lee, photocopy without permission multiple copies of a 6,000-word article every semester for classroom use in both your therapeutics and communication classes.

    e. Your colleague has written an article which is currently unpublished. He requests that you critique it and you borrow several paragraphs verbatim in your new book.

11. Which statement is accurate with regard to course packs or course management systems and copyright laws?

    a. If the course pack material is online, it is free from copyright protection.

    b. If substantial amounts are from a textbook and the intent is to save students from purchasing the textbook, this constitutes fair classroom use.

    c. If permission to use any copyrighted material in the course pack was granted and a fee was paid to the copyright holder, fair use would apply.

    d. Where the course pack is sold every semester to students and contains uncopyrightable materials for which no permission to use was obtained, copyright law is violated.

    e. None of the above are accurate.

12. Which of the following statements is ***inaccurate*** under HIPAA?

    a. Permits pharmacists to report adverse events to manufacturers and directly to the FDA without patient authorization.

    b. HIPAA allows disclosure of patient information in the handling of drug information queries but requires protection of information within the drug information center.

    c. Permits communication which discloses PHI between a pharmacist and other health care professionals with regard to a specific patient's therapy.

    d. HIPAA privacy standards do not apply to e-mail or social media communication.

    e. All the above statements are correct.

13. Which of the following actions would constitute a HIPAA violation?
   a. You publish a case report and identify the patient by his initials.
   b. You fax a response to a drug information query containing PHI to an incorrect fax number.
   c. You are conducting research using de-identified health information. You lose the flash drive containing this information.
   d. A patient you are following develops a serious, unexpected adverse drug reaction. You report the reaction to the Food and Drug Administration.
   e. a and b are HIPAA violations.

14. Which of the following is in compliance with the "PhRMA Code on Interactions with Health Care Professionals"?
   a. Gifts from pharmaceutical manufacturers of $250 or less that benefit patients or educate health care professionals are permitted.
   b. Pharmaceutical manufacturers may sponsor entertainment in university or nonprofit venues.
   c. Pharmaceutical manufacturers may sponsor meals or receptions at conferences.
   d. Consultant agreements must be in writing.
   e. c and d are true.

15. In which of the following scenarios would education be considered promotional activities?
   a. A portion of the presentation content is directed or scripted by the pharmaceutical company.
   b. Promotional activities are taking place in the educational meeting room.
   c. Disclosures do not mention that the pharmaceutical company has funded the program.
   d. Educational session evaluations report that the session was biased toward a particular product.
   e. All of the above.

REFERENCES

1. American Society of Health-System Pharmacists. ASHP supplemental standard and learning objectives for residency training in drug information practice. Practice standards of ASHP. 1995-1996. Bethesda (MD): American Society of Health-System Pharmacists; 1995.
2. Southwick AF. The law of hospital and health care administration. 2nd ed. Ann Arbor (MI): Health Administration Press; 1988.
3. Nathan JP, Gim S. Responding to drug information requests. Am J Health Syst Pharm. 2009;66:706, 710-1.

4. The Pharmacist's Patient Care Process. Joint Commission of Pharmacy Practitioners. May 29, 2014.

5. Baker K. OBRA '90 mandate and its impact on pharmacist's standard of care. Drake Law R. 1996;44:503, 508.

6. Burns K, Spies A. A pharmacist's duty to warn: trying to make sense of all the legal inconsistencies. Rx Ipsa Loquitur. 2008;35:1-2.

7. Kelly WN, Krause EC, Krowinski WJ, Small TR, Drane JF. National survey of ethical issues presented to drug information centers. Am J Hosp Pharm. 1990;47:2245-50.

8. Doppelparker Case, OLG Karllsrule GRUR 1979 P267.

9. Perkins E. Johns Hopkins' tragedy: could librarians have prevented a death? [cited 2017 Mar 18]. Available from: http://newsbreaks.infotoday.com/NewsBreaks/Johns-Hopkins-Tragedy-Could-Librarians-Have-Prevented-a-Death-17534.asp

10. 805 S.W.2d 380 (Tenn. Ct. App. 1991).

11. 453 N.Y.S.2d 121 (1987).

12. Whiting v Rite Aid Pharmacy, 2014 U.S. Dist. Lexis 87354 (D. Utah, Jun 24, 2014).

13. 544 N.W.2d 727, 731 (Mich. Ct. App. 1991).

14. Fink JL. Ignore computer alerts at your peril? Pharm Times. 2013 Jan:56.

15. 191 A.D.2d 178, 594 N.Y.S.2d 195 (1993).

16. 579 N.E.2d 1255 (Ill. App. 1991) reversed by 605 N.E.2d 557 (Ill. 1992).

17. Moore v. Memorial Hospital & Winn Dixie, 825 So.2d 658 (Miss. 2002).

18. Deed v. Walgreens, 2004 WL 2943271 (Conn. Super. Ct.).

19. K-Mart v. Chamblin, 612 S.E.2d 25 (Ga. Ct. App. 2005).

20. Brushwood DB, Belgado BS. Judicial policy and expanded duties for pharmacists. Am J Health Syst Pharm. 2002;59:455-7.

21. 780 So.2d 930 (Fla. App. 2001).

22. 1 S.W.3d 519 (Mo. App. 1999).

23. 737 N.E.2d 650 (Ill. App. 2000).

24. 30 S.W.3d 455 (Tex. App. 2000).

25. Larrimore v. Springhill Memorial Hospital. LEXIS 38:008 WL 54 2000 (Ala. 2008). CV-02-3205, 1051748.

26. 827 F. Supp. 1522 (D. Nev. 1993).

27. 598 N.Y.S.2d 592 (App. Div. 1993).

28. Hall M, Honey W. The evolving legal responsibility of the pharmacist. J Pharm Market Manage. 1994;8:27-41.

29. Brushwood DB. The pharmacist's drug information responsibility after McKee v. American Home Products. Food Drug L J. 1993;48:377-410.

30. In re Michael A. Gabert, No. 92 PHM 21 (Wis. Pharmacy Examining Bd., Dec 14, 1993).

31. Rees W, Rohde NF, Bolan R. Legal issues for an integrated information center. J Am Soc Info Sci. 1991;42:132-6.

32. Restatement (Second) of Torts, Section 311, 1982.

33. Beaird S, Coley R, Blunt JR. Assessing the accuracy of drug information responses from drug information centers. Ann Pharmacother. 1994;28:707-11.

34. Calis KA, Anderson DW, Auth DA, Mays DA, Turcasso NM, Meyer CC, Young LR. Quality of pharmacotherapy consultations provided by drug information centers in the United States. Pharmacotherapy. 2000;20:830-6.

35. McDonagh AF, Lightner DA. Attention to stereochemistry. Chem Eng News. 2003 Feb 3:2.

36. Aungst TD. Medical applications for pharmacists using mobile devices. Ann Pharmacother. 2013;47:1088-95.

37. Loy JS, Ali EE, Yap KY. Quality assessment of medical apps that target medication-related problems. J Manage Care Spec Pharm. 2016;22(10):1124-40.

38. Talwar SR, Crudele NT, Dankiewicz EH, Crudele NT, Haddox JD. Implementing a process to review product-specific misinformation in online drug information compendia. Ther Innov Reg Sci. 2015;49:262-8.

39. U.S. Food and Drug Administration. Mobile medical applications: guidance for industry and Food and Drug Administration staff. 2015 Feb.

40. In re Prempro Products, 03-CV-015070-WRW, U.S. Dist Ct., E.D. Arkansas, Jul 17, 2009.

41. Clauson KA. Pharmacists: are your drug information databases accurate? U.S. Pharmacist. 2008 Sept:54-63.

42. Gray JA. Strict liability for the dissemination of dangerous information? Law Lib J. 1990;82:497-517.

43. 694 F. Supp. 1216 (D. Md. 1988).

44. Bundesqe Richtsaf. Neue Juristische Wochenschrift (1970), 1973.

45. 110 Misc.2d 799, 442 N.Y.S.2d 945 (N.Y. Sup. 1981).

46. 938 F.2d 1033 (9th Cir. 1991).

47. 432 F. Supp. 990 (E.D.N.Y. 1977).

48. Sanofi sues decision aid maker for 'injurious falsehood.' Pharmafile. Available from: http://www.pharmafile.com/news/198126/sanofi-sues-decision-aid-maker-injurious-falsehood

49. Containment Technologies v. ASHP, 2009 US Dist LEXIS 25421 (Mar 26, 2009), 2009 US Dist LEXIS 76270 (Aug 26, 2009).

50. Talley CR. Affirming science and peer-review publishing. Am J Health Syst Pharm. 2009;66:896.

51. Prod. Liab. Rep (CCH), Section 8968 (S.D.N.Y. Feb 20, 1981).

52. Hardin v. PDX, Inc., No. A137035, 2014 WL 2768863 (Cal. Ct. App., Jun 19, 2014).

53. Restatement (Second) of Torts Sec. 324A.

54. Brannigan VM, Dayhoff RE. Liability for personal injuries caused by defective medical computer programs. Am J Law Med. 1981;122:132-3.

55. Joyce EJ. Software bugs: a matter of life and liability. Datamation. 1987 May 15:88-92.

56. Gage D, McCormick J. Case 108—we did nothing wrong. Panama's Cancer Institute. Baseline. 2004;28:32-47.

57. Cuzamanes PT. Automation of medical records: the electronic superhighway and its ramifications for health care providers. J Pharm Law. 1997;6:19.

58. Brocklesby v. Jeppesen, 767 F.2d 1288 (9th Cir. 1985), cert. denied, 474 U.S. 1101 (1986).

59. 472 U.S. 749 (1985).

60. 137 Misc.2d 94, 520 N.Y.S.2d 334 (N.Y. Civ. Ct. 1987).

61. Amerson AB. Drug information centers: an overview. Drug Info J. 1986;20:173-8.

62. 705 P.2d 1360 (Ariz. Ct. App. 1985).

63. Rumore MM, Rosenberg JM, Costa JG. The pharmacist and the law: legal aspects of providing drug information. Wellcome Trends Hosp Pharm. 1989 Dec;6-8.

64. Gallegos v. Wood, 2016 U.S. Dist. LEXIS 48150 (D. N.M. Mar 31, 2016).

65. Gough AR, Healey KM, Rupp SR. Poison control centers, from aspirin to PCBs and the scarlet runner beam: a study of legal anomaly and social necessity. Santa Clara Law Rev. 1983;23:791-809.

66. Brushwood DB, Simonsmeier LM. Drug information for patients—duties of the manufacturer, pharmacist, physician, and hospital. J Leg Med. 1986;7:279-341.

67. Curtis JA, Greenberg MI. Legal liability of medical toxicologists serving as poison control center consultants: a review of relevant legal statutes and survey of the experience of medical toxicologists. J Med Toxicol. 2009;5(3):144-8.

68. 656 P.2d 483 (Wash. 1983).

69. Collins v. Walgreen Co., 2013 U.S. Dist LEXIS 81422 (E.D. Cal. Jun 10, 2013).

70. LeFrock v. Walgreen Co., 77 F. Supp.3d 1199 (M.D. Fla. 2015).

71. Goulmamine v. CVS Pharmacy, Inc., 3:15-cv-00370-REP (U.S. Dist. VA, Oct 9, 2015).

72. Gray JA. The health sciences librarian's exposure to malpractice liability because of negligent provision of information. Bull Med Libr Assoc. 1989;77:33-7.

73. Mintz AP. Information practice and malpractice. Libr J. 1985:38-43.

74. Fidelity Leasing Corp. v. Dun & Bradstreet, Inc., 494 F. Supp. 786 (E.D. Pa. 1980).

75. Baker KR. Do people sue people who counsel? Drug Topics. 2007 Dec 3:4.

76. Food & Drug Administration [Internet]. Center for Drug Evaluation and Research, Office of Medical Policy, Division of Drug Marketing, Advertising and Communications, Comparative Advertising, Fair Balance, and the Patient-Consumer; c2003 [cited 2017 Mar 18]. Available from: http://www.fda.gov/downloads/AboutFDA/CentersOffices/OfficeofMedicalProductsandTobacco/CDER/UCM213627.pdf

77. Food & Drug Administration, Guidance for Industry: Internet/social media platforms with character space limitations—presenting risk and benefit information for prescription drugs and medical devices. Jun 2014.

78. Food & Drug Administration, Guidance for Industry: fulfilling regulatory requirements for postmarketing submissions of interactive promotional media for prescription human and animal drugs and biologics. Jan 2014.

79. Food & Drug Administration, Guidance for Industry: Internet/social media platforms: correcting independent third-party misinformation about prescription drug and medical devices. Jun 2014.

80. Food & Drug Administration, Guidance for Industry: consumer-directed broadcast advertisements. Aug 8, 1997.

81. 21 U.S.C. § 352(n).

82. 21 C.F.R. § 202.1(e).

83. Wilkes MS, Bell RA, Kravitz RL. Direct-to-consumer prescription drug advertising: trends, impact, and implications. Health Aff. 2000;19:110-28.

84. Anon. FDA officials describe agency actions on problematic drug promotion activity. BNA Pharm Law Industry Rep. 2003 Sept 19;1(35):1006.

85. Schwartz TM. Consumer-directed prescription drug advertising and the learned intermediary rule. Food Drug L J. 1991;46:829-37.

86. PDRnet. PDR network. [cited 2017 Mar 18]. Available from: http://www.pdrhealth.com

87. Food & Drug Administration, Guidance for Industry: brief summary and adequate directions for use: disclosing risk information in consumer-directed print advertisements and promotional labeling for prescription drugs. Aug 2015.

88. 161 N.J. 1, 734 A.2d 1245 (N.J. 1999).

89. Ferrelli JJ. Perez creates exception to learned intermediary doctrine. New Jersey Law J. 1999 Sept 20.

90. Gebhart F. Here comes the judge. Drug Topics. 2005 Jan 24;26-32.

91. Pharmacist's mutual [Internet]. [cited 2017 Mar 18]. Available from: https://apps.phmic .com/RMNLFlipbook/06_2011/index.html

92. Rumore MM. Direct-to-consumer advertising of prescription drugs: emerging legal and regulatory issues. Hosp Pharm. 2004;39:1058-68.

93. New Jersey Citizen Action v. Schering-Plough Corporation. 367 N.J. Super. 8, 842 A.2d 174 (App. Div. 2004). Available from: http://www.prescriptionaccess.org/ lawsuitssettlements/past_lawsuits?id=0011

94. Anderson v. SmithKline Beecham Corp., W.D. Wash. No. CV 03-2886-L, Sept 22, 2003.

95. Wyeth v. Levine 129 S. Ct. 1187, 1200 (2009).

96. Patsy BM, Furburg CD, Ray WA, Weiss NS. Potential for conflict of interest in the evaluation of suspected adverse drug reactions: cerivastin and risk for rhabdomyolysis. JAMA. 2004;292:2585-90.

97. FDC Act § 312.7.

98. 21 U.S.C. §§ 360.999, 403 (1998).

99. 21 C.F.R. § 99.101(a)(3)-(4).

100. Ward SM. WLF and the two-click rule: The First Amendment inequity of the Food and Drug Administration's regulation of off-label drug use information on the Internet. Food Drug L J. 2001;56:41-56.

101. Kennedy D. The old file-drawer problem. Science. 2004;305:451.

102. Guidance for Industry. Good reprint practices for the distribution of medical journal articles and medical-scientific reference publications on unapproved new uses of approved drugs and approved or cleared medical devices. Dept. HHS, Food and Drug Administration, Office of the Commissioner. Jan 2009.

103. Guidance for Industry. Distributing scientific and medical publications on unapproved new use—recommended practices. Dept. HHS, Food and Drug Administration, Office of the Commissioner. Feb 2014.

104. United States ex rel. King v. Solvay S.A., No. 06-2662, 2016 U.S. Dist. LEXIS 14804 (Feb 8, 2016 S.D. Tex.).

105. The medical science liaison: examining the role. CME Briefing. 2002 July-Sept;3-5.

106. Guidance for Industry. Responding to unsolicited requests for off-label information about prescription drugs and medical devices. Dept. HHS, Food and Drug Administration, Center for Drug Evaluation and Research, Center for Biologics Evaluation and Research, Center for Veterinary Medicine, Center for Devices and Radiological Health. Dec 2011.

107. American Academy of Pediatrics. Policy Statement 2002;110-1, 2002 Jul 18:1-3.

108. Fugh-Berman A, Melnick D. Off-label promotion, on-target sales. PLoS Med. 2008;5(10). [cited 2017 Mar 18]. Available from: http://www.medscape.com/viewarticle/704698

109. Understanding the approval process for new cancer treatments. Bethesda, MD: National Publications Locator. National Cancer Institute [cited 2017 Jul 27]. Available from: https://www.cancer.gov/publications

110. Brown L. Gain a solid understanding of compendia and its impact on patient access. Formulary. 2012;47:252-6.

111. Abernethy A, Raman G, Balk EM, Hammond JM, Orlando LA, Wheeler JL, Lau J, McCrory DC. Systematic review: reliability of compendia methods for off-label oncology indications. Ann Intern Med. 2009;150:336-43.

112. P.L. No. 110-275. Medicare Improvements for Patients and Providers Act of 2008. Jul 15, 2008.

113. Vivian JC. Off-label use of prescription drugs. US Pharm. 2003;28:508.

114. Beck JM, Azari ED. FDA, off-label use, and informed consent: debunking myths and misconceptions. Food Drug L J. 1998;53:71-103.

115. 21 C.F.R. pt. 50.

116. N.Y. Pub. Health L. § 2805-d(1) (McKinney 1993).

117. Institute of Medicinal Science Institute for Healthcare. Engaging patients through social media. IMS Institute Report. Parsippany, NJ: IMS Institute for Healthcare Informatics; 2014:17-25.

118. Edmunds MW, Scudder L. Using web citations in professional writing. J Prof Nursing. 2008;24:347-51.

119. Wood JM, Dorfman HL. Dot.com medicine—labeling in an Internet age. Food Drug L J. 2001;56:143-78.

120. Moberg MA, Wood JW, Dorfman HI. Surfing the net in shallow waters: product liability concerns and advertising on the Internet. Food Drug L J. 1998;53:213-24.

121. 21 U.S.C. §§ 351-354 (1994).

122. Deugan L, Powe N, Blakey B, Makary M. Wiki-Surgery? Internal validity of Wikipedia as a medical and surgical reference. J Am Coll Surg. 2007;205(Suppl):576-7.

123. Clauson KA, Poten HH, Boulos MK, Dzeno Wagis JH. Scope, completeness, and accuracy of drug information in Wikipedia. Ann Pharmacother. 2008;42:1814-21.

124. Reilly W, Jackson W, Berger V, Candelaria D. Accuracy and completeness of drug information in Wikipedia medication monographs. J Am Pharm Assoc. 2017;57(1):193-197.

125. Freeman MK, Lauderdale SA, Kendrach MG, Woolley TW. Google Scholar versus PUBMED in locating primary literature to answer drug-related questions. Ann Pharmacother. 2009;43:478-84.

126. Adams SR. Information quality—liability and corrections. Online. 2003 Sept/Oct:16-22.

127. Kane B. Guidelines for the clinical use of electronic mail with patients. White paper. JAMA. 1998:5:104-11.

128. Gulick PG. E-health and the future of medicine: the economic, legal, regulatory, cultural, and organizational obstacles. Alb L J Sci Tech. 2002;12:351-60.

129. Engstrom P. Can you afford not to travel the Internet? Med Econ. 1996;73:173-80.

130. Lopez, et al. v. Aziz, 852 S.W.2d 303, 304 (Tex. App. 1993).

131. Cubby v. CompuServe, 776 F. Supp. 135,140 (1990).

132. Stratton Oakmont Inc. and Daniel Porush v. Prodigy Services Co. & Others (NY Sup. Ct. 1995).

133. Terms of Use Agreement. HealthActCHQ™ Inc. [cited 2017 Mar 18]. Available from: http://www.healthact.com/terms.php

134. Muhlen MV, Ohno-Machado L. Reviewing social media use by clinicians. J Am Med Inform Assoc. 2012;19:777-81.

135. American Society of Health System Pharmacists. ASHP statement on use of social media by pharmacy professionals. Am J Health Syst Pharm. 2010;74:145-8.

136. Clauson KA, Seamon MJ, Fox BI. Pharmacist's duty to warn in the age of social media. Am J Health Syst Pharm. 2010;67:1290-3.

137. Update: texting orders. Jt Comm Perspect. 2016;36(5):15.

138. Kalb PE, Bass IS. Government investigations in the pharmaceutical industry: off-label promotion, fraud and abuse, and false claims. Food Drug L J. 1998;53:63-70.

139. 42 U.S.C. § 1320a-7b(b)(1) (1994).

140. Huntington S. Presentation to the American Bar Association Health Law Section, Emerging professional liability exposures for physicians on the Web. Jun 8, 2001.

141. Warnecke M. Tested IP litigation storm of '04: fair use principles prove their pluck. Patent, Trademark, Copyright J. 2005;69:369.

142. Ticketmaster Corp. v. Tickets.Com, Inc., 2003 U.S. Dist. LEXIS 6483 (C.D. Cal. 2003).

143. eBay, Inc. v. Bidder's Edge, Inc., 100 F. Supp. 2d 1058 (N.D. Cal. 2000).

144. 1998 U.S. Dist. LEXIS 17282 (E.D. Pa. 1998).

145. D Minn., No. 02-1782 ADM/JGL, 2005 Jan 28.

146. Warnecke M. Effortless nature of Web surfing makes it unlikely consumers can avoid confusion. Patent, Trademark, Copyright J. 2005;69:363-4.

147. Millstein JS, Neuberger JD, Weingart JP. Doing business on the Internet. New York: Law Journal Press, 2004, §3.02[17][a][iii].

148. Futuredontics, Inc. v. Applied Anagramics, Inc., 1998 U.S. App. LEXIS 17012 (9th Cir. 1998).

149. 17 U.S.C. § 102.

150. Eldred v. Ashcroft, 239 F. 3d 373 (D.C. Cir. 2001).

151. 17 U.S.C. § 106.

152. 17 U.S.C. § 109(a).

153. 35 U.S.C. § 107.

154. College Entrance Examination Board v. Pataki, 889 F. Supp. 554, 568 (N.D.N.Y. 1995).

155. Epstein E, Zulieve AJ. The Fair Use doctrine: commercial misappropriation and market diversion. Isaacson Raymond [Internet]. [cited 2017 Mar 18]. Available from: http://www.isaacsonraymond.com/Articles/tabid/123/articleType/ArticleView/articleId/9/The-Fair-Use-Doctrine-Commercial-Misappropriation-And-Market-Diversion.aspx

156. 471 U.S. 539 (1985).

157. Guidelines for Classroom Copying in Not-for-Profit Educational Institutions. H.R. Rep. No. 1476, 94th Cong., 1st Sess. § 68-70 (1976).

158. Latman A, Gorman R, Ginsberg JC. Copyright for the nineties. 3rd ed. Charlottesville, VA: Michie; 1989:655-6.

159. Campbell v. Acuff-Rose Music, 510 U.S. 569, 578 (1994).

160. 420 U.S. 376 (1975).

161. Perlman R. Williams & Wilkins Co. v. United States; photocopying, copyright, and the judicial process, 1975 Sup. Ct. Rev. 1976;355.

162. 74 F. 3d 1512 (6th Cir. 1996).

163. 758 F. Supp. 1552 (S.D.N.Y. 1991).

164. Copyright Clearance Center. Using course management systems. Guidelines and best practices for copyright compliance. [cited 2013 Mar 13]. Available from: http://www.copyright.com/content/cc3/en/toolbar/education/resources/reprints_and_reports.html

165. 2004 WL 1008314 (2d Cir., May 7, 2004).

166. No. 07 Civ. 09667 (S.D.N.Y. Sept 8, 2008).

167. FindLaw® for Legal Professionals [Internet]. Thomson Reuters; c2013. New York Times Co, Inc., et al vs. Tasini et al. [cited 2017 Mar 18]. Available from: http://caselaw.lp.findlaw.com/scripts/getcase.pl?court=US&vol=000&invol=00-201

168. Greenberg v. National Geographic, 201 U.S. App. LEXIS 4270 (11th Cir. 2001).

169. The Authors Guild, Inc. et al. v. Google Inc., Case No.05 CV 8136 (S.D.N.Y.).

170. Samuelson PP. The Googlebook settlement as copyright reform. Wis L. Rev. 2011;479–562. Available from: http://scholarship.law.berkeley.edu/facpubs/439

171. Persky AS. Paper or plastic? Google's plan to digitalize materials pits book lovers v. book innovators. Wash Lawyer. 2009 Jun:35-40.

172. Google begins to scale back its scanning of books from university libraries. The Higher Ed Chronicle. Mar 9, 2012. Available from: http://chronicle.Com/article/Google-Begins-to-Scale-Back/131109/

173. The National Digital Pubic Library is launched. The New York Review of Books. Apr 25, 2013. Available from: http://www.nyBooks.com/articles/archives/2013/apr/25/national-digital-public-library-launched/

174. American Libraries Association [Internet]; c 2004 [cited 2017 Mar 18]. Crews KD. New copyright law for distance education: the meaning and importance of the TEACH Act. Am Libr Assoc. Available from: http://www.ala.org/Template.cfm?Section=distanceed

175. Smedinghoff TJ, ed. Online law. New York, NY: Addison Wesley Press; 1996:139.

176. Pack R. Honest writers. Washington Lawyer. 2004 Sept:21-26.

177. Health Insurance Portability and Accountability Act of 1996, Pub. L. No. 104-191, 110 Stat. 1936 (1996) (codified as amended in scattered sections of 18, 26, 29 and 42 U.S.C.A.); 42 U.S.C.A. § 1320d to 42 U.S.C.A. § 1320d-8.

178. Barrett C. Healthcare providers may violate HIPAA by using mobile device to communicate with patients. ABA Health eSource. 2011;8(2):1-5.

179. 45 C.F.R. § 160.103.

180. 45 C.F.R. §§ 164.502(d)(2), 164.514(a) and (b).

181. Daniels JG. Health care privacy and HIPAA. In: Cronin KP, Weikers RN, editors. Data security and privacy law. Eagan, MN: West Group; 2002.

182. Clause SL, Triller DM, Bornhorst CP, Hamilton RA, Cosler LE. Conforming to HIPAA regulations and compilation of research data. Am J Health Syst Pharm. 2004;61:1025-31.

183. 45 C.F.R. § 164.512(i)(1)(i).

184. 45 C.F.R. § 164.512(b)(1)(iii).

185. Car J, Sheikh A. Email consultation in health care: 2. Acceptability and safe application. BMJ. 2004;329:439-42.

186. 42 U.S.C.A. § 290dd-2.

187. Bishop S. Interactions with individuals other than the patient, Part 2: caregivers, personnel representatives, and minors. Pharm Today. 2003 Jul;4.

188. Bishop S. Interactions with individuals other than the patient, Part 1: notice of privacy practices and medication counseling. Pharm Today. 2003 Jul;4.

189. Thompson v. CVS Pharmacy, Inc., 6:204cvo2081 (M.D. Fla. Dec 19, 2014).

190. Kolinek v. Walgreen Co., 2014 WL 3056813 (N.D. Ill. Jul 7, 2014).

191. California Healthcare Foundation [Internet]. Oakland, CA: California Health Care Foundation; 2017. Achieving the right balance: privacy and security policies to support electronic health information exchange. 2012 Jun [cited 2017 Mar 19]; [about 2 screens]. Available from: http://www.chcf.org/publications/2012/06/achieving-right-balance

192. Baker DB. Provider-patient e-mail: with benefits come risks. J Am Health Info Manage Assoc. 2003;74:22-9.

193. D. Mass, No. 00-11672-JLT, Nov 6, 2003.

194. 18 U.S.C. § 2510 *et seq.*

195. Pharmaceutical Research and Manufacturers of America Code on Interactions with Healthcare Professionals, Jul 2002. [Updated Jan 2009].

196. Health and Human Services, OIG Compliance Program for Pharmaceutical Industry, Apr 2003.

197. Accreditation Council for Pharmacy Education [Internet]. Accreditation Standards and Criteria; c2005 Jan [cited 2017 Mar 18]. Available from: https://www.acpe-accredit.org/

198. 2011 National Association of Boards of Pharmacy (NABP) Survey of Pharmacy Law. Mount Prospect, IL: NABP; 2012.

199. Cutting the strings on gifts and other questionable marketing practices: PhRMA takes a stand. CME Briefing. 2002 Jul-Sept;1-6.

200. FDA Guidance for Industry-Supported Scientific and Educational Activities, 1997.

201. Steiner JL, Norko M, Devine S, Grottole E, Vinoski J, Griffith EE. Best practices: developing ethical guidelines for pharmaceutical company support in an academic health center. Psychiatr Serv. 2003;54:1079-89.
202. Rosner F. Pharmaceutical industry support for continuing medical education programs: a review of current ethical guidelines. Mt. Sinai J Med. 1995;62:427-30.
203. 42 U.S.C. § 1320a-7b(b).
204. U.S. v. Greber, 760 F.2d 68 (3d Cir. 1985).
205. U.S. v. LaHue, 261 F.3d 993 (10th Cir. 2001).
206. *In re* Caremark Int'l, Inc. Derivative Litig., 698 A. 2d 959 (1996).
207. Drug firm settles kickback charges. The Palm Beach Post, Sept 6, 1994, p. 4B.
208. Astrue MJ, Szabo DS. Pharmaceutical marketing and the anti-kickback statutes. Food Drug Cosmet Med Device Law Dig. 1993;10(2):57-60.

SUGGESTED READINGS

1. Reilly T, Jackson W, Berge V, Candelario D. Accuracy and completeness of drug information in Wikipedia medication monographs. J Am Pharm Assoc. 2017;57(1):193-7.
2. Chew SW, Khoo CS. Comparison of drug information on consumer review sites versus authoritative health information websites. J Assoc Info Sci Tech. 2016;67(2):333-49.
3. Brand KA, Kraus ML. Drug information specialists. Am J Health Syst Pharm. 2006;63:712-4.
4. Anderson R. The difference between copyright infringement and plagiarism—and why it matters. J Periop Nursing. 2016;29(4):50-1.
5. Guidance for Industry. Responding to unsolicited requests for off-label information about prescription drugs and medical devices. Dept. HHS, Food and Drug Administration, Center for Drug Evaluation and Research, Center for Biologics Evaluation and Research, Center for Veterinary Medicine, Center for Devices and Radiological Health. Dec 2011.
6. Tyrawski J, DeAndrea DC. Pharmaceutical companies and their drugs on social media: a content analysis of drug information on popular social media sites. J Med Internet Res. 2015;17(6):e130. Published online 2015 Jun 1. Doi:10.2196/jmir.4357.
7. American Society of Health System Pharmacists. ASHP statement on use of social media by pharmacy professionals. Am J Health Syst Pharm. 2010;74:145-8.

Chapter Eleven

Ethical Aspects of Drug Information Practice

Elyse A. MacDonald • Linda K. Ohri

Learning Objectives

● *After completing this chapter, the reader will be able to*

- Explain characteristics that differentiate an ethical deliberation from other types of decision making.
- Interpret and make use of ethics rules, principles, and theories to analyze identified ethical dilemmas.
- Identify and analyze examples of ethical dilemmas that may arise for health professionals when providing drug information, in various practice settings and for various types of clients and circumstances.
- Identify micro, meso, and macro levels of ethical decision making that may occur during the provision of drug information.
- Use the described process of ethical analysis in order to propose and justify a specific decision or course of action in an ethical dilemma case.
- Describe resources and structures that can prepare, guide, and support clinicians faced with ethical dilemmas during the course of providing drug information.

Key Concepts

❶ Ethical deliberations may be differentiated by three characteristics: they are ultimate (fundamental), the issue is universal, and the welfare of all affected parties is considered.

❷ Ethical judgments may occur at micro, meso, or macro levels of health care decision making.

❸ Professional ethics is different than the law.

❹ The primary focus will be on the health care professional's identification, interpretation, specification, and balancing of pertinent ethical rules and principles.

❺ The application of a proposed process of ethical analysis is demonstrated for identifying, analyzing, and resolving ethical dilemmas that may arise during the health care professionals' provision of drug information.

❻ The first process step requires identification and evaluation of pertinent background information to ensure that the facts of the specific case are understood, and to assess whether a true ethical dilemma exists.

❼ Sometimes, the professional will find it necessary and valuable to more consciously deliberate on how various ethical theories suggest that the relevant rules and principles should be prioritized or balanced.

❽ Health care professionals need training, resources, and support to prepare them to effectively address those ethical dilemmas they confront.

Introduction

WHAT IS ETHICS AND WHAT IS NOT

The Ethics Course Content Committee of the American Association of Colleges of Pharmacy (AACP) described **ethics** as "the philosophical inquiry of the moral dimensions of human conduct."[1] They mentioned that Aristotle taught ethics as "an eminently practical discipline..." dealing "with concrete judgments in situations in which action must be taken despite uncertainty."[1] These authors indicated that the term ethical is often used synonymously with the term moral to describe an action or decision as good or right. They further stated that ethics is not the study of moral development, and it is not the law.

Veatch[2] stated that "an ethical, or moral, issue involves judgments between right and wrong human conduct or praiseworthy and blameworthy human character." This author indicated that an ❶ *ethical deliberation may be differentiated from other endeavors by three characteristics: (1) it is ultimate or fundamental, there is no higher standard against which to measure the rightness of the decision or action; (2) the issue is universal, the parties involved in the dilemma do not consider it simply a difference of opinion or taste—each party believes there is a right or wrong answer—even if they disagree about what the answer is; and (3) the deliberation takes into account the welfare of all involved or affected by the judgment at hand.* Those who provide drug information (DI) typically rely on an intuitive sense of these characteristics; they have the feeling that the situation being confronted is a big deal, and somehow anticipate that they should not address only personal preference in the matter at hand.

DIFFERENT LEVELS OF ETHICS

Over the past two decades evolving literature has described that ❷ *ethical judgments may occur at micro, meso, or macro levels of health care decision making*[3-15]: (1) traditionally recognized **micro** level of health care related decision making involves decisions made at the individual professional-patient level of health care; (2) a less commonly discussed **meso** level of decision making (with some literature using the term "organizational" for similar purpose) is variably described as occurring at the institutional/organizational level or at community/regional levels; and (3) **macro** level decision making often sets policy for the health system, as a standard established for an entire profession, or through government as law/regulation for the society as a whole.

Health care providers may be involved in ethical decision making at each of these levels related to the provision of or access to DI. Primarily micro level ethical decision making scenarios will be presented in this chapter. However, certain scenarios involving meso and macro level ethical decision making will also be addressed. For example, a physician, nurse, and pharmacist may all be participating on a pharmacy and therapeutics committee that is developing an organizational policy regarding the use of pharmaceutical samples within hospital clinics, or in a large independent clinic practice. The policy also addresses the use of in-house professionals versus industry detailers to provide information about new drug products. Each of these professionals may have competing priorities and concerns that add ethical dimensions to their decision making on this proposed policy.[11] This constitutes a meso level of ethical decision making for these professionals. A clinician participating on a national task force charged with developing policy related to **medication therapy management** services (with inherent DI access) as part of a health care reform model, will have macro level ethical decisions to make relative to balancing patient needs, professional identity, and societal economic constraints.[10]

DIFFERENCE BETWEEN ETHICS AND LAW

❸ *Professional ethics is different than the law.* Law might be defined as rules of conduct imposed by society on its members. By contrast, professional ethics has been defined as "rules of conduct or standards by which a particular group in society regulates its actions and sets standards for its members."[16] Both constitute macro level policy making, across society or across an entire profession. Law involves written rules set by the whole society (or its representatives) that address responsibilities of that society's members. Professional ethics focuses on explicit or implicit rules and standards set by a professional subgroup of society, and addresses the responsibilities of only those who are members of that subgroup. Certain ethical standards of a given profession may be institutionalized as law by society as a whole. However, professional ethical standards (e.g., do no harm or preserve life) are often impossible to fully regulate by law. Meeting an ethical standard also goes beyond legal requirements; indeed, our ethical beliefs may on occasion command our civil disobedience (e.g., a prison pharmacist who refuses to dispense drugs to be used in legal executions). On the other hand, as will be discussed further below, law also represents one aspect of the culture within which ethical decisions are made. In considering the cultural perspectives of a given dilemma, relevant legal requirements must be identified and considered when one seeks to make an ethical decision.

ETHICAL DILEMMAS WHEN PROVIDING DRUG INFORMATION

This chapter will present case scenarios representing ethical dilemmas. These scenarios will be used to demonstrate a specific method for analyzing ethical dilemmas confronted by health care professionals providing DI. The discussion will address ethical dilemmas encountered by generalist and specialist patient care providers providing DI, as well as examples drawn from the experiences of DI specialists. All health care professionals provide DI and must address the ethical dilemmas that arise in the course of providing this service. Many of these scenarios represent examples of micro level ethical dilemmas that primarily involve an interaction between a DI provider and the direct recipient of the information. Other scenarios where health care professionals may be providing or determining access to DI occur at meso (organizational) or macro (societal) levels of ethical decision making. While perhaps less immediately obvious as an ethical dilemma to some individuals involved, these may constitute dilemmas that have even further reaching impacts for both individual professionals and impacted groups. These larger dilemmas may often seem beyond the scope of individual decision making, but indeed ultimately are primarily addressed through the contributed actions or decisions of individuals, typically as they interact in some group process. Of course, all ethical dilemmas, by definition, have some implications beyond the welfare of the most immediate individuals involved. The list of example dilemmas provided in Table 11-1 includes scenarios from each of these levels. These dilemmas might arise in a wide variety of settings and circumstances where health care is practiced or health care policy is set. It is important to identify the level of ethical decision making that each example seems to represent, and consider what ethical issues might exist for each scenario.

In the fifth edition of their foundational text *Principles of Biomedical Ethics*,[17] Beauchamp and Childress address the following aspects of the moral life: principles and rules; rights, character, and virtues; and moral emotions. The responsibilities (based on principles and rules) and rights of the health care provider and other involved parties will

TABLE 11–1.   EXAMPLES OF ETHICAL SITUATIONS IN HEALTH CARE

- The hospital practitioner is asked to provide information that might be used to speed the ending of a terminal patient's life.
- The community pharmacist or physician is requested by a patient to critique another health care provider's drug therapy recommendation.
- The emergency room nurse is asked by the patient to tell his/her spouse that the treatment is for a diagnosis other than the sexually transmitted disease that is really being treated.
- The drug information specialist is confronted by an administrator, pressuring for a certain formulary recommendation that is more cost-containment than evidence-based.
- The home health care practitioner is asked to positively present questionably substantiated information on the efficacy of a given therapy, in order to support insurance reimbursement for a truly needy patient.
- The practitioners working in industry, who are asked to prepare a consumer product education and promotion piece according to directions that do not adhere to FDA or WHO guidelines for balanced presentation of both the benefits and the risks associated with the drug product being advertised.
- The health care professional practicing in any patient care setting, who experiences another episode (in a repetitious pattern) where his or her patients would benefit from additional drug information, but who finds workload demands to be an impossible barrier to providing more than the minimum, legally required information.
- The health care professional is enrolled by her professional organization to testify against a proposed health reform policy that mandates her profession to provide verbal drug information associated with a prescription refill, but does not set any requirements for third-party payer reimbursement of this service.
- The hospital pharmacist is asked to compound a medication for which there is little to no safety and efficacy data, based on the pharmacist's review of existing literature.
- The hospital only has enough of an oncology medication to treat one patient, but there are three patients who need treatment. The drug information pharmacist is asked to review literature to help decide which patient receives the medication.

be addressed briefly in this chapter as considerations that must be dealt with in the course of responding to a specific dilemma. While acknowledging their importance, this chapter will not address the roles of character, moral virtue, or emotions in ethical decision making by health care professionals. One might say that they constitute the provider's inherent moral perspective that will direct and support his or her decision making. The interested reader is referred to the text referenced above for a fascinating discussion of these factors[17]; this discussion is continued in the 2008 edition of the same text for those wishing to review updated coverage of this material.[18] The remainder of this chapter is intended to prepare and assist the pharmacist and other health care professionals providing DI to analyze and address dilemmas, such as those listed above. ❹ *The primary focus will be on the health care professional's identification, interpretation, specification, and balancing of pertinent ethical rules and principles* as he or she seeks to determine and justify what he or she considers the right decision or the best course of action.

Basics of Ethics Analysis

This section briefly presents relevant terminology and definitions used in the field of ethics, as well as an overview of a specific process of analysis that may be used in assessing ethical dilemmas. In the section following this one, specific case scenario demonstrations of this process for analysis will be presented.

DEFINITIONS USED IN THE FIELD OF ETHICS

Beauchamp and Childress[19] defined ethics as "a generic term for several ways of examining the moral life." These authors described a process of deliberation and justification that is necessary when confronting a moral dilemma. They stated, "When we deliberate...we are considering which judgment is morally justified...." They indicated that, "Particular judgments are justified by moral rules, which in turn are justified by principles, which ultimately are defended by an ethical theory." These authors presented a hierarchical diagram that depicts this approach to analysis (Figure 11-1). A later article by Beauchamp[20] further addresses the need to consider these principles and rules within the specific context of the case at hand, in order to fully realize their action-guiding potential.

The authors referred to these hierarchical levels of analysis (particularly rules and principles) as action-guides, which are used to justify a particular judgment. They describe a rule of ethics as specific to context and relatively restricted in scope; for instance, the moral rule about confidentiality that specifically addresses a patient's right to consent prior to release of privileged information.[19] Principles are more broad and fundamental in scope; for example, the principle of respect for **autonomy**, which is the patient's right to decide on personal issues. They describe ethical theories as "integrated bodies of principles and rules...that may include mediating rules that govern cases of conflicts." The prominent rules and principles guiding ethical decision making by health care professionals can generally be placed within one of two broad ethical theories: **consequentialist**

Figure 11–1. Hierarchical levels of ethical analysis.

theory or **deontological** (derived from the Greek word deon, meaning duty) theory.[19] Multiple versions exist of each of these broad categories.

Consequentialist theories describe actions or decisions as morally right or wrong based on their consequences, rather than on any intrinsic features they may have. The two cardinal principles of consequentialist theory are **beneficence** (do that which promotes a good outcome) and **nonmaleficence** (do that which minimizes bad outcomes). Consequentialist theories focus on this one feature of an act, its consequences. For example, an informed consent ethical rule can be of value within consequentialist theory because consent generally results in improved compliance and outcome—good consequences. However, if informed consent was likely to result in a bad outcome, it would not be justifiable within consequentialist theory. A mediating rule utilized by many advocates of consequentialist theory is to hold nonmaleficence as more important, or more foundational, than beneficence.

Duty-driven (deontological) theories look more to intrinsic qualities of an act or decision to assert its moral rightness or wrongness. Deontological theory considers other inherent features of an act, besides consequences, as also relevant and often of greater importance. For example, in various forms of deontological theory, the act is considered inherently wrong if it is dishonest or breaks confidentiality, or if it does not respect individual autonomy. Conflicts between different rules are mediated by appealing to more foundational, underlying principles such as adherence to justice or to respect for persons.

Conscious recognition of the pertinent action-guides, and understanding mediating rules that operate within the health professional's preferred ethical theory or theories, can help providers honestly and equitably analyze the ethical dilemma, and better comply with the imperative characteristics of ethical deliberation (see the beginning of this chapter).

OVERVIEW OF A SUGGESTED PROCESS OF ANALYSIS TO BE USED WHEN AN ETHICAL DILEMMA ARISES

In the article *Hospital Pharmacy: What is ethical?*, Veatch[2] indicated that often people reach a particular ethical decision without a great deal of conscious deliberation, through moral intuition, and without subsequent challenge from any external party. However, on occasion, when pondering a certain ethical judgment, they are called on (internally or externally) to analyze and justify the basis for their conviction. He suggested that when this occurs, it is first important to understand the facts of the specific case. He then described progression through three additional process stages of reflection (on ethical rules, principles, and theories) by which we may identify, analyze, and present reasons for our judgment. In the same report, the author also emphasized the importance in one's reflection of taking into account the points of view of all parties impacted. As stated earlier in this chapter, this is one of the key characteristics distinguishing an ethical deliberation. A survey of the text *Cross-Cultural Perspectives in Medical Ethics* (2nd ed.)[21] demonstrates that there are many commonalities, but also important differences across the ethical perspectives of different cultures. These cultural perspectives must be considered if all parties' points of view are to be taken into account.

In this section ❺ *the application of a proposed process of ethical analysis is demonstrated for identifying, analyzing, and resolving ethical dilemmas that may arise during health professionals' provision of DI.* These steps of analysis are derived from the writings of Veatch, Beauchamp, and Childress, as well as other authors.[2,19,21-23] The process may be summarized as follows:

I. Identification of relevant background information.
   A. Factual details of the issue at hand.
   B. Consideration of who is affected by the ethical issue.
   C. Learn and respectfully address the cultural perspectives (including applicable legal requirements) for those affected by the dilemma.
II. Identification and justification of the relevant moral rules and principles (action-guides) pertinent to the case.
III. Deliberation, through the use of moral intuition and application of ethical theory, on how to rank/balance the rules and principles pertinent to the case in order to resolve the ethical dilemma.

Step I: Identification of Relevant Background Information

❻ *The first process step requires identification and evaluation of pertinent background information to ensure that the facts of the specific case are understood and to assess whether a true ethical dilemma exists.* This first step deserves careful consideration and research. Once the facts of a case are known, the moral concerns may be resolved. This step has been divided into three parts: (1) data gathering, (2) consideration of the welfare of all affected parties, and (3) respect for the cultural perspectives of these parties.

Health care professionals already use data gathering when they apply a systematic approach to answering any DI question (see Chapter 2). When addressing a potential ethical dilemma, the providers must learn about the factual details of the issue, who is directly involved, and whether there is conflict in factual understanding among the involved parties in the issue. For example, does the parent who calls to ask about the medication recently prescribed for her teenager already know that the teenager is taking a birth control pill prescribed by a gynecologist (rather than a dermatologist for acne) and simply wants to know the name of the product?

If the matter still seems to involve an ethical dimension once data gathering clarifies the facts, the next step is to consider the rights and responsibilities of all affected parties.

As previously mentioned, this has been described as an essential component of any ethical deliberation.[2] The health care provider, the direct client (patient or parent in the case just described), other indirect but individual clients (e.g., any existing or unborn children, parent paying for service provided to the child patient or the patient's spouse), other health professionals (e.g., the patient's physician), other societal groups (e.g., other patients who might be harmed by an incompetent practitioner), and any higher power recognized by the health professional have rights and/or responsibilities that should be considered.

Finally, during first consideration of any potential ethical issue, the provider should take into account the cultures of the affected parties.[22] In his reviews of the foundations of modern medical ethics theories, Veatch[21,23] described how the unique perspectives of Western, Chinese, Hindu, Jewish, Catholic, Protestant, and other cultural groups have affected the formulation of their dominant medical ethics traditions. Other cultural classifications might include socioeconomic status, political affiliation, age category, and racial or ethnic group. A report by Najjar et al.[24] demonstrates some important similarities (e.g., requests to assess physician recommendations) and differences (e.g., requests to serve as a primary health care provider) in the types of ethical dilemmas that are identified by DI specialists functioning within the cultural environment of Saudi Arabia compared to those reported at U.S. centers.

In a very interesting case study, Carrese et al.[25] discussed the ethical obligations of medical professionals in caring for those of a different ethnic culture. In this case, a young Laotian mother used a traditional Mien folk cure to treat her infant. The treatment involved placing several small burns on the child's abdomen to treat *gusia mun toe*, an apparently transient, but very distressing, colic-like ailment. The cure resulted in several small scars, but no other obvious ill effects. The mother indicated that the cure worked. The physician recognized the value in supporting the positive impacts of the woman's attachment to her cultural support group. However, the physician was confronted with the dilemma of how to respond to this mother's revelation of a culturally promoted treatment measure that was not scientifically supported and could be dangerous. Sometimes, culturally based actions may conflict with the professional's goal to avoid harm and promote benefit. However, failing to consider a cultural perspective may also have harmful effects or disrupt the trust between patient and heath care professional. An extended discussion of how differing cultural perspectives affect ethical decision making is beyond the scope of this chapter. However, the health care professional should strive to be aware of and respect the cultural perspectives of the affected parties when contemplating an ethical dilemma. The interested reader is encouraged to refer to the resources cited here and above for further discussion of cultural factors in ethical analysis.[21,23]

One final issue should be addressed relative to cultural considerations. The legal requirements of the society within which an ethical dilemma occurs are part of the culture and must be identified. A specific ethical decision will not always exactly conform

to the existing legal requirements of society. The ultimate nature of ethical deliberations may result in decisions that are more demanding than the legal requirements and,
unfortunately, may even occasionally involve perceived or true conflict with specific
legal requirements. This may involve, for instance, a decision not to divulge confidential
communications between a professional and client, which may or may not be acceptable
within the law. In another case, the health professional may decide not to provide information related to abortion or capital punishment, even though these activities are acceptable within the law. Obviously, legal requirements cannot be ignored or dismissed lightly
when making a specific ethical decision.

Step II: Use of Rules and Principles (Action-Guides) to Assist in Analysis of an Ethical Dilemma

If the dilemma persists, once the available background information has been identified
and considered, proceed with the process of full ethical deliberation. Veatch[2] suggests
that the involved party/parties can proceed as far as necessary through successive stages
of general moral reflection assessing at the level of moral rules and then at the level of
ethical principles, within their accepted ethical theory. These might be described as the
action-guides referred to by Beauchamp and Childress.[19] This second process step of
analysis will look at moral rules that may apply to the specific case and more general pertinent ethical principles. Definitions are provided at the end of this section for a number of
ethical rules and principles that are considered particularly relevant to decision making
by practitioners.

Specific action-guides may be considered a rule within one ethical theory and a principle within another. For example, **veracity** (truth telling) as mentioned above, may be
considered by some ethicists to be a specific moral rule and by others to be a general
principle, depending on which ethical theory is followed. For the practitioner immediately
involved in analyzing a specific ethical dilemma, defining the relevant action-guides as
rules or principles is important only to the extent that this helps in assessing which are
more fundamental to the issue at hand. Therefore, in this chapter, both rules and principles will be included within the same process step of ethical analysis.

Examples of moral rules within biomedical ethics include a confidentiality rule dic-
tating that patient-entrusted information should not be disclosed and an informed consent
rule that addresses the individual's right to information before agreeing to a specific
medical procedure. Unfortunately, there is no definitive list universally defining all moral
rules and, sometimes, multiple pertinent rules can be in conflict. Furthermore, there are
acceptable exceptions to most moral rules. For instance, disregarding the informed consent rule might be justifiable in an acute situation to protect the life of the client, suffering
may be necessary in order to achieve cure of serious disease, and many consider killing
justified under certain circumstances. Therefore, there may not be a specific rule that
resolves a particular ethical dilemma.

When such a circumstance arises, the practitioner may begin a more general level of analysis by looking at the ethical principles that apply to the case. Sometimes, the involved parties can reach an acceptable resolution to an ethical dilemma once they recognize the broader relevant ethical principles. In a given dilemma, the professional may decide that the primary principle is to respect the autonomy of the client and that requires providing complete information enabling the client to make an informed decision. In another dilemma, if do no harm is considered the most fundamental ethical principle, decisions or acts that deny this principle would be considered unethical. It becomes immediately obvious, however, that relevant ethical principles such as these may also come into conflict. This problem can be demonstrated by the following example: The professional may believe that full disclosure will result in nonadherence by the patient, with significant risk of resultant harm. The practitioner therefore confronts two conflicting principles: respecting client autonomy by providing full disclosure versus the duty to do no harm.

Step III: Ethical Theory as a Means to Clarify or Resolve Ethical Dilemmas

This third step of ethical analysis reveals how relevant moral rules and principles interact within the preferred ethical theory to address the given dilemma. When confronted with conflicting ethical rules or principles, the practitioner may simply resolve the dilemma through his or her moral intuition of the right thing to do; even if unconsciously, this reflects the individual's at least temporary affiliation to some theory of what constitutes good versus bad or right versus wrong. ❼ *Sometimes, the professional will find it necessary and valuable to more consciously deliberate on how various ethical theories suggest that the relevant rules and principles should be prioritized or balanced.* According to Veatch,[2] this process step can lead to more rational and honest decision making or action-taking. He suggests that these ultimate deliberations at the level of ethical theory will be affected by our most basic religious and/or philosophical commitments. It is important that the practitioner recognizes and acknowledges the impact on decision making of his or her own personal ethical perspective. Those dilemmas that cannot be fully resolved can at least be viewed with greater clarity.

Veatch[23] states that, "The components of a complete theory will answer such questions as what rules apply to specific ethical cases, what ethical principles stand behind the rules, how seriously the rules should be taken, and what constitutes the fundamental meaning and justification of the ethical principles." In this reference and another text, the author reviews the foundations of consequentialist, deontological, and other ethics theories particularly relevant to health professionals, including the Hippocratic tradition; Judeo-Christian and other religious-based traditions; the philosophies of the modern secular West; and medical ethics theories outside the Anglo-American West, including Socialist, Islamic, Hindu, African, Chinese, and Japanese traditions.[21,23] Frequently, versions of the broad consequentialist and deontological theories are expressed in various ways across these traditions. Keep in mind the core of the various **Hippocratic Oaths**, since this has been the central ethical tradition of Western medicine: "Those who have stood in that (Hippocratic) tradition are committed to producing good for their patient and to protecting that patient from harm."[23] In Hippocratic tradition, there is also a special emphasis placed on the responsibility of the health care professional to the specific patient versus obligations to other less directly affected parties or to society in general. A contract theory of medical ethics has also been proposed, which describes an implicit (unwritten) contract between health professionals and patients.[23] This modern theory is of special relevance to the pharmacist providing DI as a service within an implicit pharmaceutical care contract.[23,26] First of all, this theory represents a shift in thinking for those pharmacists who might have considered their primary obligation to be to the prescriber rather than to the patient. Furthermore, this contract between patient and professional suggests an obligation for more substantive communication with patients and a higher level of caregiving than some pharmacists have previously felt obligated to offer. The reader is referred to foundational writings by Veatch, as well as those of Beauchamp and Childress, for a more in-depth discussion of various medical ethics theories.[18,19,21,23]

AN ANNOTATED LISTING OF RULES AND PRINCIPLES (ACTION-GUIDES) APPLIED IN MEDICAL ETHICS INQUIRY

The following rules and principles (action-guides) of ethical conduct will be described and subsequently used in the analysis of case scenarios provided in the next section. Their description will necessarily be brief. The reader is referred to other sources to read more about these rules and principles.[19,23]

1. *Nonmaleficence*—A basic principle of consequentialist theory; encompasses the duty to do no harm. This tenet has a long history as part of the Hippocratic tradition, where it has often been described in terms of the health care provider's duty to the individual patient. The principle is also cited as justification for actions benefiting all. Sometimes, application of the principle requires addressing conflicts between the needs of one and all.[18]
2. *Beneficence*—Another basic principle of consequentialist theory that expresses the duty to promote good. Again, conflict can arise between what constitutes good for one individual versus the larger societal group. Good or bad consequences are also of importance within deontological theories, but are evaluated along with other principles that may be considered of equal or greater importance.[18]
3. *Respecting the patient-professional relationship*—A moral rule, often referring to respect for the physician-patient relationship, but also applicable to other

professional-patient relationships, as well. This rule has been mentioned in published reports of ethical dilemmas arising during the provision of DI.[24,27-29] As expressed in Hippocratic traditions, this rule indicates that the physician's primary duty is to the patient and tends to give the physician, rather than the patient, control in the relationship, which may be judged paternalistic by some. This rule is particularly noted in duty-driven (deontological) ethical theories that consider the professional's duty to the patient, but also supports consequentialist theory to the extent that good outcomes are enhanced.

4. *Respect for autonomy*—A principle described particularly within deontological theory. This principle is founded on a belief in the right of the individual to self-rule. It speaks to the individual's right to decide on issues that primarily affect self.

5. *Consent*—A moral rule related to the principle of autonomy which states that the client has a right to be informed and to freely choose a course of action; for example, informed consent to receive a therapy or procedure.

6. *Confidentiality*—A moral rule, also related to the principle of autonomy, which specifically addresses the individual client's right to give or refuse consent relative to release of privileged information.

7. *Privacy*—Another rule within the principle of autonomy, more generally relating to the right of the individual to control his or her own affairs without interference from or knowledge of outside parties. This rule has been addressed in deliberations on the rights of individuals with AIDS versus those of their potential sexual contacts.

8. *Respect for persons*—A principle expressing duty to the welfare of the individual, particularly described within religion-based deontological theories. This principle may also be expressed within dignity of life or sanctity of human life principles. It has common elements with the respect for autonomy principle, but addresses more directly a belief in the inherent value of human life, independent of characteristics or abilities of the specific human being.

9. *Veracity*—This term addresses the obligation to truth telling or honesty. Veracity is considered an ethical principle within deontological theory. However, it is considered a useful rule within consequentialist theory, to the extent that it promotes good.

10. *Fidelity*—Another principle of moral duty in deontological theory that addresses the responsibility to be trustworthy and keep promises. This principle also relates to a duty of reciprocity—consideration of the other's point of view. Descriptions of pharmaceutical care have spoken of the need to develop an ethical **covenant** between pharmacist and client.[26] Nurses, physicians, and other health care professionals undoubtedly also have various standards that call them to such ethical relationships with their patients. This covenant details the characteristics of a

relationship requiring fidelity and reciprocity, in which each party takes on certain responsibilities and gives up certain rights in order to achieve specific good outcomes (consequentialist theory). Success of this contract depends in good measure on consideration by each party of the other's point of view.

11. *Justice*—This concept has been presented within various principles that relate to fairness and tendering what is due, resource allocation and providing that to which the individual is entitled. A number of more fundamental justice theories have also been developed to connect and justify these various principles.[18,19] Moral decision making at the meso and macro level will frequently cite justice as a main justification for particular decisions. A more thorough discussion on justice-related principles and theories is beyond the scope of this chapter. However, several texts that address this topic can provide much assistance to those health professionals preparing for roles at these levels of ethical decision making, or to those who teach such professionals.[18,30,31]

These are certainly not the only relevant rules or principles, nor are they necessarily universally accepted definitions. However, these action-guides seem particularly pertinent to medical ethics inquiry. Furthermore, several of these rules and principles have been specifically discussed in published reports that describe ethical dilemmas encountered by DI specialists.[27,28] Such dilemmas have also been described in situations where practitioners are providing DI directly to patients, either from a formal DI center or during the process of providing patient care.

DEMONSTRATION OF CASE ANALYSIS

The following examples demonstrate ethical dilemmas that might arise for professionals providing DI. These cases will be used to demonstrate the aforementioned process of analysis for the practitioner(s) addressing an ethical dilemma (Case Examples 11-1 and 11-2).

Case Example 11-1 (Micro Level Case)

Mrs. Burns, a new patient at the medical center, calls the Drug Information Center (DIC), which the medical center advertises as a resource for both patients and professionals, and asks Dr. Pike, the DI specialist, a question. She is concerned about whether she should take the amoxicillin plus clavulanate just prescribed for her by Dr. Stills, her family practitioner (who practices at the center where the DIC is located).

■ ANALYSIS

Step #1 Identification of relevant background information

A. Factual details of the issue at hand: The DI practitioner learns the following information through discussion with the patient:

1. Mrs. Burns is approximately 8 weeks pregnant; she wonders if this medication is safe for the baby.

2. She says she is being treated for acute bacterial rhinosinusitis.

3. She mentions that she has only recently begun seeing Dr. Stills as her family just moved into town about 3 months ago.

4. Mrs. Burns indicates that Dr. Stills knows she is pregnant. He is managing her pregnancy.

5. She states that she asked him about the safety of the drug, but he rather impatiently brushed off her questions by asking "don't you trust me?"

6. Dr. Pike may decide that it is necessary to consult professional resources to evaluate whether the therapy appears to be appropriate. She should not hesitate to ask the patient for some reasonable time period in which to investigate the pertinent information before providing an answer.

7. Dr. Pike will need to consider whether any identified risks are likely to be known to the physician.

8. Dr. Pike may decide that further facts must be obtained through direct discussion with Dr. Stills.

B. Identification of who is affected by any ethical issue considered to be present: As the DI provider reflects on this patient's inquiry, it is helpful to consider who might be impacted by her response:

1. Herself, relative to her own desire to do right; any relationship between her and her patient, any relationship between her and the physician.

2. Mrs. Burns relative to the consequences of any harm to her infant or of inadequate treatment of the infection, and relative to her future relationships with both the physician and the DI provider.

3. Mrs. Burns' infant, relative to the consequences of any harmful or beneficial effects of the drug, or of inadequate treatment of the mother's infection.

4. Dr. Stills, relative to the consequences of prescribing a potentially inappropriate therapy during the woman's pregnancy, and relative to the effects of any DI provided on the patient-physician relationship.

5. Mrs. Burns' family, significant others, and society in general relative to the impacts of either delivery or abortion of a child with harm from the therapy, or from inadequate treatment of the woman's infection.

C. Consideration for the cultural perspectives of those affected by the dilemma.

Dr. Pike will consciously or unconsciously act within her own cultural and religious framework, and her understanding of her legal obligations. Awareness of her own perspective, as well as consideration of the cultural perspectives of others who may be affected, is important if she is to pursue a truly ethical course of action. To repeat Veatch's words differentiating ethical deliberations, "The deliberation takes into account the welfare of all involved or affected."[1] Each involved party's welfare is affected by his or her cultural perspective. Cultural, religious, and legal perspectives that the clinician must be aware of in this case might include:

1. Perspectives regarding parental responsibility to the unborn infant versus self.
2. Perspectives and legal requirements relative to both the DI provider and physician's obligations to the patient and to her infant.
3. Perspectives about the role and authority of the physician and of the DI provider.

D. Consideration of the level of decision making involved in responding to any ethical dilemma recognized by the DI practitioners.

Within the context of this DI professional's job description, or the charge of the particular case, it should be fairly obvious whether micro, meso, or macro level decision-making activities are involved. However, a clinician may be involved in micro level decision-making activities related to individual patients, but also have obligations to the pharmacy and therapeutics committee within the health organization (meso level), or perhaps even beyond as a policy committee member for his or her national professional organization (macro level). By definition, all ethical dilemmas tend to have implications beyond the context of just two individuals (note from the first page of this chapter that ethical deliberations take into account the welfare of all involved or affected by the judgment at hand), but meso and macro level decision making will always affect various population groups, as well as the individuals within those groups.

Step #2 Identification and justification of the relevant moral rules and principles (action-guides) pertinent to the case at hand

If the background facts of Mrs. Burns' inquiry do not dismiss the DI provider's ethical concerns, Dr. Pike will find it helpful to consider the various rules and principles discussed above in order to clarify the dimensions of her concern. It is most useful to first identify all potentially pertinent action-guides, and seek an understanding of how fundamentally each applies to the situation.

Ethical action-guides that seem pertinent to this inquiry include the following:

1. *Informed consent*—A moral rule supporting Mrs. Burns' right to be informed and freely choose whether to take the amoxicillin plus clavulanate in relation to other available options.

2. *Respect for the patient-professional relationship*—This rule addresses the obligation of Dr. Pike to support the professional relationship between Mrs. Burns and Dr. Stills. It also requires Dr. Pike to respect her own professional relationship with the patient. Increasingly, professionals within all health care professional groups are interpreting this ethical rule to define their obligation to the patient as primary. Such an interpretation represents a departure for many health care providers from a historical orientation of their primary obligation being to the physician.

3. *Veracity*—Addresses the responsibility of Dr. Pike to tell the truth to Mrs. Burns. This may be considered a basic principle of obligation within deontological theory, or a useful rule within consequentialist theory (to the extent that it promotes good).

4. *Nonmaleficence*—A basic principle of consequentialist theory that would base a decision to divulge information on minimizing the potential for harm.

5. *Beneficence*—This consequentialist principle would base the decision regarding what information to divulge on the potential to promote good. Beneficence and nonmaleficence can be considered together in judging the ethical response to the dilemma faced by Dr. Pike.

Dr. Pike must consider the potential benefits of the prescribed therapy for Mrs. Burns, and address the potential harm resulting from exposure of her infant to amoxicillin plus clavulanate. Consideration of other available alternatives for therapy is also pertinent. Frequently such consideration takes place, at least initially, in the face of inadequate and conflicting information. Dr. Pike will also need to decide what constitutes harm and good for Mrs. Burns versus all others who may be affected.

6. *Fidelity/reciprocity*—A principle of obligation to an ethical covenant between Dr. Pike and Mrs. Burns (within deontological theory), which may suggest a requirement for full disclosure of information. However, to the extent that this covenant asks that each party take on certain responsibilities and give up certain rights in order to achieve specific good outcomes, full disclosure of potentially harmful information may not be required. If Dr. Pike were concerned that Mrs. Burns may decide to forgo any treatment, there could be the potential of negative consequences for both Mrs. Burns and her infant.

7. *Justice*—This principle is considered of intrinsic value within certain deontological theories, and addresses the right of Mrs. Burns (and other affected parties') to be given what is due—entitlement to information may be considered justice in this case. Certainly, the time and expertise of Dr. Pike might be legitimately considered due to her patient.

8. *Autonomy*—This principle is directly applicable to the dilemma of Dr. Pike, as was the related rule of informed consent, based on a belief in Mrs. Burns' right to

Figure 11–2. Possible hierarchy of "action-guides" in case.

decide on issues that primarily affect her. The principle of autonomy has support within both deontological (as an intrinsic good) and consequentialist (if it is likely to promote good consequences) theories. However, competing interests (e.g., Mrs. Burns and her infant), and the individual's capability to be truly autonomous (e.g., the infant in this case), are factors that often complicate the application of this principle in medical ethics.

The reader may believe that other ethical rules or principles are pertinent to this case. If so, they should also be considered as the analysis proceeds.

Step #3 How should these rules and principles be ranked or balanced against each other in order to resolve the ethical dilemma?

This step may sometimes be accomplished rather easily through the use of moral intuition. At other times, careful consideration of ethical theory can suggest the more fundamental action-guides to be applied. In some cases, it may be necessary to balance similarly weighted principles against each other, identifying when the weight of one versus another might be considered greater.

The rules and principles that Dr. Pike considers pertinent to her dilemma over how to respond to the inquiry by Mrs. Burns could be ranked as shown in Figure 11-2.

SUMMARY

In the case of Dr. Pike and Mrs. Burns, autonomy, justice, and nonmaleficence may be considered the primary principles that must be balanced against each other. Autonomy and justice are both valued principles within various deontological theories. Nonmaleficence and beneficence are the cornerstone principles of consequentialist theory. The principle of justice also seems to be inherent in the contract theory of medical ethics described by Veatch.[2] The other relevant rules and principles above support these primary principles and inform how they apply to specific ethical dilemmas. The Code of Ethics for Pharmacists (see Appendix 11-1) approved in 1994 provides further support for these fundamental principles and clearly indicates that the primary obligation of Dr. Pike is to Mrs. Burns rather than to Dr. Stills.[16,17] It may be surmised that all of the fundamental principles seem to support honestly discussing the benefits and risks of the therapy with the patient. However, if there were no good alternative therapies for Mrs. Burns' infection, and Dr. Pike was concerned that probable nonadherence constituted a greater risk to her and/or her baby, the decision would become more difficult. Once Dr. Pike has considered the facts of the case, who will be affected by her action, the cultural perspectives and legal requirements for the affected parties, and the relevant action-guides, she should have more clarity on what constitutes the ethical action. Finally, the personal beliefs and values of Dr. Pike relative to these principles of patient autonomy, promotion of justice, and the importance of potential consequences will all affect her ultimate ethical decision. It must be emphasized that she will make some response, even if only by avoiding the patient's question.

It is not likely that all will agree on the provided ranking or balancing of the pertinent rules and principles in this case, nor will there be universal agreement about what constitutes the right resolution to the ethical dilemma presented. It is necessary to remember that an ethical issue has been defined as one where most agree that there is a right answer, but cannot always agree on what that answer is.

Case Example 11–2 (Meso Level Case)

Drs. Watt, Joseph, and Stockton are a physician, a nurse practitioner, and a pharmacist, respectively. These individuals are members of a project team who work for a multinational pharmaceutical company along with advertising, communications, legal, and technical production staff. The team has just been brought together and charged to prepare a new advertisement piece for a new cholesterol-lowering drug product. The promotional piece will be targeted toward consumers in the United States and also India, therefore, two different versions will be created. One version will meet the U.S. Food and Drug Administration (FDA) guidance on drug promotion rules by including a description of safety issues. The other version will omit the safety information because it will be used in India where guideline adherence is not monitored as closely.

■ ANALYSIS

Step #1 Identification of relevant background information.

A.   Factual details of the issue at hand.

   During project group discussion, and based on their research, the health care professional members of the work group clarify their understanding of current U.S. FDA guidance on drug promotion,[32,33] and World Health Organization (WHO) criteria for ethical medicinal drug promotion that are available to the world community.[34] They confirm that the FDA educates the pharmaceutical industry and health care professionals about what constitutes misleading prescription drug promotion, and takes action in response to complaints about instances of nonadherence with promotion guidelines in the United States.[35] The health care professionals of the project group also review two published reports analyzing compliance with WHO guidelines in India.[36,37] It appears from this research and an earlier study from India[38] that there has been an ongoing history of wide noncompliance with the WHO guidelines among companies marketing drugs in India.

B.   Identification of who is affected by any ethical issue considered to be present: As these DI developers work on creating the advertisement, it is again helpful to consider who might be impacted by the included and excluded information.

   Certainly the patient will be affected by the information included and excluded in the drug advertisement. There are advocates for and opponents against direct-to-consumer advertising (DTCA).[39] Advocates of DTCA suggest increased patient knowledge aids in patient ownership of their own health care and helps them make better choices. Opponents of DTCA argue the information in the advertisements may be misleading. Additionally, opponents suggest the prescriber-patient relationship may be negatively impacted.[39]

   The medical professionals prescribing the promoted drugs may also be impacted in their ability to make evidence-based decisions on appropriate use of the drug. Their credibility may also be questioned if their prescribing practices are found to be deficient, especially if patients are demanding to be prescribed this new medication based on the placement of information in the advertisement. Furthermore, the prescriber's patients may be impacted to the extent that lack of full knowledge of the potential benefits and harms of the drug may negatively affect the outcomes of the therapy. A 2007 report from Australia[40] also notes that the cost of drugs prescribed by physicians increased for those health professionals who gave more attention to drug promotional information from pharmaceutical sales representatives. This information suggests the potential for society, in general, to be negatively impacted by drug promotional materials that encourage prescribing of higher cost drugs, and the potential for lost productivity from workers who do not gain optimal disease state management.

C. Consideration of the cultural perspectives of all those affected by the dilemma.

The professional and cultural perspectives of both the project team professionals and the prescribers/patients must be considered, as well as the overall cultural norms of populations in the two countries.

The health care professionals confronting this potential ethical dilemma will need to address the cultural and professional standards and codes that they have subscribed to as licensed members of their professions. Indeed, it might be argued that these standards, in addition to their clinical experience, are reasons for their presence on this work group. These norms may be different in India versus the United States with respect to prescriber use and dependence on promotional materials as a main source of information about new drugs available for prescribing. A 2009 report[41] evaluating drug promotional materials in Nepal commented that "unbiased and current drug references were not available in most clinical facilities for healthcare professionals," suggesting impacts of this lack resulting in use of irrational combinations of drugs, overuse of antibiotics, and other inappropriate prescribing. The typically wide gap in social and educational status between the medical practitioner in India and his/her patients may also result in a greater tendency to follow the physician's directions without question. By comparison, in the United States, attitudes are often quite different, and there is also greater access for the patient to secondary sources of information. These factors may all lead to somewhat greater risk of negative impacts felt by prescribers and patients in a country where provided promotional materials are incomplete and even misleading, but may be the only written DI available.

D. Consideration of the level of decision making involved in responding to any ethical dilemma recognized by the DI practitioners.

These authors designated the case above as one involving a meso level of ethical decision making by the concerned practitioners, because the activities involve workers within one specific drug manufacturing company. When considering the wide reach of actions taken by this group across the greater organizational system of the multinational company, and the multiple countries where the system operates, some might also appropriately judge this to involve a macro level of decision making.

Step #2 Identification and justification of the relevant moral rules and principles (action-guides) pertinent to the case at hand.

Some might claim that the charge of this work group is wholly about advertising and marketing of a product, and as such claims no particular ethical demand on the producers of the advertising piece. Such an interpretation would require an assessment of the company's and the professionals' obligations to the WHO guidelines, as well as other governmental and professional guidelines on DI. There appears to be fairly clear ethical issues for these health care professionals, as they consider their roles in determining content of the planned promotional material. A brief listing of a few ethical rules and principles is provided below that should probably be considered by them as they consider their ethical responsibilities in preparation of the advertisement.

1. *Veracity*—Does this basic principle of obligation within deontological theory constitute a duty for these professionals, impelling them to advocate for complete and truthful information to be provided, in keeping with WHO guidelines? Within consequentialist theory, veracity also holds value as an ethical rule to the extent that it promotes better prescribing by the medical professionals using the promotional materials.

2. *Nonmaleficence*—A basic principle of consequentialist theory that would base a decision to divulge more complete and accurate information on minimizing the potential for harm. This principle appears to have relevance for consideration by the project group professionals.

3. *Justice*—This principle within certain deontological theories, addresses whether it is just to provide a higher level of educational content only subject to enforced regulation and guidelines, without regard to possible innate rights of access to such information by health care providers and patients in a country with less stringent safety protections. Basic fairness would seem to be relevant when the more informative and complete materials are being prepared and could perhaps be made available without a great deal of additional cost or effort.

4. *Respect for autonomy*—The principle described in deontological theory suggests the patient has a right to self-rule and a right to be involved in his or her own health care decisions. How could the patient make an informed decision regarding the new medication if the information is incomplete?

The reader is encouraged to consider other ethical rules and principles that may apply to this case, as well as thinking about what seems to be a general tendency by some to dismiss the professional and ethical obligations of licensed health care professionals producing such materials for advertising purposes.

Step #3 How should these rules and principles be ranked or balanced against each other in order to resolve the ethical dilemma?

The reader will need to consider these rules and principles, as well as any others considered pertinent, in order to reach his or her own conclusions about the professionals' ethical responsibilities to the ultimate beneficiaries (or victims) of these information services. How does one think he or she would view his or her role and responsibilities if he or she were a health care professional providing DI in circumstances such as these?

SUMMARY

The reader is encouraged to apply this process of analysis to two additional case scenarios, found in Case Studies 11-1 and 11-2 of this chapter. Imagine a set of circumstances that might provide the background context behind each case, and carry out an ethical analysis in light of this context. The reader might perhaps then vary some important aspect of the background context to determine whether this affects the analysis of the ethical dimensions of the case. As each case is considered, also assess at what level of health care (micro, meso, or macro) does the ethical decision making seem to apply.

Case Study 11–1 (Micro Level)

A study evaluating a new medication for hypercholesterolemia includes a whole-genome sequencing component. The consent document includes a separate section for study subjects to consent to the genomic testing, but the consent document did not address what to do if there is an incidental genomic finding (IGF). During the study, there is an IGF of *BRCA* gene (indicates a substantially increased risk of developing breast cancer) in a female subject who consented to the whole-genome sequencing. Does the study team have an ethical responsibility to inform the subject of this finding?

- *Assess whether this DI request constitutes a potential ethical dilemma, based on the three characteristics that differentiate such a situation.*
- *What background information might you want to obtain to clarify this information request? (Imagine a background with details that might establish this as an ethical dilemma for you.)*
- *If you can imagine this scenario to constitute an ethical dilemma for the study team, identify whether you consider it a situation requiring decision making at a micro, meso or macro level.*
- *If, as a practitioner, this question constitutes an ethical dilemma, consider what moral rules and principles are likely to apply to this issue.*
- *Assuming that some of these relevant action-guides conflict with others, describe further deliberations by which the clinician might prioritize or balance these conflicts in order to reach a decision on how to respond to the information request.*
- *What organizational strategies might best prepare the study team to most effectively respond to ethical dilemmas such as this one?*

Refer to the article *Management and Return of Incidental Genomic Findings in Clinical Trials* by Ayuso et al.[42] for further information regarding IGF during clinical trials.

Case Study 11–2 (Micro Level)

A nurse on one of the medical-surgical units of your hospital calls you, the on-call nurse specialist who is a member of the hospital's pain management team, with a question. She has a patient who she believes is being undertreated for pain. He is a young man who was admitted from the emergency room (ER) the previous evening after a motorcycle accident. He is a frequent patient in the ER, known to have a drug problem, with use of a variety of street products. She does not believe that he is in withdrawal, but does think he is getting inadequate pain medications for the severe bruises, scrapes, and a broken leg. However, the admitting physician (coincidentally, the rather testy Chair of the Medical Staff) is quite adamant that he will not enable the patient's drug habit, and maintains that perhaps living with some pain will encourage the patient to mend his ways. The nurse asks you to intervene with the physician to convince him that additional pain therapy is indicated, medically and ethically, for this patient.

- *Assess whether this DI request constitutes a potential ethical dilemma, based on the three characteristics that differentiate such a situation.*
- *What background information might you want to obtain to clarify this information request? (Imagine a background with details that might establish this as an ethical dilemma for you.)*
- *If you can imagine this scenario to constitute an ethical dilemma for the pain management nurse, identify whether you consider it a situation requiring decision making at a micro, meso, or macro level.*
- *If, as a practitioner, this question constitutes an ethical dilemma, consider what moral rules and principles are likely to apply to this issue.*
- *Assuming that some of these relevant action-guides conflict with others, describe further deliberations by which the clinician might prioritize or balance these conflicts in order to reach a decision on how to respond to the information request.*
- *What organizational strategies might best prepare this nurse specialist to most effectively respond to ethical dilemmas such as this one?*

Refer to the article *Ethical Dilemmas: Controversies in Pain Management* by Janet Brown[43] to read the analysis of a similar case.

Case Study 11–3 (Meso Level)

Dr. Levine, who is a DI pharmacist for an academic medical center, is asked by a hospital administrator to review and strongly encouraged to recommend a medication for formulary. This medication is not as effective, is less expensive, and has a few more serious adverse events compared with a medication in its same class.

■ ANALYSIS

- *Assess whether this DI request constitutes a potential ethical dilemma, based on the three characteristics that differentiate such a situation.*
- *What background information might you want to obtain to clarify this information request? (Imagine a background context with details that might establish this as an ethical dilemma for you.)*
- *If you can envision this scenario to constitute an ethical dilemma for this health care professional, identify whether you consider it a situation requiring decision making at a micro, meso, or macro level.*
- *If, as a practitioner, this question constitutes an ethical dilemma, consider what moral rules and principles are likely to apply to this issue.*
- *Assuming that some of these relevant action-guides conflict with others, describe further deliberations by which the clinician might prioritize or balance these conflicts in order to reach a decision on how to respond to the information request.*
- *What organizational strategies might best prepare this pharmacist to most effectively respond to ethical dilemmas such as this one?*

Resources for Use by Professionals Seeking to Learn More about Medical Ethics, as Applied to Issues Involving Provision of Drug Information

❽ *Health care professionals need training, resources, and support to prepare them to effectively address the ethical dilemmas they confront.* The first goal in learning more about medical ethics should be to learn to recognize opportunities for ethical deliberation when they are confronted. Situations will arise where ethical judgments will be made that have moral consequences—with or without the conscious understanding of the parties involved. It is just as important that professionals are prepared to deal with these situations, as it is for them to learn how to address efficacy and safety concerns relative to drug therapies. This section of the chapter offers a survey of medical ethics resources that can assist practitioners who personally desire to learn how to better recognize ethical situations and how to respond to them, or who will be teaching others in formal settings or informally in the workplace.

Formal coursework, inservices, or continuing education opportunities can teach skills that will aid professionals in handling ethical dilemmas related to work responsibilities involving provision of DI. Thornton et al.[22] discussed what should be taught in basic ethics education that takes place within and outside the academic environment. Their review of important elements to be included in ethics education is worthwhile reading for anyone who may desire to participate in these teaching activities. They also refer the reader to other useful resources on the topic. In Davis's[44] manual on patient-practitioner interactions, the author presents an easy to understand description of the stages of moral development, comparing two commonly identified models proposed by Piaget and by Kohlberg. This information is valuable to assist in gaining insight into one's personal moral development, as well as that of others. This workbook, published by a physical therapist for the purpose of assisting in the professional socialization process, also offers a description of moral values associated with development as a professional. The author goes on to present a framework for resolving ethical dilemmas that has similar elements to those presented in this chapter; she also provides exercises that could be readily adapted for use in various health care professionals' education or even for professional inservices.

Haddad et al.[1] provided a comprehensive guideline on pharmacy ethics course content; this is also valuable reading for those wishing to address ethics topics in continuing education of health care professionals. This guideline describes examples of educational methods including case presentation and debate; scenario building, with identification and discussion of potential ethical issues; and role-playing activities. The authors indicate that such educational methods should involve group participation to conduct the analysis of sample cases for the ethical issue being discussed. Writing techniques, such as a 5-minute write exercise prior to discussion can serve to focus the participant's ideas and facilitate the resultant discussion.[45] The guideline also provides an extensive bibliography of resource materials. Two other texts, one edited by Haddad[46] and the updated second edition of *Case Studies in Pharmacy Ethics* by Veatch and Haddad,[47] provide further discussion of teaching methods and many case examples of ethical dilemmas confronted by pharmacists.

Pirl[16] described the use of role-playing assignments for pharmacy students. This article also listed case scenarios that could be used in continuing education programs for any practitioners who are exploring ways to resolve ethical dilemmas arising in their provision of DI. Smith et al.[48] have written a book on pharmacy ethics that also provides background discussion and case examples that relate to many target areas of health care practice, including providing responses to DI inquiries. This resource can be very useful for various practitioners who need to address ethical issues in their particular area of practice. Case discussion activities should always respect the privacy of individual practitioners and patients who have been involved in any specific case with ethical dimensions.

Students and practitioners also require education about their ethical obligations when receiving and passing on manufacturer's DI at micro, meso, or macro levels of practice. Monaghan et al.[49] addressed this issue in their report, Student Understanding of the Relationship between the Health Professions and the Pharmaceutical Industry. This cross-sectional survey of pharmacy, nursing, and medical students identified deficiencies in student knowledge and attitudes about ethical aspects of professional interactions with drug companies. Overreliance on potentially biased or incomplete promotional materials provided by industry representatives may lead professionals to make less than optimal therapeutic decisions or recommendations for their patients. It may also lead professional consultants or institutional leaders to recommend institution-wide (meso level) therapeutic policies such as formulary approvals that do not reflect the best available evidence. A 1994 report by Chren and Landefeld[50] investigated associations between physician-reported interactions with drug companies and their history of requests for additions to a hospital drug formulary. Physicians were 13 times more likely to request that drugs manufactured by specific companies be added to the formulary if they had met with industry representatives from that company. The FDA provides information and tools for health care professional education on what to expect in compliant product promotion literature, and guidance on reporting "Bad Ad" materials.[33,35]

As they prepare DI, health care professionals must also be vigilant about the potential for ethical lapses such as scientific misconduct to impact the evidence available to them from the drug therapy literature. Samp et al.[51] identified 73 drug study articles published in the general biomedical literature between 2000 and 2011 that were classified as representing scientific misconduct. Steen[52] also identified about 800 articles indexed on PubMed that were retracted for fraud or error between 2000 and 2010. Research misconduct (fabrication or falsification of data) was generally intentional with a greater number of authors and where the first author was an author in another retracted paper. While learning of such publication-related ethical lapses would not inherently constitute an ethical dilemma for the DI provider, deciding whether and how to correct faulty DI developed from such materials might indeed constitute such a dilemma.

Information technology is an integral part of the provision of DI by health care professionals. Sometimes technology is used as a tool to access literature and other information sources used by the professional responding to an inquiry. In other cases, the professional may use the Internet to offer DI to various target audiences, both professional and the lay public. Anderson and Goodman[53] authored a text *Ethics and Information Technology: A Case-based Approach to a Health Care System in Transition.* This text addresses many ethical issues of pertinence to health care professionals, related both to web-based services and DI. Case studies on topics such as provision or use of inaccurate information, conflicts of interest, issues of confidentiality and data sharing, and ethical standards that have been set for health websites are presented.

Poirier and Laux[54] have discussed redesign of a DI resources course to meet the needs of nontraditional Doctor of Pharmacy students. This report describes addition of a course section where ethical issues associated with DI questions received at the author's practice site were used to demonstrate how to deal with such situations. The authors used self-study, computer-assisted instruction, and recitations to teach the course. Published descriptions of ethical dilemmas arising during the provision of DI may be used to build case discussions. These scenarios are helpful for educators of both traditional and nontraditional students, as well as for inservices aimed at practicing health care professionals.[24,27-29]

Structures That Support Ethical Decision Making

Berger[26] describes the need for an ethical covenant between the pharmacist and the patient who is being provided pharmaceutical care. This term suggests an implicit contract between client and health care provider that broadly describes the relationship involved whenever a pharmacist provides DI. Within this contract, the service recipient has a right to receive competently provided information as well as respectful treatment. He or she also has the obligation to provide background information needed by the pharmacist. Likewise, the pharmacist has the right to adequate background information (and respectful treatment as well), and the obligation to give competent, trustworthy, and caring service. Recognition of this implicit contract can occasionally suggest corrective action to resolve or avoid perceived ethical dilemmas. Such recognition is especially helpful when there has been a failure to adequately communicate, or there has been a lack of mutual respect in the interaction. Pharmacists also have a revised Code of Ethics for Pharmacists available to them since 1994, which may serve as a general guide to those obligations implicit to the patient-pharmacist relationship.[55,56] The text of this Code is provided in Appendix 11-1. While specific documents will not be reviewed here, certainly other health care professionals practice under Codes and Ethical Standards that apply to rules of relationship with clients who are requesting DI among other services.

It is also important to establish organizational structures that guide and support the practitioner providing DI (in any setting), when he or she is faced with an ethical dilemma. Some formal structures, such as ethics committees[57,58] and other policy setting bodies (e.g., pharmacy and therapeutics committees), are generally available in larger hospitals. Formal attention to education and anticipatory planning activities on how to address ethical conflict situations is also needed within smaller hospitals and care centers, the chain pharmacy setting, or in small independent or nonprofit health care organizations (e.g., independent community pharmacies, rural hospitals). A report on a survey of medicine information pharmacists, conducted in the United Kingdom, assessed perceptions of possible ethical scenarios involving lay callers, and asked about respondents' training to address such situations.[59] The authors described considerable variation in how specific scenarios were addressed, and a minority of the respondents had received training in this area. It is also imperative that pharmacists and other health care professionals participate in policy setting that may affect how they are expected to practice.

Both the organization and the individual practitioner have an obligation to plan in advance how they will handle situations where ethical conflict might arise, particularly relative to compliance with any policy affecting the employee's patient care obligations. A February 2004 Associated Press news story demonstrates this message very clearly (and was one source for an example case analysis presented in this chapter for the third edition of this text).[60] The story describes an incident where a pharmacist on duty at a branch of the Eckerd pharmacy chain declined to fill a prescription written for an emergency contraception product for a rape victim—apparently all three pharmacists on duty refused to fill the prescription or to refer the patient to someone who would fill the prescription. One pharmacist was fired for the action by Eckerd Drugs. His stated reason for declining the prescription was that he believed the product could cause an abortion if fertilization had already occurred, expressing his unwillingness to participate in such an action. A spokesman for the Eckerd chain pharmacy indicated that their employment manual was clear that their pharmacists could not decline to fill a prescription for moral or religious reasons. The pharmacist claimed that he was not aware of the policy until he was fired; his attorney protested that such a policy violated part of the Civil Rights Act. The attorney said that this act "prohibits private companies from forcing employees to do something that violates their religious beliefs."

Yet, another article, *Promising, Professional Obligations, and the Refusal to Provide Service*, by Alexander[61] maintained that the professional "may not override the obligations derived from a prior act of promising to abide by the values, norms, and procedures that define their professional roles as instantiated within a specific practice" suggesting that the professional should leave the organization if they cannot conform to the expectations of their role within that practice. In practice, pharmacists and other practitioners may have to deal with a specific ethical dilemma very rapidly and alone in order to decide or act in a timely manner. Policies and procedures to inform and support the clinician in overall client interactions, and in ethical analysis and decision making, can better prepare the practitioner to address the real life dilemmas he or she will encounter. The emergency contraception case makes it clear that practitioners must also be involved early (whatever their side in the issue) to make their voices heard during initial policy development (a meso level activity within the organization, or perhaps a macro level one if contributing to policy development for the whole profession or in law). They must also keep themselves informed about existing organizational policies in order to protect themselves and their patients. In the opinion of these authors, after the fact controversy over unfamiliar policies does not serve the needs of practitioners, patients, or organizations.

Organizations can assist professionals by sponsoring the creation of explicit policies addressing certain issues that have demonstrated a history of ethical controversy. For example, in the American Society of Health-System Pharmacists (ASHP) *Guidelines on the Provision of Medication Information by Pharmacists* it is explicitly stated that "Consideration should be given to the ethical and legal aspects of responding to medication information requests."[62] In relation to the emergency contraception case mentioned above, a written policy might state that clinicians may refer questions (to another practice colleague or perhaps at a minimum back to the prescriber), where provision of an answer would violate their personal ethics. This could at least partially resolve a potential dilemma for the practitioner who has been asked to provide information that involves ethical conflict. A policy that states practitioners are not required to answer questions from a client who refuses to provide required background information could guide response in the dilemma of dealing with an unidentified client who wants to know how long amphetamine can be detected in the urine. Another policy might address adequate staffing requirements to ensure the community pharmacist has adequate time to perform counseling services. Of course, the legal and ethical rights of clients have to be recognized during development of such policies. These authors believe that all health care professionals, including pharmacists, should demand the right to a major role in organizational policy development that affects their practice, preferably with input from client/patient representatives. To be useful, organizational policies must be developed with attention to avoiding what constitutes infringement on the domain of personal ethics (such as a personal prohibition against euthanasia).

Finally, institutions engaged in the professional education of health care practitioners must provide foundational education in the area of ethics. Organizations employing these practitioners should continue this education through the use of various continuing education programs that foster increasing skills in application of ethical principles to practical decision making.[63]

Conclusion

Many health care professionals will be called on to provide DI. On occasion they will encounter ethical dilemmas regarding what information, if any, should be provided. It is important that the practitioner approach such moments prepared to, often quickly, identify the pertinent facts, analyze relevant points of the situation, and rank or balance the pertinent ethical rules and principles that are involved. The individual professional must recognize his or her rights and responsibilities relative to the client, to other involved individuals and populations, to society as a whole, and to any higher power to whom the practitioner feels accountable. Organizations can assist employee professionals by formal identification and orientation on certain implicit and explicit policies. Furthermore, opportunities for deliberate study and rehearsal of important analytic steps are important to help practitioners be prepared to address ethical dilemmas that arise when providing DI.

Self-Assessment Questions

1. Characteristics that differentiate an ethical deliberation from other decision making endeavors include which of the following? (Choose all that apply):
   a. The issue is universal with any parties involved agreeing that there is a right or wrong answer.
   b. The issue has been addressed in law with penalties identified for failure to comply with the legal directive.
   c. The welfare of all parties affected by the judgment at hand is taken into account.
   d. The issue is fundamental with no higher standard against which to measure the rightness of the decision.

2. A pharmacist receives a prescription for a potentially life-ending medication from a terminal patient. The pharmacist disagrees with ending one's life even with the diagnosis of a terminal illness. The pharmacist is not sure if she will fill the prescription. What level of ethical decision making would this constitute?
   a. Micro level
   b. Meso level
   c. Macro level
   d. No ethical dilemma exists

3. Assuming you decide that the case in Question #2 involves an ethical dilemma for the pharmacist, which of the following ethical rules or principles do you think would potentially apply to the situation (choose all that apply)?
   a. Respect for persons
   b. Nonmaleficence
   c. Respect for autonomy
   d. Consent

4. A new policy is presented to the pharmacy & therapeutics committee regarding medication reconciliation by pharmacy personnel. A hospital administrator approaches members of the committee regarding his distaste for the policy. He claims that it will take too much time for pharmacists to conduct thorough medication reconciliations. He thinks pharmacy personnel need to stay in the pharmacy and leave patient interaction to the nurses and physicians. One physician committee member disagrees with the administrator in theory, but she does not want to vote against him. What level of ethical decision making would this constitute for if one physician exists?
   a. Micro level
   b. Meso level
   c. Macro level
   d. None of the above

5. A practitioner is asked by administration to present an in-service for department colleagues on a recently approved drug product that may have applicability for use in the department's target population. The clinician is expected to present a set of materials provided by the administrator. What would be a first step in determining whether this is an ethical dilemma for the presenter?
   a. Considering who might be affected by the dilemma
   b. Considering the cultural perspectives of those attending the presentation
   c. Determining what ethical rules seem to be at play in this situation
   d. Seeking the factual details relative to the content provided by the administrator

6. Based on Question #5, assume the practitioner does ultimately feel that he is confronting an ethical dilemma in being asked to present DI with which he disagrees. Which of the following organization policies might be useful to support this professional in addressing his dilemma? (Choose all choices that apply)
   a. A policy that requires supervisor approval of all educational content presented by staff professionals.
   b. A policy that supports staff professional's freedom to independently develop educational content of DI provided in group settings, subject to review by designated expert reviewers.

c. A policy establishing a mediation process for resolving conflict between staff professionals and administrative supervisors.

d. A policy mandating education for administrative and professional staff on shared governance and professional rights and responsibilities.

7. Which of the following statements are true when describing ethics?

a. Philosophical inquiry on the moral dimensions of human conduct.

b. The terms ethical and moral have substantially different meaning.

c. Ethics involves the study of moral development.

d. Ethics involves concrete judgments on the legal aspects of situations.

8. Ethical issues might arise around which of the following kinds of issues in relationship to the provision of drug information?

a. Decisions by the health professional on whether to provide drug information

b. Decisions on policies related to access to drug information

c. Both answers in a and b may involve ethical issues

d. Neither answer in a or b is likely to involve ethical issues

9. Identification of relevant background information when analyzing an ethical dilemma includes which of the following statements (choose all that apply):

a. A determination of the applicable moral rules in the case

b. Determine the factual details of the issue at hand

c. Consideration of who is affected by the ethical issue

d. Identify the cultural perspectives of the dilemma

10. The purposes for identifying relevant background in analyzing a potential ethical dilemma include which of the following (choose all that apply):

a. Knowledge of available background information sometimes alleviates any moral concerns about the issue.

b. Background information typically clarifies what parties might be affected by decisions made or actions taken.

c. Background information generally leads to resolution of a recognized ethical dilemma without further analysis.

d. Background information normally facilitates the drug information provider in addressing the dilemma in a culturally sensitive manner.

11. A drug information pharmacist receives a call from a mother who wants the pharmacist to identify a pill she found in the room of her 17-year-old son. The mother says her son is not taking any medications. Which of the following moral rules or principles will likely apply to this situation? (Choose all that apply)

a. Confidentiality

b. Privacy

    c. Nonmaleficence

    d. Veracity

12. A retail pharmacist is told by a father that he has been giving his 7-year-old daughter turkey tail mushroom to help boost her immune system. The father mentioned he had started giving his daughter this product because she is always sick. What additional information is needed while addressing any ethical concerns the pharmacist may have about this situation?

    a. Potential drug-drug interactions with any other medications the child is taking

    b. Any cultural reasons for the father's use of this product

    c. Possible side effects of turkey tail mushroom

    d. All of the above

13. Considering Question #12, which of the following ethical principles or rules do you think would be most pertinent to this case?

    a. Veracity

    b. Respect for autonomy

    c. Confidentiality

    d. Respect for persons

14. A physician in the urology department of the hospital is prescribing a parenteral agent called nudrugumab for patients with a certain urological condition. There is limited data supporting the use of the agent for the urologic condition, and the product is compounded. It is unknown if the patients know this is an unlabeled use for this unapproved medication. Which of the following action-guides (rule or principle) is likely to be prioritized in this ethical dilemma?

    a. Respecting the patient-professional relationship

    b. Beneficence

    c. Consent

    d. Privacy

15. A nurse asks you, the floor pharmacist, to discuss with the attending physician the potential need for additional pain medication for a patient who has a history of addiction to opioid-like substances. The patient reports having uncontrolled pain, and his vital signs support this claim. The nurse tried, but the physician said he did not wish to support the drug habit of the patient. What level of ethical decision making would this scenario constitute if there is an ethical dilemma?

    a. Micro level

    b. Meso level

    c. Macro level

    d. None because there is no ethical dilemma

REFERENCES

1. Haddad AM, Kaatz B, McCart G, McCarthy RL, Pink LA, Richardson J. Report of the ethics course content committee: curricular guidelines for pharmacy education. Am J Pharm Educ. 1993;57(Winter Suppl):34S-43S.

2. Veatch RM. Hospital pharmacy: what is ethical? (Primer). Am J Hosp Pharm. 1989;46:109-15.

3. Wilson R, Rowan MS, Henderson J. Core and comprehensive health care services: 1. Introduction to the Canadian Medical Association's decision-making framework. Can Med Assoc. 1995;152(7):1063-6.

4. Smith L, Morrissy J. Ethical dilemmas for general practitioners under the UK new contract. J Med Ethics. 1994;20:175-80.

5. Dierchx de Casterle B, Meulenbergs T, van de Vijver L, Tanghe A, Castmans C. Ethics meetings in support of good nursing care: some practice-based thoughts. Nurs Ethics. 2002;9(6):612-22.

6. Kirby J, Simpson C. An innovative, inclusive process for meso-level health policy development. HEC Forum. 2007;19(2):161-76.

7. Martin D, Singer P. A strategy to improve priority setting in health care institutions. Health Care Anal. 2003;11(1):59-68.

8. Pentz RD. Expanding into organizational ethics: the experience of one clinical ethics committee. HEC Forum. 1998;10(2):213-21.

9. Goold SD. Trust and the ethics of health care institutions. Hastings Cent Rep. 2001;6:26-33.

10. Nunes R. Evidence-based medicine: a new tool for resource allocation? Med Health Care Philos. 2003;6:297-301.

11. Coyle SL, for the Ethics and Human Rights Committee, American College of Physicians-American Society of Internal Medicine. Physician-industry relations. Part 1: individual physicians. Ann Intern Med. 2002;136:396-402.

12. Kenny N, Joffres C. An ethical analysis of international health priority-setting. Health Care Anal. 2007;16:145-60.

13. Ruger JP. Ethics in American Health 1: ethical approaches to health policy. Am J Pub Health. 2008;98(10):1751-6.

14. Ruger JP. Ethics in American Health 2: an ethical framework for health system reform. Am J Pub Health. 2008;98(10):1756-63.

15. Khushf G. The case for managed care: reappraising medical and socio-political ideals. J Med Phil. 1999;24(5):415-33.

16. Pirl MA. An ethics laboratory as an educational tool in a pharmacy law and ethics course. J Pharm Teach. 1990;1(3):51-68.

17. Beauchamp TLC, Childress JF. Principles of biomedical ethics. 5th ed. New York, NY: Oxford University Press; 2001.

18. Beauchamp TLC, Childress JF. Principles of biomedical ethics. 6th ed. New York, NY: Oxford University Press; 2008.

19. Beauchamp TLC, Childress JF. Principles of biomedical ethics. 4th ed. New York, NY: Oxford University Press; 1994.

20. Beauchamp TL. Principles or rules? In: Kopelman L, ed. Building bioethics. Lancaster, UK: Kluwer Academic Publishers; 1999:15-24.
21. Veatch RM. Cross-cultural perspectives in medical ethics. 2nd ed. Sudbury, MA: Jones and Bartlett Publishers; 2000.
22. Thornton BC, Callahan D, Nelson JL. Bioethics education: expanding the circle of participants. Hastings Cent Rep. 1993;23(1):25-9.
23. Veatch RM. A theory of medical ethics. New York, NY: Basic Books Publishers; 1981.
24. Najjar TA, Al-Arifi MN, Gubara OA, Dana MH. Ethical requests received by drug and poison information center in Saudi Arabia. J Soc Adm Pharm. 2000;17(4):234-7.
25. Carrese J, Brown K, Jameton A. Culture, healing, and professional obligations. Hastings Cent Rep. 1993;15:7.
26. Berger BA. Building an effective therapeutic alliance: competence, trustworthiness, and caring. Am J Hosp Pharm. 1993;50:2399-403.
27. Arnold RM, Nissen JC, Campbell NA. Ethical issues in a drug information center. Drug Intell Clin Pharm. 1987;21:1008-11.
28. Kelly WN, Krause EC, Krowsinski WJ, Small TR, Drane JF. National survey of ethical issues presented to drug information centers. Am J Hosp Pharm. 1990;47:2245-50.
29. Schools RM, Brushwood DB. The pharmacist's role in patient care. Hastings Cent Rep. 1991;12:7.
30. Powers M, Faden R. Social justice: the moral foundations of public health and health policy. New York, NY: Oxford University Press; 2006.
31. Bayer R, Gostin LO, Jennings B, Steinbock B. Public health ethics: theory, policy and practice. New York, NY: Oxford University Press; 2007.
32. U.S. Food and Drug Administration. Guidance for industry presenting risk information in prescription drug and medical device promotion: Draft Guidance: Food and Drug Administration; 2009 [cited 2013 Oct 18]. Available from: http://www.complianceonline.com/articlefiles/FDA_Guidance_Presenting_Risk_Information_Labels_Drugs_Devices.pdf
33. ComplianceOnline.com. Risk information in prescription drug & medical device ads, promotional labeling—what the FDA expects. ComplianceOnline; Nov 2011 [cited 2016 Sept 15]. Available from: http://www.complianceonline.com/ecommerce/control/articleDetail?contentId=12737&catId=10002
34. World Health Organization. Ethical criteria for medicinal drug promotion. Geneva: World Health Organization; 1988 [cited 2016 Sept 15]. Available from: http://apps.who.int/medicinedocs/documents/whozip08e/whozip08e.pdf
35. U.S. Food and Drug Administration. Bad ad program: 2011-2012 year end report. Food and Drug Administration; Jul 2012 [cited 2013 Oct 18]. Available from: http://www.fda.gov/Drugs/GuidanceComplianceRegulatoryInformation/Surveillance/DrugMarketingAdvertisingandCommunications/ucm258719.htm
36. Khakhkhar T, Mehta M, Shah R, Sharma D. Evaluation of drug promotional literatures using WHO guidelines. J Pharm Negative Results [Internet]. 2013;4:33-8. Available from: http://www.pnrjournal.com/article.asp?issn=0976-9234;year=2013;volume=4;issue=1;spage=33;epage=38;aulast=Khakhkhar

37. Dhanaraj E, Nigam A, Bagani S, Singh H, Tiwari P. Supported and unsupported claims in medicinal drug advertisements in Indian medical journals. Indian J Med Ethics. 2011;8(3):170-4.

38. Lal A. Information contents of drug advertisements: an Indian experience. Ann Pharmacother. 1998;32:1234.

39. Womack CA. Ethical and epistemic issues in direct-to-consumer drug advertising: where is patient agency? Med Health Care Philos. 2013;13:275-80.

40. Spurling G, Mansfield P. General practitioners and pharmaceutical sales representatives: quality improvement research. Qual Saf Health Care. 2007;16:266-70.

41. Alam K, Shah AK, Ojha P, Palaian S, Shankar PR. Evaluation of drug promotional materials in a hospital setting in Nepal. South Med Rev. 2009;2(1):2-6.

42. Ayuso C, Millan JM, Dal-Re R. Management and return of incidental genomic findings in clinical trials. Pharmacogenomics J. 2015;15:1-5.

43. Brown J. Ethical dilemmas: controversies in pain management. Adv Nurse Pract. 1997:69-72.

44. Davis CM. Patient practitioner interaction: an experiential manual for developing the art of health care. Thorofare, NJ: Slack; 1989.

45. Coach R. 5-minutes to monitor progress. Teaching Prof. 1991;5(9):1-2.

46. Haddad AM, ed. Teaching and learning strategies in pharmacy ethics. 2nd ed. Binghamton, NY: Pharmaceutical Products Press; 1997.

47. Veatch RM, Haddad AM. Case studies in pharmacy ethics. 2nd ed. New York, NY: Oxford University Press; 2008.

48. Smith M, Strauss S, Baldwin HJ, Alberts KT. Pharmacy ethics. New York, NY: Pharmaceutical Products Press; 1991.

49. Monaghan M, Galt KA, Turner P, Houghton B, Rich E, Markert R, Bergman-Evans B. Student understanding of the relationship between the health professions and the pharmaceutical industry. Teach Learn Med [Internet]. 2009;15(1):14-20. Available from: http://www.tandfonline.com/doi/pdf/10.1207/S15328015TLM1501_04?needAccess=true

50. Chren M, Landefeld C. Physicians' behavior and their interactions with drug companies: a controlled study of physicians who requested additions to a hospital drug formulary. JAMA. 1994;271:684-9.

51. Samp JC, Schumock GT, Pickard AS. Retracted publications in the drug literature. Pharmacotherapy. 2012;32(7):586-95.

52. Steen RG. Retractions in the scientific literature: do authors deliberately commit research fraud? J Med Ethics. 2011;37:113-7.

53. Anderson JG, Goodman KW. Ethics and information technology: a case-based approach to a health care system in transition. New York, NY: Springer-Verlag; 2002.

54. Poirier TL, Laux R. Redesign of a drug information resources course: responding to the needs of nontraditional PharmD students. Am J Pharm Educ. 1997;61:306-9.

55. Vottero LD. Code of ethics for pharmacists. Am J Health Syst Pharm. 1995;52:2096-131.

56. American Pharmacists Association. Code of ethics 1994. [Updated Oct 27, 1994; Mar 26, 2010]. Available from: http://www.pharmacist.com/code-ethics

57. Mappes TA, Zembaty JS. Biomedical ethics. 3rd ed. New York, NY: McGraw-Hill; 1991.

58. Mappes TA, Degrazia D. Biomedical ethics. 5th ed. Boston, MA: McGraw-Hill; 2001.

59. Wills S, Brown D, Astubry S. A survey of ethical issues surrounding supply of information to members of the public by hospital pharmacy medicines information centres. Pharm World Sci. 2002;24(2):55-60.

60. Austin L. Emergency contraception denial raises moral, legal issues. Associate Press State and Local Wire. 2004.

61. Alexander JK. Promising, professional obligations, and the refusal to provide service. HEC Forum. 2005;17(3):178-95.

62. Ghaibi S, Ipema H, Gabay M. ASHP guidelines on the pharmacist's role in providing drug information. Am J Health Syst Pharm. 2015;72:573-77.

63. Gettman DA, Benson B, Nguyen V, Luu SN. Use of motivational techniques by drug information center personnel to respond to calls involving perceived ethical dilemmas [Abstract]. ASHP Midyear Clinical Meeting; 2000.

SUGGESTED READINGS

1. Wills S, Brown D, Astbury S. A survey of ethical issues surrounding supply of information to members of the public by hospital pharmacy medicines information centres. Pharm World Sci. 2002;24(Feb):55-60.

2. Kelly WN, Krause EC, Krowsinski WJ, Small TR, Drane JF. National survey of ethical issues presented to drug information centers. Am J Hosp Pharm. 1990;47:2245-50.

3. Beauchamp TLC, Childress JF. Principles of biomedical ethics. 6th ed. New York, NY: Oxford University Press; 2012.

4. Veatch RM, Haddad A. Case studies in pharmacy ethics. 2nd ed. New York, NY: Oxford University Press; 2008.

5. Ethical criteria for medicinal drug promotion [Internet]. Geneva: World Health Organization; 1988 [cited 2013 Oct 18]. Available from: http://apps.who.int/medicinedocs/documents/whozip08e/whozip08e.pdf

Chapter Twelve

Professional Communication of Drug Information

Patrick M. Malone • Meghan J. Malone

Learning Objectives

After completing this chapter, the reader will be able to

- State reasons both for and against writing professionally.
- Describe the various steps of professional writing.
- Identify the order for authors in a professional paper.
- Describe the importance of knowing the audience.
- Describe various writing styles and their differences.
- Explain where to find a publication's requirements for submission.
- Describe what an article proposal consists of and why it is used.
- Explain the need for continued practice to develop good writing skills.
- List the components of both a research and review paper.
- Explain the general guidelines for writing.
- Describe the peer-review process.
- Explain the absolute importance of revision.
- Explain the steps in creating a newsletter or website.
- Describe how to prepare audiovisual materials for a poster or platform presentation and place those items on a website.
- Describe techniques for creating an abstract for an article.
- Describe how to correctly cite reference materials.

Key Concepts

❶ Essentially any time a professional takes pen, pencil, word processor, or any other writing implement in hand to fulfill professional duties, it is considered professional writing.

❷ When writing, it is best to keep things as simple and direct as possible.

❸ With the probable exception of policy and procedure documents, the two most important paragraphs in any document are the first and last.

❹ If the information is taken from a particular source, even if it is reworded, the original author should be given credit via footnotes or endnotes.

❺ In many cases, revision of a document will be necessary.

❻ Instead of concentrating on the technology, it is best to concentrate on the message.

❼ Professional writing is a skill necessary for every health professional.

Introduction

A common thought when considering the topic of **professional writing** is "That doesn't apply to me, I'm not writing for a journal." But professional writing is certainly not limited to journal articles or books. It includes writing evaluations of medications for consideration on a hospital formulary, preparing written policies and procedures for the preparation of an intravenous admixture, reporting the results of the latest sales to the home office, writing on a professional website, responding to a drug information question via e-mail, preparing a written evaluation of a technician or clerk, writing in a chart, writing a term paper for a class, preparing slides or posters for a presentation, writing a letter of recommendation,[1] and many other things. ❶ *Essentially any time a professional takes pen, pencil, word processor, or any other writing implement in hand to fulfill professional duties, it is considered professional writing.* When writing, although the format changes, the general principles remain the same. So whether the objective is to write the ultimate book on the practice of medicine or to type a label for a prescription vial, a health care professional must know how to write professionally.

Although some may say the purpose of writing is to keep a job or to pass a course, there are, generally, four larger purposes for the existence of written material: to inform, instruct, persuade, or entertain. The first three items are those usually considered in professional writing, although including the fourth, whenever possible, will help convince people to read what has been written.

There are also some advantages to professional writing, besides those mentioned above. For example, writing is often used to evaluate an employee for promotion in many jobs. In academia, there is always the concept of publish or perish. Pharmacy technicians are also encouraged to write as a means of advancement.[2] Additionally, writing gives the authors the opportunity to share their knowledge or ideas,[3] obtain gratification or satisfaction,[4] and improve their knowledge. It may even lead to some fame or notoriety in a field.

Unfortunately, there are disadvantages to professional writing. The major problem is that any significant amount of writing often involves a lot of potentially frustrating work, because few people are natural writers. The author must practice to become proficient at writing, which will involve false starts, numerous drafts, roadblocks, and other problems.[5] If that is not enough, writing exposes a person to criticism and possible rejection. Although at one time authors were paid to publish articles, today it is not unheard of that authors may actually have to pay to have their article published.[6,7] At best, the direct financial rewards are likely to be few, unless a best-selling novel is produced. Indirectly, writing may lead to pay increases and promotions. However, because writing is a professional necessity, it can be made easier by following the correct procedures, which will be covered in this chapter.

Steps in Writing

As each of the steps in professional writing are covered in this section, the emphasis will be on writing items likely to be encountered in a practice setting, although additional steps that are necessary when writing for publication will be mentioned.

PREPARING TO WRITE

The first step in writing is to know the purpose—why something needs to be written in the first place. It is necessary at this time to have a good idea of the expected endpoint, which is important, no matter what is being done. For example, someone learning to mow grass with a lawn mower may be concentrating on the ground near the mower and end up wandering all over the lawn, thinking he or she is going straight. However, by concentrating on going to a specific point on the far end of the lawn, rather than looking just in front of the mower, the row will probably be mowed fairly straight. Similarly, throughout the whole writing process it is necessary to keep in mind the endpoint, to keep from wandering all over the place. If the item being written is for publication, rather than something required for work, it will also be necessary to pick the topic and, perhaps, submit an **article proposal** (see Figure 12-1). Although the writing is considered to be more important than the idea, it is still essential to have a good idea or topic that is of interest to prospective readers before starting.[8] It can even cover an old topic, as long as the topic is covered in greater depth, in a new way, or is addressed to a different group. It should also be pointed

Although relatively few professionals write articles for journals or books, those who do need to follow an occasional step in addition to those outlined in the main text of this chapter. One difference is the potential need to write an article proposal to the publisher. This simply is a letter asking the publisher whether there would be any interest in possibly publishing something on a particular topic written by the person who is inquiring. As might be expected, this step is generally not necessary if writing a description of original research, but would be important when writing a review article or even a descriptive article. The letter should contain certain information, which will be described below, and be addressed to an appropriate editor. If at all possible, it is also a good idea to talk to an editor before submitting your proposal. For example, the proposal for the first edition of this book originated after a discussion with the editor at a publisher's booth in the American Society of Health-System Pharmacists Midyear Clinical Meeting Exhibitor's Area.

In the written proposal, the prospective author should first briefly explain the basic idea that is to be covered in the article or book, including a working title. Similarly, a description of the approach the author wishes to take in covering the subject should be described. Although this description should be kept brief, it must provide enough information for the publisher to determine whether the topic and approach are even appropriate for their publication. In the case of a book, it is important to include a table of contents that is descriptive enough to be useful to reviewers who will be advising the publisher on the need for such a book. Related to that need, it is also necessary to describe why the proposed article or book will be important to the publisher's customers. This is the sales pitch. It is necessary to briefly show that there is nothing similar, or as good, currently available in the literature for the audience being addressed.

Although the above is the meat of the proposal, there are several other items that should be included. These include the time necessary to complete the article/book (be realistic), the approximate length of the work, and a statement of the authors' qualifications, including any previous publications.

There are several good reasons for submitting a proposal. The first is simply to avoid work if the editor decides that there is no need for such a publication (although an author should not hesitate to send the proposal to another publisher, if it still seems that the topic is important). Second, and perhaps most important, it allows the editor(s) to make suggestions. By following those suggestions, an author is more likely to be successful in getting work published. Finally, if the idea is accepted, the acceptance letter will provide motivation.

Figure 12–1. Article proposal to publishers.

out that in the case of clinical trial results, it can be important to publish articles showing that something did not work, although in the past such topics have often been avoided.[9]

- It is also necessary to decide whether there needs to be a **coauthor**. This may be easy to resolve, depending on who is working on the project. However, even if no one else has been involved, it may be a good idea to look for a coauthor. An inexperienced writer (e.g., a student or someone early in his or her career) would benefit from working with an experienced author.[10] Additionally, working with someone will give a different perspective (especially if working with practitioners from many disciplines) and, hopefully, lessen the work for each person. Finally, it is sometimes a necessity to include coauthors for political reasons (as in "Would you prefer to share the credit or work nights and holidays for the rest of your life?"). Although this last reason should not exist, it does. Coauthors who are not direct contributors to the written work may be considered honorary authors and are relatively common,[11] although this is considered to be inappropriate.[12] A variety of other problems with authorship credit are also seen.[13-15] The best outcome is that everyone must do part of the writing[16] and that authors be listed in the order of their contributions to the project. This does not always happen.[17,18] In some cases, pharmaceutical manufacturers may want ghostwriters to write an article for the researchers, but even they agree that original authors must prepare the first draft of editorials or opinion pieces, although non-English speaking authors may be assisted by others after that.[19] The ghostwriters should also be appropriately acknowledged.[9] Although arguments may be made,[20-26] there is no valid reason for people to be listed as an author in excess of their contribution to the writing and submission of the work for publication.[27-30] The only exception would be if the publisher has other specific rules. For example, some journals may want to list contributors with an explanation of what they contributed (e.g., writing, origination of study idea, data collection). Generally, ALL of the following must be met for an individual to be given credit as an author:[30,31]

- Conception and design of the study, or analysis and interpretation of the data in the study
- Writing or revising the article
- Final approval of the version that is published
- Agreement to be accountable for all aspects of the work, which includes ensuring questions related to accuracy or integrity are investigated and resolved

Things that do not qualify a person to be listed as an author include:[29,30,31]

- Acquisition of funding
- General supervision of the research group
- Writing assistance, editing, and proofreading

Individuals that do not meet the first qualifications should be listed in the acknowledgments section. Also, the **primary author** should be able to explain the order in which the authors are listed and journals may require one or more authors to be guarantors, who will be taking responsibility for the work as a whole, including legally.[30]

It should also be mentioned that there can be too many authors and acknowledgments.[32] Some scientific papers list many, many authors for a particular paper, and the number of authors has grown over the years.[33] It is obvious that 20 authors could not have written a three-page paper. Some of this may be a result of job requirements that include publishing a certain number of articles, leading to demands by individuals to get their name listed on any article they can. Again, authors should contribute to the written work in some significant way, as defined above. In some cases it may be necessary to just name the group performing the research, with a few of the most responsible individuals specifically named, and list others as acknowledgments, sometimes by group, institution, or type of contribution.[28,32,34] Others may be listed as clinical investigators, participating investigators, scientific advisors, data collectors, or other appropriate titles.[30] In relationship to authorship, remember the people taking credit are also taking responsibility—they need to make sure that the work is clear and not subject to misinterpretation (i.e., do not write something that is designed to mislead the reader into believing something that has not been proven).[35]

Before the first word is written, it is necessary to know the audience, which involves knowing the type of person who will be reading the final document and where it will be published. Keep in mind that the word *published* was chosen for a specific reason. Whether the final product appears in New England Journal of Medicine, the IV Room Policy and Procedure Book, or even the label on a prescription vial, it is published. It is necessary to aim the work at the audience. At a broad level, written work should not be submitted for possible publication in a journal that does not cover the topic; it is no more appropriate to submit an article on preparation of cardioplegic solutions to the Journal of Urology than it is to type a monthly fiscal report on prescription labels. So, be sure to review a journal and its Instructions for Authors before attempting to write an article for submission to that journal.[36]

More specifically, it is necessary to aim both the writing style and depth of information toward the audience. If something is written for physicians, it is not likely to be understood by laypeople. Conversely, items written for laypeople may not satisfy the needs of physicians. It is certainly appropriate to have a secondary audience in mind. For example, a report written for physicians may be of interest to pharmacists and nurses. However, make sure the secondary audience is not served at the expense of the primary audience.

In regard to writing style, there are three types of writing styles commonly used by health care professionals: **pure technical style**, **middle technical style**, and **popular technical style** (See Table 12-1).[37]

TABLE 12–1. **TYPES OF TECHNICAL WRITING**

- Pure technical style—used by professionals addressing other professionals in the same field
- Middle technical style—used by professionals addressing professionals in other fields
- Popular technical style—used by professionals addressing laypeople

Pure technical style is used by business or technical professionals when they are writing for other professionals in the same or similar fields. For example, an article published in American Journal of Health-Systems Pharmacy, American Journal of Nursing, or Journal of the American Medical Association would normally be written in this style. There are several characteristics of this style. First, the authors can use technical jargon because they can expect the readers will understand it. Second, it is written in formal English. Third, it is written in the third person; words such as I, we, us, and you are eliminated. Finally, there is a general lack of slang or contractions. The great majority of writing done by health professionals will be in this style, because it is usually other health professionals who will be reading their work.

Middle technical style is very closely related to pure technical style. This style is used by authors when they are writing for readers with a variety of technical backgrounds, with everyone having some unifying factor. For example, a report regarding a hospital's medication error reports might be presented to the hospital's pharmacy and therapeutics committee. That committee is made up of physicians, nurses, hospital administrators, pharmacists, and other professionals. Although each has a background that makes their membership on the committee appropriate, not all of them would understand what Lactated Ringer's solution is, as would most hospital pharmacists. Therefore, it is necessary to better explain, or sometimes avoid, some technical areas or specific abbreviations. Otherwise, this writing style is very similar in most respects to pure technical style.

Finally, popular technical style is used in anything meant for the general public. Common language is used throughout. For example, a patient information sheet would need to be written in this style. A widely available example would be the articles on medical subjects that have appeared in Reader's Digest over the years. Information that is written in this style will use less complicated words and be less formal in its presentation.

It should be pointed out that usual technical writing differs greatly from what most people learn in high school English class or college composition courses. Although there is often a tendency to protest the formality of professional writing styles at first, the reality of the situation is that those styles must be followed for a piece of written material to be accepted.

The next step is to know the requirements of the publisher. Whether the work is for the department's policy and procedure manual or a journal, chances are that there is a format that needs to be followed. In the case of a journal, directions on the format to follow will typically be published on the journal's website. Also, specific guidelines are followed by a number of professional journals, both for general format and statistical reporting. Many journals have approved those guidelines and expect that all work submitted for publication will follow them. Many journals follow a format called the Recommendations for the Conduct, Reporting, Editing, and Publication of Scholarly Work in Medical Journals (previously, the Uniform Requirements for Manuscripts Submitted to Biomedical Journals published by the International Committee of Medical Journal Editors [ICMJE])[30,31]. This standardization makes it easier on the prospective author; one style can be learned and followed, regardless of the journal. Other publications that can be helpful are Scientific Style and Format: The CSE Manual for Authors, Editors, and Publishers prepared by the Council of Science Editors, The American Medical Association Manual of Style, The MLA Style Manual, and the Publication Manual of the American Psychiatric Association.

In the case of reports, policy and procedure manuals, and similar documents, it is best to see what has been done in the past. If this is the first time a particular item is being prepared, it is advisable to try to see what has been done in other places, and prepare something similar that meets the perceived needs. If writing something for work, do not be afraid to try to improve the format to make it more usable. However, be aware that it may be necessary to get any changes in format approved by the appropriate individual(s) or committee(s). Whenever possible, follow the Recommendations for the Conduct, Reporting, Editing, and Publication of Scholarly Work in Medical Journals[27] format used by the medical journals, because it is the standard for biomedical writing.

GENERAL RULES OF WRITING

Once the preparation is completed, it is time to start writing. Unfortunately, there is no easy way to learn how to write professionally; it just requires a lot of practice. However, a number of rules can be followed (See Table 12-2). This section covers some of the general

TABLE 12–2. **CHECKLIST IN PREPARATION OF WRITTEN MATERIALS**

- Do research first
- Put oneself in the reader's position
- Use proper grammar and spelling
- Make the document look professional
- Keep things simple and direct
- Keep the document as short as possible
- Avoid abbreviations and acronyms
- Avoid the first person (e.g., I, we, us)
- Use active sentences
- Avoid slash construction (e.g., he/she, him/her, and/or)
- Avoid contractions (e.g., don't, can't)
- Cite other references wherever appropriate (and get permission to do so where appropriate)
- Cover things in whatever order is easiest
- Get everything down on paper before revising
- Edit, Edit, Edit!

rules, with information on how to prepare specific items (e.g., introduction, body, conclusion, references, **abstracts**) being covered later.

- **Rule 1**: Organize the information before starting to write, including preparing an outline.[5] In the past, that was an onerous task that few performed. However, with modern word processing software, the outline actually becomes part of the finished product, so it does not amount to any significant extra work. Minimally, the different sections should be listed to create some order to the layout of the work (remember, keep in mind the endpoint). Overall, the goal is to prepare a document that is clear, concise, complete, and correct. The two latter items depend, to a large part, on preparation. The former items, however, can be helped by following some simple rules.

- **Rule 2**: Do sufficient research before getting started. Research in this regard, means obtaining whatever information—whether records, articles, performance evaluations, financial reports, or anything else—necessary to prepare the item. Although it is likely that additional research will be necessary to fill in the fine points at some point in the process, most information should be gathered ahead of time. It is impossible to be organized if there is nothing collected, and a document that is not organized will generally not be worth much.

- **Rule 3**: The author should put him or herself in the reader's position. What does that reader want and how does he or she want it presented?

- **Rule 4**: Use proper spelling and grammar. This is easier than in the past because word processing programs check both; however, it is still necessary to double check because the computer is likely to overlook things. For example, a properly spelled, but incorrect, word will be missed (e.g., two instead of to, trail instead of trial, ration instead of ratio). Unfortunately for some writers, appearances count greatly. The writer may know more about a particular subject than anyone else, but if poor grammar and spelling permeate the document, it is unlikely that anyone will read or believe the information presented.[38] It will be dismissed as probably wrong, based on grammar and spelling alone. In a case where the finished product will be published in a language other than the writer's native language, the writer should have the work read and edited by someone for whom the language is their first language.

- **Rule 5**: The writing should try to be entertaining. Professional writing tends to be a bit dry; thus, an attempt should be made to make it as enjoyable and easy to read as possible while staying cautious with humor and within limits of professionalism and good taste. It should also be unpretentious, direct, and accurate.[39]

- **Rule 6**: The document should look presentable. Some students or employees are well known for turning in papers that are crumpled, creased, torn, dirty, or coffee stained. That is not professional and must be avoided. The sad truth is that people will assume that if an author was sloppy with the appearance of the document, he or she was probably sloppy with the information. That may not be so, but that assumption will kill a good, but sloppy, document.

- **Rule 7**: ❷ *When writing it is best to keep things as simple and direct as possible.*[40-43] This has been referred to as the KISS (Keep It Simple, Stupid) principle. There is a temptation to use big words that sound impressive, but doing so is more likely to confuse than impress. In the case of e-mails, it has been stated that they should be written at the third-grade reading level in order to actually get people to respond.[44]

- Related to that, keep documents as short as possible.[45] If a document is long, subheadings should be used. This can be part of the outline step, mentioned earlier. Also, consider whether tables, figures, or graphs would make the document simpler and easier to understand. This can be particularly useful with documents containing a great deal of data that may be organized through the use of tables.

- **Rule 8**: Avoid using abbreviations or acronyms. If it is necessary to do so, state the full form of the word or term the first time that it is mentioned in the document, followed by the abbreviation in parenthesis (e.g., acquired immunodeficiency syndrome [AIDS]). The only exceptions to this rule are units of measurement (e.g., mL, mg). Units of measurement should be expressed in the metric system. Clinical chemistry and hematologic measurements should be in terms of the International System of Units (SI).

- **Rule 9:** Use an appropriate "voice" in writing. Completely avoid writing in the first person, and avoid the second person wherever possible. Search via the word processor to find all occurrences of *I, me, we, us,* and *you*. If those words are found, try to rewrite the sentence to avoid them. Also, it is preferable to avoid using the passive voice throughout [46]; again, a grammar checker can help. Avoid both contractions and slash construction (i.e., *and/or, he/she* [use *he or she*], *this/that*). Finally, in this politically correct era, avoid sexism. This means to avoid using words like only *he* or *she* (both genders should be included in a statement, except where inappropriate). For example, using *he* in a case report of a patient with testicular cancer is quite appropriate. Also, it is usually considered inappropriate to use *their* instead of *his or her* to get around the problem, although there has been a recent publication saying that this is now considered to be appropriate.[47]

- **Rule 10**: Be sure to give credit where it is due. This does not mean just making sure the listed authors wrote part of the document. It includes using endnotes, or possibly footnotes, for all information obtained from one or a limited number of sources. If there is extensive quoting, permission to do so should be obtained by writing to the person or organization holding the copyright on the material. Endnotes are something everyone dreaded in the past. They waited until the end, because the articles should be cited in the order they appear in the document. By that time, it was difficult to go back and do it. Now, it is much easier with word processors; it is possible to insert the citations as the document is prepared and let the software worry about making sure they are in the correct order.

Related to the endnotes, everything that is stated should be supported by objective evidence. When writing a paper based on scientific literature, that evidence must be shown in the endnotes. To reemphasize, any unreferenced statement of fact is for all practical purposes worthless. However, it is necessary to make sure information is extracted from the original article and expressed properly. Some writers will improperly twist facts, whether inadvertently or not, to support their assertions.[48]

Rule 11: Work through the document in whatever order seems easiest.[5] In preparing a drug evaluation for a pharmacy and therapeutics committee, a stack of 50 articles might be used. At first, the stack may look like an impossible task, but after sorting the articles into groups that correspond to the sections, start with the shortest stack or the easiest information. By the time the document is finished, the writer may be surprised to find out that they were all fairly short, easy stacks.

Rule 12: Edit the document thoroughly. At first, a writer should simply try to make sure that all of the information is down on paper.[5] Once that occurs, go back and revise, and perhaps reorganize the document. Waiting a few days before revising the document can be very beneficial. After some time away from the project, errors practically jump off the page. It is also a good idea to have someone else who has not been involved with the writing, read the document. Something that seems quite clear to the author may not actually be clear at all. Also, the author may be mentally inserting words or sentences that were inadvertently omitted. Having someone edit the document can be humbling but helpful. Be sure to provide the product in a format that will make things easier for the person reviewing the document. A typed, double-spaced manuscript will make it easy to read and provide room for comments. Even better, electronic versions of a document can be reviewed directly on a computer using "comment" or "track changes" features. The reviewer can put in comments or suggested wording changes electronically and then return the document. The writer can then go through the document making changes or simply accepting proposed changes with the click of a mouse. Often, the use of the electronic reviewing mechanism will be quicker, easier, and provide much clearer suggestions.

The three most important things in real estate may be location, location, location, but the three most important things in writing are edit, edit, edit. This can be particularly important when multiple authors have contributed different sections since it will be necessary to make sure that the various contributions fit well together, including the style of writing.[49] It may be best for either the first author or most senior author to edit for consistency. Also, remember editing includes paring out unnecessary words, sentences, and larger sections. It is not sufficient to settle for good enough—do your best. Look at it this way: the boss or editor is only going to do so much editing before giving up. The trick is to make sure that the document is well prepared and does not need that much editing.

SPECIFIC DOCUMENT SECTIONS

A typical document consists of three main parts—the introduction, body, and conclusion. In the case of a clinical study, it is recommended to follow the IMRAD structure that divides a paper into Introduction, Methods, Results, and Discussion,[30] which is the standard for such papers.[50] Other parts, such as references, tables, figures, and abstracts may also be necessary. These will be discussed in later sections and in the appendices of this chapter. It should also be noted that a number of the points in Chapters 4, 5, and 6 are applicable to writing of journal articles, as are the contents of the following websites: International Committee of Medical Journal Editors (http://www.icmje.org), Consolidated Standards of Reporting Trials (CONSORT) statement (contains a checklist for contents of clinical trial to report when publishing and flow diagram illustrating recruitment, randomization, and analysis of subjects enrolled in a trial) (http://www.consort-statement.org),[51-61] Preferred Reporting Items for Systemic Reviews and Meta-Analysis (PRISMA)[62,63] (http://www.prisma-statement.org/), Conference on Guideline Standardization (COGS) standards (http://gem.med.yale.edu/cogs/), and the Good Publication Practice Guidelines (GPP3) for pharmaceutical companies (http://www.ismpp.org/gpp3).[64] A compilation of over 300 standards for reporting medical studies may be found at http://www.equator-network.org/. An example question layout that includes an introduction, body, and conclusion section is shown in Appendix 12-1.

Introduction

❸ With the probable exception of policy and procedure documents, the two most important paragraphs in any document are the first and last. It is vital to start out strong, to encourage the reader to continue reading. Otherwise, the work will end up in that stack of articles that everyone intends to read someday, but seldom does. That first paragraph should also inform the reader of what they can expect in the rest of the document; it should be similar to a road map that shows what is to be accomplished in the document. The introduction should have a clear objective for the existence of the document. Many people neglect the need to state a clear objective, which leaves the reader to flounder and wonder whether there really is a purpose to the document. In a research article, the introduction will also contain the hypothesis being investigated. In a policy and procedure document, it may simply be a description of what the remainder of the document will cover. The introduction should also contain background information about the topic that provides a good information base for the reader. The amount of background information has to be a balance—enough to show the reader that the writer has done an appropriate amount of research, but yet not so exhaustive as to bore or overwhelm the reader with unnecessary details.[65] Overall, the introduction should be short but contain properly referenced background material and show the reader where the document is headed.

The introduction should generally not be a conclusion; some people are so anxious to jump to the end that they put the conclusion first. Admittedly, the BLOT (bottom line on top) concept has its purpose in some documents (e.g., policy and procedures, formulary monographs), but that should be a conscious decision. If the introduction amounts to a conclusion, many people will read no further, making the remainder of the document a waste of time and effort.

Body

The body of the document contains all of the details. In a research article, the body may be divided into the methods, results, and, possibly, discussion sections, although the latter section may be incorporated into the conclusion. Details of what should be included are covered in Chapter 4. In other documents, the body will probably be divided into whatever sections are appropriate or logical. A number of rules can be followed in preparing the body of a document.

The first rule is that, while it is important to be concise, all necessary information must be presented. Again, keep an eye on the desired endpoint, and do not stray from the subject unless it is absolutely necessary. Including unnecessary information, even if it is interesting, will tend to confuse or obscure the important points. Also, be sure to provide a balanced coverage of the material and avoid unsupported bias.[9]

It is important to cover the information in a logical order, so that it flows easily from one point to another. A common mistake, when learning to write professionally, is to skip back and forth between subjects. For example, someone might insert a point about dosing in the middle of indications, when dosing is discussed at another point in the document.

Material that can identify patients should be left out of any work, unless it is absolutely necessary to include. If that is not possible, informed consent must be obtained[30] and pertinent legal procedures must be followed (see Chapter 10). The authors should also disclose any approval of a study by Institutional Review Boards (IRB) and their following of other rules related to protection of study subjects (both human and animal).[30]

Writers should also put the information in their own words. Perhaps out of lack of confidence, a number of professionals are tempted to simply quote other authors word for word. However, by presenting the information in their own words, writers demonstrate that they actually understand the topic. ❹ *Remember, though, that if the information is taken from a particular source, even if it is reworded, the original author should be given credit via footnotes or endnotes.*

It is necessary to expand on the topic discussed in the previous paragraph because there seems to be much confusion about it and there are many cases where the rules against copyright infringement and plagiarism are broken. Plagiarism can be considered the copying of another's words or ideas, without properly giving credit. Copyright violations consist of copying another's work, even with appropriate quotations and citation, without permission. They are similar; however, it is possible to commit either plagiarism or copyright violations without committing the other. Self-plagiarism, where an author copies material that he or she previously had published in one journal for something in another journal, is a concern and can lead to copyright violations.[66] It appears that plagiarism is becoming more frequent and many people do not understand that it is wrong to copy work without proper attribution, even something from a source written by many anonymous people (e.g., Wikipedia, Yahoo! Answers, and Answers.com).[67,68]

Sometimes those infractions are rather blatant, such as the cases documented in the newspapers about students downloading papers from the Internet and presenting them as their own or simply retyping a previously published article (an attempt to prevent this can be seen on the Internet at http://www.plagiarism.com, http://www.plagiarism.org, or http://www.turnitin.com).[69,70] Interestingly, although there might be suspicions that this is more prevalent with online classes, a study found that it was more likely to occur with traditional campus students.[71] Another website http://www.ithenticate.com/ is a resource to check if published material is plagiarized. Other times, the infringement is quite accidental. For example, it was once brought to the attention of the famous science fiction writer, Isaac Asimov, that a short story he wrote was similar to an article that had been published 10 years previously.[72] Dr. Asimov went back and found the article and read it, realizing that he had read it when it first came out and had forgotten about it. When he wrote his story 10 years later, he did not realize that portions of it could be considered plagiarism. Although he had no intention of infringing upon the other author's work, Dr. Asimov made sure that the story was never reprinted and even wrote an article discussing the problem. This shows how easy it is to inadvertently cross the line into copyright infringement or plagiarism, and there are many examples that would fall in between the extremes given above.[73] Therefore, it is necessary for the author to be on guard and to try to prevent the problem in the first place. A few general rules can act as a guide:

- Use quotations or seek permission: When copying wording directly from another's work, it should be in quotations (or otherwise shown to be a quote) and a citation should appear to give credit to the original author(s). Also, if a significant amount of a work published in the last 100 years is quoted, it is probably necessary to get permission from the copyright holder, which may require paying a fee.[74] Exactly what is a significant amount is debatable; however, it would be best to err on the side of asking for permission if a quotation is more than a few sentences. Reproducing an entire chart, table, figure, and so on should normally require asking for permission. A letter to the copyright holder will solve problems; publishers often have forms to request permission. Some special cases need to be mentioned. First, U.S. government documents are not copyrighted, so only quotation marks and citations are necessary. Second, if it is impossible to locate a copyright holder (e.g., the publisher went out of business without transferring copyrights), the writer should at least be able to document a thorough effort to obtain permission. Finally, there are special legal requirements for use of copyrighted materials in online education, covered in the Technology, Education and Copyright Harmonization (TEACH) Act. Further information on this can be found in Chapter 10.

- Extensive quotations should be avoided: If a writer cannot put something in his or her own words, does that person truly understand the material? In any writing, there really is very little reason to provide quotations. The author should try to put things in his or her own words whenever possible.
- Use original publications: Paraphrased information should have the original publication(s) cited, if it comes from one or a limited number of sources. If the material came from a review article, cite that article, not the original study that was not consulted. It is worth mentioning that in the case of unusual information, reading and citing the original study is preferable to just using a review article, because the review may be inaccurate.
- Be sure to follow publishers' rules or licenses, which may be stricter and may not allow any reproduction of material. Obtain permission from publisher, even if it is author's original work, for use in a different publication to avoid copyright violations.[66]
- Always cite everything: It is necessary to always cite others work, even on slides[75] and even if it is the author's own previously published work to avoid self-plagiarism.[66]

In preparing certain documents (e.g., written answers to questions), there may be very little information available as only one or two research articles may have been written on the topic. If so, it will often be desirable to summarize the articles in detail, including most of the information presented in an abstract (see Appendix 12-2). In general, the information presented will summarize how many and what type of patients (i.e., inclusion and exclusion criteria), the drug or procedure being investigated, the results (e.g., efficacy, adverse effects), and the conclusions of authors of referenced articles. It is also important to point out any noticeable flaws in the paper. An example would be:

> Smith and Jones performed a double-blind, randomized comparison of the effects of drug X and drug Y in patients with tsutsugamushi fever. Patients were required to be between 18 and 70 years old, and could not have any concurrent infection or disorder

that would affect the immune response to the disease (e.g., neutropenia, AIDS). Twenty patients received 10 mg of drug X, three times a day for 15 days. Eighteen patients received 250 mg of drug Y, twice a day for 10 days. The two groups were comparable, except that the patients receiving drug X were an average of 5 years younger ($p < 0.05$). Drug X was shown to produce a cure, both in terms of symptoms and cultures in 85% of patients, whereas drug Y only produced a cure in 55.5% of patients. The difference was statistically significant ($p < 0.01$). No significant adverse effects were seen in either group. Although it appears that drug X was the better agent, it should be noted that drug Y was given in its minimally effective dose, and may have performed better in a somewhat higher or longer regimen.

A list of material to be covered in a review of an article similar to that above is found in Table 12-3.

Conclusion

A conclusion should be placed at the end of the body of the document, except for certain documents (e.g., policy and procedures). This conclusion should follow logically from the information presented and should serve to summarize that information. Remember, the conclusion should also correspond with the objective stated in the introduction.[76] It is also worth noting that in clinical consultations, a common mistake is

TABLE 12–3. ITEMS TO INCLUDE IN WRITTEN REVIEW OF A JOURNAL ARTICLE

Items to Include	Examples
Main author of article and a reference number	Johnson et al.[2] Smith and associates[24]
Type of article	Clinical study, case report, case series, review, meeting abstract
Research design (if appropriate)	Blinding, randomization, experience report, descriptive report
Objective or purpose of the report	Population, disease or condition, intervention, comparison (if appropriate), outcome (primary and secondary)
Description of group studied	Size of groups, age, sex, disease state(s), other pertinent demographic characteristics, inclusion and exclusion criteria
Any important confounding factors	Smoking, age, general health
Description of treatment being studied	Drug, dose, administration route, dosing interval, treatment duration
What was measured as an indicator of effect/outcome variables	Measurements appropriately matched with outcomes
Results	Efficacy, adverse effects, safety, adherence, drop-outs (reasons)
Author conclusions	
Strengths and weaknesses of the study	See Chapters 4 and 5

to write the conclusion in a general manner, rather than addressing the specific patient in question, which is what the reader wants to hear about. The author must remember to address the specific patient's situation.

Many writers are tempted to avoid formulating a conclusion. Various reasons include not feeling qualified to make a conclusion for the reader, not wanting to restate what has already been stated, laziness, not knowing how to write one, and so on. This is improper. The readers need something to bring their thoughts together at the end, and the author is in the perfect position to provide this closure. However, the author should also be careful to avoid extrapolating beyond the information available.

Other Items

If items include endnotes, the references should be found following the conclusion (see Appendix 12-3 for more information on how to prepare a **bibliography**). Use of bibliographic software, such as EndNote (Thomson Reuters—http://www.endnote.com), or Zotero (Roy Rosenzweig Center for History and New Media—http://www.zotero.org/) can be helpful in this process.[19] Other items may also be necessary, depending on the document, such as tables, graphs, figures, and so forth. They will not be dealt with here, other than to say that those items should supplement or clarify (not distort or misrepresent), and not simply duplicate material in the text portion of a piece of written work, although there may be overlap as an author explains data or expands on the material presented.

SUBMISSION OF THE DOCUMENT

Once the document is completed, proofread, and edited, it is ready to be submitted, whether this is to a supervisor or a journal. In the latter case, you will need to include a cover letter that serves as an introduction to the document. In the former case, it will be possible to be less formal. Also, it should be noted that when submitting an item to a journal it may be necessary to include transfer of copyright forms, conflict of interest disclosures (including financial),[16,77-79] or other items, which will be found in the directions for authors for that journal (usually found in the first issue of each year and on the publication's website). The conflict of interest may be reported by the publisher in the final publication, but this is variable.[80] In addition, be sure to precisely follow the journal's Instructions for Authors to improve chances for acceptance.[81] Unless given a special circumstance, articles should not be submitted to more than one journal at the same time (note: prior publication of an abstract does not mean that submission of a full article is duplication and publication in a second language is often considered acceptable).[9,16,82] If duplicate submission is determined to be necessary, the rules outlined in the Recommendations for the Conduct, Reporting, Editing, and Publication of Scholarly Work in Medical Journals must be followed.[30] Also, the article should not be broken down into many small articles and submitted over time, unless submission as a whole would result in a publication that would be too long or complex.[83]

PEER REVIEW

If the document is to be published in a peer-reviewed publication (most biomedical journals, but not magazines), it will undergo a peer-review process as the name implies. The peer-review process is that by which **referees**, also referred to as reviewers and content experts, review, comment, and provide insights regarding the merit of the document for potential publication in the journal. On a local level, reviewers are the people that a writer may ask to look at a report before the boss gets it. Whatever arena, whether local or international, a person should also be willing to be a reviewer at that level. To be a reviewer for a journal (which produces **refereed publications**), a person usually can simply write a letter stating interests, qualifications, and experience to the editor of the journal, and ask to be considered for the journal's reviewer list. If the person has adequate credentials, the journal will usually be happy to have that person as a reviewer.

Anyone who is a reviewer should be up front about such things as lack of expertise, conflict of interest,[79] or inability to complete a review within a reasonable time, and should be willing to step aside as a reviewer of a particular paper if those are problems.[84] Also, a reviewer should treat anything submitted to him or her as a confidential document.

It should be pointed out that people who act as reviewers for papers should follow the procedures discussed in Chapters 4 and 5. Specific directions will also be received from the editor and may involve preparing comments for both the editor (to discuss matters, such as ethics, with the editor alone) and for the author(s) (this latter document is also used by the editor). It may be required that the latter be signed or unsigned. Also, as with any quality assurance procedure, the reviewer should treat it as an opportunity to provide constructive, as opposed to destructive, criticism.[85] Finally, for those who are reviewers for journals, it is recommended to get new people involved in the process, such as residents or new practitioners, so that they can learn how to be a reviewer.[86]

It is beyond the scope of this chapter, but if further information is needed on being an editor of a biomedical journal, the reader should consult the website of the World Association of Medical Editors (http://www.wame.org).

REVISION

⑤ *In many cases, revision of the document will be necessary.* This may be due to a difference in opinion or different perception of need. Although an author should never change a document to say something he or she believes is wrong, minor revisions are often necessary to improve clarity or make the document more appropriate in some other manner.

The comments given with the request for revision are likely to be helpful,[87] and they should be taken seriously. Even if it is felt that the person who read and commented on the paper is wrong, all concerns should be addressed. If a comment is truly wrong, it may still indicate that the work was not clear in a particular area and needs some other appropriate revision to clarify the material. Changes should be made, based on the comments and completed within the time limits given.

Sometimes, however, a document may be rejected entirely. This can be for any of the following reasons:[37]

- The document is not up to standards (too much work to correct or edit).
- The idea or research the document is based on is too weak.
- The idea is inappropriate for that forum of publication.
- A similar article has been recently prepared (and possibly published) by someone else in that forum.

In the case of the first item, major revisions would be necessary before resubmitting to the boss or a journal. The second reason may also prompt major revisions, or even cause an author to stop working on the document. An article submitted to a journal but rejected for the last two reasons is not necessarily bad. It may be possible to submit it to another appropriate journal after only minor changes.

GALLEY PROOFS

A term well known to authors who have published articles or books is **galley** (or page) **proofs**. This is a final copy of the article, as it is to appear when published. It is the responsibility of the author(s) to carefully check to make sure there have been no mistakes made in typesetting. Although it may seem like a lot of work, everything must be checked, including the references, which frequently contain errors.[88-93] This step is necessary to prevent problems later. Although documents ready for distribution at work are generally not referred to as galley proofs, it is still necessary to carefully check those items.

Case Study 12–1

Your boss comes to you and lets you know that you are assigned to write a new policy and procedure for a product that is to be added to the formulary; however, the product requires specific safety precautions when administered to patients (e.g., premedication of the patient, availability of resuscitation equipment, unusual preparation for administration). This is to be available for approval at the next pharmacy and therapeutics committee meeting.

- *What are your first steps?*
- *You have progressed to the point where you have the material gathered to prepare your policy and procedure. What should be done at this stage?*
- *Once the document is written, what needs to be done next?*

Specific Documents

NEWSLETTERS AND WEBSITES

Newsletters, whether printed or electronic, have been considered to be a part of any pharmacy practice, but have probably been encountered most frequently in hospitals as a method for communicating pharmacy and therapeutics committee actions and other drug-related topics to the medical, pharmacy, nursing, and other health care provider staffs. Newsletters have also been seen from community pharmacies (addressed to patients and/or physicians),[94,95] nursing homes, drug companies, pharmacy organizations, and government or regulatory bodies. Wherever newsletters are found, their reason for existence is likely to be one or more of the following: to communicate information to a target group, advertisement, and/or compliance with legal/accreditation standards. Nowadays, the electronic versions of newsletters can provide direct links to further information and even such benefits as videos.

In many cases, newsletters are now replaced by a website. Such sites can serve the same purposes, but can also have some specific advantages and disadvantages. For example, websites take very little effort for distribution, because all they take is a computer on the Internet. Also, the material can take a greater variety of forms, including audio and video. The website can actually be used to sell products. Within institutions, the material can be kept available for health care providers to review for an indefinite time period, thereby preventing problems when somebody wants another copy of an old article or when nurses are trying to make sure they have all of the publications for an accreditation visit. In regards to disadvantages, it should be noted that consulting a website does take more effort, because it does not just fall into people's hands when they open their mailboxes. Also, there are still some people who do not use the Internet and would, therefore, not be able to consult the site.

Whatever the reason for the existence of a newsletter or website, the same set of steps generally applies to their preparation.[96-100] These steps will be covered individually in the remainder of this section.

● Define the Audience

Who will, or at least should, be reading the newsletter or accessing the website? It may be physicians, pharmacists, nurses, other health care professionals, the lay public, other groups, or some combination of these. The target group(s) will have an effect on decisions made in the other steps.

● Define the Goals

The goal can be any of the reasons mentioned previously, but generally includes informing and educating the reader, and also to report news (including changes in policies and procedures, laws, etc.). With websites, it can also be to directly sell products or gather information.

Identify Constraints

● No matter what kind of newsletter or website is produced, there are always going to be constraints that will limit what it can contain and how good it will be.

●   **Constraint 1**: Time. It seems like every year people are busier and have less time to do things that they want or need to do. This includes preparing a newsletter or keeping up a website (must be done continuously), which can take a significant amount of time if it is done right. It will be necessary to have time to write, type, edit, typeset, and perform other functions in publishing the newsletter—and all of those things have to be done in time to get the finished result to the printer, so that it can be ready for distribution on time. With a website, it is necessary to write the material, figure out the layout or organization, and prepare it on the computer. It is generally best, when beginning publication of a newsletter, to have it come out at longer intervals. If the newsletter is well received, it is found that there is enough time, and there is sufficient material, publication frequency can be increased. Overall, it is better to find it necessary to speed up publication frequency, rather than spread it out (people might get the idea the newsletter ceased publication).

    Constraint 2: Manpower. People who can, or will, be involved with publishing the newsletter or website, particularly the editor-in-chief and/or webmaster, are in short supply. This is a case where the phrase, "many hands make light work" may be applicable. If a group of dependable people are willing to work together to make sure the articles get written, the job may be easier. Generally, there are two extremely hard parts to publishing a newsletter or website, neither of which is the actual writing. One of them is coming up with topic ideas; the other is to make it look good. If others are at least willing to help here, it can be a great aid to the editor of the newsletter. If at all possible, people from all groups served by the newsletter should be asked for topics, if not entire articles. If a health professional is in charge of the newsletter or website, some other possible places for help include an institution's public relations department, if available, and clerical help (to do the typing, formatting, copying, distribution, etc.). Keep an eye on the time necessary for health professional (e.g., pharmacy, nursing) staff to produce the newsletter or website, because this is likely to be the costliest item.

- **Constraint 3**: Money. As has been said, "There is no such thing as a free lunch." This also applies to newsletters and websites. There is always some cost involved. Although personnel costs are likely to be the largest expense, the computer equipment and printing or duplication charges (for printed newsletters) can be significant. If the printing is to be done by an outside agency it is best to check on such items as the effect of order size (number of copies) and type of paper (e.g., plain versus glossy, 8½ × 11 versus 11 × 17 versus A4, colors), stapling or binding on the cost. It is preferable to get bids from at least three printers, if not done by the author's company. Another item to consider is method of delivery (e.g., personal versus first-class mail versus second-class mail). All of these items do add up and, depending on the budget, it may be necessary to sell advertising space to cover the costs.

- **Constraint 4**: Resources. It is necessary to look at what equipment or resources is available. If at all possible, the use of a high-end word processing program or desktop publishing program with a laser or inkjet printer will allow production of a high-quality, professional newsletter quicker and at a lower cost. This equipment may be all that is necessary for a website, assuming that the computer has some type of Internet connection.

Newsletter/Website Design

While it might be easy to believe substance is more important than appearance, it eventually becomes noticeable that many people do not bother looking at the substance if the appearance is poor or unprofessional. Therefore, one of the most important things is to make the publication look appealing.[101,102] People tend to throw away newsletters that look sloppy or unprofessional, and do not bother with websites that are not exciting, easy to use, and neat. Even if the publication looks good it may[103-105] or may not[106,107] have any impact on health professionals; but without looking professional it is highly unlikely to even have a chance.

A few general rules can help to make a newsletter or website more appealing. These will be covered in the remainder of this section. However, for a more in-depth look at this subject, the reader is directed to references specializing in the subject.[108,109] A particularly detailed document is available on the Internet at https://guidelines.usability.gov/.

- **Rule 1**: Keep the publication consistent. This means not only from month to month, but also from page to page. This does not mean that improvements cannot be made from time to time. Nor does it mean that each page has to look exactly like the previous one. Instead, it means that it should have its own style that is recognizable by the reader, and that the various pages must fit with one another. The easiest way to do this, with either a newsletter or website, is to create a template, style sheet, or theme (these terms overlap somewhat). Many pieces of software make this possible for either type of publication. A template is a file that contains material that appears the same from issue to issue—the term is often associated with a newsletter, although there may also be template files for websites. Examples of this can be a newsletter's/website's masthead (main heading), the listing of editors, footers at the bottom of each page, number of columns, and so on. A theme should be similar to a template, but may be used more frequently when discussing a website. Style sheets define how specific paragraphs or other parts of the newsletter or websites will look (they would often be incorporated into the template or theme). For example, a style might be called "Heading 1," and by using this style for each article's title, the look remains the same from page to page, and issue to issue. This style can include such items as what the font looks like (e.g., typeface, font size, bold, italic, underlined, superscript, subscript), and what the paragraph looks like (e.g., left justified, right justified, centered, line spacing, space before or after), in addition to other items (e.g., whether the section is to be located in a particular part of the page, borders). A style manual should be established or at least a commercially available style manual, such as the American Medical Association Manual of Style, should be used. Whatever the editor(s) establish should be reasonably simple and elegant (i.e., do not get carried away—a couple of different fonts on a page are fine, but 10 fonts look terrible).

Rule 2: Use appropriate software and equipment. A high-end word processor or desktop publishing program and a laser printer can be used.[110,111] This can allow a pharmacy to turn out a product that looks typeset at a fraction of the cost. As mentioned, there are a variety of low (or no) cost website software tools. Some are specific, whereas others are incorporated into word processors, web browsers, or other software.

Rule 3: Make the newsletter or website look good. For example, use white space properly. Do not just crowd in as much material as possible on the page. The reader will have a hard time following if it is too crowded and may just give up. Layout really is a difficult problem and requires at least a little artistic ability to do well. If lack of artistic ability is a problem, it is probably a good idea to look over other newsletters or websites from various sources to try to come up with ideas concerning what looks good. Minimally, most newsletters should at least be set up in two columns to allow easier reading. Other, more artistic, items to consider are asymmetrical layout (not having the two sides of each page look the same from a distance, perhaps using a narrow column for graphics or titles along one edge), different column widths, teasers (statements taken from the text that may pique the curiosity of the reader enough to read the article), surrounding boxes and columns with rules, and artwork/graphics.[112] The programs used to prepare either newsletters or websites can also have samples that can be used to prepare a professional looking end product.

Next on the list for newsletters or websites is to design a masthead. As mentioned, the masthead is essentially the part of the first page of the newsletter that gives the name of the publication, volume, issue, date, and so on. This may be at the top of the page or down one side of the first page. On a web page, it would be material on the home page. It is a good idea to consider having this done professionally because it is a one-time expense and can be a major factor in the appearance of the newsletter. Sometimes it is good to have a multicolored masthead that is preprinted on blank stock paper, in the case of printed newsletters. The newsletter text can then just be photocopied onto the paper and look much more professional. Material to be put into the masthead, or at least be included somewhere in the newsletter includes the newsletter or website name (be descriptive, but do not get cute—remember this is a professional publication), name and address of the pharmacy/organization, names of editor and editorial staff (give credit or blame where it is due), and frequency of publication. The name of the publication, along with some way of identifying the issue and page, should be placed on every page of the newsletter, so that the source of information can be identified if the page is photocopied or torn out.

Much of the material in a masthead should also be contained on the home page, if not every page, of a website. Again, getting professional design help, at least at first, may be of value. Also, following the guidelines of the Health on the Net Foundation Code of Conduct (http://www.hon.ch/HONcode/Conduct.html) in designing the web page is appropriate.

In general, software themes available will help create a professional looking site if professional help is not available. However, some specific items that need to be considered for a website include:[113,114]

- Provide information that is good, credible, timely, and original. Share everything possible.
- Custom tailor information to take into account user preferences.
- Break up tables for readability.
- Related to the previous item, optimize the other aspects of the page to improve download times.
- Make the page easy to read—good contrast between the text and background including the colors (remember that some people are color blind and may not be able to distinguish some colors, rendering some things unreadable), not too busy.
- Use self-generating content—make the site interactive.
- Web pages should be well organized—both the pages by themselves and how the pages are interconnected on the site.
- Consider selling things, if appropriate.
- Make sure everything works, from all likely browsers.

In designing the newsletter or website, effort should also be placed in deciding on a name. A local or institutional newsletter will often have a name related to the organization and the purpose of the newsletter. A website may be similarly named, but there is an opportunity to go farther. In this case, the Uniform Resource Locator (URL) should be considered. This is the address of the website on the intranet and/or the Internet. An institution may already have a registered URL, and the department web page may simply be under that name (e.g., http://www.yourorganizationname.org/pharmacy). However, independent community pharmacies, ambulatory clinics, physician offices, etc. can also register an unused name on the Internet and have that address (e.g., http://www.johns-pharmacy.com). There is now a .pharmacy domain available, rather than just using .com.

It has been alluded to, but it is necessary to make a very specific decision on how the newsletter is to be printed, if it will be printed. While typesetting still produces the best looking newsletter, it is quite easy to get a good looking final product using a good photocopy machine. Also, even if the department produces the original copy on its computer, the file can be taken to a service bureau that can essentially produce a typeset copy. It is necessary to determine the paper to be used (glossy paper is not going to be used if you are photocopying). Most newsletters are $8\frac{1}{2} \times 11$ inches in size, but that does not mean the paper is that size. It is better to use 11×17 paper for multipage newsletters and just fold the sheets. That looks much better than simply stapling the corner. Also, it is possible to provide an electronic storage file to some professional printers for them to print good looking final copies.

Newsletter/Web Page Content

Before getting into items that a newsletter or website should or can contain, it is necessary to discuss some general rules that deal with any article.[115]

First, it is a good idea to have a number of short articles, rather than one long article.[102,116] People will take a look at a short article and mentally decide if they have the time to read it, whereas a long article may be dismissed immediately ("If I'm going to read something that long, it will be out of New England Journal of Medicine!") or put aside to read when they have time (does house dust actually come from publications on the bottom of that "read someday" pile disintegrating from old age?). As a matter of fact, some recommend that newsletters should not exceed two pages (one sheet, front and back)[115] and one hospital cut their newsletter to one page (for P&T News) and replaced the remaining articles with a page to fit into a Drug Therapy Pocket Guide that consisted of useful tables (e.g., sodium content and neutralizing capacity of different antacids).[117] Related to the above, use catchy titles to draw the reader into reading the article right then.

Use proper writing techniques, as described earlier in this chapter. Be clear, concise, and complete—do not waste the reader's valuable time. Also, be unbiased—support the article with facts. Be positive—talk about 90% adherence, rather than 10% nonadherence.

Finally, be sure the newsletter or website is properly edited. Have multiple people read and edit the newsletter or web pages before publication. Having more people read it makes it more likely that simple mistakes will be noticed and corrected. In particular, the editors should check for spelling, grammar, and readability. Also, it is a good idea to have people from each target group as editors, particularly physicians.[118]

The actual content of a newsletter or website is one of the two most difficult areas for the editor (the other being that the newsletter should look good). Coming up with new ideas on a regular basis can be rather difficult. A list of possible areas to cover is included in Table 12-4. If at all possible, material that was prepared for a different audience can be recycled for the newsletter or website readers. For example, material from

TABLE 12–4. WEBSITE OR NEWSLETTER TOPICS[96,97,102,115]

- Adherence
- Advances in therapeutics
- Adverse drug reactions
- Calendar of events
- Clinical guidelines
- Clinical pearls
- Compliance
- Drug shortages
- Drugs withdrawn from market
- Effects of external events on jobs
- FDA warnings
- Job-related information
- New information sources
- New legal or regulatory requirements
- New services
- News from other departments
- Organization's stand on issues
- Patient safety
- Personnel policies
- Pharmacoeconomics
- Pharmacogenomics
- Pharmacy and therapeutics committee actions and news
- Productivity improvement
- Professional announcements
- Review of drugs/drug classes
- Quality assurance
- Quality improvement

the pharmacy and therapeutics committee meeting might be turned into a short review of a drug. Whenever possible, the material presented should be topics not available to the audience from another source, or material that is prepared in a format that will be of greater value to the readers than that same topic area as presented by other publications. Whatever the topics used, it is a good idea to survey the readers on a regular basis to make sure their needs are being met.

Newsletter Distribution

All of the above work will be for nothing if the readers do not get the newsletter. A good distribution system must be developed. Sometimes it can be as simple as sticking the newsletters in individual mailboxes, setting out piles of newsletters, or using intraorganizational mail systems. If it is necessary to use the post office, it would be a good idea to check on the possibility of second class or bulk mail, which can save money. More often, newsletter publications are distributed by electronic mail[119] or other computerized methods.[120] It may also be useful to distribute information with QR (Quick Response) codes that will make it easier to download information via a smartphone or tablet. Whatever method used, it is important to make sure the readers actually get the newsletter. Also, make sure they get the newsletters on a regular cycle, so that they know when to anticipate the arrival of the publication.

Case Study 12–2

Your boss comes and lets you know that you are in charge of a new website for your department.

- *What are the first steps to do?*

PRESENTATIONS

A health professional may have the opportunity to give a formal presentation at some point in a career. This could be simply where the health professional works or at a national meeting. Although it is well known that fear of public speaking is an extremely common occurrence, a speaker who prepares should do well. The problem may simply be fear of the unknown and having some simple directions may be of immense help. Overall, the main concern should be to know the topic. If someone knows enough to be asked to talk, chances are that person will know quite a bit about a topic, or will be able to learn enough about the topic. Alternately, the potential presenter may volunteer to give a presentation on an interesting topic or one in which the person has done a lot of work (e.g., a new method of practice or a new practice area). After that, most of the concern will deal with looking good. This includes a variety of items, many of which involve professional writing, and will be dealt with in the remainder of this section.

In cases where a person is asking to speak, a proposal will need to be submitted. This describes the proposed topic, which should be of interest to the target audience. The directions given by the organization preparing the meeting will need to be followed. Beyond that, the skills described earlier in this chapter and appendices will need to be used.

Next, it may be necessary to write an abstract that the organization providing the presentation forum will use to inform potential attendees about the presentation. Each organization may have a format to be followed in creating the abstract. As to what should appear in the abstract, the writer might use the information presented in Appendix 12-2. Admittedly, an abstract should usually be prepared after the presentation is done to best reflect what will be said. However, abstracts may be requested more than 6 months before the presentation, so in this case it will serve more as a planning document. It may be best to create a brief outline of the presentation (at least the topics to be covered) and then write the abstract.

Along with the abstract, it may be necessary to prepare learning objectives to describe what the attendee will be able to do as a result of participating in the program. The objectives should state that behavior in objective, measurable terms. For example, an objective may state that the attendee can explain, list, or identify something. It will not say that the attendee knows, understands, or learns, because those are not measurable. The objectives should relate directly to the program and should be adequately broken down to cover the different areas of the presentation. Refer to the beginning of any of the chapters of this book for examples of objectives. Also, refer to Bloom's Taxonomy of Educational Objectives and Appropriate Verbs for more details.[121] Also, this information could be used for objectives written for other documents.[122]

Occasionally, the presenter may be requested to provide self-assessment questions. Often these will be multiple choice or true/false, to simplify assessment. Those questions should be clearly stated and measure that the attendee has met the objectives. Efforts should be made to make the questions clear. Also, they should avoid the use of NOT or EXCEPT because these terms can lead to confusion. Writing good questions can be extremely difficult, so testing the questions out on others before the presentation may help improve the quality.

The speaker may also have to prepare a brief biography to be used in the introduction. This includes a few items about the speaker's background, such as title and current position. Also, some information that gives the audience an idea of why the speaker is qualified to make a presentation is useful.

Presentations can usually be broken down into platform or poster presentations. The former is a more formal, oral presentation that typically requires some sort of audiovisual component and is often presented in a room set up for an audience. The latter requires the presenter to place a summary of the material to be presented on a poster (or series of small posters) that will be displayed on a bulletin board–type display (usually provided by the organization) that will be three to four feet high and six to eight feet wide. In that situation, the attendees can walk through a group of such presentations, stopping to look at any that appeal to them and ask the presenter questions. Also, a QR code on the poster may allow the attendee to download further information or the poster itself using a smartphone or tablet.

Many of the rules described in the main part of this chapter relate to preparing the information to be presented, including slides, posters, and other audiovisual materials. However, a few other rules need to be mentioned:

- The presenter should learn the circumstances under which the presentation is to be given. That includes whether it is a platform or poster presentation.
- The presenter should learn what equipment is to be provided (e.g., computer projector, microphone, size of board for poster presentation).
- If the presenter needs other items, they should be made clear to the organization. For example, it is common for presenters to want to use computer projection equipment, which may present certain technical requirements for both the equipment and support people. Also, the presenter may need such things as power outlet strips, extension cords, wireless microphones (many good speakers prefer to move about on the stage or in the audience and are frustrated by a podium microphone that requires them to stand in one place behind a podium), Internet connection, connections from a computer to the room sound system, Bluetooth®, USB connection, DVD player, cables, device to advance slides, audience response systems, and other items. The presenter's own needs and desires should be taken into account, in addition to those of the audience's. It is necessary to be very specific, since the people organizing the meeting may not understand the requirements. For example, a speaker requesting an Internet connection may arrive to find a connection that is too slow or one that has security restrictions preventing access to necessary Internet sites. Also, even the resolution of a computer projector or type of connector for a network may need to be specified.
- If the speaker is doing a poster presentation, it is necessary to remember to bring pushpins to mount the poster on the provided display board.
- The audience should be taken into account. One common complaint when a speaker flies in for a presentation is that they may not know anything about local circumstances, including simple social skills that are expected (e.g., foreign

countries). It is best if the speaker tries to find out more about the audience and the situation, adjusting the presentation to take those items into account.[123]

- If necessary, the setup of the room should be specified (e.g., theater style, discussion tables, screen placement).

All of the above should be double checked at the location of the presentation after arrival, but in plenty of time to correct any problems. Speakers may also want to take advantage of a Speaker Ready Room that many organizations offer to check out slides, etc. As a side note, checking in with those arranging the presentation is necessary so that they will not be worried about your arrival and they will be able to clear up any last minute items.

The speaker then needs to prepare the presentation, doing appropriate research and preparation, using skills described earlier in this chapter and in the following sections. The presentation should also be rehearsed adequately. The next steps will discuss preparation of audiovisual materials, which can enhance the audience's ability to understand and retain the material.[124,125]

Platform Presentations

When giving platform presentations, it is usually necessary to prepare audiovisual materials and, possibly, handouts. Most office software suites (e.g., Microsoft Office, Google Docs) have very powerful tools to create slides and other materials. These also have professionally designed templates that provide good layouts for materials, including color and background choices. The programs may also guide the user to follow general rules, such as avoiding a busy slide that will be unreadable from the back of a large room.[126] Also, the programs can be used to do everything from creating simple slides to multimedia extravaganzas—the former being learned in a few minutes, with the more advanced features available for those who need or desire them. Be aware, however, that it is necessary to use only those features that truly add to the presentation and to avoid having fancy effects in slides just for the sake of the effects.[126] ❻ *Instead of concentrating on the technology, it is best to concentrate on the message.*[127] This will also have the advantage of having fewer things that might go wrong in a presentation.

When starting to prepare audiovisuals, it is necessary to determine what type of equipment and situation will be found at the presentation. The most desirable type of audiovisual is the use of a computer with a projector and appropriate software to give the presentation. It is also possible to project slides from a smartphone or tablet (e.g., Android or iPad) that is properly equipped,[128] although the presentation may not be able to use some advanced features, such as the embedding of multimedia items.[129] When information or software is available on the Internet, it can be demonstrated. Also, in cases where a discussion ensues, it is possible for the presenter to use a word processor, presentation program, or other software to record items on the screen for users to read during or after the session. It is even possible to not only record the information on the screen during the presentation, but to also make it immediately available on the Internet at the end of the program, including audio and video. Some disadvantages include the cost of the equipment for the organizing group, the need for greater technical skills by both the presenter and organizing group, the potential for technological problems (e.g., a computer that refuses to boot, corrupted data, an Internet connection that does not work), and it may be necessary for the presenter to bring a notebook computer with appropriate software and data. Fortunately, the technical support people for professional meetings are familiar with the equipment and the equipment itself is often more dependable.

When preparing the slides themselves, the presenter will have to prepare an outline to guide what is to be presented and determine the information to be presented in each slide. Some general rules can be mentioned:

1. Start with an introduction that explains and gives an overview of what will be learned.[130]
2. Limit each slide to a particular topic. Sometimes this will be an **overview**, but specifics should be limited to a discrete topic. One or two minutes of presentation material per slide is appropriate. If it is necessary to refer back to a previous slide, just make a duplicate that is inserted at the appropriate location.
3. Be sure to reach a conclusion that summarizes the information, rather than just having an abrupt end.[130]
4. Keep things simple. The program may be able to do many things (e.g., 20 fonts in 16 million colors), but they may not be desirable. Typically use one font (perhaps with bold or underline in a few specific places for emphasis) and limited graphics.
5. Limit the amount of information presented on each slide.[126] A rule of thumb is no more than about five bulleted points per slide and no more than about five words per bulleted point. Any more than that quickly becomes confusing or unreadable. Generally, if someone in the back of the room has to squint or it takes more than 10 seconds to read a slide, there is too much information on it.[131] It has been theorized that a portion of the blame for the loss of the space shuttle, Columbia, was due to the information necessary for National Aeronautics and Space Administration (NASA) engineers being hidden in small print on an extremely busy slide.[132] While the consequences for most presentations are not nearly as large, it is still important that slides enhance the provision of the appropriate information, rather than obscure it.
6. Use a sans-serif font, such as Arial.
7. Consider using a theme in the program that will provide colors that go together well and contrast enough to be legible. Colors and color combinations have to be

carefully considered because they may have emotional overtones or, in cases of color-blind attendees, may not even be distinguishable.[133]

8. Consider graphics. They can make the slide more pleasing to the eye, but they also need to be as simple as possible. If cartoons are included to entertain the audience, make sure they are related to the talk and, preferably, help to make a point. Also, pictures of landscapes or the presenter's institution may be desired by the presenter, but serve only to distract from the presentation and should be avoided. Remember that if copyrighted material is to be used, it is necessary to get permission to reproduce the material.

9. Consider embedding sound or video in the presentation, if it adds to the presentation. That sounds difficult, but may be done with a few clicks of the mouse. It will be necessary in this case to make sure the computer for the presentation is connected to the room's sound system so that attendees can hear the audio.

10. Embed links to appropriate websites in the presentation. This can be particularly useful if an electronic version of the handout is provided to attendees.

11. Save the presentation in several ways. Even if it is on the computer hard drive, it may become corrupted or the computer can break. Perhaps also bring it on a USB drive so that someone else's computer can be borrowed if necessary. It is often useful to consider burning the presentation to a recordable (or read/write) CD-ROM or DVD, which will not be sensitive to magnetic fields that might have affected the original disk. Also, in case the computer to be used in the presentation does not have presentation software, it might be necessary to use the feature in many presentation software packages that creates a run-time presentation that does not require the actual software. In some cases, putting the slides on a web server in presentation format may work, although accessing the slides and web pages over the Internet can be a risky proposition. Also, as mentioned previously, the presentation might be given using a smartphone or tablet device.

Other items to consider include the following:

- Make sure to carry the presentation materials personally and do not check them as luggage, since they may be lost. Also, be careful not to damage the materials being carried.

- Make the presentation interactive—ask the audience questions and take input, or have the audience work on some project during the presentation. This is now a requirement of continuing education programs and will help the audience retain the information being presented.

- In all but a very small room, be sure to use the microphone. Speakers may not want to be bothered or may feel it is a sign of weakness to use a microphone, but they need to remember that the microphone is there to help the audience, not the speaker, and should be used so that everyone in the back of the room can hear over the ventilation system, etc.

- Keep to the slides, if at all possible, but do not read the slides—use the slides as speaking points for the oral presentation information and to organize your thoughts.[126] However, a speaker who simply reads the slides to the audience will likely be perceived as both unknowledgeable about the subject and boring.
- Do not read a prepared script, unless it is considered to be the norm in a particular environment. Actors and politicians can read such scripts and sound natural, but most speakers cannot do so. Instead use the slides (preferable) or a simple outline. The presentation program will allow easy preparation of handouts and speakers notes that can be used.
- Consider the delivery of the material, including pitch, power, pace, poise, and confidence.[134]
- Be prepared for technological disaster.[127] Even when using something as simple as a projector, the bulb can burn out. When using more equipment and more complex equipment, the potential for equipment failure rapidly increases. Whenever possible, have backup equipment, but also have a backup plan so that the presentation can proceed without any equipment. Just making sure to have a printed copy of the slides can save a presentation.
- Dress professionally.
- Be sure to make eye contact with the audience and be cheerful.
- Avoid distracting the audience with unnecessary words (e.g., um, like) or unnecessary body movements (e.g., rocking, tapping, rubbing hands) although do be sure to move around if at all possible and do not hide behind the podium.

It may be desirable to prepare a handout for the audience, in which case, the presenter can consider the following styles:[135]

- *Outline*—a reference document that gives the audience a guide to where the speaker is going in text form. This can often be prepared by importing the slide content from the presentation software to a word processor. Some presentation programs will also prepare the document itself.
- *Full text handout*—this is essentially a transcription of the speech. While helpful as a reference document, it is probably of more use to politicians when they wish to avoid being misquoted. This is seldom seen in the health care field because the presenter will not be able to make last minute changes and the audience will likely read ahead and become bored. Interestingly, a comment heard when such documents are presented is that the speaker did not know the material, because all the

person did was read the handout, even though the speaker was the one who wrote it!

- *Slide reproduction*—this is becoming more popular and easy; presentation programs allow easy slide handout preparation. This does give the attendee all of the information, including graphics, but will likely require more paper.
- *Partial text handout*—this can be something of a combination of the above, where only a portion of the presentation is on the handout.

In any of the above, it is good to consider the following:[135]

- Consider whether it is necessary to provide references or supplemental readings.
- Make sure the handout follows the order of the presentation. If it does not, the attendee may become confused and annoyed.
- Make it look good, using skills mentioned elsewhere in this chapter. By all means, allow plenty of room for the attendee to take notes.

The speaker may also use the handout as a set of speaker notes, but care should generally be taken to avoid just reading the handout to the audience, except in the case of full text handouts, for the reasons previously mentioned.

The skills necessary to give the presentation itself are beyond the scope of this chapter that deals with the preparation and distribution of written material. New presenters may wish to read a book or pamphlet on how to give effective talks. Also, Toastmasters International (http://www.toastmasters.org) is a group that will help individuals develop their speaking skills. Many organizations have a chapter of this organization. These aids will provide guidance on such skills as what level of sophistication to use in speaking, how to stand (e.g., do not hide behind the podium, make eye contact), what language to use, how to use humor and other techniques to entertain the audience, how to address questions (including so-called sniper questions that tend to disrupt speakers due to level of difficulty and how they are thrown into the middle of the presentation),[136] how to avoid distractions by having everyone turn off phones and pagers,[137] and so forth. Also, some of the references used in preparation of this chapter provide many additional suggestions.[124,135]

Poster Presentations

Preparing a poster requires the presenter to first determine what is to be included. Typically, the information will be similar to that found in an abstract, but with an expansion of the various sections. There are likely to be tables, bulleted points, and figures. Overall, the information to be presented must be brief, so that it can be read within a couple of minutes by an individual passing by the display. Therefore, large amounts of text are undesirable. A poster presentation will not likely contain nearly as much information as a formal journal article, but will contain many of the same sections. It will serve as a place for discussion to begin between the presenter and interested individuals.

Preparing posters was at one time a very difficult prospect. This has changed with the availability of presentation and high-end word processing/publishing software on computers. A large, one-piece poster that is typically about three by six feet may be made using this software. Although the final poster must be printed by a graphics firm (e.g., printer, architectural drawing firm), the cost can be reasonable to produce a very good looking poster. This may also be done over the Internet. The initial preparatory work can also be done by various firms, but it is less expensive to do this yourself. The software necessary would be either desktop publishing software (e.g., Adobe® PageMaker, Microsoft Publisher, and Microsoft PowerPoint) or a high-end word processor (e.g., Microsoft Word). Essentially, what needs to be done is to lay out the page in these programs so that it is in landscape format (i.e., sideways from the normal typed page). The top of the page will have a centered title in large print, with the author names, institution, city, and so on centered in a smaller font below the title. Often, it is desirable to place graphics to one or both sides of that information, such as the symbol(s) for the authors' institution(s). Under that, the page may be divided up into three or so columns and the information laid out in a logical order, including tables and figures, which generally read from top to bottom and left to right. It may be desirable, once finished, to print out the final copy. One can produce a copy that fits on typical 8½ × 11 inch paper that can be reproduced and distributed to interested individuals at the meeting. It may also be on larger paper (e.g., 11 × 17 inch), if there is a suitable high-quality printer available.

Some general suggestions for posters include:[138]

- Limit number of full sentences
- Use appropriate white space
- Text should be no less than 24 point
- Use a serif font (e.g., Times New Roman)
- Graphics at least 150 dpi
- Include a QR code that allows downloading of a copy of the poster or further information

Whatever method is used, the final product will need to be transported to the meeting (poster tubes are available for little or no cost from many graphics firms). It is preferable to carry such posters on airplanes, rather than to check them, because they may be crushed in the baggage areas or lost. It is also possible to have the printer send the poster directly to the location of the presentation, although this would preclude the possibility of checking it ahead of time. The presenter should also remember to bring pushpins to mount the presentation at the meeting and business cards to give to anyone requesting them. The presenter should show up early enough for the presentation to have the material mounted to the bulletin board before meeting attendees are allowed in the area and will be expected to remain with the presentation to answer questions for the assigned time. Although many people may be the authors of a presentation, it is not uncommon that only one or two actually attend the meeting and give the presentation.

Web Posting

After a presentation, consider making the material available on the Internet. Some organizations make at least some presentation materials available that way. Of course, copyright restrictions may prevent individuals from posting the material, but technology makes it easy when it is allowable. Text documents or graphic images, such as posters, are easily placed on a website. However, even full slide presentations can be placed on a website, using streaming audiovisual. A variety of software can be used to prepare such streaming presentations that can include slides and an audiovisual recording of the presenter. This can even be done concurrently with the presentation (live streaming), with a recording being made for later viewing. The equipment needs are relatively minor (i.e., computer, presentation software, microphone, inexpensive computer video capture device). For the actual Internet streaming, the appropriate streaming software, running on a file server, is necessary. For those who do not have the appropriate streaming software, just placing the slides themselves, as a downloadable file or in presentation format, can be an easy process using the original software used to prepare the slides. Even the simplest website can then be used to give access to the material.

Case Study 12–3

You are preparing a platform presentation for a national professional meeting for the first time.

- *What are some things that should be considered in slide preparation?*

Conclusion

● ❼ *Professional writing is a skill necessary for every health professional.* It simply consists of following the accepted rules for writing that have been established by the profession to prepare a written item that is clear, concise, complete, correct, and in the appropriate format.

Self-Assessment Questions

1. Which of the following items are considered to be a type of professional writing?
   a. An article published in a professional journal
   b. A budget report
   c. A label for a prescription vial
   d. A performance evaluation of a new technician
   e. All of the above

2. Which of the following is considered to be necessary for credit as an author?
   a. Writing or revising article
   b. Conception and design of the study
   c. Final approval of the version published
   d. Accountability for all aspects of the work
   e. All of the above are necessary

3. When writing a document that is intended for an audience of pharmacists, which style of writing should be employed?
   a. Pure technical style
   b. Middle technical style
   c. Popular technical style

4. Which guideline tends to be used the most in writing for medical and pharmacy journals?
   a. American Medical Association Manual of Style
   b. MLA Handbook for Writers of Research Papers
   c. Publication Manual of the American Psychiatric Association (APA)
   d. Scientific Style and Format: The CBE Manual for Authors, Editors, and Publishers
   e. Recommendations for the Conduct, Reporting, Editing, and Publication of Scholarly Work in Medical Journals

5. It is necessary to only define unusual abbreviations in a document, since nearly every reader will understand common abbreviations, such as the use of AIDS for acquired immunodeficiency syndrome.
   a. True
   b. False

6. When writing a document, it is not necessary to provide a citation to a source like Wikipedia, since that is not a refereed publication.
   a. True
   b. False

7. In most cases, when writing up an answer to a question for another health care practitioner, the first paragraph of the paper should contain the summary of the information contained in the body to make things simpler and faster to read.
    a. True
    b. False

8. Copyright violations and plagiarism are not the same. It is possible to commit one while avoiding the other.
    a. True
    b. False

9. Health on the Net Foundation provides what?
    a. A Code of Conduct for websites
    b. A web hosting site for medically related websites
    c. General drug information references
    d. b and c
    e. All of the above

10. Which of the following is an appropriate objective for a presentation? The attendee will:
    a. List the steps for preparation of the intravenous form of drug X
    b. Know the steps for preparation of the intravenous form of drug X
    c. Learn the steps for preparation of the intravenous form of drug X
    d. Understand the steps for preparation of the intravenous form of drug X
    e. None of the above are appropriate

11. When preparing slides for presentations, it is best to provide as many details on each slide as possible, even if the font has to be smaller than normal.
    a. True
    b. False

12. You are going to provide a one hour CE presentation. How many slides should you likely be preparing?
    a. 10
    b. 50
    c. 100
    d. 150

13. Which of the following is true when giving a presentation?
    a. It is best to avoid the use of a microphone, if possible, since most people do not know how to use them for the best effect and they are just another technology

that may fail. Most of the time the speaker can just raise his or her voice so that everyone can hear.

b. Microphones are placed in a room for the convenience of the audience, not the presenter. If there is a microphone present, the speaker should always use it.

c. Ask the audience whether you should use the microphone.

14. Presentation handouts should:
   a. Follow the order of the presentation
   b. Provide the full text of the speech
   c. Supplement, but not replace the presentation
   d. a and c
   e. All of the above

15. It is necessary to always send an article proposal to a publisher, prior to sending in an article.
   a. True
   b. False

REFERENCES

1. Kelley KW, Liles AM. Writing letters of recommendation: where should you start? Am J Health Syst Pharm. 2012;69:563-5.
2. Thordsen DJ. Preparing an article for publication. J Pharm Technol. 1986;Nov/Dec:268-75.
3. Generali JA. Why publish? Hosp Pharm. 2008;43(11):868.
4. Moghadam RG. Scientific writing: a career for pharmacists. Am J Health Syst Pharm. 2003 Sept 15;60:1899-900.
5. Armbruster DL. Starting the writing process. J Pediatr Pharmacol Ther. 2003;8(3): 210-1.
6. Fye WB. Medical authorship: traditions, trends, and tribulations. Ann Intern Med. 1990;113: 317-25.
7. Gannon F. Ethical profits from publishing. EMBO Rep. 2004;5(1):1.
8. Nahata MC. Publishing by pharmacists. DICP Ann Pharmacother. 1989;23:809-10.
9. Wager E, Field EA, Grossman L. Good publication practice for pharmaceutical companies. Curr Med Res Opin. 2003;19(3):149-54.
10. Morris CT, Hatton RC, Kimberlin CL. Factors associated with the publication of scholarly articles by pharmacists. Am J Health Syst Pharm. 2011;68:1640-5.
11. Dotson B, Slaughter RL. Prevalence of articles with honorary and ghost authors in three pharmacy journals. Am J Health Syst Pharm. 2011;68:1730-4.
12. Sadler TR. Publishing in academia: woes of authorship, figures, and peer review. Drug Inf J. 2011;45:145-50.
13. Wilcox LJ. Authorship: the coin of the realm, the source of complaints. JAMA. 1998;280:216-7.

14. Hoen WP, Walvoort HC, Overbeke AJ. What are the factors determining authorship and the order of the authors' names? A study among authors of the Nederlands. Tijdschrift voor Geneeskunde. 1998;280:217-8.

15. Zoog HB, Chang T. Interpretation and implementation of good publication practice. Drug Inf J. 2011;45:137-44.

16. Committee on Publication Ethics (COPE). Guidelines on good publication practice. COPE Report. 2002:48-52.

17. Shapiro DW, Wenger NS, Shapiro MF. The contributions of authors to multiauthored biomedical research papers. JAMA. 1994;271:438-42.

18. Flanagin A, Carey LA, Fontanarosa PB, Phillips SG, Pace BP, Lundberg GD, Rennie D. Prevalence of articles with honorary authors and ghost authors in peer-reviewed medical journals. JAMA. 1998;280:222-4.

19. Wager E. Raising the quality of publications: now we have GPP! Qual Assur J. 2003;7: 166-70.

20. Peterson AM, Lowenthal W, Veatch RM. Authorship on a manuscript intended for publication. Am J Hosp Pharm. 1993;50:2082-5.

21. Carbone PP. On authorship and acknowledgments. NEJM. 1992;326:1084.

22. Hart RG. On authorship and acknowledgments. NEJM. 1992;326:1084.

23. Pinching AJ. On authorship and acknowledgments. NEJM. 1992;326:1084-5.

24. Canter D. On authorship and acknowledgments. NEJM. 1992;326:1085.

25. Rennie D, Yank V, Emanuel L. When authorship fails. A proposal to make contributors accountable. JAMA. 1997;278:579-85.

26. Fathalla MF, VanLook PF. On authorship and acknowledgments. NEJM. 1992;326:1085.

27. The International Committee of Medical Journal Editors. Statement from the International Committee of Medical Journal Editors. JAMA. 1991;265:2697-8.

28. Hasegawa GR. Spurious authorship. Am J Hosp Pharm. 1993;50:2063.

29. Rennie D, Flanagin A. Authorship! Authorship! Guests, ghosts, grafters, and the two-sided coin. JAMA. 1994;271:469-71.

30. International Committee of Medical Journal Editors. Recommendations for the conduct, reporting, editing, and publication of scholarly work in medical journals [Internet]. International Committee of Medical Journal Editors; 2015 Dec [cited 2016 Jun 22]. Available from: http://icmje.org/icmje-recommendations.pdf

31. International Committee of Medical Journal Editors. Uniform requirements for manuscripts submitted to biomedical journals: writing and editing for biomedical publication [Internet]. Philadelphia, PA: International Committee of Medical Journal Editors. 2009 Nov [cited 2010 Nov 16]. Available from: http://www.icmje.org/index.html

32. Kassirer JP, Angell M. On authorship and acknowledgments. NEJM. 1991;325:1510-2.

33. Drenth JPH. Multiple authorship. The contribution of senior authors. JAMA. 1998;280:219-21.

34. Kassirer JP, Angell M. On authorship and acknowledgments. NEJM. 1992;326:1085.

35. Foote MA. Medical writing: looking back, moving forward. Drug Inf J. 2011;45:121-3.

36. Foote MA. How to write a better manuscript. Drug Inf J. 2009;43:111-4.

37. McConnell CR. From idea to print: writing and publishing a journal article. Health Care Superv. 1984;2:78-94.

38. Burnakis TG. Advice on submitting papers. Am J Hosp Pharm. 1993;50:2523.

39. Higa GM. Scientific publications and scientific style. W V Med J. 1995;91:198-9.

40. Crichton M. Medical obfuscation: structure and function. NEJM. 1975;293:1257-9.

41. Jones DE. Last word. Omni. 1980;2(12):130.

42. Hamilton CW. How to write effective business letters: scribing information for pharmacists. Hosp Pharm. 1993;28:1095-100.

43. Albert T. The fear of writing—it's not as hard as pharmacists seem to think. Pharmaceut J. 2003 Jan 11;270:55-6.

44. Tsukayama H. How to write emails if you want people to actually respond. The Washington Post [Internet]. 2016 Feb 16 [cited 2016 Jun 22]. Available from: http://washington post.com/news/the-switch/wp/2016/02/16/want-to-get-more-responses-for-your-emails-write-like-a-third-grader/.

45. Baker SJ. Getting published. Aust J Hosp Pharm. 1994;24(5):410-5.

46. Hamilton CW. How to write and publish scientific papers: scribing information for pharmacists. Am J Hosp Pharm. 1992;49:2477-84.

47. Guo J. Sorry, grammar nerds. The singular 'they' has been declared Word of the Year. The Washington Post [Internet]. 2016 Jan 8 [cited 2016 Jun 22]. Available from: http://www.washington post.com/news/wonk/wp/2016/01/08/donald-trump-may-win-this-years-word-of-the-year/.

48. Ingelfinger FJ. Seduction by citation. NEJM. 1976;295:1075-6.

49. Roederer M, Marciniak MW, O'Connor SK, Eckel SF. An integrated approach to research and manuscript development. Am J Health Syst Pharm. 2013 Jul 15;70:1211-8.

50. Sollaci LB, Pereira MG. The introduction, methods, results and discussion (IMRAD) structure: a fifty-year survey. J Med Libr Assoc. 2004;92(3):364-7.

51. Schulz F, Altman DG, Moher D. CONSORT 2010 statement: updated guidelines for reporting parallel group randomized trials. Ann Intern Med. 2010;152(11):1-7.

52. Moher D, Hopewell S, Schulz KF, Montori V, Gøtzsche PC, Devereaux PJ, Elbourne D, Egger M, Altman DG, for the CONSORT Group. CONSORT 2010 explanation and elaboration: updated guidelines for reporting parallel group randomized trials. BMJ. 2010;340:c869. doi:10.1136/bmj.c869.

53. Campbell MK, Elbourne DR, Altman DG, for the CONSORT Group. CONSORT Statement: extension to cluster randomized trials. BMJ. 2004;328:702-8.

54. Piaggio G, Elbourne DR, Altman DG, Pocock SJ, Evans SJ, CONSORT Group. Reporting of noninferiority and equivalence randomized trials. An extension of the CONSORT Statement. JAMA. 2006;295:1152-60.

55. Gagnier JJ, Boon H, Rochon P, Moher D, Barnes J, Bombardier C, CONSORT Group. Reporting randomized, controlled trials of herbal interventions: an elaborated CONSORT Statement. Ann Intern Med. 2006;144:364-7.

56. Boutron I, Moher D, Altman DG, Schulz KF, Ravaud P, for the CONSORT Group. Methods and processes of the CONSORT Group: example of an extension for trials assessing non-pharmacologic treatments. Ann Intern Med. 2008;148:W60-W66.

57. Ioannidis JP, Evans SJ, Gøtzsche PC, O'Neill RT, Altman DG, Schulz K, Moher D, CONSORT Group. Better reporting of harms in randomized trials: an extension of the CONSORT Statement. Ann Intern Med. 2004;141:781-8.

58. Hopewell S, Clarke M, Moher D, Wager E, Middleton P, Altman DG, Schulz KF, CONSORT Group. CONSORT for reporting randomized controlled trials and conference abstracts: explanation and elaboration. PLoS Med. 2008;5(1):e20. doi:10.1371/journal.pmed.0050020.

59. von Elm E, Altman DG, Egger M, Pocock SJ, Gøtzsche PC, Vandenbroucke JP, STROBE Initiative. The Strengthening the Reporting of Observational Studies in Epidemiology (STROBE) Statement: guidelines for reporting observational studies. Ann Intern Med. 2007;147:573-7.

60. Vandenbroucke JP, von Elm E, Altman DG, Gøtzsche PC, Mulrow CD, Pocock SJ, Poole C; Schlesselman JJ, Egger M, STROBE initiative. Strengthening the Reporting of Observational Studies in Epidemiology (STROBE): explanation and elaboration. Ann Intern Med. 2007;147:W163-W194.

61. Zwarenstein M, Treweek S, Gagnier JJ, Altman DG, Tunis S, Haynes B, Oxman AD; Moher D, CONSORT group. Improving the reporting of pragmatic trials: an extension of the CONSORT Statement. BMJ. 2008;227:a2390. doi:10.1136/bmj.a2390.

62. Moher D, Cook DJ, Eastwood S, Olkin I, Rennie D, Stroup DF. Improving the quality of reports of meta-analyses of randomised controlled trials: the QUOROM statement. Lancet. 1999;354:1896-900.

63. Moher D, Liberati A, Tetzlaff J, Altman DG. The PRISMA Group (2009) preferred reporting items for systematic reviews and meta-analyses. The PRISMA Statement. PLoS Med. 2009;6(7):e1000097. doi:10.1371/journal.pmed.1000097.

64. Graf C, Battisti WP, Bridges D, Bruce-Winkler V, Conaty JM, Ellison JM, Field EA, Gurr JA, Marx ME, Patel M, Sanes-Miller C, Yarker YE, International Society for Medical Publication Professionals. Good publication practice for communicating company sponsored medical research: the GPP2 guidelines. BMJ. 2009;339:b4330. doi:10:10.1136/bmj.b4330.

65. Talley CR. Perspective in journal publishing. Am J Hosp Pharm. 1993;50:451.

66. LaRochelle JM, King AR. Avoiding plagiarism. Hosp Pharm. 2011;46(12):917-9.

67. Gabriel T. Plagiarism lines blur for students in digital age. The New York Times. 2010 Aug 1 [cited 2010 Aug 2]:[4 p.]. Available from http://www.nytimes.com/2010/08/02/education/02cheat.html?_r=1&scp=1&sq=plagiarism%20lines%20blur&st=cse

68. Turnitin.com [Internet]. Oakland, CA: iParadigms, LLC; c1998-2012. Plagiarism and the web: a comparison of internet sources for secondary and higher education students; 2011 [cited 2012 Jun 13]:[about 10 p.]. Available from: http://pages.turnitin.com/rs/iparadigms/images/Turnitin_WhitePaper_SourcesSECvsHE.pdf

69. Mapes D. Net's plagiarism 'cops' are on patrol. MSNBC [Internet]. 2009 Sept 10 [cited 2009 Sept 11]:[3 p.]. Available from: http://www.msnbc.msn.com/id/32657885/ns/technology_and_science-tech_and_gadgets/.

70. Ware J. Cheat wave. Yahoo! Internet Life. 1999;5(5):102-3.

71. Stuber-McEwen D, Wiseley P, Hoggatt S. Point, click, and cheat: frequency and type of academic dishonesty in the virtual classroom. Online J Dist Learning Admin. 2009 Fall [cited 2009 Sept 17];XII(III):[10 p.]. Available from: http://www.westga.edu/~distance/ojdla/fall123/stuber123.html

72. Asimov I. Gold: the final science fiction collection. New York, NY: HarperPrism; 1995.

73. Willful infringement. [cited 2004 Aug 9]. Available from: http://www.willfulinfringement.com/.

74. Ardito SC, Eiblum P, Daulong R. Conflicted copy rights. Online. 1999 May/June:23(3):91-5.

75. Crawford M. Are you committing plagiarism? Top five overlooked citations to add to your course materials [Internet]. Message to: Patrick M. Malone. 2010 Sept 29:[4 p.].

76. Gousse G. Advice on submitting papers: I. Am J Hosp Pharm. 1993;50:2523.

77. World Association of Medical Editors. WAME policy statements [Internet]. Chicago, IL: World Association of Medical Editors; 2004 Apr 7 [cited 2004 Apr 14]. Available from: http://www.wame.org/policies-and-resources

78. International Committee of Medical Journal Editors. Conflict of interest. Am J Hosp Pharm. 1993;50:2398.

79. Davidoff F, DeAngelis CD, Drazen JM, Hoey J, Højgaard L, Horton R, Kotzin S, Nylenna M, Overbeke AJ, Sox HC, Van Der Weyden MB, Wilkes MS, International Committee of Medical Journal Editors. Sponsorship, authorship, and accountability. Lancet. 2001 Sept 15;358:854-6.

80. Krimsky S, Rothenberg LS. Financial interest and its disclosure in scientific publications. JAMA. 1998;280:225-6.

81. Laniado M. How to present research data consistently in a scientific paper. Eur Radiol. 1996;6:S16-8.

82. DeAngelis CD. Duplicate publication, multiple problems. JAMA. 2004;292:1745-6.

83. Stead WW. The responsibilities of authorship. J Am Med Inform Assoc. 1997;4:394-5.

84. Hasegawa GR. How to review a manuscript intended for publication. Am J Hosp Pharm. 1994;51:839-40.

85. Hoppe S, Chandler MJJ. Constructive versus destructive criticism. Am J Health Syst Pharm. 1995;52:103.

86. Baker DE. Peer review: personal continuous quality improvement. Hosp Pharm. 2004;39:8.

87. Garfunkel JM, Lawson EE, Hamrick HJ, Ulshen MH. Effect of acceptance or rejection on the author's evaluation of peer review of medical manuscripts. JAMA. 1990;263:1376-8.

88. Evans JT, Nadjari HI, Burchell SA. Quotation and reference accuracy in surgical journals. JAMA. 1990;263:1353-4.

89. Roland CG. Thoughts about medical writing. XXXVII. Verify your references. Anesth Analg. 1976;55:717-8.

90. Biebuyck JF. Concerning the ethics and accuracy of scientific citations. J Anesthesiol. 1992;77:1-2.

91. McLellan MF, Case LD, Barnett MC. Trust, but verify. The accuracy of references in four anesthesia journals. Anesthesiology. 1992;77:185-8.

92. de Lacy G, Record C, Wade J. How accurate are quotations and references in medical journals. BMJ. 1985;291:884-6.

93. Doms CA. A survey of reference accuracy in five national dental journals. J Dent Res. 1989;68:442-4.
94. Seltzer SM. Desktop publishing in a drug store? Am Druggist. 1987;196:64, 66.
95. Srnka QM, Scoggin JA. 10 ways to distribute newsletters to build sales volume. Pharm Times. 1984;50:71-2, 74.
96. Making the media. The pharmacy newsletter. Hosp Pharm Connection. 1986;2(3):11-2.
97. Kaldy J. Effectively creating a pharmacy newsletter. Consult Pharm. 1992;7(6):697-8, 700.
98. Goldwater SH, Haydon-Greatting S. How to publish a pharmacy newsletter. Am J Hosp Pharm. 1991;48:2121, 2125.
99. Almquist AF, Wolfgang AP, Perri M. Pharmacy newsletters—the journalistic approach. Hosp Pharm. 1988;23:974-5.
100. Schultz WL, Dendiak ST. Pharmacy newsletters: a needed service. Hosp Pharm. 1975;10(4):146-7.
101. Plumridge RJ, Berbatis CG. Drug bulletins: effectiveness in modifying prescribing and methods of improving impact. DICP Ann Pharmacother. 1989;23:330-4.
102. Appearance and content attract newsletter audience. Drug Utilization Review. 1988;4(4):45-8.
103. Lyon RA, Norvell MJ. Effect of a P&T Committee newsletter on anti-infective prescribing habits. Hosp Formul. 1985;20:742-4.
104. Fendler KJ, Gumbhir AK, Sall K. The impact of drug bulletins on physician prescribing habits in a health maintenance organization. Drug Intell Clin Pharm. 1984;18:627-31.
105. May JR, Andrusko KT, DiPiro JT. Impact and cost justification of a surgery drug newsletter. Am J Hosp Pharm. 1984;41:1837-9.
106. Ross MB, Volger BW, Bradley JK. Use of "dispense-as-written" on prescriptions for targeted drugs: influence of a newsletter. Am J Hosp Pharm. 1990;47:2519-20.
107. Denig P, Haaijer-Ruskamp FM, Zijsling DH. Impact of a drug bulletin on the knowledge, perception of drug utility, and prescribing behavior of physicians. DICP Ann Pharmacother. 1990;24:87-93.
108. Parker RC. Looking good in print. 4th ed. Scotsdale, AZ: The Coriolis Group, LLC; 1998.
109. Baird RN, McDonald D, Pittman RK, Turnbull AT. The graphics of communication. Methods, media and technology. 6th ed. New York, NY: Hartcourt Brace Jovanovich College Publishers; 1993.
110. Don't let cost prohibit publication of pharmacy-related newsletter. Drug Utilization Review. 1988;4(4):48-9.
111. Utt JK, Lewis KT. Using desktop publishing to enhance pharmacy publications. Am J Hosp Pharm. 1988;45:1863-4.
112. Pfeiffer KS. Award-winning newsletter design. Windows Mag. 1994;5(8):208-18.
113. What makes a great web site? [cited 1999 May 13]:[1 screen]. Available from: http://www.webreference.com/greatsite.html
114. Tweney D. Don't be a slow poke: keep your site up to speed or lose visitors. InfoWorld. 1999;21(12):64.

115. Tullio CJ. Selecting material for your newsletter. Hosp Pharm Times. 1992;Oct:12HPT–16HPT.

116. Journalism pro offers editing tips for effective pharmacy newsletters. Drug Utilization Review. 1988;4(4):49-50.

117. Mitchell JF, Cook RL. Pharmacy newsletters: time for a new approach. Hosp Formul. 1985;20:360-5.

118. Ritchie DJ, Manchester RF, Rich MW, Rockwell MM, Stein PM. Acceptance of a pharmacy-based, physician-edited hospital pharmacy and therapeutics committee newsletter. Ann Pharmacother. 1992;26:886-9.

119. Craghead RM. Electronic mail pharmacy newsletters. Hosp Pharm. 1989;24:490.

120. Mok MP, Castile JA, Kowaloff HB, Janousek JR. Drugman—a computerized supplement to a hospital's drug information newsletter. Am J Hosp Pharm. 1985;42:1565-7.

121. Bloom BS, editor. Taxonomy of educational objectives, handbook 1: cognitive domain. New York, NY: David McKay; 1956.

122. Medina MS. Using the three e's (emphasis, expectations, and evaluation) to structure writing objectives for pharmacy practice experiences. Am J Health Syst Pharm. 2010 Apr 1;67:516-21.

123. Speaking abroad. How to prepare when you're presenting over there. Presentations. 1999;13(6):A1-A15.

124. Spinler SA. How to prepare and deliver pharmacy presentations. Am J Hosp Pharm. 1991;48:1730-8.

125. Simons T. Multimedia or bust? Presentations. 2000;14(2):40-50.

126. Buchholz S, Ullman J. 12 commandments for PowerPoint. Teaching Prof. 2004;18(6):4.

127. Zielinski D. Technostressed? Don't let your gadgets and gizmos get you down. Presentations. 2004 Feb;28-35.

128. Malone PM. Slides, files and keeping up. Adv Pharm. 2004;2(2):175-80.

129. Goldstein M. PDA presenting has come a long way, but still has drawbacks. Presentations. 2003 Nov;22.

130. Medina MS, Avant ND. Delivering an effective presentation. Am J Health Syst Pharm. 2015;72:1091-4.

131. Endicott J. For the prepared presenter, fonts of inspiration abound. Presentations. 1999;13(4):22-3.

132. Bullet points may be dangerous, but don't blame PowerPoint. Presentations. 2003 Nov;6.

133. The psychology of presentation visuals. Presentations. 1998;12(5):45-51.

134. DeCoske MA, White SJ. Public speaking revisited: delivery, structure and style. Am J Health Syst Pharm. 2010 Aug 1;67:1225-7.

135. Engle JP, Firman SC. Perfecting pharmacist presentation skills. Am Pharm. 1994;NS34(7):60-4.

136. Simons T. For podium emergencies. Presentations. 2003 Nov;24-29.

137. Hill J. The attention deficit. Presentations. 2003 Oct;27-32.

138. McClendon KS, Sover KR. Tips for a successful poster presentation. Am J Health Syst Pharm. 2014;71:449-51.

Chapter Thirteen

Pharmacy and Therapeutics Committee

Patrick M. Malone • Mark A. Malesker • Indrani Kar • Jason E. Glowczewski • Devin J. Fox

Learning Objectives

After completing this chapter, the reader will be able to

- Describe the pharmacy and therapeutics (P&T) committee.
- Define the functions of the P&T committee.
- Describe attributes and structure of a P&T committee likely to promote its ability to function successfully.
- Describe where and how the P&T committee fits into the organizational structure of a health care institution or other groups.
- Describe how the pharmacy department participates in P&T committee activities.
- Describe and explain the concepts of drug formularies and drug formulary systems, and how pharmacy participates in their establishment and maintenance.
- Describe how P&T committee activities contribute to the quality improvement of medication use.
- Describe how to develop policies and procedures for the process of medication use.

Key Concepts

❶ A **pharmacy and therapeutics (P&T) committee**, or its equivalent, oversees all aspects of medication use within an institution.

❷ A P&T committee may determine that more than one formulary is necessary for an institution or health system.

❸ Although it is common for pharmacists to downplay or misunderstand the importance of P&T committee support in comparison to other clinical activities, such support is vital for pharmacy to impact patient care.

❹ A P&T committee may find it necessary to create ad hoc committees to address various issues, depending on their complexity and size.

❺ Typically, P&T committee functions include determining what drugs are available on **formulary**, who can prescribe specific drugs, policies and procedures regarding drug use (including pharmacy policies and procedures, clinical protocols, standard order sets, and clinical guidelines), what to do about counterfeit drugs or drug shortages, performance improvement as well as quality assurance activities (e.g., drug utilization review/drug usage evaluation/medication use evaluation, as well as compliance surveillance), adverse drug reactions/medication errors, dealing with product shortages, and education in drug use.

❻ A variety of topics regarding the quality of medication use, inclusive of applicable medication metrics, are normally part of the activities of a P&T committee.

Introduction

When considering how a pharmacist can have an impact on a patient's drug therapy, it is common to consider the individual practitioner dealing with a specific patient or, perhaps, a small group of patients. Certainly the clinician can have a deep impact this way, but he or she does have the disadvantage of dealing with a very limited number of patients. In order for pharmacists to efficiently impact a population of patients, a different approach is necessary. Fortunately, pharmacists have the opportunity to participate in the activities of ❶ *a P&T committee or its equivalent, which generally oversees all aspects of medication use in an institution.* Physicians and pharmacists have collaborated to implement cost-effective prescribing practices and assess clinical outcomes through educational initiatives, administrative programs to restrict ordering practices, use of formularies and prescribing guidelines, and financial incentives.[1] There are data to show that P&T committee actions are useful.[2,3]

Before proceeding, it must be stated that while this chapter deals with the P&T committee, which is usually the group responsible for overseeing all aspects of drug therapy in an institution, there is sometimes a similar body referred to as the formulary committee. This latter group deals strictly with determining which drugs are carried within an institution or organization, whereas, the P&T committee has numerous other tasks, covering all aspects of drug therapy (e.g., adverse drug reaction [ADR]/medication error monitoring, quality assurance, policy and procedure approval), although the exact group of functions may vary from place to place.[4] Depending on the institution or overarching health system with multiple institutions, some institutions use a formulary committee, since other bodies may perform the additional P&T committee tasks described later in this chapter, while other health care groups may use both committees. The formulary committee may function as a subcommittee reporting to the P&T committee. All structures described above apply to single institutions up to large health systems. A single institution with a formulary and/or P&T committee may address issues for the individual institution as a whole, whereas a health system representing a group of institutions addresses issues specific to the health system. In a health-system structure, a system P&T committee makes formulary decisions for the system. Individual institutions making up the health system may also employ local P&T committees to address local issues, such as restricting medications further and assessing medication safety reports. It is important to note that local P&T committees generally do not supersede system P&T committee decisions, similar to state and federal law, although in some cases the system body may cede oversight of a specific group of medications to the local body. That is because the one institution may be the only one with the specialty area that would need them and, therefore, they have the expertise to best determine which agents should be approved for formulary inclusion. In this chapter, anything discussed regarding medication availability within an institution or health system applies to both bodies, whereas all other items are for the P&T committee only (Case Study 13-1).

Case Study 13–1

You are the pharmacy manager at a community hospital in a health system. Your health system has a system P&T committee. One of your infectious disease physicians asks for a medication Alpha to be reviewed at the local P&T committee level in your hospital. The medication is on formulary for the health system and has restriction guidance available. The medication is now being discussed by your local P&T committee. The ID physician turns to you and asks the following:

- *Can you add new restrictions to the medication?*
- *Can you remove this medication from the local formulary?*
- *The system P&T committee meets a week later and removes medication Alpha from formulary. What do you do?*

It should be noted that while P&T committees have normally been associated with institutional pharmacy, other organizations have increasingly used P&T-type committees in an attempt to improve drug therapy while lowering costs. Some places where such committees are seen include **managed care organizations (MCOs)**,[5] insurance companies, pharmacy benefit management (PBM) companies, unions, employers,[6] state Medicaid boards, state departments of public institutions,[7] Medicare,[8] long-term care facilities,[9] ambulatory clinics,[10] and even community pharmacies.[11] Much of this chapter will use examples from institutional pharmacy and managed care, simply because much of the published literature deals with those areas of practice, and it is the most likely setting in which a pharmacist will be directly involved in P&T committee activities. However, the concepts covered are applicable to any P&T or equivalent committee and comply with recommendations of the American Medical Association (AMA),[12,13] the American Society of Health-System Pharmacists (ASHP),[14] The Joint Commission (TJC, formerly the Joint Commission for the Accreditation of Health Care Organizations),[15] and the Academy of Managed Care Pharmacy (AMCP).[16]

The role of the P&T committee has been continuously expanded over the years and now encompasses a great number of functions and activities that cover all aspects of overseeing drug therapy. As some of these are of sufficient size and importance, they are covered separately in other chapters (e.g., drug monographs, quality assurance). In addition, there are a number of areas (e.g., investigational drugs) in which P&T committees play a secondary role, and these too are covered in other chapters. This chapter will serve to provide a base to tie together discussion of all of these areas and a number of smaller functions or activities that will be covered as a portion of this chapter. The information is appropriate both for those just learning about the concepts and also for those individuals who are involved with P&T committee activities.

Organizational Background

ORIGIN OF P&T COMMITTEE

The concept of a P&T committee represents a unique niche within the structure of a hospital or hospital system. The current role of a hospital in Western countries[17] began about 200 years ago, at a time when very few efficacious medications were available, although drug formularies had been developed during the Revolutionary War to list the drugs available.[18] It has also been noted that a **drug formulary** was developed for all municipal hospitals in New York City at Bellevue Hospital in 1868.[19] Drug formularies were required for participation in the Medicare program in 1965.[20] The original hospital was a place to receive basic health care when a person had no extended family to provide the basic needs of good health. After infection control became a recognized concept and anesthesia for surgery evolved around 1900, the value of the modern hospital progressively became a recognized need for all segments of society. The origins for standards of how a hospital functioned subsequently developed during the first half of the twentieth century. This began with the early efforts of the American College of Surgeons in the United States to develop the first accreditation standards for hospitals. Later, the Joint Commission on Accreditation of Hospitals (JCAH), now known as TJC, evolved to centralize the basic requirements for the functional character of a U.S. hospital. The concept of the P&T committee originated and evolved to help hospitals meet various standards regarding drug therapy. The first P&T committee was formed at Bellevue Hospital in New York City in the mid-1930s.[18,21] While it dealt with true compounding formulas, it was originally founded to ensure quality and efficacy of those products, which is still a significant function of P&T committees.

In keeping with the social origins of the hospital, the legally sanctioned or licensed privilege of being a professional health care provider evolved.[17] Both the physician and pharmacist were considered unique for the needs of society. Minimum standards evolved, including the accreditation of their training as a basis for being licensed. Originally, physicians and pharmacists functioned primarily as independent professionals. The nature of a physician's independence was legally defined to further support their obligations to a patient. Many states in the United States legally prohibited a physician from being employed by a corporation. Eventually, these laws were all repealed, but they had the effect of creating the basis for a medical staff as being a separate legal entity within a hospital. The medical staff reflected the legally evolving traditions of a physician, and indirectly the pharmacist, as being independent professionals committed only to the care of a patient without unnecessary outside influences. This evolution has had a major impact on the organizational structure of hospitals.

ORGANIZATIONAL STRUCTURE OF P&T COMMITTEE

A typical hospital organization is shown in Figure 13-1. The board of directors divides the functions of its organization into two entities. First, the administration of the hospital operates as a typical business with a chief executive officer, chief operating officer, and so forth. Second, the board of directors authorizes that a medical staff be formed that reports separately to the board of directors. While the medical staff as a whole is ultimately in charge of all clinical aspects of care in the hospital, in most institutions this is unworkable without an administrative structure of some kind. Therefore, the medical staff may elect officers and either elect or appoint somebody to oversee all aspects of patient care. In this example, the term **medical executive committee** is used for that body, although the name and exact function may vary. The medical staff functions to certify the credentials

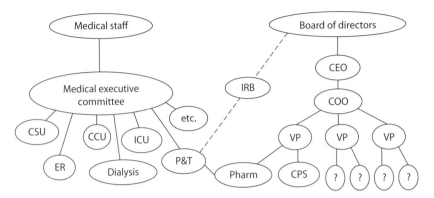

Figure 13–1. Hospital organization. CCU, critical care committee; CEO, chief executive officer; COO, chief operating officer; CPS, central processing & supply; CSU, cardiac surgery unit committee; ER, emergency room committee; ICU, intensive care unit committee; IRB, institutional review board; Pharm, pharmacy department; P&T, pharmacy & therapeutics committee; VP, vice president; ?, other hospital departments.

of its members, establish their scope of practice where appropriate, monitor the quality of health care provided by its members, and maintain the means to collaborate with the administration of the hospital.

In modern medicine, there are so many clinical areas to consider that it is unrealistic for one committee to adequately oversee all aspects of patient care, except in very small institutions. For this reason, various subcommittees of the medical executive committee are usually necessary, as can be seen in Figure 13-1. As a means to coordinate the needs of the medical staff and the operation of the hospital pharmacy, the modern P&T committee developed. From the traditions established by TJC and ASHP, the P&T committee developed as a function of the medical staff's responsibilities. This committee or related committees may have other names, such as the drug and therapeutics committee in other countries,[22,23] but the functions are the same. While the P&T committee has been referred to in TJC accreditation standards in the past, it is no longer specifically required and may be replaced by some other committee(s) or body(ies),[15,24,25] although the P&T committee concept is supported by many national and professional organizations.[26] Given the continuing growth in the number, complexity, and expense of medications, both the importance and number of functions of the P&T committee have continued to increase. Policy and procedures to set up a P&T committee are described in Appendix 13-1, but the following will serve as a general description of P&T committees and their actions.

Health-System P&T versus Local P&T

In some cases, the P&T committee may represent multiple hospitals and medical centers that comprise a health system, rather than just representing a specific institution. While the philosophy of operating one P&T committee within this corporate structure seems reasonable, this is not often accomplished without implementation obstacles, and decentralization of these efforts is one option depending on the structure.[27] Different patient populations, medication needs, cross-hospital physician participation, meeting time, length and location of meetings, and differing clinical cultures within a specific institution are examples of barriers that may be present for one committee to represent multiple hospitals with no local level committee. The P&T model may need to be revised to work with these challenges.[28-33] A hybrid model where the system-wide P&T provides oversight, structure, and manages a formulary, but local level P&T committees refine the implementation of the formulary and focus on medication safety and quality at the local level, may offer a more practical path than the elimination of local level P&T committees entirely. Alignment of a health system's individual hospitals within a system P&T structure and formulary has been a source of significant cost savings for multihospital health systems.[34]

Membership for P&T Committee

Although it is easy to assume from its name that the P&T committee is organizationally a part of the pharmacy department, such is not the case, as was mentioned above. Instead, it is usually a medical staff entity and, perhaps, only one or two pharmacists may actually be members of the committee (possibly *ex officio* members without voting privileges). Commonly, the pharmacy director or clinical coordinator, serving as the committee's secretary (e.g., taking minutes, collating, and arranging the agenda), may be the sole official pharmacy representative. Other pharmacists may also attend to act as consultants to the committee, often having great impact on the committee's decisions, even if they cannot officially vote. Fortunately, in larger hospitals, it appears that more pharmacists are now becoming full members of the P&T committee.[35]

Typically, the voting members of an institutional P&T committee are limited to members of the medical staff, although there may be a few voting or nonvoting members from other groups, including pharmacy. Membership is mostly composed of physicians (preferably a wide variety of physicians from various areas of practice), but usually includes at least one pharmacist and often members from other areas of the hospital (e.g., nursing, administration, radiology, respiratory therapy, dietary, quality assurance, medical records, laboratory, and risk management).[36] A pharmacoeconomics specialist also can be extremely helpful. There have also been recommendations to include other individuals, such as a medical ethicist or community pharmacist.[37]

Encouraging a smaller number of physician members to participate more fully may help to address a wide variety of issues, and calling in physicians to consult with the committee on an as needed basis may enhance the committee's efficiency.[38] In some cases, the pharmacy department is asked to recommend physicians for the committee. If possible, pharmacy should suggest physicians that are noted for their commitment to rational drug therapy and the institution or health-system's patients at-large.[39] As an example, the U.S. Department of Defense has procedures for appointment of members, including non-physician members, of the P&T committee. The procedures are available on the Internet.[40]

Efforts should be made to ensure that the physician chosen to be chairman of the committee is an advocate of the pharmacy department and institution or health system. It is possible for the medical executive committee of the medical staff to pass a resolution to approve a policy broadening the voting members of the P&T committee (e.g., director of pharmacy, hospital vice president) or delegating the functions of the P&T committee to the hospital. In this latter arrangement, the medical staff would reserve the right to terminate the policy if the P&T committee fails to support the needs of the medical staff. If the P&T committee is a hospital committee, rather than medical staff committee, a pharmacist or nurse might more easily obtain voting privileges, given appropriate physician quorum requirements in the authorizing policy.

The P&T committee of MCOs and government bodies often have similar membership to that in institutional committees; however, there may need to be a requirement for at least some of the members to be independent practitioners and retail pharmacists (i.e., having no financial ties to the organization or group that sponsors the P&T committee).[36,41,42] In accordance with the 2003 Medication Modernization Act, the use of formularies is an essential component to the PBM.[36]

Reporting Structure of P&T Committee

Once the general organizational setting of the P&T committee has been determined, the operating policy of the P&T committee requires careful attention to two key issues. The first key issue is obvious—to whom does the P&T committee report and to what degree can the decisions of the P&T committee be overturned by another segment of the organization. It is important to point out that, in general, the P&T committee may act only as an advisory body to the medical executive committee. Decisions of the P&T committee may not be considered final (and therefore not be implemented) until they are reviewed and approved by the medical executive committee. In this situation, a report is forwarded from the P&T committee after each meeting to the medical executive committee. In addition, an annual report of the P&T committee may be prepared for both internal review and review by the Medical Executive Committee. This annual report is time consuming in preparation, but is a very important means of tracking P&T activities and action over time.

The second issue is that the P&T committee will likely be successful based on the leadership qualities of its members and the chairperson. The role of the chairperson includes developing the respect and involvement of all members of the committee and providing leadership surrounding formulary decisions.

❷ *A P&T committee may determine that more than one formulary is necessary for an institution or health system.* As biosimilars become more prevalent or a unique service line requires special focus, a **drug formulary** may be necessary for these medications. For example, a specialty medication formulary would provide focus to a complex medication process from prescription to dispensing. Alternatively, a P&T committee may choose to focus on a smaller number of comprehensive formularies (e.g., adult and pediatrics, or academic medical center and community). The P&T committee further manages the drug formulary by providing usage guidelines, policies or procedures, or restrictions to guide medication use. These items of formulary management may be automated within the hospital's electronic medical record and drug information resource, such as Lexicomp® or Micromedex®. By incorporating medication use guidance directly into the information source at the point of prescribing, prescribers are made aware of the P&T committee's expectations for medication use. This passive display of information may be incorporated into a protocol or order set, which guides a practitioner to the appropriate medication use actively. In summary, the P&T committee provides leadership to formulary management, with the guidance of the chair.

PHARMACY BENEFIT MANAGEMENT P&T COMMITTEE ORIGIN

Evolution of PBM

The origin of the PBM organizations dates back to the late 1960s. Their primary focus was on claims administration for insurance companies. Later, it became a challenge for the insurance companies to efficiently manage the increase in drug coverage in the private sector, when the prescription volume was high and the cost per claim was low.[43] The plastic drug benefit card began in the 1970s and changed the way many prescriptions were bought and paid for by the insurance company and employee. From then on, any employee with an ID card, using a pharmacy network, only had a small copayment.[43] In addition, administrative costs for the third-party payer, whether it is the insurance company, health plan, or employer, were reduced, with the PBM creating pharmacy networks and mail service benefits. Pharmacy networks are a group of pharmacies that are under contract with the insurance company, health plan, and/or their contracted PBM partner to promote prescription services at a negotiated discounted fee.[44] Mail service is a program offered by the PBM, whereby pharmaceutical agents, both prescription and nonprescription, are offered through the mail.[44]

In the late 1980s, the introduction of real-time electronic claims processing began. Not only was there two-way communication between the pharmacy and the PBM for claim processing, but also for clinical information as well. In the 1990s, the PBMs moved toward a greater emphasis on patient health by offering a variety of new services in addition to the claims processing. Since 2000, there has been an emphasis on consumer behavior modification, enhanced patient interventions, physician connectivity, clinical consulting, disease management, and retrospective drug utilization review (DUR; see Chapter 16 for further information) to name a few.[43]

Drug Formularies in PBM

One of the key functions of a PBM is to design, implement, and administer outpatient drug benefit programs for employers, MCOs, and other third-party payers. PBMs manage prescription drug benefits separate from other health care services (i.e., physician and hospital services).[44] Determining which medications are most cost-effective, without compromising patient care, is one of the key elements for controlling the cost of a prescription drug benefit.[6,45,46] PBMs accomplish this by developing drug formularies.[6] Formularies define what medications are covered (i.e., paid for) and provide the main component of the pharmacy benefit. Specific PBM drug payment and management activities occur within this formulary structure, such as therapeutic interchange and disease management programs. Eighty to 100% of PBM covered lives receive some type of formulary management service.[6,44] The use of drug formularies is in flux due to the advantages and disadvantages identified over the last decade or so, however, they are likely to be continued for at least the foreseeable future, particularly due to the Medicare drug formulary requirements.[47]

P&T Committee in PBM

Development and maintenance of drug formularies for third-party payers is an ongoing process. The formulary must be continuously updated to keep pace with new drugs, therapies, medication shortages, prices, recent clinical research, changes in medical practice, evidence-based treatment guidelines, updated Food and Drug Administration (FDA) information,[48] and even civil rights issues.[49] PBMs use a panel of experts called the P&T committee to develop and manage their drug formularies. P&T committees may become even more important to PBMs under the Accountable Care Act.[50] Many times individuals with special clinical expertise are consulted when considering medications within a specific therapeutic class.[48] Meetings are usually held on a quarterly basis, and not only are drug formulary recommendations made, but this group also provides input into other clinical areas, such as development of disease management programs.[6,43,44,47,48]

Many PBMs establish their own P&T committee to evaluate the efficacy, safety, uniqueness, cost of therapeutic equivalent drugs, and other appropriate criteria. In addition, PBMs work with the health plan, employer, or insurance company P&T committee to develop drug formularies using the same evaluation process. This can result in drug formularies that can vary considerably in coverage.[51] In any case, if the P&T committee determines that one drug provides a clear medical benefit over the other therapeutically equivalent drugs in that same therapeutic category, the drug is usually added to the formulary.[6] However, if there are drugs in the same therapeutic category that have very similar efficacy and safety profiles and no unique properties that would make it a better drug, then the net cost becomes a deciding factor as to which drug should be added to the formulary.[6] There has been some discussion as to whether drug costs are weighted too heavily, while drug efficacy and other clinical information is weighted too lightly, when it comes to drug formulary decisions.[43,44] The committee leadership needs to recognize the potential for conflicts of interest between efficacy and economic interests of the PBM and to establish collaboration as the basis for resolving conflicts that arise.

Me-too drugs are drugs that are structurally very similar to an already known drug that has only minor differences. Many drugs come in two versions: an L-isomer (left) and an R-isomer (right). An example of a me-too drug is esomeprazole (Nexium®), the L-isomer of omeprazole (Prilosec®, the R- and L-isomers). Both drugs are used to treat gastroesophageal reflux disease (GERD). When a comparative analysis was conducted looking at drugs approved for marketing between January 2007 and July 2008, those that had a different chemical entity and a separate mechanism of action accounted for 69%; however, they offered no clinical improvement over those already on the market. Forty-four percent offered some type of new convenience, but only 13% offered greater efficacy.[52] For this reason, PBMs may include only one of the products as a covered drug.

In the case of a health plan, employer, or insurance company's own P&T committee, the drug formulary recommendations made by the PBM P&T committee are presented and reviewed by the organization's P&T committee. The PBM recommendations regarding drug formulary recommendations can be either accepted or denied by the organization's P&T committee and the organization's own decision made regarding formulary inclusion.

Pharmacy Support of the P&T Committee

ROLE OF PHARMACISTS IN P&T COMMITTEE

❸ *Although it is not uncommon for pharmacists to downplay or misunderstand the importance of P&T committee support in comparison to other clinical activities, such support is vital for pharmacy to impact patient care.* P&T committee support and participation can have far-reaching effects on the overall quality of drug therapy in an institution and must be given a great deal of attention, since the benefits of its function serves to build collaboration, transparency, and trust among the institutional divisions of authority for drug therapy within health care. While such attention is time consuming,[53] it can be of value to the pharmacy. This is an opportunity to present recommendations to a decision-making body, and P&T committees often accept pharmacists' recommendations[54,55]; therefore, pharmacy departments can have a great and far-reaching impact on drug therapy through this mechanism.

Steering Committee for Formulary Management

Some pharmacists who participate in P&T committee activities serve their function by providing information requested by physicians and considering drugs for formulary approval

TABLE 13-1. AREAS WHERE PHARMACISTS SHOULD BE SUPPORTING A PHARMACY AND THERAPEUTICS COMMITTEE

- Planning future agendas (including medications, policies and procedures, quality assurance, and other subjects to be addressed)
- Gathering data to create drug monographs and other necessary documents
- Evaluating medications for formulary adoption or deletion
- Preparing and conducting quality assurance programs (including drug usage evaluation and monitoring of adverse effects and medication errors)
- Preparing policies and procedures
- Communicating information from the P&T committee to other areas of the institution
- Creating hardcopy and/or electronic versions of the formulary
- Preparing education for individuals involved in medication use
- Collaborating with interdisciplinary groups to manage content, including safety issues
- Sharing best practices, near misses, or other safety information across a health system
- Continuously tracking new FDA drug approvals, new dosage forms, medication shortages

only following physician requests. This can rapidly deteriorate into crisis management, where the pharmacy department reacts to problems and fights each fire as it occurs. A proactive approach for a pharmacy department is more efficient and effective[56,57] and seeks to address issues (e.g., changes in drugs carried on the formulary, new policies and procedures, standard class reviews and guideline reviews, quality assurance activities) before they become problems. TJC accreditation requirements include annual evaluation of all drugs and/or drug classes.[15] Through prospective actions with the P&T committee, it is possible for the pharmacy to get physician support for their clinical activities.

In the specific instance of P&T committee support, one or more pharmacists must be identified to conduct the necessary planning. This may consist of a pharmacy-based steering committee and might include administrators, purchasing agents, or clinicians, and, particularly, drug information specialists. These people must develop and regularly evaluate data sources to anticipate physicians' needs (see Table 13-1).[58] For example, it is necessary to assess what drugs have been recently FDA-approved to identify drugs for possible formulary inclusion. FDA approval often occurs about 3 months or longer before commercial availability and is published on the FDA website (http://www.accessdata.fda.gov/scripts/cder/drugsatfda/index.cfm). Therefore, there is time for the drug to be considered for formulary addition before the first physician request or the first orders arrive from the nursing units, which necessitates a review under TJC standards.[15] In a case where it is not possible to consider a drug before it is commercially available, it has been suggested by some that drugs rated P (priority) by the FDA be made available to physicians until the drug can be fully considered (the FDA classification codes are found on Tables 13-2 and 13-3, with the priority versus standard explanation found on Table 13-3).[59]

TABLE 13–2. **FDA CLASSIFICATION BY CHEMICAL TYPE**[a]

Type	Definition
1	New molecular entity not marketed in the United States
2	New salt, ester, or other noncovalent derivative of another drug marketed in the United States
3	New formulation or dosage form of an active ingredient marketed in the United States
4	New combination of drugs already marketed in the United States
5	New manufacturer of a drug product already marketed by another company in the United States
6	New indication for a product already marketed in the United States (note: this category is no longer used)
7	Drug that is already legally marketed without an approved NDA • First application since 1962 for a drug marketed prior to 1938 • First application for DESI (Drug Efficacy Study Implementation)-related products that were first marketed between 1938 and 1962 without an NDA • First application for DESI-related products first marketed after 1962 without NDAs. In this case, the indications may be the same or different from the legally marketed product.
8	Over-the-counter switch
9	New indication submitted as separate NDA, which is consolidated with original NDA after approval
10	New indication submitted as a separate NDA, but not consolidated with original NDA

[a]Drugs@FDA frequently asked questions [Internet]. Washington, DC: Food and Drug Administration. [Updated 2015 Mar 27; cited 2016 Jul 18]. Available from: http://www.fda.gov/Drugs/InformationOnDrugs/ucm075234.htm#chemtype_reviewclass

TABLE 13–3. **FDA CLASSIFICATIONS BY THERAPEUTIC POTENTIAL**[a]

Type	Definition
P	Priority handling by FDA—before 1992 this was two categories: A—Major therapeutic gain B—Moderate therapeutic gain
S	Standard handling by FDA—before 1992 this was referred to as class C, which indicated the product offered only a minor or no therapeutic gain
0	Orphan Drug

[a]Drugs@FDA frequently asked questions [Internet]. Washington, DC: Food and Drug Administration. [Updated 2015 Mar 27; cited 2016 Jul 18]. Available from: http://www.fda.gov/Drugs/InformationOnDrugs/ucm075234.htm#chemtype_reviewclass

This latter procedure may be effective, but considering the drug before commercial availability is preferable, because if the ultimate P&T committee decision is to leave the drug off the drug formulary, there may be difficulties in helping physicians stop the use of the product.

Some P&T committees may alternatively require physician requests for medications to be reviewed for addition to the drug formulary, which is a more reactive process to market changes and available treatments, but it allows the P&T committee to remain focused on the immediate needs of the institution. A fine line between managing the immediate needs and future needs should be developed by the P&T committee. Some P&T committees review medications only after having been available on the market for 6 months or a year. In addition, class reviews, which will be discussed later in the chapter, assist with the proactive review of potential formulary opportunities in medication use guidance, cost savings, and potential additions/deletions from formulary. The P&T committee's process for reviewing medications should be determined by the committee and written into the policy and procedure governing the committee.

Tracking Medication Usage

It is also important to track older drugs at a P&T committee. For example, the use of non-formulary drugs should be tracked within the hospital (please note—a non-formulary drug is a product that has not been approved for use within an institution, or a product that has been prescribed in a particular situation for a use other than the use approved by the P&T committee when the product was added to the drug formulary).[60,61,62] If patterns of increased use are noted, a reason for that use should be identified. If the use is inappropriate, the physician(s) should be contacted and given information about alternative formulary agents. In some cases, new information may be available showing a new advantage or use for an old agent, which can lead to its reconsideration for formulary adoption. Related to this is the necessity to regularly consider the material being promoted by the drug company representatives. It is worth mentioning that some hospitals will restrict pharmaceutical representative's access to the institution or restrict the drugs that may be promoted by those representatives to only items approved for use in the hospital, in order to proactively manage this situation and facilitate compliance with the formulary (see Chapter 23 for further information).

There may also be new indications or other information that will increase demand for non-formulary items. If there are sufficient changes noted in the use(s) of a particular class of drugs, it is useful to review the class as a whole to decide which drug(s) are to be retained on the formulary. TJC now requires annual review of all medications,[10–15] which assists in reviewing new available information (e.g., labeling changes or warnings from postmarketing surveillance) that may necessitate changes in formulary items in a particular class, including additions, deletions, and therapeutic interchange opportunities. Other items, such as trends in reported ADRs in the institution or published data for new products with little information in the literature on first approval, may also be useful in determining products for P&T committee consideration or reconsideration.[63] Although there must be a mechanism by which physicians can request that drugs be added to the formulary, all of the above methods and others can help the pharmacy anticipate physician needs, allowing time for information gathering, evaluation of products, and P&T committee consideration before the need becomes too urgent to permit proper consideration.

TABLE 13–4. ITEMS THAT MAY BE ON A REQUEST FOR FORMULARY CONSIDERATION FORM

- Date and time of request
- Name of product (e.g., generic, brand, chemical)
- Source of product (e.g., manufacturer, distributor)
- Specific information about drug product (e.g., class of drug, mechanism, adverse effects, clinical studies)
- Anticipated use of drug (e.g., what type of patient, how often)
- Comparable drugs already on the formulary
- Why the product is needed
- What drugs could be removed from the formulary (medication category review)
- What restrictions, policies, cautions, etc., are necessary
- How the drug fits into any clinical guidelines
  - Evidence of unforeseen benefits, even if guidelines do not mention the medication
- Action requested (e.g., addition, deletion, restriction)
- Conflict of interest disclosure

To guide the clinician into considering the logic of requesting the addition of items to the drug formulary, a specific request form may be useful. Items that a physician may be required to fill out or attach to the form are listed in Table 13-4.[64] An example form is seen in Appendix 13-2.

Planning P&T Committee Meetings

The P&T committee should be kept advised by the above-mentioned pharmacy-based steering committee of future plans, so that it can be aware that a rational planning process is governing its agenda. Also, it is a good idea for one or more representative(s) of this steering committee to meet with the pharmacy director, chairman of the P&T committee, and a representative of the hospital administration on a regular basis to assist with planning and ensure their concerns are addressed. This meeting could be held shortly before the P&T committee actually meets to present preliminary formulary evaluations, medication use evaluation (MUE) material, and policy and procedure documents for an initial review, allowing modifications addressing physician and administration concerns to be made before formal committee review and action. During this meeting, plans for future months can be made or adjusted as the circumstances dictate. Other appropriate physicians or groups should also be consulted in order to assure that their concerns are addressed. For example, if changes to the cephalosporins carried on the drug formulary or their permitted uses (e.g., restrictions to particular uses or prescribing groups) are considered, the infectious disease specialists should be contacted to provide input. (Note: This does not necessarily mean that recommendations are changed to account for physician preferences, but that their preferences and concerns are specifically addressed in the evaluation.)

Regarding quality assurance activities, the pharmacy department should obtain data to guide the selection of upcoming quality assurance programs. This will be covered in greater detail in Chapter 16.

Guiding Medication Use Policies and Procedures

The pharmacy should also investigate which medications need specific policies and procedures developed to guide their use and monitoring. This may be done when the drug is first being evaluated for formulary addition or later if problems (e.g., increased ADR reports, medication errors, and overuse) are noted. For example, concerns about a new anticoagulant therapy leading to increased morbidity and mortality through improper use might prompt the P&T committee to approve specific protocols for the use of the agent. Policy and procedure documents are covered later in the chapter. Information on preparing policies and procedures can be found in Chapter 19.

Finally, it is extremely important for the P&T committee to make sure that physicians are informed about the actions taken. Often the pharmacy is heavily involved in providing this information to physicians. While a great deal of effort is placed on communication within the committee itself, it is also necessary to keep the entire medical staff informed. This may be accomplished through medical department meeting presentations, newsletters, e-mails, and websites (refer to Chapter 12), or other mechanisms.

AD HOC COMMITTEES

❹ *A P&T committee may find it necessary to create ad hoc committees to address various issues, depending on their complexity and size.* Some of the common committees are discussed below. Institutions may or may not use these committees (sometimes referred to as subcommittees) and their exact use varies from place to place, depending on their needs or desires.[4]

Adverse Reactions

A comprehensive ADR monitoring and reporting program is an essential component of the P&T committee (see Chapter 17 for further information about ADRs and how they are handled). A subcommittee may be helpful to review the entire ADR data for trends and any necessary actions that need to be taken. The P&T committee will usually report the ADR data on a monthly or quarterly basis. Following approval of this report, the P&T committee is responsible for the dissemination of information to the medical staff and other health professionals in the institution. This includes recommending processes to cut the rate of preventable ADRs. This subcommittee may be combined with the medication errors subcommittee.[15,65]

Anticoagulation

The anticoagulation subcommittee is responsible for policies and procedures to maintain compliance with TJC Goal 3E, now called TJC National Patient Safety Goal 03.05.01.[15] This goal is to reduce the likelihood of patient harm associated with anticoagulation therapy. The subcommittee can also participate in improvement processes to maintain standards with quality organizations, such as the National Quality Forum (NQF) and the Surgical Care Improvement Project (SCIP). Standard orders and policies to follow evidence-based guidelines of the American College of Chest Physicians (ACCP) are also developed by this subcommittee. Pharmacists have an important role on this committee. Most hospitals have pharmacists dedicated to anticoagulation monitoring and education.

Antimicrobial/Infectious Disease

Antibiotics can represent the largest category of formulary medications.[66] Frequent category review and revision is necessary and complex.[67] Cunha has defined five factors to consider when reviewing antimicrobial agents for formulary inclusion: microbiologic activity,[68] pharmacokinetics and pharmacodynamics profiles,[69] resistance patterns,[70,71] adverse effects,[72] and cost to the institution.[73] The P&T committee or a subcommittee of the P&T may be responsible for developing appropriate antibiotic selection and use in both inpatient and outpatient settings.[74,75] Some institutions may rely on input from the infection control committee regarding antimicrobial formulary management and appropriate utilization. Multidisciplinary antimicrobial use committees have limited inappropriate prescribing of antimicrobials and increased the medical staff's knowledge on appropriate antibiotic use.[73,76,77]

The main purpose of the antimicrobial/infectious disease subcommittee is to promote antimicrobial stewardship to ensure cost-effective therapy and improve patient outcomes. Antimicrobial stewardship promotes and optimizes antimicrobial therapy consistent with the hospital's/health system's antibiograms. Guideline development and education is provided to the medical staff as well as to other health care professionals. The subcommittee is also involved in the enforcement of formulary agent use, substitution policies, therapeutic interchange, and restrictions for antibiotics. In addition, review and feedback on prescribing patterns is provided to the medical staff regarding antimicrobial therapy.[78-80] Use of P&T formulary and policy decisions has been shown to be successful in controlling antimicrobial use in hospitals.[81,82] TJC now requires antimicrobial stewardship in institutions, which will allow this subcommittee to serve as a backbone for decisions and implementation of this type of program.[83]

Medication Safety

A medication safety committee (sometimes called safety committee, medication error prevention, or medication misadventure subcommittee) should be multidisciplinary in nature. This subcommittee reviews medication misadventures and medication errors that occur within the institution or health care system. They may also review adverse drug reactions (instead of an adverse reaction committee), drug-drug interactions, drug dispensing processes, medication errors (see Chapter 18 for more information), look-alike/sound-alike medications, high-alert medications, acceptable medical abbreviations, and communication errors. It may also be appropriate for them to review protocols to improve medication safety, such as the settings for intravenous (IV) fluid pumps.

A report will commonly be presented to the P&T committee on a quarterly or semi-annual basis. Following approval of this report, the P&T committee is responsible for the dissemination of information to the medical staff and other health professionals in the institution. This includes recommending processes to cut the rate of preventable medication safety issues. In some places, a medication error reduction plan (MERP) is prepared to identify process improvements that have been made and those that are planned. When evaluating drug cost strategies, patient safety should always be a priority.[84] The 2013 Joint Commission Accreditation Process Guide for Hospitals addresses the potential for adverse drug events.[15] Also, as will be explained in the next chapter, patient safety will be evaluated whenever a product is considered for formulary addition. Review of relevant policies and implementation of national safety recommendations, such as yearly best practices published by the Institute for Safe Medicine Practices (ISMP), are important functions of this subcommittee to additionally assess safety of products on formulary.[85]

Medical Devices

The P&T committee or a subcommittee may be responsible for the approval of some medical devices within an institution. This subcommittee is often multidisciplinary and is given the opportunity to review medical devices before purchases are made or contracts are signed. The committee is also responsible for reviewing the safety information associated with these devices, because adverse medical device events are an important patient safety issue. Devices that contain medications, such as topical hemostats that contain thrombin, may also be reviewed by the committee or by the transfusion service committee described below.

Nutrition

As nutrition of the hospitalized patient evolved and became more complex, the role of the pharmacist on a nutrition support team became more justified. Their role started out improving the ordering process for parenteral nutrition and communicating these changes to the pharmacy staff for proper preparation. Today, pharmacists on the nutritional team assist in the clinical management of parenteral nutrition patients, parenteral nutrition research, and continual involvement with improving the safety of parenteral nutrition use.[86] TJC, in their National Patient Safety Goals (NPSG), once addressed the safe use of parenteral nutrition feeding solutions,[87] but even though that has been removed, one of the responsibilities of the P&T committee is to oversee and approve the components of the parenteral nutrition solutions, usually in cooperation with dietitians.

Oncology Committee

Care of oncology patients is complex and requires smooth transitions between inpatient and outpatient settings. This subcommittee is charged with reviewing the use of oncology agents, appropriate restrictions for use, and need by location. An interdisciplinary group of oncologists, oncology pharmacists, oncology nurses, and electronic medical record colleagues are key to seamlessly developing and implementing formulary decisions related to oncology.

Quality Assurance of Medication Use

A subcommittee of the P&T committee may be placed in charge of planning and overseeing the plan for quality assurance regarding drug therapy. Details about this activity are found in Chapter 16. This committee may develop criteria for a drug use evaluation (DUE), collect the data, interpret the data, and develop necessary recommendations regarding the appropriate use of medication.

Transfusion Service Committee

Hospitals often have a transfusion service committee charged with reviewing the use of blood and blood derivative products. Many of these products overlap with medications and may also be classified as medications. Therefore, it is necessary for this type of committee to work with or, possibly, be combined with the P&T committee in order to oversee the proper use of such products.[88]

Frequently, departments or service lines (e.g., oncology, cardiology, critical care, psychiatry/mental health, radiology, surgery, women's health) are asked for input regarding the formulary management within their specialty area of practice.

P&T Committee Meeting

Before beginning the description of a typical P&T committee meeting, it is important to note that a smoothly functioning P&T committee has certain needs. The committee will need the support of its parent organization. A room for the meetings should be carefully selected (see Appendix 13-3). The agenda for the meeting should be prepared in advance by the committee's secretary and sent to the members. Most often, as mentioned previously, an informal meeting of the supporting pharmacists and others is required between P&T committee meetings to plan the activities necessary to support the agenda.

The chair of the committee may also attend such planning meetings to ensure that priority issues are addressed before the meeting.

Formulary reviews represent a special concern when sending out an agenda, since they may trigger the outside influences of dedicated pharmaceutical marketing efforts if companies learn from committee members that their products or their competitor's products are being evaluated. Efforts must be made to make sure the committee is not distracted by outside influences, such as the pharmaceutical industry and advertisements. This consideration should be reflected in the selection of members, and it may be necessary to avoid sending out some materials ahead of time, to lessen the chance of them being obtained by pharmaceutical company representatives. Also, if it is possible to prevent pharmaceutical representatives from knowing the membership of the committee, many of these problems may be avoided. If materials are sent out, it may be found that sending minutes from the previous P&T committee meeting is not always appropriate, since it may be difficult to adequately describe the full basis of a decision in a set of minutes. As a result, the minutes might be open to inappropriate projection regarding the basis for the P&T committee decision process. Some institutions simply make the minutes a pure recording of the decisions, eliminating any information about the discussion to avoid this problem. Though minutes pose the above challenges, some institutions use minutes as the source of truth for formulary decisions. A sample set of minutes is seen in Appendix 13-4, and a step-wise process to writing minutes is available.[89]

Along with sending an agenda to members, a reminder phone call, fax, text, and/or e-mail may be useful to facilitate attendance. Each P&T committee meeting requires extensive preparation by the pharmacists involved in its affairs. Specifically, management of the formulary requires extensive background research and the preparation of written reports for any addition or deletion. Similarly, quality-related functions require time-consuming review of patient records. Finally, the P&T committee functions are peripherally related to other affairs of the parent organization, for example, the standard order set preparation by other segments of a hospital. This requires special attention in order to prevent the use of non-formulary products. These items will be discussed in greater detail in the next section. Finally, the chairperson should be skilled at guiding an efficient meeting (see Appendix 13-5). In respect of the time commitment for members, meetings should always start and end at the scheduled times.

P&T Committee Functions

⑤ *Typically, P&T committee functions include determining what drugs are available on formulary, who can prescribe specific drugs, policies and procedures regarding drug use (including pharmacy policies and procedures, clinical protocols, standard order sets, and* *clinical guidelines—see Chapter 8 for the latter), what to do about counterfeit drugs or drug shortages (see Chapter 15), performance improvement as well as quality assurance activities (e.g., drug utilization review/drug usage evaluation/medication usage evaluation, as well as compliance surveillance—see Chapter 16), adverse drug reactions/medication errors (see Chapters 17 and 18), and education in drug use.*[15,90,91] Many of those functions are related to quality assurance activities, because they are designed to improve the quality of drug therapy. Because the functions may improve drug therapy quality, they may actually provide some legal protection for an institution, as long as the reason for decisions is not strictly based on financial considerations.[92] P&T committee functions can also include investigational drug studies; however, that is often delegated to the **Institutional Review Board (IRB)** that oversees all investigational activities in the hospital (see Chapter 21). In addition, some P&T committee functions may be delegated to subcommittees (e.g., quality assurance, antibiotic, and medication errors subcommittees)[93]; however, this can be cumbersome and is often avoided, except in larger institutions. P&T committees should recognize principles of epidemiology and pharmacoeconomics in the decision making whenever possible.[94-97] A standardized safety assessment tool has been developed to evaluate potential formulary agents.[98]

According to TJC, the medical staff, pharmacy, nursing, administration, and others are to cooperate with each other in carrying out the previously mentioned functions.[15] Although the medical staff normally takes overseeing drug therapy very seriously and expects to approve all activities of the P&T committee, it is common for the pharmacy department to complete much of the preparation work for the committee. Although pharmacists are generally charged with the preparation work, institutions may employ a specific pharmacist to manage the P&T committee functions or pay pharmacists to do this work as part of their salary. Physicians usually do not obtain any direct monetary compensation for this committee's work, although such compensation may be considered by an institution to encourage more physician participation. Physician participation in committees may be a result of medical staff bylaws to maintain credentials.

FORMULARY MANAGEMENT

Drug Formulary

Wherever a **drug formulary system** is in place, there is usually a drug formulary published, as a hardcopy book and/or more commonly in electronic format (e.g., website, intranet, or other software, particularly software used to order medications for patients). In its simplest form, the drug formulary contains a list of drugs that are available under that formulary system, which reflects the clinical judgment of the medical staff.[99,100] This list will normally be arranged alphabetically and/or by therapeutic class (e.g., American Hospital Formulary Service [AHFS] classification), and usually contains information on the dosage forms, strengths, names (e.g., generic, trade, chemical), and ingredients of combination products. Many drug formulary publications contain a great deal more material related to the drugs, including a summary of indications, side effects, dosing, use restrictions, and other clinical information.[101] Formularies may also be referred to as preferred medication lists or preferred drug lists.[18]

Definition of Formulary System

A related term, the formulary system, can be thought of as a method for developing the list, and sometimes even as a philosophy.[102] In theory, a well-designed drug formulary can guide clinicians to prescribe the safest and most effective agents for treating a particular medical problem, at the most reasonable cost.[103-108] Some people argue that the formulary system itself does not work because it is not properly implemented and recommend replacing it with counterdetailing by pharmacists or computers at the time a prescription order is written (see Chapter 23 for further information).[109] However, whether or not that is true has yet to be determined. The most well-known article indicating that formularies may ultimately result in higher patient costs was written by Horn and associates.[110] While this may be one of the best articles on the topic and the author has defended criticism of the article,[111] there are nevertheless various deficiencies in the study that make it uncertain whether it was truly the drug formulary or other factors that lead to increased costs.[112-115] Horn and associates[116] also published a similar study conducted in the ambulatory environment, which appears to have similar results and deficiencies. In the case of national drug formularies, there has been a positive[117] effect on prescribing habits shown in Canada. A study of formulary use in the western Pacific region found that they are commonly used in the hospital setting, but questioned their effectiveness, since in that area the products on the formulary are often not connected to treatment guidelines or the best evidence for treating disease.[118] Further research is needed before a definite conclusion may be reached on the effectiveness of formulary management.[119] For now, a well-constructed formulary is still believed to improve patient care while decreasing costs. It serves as a focus for building comprehensive drug therapy options.

Decision Making in Formulary System

The goal of the formulary system is to provide a decision-making process leading to the selection of medications necessary for the treatment of any disease states likely to be seen in that institution.[104] In some cases, decisions for formulary addition can be made for entire groups of institutions, for example, the U.S. Veteran's Administration has combined the formularies of all of its component parts.[120] These formulary medications should be the most efficacious, safe, and cost-effective agents with the fewest side effects or drug interactions.[15] Other factors should also be taken into consideration, such as the variety of dosage forms available for the medication, estimated use, convenience, dosing schedule, compliance, abuse potential, physician demand, ease of preparation, storage requirements, and risks.[121] Economic factors should not be the sole basis for this evidence-based process.[104] Typically, only two or, perhaps, three drugs from any drug class are added to the formulary. Some people would argue that only one agent is necessary from any class; however, some individuals will not respond and/or tolerate certain agents, so at least one secondary agent is usually desirable. Therapeutic redundancy must be minimized, however, by excluding superfluous or inferior preparations. This should improve the quality of prescribing and also lead to improved cost-effectiveness, both by eliminating less cost-effective agents that do not improve patient care and by assisting patients to become well faster. To analyze potentially conflicting literature and strength of recommendation, a grading system has been developed for review of potential formulary additions.[122]

Whether an institution has a very strict formulary with a minimum number of items or a less-restricted formulary that excludes items that are significantly inferior is sometimes a matter of philosophy. The former will cut down the pharmacy department's inventory and often save money through avoidance of highly priced products, but may only be practical in closed **health maintenance organizations (HMOs)** where the same formulary is used in both the inpatient and ambulatory environments. In cases where physicians are free to prescribe whatever products they prefer in the ambulatory environment, they have been shown to have difficulty in remembering what products are contained on the formularies of third-party payers.[123] Therefore, the increased time necessary for pharmacists to contact physicians for order changes may lead to the disruption of patient care. As a result, a less restricted formulary may be more practical. As an example, a patient is admitted to the hospital on a non-formulary medication. While there would be other satisfactory medications in the same therapeutic category on the formulary, some think it may be best to simply allow use of the non-formulary product, rather than adding another complicating factor to the patient's hospital treatment by attempting to change therapy. Pharmacist and physician time would also be saved. A more contemporary approach is available to facilities with computerized physician order entry (CPOE). The challenge of physicians remembering which medication within a class is available is reduced, and order sets can guide clinicians to formulary products. Medication orders can be programmed to list the patient's home medication if a substitution was made and a double check can be performed upon discharge medication reconciliation. Less storage space, smaller medication inventories, and significant cost savings may be achieved under this model which approaches a strict or closed formulary.

Even in cases where an institution has a strict and enforced closed drug formulary, it should be noted that there are occasions when it is necessary to prescribe a drug that is not on the drug formulary. This might be due to a patient with a rare illness, a patient who does not respond or has intolerable side effects to the formulary drugs, a patient stabilized on a non-formulary medication where it would be difficult or dangerous to change, a conflict between the institutional formulary and the patient's insurance company formulary,[124] or some other valid reason. A mechanism must be in place to promptly obtain the particular drug when it is shown to be necessary (the National Committee for Quality Assurance [NCQA] requires such a mechanism for HMOs,[125] as does TJC for other hospitals,[15] but it must try to prevent physicians from ordering non-formulary drugs "because I said so!"). Some institutions require specific requests forms to be filled out (see example in Appendix 13-2), sometimes with a cosignature from the physician's department head, or at least require a consultation between a pharmacist and the physician before the drug is obtained. Also, patients may be charged more for the non-formulary medications. In some HMOs and insurance company plans, the physicians or pharmacies may be financially penalized for use or overuse of non-formulary medications.[126] Whatever mechanism is used, it is important to make requesting non-formulary medications transparent, but difficult to obtain unnecessary medications; otherwise the benefits of the formulary system may be negated.[61] Also, it is necessary to track non-formulary drugs use and frequency, which may lead to a worthwhile addition to the drug formulary.[127]

Misconceptions about Formulary System

Some prescribers feel that a drug formulary serves only to keep costs down, at the expense of good patient care.[128] These physicians must be reassured that there is evidence to support that a good formulary does keep expenses down[129] without negatively affecting care,[130] although in some cases the costs are merely transferred to other hospital expenses.[131,132] One study demonstrated that a well-controlled formulary or therapeutic substitution (substituting a different medication that is effective for the disease being treated for the one ordered by the physician) results in 10.7% lower drug costs per patient day, and both a well-controlled formulary and therapeutic substitution together could cause 13.4% lower drug costs per day.[133]

Some prescribers do not support formularies, because they consider them to be a limitation to their authority.[128] It is necessary to keep in mind that when physicians become a part of a medical staff or sign up to participate in some managed care group, they are given privileges not rights. The privileges generally do include limitations on what medications they can prescribe, and when and how they can prescribe them. If a drug formulary system is run well there is little reason to feel there are inadequate drugs available; however, it does take some effort for the physician to learn to use the drugs available rather than the drugs they normally prescribe. An effort must be made to collaborate with physicians to reassure them that every effort is being made to ensure the best drugs are available for the patients. Additionally, all changes to the drug formulary must be quickly and effectively communicated to the physicians to avoid confusion. A lack of such communication can negate some of the benefits of the formulary and lead to poor physician/pharmacist relations.[131] Also, it is important for physicians to be aware that it is the medical staff that affirms P&T decisions, in order to avoid pharmacy being perceived as the sole participant in decisions for the institution and as a barrier to physician requests.[134]

Increasingly, prescribers will enter prescription orders into the computer, which can quickly inform the physician of formulary drug choices and guide therapeutic decisions. Currently, however, pharmacists often have to tactfully contact the physician about non-formulary drugs in order to make a formulary system work.

Similarly, pharmacies filling prescriptions for an HMO must be kept informed of the formulary status of drugs. One suggestion is to have a help desk to answer pharmacist questions and to provide information.[135]

Contents of Drug Formulary

Oftentimes, the drug formularies will have a number of other sections that may include ancillary information about the P&T committee and pharmacy department, policy and procedure information (e.g., how to obtain non-formulary drugs, how to request a drug be placed on the formulary), laboratory test information, dietary supplement charts, pharmacokinetics information, approved abbreviations, sodium content, nomograms, dosage equivalency charts, apothecary/metric equivalents, drug-food interactions, skin test directions, cost data, antimicrobial therapy charts, and any other brief clinical information tables felt to be necessary. Use of linking in websites can make such information much more readily available and usable, since users can navigate back and forth between these tables and the drug list. MCOs may need to include the procedure they use to limit choice of drugs by physicians, pharmacists, and patients.[16,136]

In institutional pharmacies, a hardcopy book was normally published once a year in the past. Often it was published in a pocket-size format that could be carried in lab coats by physicians, pharmacists, and nurses. There may also have been a larger loose-leaf binder published that could be updated regularly throughout the year. Such a book is no longer justified.[137] It is now common for this reference to be available electronically. The electronic form can be made more widely available and can be kept continually up-to-date by making changes, as necessary, at one central location. Also, the electronic formulary coupled with physician order entry may lead to the most efficient and effective way to encourage or enforce the use of formulary items,[138-140] although there is some evidence that electronic messages may be ignored by physicians.[141] Also, other information can be included to improve drug therapy. For example, this may include a requirement for a consultation by a specialist or pharmacokinetic monitoring. For outpatient drug formularies this may include quantity level limits and requirements for **prior authorizations.**

Preferably, the pharmacy can use the information on their computer system to create a formulary that is constantly up-to-date. The information can be accessed as part of the prescription order software and/or it may be interfaced with web software.[142]

The latter makes it possible to embed other information easily, but may take further work by the pharmacist. In any case, this information should be available to the physician and other health care professionals wherever necessary—even by wireless connection. As a side note, many institutions do not want information about their formularies readily available to individuals not directly associated with the institution (e.g., pharmaceutical manufacturers, pharmaceutical representatives, product vendors), but this should not be a problem using virtual private network (VPN) software and firewalls to secure the data—allowing access to only qualified individuals. Increasingly, physicians access this information using smartphones or tablets.

PBMs, in conjunction with an organization, may publish a **patient pocket formulary** or informational website in addition to the formulary published for physicians and provided online for pharmacies. These patient pocket formularies or websites may contain the top therapeutic categories and other information as well. Within these categories are the key drugs in that specific therapeutic class as well as the designated preferred products and the associated patient cost index. Patients may have access to the PBM formulary list via the plans website. Patients are encouraged to take the pocket formularies on their physician visits as a means of ensuring formulary compliance when discussing therapeutic options. Physicians may also have the capability of prescribing online, whereby the physician enters the prescription in an electronic device and instant messaging occurs alerting the physician to potential drug interactions or formulary status of the prescription, allowing the physician to change the prescription immediately and eliminating the need for a pharmacist to call.[44,143]

In addition to pocket formularies, one method whereby the pharmacist educates the physician about formulary drugs is academic detailing. Through mailings, phone conversations, and personal visits the pharmacist discusses with the physician his or her prescribing patterns and, using evidence-based medical literature, supports the rational for preferred formulary product selection and clinically appropriate, cost-effective prescribing without compromising quality (see Chapter 23 for more information).[44]

It is recommended to use a combination of methods to make sure prescribers are informed about formulary information, including electronic resources, academic detailing, educational programs, and any other available methods.[144]

Evaluating Drugs for Formulary Inclusion

The establishment and maintenance of a drug formulary requires that drugs or drug classes be objectively assessed based on scientific information (e.g., efficacy, adverse effects, cost, contribution to some critical treatment pathway,[145] ease of preparation/use, and other appropriate items), not anecdotal physician experience.[102,146] Also, it must be noted that the safety of medications is an important consideration and that decisions must not be made purely based on cost.[147] Also, when costs are considered, it needs to be an evaluation of all costs to the institution, not just the cost of the medication itself, and may include such diverse things as laboratory monitoring costs, length of therapy, nursing care demands, and rehospitalization rates.[148] Medication selection and procurement were specifically added to TJC accreditation process under medication management in the 2009 standards.[149] There is an emphasis in the literature that P&T committee activities should be a result of evidence-based decisions.[104,150] Regarding the formulary process, 2013 TJC standard MM.02.01.01 calls for written criteria for addition or deletion of medications.[15] Any health care practitioner who is involved with ordering, dispensing, administering, and monitoring medications needs to be involved with the development of the criteria.[15,149] A process must also be in place to monitor patient responses to a new medication. All formulary medications and all categories of the AHFS therapeutic classification are to be reviewed at least annually based on safety and efficacy information in order to comply with TJC standards and to maintain the most effective and safe formulary.

Evaluation Criteria

According to the 2013 TJC, the criteria used for approving addition of a drug to a formulary minimally should include the following[15]:

- Indications for use
- Effectiveness
- Risks (e.g., adverse effects, drug interactions, and potential for medication errors)
- Cost

A procedure for preparing the written evaluation of drug products is found in the next chapter, however, this section will go further into how the P&T committee should use that information and other items to do the actual evaluation.

When a P&T committee considers a drug for formulary adoption, it is quite common for the discussion to include statements such as "In my clinical experience…," which often leads the discussion into rather subjective areas. Though clinical experience adds an important component to a discussion, this should not be the sole basis for a formulary review. Additionally, physicians commonly request drugs after they have met with the pharmaceutical company representative or received compensation from the drug company (e.g., speaking fees and travel funds to a meeting).[141,152] In addition, medications may be requested and added to a formulary simply because they are new, even when they clearly are not superior and cost more.[153] Valid formulary decisions should always be based on objective evidence, particularly clinical studies,[154] rather than a few cases of clinical experience by a physician or a representative.[104] Efforts must be made to guide discussions to scientific information for an effective and comprehensive review.[103]

In some cases, this is rather difficult because many new drugs have limited published information, when they are first commercially available. The information that is available is generally placebo-controlled studies that are funded by the manufacturer. In situations such as this, the decision on formulary addition may need to be postponed until adequate information is available. It may be recommended that consideration of any new product be delayed until it has been on the market at least 1 year, unless it is a treatment that is significantly different from those already available.[155] In at least one case, it has been bluntly stated that a P&T committee should show leadership by restricting the availability of a drug product if there is no convincing evidence that the product offers meaningful benefits over other available products.[156] Sometimes the decision cannot wait, as is the case with many managed care companies, who need to review a drug before a patient picks up the drug from the pharmacy, so that appropriate coverage determination can be made, or in hospitals in response to the new TJC accreditation standards.[15,149]

The P&T committee's decision-making process needs to be structured in a manner that is objective and data driven, and takes into account the lack of data.[104] In these cases, a committee may make a decision and then place the product on a 6-month follow-up for an additional review, after which time additional prescribing and patient use data or clinical trial data may be available.

While there is a temptation to think that anything new is better, which is an attitude that is certainly advocated by pharmaceutical company representatives with new products to sell, it cannot be assumed and must be proven. In some cases, experts have determined that the new products pose no significant advantages to the patients to justify the costs.[157–159] Often, manufacturers try to get products approved and on the market that may be in a different strength or dosage form, single isomer of a product, a new indication for a product, or even an extended release version of a product (sometimes several different extended-release versions).[160] All of the products potentially need to be given consideration by a P&T committee. However, with a lack of published trials and, in many cases, objective and reliable data, the P&T committee faces the challenge of creating a sound drug formulary that represents the needs of an organization or patient population in an objective manner that encompasses current clinical practice, established guidelines of patient care, and a thorough risk-benefit analysis of the drug product.[26] Some places have even tried computerized methods to make more objective decisions[161,162]; however, there does not seem to be any data demonstrating the superiority of such a method. Similarly, there are processes called System of Objectified Judgment Analysis (SOJA), which use a computer program to score different aspects of drugs in the same class to determine the best product,[163,164] and multi-attribute utility technology.[165] An example use of technology includes a web-based tool for designing pediatric vaccine formularies that has been developed (http://www.vaccineselection.com).[166]

The 2016 Joint Commission Accreditation Process Guide for Hospitals also addresses the elements of performance for selecting and procuring medications.[15]

Elements of this performance that provide additional information to that already covered are the following:

1. Members of the medical staff, licensed independent practitioners, pharmacists, and staff involved in the ordering, dispensing, administering, and/or monitoring the effects of medications develop written criteria for determining which medications are available for dispensing or administering to patients.
2. The hospital develops and approves criteria for selecting medications, which, at a minimum, include the following—indications for use—effectiveness—drug interactions—potential for errors and abuse—adverse drug events—sentinel event advisories—populations(s) served (pediatrics, geriatrics).
3. Before using a medication new to the hospital, the hospital determines a method to monitor the response of the patient.
4. The hospital maintains a formulary, including medication strength and dosage.
5. The hospital makes its formulary readily available to those involved in medication management.
6. The hospital standardizes and limits the number of drug concentrations available to meet patient care needs.
7. The hospital has a process to select, approve, and procure medications that are not on its formulary
8. The hospital implements the process to select, approve, and procure medications that are not on its formulary.
9. Medications designated as available for dispensing or administration are reviewed at least annually based on emerging safety and efficacy information.
10. The hospital has a process to communicate medication shortages and outages to licensed independent practitioners and staff who participate in medication management (see MM.02.02.01).

Conflict of Interest

Also, it is necessary to determine whether individuals (or their spouses if applicable) involved in the discussion and decision about a drug's formulary status have a conflict of interest (i.e., would receive some direct or indirect compensation from having a drug available, e.g., stock in a company, honoraria for speaking, consulting fees, and gifts or grants from a company[91,155,167–169]) and avoid that biasing factor. Nationally, this is considered to be a significant problem.[170] The P&T committee has the responsibility to identify and address conflict of interest issues in the decision-making process.[104] A conflict of interest policy, requiring regular disclosure of any possible conflicts, should be established and declared in writing annually.[26,171,172] An example form to gather information about conflicts of interest is found in Appendix 13-6. Also, the ProPublica website (http://projects.propublica.org/docdollars/) and CMS website (http://www.cms.gov/openpayments/)

disclose payments to prescribers from some pharmaceutical companies. In certain cases, regular voting P&T committee members may have to abstain from the vote, if they disclose a possible conflict of interest, or the committee may vote to determine whether the conflict is considered to be significant enough to prevent voting by the individual in question. There is concern at a federal, state, and institutional level regarding potential conflict of interest. In 2009, some drug manufacturers made public their financial relationship with health care providers.[173] There is also concern that the PBMs P&T committees may be financially influenced by drug manufacturers.[174] Unlike the traditional health insurers, the U.S. Department of Defense solicits input from various providers and beneficiaries. In addition, they provide beneficiaries and their representatives an opportunity to comment on the committee recommendations prior to final approval. However, this has not deterred their placement in a category where they will provide the lowest reimbursement for the product.[175]

Other Aspects of Formulary Evaluation

Several other areas need to be considered, which will be explained below.

Patent Expiration

Patent expiration is a common question that should be considered for all products or drug classes undergoing formulary review, since the introduction of generic products after that date may lead to decreasing prices. Patent expiration information can be found at http://www.fda.gov/cder/ob/default.htm.

Orphan Drug Status

Similarly, whether a medication is granted orphan drug status is an issue. In 2015, over half of the novel drugs that were approved were for orphan diseases because it allows pharmaceutical companies to have high profits. This too can greatly affect the cost of medications for an institution, including for older products that might have previously been marketed for a much lower cost.[176]

High-Alert or Hazardous Medications

TJC Medication Management Standards for 2016 are focused on medication safety (see MM.01.01.03). High-alert medications are those where there is a high likelihood of errors and/or sentinel events, potential for abuse, or other adverse events. A listing of high-alert medications is available from ISMP (www.ismp.org/tools/highalertmedications.pdf). Hazardous medications by definition of exposure to animals or humans have the potential to cause cancer, developmental or reproductive toxicity, or organ damage. Lists of hazardous medications are available from NIOSH (https://www.cdc.gov/niosh/topics/antineoplastic/pdf/hazardous-drugs-list_2016-161.pdf). The definition of a medication goes beyond prescription products and the FDA classification as drugs. The following are also considered medications: herbal/alternative therapies, vitamins, nutraceuticals, nonprescription products, vaccines, diagnostic and contrast agents, radioactive agents, respiratory treatments, parenteral nutrition, blood derivatives, IV solutions, anesthetic gases, sample medications, and anything else deemed by the FDA to be a drug.[149] The pharmacist is required to review the appropriateness of all medication orders, prospectively before a medication is dispensed.[15,149,177]

Complementary and Alternative Medicine

While it is desirable to evaluate herbal or other alternative medicine products,[178–180] some institutions may instead handle them as non-formulary requests or investigational drugs.[181] Although alternative and herbal medications seem somewhat unusual to the P&T committee, they can still be treated much the same way as any drug product, perhaps with additional evaluation of the purity and composition of the products (see Dietary Supplement Medical Literature section of Chapter 5 for additional details regarding how to evaluate for these products).[182] Some pharmacies also have other policies and procedures,[183] perhaps some that are highly restrictive,[184] including requiring pharmacists to verify labeled product ingredients.[185]

Potential Medication Errors

The possibility of a new drug product leading to medication errors should also be considered in the evaluation of products. For example, difficulty in dosing or administration (including programming IV infusion pumps), boxed warnings, look-alike and sound-alike names, the need for extra monitoring, unusual storage requirements, and other issues such as Risk Evaluation and Mitigation Strategy (REMS) requirements may be considered.[186]

Patient Affordability

In addition to considering the cost of drug products in the institution, it is necessary to consider the cost to the patient, once he or she returns home. If a product is so expensive that an uninsured or underinsured patient cannot afford it in the ambulatory environment, it may not be appropriate to place the patient on that drug in the hospital. However, in some cases pharmaceutical companies may offer assistance to this type of patient.

A newer concept that needs to be considered is "Right to Try" laws being adopted by some states that allow patients to try experimental medications without approval of the FDA.[187] This may be more of an issue for the IRB in an institution, but the P&T committee may be involved.

Open versus Closed Formularies

When setting up a drug formulary there are several things to consider. First is whether it will be an open or **closed formulary**.[188] The **open** (or voluntary) **formulary** is defined as including any drug on the market is available, and some would argue that the term open formulary is really an oxymoron.[103] One exception to this definition is that the NCQA states that an open formulary for an MCO can be a list of recommended drugs, as long as there are no requirements concerning its use.[189] A closed (or restricted) formulary means that only a limited number of agents are available.[99] This is certainly preferable, because such agents should be chosen by objective evidence in the scientific literature. The evidence should support the superiority of the agents over other similar drugs, and can result in cost savings.[190] Closed formularies are becoming much more common in HMOs.[191,192] In some instances of closed formularies, patients may have access to non-formulary or nonpreferred drug products by paying a substantially higher copayment, by paying the difference between the formulary and non-formulary products in addition to the copayment, or by paying for the non-formulary drug in its entirety unless there is a prior authorization to allow this drug.[43]

Issues may arise with a closed or restricted formulary in that it may be too restrictive for those patients who cannot afford the drug, even though the drug is still available on a closed formulary. A growing health policy concern is the ability to successfully appeal for coverage of a non-formulary product. Newer breakthrough medications and biotechnology products are making their way onto the market. Although clinically valuable, they are very expensive. In addition, PBMs have managed or preferred formularies. In a managed or preferred formulary, interventions may be used to encourage physicians to use the preferred products. Some of these interventions for physicians include academic detailing, prior authorizations, and coverage rules. For pharmacies this may mean a higher dispensing fee for formulary compliance. For the patient this may mean higher copayments if the formulary or preferred product is not used.

Unlike hospitals, PBMs along with their clients (i.e., health plans) place their formulary and non-formulary medications into tiers with an associated copayment with each tier. This tier copayment structure came about in response to the rising cost of prescription drugs. The first tier is generally reserved for generic drug products. This tier usually has the lowest copayment (e.g., $15.00). The second tier is usually reserved for those name brand drugs that are formulary (e.g., $40.00). This tier has a higher copayment than the first tier due to the added cost of the brand name drug. The third tier is reserved for those drug products that are non-formulary brand names. This copayment is significantly higher than the other two tiers (e.g., $80). However, some third-tier copayments may be calculated as a proportion of the drug cost, even as much as one-third as a form of coinsurance, or require paying for the drug in its entirety. The reason for the copayment structure is to encourage the patient to use the most clinically appropriate, cost-effective drug without compromising quality care.[43] Decisions as to the tier placement of a drug product may be dependent on comparative effectiveness research.[193]

The closed formulary can also be broken down into what is referred to as positive or negative formularies. This is the method by which the formulary is developed.

A positive formulary effectively starts with a blank sheet of paper and specifically adds agents. While this is probably the best method to limit the number of drugs available, it is often not very popular when first implementing the formulary because every agent must be considered. That means the physicians must even make specific decisions on whether they should add such things as acetaminophen and amoxicillin to the formulary. Therefore, in hospitals just establishing a formulary, it is often more popular and easier to use a negative formulary system. This essentially starts with the current hospital drug stock, with each drug class being evaluated to eliminate agents that are not necessary.[194] The first steps in this process may be as simple as eliminating multiple salts/esters of the same drug. Then classes of drugs with multiple similar products could be addressed (e.g., analgesics, antacids, laxatives, vitamins, and topical steroids). While in some ways this process is easier, it is also likely to result in a much bigger formulary, since the decision will be made as to what drugs are definitely not needed, rather than which drugs the institution definitely needs. However, the specific institution's situation will need to be assessed before the method of determining the formulary items can be decided on. Overall, the goal is to provide an optimal array of agents; it is easy to end up with too many duplicative agents; however, having a greater number of agents to choose from can lead to better patient care in some areas.[195,196]

It also needs to be mentioned that while a drug formulary provides medication use guidance, a drug formulary does not require a hospital to stock the product. A formulary medication may not always be available in the pharmacy for a variety of reasons. The P&T committee should work closely with pharmacy management to maintain an expectation of medication stock, if stock specifically affects the safety and need of patients. For example, an antidote for snake bites on formulary should be available at the hospital, if snake bites are common in the community the hospital serves.

Regardless of which formulary type a P&T committee maintains, managing the use of medications on formulary is accomplished in a number of ways. Particularly, restriction criteria surrounding service type, patient type, medication criteria, etc., provide the means by which a P&T committee guides practitioners to appropriate medication use. The types of restrictions allowed by a P&T committee should be developed by the voting membership. In addition to restrictions in one or more formularies, a P&T committee may choose to maintain an emergency review process for non-formulary medications for documentation of non-formulary use.

Therapeutic Interchange

Definition of Therapeutic Interchange

The AMA[12,188] defines therapeutic interchange as "authorized exchange of therapeutic alternatives in accordance with previously established and approved written guidelines or protocols within a formulary system." An example would be the use of cefazolin in specific doses whenever any other first-generation injectable cephalosporin is ordered.

Note that therapeutic interchange is different from biosimilar substitution in which the FDA has determined that specific biologic products (i.e., not drugs in general) are similar except for minor differences in clinically inactive components, with no meaningful differences between the biologics in safety, purity, and potency.[197] Biosimilar substitution may allow something very similar to therapeutic interchange, even in community pharmacies, depending on state laws that are being updated to allow for it.[198] A P&T committee can assess biosimilars as a candidate for therapeutic substitution and approve the protocol within the formulary system, regardless of state law. It is important to note that the evaluation of a biosimilar should follow the normal process of evaluating a product for formulary. There are unique items to consider during this review, such as indications for use, immunogenicity, transitions of care, and nomenclature.[199]

Benefits of Therapeutic Interchange

Therapeutic interchange is used in nearly 90% of U.S. hospitals[200] to take advantage of cost savings,[201–203] improved patient outcomes, decreased adverse effects, decreased inventory, fewer medication errors,[204] or other benefits. Therapeutic interchange has been shown to decrease costs without adversely affecting patient outcomes.[57,205] There is even reason to believe that when therapeutic interchange is properly performed, and not entirely based on financial considerations, it may produce lower legal liability on an institution,[92] although there are no published legal cases regarding therapeutic interchange to demonstrate either increased or decreased legal liability.[206] Interdisciplinary teams should develop protocols and comprehensive therapeutic assessments in collaboration to result in an effective and supported therapeutic interchange.

Several medication classes may be the target of therapeutic interchange, and an aggressive IV to oral conversion may be part of this process.[207] The most common classes of drugs for therapeutic interchange are, in order: H_2 antagonists, proton pump inhibitors, antacids, quinolones, potassium supplements, cephalosporins, and hydroxymethylglutaryl-coenzyme A reductase inhibitors.[208] Some drugs classes, such as low-molecular-weight heparins, that at first glance may appear to be possible places for therapeutic interchange, may be found to be unacceptable after a closer inspection.[208]

Therapeutic interchange is considered acceptable to the AMA, unlike therapeutic substitution, which they define as the "act of dispensing a therapeutic alternative for the drug product prescribed without prior authorization of the prescriber" (note: prior authorization may be a blanket authorization, not a specific authorization for each case[209]).[210] Therapeutic interchange has also been found to be acceptable by other organizations, including the American College of Clinical Pharmacy (ACCP), American College of Physicians (ACP),[211] ASHP, American Pharmacists Association (APhA), American Association of Colleges of Pharmacy (AACP), AMCP,[212] and the American Society of

Consultant Pharmacists (ASCP).[213,214] The ACCP spells out the concept of therapeutic interchange in great detail and suggests that it not only be conducted under the auspices of a P&T-type committee, but also that it specifically include DUE, a set method for informing the physicians and other staff that interchange is taking place (should be well planned and thorough[215]), and a mechanism under which the therapeutic interchange policies may be overridden in specific cases.

Decisions for Therapeutic Interchange

Evaluations for therapeutic interchange should also consider medical, legal, and financial evaluations.[208] Other practical aspects, such as communication forms, policies and procedures, medical staff bylaw changes, and other items may need to be addressed by the institution.[216] Electronic means to provide authorization for a therapeutic interchange may be an option.[217] Outside of an institution (e.g., ambulatory environment), therapeutic interchange may not be as easy to implement due to practical procedure methods and because patients are not as closely monitored; however, it may still be possible.[218,219] In the ambulatory situation, the AMA states that therapeutic interchange recommendations must be approved by the majority of physicians affected and must otherwise follow similar standards to that described for inpatient settings.[188]

The consideration of certain therapeutic agents for interchange may result in strong differences of opinion among medical staff members regarding their appropriate use. The process for evaluating any product should be followed, along with efforts being made by committee members to actively approach appropriate influential individuals to manage expectations and assess individual thoughts on an interchange prior to formulary discussion. Through anticipatory, structured negotiation, it is more likely that rational and balanced decisions will be made. Also, it is necessary to take into consideration whether a short-term interchange of products, while the patient is in a hospital, may cause confusion or other difficulties when the patient returns to the outpatient environment and may be restarted on the original agent.[220] Working with the physicians to resolve this issue is a necessity for the long-term care of patients.

Generic substitution can also be considered by the P&T committee, but many pharmacies consider generic substitution to be one of their responsibilities and do not take such decisions to a P&T committee for approval. An exception may be drugs with narrow therapeutic indexes (e.g., anticonvulsants), where a P&T committee may determine a list of products where generic substitution is not allowed,[221] although the FDA insists that such precautions are unnecessary.[222] In relation to generic substitution, it must be mentioned that pharmacies must determine quality suppliers. The ASHP has guidelines for this function.[223] Also, states may have a variety of laws governing generic substitution. They may also publish so-called positive and negative formularies, which differ in definition from those terms used elsewhere in this chapter in that they are lists of drugs that may or may not be substituted for one another, respectively.[206]

In some instances, physicians may prefer that no generic substitution or therapeutic substitution occur on a written order or prescription by indicating "Dispense as Written" (DAW) on that document. This can occur in the inpatient setting as well as the outpatient setting. Depending on the state, DAW is synonymous with the following: no substitution, do not substitute, medically necessary, brand necessary/medically necessary, no drug product selection, brand medically necessary, substitution prohibited without permission of physician or patient, or no substitution/brand necessary.

In most states, the law provides that pharmacists can use a generic version of any medication on a prescription or medication order if the physician has not precluded that action by indicating DAW. In the outpatient setting, in general, if a patient wants a generic medication, they should be sure that their pharmacist knows of their desire.

In some benefit plans, if the physician requests a brand name medication when a generic equivalent is available, the patient member may be responsible to pay the difference in cost in addition to the generic copayment. In some instances, members may not be required to pay this cost difference, if their physician documents that the brand name medication is necessary (Case Study 13-2).

Case Study 13–2

You are the only pharmacist assigned to work the evening shift in the main pharmacy doing electronic order entry. The physician writes an order for dexlansoprazole. From the order you cannot tell if the dexlansoprazole is a patient's home medication or a new order. The clinical pharmacist on that particular floor has gone home for the day. The hospital where you practice has a closed formulary. Your formulary agent is pantoprazole. Your hospital has a policy and procedure for non-formulary drug orders as well as a therapeutic interchange program that includes this class of drugs. You call the physician and explain to him that pantoprazole is the formulary agent. He states that dexlansoprazole is what he prefers for this patient.

- *In order for dexlansoprazole to be dispensed, what form does the physician have to fill out?*
- *Upon receiving the non-formulary request, you notice the reason for the dexlansoprazole order is efficacy. Is this consistent with what you know about the products?*
- *You call the physician and explain what you found and the approved therapeutic interchange. You inform the physician that, per the non-formulary medication policy, it may*

take 24 hours or longer to obtain the non-formulary medication. The physician approves the interchange this time but wants a formal review of the drug at P&T. How would you document the therapeutic interchange?

- *Knowing that the physician wants a formal review of dexlansoprazole, how do you proceed with the request in the pharmacy records or medical records?*

Non-Formulary Usage

Many institutions track the drug use patterns of prescribers, as was mentioned previously in describing the tracking of non-formulary drug products.[224] Annually, a listing of non-formulary products and expenses should be made available to the P&T committee. It is helpful if the pharmacy director can report the total cost of non-formulary items as a percent of the total budget, particularly since the cost can exceed the cost of carrying the non-formulary product on the formulary.[225] Also, it is important to include whether non-formulary drug usage has led to medication errors, since there was at least one report that such non-formulary use resulted in a 28% error rate.[224] Ideally, a report of the number involved and costs of non-formulary orders will be made available to each prescriber. This process is helpful in improving the appropriate use of medications and has also been linked to the prescriber credentialing process.[226] The process can also be used to reevaluate whether non-formulary items should be made available on the drug formulary.

Unlabeled Uses

While some third-party payers may attempt to limit the use of drugs to only FDA-approved indications, this may unnecessarily restrict use of products for indications that may have significant literature support. This should not be supported.[227] However, as will be discussed in more detail in the next chapter, it is sometimes necessary for institutions to specifically restrict drugs to specific uses, if there is a high probability they may be used inappropriately. Such restrictions may be totally unrelated to approved labeling, since product use may be permitted for unlabeled indications if there is adequate literature support and, conversely, may not be permitted at least without special approval within the institution, for FDA indications when there may be more appropriate drugs available. An institution may use monitoring of off-label use of medications to determine if they should be allowed or otherwise addressed.[228]

New Product Introductions

When new drug products are added to the formulary, it is best to prepare physicians, nurses, and others.[141] Initially, it is necessary to inform affected individuals that the drug will be available as of a specific date. That could be immediately or at some time in the near future. There are various reasons for a delay. For example, a drug may have been approved by both the FDA and the P&T committee, but the company may not have yet made it commercially available because they have not yet produced a sufficient supply or they are not yet ready to start their marketing efforts. In some cases, it is necessary for specific equipment to be obtained and installed. Such was the case a number of years ago, when Fluosol®-DA was made available for a limited period of time. This parenteral product required very specialized preparation method involving a warm water bath and percolating a mixture of gases through an IV bag under sterile conditions. Few, if any, pharmacies had the necessary equipment at the time of introduction, and it would have taken some time to get the equipment, set it up, and train pharmacists and technicians in its use, requiring a delay in making the product available in an institution.

In addition to equipment acquisition time, hospitals using electronic medical records, smart pump technology, patient education tools, and formulary management software to electronically list formulary changes may need time for those items to be updated. This includes building automated formulary restrictions into an electronic medical record; thereby providing prescribers the information at the point of prescription. Each of these areas may have their own processes to update each system. Another important reason for the delay includes the time it takes to inform all individuals who will be involved in prescribing, preparing, and administering the drug of drug availability and education in proper use. These education efforts may be provided through newsletters, websites, portals, e-mail, memos, educational programs, RSS (Really Simple Syndication) **aggregators** (programs that pull together information from a variety of sources, such as news resources—an example is Google Reader), or other methods. The method chosen should generally be a standard method used within the institution and should be appropriate for the specific medication product introduction. In cases where a product is particularly complicated, dangerous, or prone to misuse, several methods of instruction, perhaps along with prescribing restrictions, should probably be employed. Further information about newsletters and websites is found in Chapter 12.

POLICIES AND PROCEDURES

Occasionally, policies and procedures must be developed to support the rational use of medications. While the pharmacy department may decide they need to have their own policies and procedures for internal functions, that is not the focus of this discussion.[229] Instead, policies and procedures for the use of medications in an institution, clinic, and so forth will be discussed, since that is often provided through a P&T committee.

TJC recognizes the potential for medication errors and promotes written policy to minimize errors (see MM.04.01.01). TJC has specifically stated that they expect policies and procedures for the following types of orders[15]:

- As needed (prn) medications
- Standing orders
- Automatic stop
- Titrating
- Taper
- Range
- Compounded or admixed drugs
- Medication-related devices
- Investigational medications
- Herbal products
- Medications at discharge or transfer[60]

Definitions of Policies and Procedures

To begin this discussion, the definitions for policies and procedures should be considered.[230] A policy is a broad general statement that describes the goals and purposes of the document. The procedures are specific actions to be taken. In some ways, policies and procedures may resemble a cookbook-type approach, in that a set of steps to be accomplished are described in order. Taken together, these policies and procedures may be a logical, step-by-step explanation of why and where a product may be used, how to use it, and who is to follow the policy (i.e., there may be different portions of the document addressed to pharmacists, technicians, nurses, and prescribers),[231] along with a brief introductory statement describing why the process is necessary.

Before developing a specific policy and procedure, the first step should be deciding whether it is necessary at all. This can be looked at as a risk-benefit decision. For example, is there sufficient risk that a particular medication will be used incorrectly (e.g., prepared wrong, administered wrong, and used for an inappropriate indication) to make it worthwhile to develop a policy and procedure? Generally, the answer will be no, but in a certain number of cases, policies and procedures may be necessary. Examples of where a policy and procedure may be necessary include thrombolytic agents (where the drug can cause serious or fatal effects if used improperly), antibiotics (where it is found that expensive, broad-spectrum antibiotics are being used where amoxicillin should suffice), injectable drugs (where specific individuals who will administer the medication and the process, including programming infusion devices, will be defined),[232] and even for drugs where reimbursement may be a problem. All policies and procedures may be surveyed by CMS and TJC. As such, P&T

committees may choose to develop guidelines, which at times are incorrectly called policies and procedures, as opposed to policies and procedures to guide appropriate medication use. The challenges of education and availability of these guidelines apply.

Developing Policies and Procedures

Once a decision is reached to develop the policy and procedure or guideline, a logical and orderly course should be followed. A proactive, rather than reactive, approach should be employed, when determining if a policy is needed. The policy should be reviewed by the normal drug formulary process, where a mechanism is set up to help determine policy need, evaluate content, and approve the policy. In many cases, a policy and procedure for use of drugs likely to be misused may be developed in conjunction with its consideration for addition to the drug formulary.

As in any process, it is first necessary to decide who will be coordinating the effort and the likely endpoint. That person, or designee, will then need to investigate various sources for background material necessary to develop the policy and procedure. This might include completing a literature search, talking to experts in the field, collaborating with other institutions who have already developed policies on the same topic, reviewing published professional material (e.g., http://www.ashp.org/menu/PracticePolicy/PolicyPositionsGuidelinesBestPractices.aspx) or clinical guidelines (e.g., http://www.guideline.gov), and checking the institution's requirements for developing policies and procedures. If the policy and procedure is for a hospital group, other institutions in the group must also be involved. In particular, it is necessary for the person developing the policy and procedure to have good communications with those who will be affected to avoid confusion and enhance likelihood of policy and procedure utilization. Where the policy and procedure fits in relation to other institutional policies and procedures will also have to be evaluated. Finally, a document should be written, reviewed, and revised, using many of the skills outlined in Chapter 12.

As part of the process of preparing the policy, it is important to be clear how the policy will be applied, and if there may be exceptions. For example, institutions have policies for the automatic stop of specific medications (e.g., stopping an antibiotic after 7 days). The policy should only be applied in cases where it will improve drug therapy. There also needs to be a mechanism to make sure that such an automatic stop, which may be programmed into the computer system, does not cause harm to particular patients (e.g., patients with osteomyelitis receiving antibiotics for an extended period of time).

Implementation of Policies and Procedures

Once the policy and procedure is finished, it will need to be approved by the same process that drug formulary changes go through (i.e., P&T committee, medical executive committee). Some facilities or organizations also have policy approval bodies that have other reporting structures. It is important to understand the appropriate process for policy approval.

The approval and/or effective date for the policy and procedure should be recorded on the document itself to ensure it is not confused with earlier or later documents. A plan for implementing the policy and procedure and educating those involved should also be developed. Forms may need to be prepared and distributed. The policy and procedure should be made available to all people affected by the policy (preferably on the computer network or intranet), and educational programs will need to be planned and given.

Once the policy and procedure is implemented, perhaps in conjunction with the first appearance of a particular agent on the drug formulary, the policy and procedure should be evaluated to determine if it is being properly followed and having the desired effect as a part of a quality assurance plan. A method to enforce compliance with the policies and procedures is required, and it is necessary for legal reasons to demonstrate that this enforcement method is used.[231] Also, the policy and procedure will need to be reviewed, revised (if necessary), and reapproved on a regular basis (preferably once a year). As part of that process, the actual need for the policy and procedure should be reconsidered. The policy and procedure should be eliminated if no longer needed. One way to determine whether the policy and procedures are consulted is if they are on a web server, where the number of times the specific page is opened is recorded. Superseded copies (i.e., previous versions) of the policies and procedures should be kept on file for background and for legal purposes, but should not be available as live documents for use.

It is also necessary to have policies and procedures for the operation of the P&T committee itself (see Appendix 13-1 for policies and procedures for setting up a P&T committee). Some examples of other policies and procedures that may need to be developed include how new drugs are requested for addition to the formulary, how non-formulary drugs can be used, what procedure is used to evaluate new drugs,[149] the composition of the committee, and other committee functions (e.g., conflict of interest). These have been discussed elsewhere in the chapter and will not be dealt with further at this point. For more information on writing policies and procedures, please refer to Chapter 19.

CLINICAL GUIDELINES

P&T committees may be involved with the development, alteration (to fit local circumstances), and/or approval of evidence-based clinical guidelines. The reader is directed to Chapter 8 to obtain further information.

STANDARD ORDER SET DEVELOPMENT

Many prescribers, both in their offices and in institutions (e.g., hospital and nursing home), make use of something called standard orders. This usually consists of a form, preprinted hardcopy, or electronic checklist, which lists orders that are often written for specific patients under certain circumstances. This can include medications, laboratory tests, x-rays, other diagnostic tests, diet restrictions, preoperative preparation, restrictions, and many other things. For example, there may be a specific set of orders for all patients a prescriber admits to the hospital in general or for a specific diagnosis, or a set of orders for a patient who is scheduled to undergo a specific procedure, such as an operation. Standard order sets are commonly used for some medications, such as total parenteral nutrition solutions and oncology agents, where the order can be complex and confusing, perhaps resulting in potential medication errors. The prescribers using the standard order sets can simply indicate which of the items they wish their patients to receive and provide various necessary details, such as dose or duration. The use of standard order sets can be a very good practice, since they act like checklists used by pilots or astronauts—saving time and ensuring that important items are not inadvertently missed or misused. This can be particularly important in the use of drugs that can be dangerous or ineffective if not properly used, such as chemotherapeutic regimens in oncology patients. However, the disadvantage is that the standard order sets do take time to establish and maintain, and may not keep up with actual practice standards depending on review/update process, therefore, contributing to the perpetuation of outdated or inappropriate practices.

While many P&T committees do not address standard order sets directly, leaving them to the individuals or groups that use them or collaborating with other groups specifically designed to look at order sets, it is something that still needs to be considered for several reasons. First, P&T committees are responsible for overseeing all things related to medication use in an institution. Second, the standard order sets include medications, which should only be medications on formulary. If medications are included in standard order sets and are medications that have been removed from formulary, P&T committees should integrate into those discussions to prevent error. The same thought process applied to adding medications to standard order sets that are not yet added to formulary. These situations require the P&T committee to make a special effort to communicate with those individuals or groups with standard order sets. This communication should begin prior to medication-related recommendations. This formulary and order set processes are likely separate, which may delay the frequency of changes based on meeting times of the affected groups, the time it takes to have new standard order set sheets either printed or put on the computer system, and the necessity to adequately train personnel in the use of the updated order sets. In all likelihood, it may take several months after a decision by the P&T committee before the changes can be put into effect. Practitioners should be made well aware of the expected timeline for completion, when such a time difference exists in formulary approval and actual implementation of operations for a formulary change that affects a standard order set. Finally, P&T committees may find that products on standard order sets may be used in ways that are not supported by the medical literature and/or hospital policy, which means that they need to make sure the prescribers or groups that use those orders make necessary changes.

Optimally, individuals or groups using standard orders should be required to review and reapprove their use on a regular basis (probably at least once a year). These standard order sets usually go through an institutional standard order sets committee. In any case, TJC requires a specific policy and procedure for how institutions handle standard order sets.[149] Any changes should be reported to the affected groups (e.g., nursing units, pharmacy, and information technology) and to the P&T committee in cases where the standard order sets include drugs. All standard order sets should include their revision date, to make sure that that old copies are not inadvertently used. Old copies of the orders must be maintained for medicolegal purposes, with the length of time for keeping such records to be determined by the institution's legal counsel.

CREDENTIALING AND PRIVILEGES

Health care institutions are required by various groups to verify that physicians and other health care professionals have the credentials to practice.[234] This can include degrees, licenses, training, and experience. Based on the credentials, professionals may be given privileges to practice within that institution and perform certain activities.[235] Please note that this term is privilege, not right. For example, while all physicians may have the same license, only those trained in surgery may be allowed to do more than very minor surgical procedures (e.g., suturing lacerations and removing minor skin growths). There may be even more specific rules, such as those preventing a chest surgeon from performing neurosurgery. These privileges can also extend to drugs. For example, it may be decided within the P&T committee that only oncologists have privileges to prescribe most antineoplastic agents. This type of policy and procedure is the basis for some restrictions that may be placed when a drug is considered for formulary addition. In addition to restrictions placed within an institution, restrictions may be enforced from outside the institution.

It also must be mentioned that policies and procedures may be in place within an institution to require pharmacists to perform certain operations, whether that is the preparation of particular agents or performing specific clinical functions (e.g., pharmacokinetics and warfarin dosing).[234] Institutions may have a method by which pharmacists are credentialed to perform such services. Further credentialing of pharmacists may be necessary in the future as pharmacist interdependent prescribing becomes more common.[236]

QUALITY IMPROVEMENT WITHIN THE P&T COMMITTEE—INTERNAL AUDIT

❻ *A variety of topics regarding the quality of medication use, inclusive of applicable medication metrics, are normally part of the activities of a P&T committee*, especially timely communication issues. Many of these activities are covered in Chapter 16, however, the items described in the following sections may be considered to be specific to the P&T committee.

Medication Quality Assurance

In addition to determining which medications are available and providing direction in their use, it is required that the quality of use is regularly measured in whatever areas are felt to be necessary, including MUE, DUE, and other similar activities. The P&T committee will likely be involved in this, although coordination of such efforts, including preparing an annual plan of quality assurance activities, may be through other groups, such as a quality assurance committee. The initial plan may be developed by pharmacists, but multidisciplinary feedback is essential before the focused areas of evaluation are finalized. Ideally, all practice areas of the medical staff are given opportunity for input into these focused evaluations. The project list should be continually reviewed and allow for special urgent projects when necessary. If a project is not completed during the year, it may be reconsidered for the next year. DUE criteria selected for continuous improvements should meet TJC accreditation requirements. DUE activities may be used to identify ADRs, contain cost, and expand clinical pharmacy activities.[237] Even if the P&T committee does not direct quality assurance efforts, they must be kept informed of the information gathered and the medication-related quality improvement efforts that are being instituted. This way the P&T committee can be supportive of such efforts directly (e.g., making changes to the drug formulary or policies and procedures to improve medication use) or less directly (e.g., providing statements supporting such activities). Quality assurance is a large topic and further information is available in Chapter 16.

Adverse Drug Reactions

The P&T committee has a responsibility to review adverse reaction data in an institution to identify trends. One tool they can employ is to monitor the use of medications, sometimes referred to as tracer drugs, to treat the symptoms and side effects of other medications.[238] For example, the monitoring of epinephrine, flumazenil, phytonadione, or protamine to try to detect allergic responses, benzodiazepine overdoses, warfarin overdoses, or heparin overdoses, respectively. The topic of ADRs is covered more in Chapter 17.

Medication Error Incidents

Data collected regarding medication errors may be reported to the P&T committee and, probably, for investigational drugs, to the IRB. A systematic method to collect data about medication errors must be set up within an institution, perhaps using internal incident report forms employed by the institution to track all unusual occurrences regarding patients. All incidents are reviewed by severity (e.g., none, minimal, moderate, major, death) and by process (e.g., prescribing, transcription, dispensing, administration, other). A multidisciplinary review of all incidents should take place and trends in the specific quality indicators should be shared with the entire professional staff. High-alert medications (e.g., narcotics, patient-controlled analgesia, insulin, anticoagulants, electrolytes, neuromuscular blockers, thrombolytics, and chemotherapy) should be benchmarked and followed to identify trends to improve the medication management system and ultimately enhance patient safety.

Another monitoring consideration is related to errors with medical devices and may also be monitored by these committees. A study completed in a 520 bed tertiary teaching institution demonstrated that more intensive surveillance methods yielded higher rates of medical device problems as compared to voluntary reporting.[239]

The topic of medication errors is covered in more detail in Chapter 18.

Illegible Handwriting, Transcription, and Abbreviations

It is important to work with the medical staff and all other health professionals regarding illegible handwriting and transcription errors in places where computerized electronic order entry is not utilized. Typically, a task force assigned by the P&T committee is given the charge of evaluating and trending illegible handwriting, followed by developing process improvement measures. A report can be made to the P&T on an ongoing or quarterly basis. An education process must be in place for those individuals who consistently demonstrate poor handwriting. Hands-on reminders have been helpful or, in some extreme cases, handwriting school is recommended. In addition, institutions have adapted TJC unapproved abbreviation list.[15] Unacceptable abbreviations may have an intended meaning but often are potentially misinterpreted and can lead to serious complications. In many institutions, the nurse or pharmacist must clarify the order with the prescriber, when an unapproved abbreviation is written. In some cases, the only effective prevention of this problem has been when the medical staff has determined through the P&T committee that orders containing unapproved abbreviations are completely invalid and must be rewritten by the physician without the inappropriate abbreviation.[240] The addition to the formulary of look-alike, sound-alike medications is discouraged.[241-244] Increasingly, institutions are implementing CPOE, which eliminates the problem of illegible handwriting and decimal point errors, thus reducing medication errors,[245] although implementation costs are considerable, and some institutions may currently feel that it is not yet worth the effort and expense.[246] Also, CPOE may lead to other errors that may turn up in the monitoring for medication errors.

Timeliness

The time for medication orders to be filled and sent to the floor may be tracked by the P&T committee. One area of importance is the response time sequence for a stat (immediate) order. The time should be evaluated from the time the order was written, to when the order was filled, to when the patient receives the medication. There are many obstacles in the order process and getting the medication to the patient. Each institution should have a standard expectation of the turnaround time for stat orders and a policy that will assure that the medication is dispensed and administered promptly. Benchmarking should be done to make sure the policy is followed.

Although not quite as imperative, the timeliness of ordinary order fulfillment must also be evaluated for appropriateness.

Counterfeit Drug Products

Counterfeit drugs can be considered to be those that do not contain the ingredients claimed on the labeling, perhaps having no active ingredients, incorrect dose, or even other drugs.[247] Counterfeit drugs appear to be an increasing problem, although the actual incidence is unknown.[248] The ASHP announced in February 2004 that it would partner with the FDA in a program to keep pharmacists informed about entrance of counterfeit drug products into the nation's drug supply. The ASHP planned to provide rapid alerts to hospital pharmacy departments about counterfeit drug incidents.[249] Also, there are methods being developed or implemented that will help to ensure the pedigree of products, particularly those imported from foreign countries, to help avoid counterfeit products. This may include the use of radio frequency identification (RFID) tags to help track products.[250]

The FDA website may be consulted at http://www.fda.gov/Safety/MedWatch/SafetyInformation/SafetyAlertsforHumanMedicalProducts/default.htm for an updated list of counterfeit products. Because of the potential problems associated with counterfeit drug products, the P&T committee must be kept informed of any situations that affect the institution, as should the medical staff as a whole.[248] This topic also may be handled with medication errors, since it leads to such errors. With the approval of the Drug Supply Chain Security Act (DSCSA), several requirements are now in place to prevent counterfeit product from reaching a hospital. A number of companies have developed software to collect the required medication tracking data for auditing purposed by the FDA or other organizations attempting to reduce medication counterfeiting. Hospitals need to evaluate their suppliers to ensure compliance with DSCSA standards and to implement procedures to restrict access for staff to place orders through less reputable, or gray market, vendors. Staff education on how to detect potentially counterfeit medication products is another risk mitigation strategy that can be coordinated with the P&T committee as drug procurement can involve other departments like radiology, supply chain, and physician offices. Additional information on this topic may be found in Chapter 15.

Safety Alert

A variety of other safety-related items are also important to P&T committees, including recalls, black box warnings, REMS (see Chapter 22),[147] and product shortages, which will be covered in the following subsections and in Chapter 15. The items covered in this section can also be considered related to ADRs and medication errors, since some portions fit under those categories.

Recalls

The 2013 Joint Commission Accreditation Process Guide for Hospitals requires that a policy and procedure be in place, and be implemented when necessary, to retrieve recalled or discontinued medications. This policy must involve notification of prescribers and patients.[15] The pharmacy department constantly reviews medication products recalled by the manufacturer or the FDA due to a safety issue.[251] This information is provided to the pharmacy by the wholesaler and the manufacturer. If a product lot number involved in the recall is found in the pharmacy inventory, that product should be removed from the inventory immediately and recalled from other areas of the institution that may stock it.[149] In the outpatient environment, a recall from consumers may be necessary. A report of medications that have been pulled from the pharmacy inventory should be made available to the P&T committee and the committee may need to decide whether or not to identify patients who may have been affected by the safety issue. Further actions would be based on these findings. The P&T committee chair should be contacted when a patient has significant consequences in relation to a product recall. When a product recall requires the removal of a product treating a disease with limited alternative treatments from the pharmacy inventory, therapeutic alternatives must be made known to the prescribers.[10]

The safety of medications is under constant evaluation, and the safety of new agents cannot be known until the product has been on the market for a period of time.[252] Some newly reported serious adverse effects result in black box warnings being inserted in the product labeling or REMS requirements, which may necessitate action up to the withdrawal of the medication from the market, as was done with propoxyphene.[253] The reason for this name is that the warning is set off from the rest of the information in the package insert by a thick black box that is drawn around it. It is the responsibility of the P&T committee to review safety data for every medication on the formulary. Many P&T committees have a standing agenda item to review all new black box warnings or newly released FDA safety alerts for medications (obtainable from http://www.fda.gov/Safety/ MedWatch/default.htm). The P&T committee needs to review the safety data and make any formulary, policy and procedure, and/or other changes as required. The black box safety data of formulary products need to be disseminated to the medical staff, including any special restrictions or actions taken on a specific product.[15]

Product Shortages

Product shortages should be continuously monitored by the pharmacy department in an organized fashion; this is a TJC requirement.[91,149,251] Information on this can be found at https://www.fda.gov/drugs/drugsafety/drugshortages/default.htm or https://www. ashp.org/drug-shortages/current-shortages. It is possible to get a free e-mail of these shortages or subscribe to an RSS feed. In recent years, there has been a trend toward more frequent medication shortages.[254] In some cases, evaluation of information may show that acceptable alternative products or treatments may be interchanged for products affected by a shortage. The appropriate health care professionals (e.g., physicians, drug information service, pharmacy director, and buyer) need to be immediately notified of product shortages that may have an effect on therapeutic outcomes, along with plans or recommendations on how to address the situation.[255] In some instances, the chief of the medical staff and even the ethics committee may be consulted when policies need to be put into place to ration drug supplies. The shortage of intravenous immunoglobulin (IVIG) in the 1990s necessitated a complete medical staff and pharmacy department agreement for appropriate patient selection for treatment.[256] This shortage required product rationing with the available supply. Unfortunately, no therapeutic alternatives were available for the IVIG shortage. Methods of alerting medical staff of shortages include personal communication, the use of posters or message boards in key areas of the hospital (e.g., medical staff lounge, dictation area, parking garage, and high traffic areas), e-mail, smartphone notification, computer/tablet notification during physician order entry, and the use of newsletters or faxes. A guideline is available from the ASHP to aid in determining how to handle a variety of types of shortages.[251]

In today's health care environment, it is essential to keep medication shortages as a standard agenda item for each P&T meeting. Products with limited availability and products that are not available need to be evaluated constantly. Formulary alternatives for these product shortages then need to be communicated to the medical staff. Further information on this topic may be found in Chapter 15 (Case Study 13-3).

Case Study 13–3

You are the pharmacist medication buyer for the health system. Your wholesaler has notified you that there is a product shortage of IV furosemide and there is no timeframe when it will be available. You check the FDA website as well as the ASHP website for further information. Information is available for estimated resupply dates, implications for patient care, safety and alternative agents, and management of this shortage. You are asked to develop a plan to manage this shortage.

- *What health care personnel should be notified of this shortage?*
- *What methods should be used to alert the medical staff?*
- *What information should you provide to the P&T committee regarding this drug shortage?*
- *What steps do you need to develop a plan to manage this shortage and ensure that patient care is not compromised?*

Communication Within an Organization

INVESTIGATIONAL REVIEW BOARD ACTIONS

While P&T committees are generally responsible for overseeing all aspects of medication use in a hospital, they often turn the major responsibility for overseeing investigational drug use over to an IRB. The IRB should provide a regular overview of its actions to the P&T committee for review, but oftentimes this is all that is done. Further information about IRBs can be found in Chapter 21.

COST, BUDGET, AND FORECASTING

How does the P&T committee actively balance its quality promoting activities as well as the economic requirements of its parent organization? For an individual hospital, this is probably an easier task as long as the economic pressures on the hospital's margin are manageable. As previously mentioned, a closed formulary can result in lowered costs within an institution.[190] However, the P&T committee decisions will be more difficult for the PBM function of a health insurance company or HMO. In the latter situation, the pressures of cost containment, the contents of an insurance plan's Certificate of Benefits, and the applicable payer regulations represent formidable obstacles for building broad support for the decisions of a PBM's P&T committee. In comparison to institutional formularies, PBMs have instituted tier-based formularies that encourage the use of more cost-effective agents to control prescription costs and improve therapy.[257,258] In spite of the economic influences on the P&T committee functions of a PBM, there is no end to opportunities for quality improvement by a PBM since there is no other organization that has the ability to access outpatient medication use to the same extent. Regardless of the organizational setting, the requirements for quality as a basis for decisions should be the chief focus of a P&T committee. Obviously, this is a potentially moving target because of the need to achieve a balance between the ethical standards involved in health care. The vested interests of the parent organization, patient's needs and expectations, the professional activities of physicians, pharmacists and nurses, the pharmaceutical companies, and the requirements of society may be very difficult to reconcile.

National drug expenditure projection data, and the factors likely to influence drug costs for a particular year, can be reviewed by the P&T committee on a yearly basis. Also, it is necessary to keep hospital administrators informed of drug costs and the measures in place to contain costs.[259] An opportunity to inform frontline prescribers of increased drug costs exists in integration with the electronic medical record. In CPOE, a medication order not only can list medication use guidance (i.e., restriction, guideline, order set) to coach appropriate use, but also include cost information. An institution includes dollar signs next to high-cost medications in the CPOE system in order to inform prescribers of high-cost items.[260,261] An understanding of current trends is also essential for formulary management.[262-264] With knowledge of cost trends, available resources and reports from group purchasing organizations, and historical purchase data from the hospital, pharmacy leaders must attempt to request a rational drug budget and justify the request.

LIAISON WITH OTHER ELEMENTS OF THE ORGANIZATION

Within any organization, it is often found that the root of problems is communications or, perhaps more often, a lack thereof. Unfortunately, the solution is not simply an increase in communication efforts in general. Instead, the need is for increasing appropriate communication, along with decreasing inappropriate communication. Some specific things have to be kept in mind.

All individuals involved in drug therapy should receive concise and effective communication about medication-related matters.[169,265] Often, this may simply be a list of new drugs available to practitioners, along with any policies and procedures. Newsletters and educational presentations may also be valuable, depending on the circumstances. Electronic methods of communication are increasingly important, but the use of in-person counterdetailing may be necessary (see Chapter 23).[144]

In addition to making sure that information is provided to those needing it, be sure the amount of material is not overwhelming, otherwise it will be ignored. A news program on television a number of years ago described a situation that the military found regarding its pilots in Vietnam. They had a tape from the cockpit of an aircraft that had been shot down. Those listening to the tape could clearly hear the warning alarm letting the pilot know that a radar missile was locked on his aircraft and posing an imminent danger, however, it was also clear that the pilot did not even realize that warning was happening because of everything else going on. He mentally tuned out the warning and was shot down as a result. It became clear to those training pilots that it was necessary to limit the amount of information to whatever is most important, so that those items were noticed. This is also important in communicating P&T committee materials.

In addition, it is important to keep certain materials confidential for various reasons. In the case of quality assurance materials, keeping materials suitably confidential may protect that data from legal discovery in court (see Chapter 10 and consult attorneys for specifics). Also, some P&T committees keep the agenda and handouts confidential by not sending them to committee members in advance and by collecting the materials at the end of the meeting in order to destroy them. By doing so, they can often avoid pressure put on the committee by pharmaceutical company representatives, who may be trying to have their products included on the formulary, while having their competitor's products excluded. The disadvantage, of course, is that committee members are not able to prepare for a meeting in advance. In relationship to this, it is often a good idea to make sure the pharmaceutical company representatives do not know the members of the committee and who is preparing the evaluation of a particular product, since that can lead to the evaluator being pressured to sway his or her opinion about a particular product. Many hospitals even fully ban pharmaceutical representatives from the hospital to avoid issues.

Finally, an annual report of the P&T committee may be prepared for both internal review and review by the medical executive committee. This annual report is time consuming in preparation but is a very important means of tracking P&T activities and actions over time.

Overall, it is necessary for the chairperson and secretary of the P&T committee to work in cooperation with other appropriate individuals and groups to make sure that essential information is provided wherever needed, while minimizing the amount of extraneous material.

SYNCHRONIZATION OF DATABASES

Although it is more common to think of communication in regard to people, another important area of communications to be addressed is that between electronic databases. The pharmacy computer system may have to communicate with a whole hospital system or other computer systems. It is important to make sure all of these electronic systems are also synchronized, preferably automatically, although the interfaces required to facilitate synchronization may be cost or time prohibitive.[266] In addition, they may introduce medication errors if they are not done properly (Case Study 13-4).

Case Study 13–4

You are the clinical pharmacist assigned to be the secretary of the pharmacy and therapeutics committee (P&T). You are asked to develop an agenda for each monthly meeting, prepare each agenda topic, present each agenda item in a presentation, take notes, and provide follow-up to the meeting.

- *What steps do you need to take to prepare an agenda?*
- *What steps are needed to prepare a medication monograph, including the summary page?*
- *What items are included in meeting minutes?*

- *What methods are used to disseminate the information once approved by the committee?*
- *What steps are needed to operationalize a formulary change?*
- *What steps are needed to further evaluate the formulary change?*

Conclusion

The pharmacy department can have a major impact on the quality of drug therapy in an institution through participation in P&T committee functions and activities described in this chapter, many of which are related to the management of information or are commonly performed by drug information practitioners. While there are many appropriate ways that may be used in addition to those outlined above, those described can be successfully used to improve drug therapy.

Study Questions

1. What is the P&T committee, what are its functions, and how does the committee relate to a pharmacy department?
2. How should a pharmacy/pharmacist be involved in supporting a P&T committee?
3. Define drug formulary and formulary system. How do those items relate to one another?
4. Define open versus closed formularies, including the specific types of closed formularies.
5. What methods can a P&T committee employ to manage and disseminate information about appropriate medication use?
6. Define a restriction and provide an example.
7. How does a P&T committee improve the quality of medication use in a hospital?
8. Define policy. Define procedure.
9. What are the steps in preparing a policy and procedure?
10. Name and briefly explain four policies and procedures that may be implemented by a P&T committee.
11. How does an institutional P&T committee differ from one in a PBM?
12. Who must a P&T committee communicate with? What should they communicate and how should they communicate?
13. What is considered a conflict of interest?
14. What other areas of a hospital need to be updated after a medication has been added to formulary?

Self-Assessment Questions

1. The pharmacy and therapeutics (P&T) committee can be defined as:
   a. A committee that oversees all aspects of medication therapy in an institution
   b. A committee that oversees all procedures of the institution
   c. A committee that oversees only the medications that are carried in a hospital
   d. A committee that oversees only the quality of medication utilization

2. The P&T committee may act only as:
   a. An advisory body to the medical executive committee
   b. An advisory body to the administration
   c. An advisory body to the board of trustees
   d. An advisory body to the pharmacy

3. The functions of a P&T committee include:
   a. Determining what medications are available
   b. Providing medication use guidance at point of dispensing
   c. Quality assurance activities
   d. Policies and procedures regarding drug use
   e. All the above

4. Pharmacy/pharmacists support the P&T committee by:
   a. Having the P&T committee part of the pharmacy department
   b. Serve as chairperson
   c. Involvement in the rational planning process for each meeting agenda
   d. Only addressing medications to be carried on the formulary

5. A drug formulary and a formulary system relate to each other in that:
   a. A drug formulary is a list of available medications under the formulary system which is the method for developing the drug list that reflects the clinical judgment of the medical staff.
   b. A drug formulary comes before a formulary system.
   c. The formulary system provides for a drug formulary that serves only to keep costs down at the expense of patient care.
   d. Where there is a drug formulary system in place there is never a drug formulary published.

6. A closed formulary differs from an open formulary in that:
   a. A closed formulary includes all medications on the market
   b. Closed formularies may not result in cost savings
   c. Only certain medication classes are available in a closed formulary
   d. It is restrictive

7. Which of the following does not describe the benefits of a therapeutic interchange:
   a. Decrease cost
   b. Improve patient outcomes
   c. Decrease inventory
   d. Increased medication errors

8. The P&T committee improves the quality of medications used in the hospital by:
   a. Objectively assessing medications based upon the scientific evidence
   b. By anecdotal physician experience
   c. By manufacturer sponsored information
   d. Occasional review of formulary medications

9. A conflict of interest is considered when people involved in the drug decision process:
   a. Receive direct or indirect compensation from having the drug available
   b. Have stock in the company
   c. Receive honoraria for speaking, consulting fees and gifts or grants from the company
   d. All the above

10. Pharmacy networks are a group of pharmacies that are under contract with insurance companies, health plans, and/or contracted PBM parties to promote pharmacy services at negotiated discount fees.
    a. True
    b. False

11. A drug formulary that provides a list of approved medications with usage guidance for many institutions that are governed by one P&T committee is called a system formulary.
    a. True
    b. False

12. A P&T committee always manages one formulary.
    a. True
    b. False

13. Common formulary management software programs include:
    a. Lexicomp®
    b. Micromedex®
    c. All of the above
    d. None of the above

14. A drug formulary cannot include restriction criteria as a method for guiding appropriate medication use.
    a. True
    b. False

15. Individuals that you would commonly expect to attend a P&T committee meeting include:
    a. Nurse leaders
    b. Quality management
    c. Laboratory technicians
    d. All of the above

Acknowledgment

Paul Nelson, MD is acknowledged for his assistance on previous editions of this book.

REFERENCES

1. Shulkin DJ. Enhancing the role of physicians in the cost-effective use of pharmaceuticals. Hosp Formul. 1994;29:262-73.
2. Nair KV, Ascione FJ. Evaluation of P&T committee performance: an exploratory study. Hosp Formul. 2001;3:136-46.
3. Zellmer WA. Dr. Avorn's wake-up call to pharmacy. Am J Health Syst Pharm. 2004;61:2010.
4. Nair KV, Coombs JH, Ascione FJ. Assessing the structure, activities, and functioning of P&T committees: a multisite case study. P&T. 2000;25(10):516-28.
5. Redman RL, Mays DA. Data analysis. Drug information services in the managed care setting. Drug Benefit Trends. 1997;9:28-40.
6. Sroka CJ. CRS report for Congress: pharmacy benefit managers. Washington, DC: Library of Congress; 2000 Nov 29.
7. Gourley DR, Halbert MR, Hartmann KM, Malone PM. Development and implementation of a P&T committee for state institutions. Hosp Formul. 1981;16(2):143-4, 149-51, 154-5.
8. McCutcheon T. Medicare prescription drug benefit model guidelines. Washington, DC: United States Pharmacopeial Convention; 2004.
9. Stefanacci RG. The expanding role of P&T committees in long-term care. P&T. 2003;28:720-3.
10. Feldman L. Pharmacists' role in the pharmacy and therapeutics committee. Pharma Times. 2004 Feb:26.
11. Jenkins A. Formulary development by community pharmacists. Pharm J. 1996;256:861-3.
12. AMA Board of Trustees. Drug formularies and therapeutic interchange. Recommendations adopted at the American Medical Association (AMA) House of Delegates Interim Meeting 1993. Chicago, IL: American Medical Association; 1993.

13. H-125.991 drug formularies and therapeutic interchange [Internet]. Chicago, IL: American Medical Association; 2000 [cited 2004 Mar 9]:[2 p.]. Available from: http://www.ama-assn.org/apps/pf_new/pf_online?f_n=browse&doc=policyfiles/HnE/H-125.991.HTM

14. Formulary management (medication-use policy development) [Internet]. Bethesda, MD: American Society of Health-System Pharmacists; 2004 [cited 2004 Mar 9]:[1 p.]. Available from: https://www.ashp.org/-/media/assets/policy-guidelines/docs/browse-by-document-type-formulary-management.ashx?la=en&hash=17B045C95B23D1D042242 67874354296BCB25859

15. TJC—The Joint Commission comprehensive accreditation and certification manual [Internet]. Accreditation requirements for hospitals [Internet]. Oakbrook Terrace, IL: The Joint Commission; 2013 Jan 1 [cited 2012 Dec 14]. Available from: https://edition.jcrinc.com/MainContent.aspx

16. Format for formulary submissions. Version 4.0. Alexandria, VA: Academy of Managed Care Pharmacy; 2016.

17. Raffel MW, Barsukiewicz CK. The US health system: origins and functions. Albany, NY: Delmar; 2002.

18. Balu S, O'Connor P, Vogenberg FR. Contemporary issues affecting P&T committees. Part 1: the evolution. P&T. 2004;29:709-11.

19. Worthen DB. The amazing Charles Rice and Bellevue Hospital [Internet]. Pharm Pract News. 2010;37(06):[2 p.]. Available from: http://pharmacypracticenews.com/index.asp?section_id=402&show=dept&issue_id=643&article_id=15339

20. Condition of participation: pharmaceutical services. Fed Regist. 1986;51:22042.

21. Millano C. Bellevue Hospital: the birthplace of formulary medicine? Pharm Pract News. 2004;31:14.

22. Plumridge RJ, Stoelwinder JU, Rucker TD. Drug and therapeutics committees: the relationships among structure, function, and effectiveness. Hosp Pharm. 1993;28:492-3, 496-8, 508.

23. World Health Organization, Management Sciences for Health. Drug and therapeutics committees—a practical guide. Geneva, Switzerland: World Health Organization; 2003.

24. Doherty EC. The JCAHO agenda for change: what changes in pharmacy and P&T activities do you need to prepare for in 1994. Hosp Formul. 1994;29:54-68.

25. The Joint Commission on Accreditation of Health Care Organizations. 1995 Comprehensive Accreditation Manual for Hospitals. Oakbrook Terrace, IL: Joint Commission on Accreditation of Healthcare Organizations; 1994.

26. Academy of Managed Care Pharmacy. Principles of a sound drug formulary system. 2000 [cited 2004 Mar 18]. Available from: http://www.amcp.org/WorkArea/DownloadAsset.aspx?id=9280

27. Eavy GR, Swinkey NJ, Rehan A. Decentralizing the P&T committee: rationale and successes. Formulary. 2000;35:752-69.

28. Mubarak-Shaban H, Billups SJ. The pharmacy and therapeutics committee within a hospital corporation: challenges and solution. P&T. 1998;23(6):309-10, 332.

29. Herbert WJ, Mahaney LM. Consolidating P&T committees in an integrated health care system. Formulary. 1996;31:497-504.

30. Cano SB. Formularies in integrated health systems: Fallon Health Care System. Am J Health Syst Pharm. 1996;53:270-3.

31. Rizos AL, Levy E, Furnier J, Crowley K. Formularies in integrated health systems: Sharp HealthCare. Am J Health Syst Pharm. 1996;53:274-8.

32. Barkley GL, Krol G, Anandan JV, Isopi M. An integrated health care system's attempt to create a unified formulary. Formulary. 1997;32:60-74.

33. Jarry PD, Fish L. Insights on outpatient formulary management in a vertically integrated health care system. Formulary. 1997;32:500-14.

34. Glowczewski JE, Osborne SM. Aligning health system formularies for cost savings. Pharmacy Purchasing & Products. 2015;12(11):4-8.

35. Mannebach MA, Ascione FJ, Gaither CA, Bagozzi RP, Cohen IA, Ryan ML. Activities, functions, and structure of pharmacy and therapeutics committees in large teaching hospitals. Am J Health Syst Pharm. 1999;56:622-8.

36. Balu S, O'Connor P, Vogenberg FR. Contemporary issues affecting P&T committees. Part 2: beyond managed care. P&T. 2004;29:780-3.

37. Solow BK. P&T committees today: ensuring they bring value to your organization. Am J Pharm Benefits. 2009;1(4):189-90.

38. Teagarden JR. How many members should be on a P&T committee. P&T Society. 2003 Fall.

39. Miller WA. Making the pharmacy and therapeutics committee more effective. Curr Concepts Hosp Pharm Manage. 1986;Summer:10-5.

40. Bono RC. Charter Department of Defense pharmacy and therapeutics committee [Internet]. Washington; 2015 Dec 18 [cited 2016 Jul 19]:[5 p.]. Available from: http://www.health.mil/Policies/2015/12/18/DoD-Pharmaceutical-and-Therapeutics-Committee-Charter

41. Barlas S. Role of P&T committees in Medicare: how much authority, accountability? P&T. 2004;29:678.

42. Cross M. Increased pressures change P&T Committee makeup. Managed Care. 2001;10(12):18-30.

43. The ABCs of PBMs. A discussion featuring Peter D. Fox, Ph.D., Terry S. Latanich, Chris O'Flinn, J.D. LLM, and Phonzie Brown. Washington, DC: The George Washington University. National Health Policy Forum. Issue Brief No. 749; 1999 Oct 27.

44. Lipton HL, Kreling DH, Collins T, Hertz KC. Pharmacy benefit management companies: dimensions of performance. Annu Rev Public Health. 1999;20:361-401.

45. Cross M. Do P&T committees have enough power? Managed Care. 2007;16(4):28-30.

46. Reinke T. PBMs just say no to some drugs—but not to others. Managed Care. 2015 Apr;24(4):24-6.

47. Teagarden JR. Perspectives on prescription drug benefit formularies. Hosp Pharm. 2004;39:1102-25.

48. PricewaterhouseCoopers. The value of pharmacy benefit management and the national cost impact of proposed PBM legislation. Pharmaceutical Care Management Association; 2004 Jul.

49. Barlas S. Formulary policies a battleground in HHS proposal on nondiscrimination. Are tiering and cost sharing civil rights issues? P&T. 2016 Mar;41(3):173-5, 193.

50. Barlas S. HHS proposes formulary changes for marketplace health plans. P&T committees would take on a more visible role. P&T. 2015 Feb;40(2):119-22.

51. Regnier SA. How does drug coverage vary by insurance type? Analysis of drug formularies in the United States. Am J Manag Care. 2014 Apr;20(4):322-31.

52. Carroll J. Plans look askance at me-too medications. Managed Care. 2008;17(1):37-42.

53. Butler CD, Manchester R. The P&T committee: descriptive survey of activities and time requirements. Hosp Formul. 1986;21:89-98.

54. Chi J. When R.Ph.s talk P&T committees listen. Hosp Pharm Rep. 1994;8(5):1, 7-8.

55. Gannon K. More power to you. Pharmacists flex their muscles and exert greater influence on P&T committees. Hosp Pharm Rep. 1998;12(2):18-20.

56. Chase P, Bell J, Smith P, Fallik A. Redesign of the P&T committee around continuous quality improvement principles. P&T. 1995;20(10):25-26, 29-30, 32, 34, 37-8, 40.

57. Croft CL, Crane VS. Redesign of P&T committee functions and processes: a model. Formulary. 1998;33:1105-22.

58. Crane VS, Gonzalez ER, Hull BL. How to develop a proactive formulary system. Hosp Formul. 1994;29:700-10.

59. Poirier TI, Vorbach M, Bache T. Linking a policy on nonformulary drugs to the FDA's therapeutic–potential classification system. Am J Hosp Pharm. 1994;51:2277-8.

60. Rich DS. Pharmacies' noncompliance with 2009 Joint Commission hospital accreditation requirements. Am J Health Syst Pharm. 2009;66:e27-30.

61. Green JA, Chawla AK, Fong PA. Evaluating a restrictive formulary system by assessing nonformulary-drug requests. Am J Hosp Pharm. 1985;42:1537-41.

62. Hailemeskel B, Kelvas M. Nonformulary drug requests as a guide in formulary system management. Am J Health Syst Pharm. 1999;56:818, 820.

63. Adding drugs to the formulary: your work is never done. Hosp Pharm. 1999;34(7):828.

64. Shea BF, Churchill WW, Powell SH, Cooley TW, Maguire JH. P&T committee overview: Brigham and Women's Hospital. Pharm Pract Manag Q. 1998;17(4):76-83.

65. McCain J. P&T Committees in position to reduce medication errors. Managed Care. 2004;13(6):39-42.

66. Cunha BA. Principles of antibiotic formulary selection for P&T committees. P&T. 2003;28(6):396.

67. Empey KM, Rapp RP, Evans ME. The effect of an antimicrobial formulary change on hospital resistance patterns. Pharmacotherapy. 2002;22(1):81-7.

68. Cunha BA. Principles of antibiotic formulary selection for P&T committees. Part 1: antimicrobial activity. P&T. 2003;28(6):397-9.

69. Cunha BA. Principles of antibiotic formulary selection for P&T committees. Part 2: pharmacokinetics and pharmacodynamics. P&T. 2003;28(7):468-70.

70. Cunha BA. Principles of antibiotic formulary selection for P&T committees. Part 3: antibiotic resistance. P&T. 2003;28(8):524-7.

71. Polk RE. Antimicrobial formularies: can they minimize antimicrobial resistance? Am J Health Syst Pharm. 2003;60(Suppl 1):S16-S19.

72. Cunha BA. Principles of antibiotic formulary selection for P&T committees. Part 4: antimicrobial side effects. P&T. 2003;28(9):594-6.

73. Cunha BA. Principles of antibiotic formulary selection for P&T committees. Part 5: the cost of antimicrobial therapy. P&T. 2003;28:662-5.

74. Motz JC. Influence of the P&T committee on antibiotic selection in a staff model HMO. P&T. 1998;23(8):411-8.

75. DiLiegro N, Groves AJ, Caspi A. Cost savings from an antimicrobial-monitoring program. P&T. 1998;23(8):419-24.

76. Carlson JA. Antimicrobial formulary management: meeting the challenge in a health maintenance organization. Pharmacotherapy. 1991;11(1 Pt 2):32S-35S.

77. Quintiliani R, Quercia RA. How to create a therapeutics committee that is scientifically and economically sound. Formulary. 2003;38:594-602.

78. Owen RC, Shorr AF, Deschambeault AL. Antimicrobial stewardship: shepherding precious resources. Am J Health Syst Pharm. 2009;66(Suppl 4):S15-S22.

79. Lesprit P, Brun-Buisson C. Hospital antibiotic stewardship. Curr Opin Infect Dis. 2008;21:344-9.

80. Drew RH. Antimicrobial stewardship programs: how to start and steer a successful program. J Manag Care Pharm. 2009;15(2 Suppl):S18-S23.

81. Chen AWJ, Khumra S, Eaton V, Kong DCM. Snapshot of antimicrobial stewardship in Australian hospitals. J Pharm Pract Res. 2010;40(1):19-25.

82. Deuster S, Roten I, Muehlebach S. Implementation of treatment guidelines to support judicious use of antibiotic therapy. J Clin Pharm Ther. 2010;35:71-8.

83. Approved: new antimicrobial stewardship standard [Internet]. The Joint Commission. 2016; [cited 2017 Sept 18]. Available from: https://www.jointcommission.org/assets/1/6/New_Antimicrobial_Stewardship_Standard.pdf

84. Culley CM, Carroll BA, Skledar SJ. Formulary decisions for pre-1938 medications. Am Health Syst Pharm. 2008;65(15):1368-83.

85. Targeted medication safety best practices for hospitals [Internet]. Institute for Safe Medication Practices. c2016 [cited 2016 Jun 29]. Available from: http://www.ismp.org/Tools/BestPractices/default.aspx

86. Mirtallo JM. Advancement of nutrition support clinical pharmacy. Ann Pharmacother. 2007;41:869-72.

87. The Joint Commission. 2010 Provision of Care, Treatment and Services. The Joint Commission Web. Available from: https://www.jointcommission.org/. Accessed Oct 21, 2010.

88. Fagan NL, Malone PM, Baltaro RJ, Malesker MA. Applying the principles of formulary management to blood banking. Transfusion. 2013 Sept;53:2094-7.

89. Anagnostis E. Writing meeting minutes for a pharmacy and therapeutics committee and its subcommittees. Am J Health System Pharm. 2015;72:95-9.

90. ASHP statement on the pharmacy and therapeutics committee. Am J Hosp Pharm. 1992;49:2008-9.
91. Ventola CL. An interview series with members of the ASHP Expert Panel on Formulary Management. Part 1: Linda S. Tyler, Pharm.D. P&T. 2009;34(11):623-31.
92. Brushwood DB. Legal issues surrounding therapeutic interchange in institutional settings: an update. Formulary. 2001;36:796-804.
93. Mutnick AH, Ross MB. Formulary management at a tertiary care teaching hospital. Pharm Pract Manag Q. 1997;17(1):63-87.
94. Dore DD, Larrat EP, Vogenberg FR. Principles of epidemiology for clinical and formulary management professionals. P&T. 2006;31(4):218-26.
95. Suh D, Okpara I, Agnese WB, Toscani M. Application of pharmacoeconomics to formulary decision making in managed care organizations. Am J Manag Care. 2002;8(2):161-9.
96. Odedina FT, Sullivan J, Nash R, Clemmons CD. Use of pharmacoeconomic data in making hospital formulary decisions. Am J Health Syst Pharm. 2002;59:1441-4.
97. Getting the most out of formularies involves a bit of economic training. Managed Care. 2015;24(4):9-10.
98. Pick AM, Massoomi F, Neff WJ, Danekas PL, Stoysich AM. A safety assessment tool for formulary candidates. Am J Health Syst Pharm. 2006;63:1269-72.
99. Barr B. Open and closed. Pharmaceutical Representative[Internet]. 2007 May 1 [cited 2008 Jul 14]:[4 p.]. Available from: http://www.pharmexec.com/open-and-closed
100. ASHP statement on the formulary system. Am J Hosp Pharm. 1983;35:326-8.
101. ASHP technical assistance bulletin on drug formularies. Am J Hosp Pharm. 1991;48:791-3.
102. ASHP guidelines on formulary system management. Am J Hosp Pharm. 1992;49:648-52.
103. Rucker TD, Schiff G. Drug formularies: myths-in-formation. Med Care. 1990;28:928-42.
104. Tyler LS, Cole SW, May JR, Millares M, Valentino MA, Vermeulen LCJr, Wilson AL. ASHP guidelines on the pharmacy and therapeutics committee and the formulary system. Am J Health Syst Pharm. 2008;65:1272-83.
105. Grissinger M. The truth about hospital formularies Part I. P&T. 2008;33(8):441.
106. Lehmann DF, Guharoy R, Page N, Hirschman K, Ploutz-Snyder R, Medicis J. Formulary management as a tool to improve medication use and gain physician support. Am J Health Syst Pharm. 2007;64:464-6.
107. ASHP statement on the pharmacy and therapeutics committee and the formulary system. Am J Health Syst Pharm. 2008;65:2384-6.
108. Rubino M, Hofman JM, Koseserer LJ, Swendryznski RG. ASHP guidelines on medication cost management strategies for hospitals and health systems. Am J Health Syst Pharm. 2008;65:1368-84.
109. Chi J. Hospital consultant foresees dim future for drug formularies. Drug Topics. 1999 April 19:67.
110. Horn SD, Sharkey PD, Tracy DM, Horn C, James B, Goodwin F. Intended and unintended consequences of HMO cost-containment strategies: results from the managed care outcomes project. Am J Manag Care. 1996;2:253-64.

111. Horn SD. Unintended consequences of drug formularies. Am J Health Syst Pharm. 1996;53:2204-6.

112. Goldberg RB. Managing the pharmacy benefit: the formulary system. J Manag Care Pharm. 1997;3(5):565-73.

113. Formulary effectiveness: many questions, but few clear answers. Consult Pharm. 1996;11(7):635.

114. Curtiss FR. Drug formularies provide a path to best care. Am J Health Syst Pharm. 1996;53:2201-3.

115. Formularies and generics drive up health resource use, study suggests. Am J Health Syst Pharm. 1996;53:971-5.

116. Horn SD, Sharkey PD, Phillips-Harris C. Formulary limitations and the elderly: results from the managed care outcomes project. Am J Manag Care. 1998;4:1105-13.

117. Marra F, Patrick DM, White R, Ng H, Bowie WR, Hutchinson JM. Effect of formulary policy decisions on antimicrobial drug utilization in British Columbia. J Antimicrob Chemother. 2005;55:95-101.

118. Penm J, Chaar B, Dechun J, Moles R. Formulary systems in the Western Pacific Region: exploring two Basel Statements. Am J Health Syst Pharm. 2013;70:967-79.

119. Hepler CD. Where is the evidence for formulary effectiveness. Am J Health Syst Pharm. 1997;54:95.

120. VHA formulary management process. Washington, DC: Department of Veterans Affairs; 2009.

121. Kelly WN, Rucker TD. Considerations in deciding which drugs should be in a formulary. J Pharm Pract. 1994;VII(2):51-7.

122. Corman SL, Skledar SJ, Culley CM. Evaluation of conflicting literature and application to formulary decisions. Am J Health Syst Pharm. 2007;64:182-5.

123. Shih Y-C T, Sleath BL. Health care provider knowledge of drug formulary status in ambulatory care settings. Am J Health Syst Pharm. 2004;61:2657-63.

124. Muirhead G. When formularies collide. Hospitals vs. health plans. Hosp Pharm Rep. 1994;8(10):1, 8.

125. 1999 accreditation standards address public concerns, says NCQA. Am J Health Syst Pharm. 1998;55:2221, 2225.

126. Bruzek RJ, Dullinger D. Drug formulary: the cornerstone of a managed pharmacy program. J Pharm Pract. 1992;V(2):75-81.

127. North GLT. Handling nonformulary requests for returning or transfer patients. Am J Hosp Pharm. 1994;51:2360, 2364.

128. Davis FA. Formularies: a dangerous concept for patients. Priv Pract. 1991 Sept:11-17.

129. Palmer MA, Hartman SK, Gervais S. Introducing a formulary system in long-term care facilities: initial experience. Consult Pharm. 1994;9:307-14.

130. Shulkin DJ. Enhancing the role of physicians in the cost-effective use of pharmaceuticals. Hosp Formul. 1994;29:262-73.

131. Pearce MJ, Begg EJ. A review of limited lists and formularies. Are they cost-effective? Pharmacoeconomics. 1992;1:191-202.

132. Sloan FA, Gordon GS, Cocks DL. Hospital drug formularies and use of hospital services. Med Care. 1993;31:851-67.

133. Hazlet TK, Hu T-W. Association between formulary strategies and hospital drug expenditures. Am J Hosp Pharm. 1992;49:2207-10.

134. Pickette S, Hanish L. Dealing with demands for nonformulary drugs. Am J Hosp Pharm. 1992;49:2920, 2923.

135. Corliss DA. Computer-assisted help desk for handling drug benefits. Am J Health Syst Pharm. 1997;54:1941-42, 1945.

136. NCQA draft accreditation standards for 2000 address formularies. Am J Health Syst Pharm. 1998;55:1266-7.

137. Le AG, Generali JA. From printed formularies to online formularies. Hosp Pharm. 2004;38:1003.

138. Navarro RP. Electronic formulary control. Med Interface. 1997;10(8):74-6.

139. Drug czars, electronic formulary systems increase formulary compliance. Formulary. 1997;32:171-2.

140. Ukens C. Hospital finds computer carrot can save drug dollars. Hosp Pharm Rep. 1994;8(6):20.

141. Computerized drug cost information fails to sway physician prescribing. Am J Health Syst Pharm. 1999;56:1183-4.

142. Sears EL. Development and maintenance of an online formulary for a large health system. Am J Health Syst Pharm. 2008;65:510,512.

143. E-prescribing applications help physicians with Vioxx recall. Pharm Pract News. 2004;31(11):67.

144. Patel B, Pichardo RV. Improve formulary adherence through effective provider engagement. Formulary. 2012;47:400-1.

145. McCaffrey S, Nightingale CH. How to develop critical paths and prepare for other formulary management changes. Hosp Formul. 1994;29:628-35.

146. Current formulary decision-making strategies and new factors influencing the process. Formulary. 1995;30:462-70.

147. Raber JH. The formulary process from a risk management perspective. Pharmacotherapy. 2010;30(6 Pt 2):42S-47S.

148. Shulkin D. Reinventing the pharmacy and therapeutics committee. P&T. 2012 Nov;37(11):623-4, 649.

149. Rich DS. New JCAHO medication management standards for 2004. Am J Health Syst Pharm. 2004;61:1349-58.

150. Neumann PJ. Evidence-based and value-based formulary guidelines. 2004;23(1):124-34.

151. Murri NA, Somani S. Implementation of safety-focused pharmacy and therapeutics monographs: a new University Health System Consortium template designed to minimize medication misadventures. Hosp Pharm. 2004;39:654-60.

152. Chren M-M, Landefeld CS. Physicians' behavior and their interactions with drug companies. JAMA. 1994;271:684-9.

153. Bach PB, Saltz LB, Wittes RE. In cancer care, cost matters. New York Times. 2012 Oct 14:A25.

154. Haslé-Pham E, Arnould B, Späth H-M, Follet A, Duru G, Marquis P. Role of clinical, patient-reported outcome and medico-economic studies in the public hospital drug formulary decision-making process: results of a European survey. Health Policy. 2005;71:205-12.

155. Ventola CL. An interview series with members of the ASHP Expert Panel on Formulary Management. Part 3: Sabrina W. Cole, Pharm.D. P&T. 2010;35(1):24-8.

156. Shrank WH. Change we can believe in: requiring better evidence for formulary coverage. Am J Pharm Benefits. 2009 Fall:134-6.

157. Asmus MJ, Hendeles L. Levalbuterol nebulizer solution: is it worth five times the cost of albuterol? Pharmacotherapy. 2000;20:123-9.

158. Desloratadine (Clarinex). Med Lett. 2002;44(W1126B):27-9.

159. Escitalopram (Lexapro) for depression. Med Lett. 2002;44(W1140A):83-4.

160. Most medications approved in the 1990s not new, but modified versions of older drugs, report states [Internet]. Menlo Park, CA: kaisernetwork.org; 2002 May 29 [cited 2004 Apr 22]. Available from: http://khn.org/morning-breakout/dr00011414/

161. Senthilkumaran K, Shatz SM, Kalies RF. Computer-based support system for formulary decisions. Am J Hosp Pharm. 1987;44:1362-6.

162. Computer tool lets P&T members assess Tx classes with their own weightings, product ratings. Formulary. 2000;35:603.

163. Janknegt R, Steenhoek A. The system of objectified judgement analysis (SOJA). A tool in rational drug selection for formulary inclusion. Drugs. 1997;53(4):550-62.

164. Janknegt R, van den Broek PJ, Kulberg BJ, Stobberingh E. Glycopeptides: drug selection by means of the SOJA method. Eur Hosp Pharm. 1997;3(4):127-35.

165. Zachry WM III, Skrepnek GH. Applying multiattribute utility technology to the formulary evaluation process. Formulary. 2002;37:199-206.

166. Jacobson SH. A web-based tool for designing vaccine formularies for childhood immunization in the United States. J Am Med Inform Assoc. 2008;15(5):611-9.

167. Berghelli JA. Conflict of interest policy approved. P&T. 1995;20:497.

168. Alpert JS. Doctors and the drug industry: how can we handle potential conflicts of interest? Am J Med. 2005;118:88-100.

169. Ventola CL. An interview series with members of the ASHP Expert Panel on Formulary Management. Part 2: J. Russell May, Pharm.D. P&T. 2009;34(12):671-7.

170. Campbell EG. Doctors and drug companies—scrutinizing influential relationships. NEJM. 2007;357(18):1796-7.

171. Palmer MA. Developing a conflict-of-interest policy for the pharmacy and therapeutics committee. Am J Hosp Pharm. 1987;44:2012-4.

172. Fredrick DS, Maddock JR, Graman PS. Hashing out a policy on conflicts of interest for a P&T committee. Am J Health Syst Pharm. 1995;52:2791-2.

173. Campbell EG. A national survey of physician-industry relationships. NEJM. 2007;356:1742-50.

174. Barlas S. Inspector General cautions PBMs on formulary decision making. P&T. 2003;28(6):367.

175. Trice S, Devine J, Mistry H, Moore E, Linton A. Formulary management in the Department of Defense. J Managed Care Pharm. 2009;15(2):133-46.

176. Johnson CY. High prices make once-neglected 'orphan' drugs a booming business. [Internet]. The Washington Post. 2016 Aug 4 [cited 2016 Aug 10]. Available from: https://www.washingtonpost.com/business/economy/high-prices-make-once-neglected-orphan-drugs-a-booming-business/2016/08/04/539d0968-1e10-11e6-9c81-4be1c14fb8c8_story.html

177. JCAHO unveils medication-management standards. Am J Health Syst Pharm. 2003;60:1400-1.

178. Cardinale V. Alternative medicine: the law, the marketplace, the formulary. Hosp Pharm Rep. 1999;13(7):15.

179. Is alternative medicine poised for hospital formularies. Drug Util Rev. 1999;15(5):65-8.

180. Brubaker ML. Setting up the herbal formulary system for an alternative medicine clinic. Am J Health Syst Pharm. 1998;55:435-6.

181. Beal FC. Herbals and homeopathic remedies as formulary items. Am J Health Syst Pharm. 1998;55:1266-7.

182. Johnson ST, Wordell CJ. Homeopathic and herbal medicine: considerations for formulary evaluation. Formulary. 1997;32:1166-73.

183. Malesker MA, Meyer RT, Kuhlenengel LJ, Galt MA, Nelson PJ. Development of an alternative medication use policy [abstract]. ASHP Midyear Clinical Meeting. 1998;33(Dec):P-406R.

184. Walker PC. Evolution of a policy disallowing the use of alternative therapies in a health system. Am J Health Syst Pharm. 2000;57:1984-90.

185. Ansani NT, Ciliberto NC, Freedy T. Hospital policies regarding herbal medicines. Am J Health Syst Pharm. 2003;60:367-70.

186. Pick AM, Massoomi F, Neff WJ, Danekas PI, Stoysich AM. A safety assessment tool for formulary candidates. Am J Health Syst Pharm. 2006;63:1269-72.

187. Dennis B, Cha AE. 'Right to Try' laws spur debate over dying patients' access to experimental drugs [Internet]. The Washington Post. 2014 May 16 [cited 2016 Aug 10]. Available from: https://www.washingtonpost.com/national/health-science/right-to-try-laws-spur-debate-over-dying-patients-access-to-experimental-drugs/2014/05/16/820e08c8-dcfa-11e3-b745-87d39690c5c0_story.html

188. H-125.911 Drug formularies and therapeutic interchange [Internet]. Chicago, IL: American Medical Association [cited 2004 Apr 23]. Available from: http://www.ama-assn.org/apps/pf_new/pf_online?f_n=browse&doc=policyfiles/HnE/H-125.991.HTM

189. NCQA draft accreditation standards for 2000 address formularies. Am J Health Syst Pharm. 1999;56:846.

190. Chiefari DM. Effect of a closed formulary on average prescription cost in a community health center. Drug Benefit Trends. 2001;13:44-5, 52.

191. Survey reveals continued HMO shift toward closed and partially closed formularies. Formulary. 1997;32:781-2.

192. Survey finds HMOs, PBMs still moving to restricted formularies, quickly advancing in informatics. Formulary. 1998;33:622, 625.

193. Doyle JJ. The effect of comparative effectiveness research on drug development innovation: a 360° value appraisal. J Comp Eff Res. 2011;1:27-34.

194. Abramowitz PW. Controlling financial variables—changing prescribing patterns. Am J Hosp Pharm. 1984;41:503-15.

195. Open formularies improve oncology outcomes in capitated care system. Formulary. 1996;31:878, 881.

196. TennCare formulary restrictions hurt patient care, survey says. Formulary. 1996;31(6):443.

197. Traynor K. Virginia passes nation's first biosimilar substitution law. Am J Health Syst Pharm. 2013 May 15;70:834-6.

198. Blank C. Arizona passes pharmacy biosimilar law [Internet]. Drug Topics. 2016 Jun 2 [cited 2016 Aug 10]. Available from: http://drugtopics.modernmedicine.com/drug-topics/news/arizona-passes-pharmacy-biosimilar-law

199. Ventola CL. Evaluation of biosimilars for formulary inclusion: factors for consideration by P&T committees. P&T. 2015;40:680-9.

200. Schachtner JM, Guharoy R, Medicis JJ, Newman N, Speizer R. Prevalence and cost savings of therapeutic interchange among U.S. hospitals. Am J Health Syst Pharm. 2002;59:529-33.

201. Bowman GK, Moleski R, Mangi RJ. Measuring the impact of a formulary decision: conversion to one quinolone agent. Formulary. 1996;31:906-14.

202. Chase SL, Peterson AM, Wordell CJ. Therapeutic-interchange program for oral histamine H_2-receptor antagonists. Am J Health Syst Pharm. 1998;55:1382-6.

203. Therapeutic substitution could lower prescription drug spending. Avoidable brand-name costs reached $73 billion in three years, study finds [Internet]. Managed Care. 2016 May 10 [cited 2016 Aug 10]. Available from: http://www.managedcaremag.com/news/therapeutic-substitution-could-lower-prescription-drug-spending

204. Stoysich A, Massoomi F. Automatic interchange of the ACE inhibitors: decision-making process and initial results. Formulary. 2002;37:41-4.

205. Frighetto L, Nickoloff D, Jewesson P. Antibiotic therapeutic interchange program: six years of experience. Hosp Formul. 1995;30:92-105.

206. Vivian JC. Legal aspects of therapeutic interchange [Internet]. 2004 Aug 15 [cited 2004 Oct 22];[6 screens]. Available from: http://www.uspharmacist.com/index.asp?show=article&page=8_1129.htm

207. Janifer AN, Chatelain F, Goldwater SH, Mikovich G. Reengineering hospital pharmacy through therapeutic equivalency interchange while maintaining clinical outcomes. P&T. 1998;23(2):78-82, 85-8, 90-2.

208. Merli GJ, Vanscoy GJ, Rihn TL, Groce JBIII, McCormick W. Applying scientific criteria to therapeutic interchange: a balanced analysis of low-molecular-weight heparins. J Thromb Thrombolysis. 2001;11(3):247-59.

209. Reich P. Therapeutic drug interchange. Med Interface. 1996;9(5):14.

210. H-125.995 Therapeutic and pharmaceutical alternatives by pharmacists [Internet]. Chicago, IL: American Medical Association [cited 2004 Apr 23]. Available from: http://www.ama-assn.org/apps/pf_new/pf_online?f_n=browse&doc=policyfiles/HnE/H-125.995.HTM

211. American College of Physicians. Therapeutic substitution and formulary systems. Ann Intern Med. 1990;113:160-3.

212. Therapeutic interchange [Internet]. Alexandria, VA: Academy of Managed Care Pharmacy; 2012 June [cited 2014 Feb 17]. Available from: http://www.amcp.org/Tertiary.aspx?id=8749&terms=therapeutic%20interchange

213. American College of Clinical Pharmacy. Guidelines for therapeutic interchange. Pharmacotherapy. 1993;13(2):252-6.

214. Massoomi F. Formulary management: antibiotics and therapeutic interchange. Pharm Pract Manag Q. 1996;16(3):11-8.

215. Heiner CR. Communicating about therapeutic interchange. Am J Health Syst Pharm. 1996;53:2568-70.

216. Rosen A, Kay BG, Halecky D. Implementing a therapeutic interchange program in an institutional setting. P&T. 1995;20:711-7.

217. Kielty M. Improving the prior-authorization process to the satisfaction of customers. Am J Health Syst Pharm. 1999;56:1499-501.

218. Carroll NV. Formularies and therapeutic interchange: the health care setting makes a difference. Am J Health Syst Pharm. 1999;56:467-72.

219. Nelson KM. Improving ambulatory care through therapeutic interchange. Am J Health Syst Pharm. 1999;56:1307.

220. D'Amore M, Masters P, Maroun C. Impact of an automatic therapeutic interchange program on discharge medication selection. Hosp Pharm. 2003;38:942-6.

221. Banahan BFIII, Bonnarens JK, Bentley JP. Generic substitution of NTI drugs: issues for Formulary Committee consideration. Formulary. 1998;33:1082-96.

222. FDA comments on activities in states concerning narrow-therapeutic-index drugs. Am J Health Syst Pharm. 1998;55:686-7.

223. ASHP guidelines for selecting pharmaceutical manufacturers and suppliers. Am J Hosp Pharm. 1991;48:523-4.

224. Pummer TL, Shalaby KM, Erush SC. Ordering off the menu: assessing compliance with a nonformulary medication policy. Ann Pharmacother. 2009 July/Aug;43:1251-7.

225. Sweet BV, Stevenson JG. Pharmacy costs associated with nonformulary drug requests. Am J Health Syst Pharm. 2001;58:1746-52.

226. Tse CST, Roecker W, Benitez M, Musabji M. How to tie a drug therapy improvement program to physician credentialing. Hosp Formul. 1994;29:646-56.

227. ASHP statement on the use of medications for unlabeled uses. Am J Hosp Pharm. 1992;49:2006-8.

228. Skledar SJ, Corman SL, Smitherman T. Addressing innovative off-label medication use at an academic medical center. Am J Health Syst Pharm. 2015;72:469-77.

229. Steinberg SK. The development of a hospital pharmacy policy and procedure manual. Can J Hosp Pharm. 1980;XXXIII(6):194-5, 211.

230. Ginnow WK, King CMJr. Revision and reorganization of a hospital pharmacy and procedure manual. Am J Hosp Pharm. 1978;35:698-704.

231. Van Dusen V, Pray WS. Issues in implementation and enforcement of hospital pharmacy policies and procedures. Hosp Pharm. 2001;36(4):398-403.

232. Piecoro JJ Jr. Development of an institutional I.V. drug delivery policy. Am J Hosp Pharm. 1987;44:2557-9.

233. Grissinger M. Eliminating problem-prone, automatic stop-order policies. P&T. 2004;29:344.

234. Galt KA. Credentialing and privileging for pharmacists. Am J Health Syst Pharm. 2004;61:661-70.

235. Galt KA. Privileging, quality improvement and accountability. Am J Health Syst Pharm. 2004;61:659.

236. Abramowitz PW, Shane R, Daigle LA, Noonan KA, Letendre DE. Pharmacist interdependent prescribing: a new model for optimizing patient outcomes. Am J Health Syst Pharm. 2012;69:1976-81.

237. Sass CM. Drug usage evaluation. J Pharm Pract. 1994;7(2):74-8.

238. Orsini MJ, Funk Orsini PA, Thorn DB, Gallina JN. An ADR surveillance program: increasing quality, number of incidence reports. Formulary. 1995;30:454-61.

239. Samore MH, Evans RS, Lassen A, Gould P, Lloyd J, Gardner RM, Abouzelof R, Taylor C, Woodbury DA, Willy M, Bright RA. Surveillance of medical device-related hazards and adverse events in hospitalized patients. JAMA. 2004;291:325-34.

240. Traynor K. Enforcement outdoes education at eliminating unsafe abbreviations. Am J Health Syst Pharm. 2004;61:1314, 1317, 1322.

241. Baker De. Sound-alike and look-alike drug errors. Hosp Pharm. 2002;37:225.

242. Vaida AJ, Peterson J. Common sound-alike, look-alike products. Pharma Times. 2002;68:22-3.

243. Starr CH. When drug names spell trouble. Drug Topics. 2000;144:49-50, 53-4, 57-8.

244. Cohen M. Medication error update. Consult Pharm. 1997;12:1328-9.

245. Soulliard D, Hong M, Saubermann L. Development of a pharmacy-managed medication dictionary in a newly implemented computerized prescriber order-entry system. Am J Health Syst Pharm. 2004;61:617-22.

246. First Consulting Group. Computerized physician order entry: costs, benefits and challenges. A case study approach. Long Beach, CA: First Consulting Group; 2003.

247. FDA's counterfeit drug tasks force interim report [Internet]. Washington, DC: U.S. Department of Health and Human Services; 2003 Oct [cited 2004 Mar 8]. Available from: http://www.fda.gov/oc/initiatives/counterfeit/report/interim_report.html

248. Generali JA. Counterfeit drugs: a growing concern. Hosp Pharm. 2003;38:724.

249. Young D. FDA urges adoption of anticounterfeit technologies by 2007 [Internet]. Bethesda, MD: American Society of Health-System Pharmacists; 2004 Feb 19 [cited 2004 Mar 8]. Available from: https://www.ashp.org/news/2004/02/19/fda_urges_adoption_of_anticounterfeit_technologies_by_2007

250. Redwanski J, Seamon MJ. Impact of counterfeit drugs on the formulary decision-making process. Formulary. 2004;39:577-9, 583.

251. ASHP guidelines on managing drug product shortages. Am J Health Syst Pharm. 2001;58:1445-50.

252. Lasser KE, Allen PD, Woolhandler SJ, Himmelstein DU, Wolfe SM, Bor DH. Timing of new black box warnings and withdrawals for prescription medications. JAMA. 2002;287:2215-20.

253. Gandey A. Propoxyphene withdrawn from US market [Internet]. Medscape. 2010 Nov 19 [cited 2010 Nov 19]:[2 p.]. Available from: http://www.medscape.com/viewarticle/732887_print

254. Fox ER, Tyler LS. Managing drug shortages: seven years' experience at one health system. Am J Health Syst Pharm. 2003;60:245-53.

255. Leady MA, Adams AL, Stumpf JL, Sweet BV. Drug shortages: an approach to managing the latest crisis. Hosp Pharm. 2003;38:748-52.

256. Schrand LM, Troester TS, Ballas ZK, Mutnick AH, Ross MB. Preparing for drug shortages: one teaching hospital's approach to the IVIG shortage. Formulary. 2001;36:52-9.

257. Huskamp HA, Deverka PA, Epstein AM, Epstein RS, McGuigan KA, Frank RG. The effect of incentive-based formularies on prescription-drug utilization and spending. NEJM. 2003;349:2224-32.

258. Thomas CP. Incentive-based formularies. NEJM. 2003;349:2186-8.

259. Crane VS, Hull BL, Hatwig CA, Teresi M, Croft CL. Presenting drug cost information to a board of directors: a case example. Formulary. 2001;36:857-64.

260. Helmons PJ, Coates CR, Kosterink JGW, Daniels CE. Decision support at the point of prescribing to increase formulary adherence. Am J Health Syst Pharm. 2015;72:408-13.

261. Rattles by drug price increases, hospitals seek ways to stand guard [Internet]. The Washington Post [cited 2016 Jun 29]. Available from: https://www.washingtonpost.com/national/health-science/rattled-by-drug-price-increases-hospitals-seek-ways-to-stay-on-guard/2016/03/13/1c593dea-c8f3-11e5-88ff-e2d1b4289c2f_story.html

262. Hoffman JM, Shah ND, Vermeulen LC, Hunkler RJ, Hontz KM. Projecting future drug expenditures-2004. Am J Health Syst Pharm. 2004;61:145-58.

263. Shah ND, Vermeulen LC, Santell JP, Hunkler RJ, Hontz K. Projecting future drug expenditures—2002. Am J Health Syst Pharm. 2002;59:131-42.

264. Shah ND, Hoffman JM, Vermeulen LC, Hunkler RJ, Hontz K. Projecting future drug expenditures—2003. Am J Health Syst Pharm. 2003;60:137-49.

265. Mora MW. How P&T committees can be effective change agents: part 1. Am J Pharm Benefits. 2010;2(2):99-100.

266. Brookins L, Burnette R, De la Torre C, Dumitru D, McManus RB, Urbanski CJ, et al. Formulary and database synchronization. Am J Health Syst Pharm. 2011 Feb 1;68:204, 206.

Chapter Fourteen

Drug Evaluation Monographs

Patrick M. Malone • Mark A. Malesker • Indrani Kar • Jason E. Glowczewski • Devin J. Fox

Learning Objectives

● *After completing this chapter, the reader will be able to*

- Describe and perform an evaluation of a drug product for a drug formulary.
- List the sections included in a drug evaluation monograph.
- Describe the overall highlights included in a monograph summary.
- Describe the recommendations and restrictions that are made in a monograph.
- Describe the purpose and format of a drug class review.
- Describe and perform an evaluation of a therapeutic interchange.

Key Concepts

1 The establishment and maintenance of a drug formulary requires that drugs or drug classes be objectively assessed based on scientific information (e.g., efficacy, safety, uniqueness, cost), not anecdotal prescriber experience.

2 The drug evaluation monograph provides a structured method to review the major features of a drug product.

3 A definite recommendation must be made based on need, therapeutics, side effects, cost, and other items specific to the particular agent (e.g., evidence-based treatment guidelines, dosage forms, convenience, dosage interval, inclusion on the formulary of third-party payers, hospital antibiotic resistance patterns, potential for causing medication errors), usually in that order.

4 The recommendation must be supported by objective evidence.

❺ The most logical decision to benefit the patient and the institution should be recommended to the pharmacy and therapeutics (P&T) committee.

❻ Cost is heavily emphasized in formulary decisions and must be properly accounted for given the complexities of drug acquisition pricing and reimbursement.

❼ Preparation of a drug evaluation monograph requires a great amount of time and effort, using many of the skills discussed throughout this text to obtain, evaluate, collate, and provide information. However, the value of having all of the issues evaluated and discussed can be invaluable in providing quality care.

Introduction

❶ *The establishment and maintenance of a* **drug formulary** *requires that drugs or drug classes be objectively assessed based on scientific information (e.g., efficacy, safety,[1] uniqueness, cost), not anecdotal prescriber experience.* A rational evaluation of all aspects of a drug in relation to similar agents provides the most effective and evidence-based method in deciding which drug is appropriate for formulary addition. In particular, it is necessary to consider need, effectiveness, risk, and cost (overall, including monitoring costs, discounts, rebates, and so forth)—often in that order. Some other issues that are evaluated include dosage forms, packaging, requirements of accrediting or quality assurance bodies, evidence-based treatment guidelines, prescriber preferences, regulatory issues, patient/nursing convenience, advertising, possible discrimination issues,[2] and consumer expectations.[3] There is increasingly more emphasis on evaluating clinical outcomes from high-quality trials, continuous quality assurance information, comparative efficacies,[4] pharmacogenomics, and quality of life.[5]

PURPOSE OF DRUG EVALUATION MONOGRAPH

When completing an evaluation, special consideration should be given to how a drug, if added to formulary, will safely be implemented at the institution. Example questions should be considered (e.g., Does the medication need an order set? Will the medication be stocked? Does the medication need to be added to tools like a smart pump? Does the institution require a medication use guideline for this medication? What restrictions should be considered and why?). Even the potential effect that a drug addition to formulary may have on the public image of the institution may impact the pharmacy and therapeutics (P&T) committee's decision. An in-depth **drug evaluation monograph** can be prepared to assist in this process as described below. **❷** *The drug evaluation monograph* *provides a structured method to review the major features of a drug product.* Once a monograph is prepared, it can easily be used as a structured template or overview of a drug product. That allows for easy comparison or contrast to other products that may be used for the same indication or that are in the same product class.

When a P&T committee reviews an entire class of drugs, the drug class review is prepared instead of one drug evaluation monograph. **Drug class reviews** are often lengthier than a single product drug evaluation monograph; however, they can also use a similar structure and format. Hospitals, health systems, and managed care organizations review an entire class of drugs on a scheduled basis, which must be at least annually, according to accreditation standards.[6] This gives an organization the opportunity to reevaluate the formulary status of products in light of new publications or trials, new products that have entered the market, safety warnings from the FDA, or the potential to delete particular products from the class. Samples of drug class reviews prepared by the Veterans Administration are available on the Internet at http://www.pbm.va.gov/clinical-guidance/drugclassreviews.asp. Similar to drug class reviews, developing a therapeutic interchange or removal from formulary recommendation can follow the same structure and format as a drug monograph. This structure allows for appropriate efficacy, safety, and cost review to be completed. Presentation of all formulary reviews to the P&T committee is essential. These types of reviews, as outlined above, include (a) addition to formulary, (b) removal from formulary, (c) therapeutic interchange, and (d) drug class review considerations.

SOURCES OF DRUG MONOGRAPH

Commercially prepared monographs can be obtained from several sources and can be used as is or with modifications to suit the needs of the institution. If this latter method is used, be aware that the quality of the commercial monographs may vary, even from the same publisher, and they may need extensive updating. Often, writing a new drug evaluation monograph may be easier than improving a commercial monograph. Whether or not the monograph is commercially available or prepared by a member from within the organization, the material should reflect the local conditions or current prescribing practices. As such, this material is owned by the P&T committee as a means of executing its functions per policy and procedure. In order to prevent unwarranted dissemination of institution- and committee-owned materials (especially related to drug company representatives or others), some institutions distribute this material for review during a P&T committee meeting, and then require the materials to be returned at the end of the meeting, rather than providing materials ahead of time. Some institutions even number each monograph with a unique numbering system to assist in tracking the return of P&T committee documents.

CONTENTS OF DRUG MONOGRAPH

Although there are recommendations concerning monograph contents,[3,7] information that may be valuable and specific to an institution and necessary for an objective review of the product is commonly missing.[8] An outline of a sample monograph is found in Appendix 14-1. Each of the sections of this monograph will be discussed below. An example of some of the information found in the various parts of a monograph is seen in Appendix 14-2. This sample monograph meets or exceeds the recommendations of the American Society of Health-System Pharmacists (ASHP),[7] and should serve as a good example for most circumstances. Guidelines published by the Academy of Managed Care Pharmacy (AMCP)[3,9] and The Joint Commission (TJC)[6] are also noted and discussed for situational applicability. The AMCP format is the recommended standard for manufacturers to submit data to managed care organizations. It is designed to restrict the marketing impact of the company in providing information. While it has applicability as to how an institution may evaluate a drug, it also has restrictions as to the amount of information that it can cover, which may make it undesirable in some cases. However, it may be worthwhile for institutions or other organizations to request this information from the drug company, preferably, well in advance of the time it is needed. Note, in some cases this request may require signing a nondisclosure agreement, since it may contain proprietary information.[3]

Overall, the precise monograph should be tailored to the institution, organization, patient population, clinic, and so forth. Several sections not recommended by ASHP have been added to increase the utility of the monograph for other sites of practice, including ambulatory clinics, pediatric institutions, long-term care facilities, managed care or pharmacy benefit managers, or even Medicare or Medicaid formularies. Also, in some cases, the information has been divided into multiple sections or subsections to increase clarity. This format can also be used to evaluate whole classes of drugs. In most cases, a specific drug is compared with others in the same class. The only difference in a class review is that one drug is not receiving the greatest attention; all drugs are being compared with equal attention. Comparative charts and tables are often more prevalent in drug class reviews, as they can serve as a concise method to provide an overview of comparative features for the products in a particular drug class. This format can also be used to evaluate a therapeutic interchange and a potential removal from formulary. Monograph expectations on length and depth vary greatly between institutions. Regardless of these factors, the monograph is a tool to effectively review information in a manner that assists the P&T committee in evaluating the evidence for a recommendation.

Specific formats, differing somewhat from the one presented here, may be required by organizations or governments. For example, Australia (http://www.tga.gov.au/industry/pm-argpm.htm),[10] Ontario, Canada (http://www.health.gov.on.ca/en/pro/programs/drugs/dsguide/docs/dse_guide.pdf),[11] and the United Kingdom (https://www.nice.org.uk/process/pmg19/chapter/1-acknowledgements)[12] have specific, published guidelines that need to be followed for a drug product to be considered for their formularies. The process recommended in this chapter appears to be common in both Canada and the United States, and has been recommended in Australia.[13] Where appropriate, features of these formats have been incorporated into the description presented in this chapter. While the format described in this chapter does provide much of the information in those government standards, with the exception of details about product manufacturing and specific pricing for the particular country, the order and amount of information is often different, and the reader is referred to those standards for details.

IMPORTANCE OF DRUG MONOGRAPH

Before discussing details about monograph preparation, it should be emphasized that the drug monograph is a powerful tool for the pharmacy to guide the rational development of a drug formulary. Although the pharmacy department or an individual pharmacist may have few, if any, votes in the ultimate adoption of a formulary agent, the monograph guides the evaluation process and is likely to be a major factor in the final decision. While monograph preparation can be very time consuming, it is extremely important and should be given proper attention. The structured evaluation process of a drug monograph, in many cases, is the only time a full, fair, and balanced review of a drug that may be presented to a practitioner. Pharmacists have a unique role in the preparation of a monograph in that they view the drug product from a whole and macroeconomic view—all aspects of the drug product are objectively reviewed in a monograph, whereas, oftentimes when a prescriber is presented information about a new drug product, they may be basing their use or nonuse of the product on a single study, package insert data, pharmaceutical representative information, or some other microeconomic view of a drug product that may or may not represent the full utility of the drug product.[14,15]

In addition to FDA-regulated drug products, health care professionals need to be aware of complementary/alternative medicine use, along with the responsibilities and implications that it has for pharmacy services. These products can only be marketed as dietary substances, since the FDA does not regulate herbal products, so manufacturers and distributors cannot make specific health claims. Although there may be minimal scientific evidence regarding efficacy and safety of these products, pharmacists must provide information relating to all therapeutic agents that patients are receiving, preparing a drug monograph for the P&T committee, much the same as for any FDA-approved product. This can also follow the format described in this chapter.[16]

The following sections describe the parts of the drug monograph, as shown in the appendices. Please note that skills in information retrieval (see Chapter 3), drug literature evaluation (see Chapters 4 and 5), professional writing (see Chapter 12) and areas covered in various other chapters must be employed when preparing a drug evaluation monograph.

SUMMARY PAGE

The first page of the monograph is essentially a summary of the most important information concerning the drug, and includes a specific recommendation of the action to be taken on the product. The summary itself is a brief overview of the important aspects of the drug product. Some P&T committees only review this first sheet; however, the remainder of the document should be prepared in order to completely evaluate a drug product and to provide a record of all that was taken into consideration. The summary and recommendation could be placed at the end of the monograph, but it is probably best to keep it on the front to make it easier to refer to during the P&T committee meeting.

FORMAT OF SUMMARY PAGE

The format of the summary page usually begins with general institutional information. Following the name header, specific introductory information about the product is included. The generic name, trade name, and manufacturer are self-explanatory, but the classification may require some explanation. This is meant to give the readers a quick way of classifying the agent.

Determining Drug Classification

The summary page includes the drug's prescription or controlled substance status, **American Hospital Formulary Service (AHFS) classification**, and FDA classification. It may also contain other classification schemes used by particular organizations, such as the Veterans Administration. Managed care organizations may use more detailed drug product identification scheme, such as those established by First DataBank (http://www.fdbhealth.com).

The AHFS classification can be found in the *AHFS Drug Information* reference book, published by the ASHP. This classification can help the reader determine where a new agent falls in therapy. Most of the time, new drugs will be evaluated for possible formulary addition before they are actually placed in that book, so it will be necessary to consult the therapeutic classification table in the front of the *AHFS Drug Information* reference book to decide where the product fits. The classification of similar products listed in *AHFS Drug Information* can also be checked before deciding where to categorize the new product. One AHFS category often overlooked is blood products. FDA classifies blood and blood derivatives as medications. Even if these products are stored in the blood bank, TJC recognizes oversight responsibility by the pharmacy department.[17]

The FDA classification is given to nonbiologic products during the review process and is finalized when the new drug application (NDA) is approved. This classification gives some idea of the importance of the product. The classification consists of chemical type classification (see Table 14-1) and therapeutic rating classification

TABLE 14–1. FDA CLASSIFICATION BY CHEMICAL TYPE*

Type	Definition
1	New molecular entity (NME) not marketed in the United States
2	New salt, ester, or other noncovalent derivative of another drug marketed in the United States
3	New formulation or dosage form of an active ingredient marketed in the United States
4	New combination of drugs already marketed in the United States
5	New manufacturer of a drug product already marketed by another company in the United States
6	New indication for a product already marketed in the United States (note: this category is no longer used)
7	Drug that is already legally marketed without an approved NDA • First application since 1962 for a drug marketed prior to 1938 • First application for DESI (Drug Efficacy Study Implementation)-related products that were first marketed between 1938 and 1962 without an NDA • First application for DESI-related products first marketed after 1962 without NDAs. In this case, the indications may be the same or different from the legally marketed product.
8	Over-the-counter switch
9	New indication submitted as separate NDA, which is consolidated with original NDA after approval
10	New indication submitted as a separate NDA, but not consolidated with original NDA

*Drugs@FDA frequently asked questions [Internet]. Washington, DC: Food and Drug Administration. [Updated 2015 Mar 27; cited 2016 Jul 18]. Available from: http://www.fda.gov/Drugs/InformationOnDrugs/ucm075234.htm#chemtype_reviewclass

TABLE 14–2. FDA CLASSIFICATIONS BY THERAPEUTIC POTENTIAL*

Type	Definition
P	Priority handling by FDA—before 1992 this was two categories: A—Major therapeutic gain B—Moderate therapeutic gain
S	Standard handling by FDA—before 1992 this was referred to as class C, which indicated the product offered only a minor or no therapeutic gain
O	Orphan drug

*Drugs@FDA frequently asked questions [Internet]. Washington, DC: Food and Drug Administration. [Updated 2015 Mar 27; cited 2016 Jul 18]. Available from: http://www.fda.gov/Drugs/InformationOnDrugs/ucm075234.htm#chemtype_reviewclass

(see Table 14-2). An FDA classification of 1P (or 1A prior to 1992) would indicate a drug that was given a priority review status by the FDA. This means that the product offered a therapeutic advance over existing products in the market, may be for a new disease state, or may represent a new drug class. The FDA generally reviews these products in an expedited manner, often not requiring as many clinical trials or a lower number of patients enrolled in the trials before the drug is approved to be on the market. In contrast, a classification of 3S (or 3C prior to 1992) is likely a me-too product, meaning that it is an additional product in a class of medications that is already on the market and is similar in many ways to the other products already marketed. These products are generally reviewed by the FDA in a standard review manner and do not receive an expedited review process.

Knowing and understanding the FDA classification status of a product can assist a reviewer in preparing the drug evaluation monograph in several ways. First, if the reviewer knows that the product being reviewed has an FDA classification status of 1P, the reviewer will often have to compare the product to a drug outside of the class of the product being reviewed. For example, if a new class of antibiotics was developed and called ketolides, the reviewer will not have any other drugs in the class with which the product can be compared, and therefore he or she may need to search for studies or review articles of products that fall in other classes of antibiotics, such as the macrolides. Oftentimes in cases in which cancer chemotherapy medications are approved for a treatment that was previously treated by nondrug therapy, a surgical procedure or radiation therapy may be the best comparator for the product. In the case of products that are given an FDA classification status of 3S, the reviewer generally will be able to prepare a head-to-head comparison of the product to another product that is in the same drug class. For example, if a new hydroxymethylglutaryl-coenzyme A (HMG-CoA) reductase inhibitor was approved by the FDA, the reviewer would normally want to the compare the product with other HMG-CoA reductase inhibitors. Sometimes, when 3S or standard review products enter the market, if there are already a number of similar products available in the market, the manufacturer will conduct trials with the product compared with others in the same class. This product is generally then referred to as the comparator or gold standard product. The reviewer will want to discuss the comparator product and any other similar agents in the class. This can assist the decision makers in the P&T committee in reviewing the new product if they are already familiar with other products in the class.

Comparative Analysis

A particular institution may request additional or specific information that may be relevant to include in the introductory information. Additional product introductory information may include the product's patent exclusivity date and/or the product's patent expiration date. This information can generally be located on the FDA's website at http://www.accessdata.fda.gov/scripts/cder/drugsatfda/index.cfm. It is also common to provide a list of similar agents.

The summary itself is a brief overview of the important aspects of the drug product. If there are similar products or different drugs used for the same indication, it is important to state how the drug being reviewed compares to those products. If a comparison between the agent in question and some other treatment is possible, that comparison must make up the bulk of the section, just as the comparison must be a prominent feature in every other section of the document. The summary will include information on the efficacy, safety (e.g., adverse effects and drug interactions[18]), uniqueness, cost, treatment need in the institution, inpatient versus outpatient needs, potential for inappropriate use,[19] and other factors, such as the likelihood patients would be more compliant with one agent or another[20,21] or how the therapy fits into published clinical guidelines. Information should be limited in this section to those items where a drug has a definite advantage/disadvantage or, if products are similar, where there would be concerns about the possibility of a clinically significant difference. Items that are not clinically significant and not likely to be of concern should be left out of the summary to avoid distractions. In cases where the new drug under evaluation is indicated for a disease that has normally received nondrug treatment (e.g., surgery, radiation, physical therapy), the drug should be compared to that standard treatment. It is worth pointing out that the summary should be just that—a summary of the material presented in the body of the document. Similar to the conclusion of a journal article, this is not the place to put new material or, for that matter, to provide citations; both of those items belong in the body.

● FORMULARY RECOMMENDATION

❸ *Finally, a definite recommendation must be made based on need, therapeutics (including outcome data and the use of evidence-based clinical guidelines), adverse effects, cost (full pharmacoeconomic analysis, if possible), and other items specific to the particular agent (e.g., evidence-based treatment guidelines, dosage forms, convenience, dosage interval, inclusion on the formulary of third-party payers, hospital antibiotic resistance patterns, potential for causing medication errors[22]), usually in that order.*[23,24] Recommendations should be specific to the circumstances in the institution, hospital system, third-party payer plan, and/or other organization in which it is being considered. In hospitals, an accreditation requirement makes it necessary to list the indications for use that the drug the P&T committee is approving; this must be a specific list, although it is acceptable to give a blanket authorization to FDA-approved indications in general.[25] Note that the requirement that drugs be approved for specific indications may be practical only in hospitals where computerized prescriber order entry is available and the prescriber has to enter to state the indication when ordering.

● Tiered Formulary Decisions by Third-Party Payers

When making formulary recommendation as it pertains to third-party payers (e.g., insurance companies), consideration should also be given to the placement of the formulary agent into a multitiered copayment system, where the copayment varies according to the cost of the drug and/or formulary status. The patient member is required to pay these varying amounts of copayment out-of-pocket at the time when the prescription is filled. In general, if the drug is a generic, the placement is at the first tier that has the lowest copayment. If the drug is a brand name drug preferred by the health plan, it is usually placed in the second tier with a higher copayment. All other brand name, nonpreferred drugs are usually placed in the third tier with the highest copayment. Drugs in the third tier, the nonpreferred agents, usually have therapeutic alternatives in either the first or second tier. Patient members are encouraged to talk to their prescribers about switching to the more cost-effective, therapeutic alternative drugs in the lower tiers.[26,27]

Tier designation or formulary status may change, based on the discretion of the health plan and/or pharmacy benefits management (PBM), in the absence of significant new clinical evidence.[28] Quality-of-life information and patient preferences should be considered, if possible. Recommendations for third-party payers may also include a step-therapy approach, quantity limits on the prescription, prior authorization, and coverage rule criteria in order for the drug to be covered. Third-party payers may require some drugs to have a prior authorization before being dispensed. In the community pharmacy setting, prior authorization (also known as prior approval) is usually required for those drugs that are of high cost and/or are likely to be used inappropriately. Examples include tumor necrosis factor blocking agents, compounded medications, newer long-acting opioids, newer atypical antipsychotics, and growth hormones. Prior authorization requires that predetermined guidelines must be met by the member before the drug can be covered by the third-party payer. As an example, the member may be required to try an established, less expensive drug therapy first. If this drug therapy proves to be ineffective or if the patient is unable to tolerate the therapy, then the third-party payer may cover a newer, more expensive therapeutically equivalent drug.[29]

In some cases, an institution may have a subformulary that is available for only a specific group of patients (e.g., Medicaid).[30] Recommendations to conduct drug use evaluation on the drug (see Chapter 16), clinical guidelines to be followed (see Chapter 8), how prescribers are to be educated about the new drug, and other items may also be necessary. Education may range from a simple newsletter or web page, to a specific educational program and certification required before a prescribing.[31]

Some people strongly object to the presence of specific recommendations being placed in the document, because the recommendation in a monograph may differ from the final recommendation approved by the P&T committee. Others do not feel it is appropriate for them to make these recommendations before committee review; however, the person preparing the monograph is in the best situation to advance a logical recommendation. Second, without a recommendation, the discussion does not have a foundation to begin with. Third, the lack of a specific recommendation allows emotion and conjecture to overcome evidence and science. From the pharmacists' perspective, the expectations that a prepared monograph include a formulary recommendation can vary with the culture of the specific organization. This opportunity is welcomed because provision of a specific recommendation is one of the best opportunities for pharmacists to have a deep and wide-ranging impact on patient care, and should not be neglected.

Input and Support from Nonmember Expertise

❹ *The recommendation must be supported by objective evidence* (presented in the summary). Subjective factors that are likely to be significant from the point of view of all involved parties (i.e., physicians, pharmacists, nurses, and patients) should also be considered. Dieticians and respiratory therapists may not be regular members of the P&T Committee; however, they may be called upon for input regarding nutritional supplements or respiratory medications. Decision analysis can be used to show the best drug at the least cost (effectively, this is pharmacoeconomic analysis—see Chapter 7 for details).[29,32-35] Other factors may also be considered and given weight to indicate importance (e.g., multi-attribute utility theory[36]). These methods may be commonly seen in managed care.[37] They look at the possible decisions and their likely outcome, allowing a decision to be made that is likely to lead to the most desirable outcome. Meta-analysis may also find a place in the decision-making process[38]; however, appropriate evaluation of a meta-analysis is important if being utilized. Tentative recommendations should be discussed with appropriate physicians and any clinical pharmacists specializing in that area of therapy before the recommendation is finalized. For example, if a cardiac medication is being evaluated, one or more cardiologists should be consulted to identify their concerns and desires. That does not mean the recommendation should necessarily be changed to what a prescriber wants. If the objective evidence supports the original recommendation, that is the one that should be made; however, it is necessary to demonstrate that the prescribers' concerns were addressed. In a health system, considerations should be given to concerns that effect the entire system, when creating a recommendation. This may include reviewing the recommendation with specialists in the appropriate areas from all hospitals in the system that may have a need for the agent(s). This can be challenging, so the need to leverage physician, pharmacy, and nursing leadership to build consensus is essential.

It is important to minimize opportunities for pharmaceutical representative to influence any decision, so that clinical evidence is the basis of a recommendation. Overall, the items most likely to be added to the formulary include those that are unique, that serve the specific population, that are most cost-effective and, unfortunately, those with the biggest marketing drive by the marketer. Multiple ingredient products or products that are the extended-release or other variations on the patent of a product are least likely to be added in the institutional setting.[39]

Types of Formulary Recommendation

The recommendation should be a logical conclusion supported by the objective evidence and the needs of the health care system, including health care staff needs, distribution concerns, drug administration, and drug availability. Whenever possible, at least for recommendations prepared for an institutional pharmacy, it is best to follow or adapt the

ASHP guidelines for recommendations, which would place the drug into one or a combination of the following groups[7]:

- Added for uncontrolled use by the entire medical staff.
- Added for monitored use—No restrictions placed on use, but the drug will be monitored via a quality assurance study (e.g., drug usage evaluation, medication usage evaluation) to determine appropriateness of use. This is a tie-in to the institution's quality assurance/drug usage evaluation process.[40] Note: this category does not mean that the patient is monitored, since that is necessary for every drug. It means that the quality and appropriateness of how the drug is used is monitored.
- Added with restrictions—The drug is added to the drug formulary, but there are restrictions on who may prescribe it and/or how it may be used (e.g., specific indications, certain physicians or physician groups, certain policies to be followed, specific locations for use, certain medication use guidelines).
- Conditional—Available for use by the entire medical staff for a finite period of time. This may be particularly important during a heightened market, where shortages are common.
- Not added/deleted from formulary—Non-formulary medications are not routinely stocked and, when ordered, the prescriber needs to provide justification for use and recognize procurement may take 24 hours or longer.
- Therapeutic interchange with a preferred agent for the institution's formulary.

Note, there may be different recommendations presented for specific strengths, forms, sizes, and so forth of a drug being reviewed. However, being that specific may not result in any real benefit and may only make things more complicated to manage, with little improvement in drug therapy or decrease in costs.[41] Also, remember that, in any of the above, there is now a requirement to provide a specific list of approved indications for which the drug may be used.[6]

Most drugs should be added for uncontrolled use or, at the other extreme, not be added, simply because the three other categories cause greater work for the pharmacy or other departments. As a side point, if a recommendation to not add the drug to the formulary is approved, it is often good to require a time period before the drug can be considered again (typically 6 months) to prevent political pushback and subsequent approval of a less-than-desirable drug, due to a request for review every month. Monitored use is occasionally needed if there is concern that a drug might be used in some inappropriate manner or has a great risk for adverse events. A limited drug usage evaluation would be conducted until it is evident that the drug is being appropriately used or not causing adverse events. One example where monitored use might be considered is an expensive biotechnology product that only has one normal dose, but multiple investigational doses, where it could be inappropriately prescribed without an investigational protocol. Also, a toxic product might be monitored to see if adverse effects are appropriately addressed by the prescriber. As electronic drug usage evaluation becomes standard, monitoring will be used to a greater extent, but is seldom justified in systems requiring the pharmacist to manually collect data. Instead, frequent drug usage evaluations will necessitate the importance of data availability as opposed to a manual collection process. Newer products, such as interfaced clinical surveillance software systems, can gather data without a manual chart review. A true chart review's importance should not be minimized; instead, because it takes substantial time to complete, a manual chart review should be used to evaluate medication use of an item when the data cannot be obtained any other way.

Conditional addition to the formulary is a recommendation of last resort, simply because it is much easier to keep a drug off the formulary rather than try to delete an inappropriate drug that is being used by prescriber. This type of approval might be used when it is very difficult to clearly determine whether an agent will benefit the institution, if available data are limited at the time of the P&T meeting, or if there is a shortage situation where a normally non-formulary medication needs to become the formulary agent of choice, while the current formulary agent of choice is on shortage. If conditional approval is given, it is absolutely necessary to specify when the P&T committee will reconsider whether the drug should be retained on the formulary.

Recommendations to Add with Restrictions

The recommendation to add with restrictions deserves more explanation. Occasionally, there are drugs that should be added to a drug formulary, but are dangerous[42] or prone to misuse or overuse. This could include agents such as antineoplastics, thrombolytics, and fourth- or fifth-generation cephalosporins.[43] In such cases, it may be desirable to limit the use of the drugs in some manner.[44] For example, the antineoplastics might be limited to prescriptions from oncologists or a defined group that might include a few physicians who are not oncologists (e.g., rheumatologists using methotrexate), and may be required to have written or electronic orders (i.e., verbal orders not being accepted) to eliminate errors and for dose verification. Specific antibiotics might be limited to either infectious disease physicians or to specific, culture-proven diagnoses (this could be done in conjunction with the TJC requirement to approve drugs for specific indications[6]). Often antibiotics may be restricted to a specific length of therapy, after which a new order must be provided or the original order will automatically be discontinued. Other restrictions could include specific floors/areas of the institution or that the physician must receive counterdetailing by the pharmacist before the drug is dispensed.[45]

Relatively new methods of restriction involve formularies for managed care organizations, where they may employ any number of restrictions. There may be a cap or limitation on the price, quantity, or on how many times a patient may receive a drug (e.g., one-time use for nicotine patches to quit smoking) or on how much a patient may receive at one time (e.g., 3-month supply). A medication may be subject to prior authorization or precertification before the drug can be made available to a patient. There may be step therapy or medications, which have to be tried and failed before a specific agent may be available for coverage for a patient. Additionally, practitioners (e.g., prescribers, pharmacists) may receive financial or other incentives to cut back on the use of specific products.[46] Whenever possible, these types of restrictions should be based on objective data, such as the FDA-recommended maximum dose limitations or prescribing contraindication that can be obtained from medication use evaluation.

Some prescribers will object to restrictions, but remember that the prescribers are given privileges to prescribe specific drugs and not rights, which allows the use of restrictions. Usually, this is not an issue, because good prescribers realize there is a reason for the restrictions. The real problem, however, is the desire to use this category much too often in an attempt to ensure proper use of all drugs. While restrictions can be effective in changing usage of specific formulary agents,[47] every time a restricted drug is prescribed, more time and effort by the pharmacy, managed care organization and, perhaps, the prescriber is required to ensure compliance with restrictions. At the very least, a policy and procedure or guideline, and probably appropriate forms or computer restriction methods, will need to be developed or adapted and be presented as part of the drug recommendation to the P&T committee. A cost-benefit analysis may also need to be conducted to ensure that the restriction is valid, meaning that it does assist in curbing inappropriate prescribing or use of an agent. A drug use evaluation may also be performed to assess the usefulness of the restriction. If the results of the drug usage evaluation suggest an acceptable level of appropriate use, the P&T committee may need to reconsider the restriction placed on the product or the restriction could be costing the institution more to administer and monitor than it is saving or avoiding. Therefore, unless the computer system can eliminate much of the effort, there needs to be great restraint used when deciding to recommend that a drug be added to the drug formulary with restrictions.

Oftentimes, adding with monitoring may be a viable alternative. A twist to the restrictions or monitoring types of approval is the use of critical or clinical pathways.[48,49] In this case, a drug may be approved for use in a particular manner for the treatment of a particular disease. These critical pathways may be established for several target populations or target diseases, where additional guidance of patient treatments can result in significant improvement in patient care and/or significant decreases in costs. Because a great deal of time is necessary to develop and manage these critical pathways, they will most likely only be seen in a few areas of any institution at any given time. The recommendation should state if the drug is to be used as part of some clinical guidelines or disease state management (DSM) program.[50] The reader is referred to Chapter 8 for further information. In managed care organizations, critical pathways may be incorporated into the use parameters of a drug, through prior authorization or precertification criteria. These are specific criteria that must be met, based on clinical guidelines, current medical practices, and product prescribing information before a product is deemed medically necessary for use.

Considerations for Formulary Deletion

While the decision to add or delete a drug from the formulary is seldom black or white, a general guideline may be helpful. If the drug is less expensive or the same price as others and is more efficacious or safer—addition to the formulary is appropriate. If the drug is more expensive without added benefit, such as increased safety or effectiveness—do not add to the formulary (or deletion from the formulary is appropriate). The problem comes when the drug is more expensive and also has more benefits. In that case, the careful analysis of the literature and weighing of the institution's needs must be carried out. This is the gray area that has no right answer, but the most appropriate decision must be found. This latter decision may also involve conditional or monitored use. For medications administered primarily in an outpatient setting, reimbursement for the medication, the cost to the patient, and any current or potential bundled-pricing contracts also must be factored into the decision.

Whenever a recommendation is made to add a new agent, consideration should be given to the possibility of removing agents that will no longer be necessary or, in the case of a PBM, moving the agent to a different classification for reimbursement. This whole process can be used as a way of removing extraneous agents on the formulary; however, removal of agents can be difficult if the products are frequently prescribed. (Note: it is often worthwhile to annually review a list of products that have seen little or no use in the previous year in an attempt to remove these products from the formulary.[51]) Whether removing agents individually or through a review of an entire therapeutic class, there needs to be adequate information presented to the P&T committee to show that the product is no longer necessary.

The reasons for removal may include superior agent(s) on the formulary, safety, low or no use, and/or high cost.[52] A timetable for deleting these agents from the formulary must then be developed, and the prescribers must be informed when the agent will no longer be available. The TJC medication management standards require health care organizations to review medications that are available for dispensing or administration on at least an annual basis for safety and efficacy information.[6] Many managed care organizations, health systems, and individual hospitals accomplish this via the use of the drug class review on a scheduled basis. The drug classes may be placed on a schedule for review in which all classes are reviewed over the course of the year. No matter what system an institution chooses to use to delete or review agents, the use should be monitored and follow-up is necessary to ensure the formulary deletions proceed smoothly.[53]

Communication of these deletions can generally appear in newsletters, e-mails, websites, and intranet. If a product is used by only one particular prescriber who is the only one utilizing a product, personal contact may be best to communicate the change as well as to provide information to the prescriber of alternative products.

Consideration for Therapeutic Interchange

Finally, therapeutic interchange must be considered (see Chapter 13).[54,55] If this concept is acceptable to the institution, and legal in the state, it may be appropriate that the new drug be used to substitute for a less desirable agent, or vice versa. In that case, a separate policy and procedure or guideline for handling that interchange needs to be prepared and considered at the same time. Please refer to Chapter 13 for further information on this subject. Also, there may be other policies and procedures or clinical guidelines that may need approval as part of the recommendation, including the requirement for availability and use of concomitant drug therapy (e.g., perhaps a requirement that antiemetic therapy needs to be given prophylactically prior to the administration of a new cancer chemotherapy agent). It is worth noting that therapeutic interchange is perhaps the least expensive method to deal with orders for non-formulary drug products.[56]

All of the material on recommendations presented above may be confusing. ❺However, to state it simply, *the most logical decision to benefit the patient and the institution should be recommended to the P&T committee.*

BODY OF THE MONOGRAPH

Considerations for Monograph Preparation

Many parts of the body of the monograph are self-explanatory from their names and will not be discussed in detail. Some specific points, however, do need to be made about the body. First, the body may not always be reviewed by the P&T committee and, even if presented, it may be covered only briefly. The body needs to be written as a means to compile the information for reference and further information. Importantly, it serves as a way of bringing all of the information together in a logical order for preparation of the summary. Some P&T committees will want to review the data presented in the body of the monograph, but all need to know that the clinical data were reviewed adequately. Other times, an abbreviated monograph may be presented to the P&T committee, and the full monograph is presented to the chairman.

Second, efforts must be made to ensure that the drug in question has been adequately compared with other therapies (whether drug, surgical, radiation, or something else). The person preparing a monograph must go through each section and ask "Have comparisons been made between this drug and the appropriate alternative therapy?" If not, there should either be a good reason for the lack of comparison or some explanation must be put in the section. Sometimes, there will be no published comparison with other drugs or therapies. For example, when anistreplase was first marketed, there were only comparisons to streptokinase available, but physicians wanted to know how the drug compared to alteplase. In that case, information comparing both drugs to streptokinase was used to discern how the drugs would compare to each other. Scientifically, this leaves much to be desired, but sometimes there is no alternative. Other indirect methods of comparison may also be necessary. If at all possible, studies directly comparing the drug being evaluated to the standard of therapy should be used. Also, if there are outcome studies data, that can be important to put in the evaluation, including such hard to quantify items as quality of life.[57] Third, every item should be addressed, even if only to state that information was not available or that it is not applicable (e.g., absorption of intravenous [IV] drugs). This follows the rule that "if it was not written down, it was not done," or in this case was not reviewed.

Finally, the source of the information should be mentioned—any important statement of fact must be referenced, or must be suspected of being inaccurate. The package insert (now often available from http://www.accessdata.fda.gov/scripts/cder/drugsatfda/index.cfm for newly approved products) will serve as a basis for some of the information, particularly to define what is the FDA-approved information, but other references must be used to fill in the gaps and to back up that information. Other information can be obtained from the manufacturer, as stated in the Format for Formulary Submissions, Version 4.0 by the AMCP[3] (an example letter requesting such information is available as a part of that document), but the person preparing the monograph should also personally complete an adequate literature search to identify clinical trials related to the medication for review.

Sections of Drug Monograph

Pharmacologic Data

The Pharmacologic Data section is often one of the shortest. A simple one-paragraph explanation of the proposed mechanism of action and how it differs from the comparator agent(s) usually will suffice for the drug in question. More may be needed if the agent is being compared to a drug with an entirely different mechanism of action (e.g., comparing a new angiotensin-converting enzyme [ACE] inhibitor to a calcium channel blocking agent). If the agent under consideration is an antibiotic, the spectrum of activity should be discussed, which will be much longer.

Therapeutic Indications

The Therapeutic Indications section normally requires the most work. This section may be broken into three main subsections. The first is a brief coverage of the indications that the drug has been used to treat. It is necessary to clearly indicate which uses are FDA approved, non-FDA approved but reasonably supported and likely to be seen, and those that are early in investigation. Non-FDA-approved indications or possible uses may be

difficult to find for new drugs; however, a literature search may be conducted to determine if any abstracts or case reports have been published for uses that were not approved
by the FDA. It is important to note these non-FDA-approved uses as they may be helpful
in determining possible restrictions to place on the drug in the recommendations section
of the monograph, and it will be necessary to consider which, if any, of those uses will be
approved for orders in an institutional pharmacy or health system.[58]

An example would be a new agent that is approved for a single indication. If it is
a relatively new alternative to another agent, many prescribers may want to use it for
investigational uses in patients in which the other agent is indicated, but not tolerated.
Doses may be different in those indications. The P&T committee should review available
data to determine if these investigational uses will be allowed if the new agent is on formulary. Also, non-FDA-approved uses are vital when evaluating medications in a pediatric
institution or various other subpopulations. Often, if non-FDA-approved uses are found
to have therapeutic benefit, they will be studied further and manufacturers will submit
a request to the FDA to add indications for the product. Therefore, the consideration of
other uses is important when considering possible future use of the product. They can
have an impact on use of an agent for an institution. If no off-label uses are noted when the
reviewer is researching the product, it is appropriate to note that fact in the evaluation.[59]

The second subsection will explain how the product and any comparison products fit
into any published clinical guidelines. This should include methods for treatment of the
condition, both pharmacologic and nonpharmacologic treatment approaches. An excellent source of these guidelines is the National Guidelines Clearinghouse (http://www.
guideline.gov/). The reader may also consult Chapter 8 for further information. The use
of clinical guidelines is important for a P&T committee's consideration. The inclusion of
clinical guidelines allows the reader to see the product's anticipated place in therapy. If
the product will be a new first-line agent, an agent should often be available for second-
or third-line therapy after other agents have failed. The product's place in therapy for a
particular disease or indication can play an important role in budgetary decisions when
determining the usage potential of a particular product. A pharmacy department may
want to increase their budget in anticipation of a new drug that will see a lot of usage for
a particular condition. For example, if a new vaccine was developed to help reduce or
prevent Alzheimer's disease, a nursing home or long-term care pharmacy provider may
want to increase their medication budget to allow for a larger supply of the product to be
on hand. However, if a product is for an indication that occurs in less than 1% of a specific
gender of a particular ethnic group, the recommendation for the product may be to not
add it to the formulary.

The third subsection will be abstracts of clinical studies supporting the various uses
(see Chapter 12 for further information on how to prepare an abstract of a study). In
the rare case where a product only has one indication, data from several studies on that

indication should be reviewed in the monograph. If there are multiple indications, at least one well-conducted study for each FDA-approved or the most used indication is usually reviewed. More can be added, but may be redundant and provide no added benefit. If there are several similar studies, one may be covered in depth with a statement at the end of the paragraph that the use is supported by other studies, providing citations. If one well-conducted study for an indication cannot be found, several lower-strength studies may be needed to provide sufficient information. Whenever possible, clinical comparison studies should be used. When reviewing newly approved drugs, it is not unusual to find that no comparison studies have been published. In that case, a simple efficacy study should be used. In some cases, it may be necessary to use a meta-analysis or case report, simply because the disease state is rare, and a typical clinical study cannot be performed. Overall, the quality of the information needs to be evaluated, using the skills described in Chapters 4 and 5.

In cases where no human trials are available, unless there are extenuating circumstances, the drug should generally not be added to a drug formulary until sufficient published information is available. An example of extenuating circumstances would be when a new drug is available for a previously untreatable illness. In that case, the philosophy of anything-is-better-than-nothing may apply. Also, products are sometimes approved on a fast track through the FDA because they treat a very serious, but relatively untreatable disease (e.g., certain cancers, Alzheimer's disease). These drugs may be approved based on a surrogate endpoint (i.e., not the ultimate desirable endpoint, such as length of life in cancer patients, but something that is more easily measured) or with an agreement that further studies be conducted. In cases like this, it may be desirable for the P&T committee to wait until further studies are conducted. Information about requirements for individual agents may be found on the FDA website at http://www.accessdata.fda.gov/scripts/cder/pmc/index.cfm.[60] Orphan drugs are approved with little clinical data for small populations of patients with rare diseases (200,000 or fewer Americans). Approximately 6,800 rare diseases have been identified affecting 30 million people. In 2015, 47% of new drug approvals were for orphan drugs (http://www.fda.gov/ForIndustry/DevelopingProductsforRareDiseasesConditions/ucm2005525.htm).

The information should be presented in a manner that is similar to the description of abstracts given in the appendices to Chapter 12, making sure all information is covered. When reviewing the clinical study, the person writing the drug evaluation monograph should point out strengths and weaknesses of the studies, along with applicability of the information to the patients that are covered by the drug formulary. This evaluation may be vital in arriving at the final recommendation. In some cases, the quality, quantity, and consistency of the literature are formally graded and given a score, in a way similar to the described evaluation of articles in Chapter 8 on evidence-based clinical guidelines, which is then used in the final evaluation of the product.[61]

A new item to consider in this section is pharmacogenomics. Pharmacogenomics has been defined as the individualization of drug therapy based on individual's genetic information.[62,63] Numerous articles have been cited showing the benefits of pharmacogenomics in potentially improving therapy and reducing adverse drug reactions.[64–66] If the genetic makeup of patients is a factor in how the medication is to be used,[67] such clinical study information should be presented in this section. In addition, where appropriate, pharmacogenomic information should be presented in other appropriate sections, such as pharmacokinetics, adverse effects, summary, and so forth. It has been postulated that by the year 2020 pharmacogenomics may become a standard of practice for many disease states and drugs. The FDA's website contains a table that includes genes and affected drug products.[68] The National Institutes of Health (NIH) and the FDA have announced a joint venture regarding the scientific and regulatory structure needed to support advancements in personalized medicine. Other sources of information include the Evaluation of Genomic Applications in Practice and Prevention (EGAPP) (http://www.egappreviews. org/), the International Society for Pharmacoeconomics and Outcomes Research (ISPOR) (http://www.ispor.org), and The Pharmacogenomics Knowledgebase (http://www.pharmgkb.org/). There are no specific methods for incorporation of pharmacogenomic information in a drug evaluation monograph. Since the information can be limited to various areas of the evaluation, it can be placed in the therapeutic information or other sections wherever it best fits. Quite often, if any information is available, it will be under all three subsections of the therapeutic information section and perhaps other places.[69]

In cases of pediatric drug use, studies may focus on adult literature and the data for pediatric literature may be available in abstracts or poster presentations only. The situation may be the same in other areas where there may not be a great deal of information on the use of the product under review. For these cases, a summary of evidence table, such as the one in Table 14-3, may be beneficial to include in the product review, which should cover material whether it is positive or negative. This provides a concise overview of all the available literature, as well as a rating system for the weight of evidence that is available for a particular indication in the pediatric population. It also contains a comparative summary, in a tabular formation, of the literature and evidence available in the adult population. In cases in which published clinical trials are not available, the summary of evidence table serves to provide the P&T committee with an overview of the data available (Table 14-4).

Another new type of publication that may be of interest in this section is comparative effectiveness research, which helps in analyzing competing treatments for specific illnesses[4] and may be available in the FDA-approval packages for as many as half of all new drug products that are approved.[70] This is different from efficacy trials in that it often consists of a great number of patients who are typical of the patients receiving the medications in normal practice (i.e., they are considered to be real-world patients and may have other

TABLE 14–3. SUMMARY OF EVIDENCE TABLE

Summary of Evidence (Place Drug Name Here)		
Literature Type	**Comments**	**Weight of Evidence***
Pediatric Evidence		
Efficacy		
Controlled trials		
Published reports		
Abstract		
Uncontrolled trials		
Published reports		
Abstract		
Experience reports		
Published reports		
Abstracts		
Local specialist experience		
Safety		
Published		
Abstract		
Local specialists' experience		
PK/Dosing		
Published		
Abstract		
Adult Evidence		
Efficacy		
Evaluative reviews		
Controlled trials		
Other		
Summary comments		

*Levels of evidence: Good; fair; poor; none.
Abbreviations: Ra = randomized; DB = double-blind; PC = placebo controlled; F/U = follow-up studies.
Linda K. Ohri, PharmD

confounding disease states, etc.). Often this information is developed from cohort studies, systematic reviews, observational studies, or meta-analyses, using large numbers of patients. Insurance company data may be used for obtaining information to conduct these trials, and it is worth noting that these studies are much less likely to be commercially funded than normal efficacy trials.[71] While these studies are useful for practical data and to help discover rare adverse effects, they also do suffer from the weaknesses inherent in any cohort trial or meta-analysis (see Chapter 5 for further information). They are also relatively rare in the literature, even though it is believed that they can help to obtain formulary

TABLE 14–4. EXAMPLE SUMMARY OF EVIDENCE TABLE

Summary of Evidence (Zonisamide [Zonegran®])		
Literature Type	**Comments**	**Weight of Evidence***
Pediatric Evidence		
Efficacy		
Controlled trials		
Published reports	2 trials; total $n=333$ subjects; generalized & partial; intellectual disability and/or refractory	Good documentation of efficacy
Abstract		
Uncontrolled trials		
Published reports	1 review/study and 2 study reports on use for infantile spasms; total $n= {\sim}109$	Good documentation for efficacy; poor for safety
Abstract	(Much of the pediatric literature is from Japan, with limited availability in English language)	Poor documentation
	14 prospective, open-label Japanese trials involving 1,237 subjects were reviewed in an *Epilepsia* abstract.	Response ($\downarrow$ by $>50\%$):
	Direct study review available for some trials.	Generalized: 47%, 152/325
		Partial: 63%, 578/912
Experience reports		
Published reports	2 reports; total $n=4$ infants with infantile spasms	Good documentation for these cases
Abstracts	8 abstracts; total $n=135$; most were pediatric	Poor documentation of varied experience from multiple independent groups
Local specialist experience	Not Indicated (NI)	
Safety		
Published	10 case/case series reports published, with extensive description of adverse events	Good documentation of ADR experience reports
Abstract	2 U.S. summaries of Japanese safety experience; 1st—4 data sources, $n=2,574$; 2nd—14 studies, $n=1,237$. Likely overlap between 2 reports.	Poor documentation; rather extensive experience
Local specialists' experience	NI	
PK/Dosing		
Published	2 reports; total $n= 194$; children & adults	Good documentation; limited data
Abstract	~6 reports; children and/or adults; drug interaction effects on PKs	Poor documentation of limited data

continued

TABLE 14–4. EXAMPLE SUMMARY OF EVIDENCE TABLE (*CONTINUED*)

Summary of Evidence (Zonisamide [Zonegran®])		
Literature Type	**Comments**	**Weight of Evidence***
Adult Evidence		
Efficacy		
Evaluative reviews	Cochrane Review of adjunctive use for refractory partial epilepsy in 3 Ra studies; total $n = 499$; 12-wk duration	Reviewer conclusions:
	An assessment of Japanese experience was compared against clinical guidelines for AED use (established by the International League Against Epilepsy); $n=1,008$ (ped $n=403$)	Effective as adjunctive treatment for refractory partial seizures. Authors concluded that zonisamide was effective against both partial and refractory generalized seizures.
Controlled trials	Deferred review; FDA approved for adjunctive therapy of partial seizures in adults	Good documentation, based on FDA approval
Other		
Summary comments	Extensive, independent pediatric reports of efficacy in a variety of seizure types, both published and abstracts; demonstrated benefit in refractory seizure types, including infantile spasms; substantial published experience literature on a variety of adverse events, generally documenting reversibility with dosage adjustment or discontinuation. Limitations in evaluation: multiple publications representing the same subjects.	

*Levels of evidence: Good; fair; poor; none.
Abbreviations: Ra = randomized; DB = double-blind; PC = placebo controlled; F/U = follow-up studies.

admission for drug products[72] and are more commonly being used for formulary decisions made by national committees in countries such as Britain, Australia, and Canada.[73] They may also be used by third-party payers to determine the payment-tier placement of products.[74] Overall, it is hoped that these trials will help to identify overuse, misuse, and underuse of various treatments,[75] and may be seen more commonly in the future.

In preparing the therapeutic use section, it may also be useful to review materials that were presented to any FDA Advisory Committees, which may be found at http://www.fda.gov/AdvisoryCommittees/CommitteesMeetingMaterials/Drugs/default.htm.

Other information may also be covered in the therapeutics section, including quality-of-life studies.

● *Pharmacokinetics*

The Bioavailability/Pharmacokinetics section is similar to what would be found in most publications, but the information may be difficult to find for some new drugs. In some cases, a new dosage form may be considered in a drug evaluation. For example, when a drug is released in IV form, its use may be entirely different from the oral form, so the P&T committee might separately consider it. A change in route, however, does not necessarily mean that elimination is significantly different in the same patient population. Therefore, oral data may be more useful than no information. Whenever possible, a table comparing the drug in question to other products or formulations may be helpful.

● *Dosage, Administration, and Supply*

The Dosage Form section is a good place to point out the limitations in dosage forms available for some drugs. For example, perhaps the drug in question is available only as an oral solid, but its comparator agent is available in oral solid, oral liquid, and injectable forms, which could be an advantage. This section can also be used to discuss unusual preparation directions or pointing out which product would be easier, quicker, and less expensive to prepare. Additionally, this section should state if the product has any limitations on access (i.e., the product is only available from a registry or available to select facilities), distribution, supply limitations, or possible anticipated shortages.[76] This section can also cover the handling of medications that have a high risk for serious injury if misused. In addition, the Dosage Form section should also address special provisions for the procurement, storage, ordering, dispensing, and monitoring of these high-risk agents. Medication error problems in this area may be addressed by professional practice procedures describing product labeling and packaging, nomenclature, compounding and dispensing, education, administration, monitoring, and use. Specific recommendations are available regarding antineoplastic agents that address health care professionals, organizations, and patients.[77]

Known Adverse Effects/Toxicities

When presenting the information in the Known Adverse Effects/Toxicities section, serious and/or common adverse effects for both the specific drug and the drug class should be the focus. Whenever possible, incidence and severity should be included. An incidence comparison table listing the agent under consideration and other similar agents may be an efficient and informative method to show the material. If there are many rare, minor adverse effects, a statement to that effect can be listed at the end of the discussion. Conversely, other agents may have very little information available on adverse effects, simply because they are too new. In that case, it may be necessary to discuss adverse effects common to that class of agent, making it clear that they have not yet been seen with the new drug, but are possible. The new agent should be compared to other agents used for the same indication to determine whether there are any advantages. Keep in mind that these tables can be deceiving, because older agents may have 20 years of side effect reports, whereas, a number of adverse effects of the new agent may not yet be discovered.

Also, TJC now requires patient safety information to be addressed in all monographs, including sentinel event advisories.[6] It has been recommended that a list of possible safety problems be compiled. This may include concerns in such areas as ordering, transcribing, order entry, storage, order verification, compounding, dispensing, administration, and monitoring.[78] It may be good to consider **Risk Evaluation and Mitigation Strategies (REMS)** information from the FDA in this section.[79] Some drugs may be added to the formulary simply because of improved patient safety, even though that comes at an increased cost.[1] Besides the package labeling, other sources of this information can be found at:

- Institute for Safe Medication Practices (ISMP): http://www.ismp.org
- MedWatch: http://www.fda.gov/medwatch
- United States Pharmacopeia Patient Safety Program: http://www.usp.org/

Once the list of possible safety concerns has been compiled, even a tally of the number of items can be helpful, but it also may be that specific items cause an overriding concern. In response, P&T committees are implementing safety-focused drug monographs, which include information regarding medication errors.[80]

The Patient Information section complies with the Omnibus Budget Reconciliation Act (OBRA) '90 standards for prospective drug utilization review (DUR).

The Patient Monitoring Guidelines and Patient Information sections listed are items not suggested by ASHP. These sections were originally added for use in the ambulatory care environment, although they can be quite informative in any practice area.

Cost Comparison

The final section is the cost comparison, where the product being reviewed is compared in price to other similar products. Typically, three or four medications (possibly including both trade name and generic products) are compared, although sometimes it is necessary to compare a dozen or more products or dosage forms. Preferably, a pharmacoeconomic analysis should be prepared[81] (see Chapter 7), because the seemingly more expensive agent may turn out to be less expensive, as it decreases the length of hospitalization, degree of monitoring, or number of adverse events that would otherwise occur.[82,83] Such an analysis is considered to be important by the majority of institutions[84] and managed care organizations.[85] It may, however, take a considerable amount of time to prepare and sometimes the assumptions made in preparing the analysis will be challenged by attendees.[86] Sometimes, it may even be necessary to provide a spreadsheet to show what effect changes in assumptions may have on the economic analysis. In the case of drug evaluation monographs prepared in the method of the AMCP guidelines, the information in this section may provide detailed abstracts of pharmacoeconomic studies, in a manner similar to that seen for clinical studies in the Therapeutics section.[3] Overall, the items included in the analysis should make sense to those doing the evaluation.[87] It should be noted that the assumptions intrinsic in any pharmacoeconomic analysis are considered pseudoscience by some and are discouraged,[88,89] even though they may be the best information available on which to make important financial decisions.

Often, a full pharmacoeconomic review is not practical because of lack of time or expertise, although most large hospitals do report doing a formal economic analysis of some kind for each drug reviewed for possible formulary addition.[90] With particularly expensive products, a comprehensive pharmacoeconomic analysis becomes necessary.[91,92] Even when a full pharmacoeconomic analysis is not practical, any pertinent information that could be used in a full analysis should be included. After all, it sometimes can be determined that the most expensive (per dose) drug product may actually be much less expensive in the long run, because of increased or faster efficacy, decreased incidence of adverse effects, or lower monitoring costs.

In some cases, a simple price comparison can be prepared using the cost of the drugs and the frequency of administration. Health systems may be challenged with a medication cost analysis, since each hospital comprising the health system may purchase the medication at a different price. System-wide contracting agreements may mitigate this issue, but there will likely remain a gap for facilities that have **340b** program pricing and for those that do not. In these cases, the unique costs and current or estimated purchase volume must be evaluated to make sure that a rational decision is made. Such a price comparison must also consider that the patient may be getting medications both within an institution and after returning home, because institutional pharmacies may get considerable discounts. Therefore, both the institution's cost for the medication, likely **group purchasing organization (GPO)** pricing, and the average wholesale price (AWP) should be considered. Some medications are extremely inexpensive to the institution, making it tempting to include those agents on the formulary instead of similar therapeutic agents. However, if the AWP is excessively high, the patient may not be able to afford the product in the community, which could quickly lead to readmission into the hospital, when the patient's disease is no longer being treated. In those cases, it may not be an appropriate product to carry on the formulary. Also, the differences in package sizes and frequency of administration must be considered. In most cases, products can be compared on the cost of a typical day's therapy at a relatively normal dose; however, in some cases, a different approach may be necessary. For example, an antineoplastic agent may need to be compared with other agents based on a per-cycle or per-cost of therapeutic regimen basis. Another example that results in unusual cost comparisons is Nexplanon® (an implantable contraceptive agent). The cost of both the drug and the implantation procedure need to be compared to a 3-year supply of other contraceptive agents. In cases like this, over a period of years, it may be necessary to include calculations of inflation or other factors likely to change over the time period.[93]

Other costs should also be considered when possible, such as drug preparation costs, administration costs, laboratory tests, monitoring requirements, and changes of length of stay/therapy—after all, it is not a savings overall if costs are simply shifted from the pharmacy (i.e., drug price) to the laboratory (i.e., monitoring costs).[94] In the future, theranostics (also known as pharmacodiagnostics—which is defined as the analysis of a patient's genome in order to personalize medical treatment using pharmacogenomics) will be a substantial cost that needs to be included in the analysis.[95] Some pharmacies even include such items as the cost to order and hold the drug, and the cost of preparing the evaluation of the drug for the P&T committee.[96] Also, it is becoming more common to take into account some items more difficult to assess, such as the probability and cost of therapeutic failure in comparison to other similar agents, impact of specific drug therapy on other health care costs (a drug may be cheaper, but require an increase in the cost of other nondrug therapy for the patient), and the cost of adverse drug effects.[97] Because these items may depend on the characteristics of the patients (e.g., age, socioeconomic status, education level), the figures used are necessarily going to be uncertain. In some cases, however, they will be important in the final formulary decisions. A drug that at first glance appears more expensive may be found to actually cost the institution less in the end.[82] Also, it is necessary to consider nondrug therapy (e.g., surgery, radiation therapy, physical therapy) in the comparison, when they are legitimate alternatives to drug therapy. Overall, the goal is to ensure that the comparison makes sense and takes into consideration all of the relevant economic factors. ❻ *Cost is heavily emphasized in formulary decisions and must be properly accounted for given the complexities of drug acquisition pricing and reimbursement.* Some drugs cost thousands of dollars per dose, and that can quickly deplete a pharmacy department's budget and significantly affect the economic status of an institution.

Of importance, a drug evaluation monograph follows a general pattern and sequence of content as outlined in this chapter. The depth, length, and expected template for use will differ between institutions, but should be appropriate and approved for use at the institution. For example, some places prefer bullet points and tables to present information, while others expect a longer paragraph review. Refer to the institution for the guidance on a drug evaluation monograph.

Conclusion

❼ *Preparation of a drug evaluation monograph requires a great amount of time and effort, using many of the skills discussed throughout this text to obtain, evaluate, collate, and provide information. However, the value of having all of the issues evaluated and discussed can be invaluable in providing quality care* (Case Studies 14-1, 14-2, and 14-3).

Case Study 14–1

You are a recent graduate who just completed a PGY1 residency. You have accepted a position at a local hospital medical center as a clinical pharmacist. One of your first assignments is to prepare and present a medication monograph on a new oral direct thrombin inhibitor that was just approved by the FDA. You will have 10 minutes to present at the next pharmacy and therapeutics committee meeting that will be held next week. The only piece of information that you are given is the non-formulary request to add this drug to formulary. All medications are reviewed for the outpatient pharmacy as well.

- *Having reviewed the non-formulary request, what are the steps to add this drug to the formulary?*
- *What are the essential elements of a medication monograph?*
- *What sources of information do you need to develop a complete evidence-based medication monograph?*

Case Study 14–2

Following the development of the drug evaluation monograph, you are then asked to prepare a concise high-level summary page of this medication monograph.

- *What are the elements of a high-level summary page?*
- *You are planning to use this monograph for your inpatient as well as the outpatient pharmacies. What information should be included as it relates to the outpatient dispensing of this medication?*
- *What are the different types of formulary status recommendations and how do they differ?*

Case Study 14–3

After your success with the drug evaluation monograph and the high-level summary, you have now been asked to evaluate the cost of a new chemotherapy medication that has just received FDA approval. Your work will then be turned over to others for the creation of a full drug evaluation monograph. It is important to be aware that your hospital is part of a health system with a system-wide formulary so the following information will be important for your analysis of the cost of the new medication "Chemotherapy 1":

- GPO price: $10,000 per 100 mg vial
- 340b price: $9,000 per 100 mg vial
- 10 hospitals in the health system and 2 qualify for 340b pricing
- Anticipated annual use will be in 70 patients
- Average dose is 300 mg per patient × 28 doses
- Medicare reimbursement is $950 per 10 mg
- Your hospital markup for drug prices is 2 times cost
- Private insurance companies on average pay 53% of what they are charged for outpatient medications
- Medicare accounts for 50% of patient volume and the other 50% is private insurance
- 304b facilities account for 10% of health system oncology volume
- The health system charges all patients the GPO price for medications and passes on the 340b savings in other ways
    1. *What is the annual cost impact if this medication is added to formulary?*
    2. *How will the health system be reimbursed for this medication?*
    3. *What other considerations are important as the cost data is prepared for the monograph?*

Self-Assessment Questions

1. Medications or medication classes considered for a medication formulary should be objectively assessed based on:
    a. Scientific information
    b. Anecdotal prescriber experience
    c. Manufacturer information
    d. Published review
    e. All of the above

2. The summary page of a medication monograph:
   a. Provides a summary of the most important information concerning the medication
   b. Completely evaluates a medication product
   c. Provides a record of all that was taken into consideration
   d. Includes items that are not clinically significant

3. Included on the summary page is a definite recommendation primarily based upon:
   a. Objective outcome data and the use of evidence-based clinical guidelines
   b. Cost
   c. Anecdotal prescriber experience
   d. Other items specific to the particular agent

4. The body of the monograph does which of the following:
   a. Brings all the information together in a logical order
   b. Adequately compares the medication to other therapies
   c. Only addresses certain items
   d. Includes the source of the information
   e. a and b

5. Hospitals and health systems review an entire class of medications on a scheduled basis which must be at least annually according to The Joint Commission.
   a. True
   b. False

6. A medication monograph provides a tool for the pharmacy to:
   a. Guide the rational development of a medication formulary
   b. Provide a full, fair, and balanced review of a medication
   c. View medications from a whole and macroeconomic view
   d. All the above

7. Pharmacogenomics is the study of:
   a. Medication indications and nonapproved indications
   b. Medication cost
   c. Medication tier placement
   d. Individualized drug therapy based on an individual's genetic makeup

8. Pharmacoeconomics is primarily the study of:
   a. Medication cost
   b. Medication indications

    c. Medication adherence

    d. All of the above

9. When making formulary recommendations as it pertains to third-party payers, consideration should be given to the placement of the formulary agent into a multitiered copayment system where the copayment varies according to the cost of the drug and/or formulary status.

    a. True

    b. False

10. Future medication monographs may be expected to include clinical outcomes, continuous quality assurance information, pharmacogenomics, and quality of life issues.

    a. True

    b. False

11. A drug evaluation monograph cannot be used to evaluate a therapeutic interchange.

    a. True

    b. False

12. A drug use evaluation should include manual chart review data, if necessary, and aggregate data from reporting tools available to the institution.

    a. True

    b. False

13. There is only one format, length, and style that a drug evaluation monograph should follow.

    a. True

    b. False

14. When evaluating the price of a medication for a monograph to be used for a health system, the following must be considered:

    a. Each hospital's individual price

    b. 340b status of the hospital

    c. If the medication will primarily be used inpatient our outpatient

    d. All of the above

15. All hospitals qualify for 340b medication pricing and it should be consistently used when evaluating medication costs:

    a. True

    b. False

Acknowledgment

The assistance of Linda K. Ohri, PharmD, MPH in preparation of this chapter in previous editions is acknowledged with thanks.

REFERENCES

1. Raber JH. The formulary process from a risk management perspective. Pharmacotherapy. 2010;30(6 Pt 2):42S-47S.
2. Barlas S. Formulary policies a battleground in HHS proposal on nondiscrimination. Are tiering and cost sharing civil rights issues? P&T. 2016 Mar;41(3):173-5, 193.
3. Format for formulary submissions, version 4.0. Alexandria, VA: Academy of Managed Care Pharmacy; 2016.
4. Schumock GT, Pickard AS. Comparative effectiveness research: relevance and applications to pharmacy. Am J Health Syst Pharm. 2009;66:1278-86.
5. Wade WE, Spruill WJ, Taylor AT, Longe RL, Hawkins DW. The expanding role of pharmacy and therapeutics committees. The 1990s and beyond. PharmacoEconomics. 1996;10(2):123-8.
6. TJC—The Joint Commission comprehensive accreditation and certification manual. Accreditation requirements for hospitals [Internet]. Oakbrook Terrace, IL: The Joint Commission; 2013 Jan 1 [cited 2012 Dec 14]. Available from: https://e-dition.jcrinc.com/MainContent.aspx
7. ASHP technical assistance bulletin on the evaluation of drugs for formularies. Am J Hosp Pharm. 1991;48:791-3.
8. Majercik PL, May JR, Longe RL, Johnson MH. Evaluation of pharmacy and therapeutics committee drug evaluation reports. Am J Hosp Pharm. 1985;42:1073-6.
9. Academy of Managed Care Pharmacy. Therapeutic interchange. 2003 Feb [cited 2010 Nov 5]:[2 p.]. Available from: http://www.amcp.org/WorkArea/DownloadAsset.aspx?id=18745
10. Australian regulatory guidelines for prescription medicines [Internet]. Woden, Australia: Australian Government, Department of Health and Ageing, Therapeutic Goods Administration; 2015 Dec 22 [cited 2016 Jul 14]. Available from: https://www.tga.gov.au/publication/australian-regulatory-guidelines-prescription-medicines-argpm
11. Ontario guidelines for drug submission and evaluation. Toronto: Ministry of Health and Long-Term Care; 2000.
12. Guide to the process of technology appraisal [Internet]. London: National Institute for Clinical Excellence; 2014 [cited 2016 Jul 13]. Available from: https://www.nice.org.uk/process/pmg19/chapter/1-acknowledgements
13. Duguid MJ. Evaluating new medicines for use in Australian hospitals: lessons from North America. J Pharm Pract Res. 2010;40(2):124-9.
14. Groves KE, Fanagan PS, MacKinnon NJ. Why physicians start or stop prescribing a drug: literature review and formulary implications. Formulary. 2002;37(4):186-8, 190-4.

15. Strite S, Stuart ME, Urban S. Process steps and suggestions for creating drug monographs and drug class reviews in an evidence-based formulary system. Formulary. 2008;43:135-6, 139-40, 142, 144-5.

16. Cohen KR, Cerone P, Ruggiero R. Complementary/alternative medicine use: responsibilities and implications for pharmacy services. P&T. 2002;27(9):440-6.

17. Fagan NL, Malone PM, Baltaro RJ, Malesker MA. Applying principles of formulary management to blood banking. Transfusion. 2013;53(9):2094-7.

18. Chan L-N. Consider potential for drug interactions during formulary review. Am J Health Syst Pharm. 2000;57:391.

19. Schiff GD, Galanter WL, Duhig J, Koronkowski MJ, Lodolce AE, Pontikes P, Busker J, Touchette D, Walton S, Lambert BL. A prescription for improving drug formulary decision making. PLoS Med. 2012 May;9(5):e1001220.

20. Feldman JA, DeTullio PL. Medication noncompliance: an issue to consider in the drug selection process. Hosp Formul. 1994;29:204-11.

21. Sesin GP. Therapeutic decision-making: a model for formulary evaluation. Drug Intell Clin Pharm. 1986;20:581-3.

22. Cohen MR. Adding drugs to the formulary: your work is never done. Hosp Pharm. 1999;34:828.

23. Hedblom EC. Pharmacoeconomic and outcomes data in the managed care formulary decision-making process. P&T. 1995;20:462-4, 468, 471-3.

24. Klink B. Formulary influences. Drug Top. 1998;142(20):72.

25. Rich DS. Pharmacies' noncompliance with 2009 Joint Commission hospital accreditation requirements. Am J Health Syst Pharm. 2009;66:e27-30.

26. Abourjaily P, Kross J, Gouveia WA. Initiatives to control drug costs associated with an independent physician association. Am J Health Syst Pharm. 2003;60:269-72.

27. Gleason PP, Gunderson BW, Gericke KR. Are incentive-based formularies inversely associated with drug utilization in managed care? Ann Pharmacother. 2005;39:339-45.

28. Reissman D. Issues in drug benefit management. Drug Benefit Trends. 2004; Dec:598-99.

29. Sroka CJ. CRS report for Congress: pharmacy benefit managers. Washington, DC: Library of Congress; 2000.

30. Tyler LS, Cole SW, May JR, Millares M, Valentino MA, Vermeulen LC Jr, Cole SW. ASHP guidelines on the pharmacy and therapeutics committee and the formulary system. Am J Health Syst Pharm. 2008;65:1272-83.

31. Dedrick S, Kessler JM. Formulary evaluation teams: Duke University Medical Center's approach to P&T committee reorganization. Formulary. 1999;34:47-51.

32. Kresel JJ, Hutchings HC, MacKay DN, Weinstein MC, Read JL, Taylor-Halvorsen K, Ashley H. Application of decision analysis to drug selection for formulary addition. Hosp Formul. 1987;22:658-76.

33. Szymusiak-Mutnick B, Mutnick AH. Application of decision analysis in antibiotic formulary choices. J Pharm Technol. 1994;10:23-6.

34. Basskin L. How to use decision analysis to solve pharmacoeconomic problems. Formulary. 1997;32:619-28.

35. Kessler JM. Decision analysis in the formulary process. Am J Health Syst Pharm. 1997;54(Suppl 1):S5-S8.

36. Schumacher GE. Multiattribute evaluation in formulary decision-making as applied to calcium-channel blockers. Am J Hosp Pharm. 1991;48:301-8.

37. Barner JC, Thomas J III. Tools, information sources, and methods used in deciding on drug availability in HMOs. Am J Health Syst Pharm. 1998;55:50-6.

38. Gibaldi M. Meta-analysis. A review of its place in therapeutic decision-making. Drugs. 1993;46:805-18.

39. Gannon K. Uniqueness of a drug key to formulary inclusion. Hosp Pharm Rep. 1996;10:27.

40. Chase P, Bell J, Smith P, Fallik A. Redesign of the P&T committee around continuous quality improvement principles. P&T. 1995;20(1):25-6, 29-30, 32, 34, 37-8, 40.

41. Ain KB, Pucino F, Csako G, Wesley RA, Drass JA, Clark C. Effects of restricting levothyroxine dosage strength availability. Pharmacotherapy. 1996;16(6):1103-10.

42. Limit potential dangers by restricting problem drugs on formulary. Drug Util Rev. 1997;13(4):49-51.

43. Anassi EO, Ericsson C, Lal L, McCants E, Stewart K, Moseley C. Using a pharmaceutical restriction program to control antibiotic use. Formulary. 1995;30:711-4.

44. Berndt EM. Drug expenditures. A medical center's experience with antibiotic cost-saving measures. Drug Benefit Trends. 1997;9:32-6.

45. McCloskey WW, Johnson PN, Jeffrey LP. Cephalosporin-use restrictions in teaching hospitals. Am J Hosp Pharm. 1984;41:2359-62.

46. Goldberg RB. Managing the pharmacy benefit: the formulary system. J Manag Care Pharm. 1997;3(5):565-73.

47. Hayman JN, Sbravati EC. Controlling cephalosporin and aminoglycoside costs through pharmacy and therapeutics committee restrictions. Am J Hosp Pharm. 1985; 42:1343-7.

48. McCaffrey S, Nightingale CH. The evolving health care marketplace. How to develop critical paths and prepare for other formulary management changes. Hosp Formul. 1994;29:628-35.

49. Dana WJ, McWhinney B. Managing high cost and biotech drugs: two institutions' perspectives. Hosp Formul. 1994;29:638-45.

50. Armstrong EP. Disease state management and its influence on health systems today. Drug Benefit Trends. 1996;8:18-20, 25, 29.

51. Persson EL, Miller KS, Nieman JA, Sgourakis AP, Akkerman SR. Formulary evaluation using a class review approach. Experience and results from an academic medical center. P&T. 2013 Apr;38(4):213-6.

52. Kelly WN, Rucker TD. Considerations in deciding which drugs should be in a formulary. J Pharm Pract. 1994;VII(2):51-7.

53. Lemay AP, Salzer LB, Visconti JA, Latiolais CJ. Strategies for deleting popular drugs from a hospital formulary. Am J Hosp Pharm. 1981;38:506-10.

54. Boesch D. Formularies and therapeutic substitution: gaining ground in long-term care. Consult Pharm. 1994;9:284-97.

55. Therapeutic interchange [Internet]. Alexandria, VA: Academy of Managed Care Pharmacy; 2012 Jun [cited 2017 Sept 22]:[2 p.]. Available from: http://www.amcp.org/WorkArea/DownloadAsset.aspx?id=18745

56. Helmons PJ, Kosterink JW, Daniels CE. Formulary compliance and pharmacy labor costs associated with systematic formulary management strategy. Am J Health Syst Pharm. 2014 Mar 1;71:407-15.

57. Lewis BE, Fish L. Drug approvals. Formulary decisions in managed care: the role of quality of life. Drug Benefit Trends. 1997;9:41-7.

58. Skledar SJ, Corman SL, Smitherman T. Addressing innovative off-label medication use at an academic medical center. Am J Health Syst Pharm. 2015;72:469-77.

59. ASHP statement on the use of medications for unlabeled uses. Am J Hosp Pharm. 1992;49:2006-8.

60. Marchand HC, Rose BJ, Fine AM, Kremzner ME. The U.S. Food and Drug Administration: drug information resources for formulary recommendations. J Manage Care Pharm. 2012 Nov/Dec;18(9):713-8.

61. Corman SL, Skledar SJ, Culley CM. Evaluation of conflicting literature and application to formulary decisions. Am J Health Syst Pharm. 2007 Jan 15;64:182-5.

62. Feero WG, Guttmacher AE, Collins FS. Genomic medicine—an updated primer. N Engl J Med. 2010;363:301-4.

63. Hamburg MA, Collins FS. The path to personalized medicine. N Engl J Med. 2010;363:301-4.

64. Philips KA, Veensta DL, Oren E, Lee JK, Sadee W. Potential role of pharmacogenomics in reducing adverse drug reactions: a systemic review. JAMA. 2001;286:2270-9.

65. Meyer UA. Pharmacogenetics and adverse drug reactions. Lancet. 2000;356(9242):1667-71.

66. Empey PE. Genetic predisposition to adverse drug reaction in the intensive care unit. Crit Care Med. 2010;38(6):S106-S116.

67. Morrow TJ. Implications of pharmacogenomics in the current and future treatment of asthma. J Managed Care Pharm. 2007;13(6):497-505.

68. U.S. Food and Drug Administration. Table of valid genomic biomarkers in the context of approved drug labels. 2009 [cited 2010 Aug 4]. Available from: http://www.fda.gov/Drugs/ScienceResearch/ResearchAreas/Pharmacogenetics/ucm083378.htm

69. Poppe LB, Roederer MW. Global formulary review: how do we integrate pharmacogenomics information. Ann Pharmacotherapy. 2011 April;45:532-8.

70. Goldberg NH, Schneeweiss S, Kowal MK, Gagne JJ. Availability of comparative efficacy data at the time of drug approval in the United States. JAMA. 2011 May 4;305(17):1786-9.

71. Hochman M, McCormick D. Characteristics of published comparative effectiveness studies of medications. JAMA. 2010 Mar 10;303(10):951-8.

72. Brixner DI, Watkins JB. Can CER be an effective tool for change in the development and assessment of new drugs and technologies. J Manage Care Pharm. 2012 June;18(5):S6-S11.

73. Clement FM, Harris A, Li JJ, Yong K, Lee KM, Manns BJ. Using effectiveness and cost-effectiveness to make drug coverage decisions. A comparison of Britain, Australia, and Canada. JAMA. 2009;302(13):1437-43.

74. Doyle JJ. The effect of comparative effectiveness research on drug development innovation: a 360° value appraisal. J Comp Eff Res. 2011;1:27-34.

75. Comparative effectiveness research: paving the way for evidence-based decision making. Managed Care. 2011 Aug;20(7 Suppl 4):2-7.

76. Leady MA, Adams AL, Stumpf JL, Sweet BV. Drug shortages: an approach to managing the latest crisis. Hosp Pharm. 2003;38:748-52.

77. ASHP guidelines on preventing medication errors with antineoplastic agents. Am J Health Syst Pharm. 2002;59:1648-68.

78. Pick AM, Massoomi F, Neff WJ, Danekas PI, Stoysich AM. A safety assessment tool for formulary candidates. Am J Health Syst Pharm. 2006;63:1269-72.

79. Milenkovich N. Ready or not, here come the REMS. Drug Top. 2009 Oct:65. Available from: https://www.questia.com/magazine/1P3-1901981141/ready-or-not-here-come-the-rems

80. Murri NA, Somani S, University HealthSystem Consortium Pharmacy Council Medication Management/Quality Improvement Committee. Implementation of safety-focused pharmacy and therapeutics monographs: a new University HealthSystem Consortium template designed to minimize medication misadventures. Hosp Pharm. 2004;39(7):653-60.

81. Sanchez LA. Pharmacoeconomics and formulary decision-making. PharmacoEconomics. 1996;9(Suppl 1):16-25.

82. Heiligenstein JH. Reformulating our formularies to reflect real-world outcomes. Drug Benefit Trends. 1996;8:35, 42.

83. Shulkin D. Reinventing the pharmacy and therapeutics committee. P&T. 2012 Nov;37(11):623-4, 649.

84. Odedina FI, Sullivan J, Nash R, Clemmons CD. Use of pharmacoeconomic data in making hospital formulary decisions. Am J Health Syst Pharm. 2002;59:1441-4.

85. Suh D-C, Okpara JRN, Agnese WB, Toscani M. Application of pharmacoeconomics to formulary decision making in managed care organizations. Am J Manage Care. 2002;8(2):161-9.

86. McCain J. System helps P&T committees get pharmacoeconomic data they need. Managed Care [Internet]. 2001 Apr [cited 2007 Jul 17]:[14 p.]. Available from: http://www.managedcaremag.com/archives/0104/0104.amcp.html

87. Getting the most out of formularies involves a bit of economic training. Manage Care. 2015 Apr;24(4):9-10.

88. Langley PC. Supporting formulary decisions: the discovery of new facts or constructed evidence? Inov Pharm [Internet]. 2016;7(2): Article 15. Available from: http://pubs.lib.umn.edu/innovations/vol7/iss2/15

89. Langley PC. Modeling imaginary worlds: Version 4 of the AMCP format for formulary submissions. Inov Pharm [Internet]. 2016;7(2): Article 11. Available from: http://pubs.lib.umn.edu/innovations/vol7/iss2/11

90. Mannebach MA, Ascione FJ, Gaither CA, Bagozzi RP, Cohen IA, Ryan ML. Activities, functions, and structure of pharmacy and therapeutics committees in large teaching hospitals. Am J Health Syst Pharm. 1999;56:622-8.

91. Shepard MD, Salzman RD. The formulary decision-making process in a health mainte-nance organisation setting. PharmacoEconomics. 1994;5:29-38.

92. Johnson JA, Bootman JL. Pharmacoeconomic analysis in formulary decisions: an interna-tional perspective. Am J Hosp Pharm. 1994;51:2593-8.

93. Basskin L. Discounting in pharmacoeconomic analyses: when and how to do it. Formulary. 1996;31:1217-27.

94. Macklin R. Understanding formularies. Drug Store News Pharmacist. 1995;5:82-8.

95. Vogenberg FR, Barash CI, Pursel M. Personalized medicine. Part 1: evolution and devel-opment into theranostics. P&T. 2010 Oct;35(1):560-2, 565-7.

96. Myers CE, Pierpaoli P, Smith MA. Measurement of formulary inclusion costs. Hosp Formul. 1981;16:951-3, 957-8, 967-8, 970-1, 975-6.

97. Crane VS, Gonzalez ER, Hull BL. How to develop a proactive formulary system. Hosp Formul. 1994;29:700-10.

Chapter Fifteen

Drug Shortages and Counterfeit Drugs

Erin R. Fox

Learning Objectives

● *After completing this chapter, the reader will be able to*

- Describe the reasons why drug shortages occur.
- Describe actions taken to ameliorate the drug shortage problem.
- Formulate management strategies for drug shortage situations.
- Analyze drug shortage situations for potential medication safety implications.
- List methods for identifying and reporting potential counterfeit drugs.

Key Concepts

❶ Drug shortages are a significant public health problem, affecting patients, clinicians, and all aspects of the medication supply chain.

❷ The leading cause of drug shortages is manufacturing problems, mostly related to quality or not following FDA's Current Good Manufacturing Practices (CGMPs).

❸ The FDA works to prevent shortages by expediting reviews of new manufacturing sites, processes, or new products.

❹ Every health care setting should have a plan that addresses how drug shortages are managed.

❺ Managing drug shortages requires complex problem-solving skills. Health care professionals must assess how a shortage will impact patient care, medication safety, and workflow in order to develop the best management plan.

❻ Drug shortages increase the risk of medication errors and can result in delayed patient care or adverse patient outcomes.

❼ Most counterfeit medications found in the United States are purchased over the Internet, or from unlicensed or foreign suppliers.

Introduction

❶ *Drug shortages are a significant public health problem, affecting patients, clinicians, and all aspects of the medication supply chain.*[1] Defining a drug shortage is not easy as the definition can differ depending on perspective. At the most basic level, a shortage exists if a medication is not available for a patient. However, there can be many reasons besides a shortage that a medication may not be available. Short-term situations where a medication is not ordered or delivered on time are common. Most health care organizations use just-in-time inventory systems to prevent the cost burden of excess inventory, but this system can result in short-term shortages. Likewise, weather delays can prevent deliveries from wholesalers, also resulting in short-term shortages. This chapter will address longer-term drug shortages that impact the entire supply chain on a national scale.

Drug Shortages

DEFINITION OF A DRUG SHORTAGE

There are two key sources of information regarding drug shortages. The Food and Drug Administration (FDA) and the American Society of Health-System Pharmacists (ASHP) both provide information about drug shortages on frequently updated websites. The University of Utah Drug Information Service (UUDIS) provides drug shortage content for ASHP.[2] These data are recognized by the Government Accountability Office (GAO) as the most comprehensive source of drug shortage information.[3,4] Both sources differ with regard to their definition of a drug shortage. The FDA defines a shortage as "a situation in which the total supply of all clinically interchangeable versions of an

FDA-regulated drug is inadequate to meet the current or projected demand at the patient level."[5] The UUDIS and ASHP define a shortage as "a supply issue that affects how the pharmacy prepares or dispenses a drug product or influences patient care when prescribers must use an alternative agent."[6] The differences in definitions mean that ASHP reports higher drug shortage totals than the FDA. National tracking of drug shortages began in 2001.

Figure 15-1 shows the historical trends of the number of drug shortages on an annual basis. Figure 15-2 shows the number of active and ongoing shortages by quarter. These

Figure 15–1. Number of new national drug shortages starting in each calendar year, January 2001 to June 30, 2016. Data are from the University of Utah Drug Information Service.

Figure 15–2. Number of active drug shortages by quarter through June 30, 2016. Q1-12 indicates January through March 2012; Q2-12, April through June 2012; Q3-12, July through September 2012; Q4-12, October through December 2012. Data are from the University of Utah Drug Information Service.

figures are updated quarterly on the ASHP Drug Shortage Resource Center (https://www.ashp.org/Drug-Shortages). The current trend at the end of 2016 is a decrease in the number of total new drug shortages occurring each year and a gradual decrease in the number of ongoing active drug shortages (Case Study 15-1).

Case Study 15–1

During rounds, one of the team members mentioned that they read on a listserv that amikacin was in short supply. The team is concerned because results from the patient's blood sample show an infection that is only susceptible to amikacin. You volunteer to find out if the medication is available.

• *What sources are available to determine if a product is in short supply?*

CAUSES OF DRUG SHORTAGES

● The reasons for drug shortages are complex and, to a certain degree, remain unknown. Prior to the publication of *A Review of FDA's Approach to Medical Product Shortages*, few specifics were known regarding the key causes of drug shortages.[2] Drug manufacturers do not have to provide specific reasons for shortages. The FDA may know the reasons but cannot always provide detailed information as the manufacturer may consider the information to be proprietary. ❷ *According to the FDA, the leading cause of drug shortages is manufacturing problems, mostly related to quality or not following FDA's Current Good Manufacturing Practices (CGMPs).*[2] Injectable products are particularly susceptible to quality problems and therefore may cause drug shortages due to the increased difficulty in manufacturing. In 2012, 77% of injectable shortages were caused by quality problems.[1] The specific reason for a shortage is almost never known. For example, a drug company may state that manufacturing problems are causing a shortage but the company does not reveal the root cause of the manufacturing problem.

Clinicians can follow the quality data that the FDA provides regarding manufacturers, by reviewing FDA-issued **warning letters** and **483 inspection reports** (http://www.fda.gov/ICECI/EnforcementActions/WarningLetters/). These data can provide a limited picture of a manufacturer's quality and may potentially be used to identify additional reasons for drug shortages. The reason for the limited information is that drug manufacturers consider many things propriety and therefore the reports redact this information. Examples of items that are considered to be proprietary include the list of products manufactured at a specific factory and the manufacturer of the product. U.S. labeling laws do not require that prescribing information (i.e., package insert) should include the name of the manufacturer or location of the factory. Despite these limitations, clinicians who are interested in the quality of drug manufacturing and drug shortages should sign up on the FDA's website to receive FDA's alerts regarding warning letters and 483 inspections (http://www.fda.gov/ICECI/EnforcementActions/ WarningLetters/).

PREVENTING DRUG SHORTAGES

The FDA works diligently to prevent shortages from happening in the first place. A key aspect in their work is advanced notice that is required for successful prevention. ❸ *The key ways that the FDA prevents shortages is to expedite reviews of new manufacturing sites, processes, or new products.*[2] The FDA can also prevent shortages by using their regulatory discretion to allow a product with a minor problem to be distributed. Examples of this type of prevention strategy include allowing sodium phosphate to be distributed even though it contained particles. To prevent a shortage, the FDA allowed the product to be distributed with filters and a **Dear Health Care Provider letter**. Once a shortage has started, it is more difficult for the FDA to ameliorate the situation, but they can allow companies to import products that meet FDA standards. Importing products is not always an available strategy as the FDA often cannot find another supplier with sufficient supplies to share with the United States. The FDA posts information about the availability of imported products on their drug shortage website. Examples of past imports include saline, propofol, and bleomycin.

A number of actions have occurred to attempt to improve the drug shortage problem. One of the key actions occurred on July 12, 2012, when the FDA Safety and Innovation Act was passed by Congress.[7] This legislation requires manufacturers to provide the FDA with advanced notice (6 months or as soon as possible) of any potential supply disruption. Ever since this law was passed, the FDA has been able to prevent more shortages, and the overall number of drug shortages has decreased. The International Society for Pharmaceutical Engineering (ISPE) has also been working on the drug shortage problem.[8] This organization is focusing on helping manufacturers improve their overall quality systems.

TABLE 15–1. KEY ACTIVITIES DRUG SHORTAGE TEAM MEMBERS MUST ACCOMPLISH

- Gather data on amount of product on hand, typical usage, and monitor drug shortage information
- Contact wholesaler or manufacturers to ensure backorders are in place
- Purchase alternatives
- Make decisions such as changing the stocking location to a centralized location, or changing preparation or dispensing methods
- Evaluate medication safety risks
- Make changes to technology
- Facilitate conservation and rationing decisions by contacting the Ethics Committee or Pharmacy and Therapeutics Committee
- Communicate shortage management plan to all stakeholders

MANAGING DRUG SHORTAGES

Despite advocacy by health care professionals and prevention strategies from the FDA, drug shortages impact health systems on a daily basis. ❹ *Every health care setting should have a plan that addresses how drug shortages are managed.* Some accrediting bodies such as The Joint Commission require policies for managing drug shortages. The first step is to build a team of health care professionals to manage drug shortages. The team should include people who can make decisions and quickly access information, such as purchase history or usage. Team members should understand the organization's process for change as well as how to expedite that process if needed. One person may be delegated to lead the team, but an effective drug shortage management team will include both decision makers in the administration and informal leaders, such as clinical specialists or front-line staff. This group should also develop a list of stakeholders for specific clinical areas that can be called upon to weigh in on potential management strategies for specific situations. For example, identify key clinicians in specific clinical areas that frequently suffer drug shortages such as Anesthesia and Infectious Diseases. Communication is an essential component of the drug shortage management team. Make sure each member understands their role and shares information with the rest of the team in a timely manner. Table 15-1 identifies key actions required of drug shortage team members. Ensure each activity has a designated person to follow through on these actions.

❺ *Managing drug shortages requires complex problem-solving skills. Health care professionals must assess how a shortage will impact patient care, medication safety, and workflow in order to develop the best management plan.* Table 15-2 outlines key steps to developing a drug shortage management plan. For example, is this a shortage of a product that has clear and effective alternatives, or is this a shortage that may delay treatments or cause patient harm. Analyze which patients and clinicians will be impacted the most by the shortage. Review potential medication safety concerns that this shortage may pose (Case Study 15-2).

TABLE 15–2. STEPWISE APPROACH TO DEVELOPING A DRUG SHORTAGE MANAGEMENT PLAN

Action	Resources for Information
Determine the amount of product on hand. • Estimate how long that product will last • Estimate quantity and timing of next delivery	• Purchasing staff • ASHP and FDA shortage websites
Determine the clinical impact of the shortage. • How essential is the product? Is it lifesaving or curative? Can treatment be postponed? • Are there clear alternatives? • Which clinicians or patients are most impacted?	• Clinical knowledge • Front-line staff • ASHP website for alternatives
Determine any potential medication safety risks posed by the drug shortage. • If using an alternative, identify any differences in dosing, adverse effects, or drug interactions. • Is a different strength or formulation being used? • Are there potential look-alike or sound-alike differences?	• Clinical knowledge • Medication safety officer
Determine whether any changes are needed to the overall workflow. • Should the shortage item be stored in a central location to ease tracking? • Does the shortage affect any technology?	• Operations managers • Informatics
Determine how remaining product should be utilized. • Is conservation or rationing the best strategy?	• Ethics committee • P&T committee • Stakeholder clinicians

Case Study 15–2

Your organization has discovered that a shortage of amikacin exists. The purchasing staff states that there is approximately a 20-day supply left at current usage rates. The next delivery date is unknown.

- *What are the next steps in managing this drug shortage? Which clinicians should you contact first?*

Once a plan is in place, it is essential to communicate effectively based on your audience. Target communications when possible to avoid information overload. Share information in formal and informal ways. Use multiple methods to share the message such as rounds, team huddles, e-mail, intranet blogs, or even paper or white boards. Make sure the communication provides details about the management strategy. If an alternative is recommended, make sure to include any differences in dosing, adverse effects, or drug interactions. If the product is going to be reserved for specific patients to conserve supplies, make sure to include criteria for use and a method for clinicians who would like an exception. The health system's ethics committee should be involved in decisions to ration drug products.[9] See Chapter 11 for additional information on ethical dilemmas in pharmacy practice.

IMPACT OF DRUG SHORTAGES

● Drug shortages impact patient safety in two major ways. ❻ *Drug shortages increase the risk of medication errors and can result in delayed patient care or adverse patient outcomes.* Drug shortages pose high medication-safety risks because they can affect each step of the medication use process. Clinicians have attempted to identify the key safety risks of drug shortages through a failure modes and effects analysis. These data show that the highest risk points during a shortage are using a different concentration or using an alternative.[10] Medication errors and deaths have occurred when clinicians were unfamiliar with the dosing of an alternative agent.[11,12] Patient safety is also at risk when shortages cause treatment delays. For example, there may be missed opportunities to immunize, clinical trials may be delayed when the standard of care is not available, and delays in obtaining antimicrobials or chemotherapy agents may be life-threatening or affect the potential chance for a cure[13-16] (Case Study 15-3).

Case Study 15-3

Your organization has suffered multiple shortages in the past week. You speak with the purchasing staff who provide you with and update on what products they have been able to obtain. They tell you about how they have purchased heparin vials since the premixed bags are not available. They have also purchased dopamine 200 mg/250 mL premixed bags because it was the only strength available and you are almost out of dopamine 800 mg/250 mL premixed bags.

- *What patient safety concerns do you have? What technology may be affected by these substitutes?*

Counterfeit Drugs

The World Health Organization (WHO) notes that **counterfeit drugs** affect every region of the world.[17] The WHO defines these products as "substandard, spurious, falsely labelled, falsified, and counterfeit" (SSFFC) products. The medications may not contain the right amount of **active pharmaceutical ingredient**, or may not contain the correct active ingredient at all. Products might contain fillers like chalk or even toxic chemicals. All types of medicines are falsified including expensive medications as well as generics. The most commonly reported counterfeit medications worldwide are antimicrobials.

❼ *Most counterfeit medications found in the United States are purchased over the Internet or from unlicensed or foreign suppliers.* In 2015, the FDA found a counterfeit version of Botox® that was sold by an unlicensed, foreign supplier. The FDA also found counterfeit Cialis® in 2015 that had been purchased by a single consumer from an Internet pharmacy (http://www.fda.gov/Drugs/ResourcesForYou/Consumers/BuyingUsingMedicineSafely/CounterfeitMedicine/). The FDA recommends patients or health care providers to purchase medications only from state licensed pharmacies or Internet pharmacies with the Verified Internet Pharmacy Practice Sites accreditation program seal (https://nabp.pharmacy/programs/vipps/). The WHO provides recommendations to help identify counterfeit medications such as ensuring the package is in good condition, reviewing security seals, and checking that batch numbers and expiration dates match between the internal and external packages (http://www.who.int/medicines/regulation/ssffc/en/).[17] Health care providers can report potential counterfeit medications to FDA via **MedWatch** (http://www.fda.gov/Safety/MedWatch/). Ways of tracking medications within the medication supply lines to prevent the substitution of counterfeit products have been investigated, including the use of radio-frequency identification (RFID) tags.

Conclusion

Drug shortages and counterfeit drugs pose significant public health risks. Clinicians can minimize the impact of drug shortages on their patients and practices by developing clear plans to manage the shortages. Health care providers can minimize the potential risks of counterfeit medications by purchasing medications from recommended sources and reviewing medication packaging for potential tampering or falsification.

Self-Assessment Questions

1. The trend in drug shortages for 2016 is one of:
   a. Decreasing new shortages and increasing active shortages
   b. Increasing new shortages but decreasing active shortages
   c. Slight increase in new shortages and decreasing active shortages
   d. Decreasing new shortages and a gradual decrease in active shortages

2. Most shortages have occurred due to:
   a. Raw material shortages
   b. Natural disasters
   c. Manufacturing or quality problems
   d. Corporate decisions

3. Package inserts must include which of the following items:
   a. Name of the company that manufactured the drug
   b. Location of the factory
   c. Country of origin for the active pharmaceutical ingredient (API)
   d. None of the above

4. FDA can help prevent drug shortages by:
   a. Prioritizing approvals of new products
   b. Forcing companies to increase production
   c. Forcing companies to continue to produce a drug
   d. Decreasing drug prices

5. FDA can help alleviate an ongoing drug shortage by:
   a. Requiring companies to manufacture additional product
   b. Fine companies that don't provide advanced notice of a shortage
   c. Allowing companies to import products that meet FDA criteria
   d. Override patents and approve new formulations

6. The FDASIA bill was signed in July 2012 and gave FDA what new authority with regard to drug shortages?
   a. Allows FDA to make their own products to prevent shortages
   b. Allows FDA to require manufacturers to notify them in advance about shortages
   c. Allows FDA to fine companies for causing shortages
   d. Allows FDA to require manufacturers to continue to produce medically necessary drugs

7. A drug shortage policy has which of the following characteristics?
   a. Required by the Joint Commission
   b. Required by the FDA
   c. Required by wholesalers
   d. Required by group purchasing organizations

8. Members of a drug shortage team should do which of the following?
   a. Put a positive spin on communications by overestimating the supply on hand
   b. Consider making changes to the stocking locations
   c. Remove the product from formulary
   d. Rely on word of mouth to get the message out

9. Clinicians should exercise particular care at what point during a shortage?
   a. After the P&T committee decides on an allocation strategy
   b. Selecting when to remove stock from the automated dispensing cabinets
   c. Selecting when to begin drawing up doses to conserve product
   d. At the beginning and ending of a shortage

10. What information is necessary when assessing the potential impact of a drug shortage at an individual health system?
    a. Amount and location of inventory on hand
    b. Status of drug in short supply—unapproved or approved
    c. Whether or not FDA considers the drug medically necessary
    d. Whether the drug is available as a brand or generic product

11. The FDA's drug shortage information is different from that of the ASHP's because:
    a. FDA provides detailed alternatives
    b. ASHP does not include vaccines or biologics
    c. FDA focuses on medically necessary drugs and information provided by the manufacturer
    d. The ASHP website is only updated monthly

12. Important considerations in determining the potential clinical impact of a shortage include:
    a. Whether an alternative is available
    b. Identifying which patients will be most impacted
    c. Determining if the product is lifesaving or curative
    d. All of the above

13. A failure modes and effects analysis identified which of the following items as the greatest medication safety risks during a drug shortage?
    a. Using different concentration or an alternative drug
    b. Purchasing a more expensive product that is not on contract
    c. Dispensing the product in a syringe instead of a vial
    d. Changing the storage location of a product

14. Clinicians should report suspected counterfeit drugs to:
    a. FDA's MedWatch program
    b. The Federal Bureau of Investigation
    c. The Federal Trade Commission
    d. The wholesaler

15. Patients who purchase medications on the Internet should look for the following to ensure that they do not receive counterfeit medications:
    a. Consumer star ratings
    b. Pharmacies with best customer service ratings
    c. Pharmacies with the Verified Internet Pharmacy Practice Sites accreditation program seal (VIPPS)
    d. Pharmacies with locations listed in Canada

REFERENCES

1. Fox ER, Sweet BV, Jensen V. Drug shortages: a complex health care crisis. Mayo Clin Proc. 2014;89(3):361-73.
2. A review of FDA's approach to medical product shortages. U.S. Food and Drug Administration Web 2011, 2011 Oct [cited 2016 Nov 10]. Available from: http://www.fda.gov/aboutfda/reportsmanualsforms/reports/ucm277744.htm
3. American Society of Health-System Pharmacists. ASHP guidelines on managing drug product shortages in hospitals and health systems. Am J Health Syst Pharm. 2009;66(15):1399-406.
4. Fox ER, Tyler LS. Managing drug shortages: seven years' experience at one health system. Am J Health Syst Pharm. 2003;60(3):245-53.
5. Drug shortages: FDA's ability to respond should be strengthened. United States Government Accountability Office, 2011 Nov [cited 2016 Nov 10]. Available from: http://www.gao.gov/assets/590/587000.pdf
6. Drug shortages: public health threat continues, despite efforts to help ensure product availability. United States Government Accountability Office Web 2014, 2014 Feb [cited 2016 Nov 10]. Available from: http://www.gao.gov/products/GAO-14-194
7. U.S. Food and Drug Administration Safety and Innovation Act (FDASIA) U.S. Food and Drug Administration, 2015 Oct [cited 2016 Nov 10]. Available from: https://www.fda.gov/RegulatoryInformation/LawsEnforcedbyFDA/SignificantAmendmentstotheFDCAct/FDASIA/ucm20027187.htm

8. ISPE drug shortages initiative: FAQs. International Society for Pharmaceutical Engineering (ISPE) Web 2015 [cited 2016 Sept 10]. Available from: http://www.ispe.org/drug-shortages-initiative/faqs

9. Unguru Y, Fernandez CV, Bernhardt B, Berg S, Pyke-Grimm, Woodman C, Joffe S. An ethical framework for allocating scarce life-saving chemotherapy and supportive care drugs for childhood cancer. J Natl Cancer Inst. 2016 Jan 29;108(6):djv392. doi: 10.1093/jnci/djv392. Print 2016 Jun. PubMed PMID: 26825103.

10. MacDonald EA, Fox ER, Tyler LS. Drug shortages: process for evaluating impact on patient safety. Hosp Pharm. 2011;46(12):943-51.

11. Institute for Safe Medication Practices. Drug shortages: national survey reveals high level of frustration, low level of safety. ISMP Medication Safety Alert! Acute Care. 2010;15(15).

12. Institute for Safe Medication Practices. A shortage of everything except errors: harm associated with drug shortages. ISMP Medication Safety Alert! Acute Care. 2012;17(8).

13. McBride A, Holle LM, Westendorf C, Sidebottom M, Griffith N, Muller RJ, Hoffman JM. National survey on the effect of oncology drug shortages on cancer care. Am J Health Syst Pharm. 2013; Apr 1;70(7):609-17. doi: 10.2146/ajhp120563. PubMed PMID: 23515514.

14. Goozner M. Drug shortages delay cancer clinical trials. J Natl Cancer Inst. 2012;104(12):891-2.

15. Griffith MM, Gross AE, Sutton SH, Bolon MK, Esterly JS, Patel JA, Postelnick MJ, Zembower TR, Scheetz MH. The impact of anti-infective drug shortages on hospitals in the United States: trends and causes. Clin Infect Dis. 2012 Mar 1;54(5):684-91. doi: 10.1093/cid/cir954. Epub 2012 Jan 19. PubMed PMID: 22267747.

16. Gogineni K, Shuman KL, Emanuel EJ. Survey of oncologists about shortages of cancer drugs. N Engl J Med. 2013;369(25):2463-4.

17. Substandard, spurious, falsely labelled, falsified and counterfeit (SSFFC) medical products. World Health Organization website 2016 Jan [cited 2016 Sept 13]. Available from: http://www.who.int/mediacentre/factsheets/fs275/en/

SUGGESTED READINGS

1. American Society of Health-System Pharmacists Drug Shortage Resource Center. Available from: https://www.ashp.org/Drug-shortages

2. U.S. Food and Drug Administration—drug shortages. Available from: http://www.fda.gov/Drugs/DrugSafety/DrugShortages/

3. American Society of Health-System Pharmacists Guidelines for Managing Drug Product Shortages. Available from: https://www.ashp.org/Drug-Shortages/Shortage-Resources

4. The World Health Organization Substandard, Spurious, Falsely labelled, Falsified and Counterfeit (SSFFC) medical products. w from: http://www.who.int/medicines/regulation/ssffc/en/

5. National Association of Boards of Pharmacy's Verified Internet Pharmacy Practice Sites (VIPPS) program. Available from: https://nabp.pharmacy/programs/vipps/

Chapter Sixteen

Quality Improvement and the Medication Use System

Jennifer K. Thomas • David P. Nau

Learning Objectives

After completing this chapter, the reader will be able to

- Explain the changing environment for quality measurement and performance reporting in health care.
- Define quality and value in the context of health care services.
- Define quality measures and explain their development.
- Delineate the concepts of structure, process, and outcomes for quality assessment.
- Describe a systematic method for quality improvement.
- Define health equity and health disparities and how to improve health quality for all groups.
- Explain the role of performance indicators in quality improvement.
- Draft a performance indicator related to the medication use system.
- Discuss quality improvement techniques applied in drug information practice.

Key Concepts

❶ The term value has been assigned many definitions, but within health care, it usually reflects the ratio of quality and costs (value = quality/cost).

❷ Significant drivers for greater transparency in the quality and value of health care services include the federal government, employers that provide health care benefits, and accreditation organizations such as The Joint Commission (TJC).

❸ Quality improvement is prospective, continuous, team oriented, nonpunitive, systems oriented, customer focused, and data driven.

❹ A common methodology for quality improvement is known as FOCUS-PDCA (Find, Organize, Clarify, Understand, Select, Plan, Do, Check, Act).

❺ Donabedian's framework for quality assessment in health care includes the key elements of structure, process, and outcomes.

❻ Performance indicators are used to measure quality as part of the check function of quality improvement. The indicators typically focus on the process or outcomes of a care system.

❼ Performance indicators can be subdivided into sentinel (occurrence of a serious event) or aggregate categories. Aggregate indicators are further divided into continuous or rate-based indicators.

❽ Focus on health equity and elimination of health disparities are necessary to achieve quality health care for all.

❾ Medication use evaluation is often part of an organization's overall performance improvement program that uses definitions of safe and effective use of medications to assess components of the medication use process.

❿ Performance, as demonstrated by data collected in the performance improvement process, not meeting the defined standard or threshold or falling outside the control limits (for ongoing or follow-up assessments) indicates that intervention to improve performance is necessary.

Introduction

● Value-driven health care is being touted as the future model for health care in the United States.[1] ❶ *The term, value, has been assigned many definitions, but within health care, it usually reflects the ratio of quality and costs (value = quality/cost)*. Thus, value is optimized by enhancing quality while minimizing cost. Although it was traditionally assumed that higher quality would only be possible through higher expenditures, the medical community has learned that improving the quality of care may lead to long-term control of health care costs. Health care administrators have long been attentive to measuring expenditures on care and have developed cost-accounting systems that have allowed determination of costs of procedures, drugs, and various care models. However, the health care system has only recently developed explicit measures of quality. By measuring this missing piece of the value equation, it is now possible to achieve a more balanced perspective on health system performance.

The Changing Environment for Health Care Quality

● The measurement of quality within health care settings has expanded rapidly during the previous two decades. ❷ *Significant drivers for greater transparency in the quality and value of health care services include the federal government, employers that provide health care benefits, and accreditation organizations such as The Joint Commission (TJC).* Accreditation standards for many providers have been amended to require providers to collect performance data. The federal government is the major driver of health care quality measurement and is accelerating change through implementation of the value-based model of care defined by the Affordable Care Act (ACA) with identified priorities from the National Quality Strategy.[2] Specifically, goals are identified that tie payment to performance in the Medicare Fee-for-Service (FFS) program with an invitation to private payers to match or exceed these goals. Goals for FFS payments include "Goal 1: 30% of Medicare payments are tied to quality or value through alternative payment models by the end of 2016, and 50% by the end of 2018. Goal 2: 85% of all Medicare FFS payments are tied to quality or value by the end of 2016, and 90% by the end of 2018."[3] An example of Medicare FFS payments that may impact pharmacy practice are immunizations, influenza and pneumococcal vaccines, reimbursed for Medicare enrollees under Medicare Part B FFS. The above quality goals are primarily accomplished through (1) hospital payment adjustments for Medicare in-patient services in the Hospital Value-Based Purchasing program[4]; (2) transition of physicians FFS payment away from volume, ending the sustainable growth rate formula of payment, to payment for quality; and (3) accountable care organizations (ACOs). The latter two are included in the Merit-Based Incentive Payment System (MIPS) and Alternative Payment Model (APM) as defined in the Medicare Access and CHIP Reauthorization (MACRA) legislation.[5] This program began in January 2017, that is referred to as the Quality Payment Program (QPP), allows eligible professionals (physicians, physician assistants, nurse practitioner, clinical nurse specialist, nurse anesthetist) to select either MIPS, if they bill Medicare Part B above a specific threshold ($30,000) and have greater than 100 FFS patients, or APM if they are part of a group using an inno-

● vative payment model, such as ACOs. The Centers for Medicare & Medicaid Services (CMS) value-based payment models include not only hospitals, but other health care settings including end-stage renal disease care, skilled nursing facilities (nursing homes), and home health agencies.[6] CMS displays publically available reports on the quality of care across multiple care settings: hospitals,[7] long-term care facilities,[8] health plans,[9,10] home health agencies,[11] dialysis facilities,[12] and physicians.[13,14] Additionally, many public and private purchasers (e.g., insurance companies) of health care services have begun to demand evidence of quality and value,[15,16] and consumers selecting plans in the recently established ACA Health Insurance Marketplace (also known as Health Insurance Exchange) may select their plan based on quality "star ratings" through a limited pilot program in two states, Virginia and Wisconsin. These pilot states included star ratings for the 2017 enrollment year based on 2016 quality data provided by the plans.[17] While many care settings and providers are being directly measured with attribution of their quality of care, pharmacies and pharmacists are currently only indirectly assessed. For example, there is no pharmacy compare website at this time. However, measuring pharmacy/pharmacist performance with attribution of the quality of pharmacy provided care, is moving forward.

In 2006, CMS facilitated the creation of the Pharmacy Quality Alliance (PQA) to create standards for performance measurement and reporting for prescription drug plans and community pharmacies.[18] The initial testing of these performance measures took place in 2007,[19] and several demonstration projects have been conducted to show how community pharmacies can be included in performance measurement systems.[20] Although CMS is not publicly reporting on the quality of individual pharmacies, it has included several PQA-developed quality measures within the Medicare Part D Plan ratings.[21] As the scrutiny of prescription drug plans increases, plans are beginning to require participation of their preferred network pharmacies in quality measurement programs, including medication adherence, medication therapy management, and generic medication utilization. These plan sponsors are determining pharmacy performance[22,23] and may report this data to the public. Thus, all sectors of health care will be affected by the rapidly expanding trend of quality measurement and public reporting of performance data.

This chapter will focus on the measurement of quality in the medication use system and the use of these measures in improving the quality of medication use. The term performance will be used interchangeably with quality within this chapter, although understanding that performance can also refer to the overall value of the health care system is important.

Purpose of Measuring Quality

Quality, like value, has been defined in many different ways. Although the definitions for quality may vary, the purpose of measuring quality is to identify problems in a system (also known as opportunities for improvement) and to monitor improvements in quality as systems are modified.[24] Although quality improvement is the goal of collecting performance data, the mechanisms for using performance data in achieving quality improvement may vary. For example, the performance data may be used directly by a health care organization to identify opportunities for improvement and to gauge the impact of changes in its policies or procedures.

Performance data may also be used by external entities (e.g., a regulatory or accrediting body) to determine whether a health care organization should retain its accreditation or certification. The data may also be used to determine payments to providers (e.g., pay for performance), or the data may be used by employers, governments, or the public for determining which providers to use.

When comparative data on the performance of health care providers are released to payers and patients, it is presumed that the providers in a competitive environment will improve quality to maintain market share.

Quality Measures

Use of **quality measures**, specifications developed for measuring different aspects of health care provided by practitioners in different care settings, allows us to quantify performance compared with thresholds on processes, outcomes, and performance by providers, and patient perceptions of care.[25,26] Various stewards or measure developers such as CMS, the National Committee for Quality Assurance (NCQA), and PQA to name a few, submit their measures for consideration of endorsement by the National Quality Forum (NQF). NQF, under contract of the U.S. Department of Health and Human Services, is responsible for creating, prioritizing, and maintaining a portfolio of quality and efficiency measures across care settings and providers. Measure stewards invite participating experts, representatives from areas of practice, organizations, and stakeholders, including patient and family advocacy groups to reach consensus in developing applicable measures. The measures are submitted to NQF for endorsement; if endorsed the steward maintains and updates the measures as necessary. NQF currently categorizes measures into clinical conditions/topic areas, by care setting, and into one of the six NQS priorities: affordable care, effective communication and care coordination, health and well-being, patient safety, person and family-centered care, and prevention and treatment of cardiovascular disease (diseases as leading causes of mortality). An example of a cross-cutting medication safety and care coordination measure is the medication reconciliation post-discharge measure (measure steward: NCQA, NQF #0097). A searchable listing of measures, the Quality Positions System (QPS), is available under the measures, reports, and tools of the NQF website.[27]

Quality Improvement

Practitioners are sometimes confused when faced with the myriad of quality-related acronyms being used today, such as CQI (continuous quality improvement), QI (quality improvement), QA (quality assurance), QAPI (quality assurance, performance

TABLE 16-1. ATTRIBUTES OF CONTINUOUS QUALITY IMPROVEMENT

Characteristic	Description
Prospective	Forward thinking; always looking for better ways to provide care.
Continuous	A standard element of practice rather than a one-time effort.
Team oriented	A collaborative effort of all employees and management; recognizes the unique and valuable knowledge of each team member.
Nonpunitive	Employees should be rewarded for identifying problems/mistakes and not be fearful of discussing operational problems.
Systems oriented	Focus of improvement efforts is on the process or system of care rather than the elimination of bad employees.
Customer focused	All team members are focused on fulfilling the needs of the customer (e.g., patient, physician, other team members).
Data driven	Evaluates performance based on objective data.

improvement), TQM (total quality management), SPC (statistical process control), and PDCA (plan, do, check, act). Things become even murkier when many different quality-related philosophies are added, along with blurry distinctions between quality improvement, quality assurance, and quality control.

Quality improvement can generally be characterized by certain attributes, which are listed in Table 16-1. Concisely stated, ❸ *quality improvement is prospective, continuous, team oriented, nonpunitive, systems oriented, customer focused, and data driven.* Although there are a variety of methods, the quality improvement process is typically implemented via the PDCA or PDSA cycle, also called the Deming cycle (although Deming referred to it as the Shewhart cycle).[28,29] This cyclical process involves four key elements: *Plan, Do, Check (or Study),* and *Act.*

To apply PDCA to a new health care service, *Plan* would entail designing a new approach for providing the service that leads to an improvement in quality. This approach would include guidelines or procedures for how care will be provided and also plans for how the care process will be evaluated. The *Do* step in the cycle concerns the implementation of the new plan, while *Check* refers to an objective evaluation of the plan. Once the performance of the plan has been checked, the performance data can be *Acted* upon to standardize the new plan (assuming that it led to improvement) or the existing plan can be further revised and the PDCA cycle can be repeated.

❹ *A common methodology for quality improvement is known as FOCUS-PDCA (Find, Organize, Clarify, Understand, Select, Plan, Do, Check, Act). It is an extension of the PDCA cycle* (Figure 16-1).[30] *This approach was developed by the Hospital Corporation of America to facilitate quality improvement efforts in their hospitals.* The first step of FOCUS-PDCA is to *Find* the process that will be targeted for improvement (e.g., the pharmacokinetic

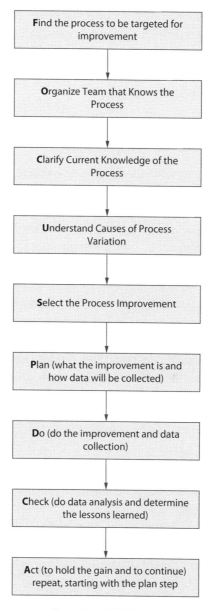

Figure 16–1. FOCUS-PDCA®.

service referral process). The second step is to *Organize* a team to study the problem (e.g., pharmacists, physicians, nurses, unit clerks). Next, *Clarify* the team's understanding of the process (i.e., ensure that everyone has a common understanding of how the referral process is actually being carried out, perhaps through the use of a flow diagram). Then, seek to *Understand* the root causes of variation in performance (i.e., identify problems such as a poorly designed workflow, inadequate training, or unclear roles and determine why they occur). Finally, *Select* the parts of the structure or process to change. Once the target for change has been selected, a new *Plan* can be formulated for how the process will change and then continue the PDCA cycle through the *Do*, *Check*, and *Act* steps.

MEASURING QUALITY IN THE MEDICATION USE SYSTEM

• One of the most challenging elements of quality improvement is measuring the quality of care. Donabedian[31] suggested that the evaluation of medical care quality could be best accomplished by subdividing care into three parts. ❺ *Donabedian's framework for quality assessment in health care includes the key elements of structure, process, and outcome.* The Donabedian framework also can be used to evaluate the quality of the medication use system.[32]

• *Structure* refers to the characteristics of providers, the tools and resources at their disposal, and the physical or organizational settings in which they work.[30] Examples include professional licensure or certification, computer systems for tracking patient information, patient counseling areas, and human resource policies. The elements of structure create the environment for care. These structural elements may be necessary to provide optimal care, but their presence does not ensure optimal care.

• *Process* refers to the set of activities that occur between patient and provider, encompassing the services and products that are provided to patients and the manner in which the services are provided. Experts often group the specific elements of care processes within two domains: *technical* or *interpersonal*. The technical domain of patient care may include gathering patient information, entering prescription information into computers, reviewing patient records, checking prescription labels, evaluating a patient's laboratory results, identifying and resolving potential drug-related problems, and answering patient questions. The interpersonal domain of patient care includes the ability of the practitioner to express empathy, listen attentively, and develop a caring relationship with the patient.[31] The process of care is often the primary focus of quality improvement efforts as practitioners strive to do what is best for patients. Care processes can be directly evaluated by using the norms or standards that exist across the health care system (e.g., what is commonly accepted as good care) or indirectly evaluated by determining their impact on outcomes.

• The term *outcomes* was originally defined by Donabedian as "a change in a patient's current and future health status that can be attributed to antecedent health care."[31] Lohr[33] also characterized outcomes in terms of the consequences of medical care for patients (death, disability, disease, discomfort, and dissatisfaction). In later years, the use of this term has broadened to encompass the economic, clinical, and humanistic consequences of health care processes (ECHO model).[34] In the ECHO model, outcomes may include:

- Economic consequences (e.g., costs of care)
- Clinical measures or endpoints (e.g., blood pressure, glycosylated hemoglobin [HgbA1c], pain, mortality—see Chapters 4 and 5)
- Humanistic issues (e.g., patient satisfaction, health-related quality of life)

Outcomes are sometimes classified as *intermediate* or *long term*.[35] This terminology results from considering the link between process and numerous outcomes as a causal chain of events. Intermediate outcomes may occur between the health care process and long-term or ultimate outcomes. For example, providing patient counseling services regarding the appropriate use of blood glucose meters (the process) will lead to better adherence to the meter (an intermediate outcome), which leads to more appropriate adjustments of medications (another intermediate outcome) that leads to better glycemic control (another intermediate outcome) that could, in turn, lead to better health-related quality of life (the long-term outcome). Thus, when evaluating the linkage of the *process* with long-term *outcomes*, identifying potential intermediate outcomes along the causal path between the process and long-term outcomes may be useful.

Performance Indicators

Within the cycle for continuous quality improvement, quality is often monitored through the use of performance indicators.[36] ❻ *Performance indicators are used to measure quality as part of the check function of quality improvement. The indicators typically focus on the process or outcomes of a care system* although they can also focus on structure. Typically, they measure specific processes or steps within a process that are known to be associated with an important outcome. For example, to evaluate the process of responding to a drug information request, one could identify a few key steps within the process that can be easily measured (e.g., in what percentage of cases was the desired timeline for a response documented, in what percentage of cases was the desired timeline met?).

Although one might think that outcomes are the ideal indicator of health care performance, they are often more difficult to measure than specific health care functions and may not always be directly, or independently, caused by the process of interest. Process indicators are useful for quality improvement when the:

- Outcome is difficult to measure.
- Outcome is far removed in time from the process (e.g., 10-year survival in cancer).
- Outcome is influenced by many factors other than the process.
- Process, by itself, is of interest (e.g., it is required to be measured for accreditation by TJC or reflects an issue of social justice, such as racial inequities in receiving specific elements of care).

Therefore, if one wanted to improve the quality of care for patients with diabetes, it may be more useful to assess the appropriateness of adjustments in insulin doses than to measure the rate of hospitalizations during a 5-year period for patients in the diabetes care program. This is not to suggest that evaluating outcomes is unwise. If outcomes can be directly linked to the process and can be evaluated in a timely, efficient, and reliable manner, they become powerful tools for quality improvement.

❼ *Performance indicators are typically categorized as either sentinel or aggregate measures.*[36] **Sentinel indicators** *reflect the occurrence of a serious event that requires further investigation (e.g., adverse drug-related event, death), whereas* **aggregate indicators** *provide a summary of the frequency, or timeliness, of a process by aggregating numerous cases. Aggregate indicators are further divided into continuous or rate-based indicators.* **Continuous indicators** provide a simple count, or time estimate, related to a process (e.g., average turnaround time on medication orders), whereas **rate-based indicators** usually measure the proportion of activities, or patients, that conform to a desired standard (e.g., the proportion of stat orders that are dispensed within 15 minutes). Thus, the rate-based indicators are generally expressed as a ratio. The denominator within the ratio should be the total number of patients within the target population, while the numerator should be the number of patients who received (or failed to receive) the desired test or who achieved a specified goal. For example, if it is necessary to construct an indicator for medication errors, the numerator would be the number of medication errors within a defined time period and the denominator would be the total number of error opportunities (e.g., number of prescriptions filled) during the same time period. This facilitates the comparison of error rates over time even as prescription volume fluctuates.

Selecting and Defining an Indicator

Characteristics for an ideal indicator have been proposed by several authors and organizations.[36-38] In general, it is necessary to seek indicators that are clearly defined, quantitative, reliable, clinically meaningful, and actionable. Kerr and associates[39] also suggest using indicators where the link between process and outcome is clearly established and the link between an indicator and a potential quality improvement response is evident. Thus, the indicator provides clinically meaningful and actionable information. Indicators should be selected on the basis of their usefulness to quality improvement efforts. The indicator should help determine where potential problems are occurring within the process. For example, it may be useful to know that only 30% of patients reported that they were provided with adequate answers to their questions about medications. The method with which drug-related information is provided to patients can then be changed. However, knowing that only 30% of patients with diabetes had received a microalbumin test would not be as helpful if there is no control of when that test is ordered.

Providing definitions for any variables that are not intuitive will also be necessary. **Medication error** means different things to different people; therefore, if it is necessary to construct an indicator for medication errors, the staff would need to be informed what constitutes an error (see Chapter 18). It is also necessary to identify inclusion or exclusion criteria. The patients to be included within an indicator must be determined. Even for disease-specific indicators, it is necessary to decide whether to combine data for all patients with the disease or to subdivide the analyses for different types of patients with that disease. For example, it may be possible to divide patients with diabetes into at least three subgroups: Type 1, Type 2, and gestational. Other questions include the following: are people of all ages included? Are only those who attended all diabetes education sessions or anyone who completed even a portion of the program included? The answers to these questions may depend on the particular indicator. The key is to compare apples to apples. If, for example, the standard for HgbA1c testing is different for patients with gestational diabetes compared with Type 1 or Type 2 diabetes, then a person would not want to combine HgbA1C data from all these patients into a single indicator.

To judge the quality of performance from the indicator data, having a frame of reference will be necessary. Thus, current performance data can be compared with previous performance (i.e., was there an improvement over time?) or with an external criterion or standard (i.e., benchmark); both comparisons can be useful. For example, it is possible to track the proportion of patients who reached the target HgbA1C during the previous 2 years (e.g., 45% of patients last year versus 62% of patients this year). However, whether this year's result, 62% of patients reaching the target, is considered good, fair, or poor performance is less clear. To determine this, compare the success rate with that of other programs. If the latest data from surrounding health plans indicate that 60% of their enrollees with diabetes have achieved the same target for HgbA1C, the person could assert that performance is at least as good as the standard. Ideally, the goal will be to continually improve success rate, regardless of the minimal standard.

Sources for Indicator Data

Data for constructing indicators can come from numerous sources. The most common sources of performance data are (1) medical or prescription records, (2) administrative claims, (3) operations records, and (4) patient reports. Each of these sources has strengths and weaknesses. Medical records provide rich information about an individual patient; however, the aggregation of data from written documents can be very slow and labor intensive. As advances in health information technology lead to widespread adoption of electronic medical records, the use of medical records for performance review will become increasingly attractive.

Administrative claims are available in electronic format, so data across providers and across an entire patient population can be easily aggregated and analyzed. However, administrative claims lack in-depth information and may contain some inaccuracies in coding. Thus, indicators built solely on administrative claims are limited in their usefulness for problem solving.

Operations records refer to data that are collected as part of the process of care. For example, a hospital pharmacy may document the time that a medication order was received and the time that the medication was dispensed. If the pharmacy has a predetermined standard for the timeliness of medication-order turnaround, then a performance indicator could be developed to show the proportion of medications that were dispensed within the designated timeframe.

Patient-reported data can also be valuable in assessing several subdomains of quality. Patient satisfaction measures are the most common way of collecting patient feedback on care. Satisfaction is an important outcome of care because patients who are dissatisfied with services are more likely to complain to external entities (e.g., regulatory agencies, employers) and are more likely to discontinue using services. Patients can also be asked questions about specific steps in the process of care to identify the source of quality deficits (e.g., were you asked if you had any questions about your medication?). The most commonly used tools for gathering patient feedback are within the Consumer Assessment of Healthcare Providers and Systems (CAHPS) family of surveys (http://www.ahrq.gov/cahps/index.html).[40] CAHPS contains surveys for health systems, physicians, and other facilities and clinicians. PQA has developed a CAHPS-like survey tool to gather patient feedback on ambulatory pharmacy services.[41]

The best method for collecting performance data is to use a hybrid approach wherein several different sources of data are used to examine the same care process. This allows for a more reliable and broad-based perspective on performance. This is important because different data sources have been found to provide different estimates of the quality of care.[42,43]

Interpreting Indicator Data

The collection of performance data is good, but data are most useful when transformed into interpretable and actionable information. Several tools can help to transform data into easily interpreted information. These tools include Pareto charts, bar charts, scatter diagrams, regression analyses, run charts, and control charts. Detailed information on the use of these tools can be found elsewhere, including Appendix 16-1[44]; however, examples for a few of the tools are shown in Figures 16-2 through 16-6.

Pareto charts are vertical bar graphs with the data presented so that the bars are arranged from left to right on the horizontal axis in their order of decreasing frequency. This arrangement helps to identify which problems to address in what order. By addressing the data represented in the tallest bars (e.g., the most frequently occurring problems or contributing factors) efforts can be focused on areas where the most gain can

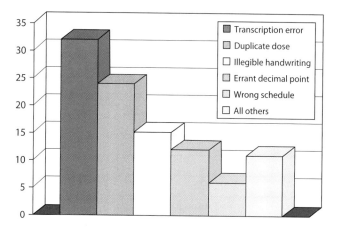

Figure 16–2. Pareto chart: factors contributing to improper dose errors.

be realized. Pareto charts are commonly used to identify issues to address, delineate potential causes of a problem, and to monitor improvements in processes. An example of a Pareto chart is shown in Figure 16-2. This example illustrates frequently occurring factors contributing to improperly dosed medication errors. By looking at transcription errors as a contributing factor on which to focus quality improvement efforts, the quality improvement team will generally gain more than by tackling the smaller bars.

Bar charts and scatter diagrams are particularly useful for displaying data for sentinel events. If a pharmacy wanted to evaluate data on medication errors, a bar chart could show the distribution of errors by day of the week or by time of day (Figure 16-3). Displaying the rate (i.e., percent of doses dispensed in error) rather than a simple count

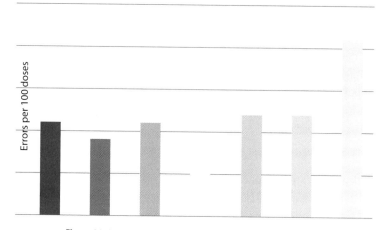

Figure 16–3. Bar chart showing percentage of doses dispensed in error.

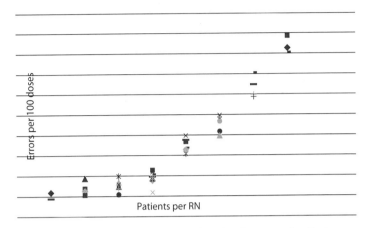

Figure 16–4. Scatter diagram to depict relationship of error rate and workload.

of errors helps to control for fluctuations in the workload across days of the week. This might help to pinpoint whether errors were more likely to occur during particular days or shifts. If so, the staff could then investigate why the errors were higher at particular times. The frequency of errors could also be depicted on a scatter diagram. A scatter diagram illustrates the relationship of two variables. For example, a nursing home might be interested in whether the frequency of errors is related to staffing levels. A scatter diagram could be constructed wherein the number of errors was shown on the vertical (y) axis and the staffing level on the horizontal (x) axis (Figure 16-4). The data points are plotted to show the number of errors at each level of staffing.

Run charts and control charts are useful for depicting trends in rate-based indicators. Both charts illustrate the trend in a variable over time; however, the control chart also shows the extent of variation in the trend by placing control limits above and below the trend line (typically at two standard deviations from the mean). In most cases, a simple run chart will suffice for visualizing a trend. For example, if a health system wanted to examine the impact of changing the medication delivery process on the rate of missing doses of medications, the rate could be calculated for each month and trended over time (Figure 16-5).

Constructing Process Indicators

A stepwise approach to constructing a rate-based, process indicator is outlined here.[45]

1. **Identify an area of concern.** The area of concern may be identified from internal reports of quality-related problems or from external mandates (e.g., requirements for accreditation). Often, these concerns relate to areas in which errors have occurred with great frequency or in which the clinical consequences of

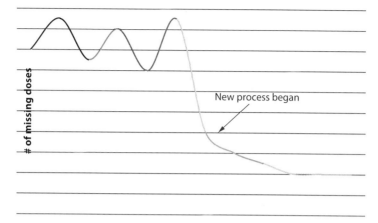

Figure 16–5. Run chart depicting rate of missing doses over time.

suboptimal quality are substantial. For illustrative purposes, patient's understanding of a medication regimen will be used as the area of concern for a community pharmacy.

2. **Select the process, or segments of a process, to study.** The process most directly related to the area of concern should be examined, and a specific segment of the process may be selected for performance measurement. For patient's understanding of a medication regimen, the relevant process within a community pharmacy may be the dispensing process and the specific segment of the process for assessment may be patient counseling.

3. **Determine what can be measured to evaluate the process.** For patient counseling, it is possible to measure the frequency of patient counseling events, the accuracy of information provided to patients, or the patient's knowledge about the medication regimen. Those performing the assessment should then select the measures that are most likely to be reliable, are feasible to collect, and facilitate a valid assessment of the quality of the counseling segment of the dispensing process. In this example, the rate of patient counseling might first be selected for measurement because it should be easily and reliably collected and will provide a valid assessment of whether counseling was occurring (although it would not tell the effectiveness of counseling).

4. **Define the numerator for your indicator.** For an indicator, the numerator should reflect the number of times that a selected event occurred. For the patient counseling indicator, the numerator could be the number of patient counseling events within a specified time interval (e.g., 1 month). To accurately determine the number of counseling events, defining what is and what is not a counseling event

is important. For example, must a counseling event involve oral communication between patient and pharmacist or will the provision of a written pamphlet suffice? If oral communication is required, how much communication is necessary to be considered a counseling event? Do certain elements of drug information need to be conveyed for the event to be counted? Ensuring that all employees have a clear understanding of the definition of counseling is important to reduce inaccuracies in counting the events.

5. **Define the denominator for your indicator.** For an indicator, the denominator should represent the eligible population or the total number of opportunities in which the numerator could have occurred. For the counseling indicator, the denominator could simply be defined as the number of prescriptions dispensed in a time period (e.g., 1 month). However, it is necessary to refine this number to enhance the validity of our inferences about the quality of counseling. Should both new and refill prescriptions be included in the denominator? If the patient declines the offer to counsel, should they be included in the denominator? If the patient receives five prescriptions at one time, will they be counted as one counseling opportunity or as five counseling opportunities? Having clear inclusion and exclusion criteria will be important to the interpretability of the indicator.

6. **Determine the method for data collection.** Numerous methods may exist for collecting data for a specific indicator. For the counseling indicator, the denominator could be derived from automated reports of new (and perhaps refill) prescriptions. If the pharmacy has a mechanism for tracking patients who were offered but declined counseling, then the prescriptions for those patients could be subtracted from the denominator. The numerator in the counseling indicator could be measured in several ways. A pharmacist could record on a notepad, or electronic record, whether he or she counseled the patient. Alternatively, the pharmacy could select a time period during which an external data collector would document the frequency of counseling. This could entail direct observation of the pharmacist-patient encounters or could entail the data collector asking the patients whether they had been offered counseling and had received counseling about their medications. In the latter approach, the patient could also be asked whether he or she understood the information that they were provided. A step further would be to assess the patient's understanding, although that would take more time and, therefore, may not be possible. Each of these methods has strengths and limitations.

7. **Select tools to display the indicator data.** After the data are collected, displaying the results in a manner that provides an efficient assessment of quality would be helpful. This can be accomplished by comparing the results with an external

benchmark or by comparing the most recent results with previous results for the same provider. Currently, the only external benchmark that exists may be a regulatory requirement for counseling. For example, the state of Michigan requires pharmacists to counsel 100% of patients who receive a new prescription unless the patient meets certain exemption criteria. However, a more useful comparator may be the prior performance of the pharmacy. Thus, plotting the counseling rate on a run chart each month may eventually provide the pharmacy with insight on whether the counseling rate is improving or declining. If the rate is declining, then further investigation could reveal the potential causes of the change in performance and actions taken to improve performance.

Quality Indicators and Measures Evaluation

A quality indicator or measure may be identified and defined internally by the health care provider, the facility, the system, or plan. However, more frequently providers are assigned specific nationally recognized indicators or measures by which their performance will be determined. As previously mentioned the NQF and the NCQA and PQA are two sources of developed endorsed quality measures. These endorsed measures are included by agencies, health insurers, and others to assess performance of providers, facilities, care settings, or plans. Several examples of medication-related measures with descriptions are provided in Table 16-2.

Multiple PQA endorsed measures have been adopted over time by CMS for inclusion in the Medicare Part D 5-star rating evaluation. In 2017, there are five PQA measures used for evaluating Part D and three PQA measures are included in the Quality Rating System in the Health Insurance Marketplace. Three of the five Part D measures and the three Marketplace measures are medication adherence measures assessed by use of the proportion of days covered (PDC) formula. The adherence measures are: PDC for oral diabetes medications, PDC for renin angiotensin system antagonists (RASA), and PDC for the cholesterol HMG-CoA inhibitors (statin) use. The PDC rate of >80% is considered high adherence. The other two Part D measures are: the completion rate for the comprehensive medication review (CMR) for beneficiaries eligible for medication therapy management and the percent of beneficiaries that receive a high-risk medication.[18]

Other programs include a myriad of different medication measures for specific disease states for quality of care assessment. One example is the hospital value-based purchasing program.[46] A process measure of clinical care, for the disease acute myocardial infarction, includes evaluation of receipt of fibrinolytic therapy within 30 minutes of hospital arrival and for another process, prevention management, receipt of an immunization (influenza vaccine). The hospital is evaluated based on a total performance score and the clinical care

TABLE 16–2. MEDICATION MEASURES AND EVALUATION

Measure Name	Measure Description	Setting, Evaluation Domain
High-risk medication	Percent of plan members who got prescriptions for certain drugs with a high risk of serious side effects, when there may be safer drug choices.	Medicare Part D star rating, drug pricing patient safety
Medication adherence for diabetes medications	Percent of plan members with a prescription for diabetes medication who fill their prescription often enough to cover 80% or more of the time they are supposed to be taking the medication.	Medicare Part D star rating, drug pricing patient safety
Medication adherence for hypertension renin angiotensin system antagonists	Percent of plan members with a prescription for a blood pressure medication who fill their prescription often enough to cover 80% or more of the time they are supposed to be taking the medication.	Medicare Part D star rating, drug pricing patient safety
Medication adherence for cholesterol (statins)	Percent of plan members with a prescription for a cholesterol medication (a statin drug) who fill their prescription often enough to cover 80% or more of the time they are supposed to be taking the medication.	Medicare Part D star rating, drug pricing patient safety
Medication Therapy Management program completion rate for comprehensive medication review (CMR)	Some plan members are in a program (called a Medication Therapy Management program) to help them manage their drugs. The measure shows how many members in the program had an assessment of their medications from the plan. The assessment includes a discussion between the member and a pharmacist (or other health care professional) about all of the member's medications. The member also receives a written summary of the discussion, including an action plan that recommends what the member can do to better understand and use his or her medications.	Medicare Part D star rating, drug pricing patient safety
Fibrinolytic therapy received within 30 minutes of hospital arrival	Acute myocardial infarction (AMI) patients receiving fibrinolytic therapy during the hospital stay and having a time from hospital arrival to fibrinolysis of 30 minutes or less.	Hospital value-based purchasing, clinical care process measures

Measure Name	Measure Description	Setting, Evaluation Domain
Influenza immunization	This prevention measure addresses acute care hospitalized inpatients age 6 months and older who were screened for seasonal influenza immunization status and were vaccinated prior to discharge if indicated.	Hospital value-based purchasing, clinical care process measures
Coronary artery disease (CAD) antiplatelet therapy	Percentage of patients aged 18 years and older with a diagnosis of coronary artery disease (CAD) seen within a 12-month period who were prescribed aspirin or clopidogrel.	Practices Merit-Based Incentive Payment System (MIPS), quality
Avoidance of antibiotic treatment in adults with acute bronchitis	The percentage of 18–64 years of age with a diagnosis of acute bronchitis who were not dispensed an antibiotic prescription.	Practices MIPS, quality
Medication management for people with asthma	The percentage of patients 5–64 years of age during the measurement year who were identified as having persistent asthma and were dispensed appropriate medications that they remained on for at least 75% of their treatment period.	Practices MIPS, quality
Atrial fibrillation and atrial flutter: chronic anticoagulation therapy	Percentage of patients aged 18 years and older with a diagnosis of nonvalvular atrial fibrillation (AF) or atrial flutter whose assessment of the specified thromboembolic risk factors indicate one or more high risk factors or more than one moderate risk, as determined by CHADS2 risk stratification, who are prescribed warfarin OR another oral anticoagulant drug that is FDA approved for the prevention of thromboembolism.	Practices MIPS, quality
Adherence to antipsychotic medications for individuals with schizophrenia	Percentage of individuals at least 18 years of age as of the beginning of the measurement period with schizophrenia or schizoaffective disorder who had at least two prescriptions filled for any antipsychotic medications and who had a proportion of days covered (PDC) of at least 0.8 for antipsychotic medications during the measurement period (12 consecutive months).	Practices MIPS, quality

779

process measures constitute a percentage (in 2017, 5%) of the total (100%) performance composite score. Weighted scoring changes occur over the years of the program.

In the MIPS program for eligible providers there are four categories that are part of a composite performance score, each category contributes to the total performance score.[47] The four categories and the associated 2017 percentages contributions include: (i) quality (60%), (ii) improvement activities (15%), (iii) advancing care information (25%), and (iv) cost. Within the first three categories there are multiple options for providers to select the measures they want to be assessed for performance, and many of these options include medication measures. Under the category quality, there are over 270 measures and a provider must select six. Many of quality measures are medication related, such as chronic stable coronary artery disease (CAD) patients who were prescribed antiplatelet therapy, aspirin, or clopidogrel within a 12-month period; antibiotic avoidance in patients with bronchitis; or the percentage of asthma patients dispensed appropriate asthma controller medications. Overall provider performance will be determined by the performance within each category as part of the composite score.

MEASURING HEALTH EQUITY

In determining quality and performance, the development of indicators, measurement, and collection of data must take into consideration the distinguishing characteristics of all people. Despite advances in health care quality and access, there are numerous reports of minority groups experiencing differences in care and worse outcomes. The CMS Office of Minority Health (CMS OMH) has one-page fact sheets on several chronic conditions – such as atrial fibrillation to osteoporosis to stroke – with a focus on health disparities in the Medicare population. https://www.cms.gov/About-CMS/Agency-Information/OMH/OMH-DataSnapshots.html.[48]

Definition of Health Equity

❽ *Focus on health equity and elimination of health disparities are necessary to achieve quality health care for all.* **Health equity** is defined as the attainment of the highest level of health for all people. To achieve health equity, the health care system must focus on valuing each patient or customer equally, regardless of what group(s) they are assigned. When measuring health equity, an identified health disparity may be associated with one or more social, economic or environmental factors. Health disparities indicate differences associated with being a member of a group or groups that have historically experienced systematic obstacles to optimal health due to conditions of their birth, or how they live, work, grow, and age, to include: race and/or ethnicity; religion; socioeconomic status; gender; age; mental health, cognitive, sensory, or physical disability; sexual orientation or gender identity; geographic location; or other characteristics of discrimination or exclusion.[49]

Measurement Standards

Our ability to measure health disparities is dependent on the collection of data for applicable groups through standardized, structured data elements. National data collection standards for documenting information by different groups was authorized by the ACA.[50] Health care settings use electronic health records, as part of Stage 2 meaningful use, to capture these data elements, such as REAL (race, ethnicity, preferred language), gender, and date of birth to inform our understanding of how well we provide care to patients assigned to different groups.[52] However, not all data elements – for example, gender identification and sexual preference – can be readily captured in the current electronic health records. To achieve health equity, the plan step of the PDCA must include demographic data collection for all groups, thorough and objective assessment, and focused interventions that address observed differences in care. The Institute of Healthcare Improvement (IHI) Guide to Achieving Health Equity includes the business case, a case study, tools, and a description of measurement by different subpopulations identifying measures in two categories, summary or aggregated and stratified or disaggregated, to assist organizations to successfully address health disparities.[53] Pharmacy information systems and prescription drug claims will require data element capture for the different groups to determine if health disparities exist with regard to prescription drugs and pharmacy services. Recently, CMS reported on Medicare Advantage differences in race/ethnicity groups from 2014 data for two patient experience measures: obtaining needed prescription drugs and obtaining information about prescription drugs. Results for the two measures were highest for Whites 91.1% and 82.2% and lowest in Asian or Pacific Islanders (API) 85.1% and 72.7%, respectively. For Blacks, results for the two measures were 90% and 77.7%, for American Indians or Alaska Natives 87.3% and 79.9%, and for Hispanics 88% and 76.8%, respectively.[54] These results are similar to a 2008 study of surveyed Medicare Part D beneficiaries for the same measures; Blacks, Hispanics, and API results were 2 to 11 points lower as compared to Whites[55] (Case Study 16-1).

Case Study 16–1

In evaluating medication reconciliation at admission in a nursing home, the medical director believes there are differences in medication discrepancies based on patient demographics and would like the nursing staff and consultant pharmacist to present data to refute or confirm. What steps should the nursing home take to assess the medication discrepancies by patient subgroups?

MEDICATION USE EVALUATION

- Medication use evaluation (MUE) is often included in the overall performance improvement programs within institutional settings to provide in-depth assessment of the medication use process. MUE programs should, over time, examine all aspects of medication use and require direct involvement of pharmacists.[56,57] ❾ *MUE is often part of an organization's overall performance improvement program that uses definitions of safe and effective use of medications to assess components of the medication use process.* These definitions are usually described as **criteria** and are endorsed by the organization within which they are to be applied. Criteria summarize an organization's definition of appropriate or acceptable use of the medication. The manner in which medications are actually used, administered, and monitored within the organization is compared with the criteria to determine if actual practice matches the best (or at least acceptable) practice as stated with the criteria. For example, based on evidence that slowing the infusion rate of an intravenous medication reduces the risk of serious adverse events, the criteria may state that the medication should be infused over at least 60 minutes. However, when actual practice is accessed as part of an MUE, results indicate that the medication is infused over 30 minutes or less in 50% of cases, and adverse effects were noted in most of these cases. These results indicate that best practice is not occurring (Case Study 16-2).

Case Study 16–2

In a situation where an intravenous antibiotic was administered more rapidly than recommended, what factors could be contributing to this problem?

- Endorsement of criteria is usually provided by a multidisciplinary group that includes medical staff (e.g., the pharmacy and therapeutics [P&T] committee). The goal of MUE is to provide all patients with the most rational, safe, and effective drug therapy through the assessment and improvement of specific medication use processes. MUE may focus on a specific medication (e.g., alteplase), a class of medications (e.g., thrombolytics), medications used in the management of a specific disease state or clinical setting (e.g., thrombolytics in acute myocardial infarction), medications related to a clinical event (e.g., drug therapy within the first 24 hours for patients admitted with acute myocardial infarction including aspirin, beta blockers, thrombolytics), a specific component of the medication use process (e.g., time from admission to administration of thrombolytic), or can be based on specific outcomes (e.g., vessel patency following thrombolytic administration). MUE is not designed to address if-then questions (such as if one dose is used instead of another, then will outcomes be affected), but simply determines if the actual use of a medication is consistent with the standards established within the criteria. Although MUE is no longer explicitly addressed within TJC Standards, it remains an important component of broader requirements related to performance improvement within organizations. In order to be effective, challenges such as a lack of resources or authority, politics, difficulty in identifying issues (e.g., high-use, high-risk, or problematic medications or processes) or in acting upon data to improve performance, and cumbersome or ineffective reporting structure or processes must be addressed. For example, unless the organization has a functional process to use the information generated by MUE to improve patient care, outcomes are unlikely to improve. If a minority of prescribers or any single group (e.g., nursing, clinical laboratory, pharmacy, respiratory therapy) can unilaterally disagree with the recommendations from an MUE and successfully block efforts to implement process improvement initiatives, efforts will fail. In order for MUE to effectively improve patient care, the organization must have a commitment to improving medication use and a committee structure that facilitates multidisciplinary collaboration and cooperation.

The Medication Use Process

In 1989, a multidisciplinary task force was organized by TJC to describe the medication use process as a component of their effort to develop tools to assess medication use. The medication use process is the outline of the steps involved in providing medications to patients (e.g., prescribing, dispensing) and what happens after the medication is administered (e.g., monitoring). The original definition of the medication use process included prescribing, transcribing, dispensing, administering, monitoring, and systems and management control (see Table 16-3 for the full definition). This description serves as the basis for MUE.[58,59] Currently, systems and management control is often not included within the description of the medication use process as it applies to virtually all aspects of patient care. Medication acquisition, storage, distribution, and disposal may also be assessed if pertinent.

It is important to note that this description outlines a process more multidisciplinary than the categories might imply. For example, while the prescribing category may imply a physician function, pharmacists are often involved as they assist in drug selection and individualization of the therapeutic regimen.

Medication Use Evaluation and The Joint Commission

The terminology used to describe MUE has changed over time and can be confusing. MUE, DUE, DUR, and AUR (antibiotic use review) were often used interchangeably

TABLE 16-3.   DESCRIPTION OF THE MEDICATION USE PROCESS

Function	Description
Prescribing	Assessing the need for/selecting the correct drug
	Individualizing the therapeutic regimen
	Designing the desired therapeutic response
Dispensing	Reviewing the order for correct dose and indication for use
	Processing the order
	Compounding/preparing the drug
	Dispensing the drug in a timely manner
Administering	Administering the right medication to the right patient
	Administering the medication when indicated
	Informing the patient about the medication
	Including the patient in administration
Monitoring	Monitoring and documenting the patient's response
	Identifying and reporting adverse drug reactions
	Reevaluating the drug selection, drug regimen, frequency, and duration
Systems/Management control	Collaborating and communicating among caregivers
	Reviewing and managing the patient's complete therapeutic drug regimen

despite being different in their approach and application (Table 16-4). Greater consistency in terminology and standards were established with an initiative called the *Agenda for Change* from TJC in 1986.[60,61] It was intended to improve standards by focusing on key functions of quality of care, to monitor the performance of health care organizations using indicators, to improve the relevance and quality of the survey process, and to enhance the accuracy and value of TJC accreditation. Indicators are quantitative measures of an aspect of patient care and are used to screen for potential problems; indicators will be discussed in detail later in the chapter. The revised process was to focus on actual performance versus the capability to perform well. An organization could no longer hide behind having well-designed processes or policies and procedures on paper; TJC surveyors would now be looking at how processes were actually carried out. Within this initiative, TJC endorsed the concept of CQI, whereby data would be used to uncover problems and use that information to correct issues and avoid problems in the future, and included CQI within its standards beginning in 1994.

As part of this process, the Accreditation Manual for Hospitals (AMH) was significantly modified and much of the definition of expectations related to organization performance was deleted.[62] Multidisciplinary involvement in the evaluation of medication use was emphasized. Eventually, the standards were moved from the Medical Staff chapter of the AMH to the Care of Patients and Performance Improvement chapters. In 1992, the

TABLE 16–4. ACRONYMS ASSOCIATED WITH THE EVALUATION OF MEDICATION USE

Term	Origin	Description
Drug use review (DUR)	1969 Task Force on Prescription Drugs	Retrospective evaluation to monitor medication use patterns. Usually quantitative and limited to trending.
	1990 Medicaid Anti-Discriminatory Drug Price and Patient Benefit Restoration Act (*Pryor II*)	Usually retrospective evaluation based on claims data. Results used to direct education and to reduce fraud, abuse, overuse, and inappropriate or unnecessary care.
Antibiotic use review (AUR)	1978 JCAHO Standards	Retrospective evaluation of antibiotic use. Usually quantitative and limited to identifying patterns of use.
Drug use evaluation (DUE)	1986 JCAHO Standards	Expansion of AUR to all drugs. Concurrent evaluation of prescribing and outcome only. Multidisciplinary involvement.
Medication use evaluation (MUE)	1992 JCAHO Standards	Expansion of DUE to include all medications and all aspects of medication use including prescribing, dispensing, administering, monitoring, and outcome.

terminology was also changed from drug use evaluation to MUE to reflect that all medications and all medication-related functions are included in the standard. This change also broadened the scope to reflect TJC's expanded reach into non-acute care settings (such as clinics and intravenous infusion centers) and clarified that the process did not focus on illicit drug use. MUE standards first appeared in the 1992 AMH and were required of all institutions beginning in 1994.

Current standards focus on performance improvement, but no longer require that a specific approach be used. The organization is allowed to select, based on its characteristics and structure, a performance-improvement approach (e.g., FOCUS-PDCA, Six Sigma) that best meets their needs and that of its patients. Standards state that MUE should be a systematic, multidisciplinary process focusing on continual improvement in the medication use process and patient outcomes. The use of data for reappointment or re-credentialing is still required, but the emphasis is on continuous performance improvement.

Priorities should be established based on:

- effect on performance and improved patient outcomes
- selected high-volume, high-risk, or problem-prone processes
- resources and organizational priorities

Evaluation of the use of high-cost medications is often a priority within organizations hoping to optimize use of available financial resources. However, in the past, many organizations based their topic selection solely on cost-saving initiatives rather than on improving the quality of medication use. As a result, this category, when stated as a sole rationale for topic selection, is no longer considered to be consistent with the goals of MUE. High-cost medications continue to be a focus of evaluation, but organizations are careful to justify the evaluation based on other criteria, such as the use of the medication being problem-prone or its importance in determining patient outcome.

The pharmacist plays a key role within the multidisciplinary MUE process. Although not always involved in specific initiatives, all pharmacists should actively identify opportunities for improvement in processes.[63] Although many pharmacists within the organization will have some role in the MUE process, those responsible for coordination and implementation of MUE initiatives are often those with drug information or performance improvement responsibilities, as well as those with specialized knowledge or experience in the component of medication use under assessment. The American Society of Health-System Pharmacists (ASHP, http://www.ashp.org) has developed guidelines for pharmacist's participation in MUE.[57] These guidelines can serve as a resource to those developing or revising an MUE program or for practitioners new to the process.

The MUE Process

The process of MUE has often been implemented through a 10-step process described by TJC in 1989.[62,64] Although this specific process is no longer mandated by TJC, it does offer a reasonable model for MUE. The 10 steps are:

1. Assign responsibility for monitoring and evaluation
2. Delineate scope of care and service provided by the organization
3. Identify important aspects of care and service provided by the organization
4. Identify indicators, data sources, and collection methods to monitoring important aspects of care
5. Establish means to trigger evaluation (e.g., trends or patterns of use, thresholds)
6. Collect and organize data
7. Initiate evaluation of care (as indicated by triggers set in step 5)
8. Take actions to improve care and service
9. Assess the effectiveness of actions and maintain the improvement, document improvements in care
10. Communicate results to relevant individuals and groups

Please note, as these steps are described below, that they are often concurrent and overlapping. For example, the final step of communication is important throughout the other steps.

Responsibility for the Medication Use Evaluation Function

The 10-step process begins with the organization defining which group or groups will participate in and be responsible for the evaluation of medication use. These groups oversee the process, since it has to be assumed that everyone will provide effort toward actually performing or implementing quality assurance activities. Although TJC standards no longer assign the responsibility for MUE to the P&T committee, nor do they require a P&T committee at all, the function is well suited to this group as well as to a performance/quality improvement committee. *Performance improvement committees* are usually multidisciplinary, but may lack medical staff participation. Their focus may be quite broad and may include oversight for a wide variety of performance improvement functions throughout the organization. Some organizations have formed an MUE subcommittee to the P&T group, while others have distributed the responsibility for MUE along patient population or product lines. Subcommittees are generally assigned responsibility for a specific set of responsibilities or information and report to the larger committee. They serve as a platform to work through the details of an issue or process and generate recommendations to the parent committee. A patient safety committee may also play a role in identification of topics, evaluation of findings, and implementation of corrective actions. The entire committee may participate in evaluations or working groups, consisting of committee members, may be established; nonmembers may be appointed to address specific issues. The size, scope, and makeup of the health care organization and its approach to performance improvement should determine the approach to be used. The participants in the group charged with overseeing MUE must have a clear understanding that the purpose is that of improving the quality of the medication use process and that each member is expected to actively participate. Newly formed groups may benefit from an overview of the organization's overall approach to quality improvement and how MUE contributes to overall goals.

Topic Selection

Topic selection should be based on the mission and scope of care of the organization and should focus on high-volume, high-risk, or problem-prone medication-related processes. Topics may also focus on institutional priorities (e.g., initiation of new clinical programs or services). Several sources of information are commonly used to identify these agents and issues. They include medication error reports, adverse drug reactions (ADRs), advances in patient care modalities that involve changes in optimal pharmacotherapy, disease- or diagnosis-based length of stay or cost outliers within an organization, purchasing reports indicating a significant increase in the use of an agent (without a related shift in patient population), medications that are a key component of a process or procedure (e.g., thrombolytics, glycoprotein IIb/IIIa receptor inhibitors), and more. It is essential that the topics selected reflect the overall scope of medication use throughout the organization, including inpatients, outpatients, emergency care, and short-stay settings, rather than always centering on a finite area.

The inclusion of specific requirements within TJC's Medication Management Standards and National Patient Safety Goals related to identification and monitoring of medications described as high-risk or high-alert within the organization provides another mechanism to target specific medications for additional assessment. High-risk or high-alert medications are those that are most likely to result in adverse outcomes if used inappropriately or if errors are made.

Ideally, the group charged with MUE should develop an annual plan that will establish goals for new topics to be assessed and provide for follow-up on previous evaluations. Priorities should be reevaluated and the scope and breadth of recent evaluations should be assessed relative to the scope of care provided within the organization. For example, if recent MUE efforts focused primarily on issues related to antibiotic use, the plan for the upcoming year should deemphasize assessment of this class in favor of a more balanced topic selection. The planning process can identify follow-up assessments (used to assess and document that previous efforts were successful in improving performance) that remain to be performed. The failure to perform and document these follow-up evaluations is problematic in many organizations, but is a key component of the quality improvement process. Development of an annual plan also allows an opportunity to discontinue activities that are no longer useful, such as an ongoing assessment that has demonstrated sustained improvement and can now be replaced by periodic rechecks to assure continued compliance.

Criteria, Standards, and Indicators

Criteria are statements of the activity to be measured and standards define the performance expectations. For example, criteria for the management of patients with pneumonia might state that the first dose of antibiotic must be administered within 2 hours. The standard for this criteria statement would be set at 100% if there were no acceptable exceptions to this timeframe. Criteria should be based on current best or at least accepted practice or available organization-based clinical care plans, appropriate for the target patient population(s), and be supported by current literature. Ideally, a multidisciplinary group develops the criteria. The membership of this group (e.g., prescribers, nurses, pharmacists, respiratory therapists, social workers, clinical laboratory and information systems personnel, discharge planners) should be determined by the nature of the process under evaluation. Inclusion of all involved disciplines initially will also facilitate implementation of corrective actions, if deficiencies are identified. However, criteria are most often developed by one or two of the involved disciplines and are subsequently approved by a multidisciplinary group with representation from all applicable practice groups (e.g., prescribers, pharmacists, nurses). Explicit (objective) criteria are preferred in that they are clear cut, based on specific measurable parameters, and are better suited for automation. Implicit (subjective) criteria require that a judgment be made and require appropriate clinical expertise to be effective. They are often too subjective to be consistently evaluated (i.e., different people would interpret them differently). Table 16-5 compares implicit and

TABLE 16–5. EXAMPLES OF IMPLICIT AND EXPLICIT CRITERIA STATEMENTS

Implicit Criteria Statements	Explicit Criteria Statements
Blood work ordered	Pretreatment WBC with differential ordered and completed within 48 hours prior to the initiation of therapy
Renal function assessed routinely	Serum creatinine evaluated every 3 days during therapy
Neutropenic patients	Patients with WBC $<1,000/mm^3$

explicit criteria statements. Appendix 16-2 provides an example of criteria. It is imperative that the appropriate oversight group approves the criteria prior to initiation of data collection (Case Study 16-3).

Case Study 16–3

The antibiotic that was being infused too rapidly is used to prevent surgical infections and for infections caused by gram+ organisms. There is some evidence of other issues with the use of this antibiotic and an MUE is planned. The preoperative dose is given in the surgical area and the postoperative doses and treatment doses are given throughout the health system and in home care patients. Who would you invite to participate in an evaluation of the use of this antibiotic?

Criteria should be phrased in yes/no or true/false (along with not applicable as appropriate) formats and should avoid interpretation on the part of data collectors. They should assess important aspects in the use of the medication or therapy under evaluation and focus on aspects most closely related to outcomes of the care provided. Definition of outcome should also be established within the criteria based on the scope of care provided by the organization. For example, in a truly acute care setting, the outcome assessment of antibiotic management of pneumonia may be limited to a decrease in clinical signs and symptoms indicating a response to therapy and the ability to be discharged on an oral antibiotic(s). However, in an integrated system that includes both acute and ambulatory or long-term care, the evaluation could continue through the entire treatment course and outcome could be assessed based on cure or control of the disease state at the conclusion of therapy.

As the criteria are finalized, it is helpful to consider how opportunities for improvement identified via a criteria statement could be addressed. For example, could the computer system be used as a tool to improve prescribing, would a double check by a nurse and a pharmacist help to prevent errors, or could the dispensing process be modified to improve delivery time? If the corrective action would involve participation of a group not represented in the development process, it may be wise to add them to the team at this point.

Validity should be assessed as part of the development process. Validity assessments consider how effective the criteria will be in providing the information necessary to obtain an actual comparison of what is happening to the expectations outlined in the criteria. Table 16-6 outlines several questions to test the validity of criteria or indicators.[65-68] A short pilot of data collection with an analysis of resulting information is often a good way to test the validity of criteria and its utility in assessing medication use.

Although general guidelines related to criteria are available, most texts providing example criteria are no longer published.[35,69,70] Many group purchasing organizations and other networks have systems to facilitate sharing of MUE materials (e.g., criteria, data collection forms) and methods of comparing results with those from similar organizations. The advantages to using predeveloped criteria include prior expert review and assessment, and time savings. However, criteria developed outside the organization must be adapted to the practice setting and patient population as appropriate and must be approved by the designated multidisciplinary group prior to data collection. For example, criteria intended for use in a general adult population may not be appropriate for geriatric

TABLE 16–6.   TESTS OF VALIDITY OF CRITERIA OR INDICATORS

Types of Validity	Tests
Face validity	Are they important to patient outcome?
	Do they assess a problematic area?
	Do they have some utility in improving patient care?
	Do they reflect system-wide performance?
	Are they appropriate, based on current practice standards and literature?
External validity	Have they been thoroughly reviewed by practitioners with expertise in the use of the medication?
	Are they applicable within organization?
	Has the review process clarified and improved the criteria/indicators without weakening their intent?
Feasibility of data collection and retrieval	Are they clear and not subject to interpretation?
	Are data available?
	How many cases will need to be evaluated in order to provide adequate data?
	How difficult or complex will the data collection process be?
	What benefits will be gained versus the effort for data collection?
	Will data collection methods be consistent?

patients without modification. Also, predeveloped criteria may include uses of a medication not applicable to certain settings or aspects of use that are not a priority for assessment within the organization. For example, criteria for the use of midazolam that address its use for conscious sedation in a setting where conscious sedation is not performed can be streamlined by eliminating criteria related to conscious sedation. Criteria related to the use of antibiotics to treat infection, when the concerns prompting the evaluation relate solely to perioperative use, should be streamlined to focus solely on perioperative use. Criteria may also be derived from guidelines for use developed or adopted within the organization. For example, the P&T committee may agree to add a medication to the formulary for specific indications and require that the use of the agent and patient outcomes be concurrently evaluated based on these guidelines. In this situation, the criteria for use of the medication would reflect the indications approved by the committee and the MUE would assess the desired outcomes as defined by the committee. Data collection would begin as the medication is first used with results reported to the P&T committee at specific intervals (e.g., quarterly) or after a defined period of time (e.g., for the first 6 months) (Case Study 16-4).

Case Study 16–4

Within your organization, warfarin is responsible for more adverse events than any other medication. The P&T committee wants to do an MUE to identify opportunities to reduce the number and severity of adverse effects associated with warfarin. How would you identify existing guidelines or standards for warfarin use to assist in drafting criteria for this MUE?

Performance indicators can also be used to evaluate medication use. As described previously, an indicator is a quantitative measure of an aspect of patient care that is used as a screening tool to detect potential problems in quality.[36] For example, the number of doses of naloxone administered to reverse the effects of opioids administered in a procedure area or in outpatient areas could serve as an indicator of the appropriateness of opioids in clinical management. While the criteria used in MUE are focused and assess specific important components of medication use, indicators measure symptoms of a medication use system that could indicate that something is not working well, but there is no assurance that there really is a problem when an indicator is not met. They can serve as a tool to identify potentially problematic aspects of care, but require more focused assessment (such as an MUE) to identify the cause.

Within the MUE process, standards are used to define optimal performance and are usually set at 0% (should never happen) or 100% (should always happen). Thresholds are similar to standards but they specify an acceptable level of compliance or performance is usually set higher than 0% or lower than 100% based on acceptable variation, standards of practice, or benchmarks.[71] Thresholds are sometimes used instead of standards to allow limited noncompliance with the criteria when the clinical impact of noncompliance is felt to be of low risk. They should not be used to avoid intervention. Thresholds are useful when the group overseeing the MUE process is most interested in addressing performance that is clearly unacceptable, while allowing some variation from best practice.

Control limits can be used when measurements continue over an extended period of time (e.g., weeks or months). Unlike standards and thresholds, they are usually not applied in the initial MUE but can be used to follow a process over time. For example, an MUE was conducted and action taken to improve the use of the medication. Control limits could be used to monitor the ongoing use of the medication to assure that the improvement was sustained over time. Control limits define the limits of allowable or expected variation in performance (often two to three times the standard deviation from the mean initially) and may be used to assess the results on ongoing monitoring. As long as performance remains between the upper and lower control limits, action is not necessary to address the variations that occur over time. However, performance above or below the control limits is referred to as special variation and prompts assessment as to what factor(s) resulted in the special variation and should result in actions being taken to address the impact of these factors over time. For example, within an organization training medical residents, the number of pharmacists' interventions as documented on a control chart, might spike upward around July 1, corresponding to the start date for the new residents. While the organization may have limited opportunity to stagger starting dates, specific aspects of their orientation process could be enhanced to improve initial performance. As actions are taken to address factors resulting in special variations and the overall variability are reduced, control limits should narrow.[35] An example of a control chart with limits appears in Figure 16-6.

⑩ *Performance, as demonstrated by data collected in the performance improvement process, not meeting the defined standard or threshold or falling outside the control limits (for ongoing or follow-up assessments) indicates that intervention to improve performance is necessary.* In some cases, performance outside the defined parameters may, upon review, be acceptable to the oversight group. This usually results from expectations being set too high (e.g., that the rate of adverse effects with any agent will be 0%) or when the criteria fail to include the appropriate exceptions. When this occurs, the multidisciplinary oversight group must agree that the level of performance is acceptable and that intervention is not necessary. These decisions must be clearly documented in meeting minutes or summaries of results. If this is not done, regulatory bodies may infer that the organization

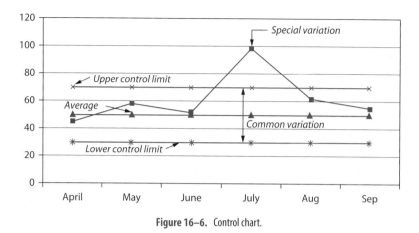

Figure 16–6. Control chart.

chose to ignore the findings of the evaluation, thus failing to meet the quality improvement requirements.

Data Collection

- Prior to the initiation of data collection, the multidisciplinary oversight group must approve the topic selection, criteria, patient selection process, sample size, sampling method (e.g., all consecutive patients, intermittent sampling, random sampling), evaluation timeframe, data collection method, and standards of performance.[57] It may be appropriate to distribute the approved criteria as an educational tool prior to data collection. Although this may address some performance issues prior to data collection and result in less dramatic results, it may support the ultimate goal of improving care and do so in a more expedient manner. In this situation, if there is a need to document the overall impact of an MUE effort, collection of baseline performance data even as criteria are being finalized and

- approved can provide a more accurate representation of before and after. If at any point problems are identified in the criteria or indicators or with any component of the evaluation, the issue should be brought back to the oversight group and modifications made as appropriate. Bringing necessary modifications back to the oversight group ensures that the MUE is conducted based on their guidance and approval and helps to assure their support of the results and recommendations resulting from the MUE. This step is not unusual but can often be avoided through careful preparation and review of criteria early in the MUE process.

- The timing of data collection can be influenced by seasonal variations in the types of care provided (e.g., increased frequency of pneumonia in the winter months), systems issues (e.g., construction, implementation of new computer systems, initiation of new services), and personnel issues (e.g., the influx of new health professional graduates and medical house staff that occurs during the summer months, staff absences during vacation or flu seasons). Therefore, the timeframe for data collection, both in duration and time of year, should be considered in the planning process. For example, an assessment of care provided to patients with pneumonia is usually best performed during the winter months when this diagnosis is more frequent, while an assessment of the management of near-drowning may be more appropriate during the summer months. The longer the data collection period, the more likely various fluctuations in quality of care will be identified.

• Retrospective data collection was used primarily in the era of AUR and DUR. This method involved reviewing the patient's medical record after discharge. It allowed data collection to be scheduled when convenient or when staff was available, but was totally dependent on documentation in the medical record. If an opportunity for improvement was identified, there was no opportunity to improve that particular patient's care; it would only help future patients.

• Concurrent data collection occurs while the patient is still actively receiving the medication, but after the first dose is dispensed or administered. Data sources other than the medical record are available (e.g., staff or patient interviews) and there is an opportunity to improve patient care while the patient is receiving it. Based on complete information, results may be more complete as well as more accurate.[72] However, the need for data collection is constant and must occur within a specific timeframe, which is not always convenient. This often results in an increased number of personnel being involved in the data collection process and increased inconsistency.

• Prospective evaluation occurs before the patient receives the first dose of medication and is initiated whenever an order for the medication is generated. Simple prospective evaluations can be at least partially automated and are likely to become more common. An example of this is a clinical information system that generates a warning to the pharmacist or prescriber if the dose of a drug is outside the normal limits based on a patient's organ function. Clinical judgment must also be applied in many of these settings.

• In systems with computerized prescriber order entry, the system itself can drive prescribing to comply with guidelines and standards by limiting prescribing options or directing users to specific therapy, such as appropriate dosing, stop notices, and IV to PO changes for antimicrobial stewardship.[73] In some cases, the system can report instances where prescribers attempt to prescribe a medication outside established limits. These limits are usually developed by the P&T committee, optimally as the agent is being considered for addition to the formulary, and fall into three general categories: diagnosis, prescriber, and medication specific. Diagnosis-based limits may define the allowable indications for use or may drive the use of an agent under a specific protocol approved by the committee. Prescriber limits may restrict the use of an agent to a specific subset of prescribers (e.g., infectious disease or critical care specialists). Medication-specific limits can designate approved dosage regimens (e.g., disallow intravenous push promethazine), frequency of administration (e.g., once-daily dosing of ceftriaxone), and duration of therapy (e.g., no more than 10 doses or days of therapy).

Prospective evaluations that are not automated are the most cumbersome to implement because the evaluation must occur promptly every time an order is initiated to avoid therapy delays. This requires personnel to be available to collect data and report results at all times and force immediate interaction between practitioners. This approach offers the greatest opportunity for intervention and education, but also increases the risk for potentially negative interactions with prescribers and other health professionals, and can result in therapy delays. Furthermore, it is essential that the interventions made as part of the prospective evaluation are documented in order to evaluate workload and effectiveness of the interventions, and that outcomes are assessed in some manner.

Limiting the number of data collectors or automating data collection is valuable in maintaining consistency. When multiple data collectors are involved, it becomes even more important to have clear, explicit criteria that are not subject to interpretation. For example, a data dictionary to define each data element and identifying the location(s) in the record to gather the data should be developed and utilized to obtain consistent results.

The selection of patients or cases for inclusion in the evaluation should be determined and approved by the oversight group prior to data collection. It is essential that the selection be unbiased, consistent, and representative of the care provided. Sample size should be based on the size of the patient population. It has been suggested that, for frequently occurring events, a sample of at least 5% of cases be used, and for events occurring less frequently that a minimum of 30 cases be assessed.[74]

Data Analysis

Reports should compare actual performance with expectations defined by the standards (or thresholds or control limits) established and approved prior to data collection. Performance not meeting standards (or threshold or control limits) may be considered opportunities for improvement. The multidisciplinary oversight group does not usually conduct the actual analysis, but should be involved in interpreting the results. This group may determine that the standards were too rigorous, that unforeseen exceptions were encountered, and/or that actual performance falls within current acceptable standards of practice. Specific corrective actions should be recommended for all identified opportunities for improvement (e.g., for all criteria statements for which the standard of performance was not met) whenever possible. The need for and nature of follow-up should also be assessed based on the frequency, prevalence, and/or severity of the issue. For example, if an evaluation of the management of pneumonia identified no issues with drug selection, but did identify an unacceptable delay in time to first dose of antibiotic (e.g., greater than 2 hours after admission), the follow-up evaluation could focus on the time to first dose and not assess antibiotic selection. Furthermore, if this issue was identified in patients admitted to a particular unit, then the follow-up could focus on assessing and documenting improvement in only that unit.

Computer software programs (e.g., relational databases and spreadsheets) can be very helpful in collecting data, managing data, providing alerts, mitigating adverse events, and reporting results.[75-78] Handheld devices, bar code technology, proprietary software products, and computer systems used within the organization's clinical departments can be employed as tools to assist in patient identification, data collection and analysis, and documentation.[79,80]

The report to the oversight group should contain: (1) the rationale for the topic selection, (2) team members involved in the evaluation, (3) a description of the patient population evaluated, (4) any selection criteria used, (5) a copy of the criteria/indicators, (6) discussion of the results, (7) identification of likely causes for performance improvement opportunities identified, and (8) recommendations for corrective action and follow-up evaluation. An example is provided in Appendix 16-3. In most settings, delineation of results on a practitioner specific basis is not appropriate at this level. The exception would be if a subset of practitioners consistently fell outside the criteria.

Interventions and Corrective Actions

The key to quality improvement is improving the process and outcomes, not blaming an individual or group of individuals. Steps to improve performance or avoid similar outcomes in the future fall into three categories: educational, restrictive interventions, and process changes. Educational interventions are most appropriate when knowledge deficits contribute to performance outside the criteria. They are most effective when they are directed personally, take place soon after the problem occurs, the educator is a peer or superior of the person being educated, and when the education is supported in the literature or by practice standards.[81] One-on-one or group discussion of results, letters, e-mails, newsletters, and presentation via quality improvement channels are examples of educational approaches. Generally, educational interventions incorporated into ongoing processes (e.g., education screens in computer order entry systems) are more effective while one-time efforts (e.g., newsletters) may not have a sustained effect. In many situations, educational interventions are the most palatable.

Restrictive approaches may involve special ordering procedures, compliance with guidelines for use, consultation with a specialty service, or formulary restrictions. The impact of restrictive interventions often reverses when the restrictions are removed.[82,83] Restrictive interventions are perhaps most effective when used to establish appropriate practice patterns when an agent is first made available for use within the organization.

Process changes incorporate the correction into routine practice. This approach may involve changes in policy or procedures, implementation of new services, acquisition of new equipment, changes in staffing, or generation of regular notifications etc., when practice does not appear to meet standards. As clinical information and physician order entry systems become more sophisticated, process changes can be built directly into the prescribing, dispensing, and administering processes.

Disciplinary actions against individuals are not commonly employed as an intervention; however, when individuals refuse to modify their behavior, discipline may eventually be required. Discipline may include placing limits on an individual's activities and responsibilities or termination of employment. When possible, punitive actions should be avoided, since they can result in loss of acceptance of quality improvement efforts and fear of retribution.[84,85] Generally, the concept of Just Culture is useful to consider. Greater information on Just Culture is found in Chapter 18.

Communication of MUE-related information is important and must be done carefully. Communication of the purpose of the evaluation and the significance of its outcomes should be reported to all groups involved in or impacted by the process. If a process is changed based on MUE results, the reason for the change should be explained. If, as a result of an MUE, a prescriber will be required to change the way they prescribe a medication or a nurse will no longer be able to access a medication as they had in the past, the reason for the change should be communicated along with the announcement of the change. Confidentiality of patient information (e.g., names and other identifiers) must be maintained. The identity of practitioners (physicians, pharmacists, nurses) must be revealed only in information provided for use by managers or designated peer-practitioners for assessment of personal performance.

Follow-up

Follow-up evaluation should occur within a reasonable timeframe after completion of the initial evaluation and completion of the corrective action. Follow-up is designed to assess the effectiveness of the intervention. The same criteria, standards, and sample should be used for the follow-up assessment as in the initial evaluation. Exceptions to this rule should be made if there was a problem with the initial criteria, standards, and sample, if the standard of practice changes in the interim, or if there is an opportunity to focus on a subset of the original data elements or patient population. For example, if issues were only found in the administration component of the use of a medication (and not in the prescribing, dispensing, or monitoring components) or only in a specific age group, follow-up evaluation could focus on these issues or populations rather than repeating the broader assessment performed initially.

MUE has been criticized as being heavy-handed, non-patient-focused, and for not addressing the issue of accountability for provision of care based on a unique body of knowledge. If the approach termed MUE is utilized in its true spirit, many of these challenges are addressed. MUE is a truly multidisciplinary, process-oriented approach to evaluate the quality of medication use. The process goes beyond numbers and percentages to identify opportunities for improvement and more importantly, to improve the quality of care.

Quality in Drug Information

Quality standards for drug information practice have not been established to date, and quality assessment techniques used in drug information practice vary greatly among practice sites.[86-88] Several studies have found inconsistencies in the quality of drug information practice and have called for increased emphasis on quality and the development of practice standards.[89-92] Most drug information services conduct some form of quality assessment based on the scope of service provided by that center and preestablished levels of acceptable performance. Quality assessment is usually conducted on the responses provided to drug information requests, medical literature search and evaluation processes, availability, accuracy and timeliness of drug information resources, and the quality of materials produced by the drug information service staff (e.g., monographs, newsletters, continuing education programs). Although some quality assessment processes are conducted concurrently, most assessments are done retrospectively, often by randomly sampling of drug information requests, monographs, and so forth. Furthermore, assessments may be performed via peer review or by the director of the service. Currently, no standards have been developed for this process.[93]

Assessment of the quality of responses to drug information inquiries may include components such as timeliness, completeness and appropriateness of response, and the method of communication of the response. Additionally, aspects such as documentation of search terms, references utilized, and the availability of appropriate background or patient-specific information may also be assessed. This assessment may be carried out internally based on standards of practice at the site. This usually offers the advantage of peer review by practitioners skilled in these functions. Another method is to poll those using the service about the quality of service and response received. This approach is hampered because consumers of the response are rarely able to assess the quality or appropriateness of the search strategy utilized to formulate the response that they received in lieu of performing the search themselves or being present while the search is performed. An example assessment tool is provided in Appendix 16-4. Questions that are often asked in the process of assessing drug information responses include:

- Is the response correct and appropriate to the situation presented?
- Is the response provided promptly?
- Does the response completely address the question posed?
- Is the response communicated appropriately?
- Are search terms and references appropriately documented?
- Is the response clear, concise, and appropriate for the clinical situation?
- If follow-up was warranted, was it provided?

The search process itself can be assessed by evaluation of the appropriate depth and breadth of resources used, the timeliness of the resources accessed, and the search strategy. This process can also assess documentation issues, the application of literature evaluation skills to the information, and resources used by the practitioner completing the search.

Drug information practitioners are often responsible for assessing and recommending drug information resources available within the organization. These resources may include printed references such as handbooks, textbooks, educational materials, or electronic resources such as large search engines or Internet websites. This process should assess whether the appropriate information resources are available based on the scope of care provided and expertise of the practitioners and whether the resources contain accurate and timely information that can be applied in clinical situations. Available primary, secondary, and tertiary resources should be evaluated based on established standards. The explosion of medical information on the Internet has created new challenges in evaluating drug and medical information resources. Because there are currently no regulations of content on Internet sites, caution must be used when utilizing these resources to support clinical decision making. With the number of websites expanding faster than most practitioners can assess their content and editorial policies (if any), it has become increasingly difficult for drug information practitioners to stay abreast of those sites that offer legitimate and validated information compared to those offering only conjecture and opinion. Information obtained from other sources including manufacturer's drug information services should also be assessed. See Chapters 3, 4, and 5 for further information on assessing information.

A final component of quality relates to material produced by the drug information service. This includes newsletters, websites, drug monographs, and clinical guidelines developed by the service. Most measure quality related to the accuracy, timeliness, and clinical applicability of such documents. Unfortunately, more time is often spent on assessing quality of grammar and writing style than is devoted to clinical content and interpretation. Once again, Chapters 4 and 5 provide further information on assessing the quality of the material itself.

Publication of Quality Improvement Studies

Individuals or organizations interested in reporting their quality improvement interventions and results should use the SQUIRE 2.0 (Standards for Quality Improvement Reporting Excellence). SQUIRE was developed to provide authors guidance in reliably and consistently reporting their improvement work and for contributing knowledge to the "science of improvement."[94] Peer-reviewed journals will request the SQUIRE format for quality improvement manuscripts. The question of whether the organization's Institutional Review Board (IRB) submission and approval is required should be addressed with your IRB prior to submission of reports; generally quality improvement work, not intended for publication outside the organization, is provided an exemption. The importance of quality improvement publication is described by the SQUIRE authors as essential for others to learn about successes and failures in health care quality improvement work.[91]

Conclusion

The health care system continues to move toward greater transparency of quality as part of an overall shift toward value-driven health care. Government agencies and private purchasers of health care are demanding more evidence on quality and safety in the use of medications, and a growing number of accreditation programs are also scrutinizing performance indicators as a means for reaccreditation of organizations and providers. Thus, it is imperative that all practitioners involved in the medication use system understand how to measure and improve quality in the use of medications. As the American health care system continues to evolve, health care practitioners should maintain awareness and be ready to quickly adjust to the changes that will occur in measuring quality and performance for medication use.

Self-Assessment Questions

1. The major driver for quality measurement in U.S. health care today is:
   a. State Marketplace Health Insurance Plans
   b. The International Organizations for Standardization (ISO) 9000
   c. Consumers that purchase their own health insurance
   d. Federal government, Centers for Medicare & Medicaid Services

2. The PDCA model of quality improvement stands for:
   a. Prepare, Develop, Calculate, Assess
   b. Produce, Design, Cost-control, Act
   c. Plan, Develop, Check, Assess
   d. Plan, Do, Check, Act
   e. None of the above

3. Which of the following is NOT a characteristic of continuous quality improvement?
   a. Systems oriented
   b. Data driven
   c. Team oriented
   d. Punitive
   e. a and d

4. Which of the following are common purposes for measuring quality?
   a. Identify problems within a system
   b. Monitor improvements within a system
   c. Public reporting on providers
   d. Removal of bad employees
   e. a, b, and c

5. Within the Donabedian framework for quality assessment, which of the following indicators pertain to **STRUCTURE**:
   a. Percent of pharmacies with a patient counseling area
   b. Percent of patients with diabetes who received an annual eye examination
   c. Death of a patient due to an adverse drug-related event
   d. Percent of patients who received counseling on medications prior to discharge
   e. a and d

6. Within a Donabedian framework for quality assessment, which of the following indicators pertains to **OUTCOMES**:
   a. Percent of pharmacies with a patient counseling area
   b. Percent of patients who received an annual eye examination
   c. Death of a patient due to an adverse drug-related event
   d. Percent of patients who received counseling on medications prior to discharge
   e. b and c

7. When is it useful to directly measure aspects of the process of care?
   a. Outcome is difficult to measure
   b. Outcome is far removed in time from the process
   c. Outcome is affected by many different processes
   d. All of the above
   e. None of the above since outcomes are the only valid indicator of quality

8. A sentinel indicator:
   a. Reflects the occurrence of a serious event that requires further investigation
   b. Can be subdivided into rate-based or aggregate indicators
   c. Could be a death from an adverse drug-related event

    d. Is typically expressed as a percentage

    e. a and c

9. A rate-based indicator:
    a. Is typically expressed as a percentage
    b. Is a type of aggregate indicator
    c. Is typically expressed as a count of events over time
    d. Can only be used to track safety events in hospitals
    e. a and b

10. Public reporting of quality is available for all of the following *except:*
    a. Nursing homes
    b. Pharmacies
    c. Home health agencies
    d. Dialysis facilities

11. Value-based purchasing refers to:
    a. Purchase or payment of health care services based on performance
    b. Only hospital value-based purchasing
    c. Incentive payments to hospitals and physicians based on performance
    d. a and c
    e. None of the above

12. Medication measures (pharmacy) quality reporting occurs through which of the following:
    a. Pharmacy Compare
    b. Pharmacy Quality Alliance
    c. Medicare Part D insurance plans
    d. Pharmacy benefits managers

13. The acronym REaL represents the following in terms of health disparities?
    a. Respect, equality, and laws
    b. Race, ethnicity, and language
    c. Report, examine, and language
    d. Rates, evaluate, attribute, and limits

14. Quality measures development under the National Quality Forum includes:
    a. Stewards develop, maintain, and update measures
    b. Categorization of measures by National Quality Strategies priorities
    c. A searchable measures repository, the Quality Positioning System
    d. All of the above
    e. None of the above

15. To ensure health equality, health care organizations will provide all of the following except:
    a. Collect data using standard elements of groupings such as age, race, ethnicity, sex, (gender), gender identity, payers, socioeconomic
    b. Health disparities awareness training for all staff
    c. Inform stakeholder employers of services provided
    d. Outcomes analysis of services by subgroups

REFERENCES

1. Centers for Medicare & Medicaid Services. Roadmap for implementing value-driven health care in the traditional Medicare fee for service program [Internet]. Baltimore, MD: Centers for Medicare & Medicaid Services. 2012 Nov 25 [cited 2013 Oct 2]. Available from: http://www.cms.gov/Medicare/Quality-Initiatives-Patient-Assessment-Instruments/QualityInitiativesGenInfo/Downloads/VBPRoadmap_OEA_1-16_508.pdf

2. VanLare JM, Conway PH. Value-based purchasing—national programs to move from volume to value. N Engl J Med. 2012;367:292-5.

3. CMS.gov. CMS quality strategy 2016 [Internet]. Baltimore, MD: Centers for Medicare & Medicaid Services. [cited 2016 Aug 15]. Available from: https://www.cms.gov/Medicare/Quality-Initiatives-Patient-Assessment-Instruments/QualityInitiativesGenInfo/Downloads/CMS-Quality-Strategy.pdf

4. CMS.gov. Hospital value-based purchasing [Internet]. Baltimore, MD: Centers for Medicare & Medicaid Services. 2016 Oct 30 [cited 2016 Aug 15]. Available from: https://www.cms.gov/Medicare/Quality-Initiatives-Patient-Assessment-Instruments/hospital-value-based-purchasing/index.html?redirect=/Hospital-Value-Based-Purchasing/

5. Federal Register. Medicare program; merit-based incentive payment system (MIPS) and alternative payment model (APM) incentive under the physician fee schedule, and criteria for physician-focused payment models. 2016 May 9 [cited 2016 Aug 15]. Available from: https://www.federalregister.gov/articles/2016/05/09/2016-10032/medicare-program-merit-based-incentive-payment-system-mips-and-alternative-payment-model-apm

6. CMS.gov. What are the value-based programs? [Internet]. Baltimore, MD: Centers for Medicare & Medicaid Services. [cited 2016 Aug 15]. Available from: https://www.cms.gov/Medicare/Quality-Initiatives-Patient-Assessment-Instruments/Value-Based-Programs/Value-Based-Programs.html

7. Medicare.gov. Hospital compare [Internet]. Baltimore, MD: Department of Health & Human Services. 2012 Nov 25 [cited 2013 Oct 2]. Available from: http://www.hospitalcompare.hhs.gov/hospital-search.aspx

8. Medicare.gov. Nursing home compare [Internet]. Baltimore, MD: Department of Health & Human Services. 2009 Jan 11 [cited 2013 Oct 2]. Available from: http://www.medicare.gov/NursingHomeCompare/search.aspx

9. Report cards [Internet]. National Committee for Quality Assurance (NCQA). [cited 2016 Jul 31]. Available from: https://reportcards.ncqa.org/#/.

10. Medicare.gov. Medicare plan finder [Internet]. Baltimore, MD: Department of Health & Human Services. [cited 2016 Jul 31]. Available from: https://www.medicare.gov/find-a-plan/questions/home.aspx

11. Medicare.gov. Home health compare [Internet]. Baltimore, MD: Department of Health & Human Services. [cited 2016 Jul 31]. Available from: https://www.medicare.gov/home healthcompare/search.html

12. Medicare.gov. Dialysis facility compare [Internet]. Baltimore, MD: Department of Health & Human Services. [cited 2016 Jul 31]. Available from: https://www.medicare.gov/dialysisfacilitycompare/

13. Medicare.gov. Physicians compare [Internet]. Baltimore, MD: Department of Health & Human Services. [cited 2016 Jul 31]. Available from: https://www.medicare.gov/physician compare/search.html

14. Massachusetts health quality partners [Internet]. Watertown, MA: Massachusetts Health Quality Partners. 2012 Nov 25 [cited 2013 Oct 2]. Available from: https://www.mhqp.org

15. The Leapfrog Group [Internet]. Washington, DC: The Leapfrog Group. 2012 Nov 25 [cited 2013 Oct 2]. Available from: www.leapfroggroup.org

16. Robert Woods Johnson Foundation Aligning forces for quality. How employers can improve value and quality in health care [Internet]. Princeton, NJ: Robert Woods Johnson Foundation. 2013 Jan 1 [cited 2016 Jul 31]. Available from: http://www.rwjf.org/content/dam/farm/reports/issue_briefs/2013/rwjf403361

17. HealthCare.gov. Quality ratings of health plans on Healthcare.gov [Internet]. Baltimore, MD: Department of Health & Human Services. 2013 Jun 21 [cited 2016 Dec 23]. Available from: https://www.healthcare.gov/quality-ratings/

18. PQA Pharmacy Quality Alliance. PQA performance measures [Internet]. Springfield, VA. 2017 [cited 2017 Feb 19]. Available from: http://pqaalliance.org/measures/default.asp

19. Pillittere-Dugan D, Nau DP, McDonough K, Zakiya P. Development and testing of performance measures for pharmacy services. J Am Pharm Assoc. 2009;49:212-9.

20. Doucette WR, Conklin M, Mott DA, Newland B, Plake KS, Nau DP. Pharmacy Quality Alliance Phase I Demonstration Projects: descriptions and lessons learned. J Am Pharm Assoc. 2011;51:544-50.

21. CMS.gov Medicare 2017 Part C & D Star Rating Technical Notes, First Plan Review Draft [Internet]. Baltimore, MD: Centers for Medicare & Medicaid Services. 2016 Aug 3 [cited 2016 Aug 15]. Available from: https://www.cms.gov/Medicare/Prescription-Drug-Coverage/PrescriptionDrugCovGenIn/Downloads/2017_Technical_Notes_preview_1_2016_08_03.pdf

22. Reinke T. Preference for preferred networks grows along with community pharmacist anger. Managed Care. 2015 Mar [cited 2016 Aug 15]. Available from: http://www.managedcaremag.com/archives/2015/3/preference-preferred-networks-grows-along-community-pharmacist-anger

23. How health plans and PBMs evaluate pharmacy performance. 2014 Mar 12 [cited 2016 Aug 15]. Available from: http://smartretailingrx.com/patient-care-counseling/health-plans-pbms-evaluate-pharmacy-performance/

24. McLaughlin CP, Kaluzny AD. Continuous quality improvement in health care. 2nd ed. Gaithersburg, MD: Aspen Publishers; 1999.

25. CMS.gov. Quality measures [Internet]. Baltimore, MD: Centers for Medicare & Medicaid Services. [cited 2016 Aug 15]. Available from: https://www.cms.gov/Medicare/Quality-Initiatives-Patient-Assessment-Instruments/QualityMeasures/index.html

26. National Quality Forum. Measuring performance [Internet]. Washington, DC. [cited 2016 Aug 15]. Available from: http://www.qualityforum.org/Measuring_Performance/Measuring_Performance.aspx

27. National Quality Forum. Measures, reports & tools [Internet]. Washington, DC. [cited 2016 Aug 15]. Available from: http://www.qualityforum.org/measures_reports_tools.aspx

28. Deming WE. Out of the crisis. Cambridge, MA: Massachusetts Institute of Technology, Center for Advanced Engineering Study; 1986.

29. Deming WE. The new economics for industry, education, government. Cambridge, MA: Massachusetts Institute of Technology, Center for Advanced Engineering Study; 1993.

30. Edmonds J, Zagami M. QI team shares ownership and gets results. J Health Qual. 1992;14:24-8.

31. Donabedian A. Explorations in quality assessment and monitoring. In: The definition of quality and approaches to its assessment. Ann Arbor, MI: Health Administration Press; 1980:79-128.

32. Farris KB, Kirking DM. Assessing the quality of pharmaceutical care. II. Application of concepts of quality assessment from medical care. Ann Pharmacother. 1993;27: 215-23.

33. Lohr KN. Outcomes measurement: concepts and questions. Inquiry. 1988;25:37-50.

34. Kozma CM, Reeder CE, Schulz RM. Economic, clinical and humanistic outcomes: a planning tool for pharmacoeconomic research. Clin Ther. 1993;15:1121-32.

35. Lipowski EE. Evaluating the outcomes of pharmaceutical care. J Am Pharm Assoc. 1996;NS36:726-34.

36. Angaran DM. Selecting, developing and evaluating indicators. Am J Hosp Pharm. 1991;48:1931-7.

37. Joint Commission on Accreditation of Healthcare Organizations. A guide to performance improvement for pharmacies. Oakbrook Terrace, IL: Joint Commission; 1997.

38. Hepler CD, Segal R. Preventing medication errors and improving drug therapy. Boca Raton, FL: CRC Press; 2003.

39. Kerr EA, Krein SL, Vijan S, Hofer TP, Hayward RA. Avoiding pitfalls in chronic disease quality measurement: a case for the next generation of technical quality measures. Am J Manag Care. 2001;7:1033-43.

40. Agency for Healthcare Research & Quality. Consumer Assessment of Healthcare Providers & Systems (CAHPS) [Internet]. Rockville, MD: Agency for Healthcare Research & Quality. 2012 Nov 25 [cited 2013 Oct 2]. Available from: http://cahps.ahrq.gov/

41. Blalock SJ, Keller S. Consumer assessment of pharmacy quality. In: Warholak T, Nau DP, editors. Quality and safety in pharmacy practice. New York, NY: McGraw-Hill; 2010.

42. Kerr EA, Smith DM, Hogan MM, Krein SL, Pogach L, Hofer TP, Hayward RA. Comparing clinical automated, medical record, and hybrid data sources for diabetes quality measures. Jt Comm J Qual Improv. 2002;28:555-65.

43. Kerr EA, Smith DM, Hogan MM, Hofer TP, Krein SL, Bermann M, Hayward RA. Building a better quality measure: are some patients with 'poor quality' actually getting good care? Med Care. 2003;41:1173-82.

44. Moczygemba LR, Holdford DA. Statistical process control. In: Warholak T, Nau DP, editors. Quality and safety in pharmacy practice. New York, NY: McGraw-Hill; 2010.

45. Nau DP. Measuring pharmacy quality. J Am Pharm Assoc. 2009;49:154-63.

46. QualityNet. Fiscal Year 2017 measures. Hospital value-based purchasing [Internet]. Baltimore, MD: Centers for Medicare & Medicaid Services. 2017 Jan [cited 2017 Feb 19]. Available from: http://www.qualitynet.org/dcs/ContentServer?c=Page&pagename=QnetPublic%2FPage%2FQnetTier3&cid=1228775522697

47. Quality payment program [Internet]. Baltimore, MD: Centers for Medicare & Medicaid Services. 2017 Jan [cited 2017 Feb 19]. Available from: https://qpp.cms.gov/

48. CMS.gov. CMS OMH data snapshots [Internet]. Baltimore, MD: Centers for Medicare & Medicaid Services Office of Minority Health. 2016 Jun 16 [cited 2016 Aug 25]. Available from: https://www.cms.gov/About-CMS/Agency-Information/OMH/OMH-DataSnapshots.html

49. National Partnership for action to end health disparities. National Stakeholder Strategy for Achieving Health Equity [Internet]. Rockville, MD: U.S. Department of Health & Human Services, Office of Minority Health. 2016 Mar 25 [cited 2016 Aug 25]. Available from: http://minorityhealth.hhs.gov/npa/templates/content.aspx?lvl=1&lvlid=33&ID=286

50. Data collection standards for race, ethnicity, primary language, sex, and disability status [Internet]. Rockville, MD: U.S. Department of Health & Human Services, Office of Minority Health. 2016 Jun 16 [cited 2016 Aug 25]. Available from: http://minorityhealth.hhs.gov/omh/browse.aspx?lvl=2&lvlid=23

51. Health Research & Educational Trust. Reducing health care disparities: collection and use of race, ethnicity and language data. Chicago, IL: Health Research & Educational Trust. 2013 Aug [cited 2016 Aug 25]. Available from: http://www.hpoe.org/Reports-HPOE/Equity_Care_Report_August2013.PDF

52. HealthIT.gov. Step 5: achieving meaningful use Stage 2. Record demographics [Internet]. Washington, DC: Department of Health & Human Services. 2014 Feb 14 [cited 2016 Aug 25]. Available from: https://www.healthit.gov/providers-professionals/achieve-meaningful-use/core-measures-2/record-demographics

53. Wyatt R, Laderman M, Botwinick L, Mate K, Whittington J. Achieving health equity: a guide for health care organizations. IHI White Paper. Cambridge, MA: Institute for Healthcare Improvement. 2016 [cited 2016 Aug 25]. Available from: http://www.ihi.org/resources/Pages/IHIWhitePapers/Achieving-Health-Equity.aspx

54. CMS.gov. Racial and ethnic disparities in health care in Medicare advantage [Internet]. Baltimore, MD: Centers for Medicare & Medicaid Services Office of Minority Health. 2016 Apr [cited 2016 Aug 25]. Available from: https://www.cms.gov/About-CMS/Agency-Information/OMH/Downloads/National-Level-Results.pdf

55. Haviland AM, Elliott MN, Weech-Maldonado R, Hambarsoomian K, Orr N, Hays RD. Racial/ethnic disparities in Medicare Part D experiences. Med Care. 2012;50:S40-7. [cited 2016 Aug 25]. Available from: https://www.ncbi.nlm.nih.gov/pmc/articles/PMC4801234/

56. Stolar MH. Drug use review: operational definitions. Am J Hosp Pharm. 1978;35:76-8.

57. American Society of Health-System Pharmacists. ASHP guidelines on medication-use evaluation. Am J Health Syst Pharm. 1996;53(16):1953-5.

58. Nadzam DM. Development of medication-use indicators by The Joint Commission on Accreditation of Healthcare Organizations. Am J Hosp Pharm. 1991;48:1925-30.

59. Cousins DD. Medication use: a systems approach to reducing errors. Chicago, IL: Joint Commission on Accreditation of Healthcare Organizations; 1998.

60. New accreditation process model for 1994 and beyond. Am J Hosp Pharm. 1993;50:1111-2, 1121.

61. Ente BH. The Joint Commission's agenda for change. Curr Concepts Hosp Pharm Manage. 1989 Summer:11(2): 6-14.

62. The Joint Commission on Accreditation of Hospitals. 1990 AMH. Accreditation Manual for Hospitals. Chicago, IL: Joint Commission on Accreditation of Hospitals; 1989.

63. Flagstad MS, Williams RB. Assuming responsibility for improving quality. Am J Hosp Pharm. 1991;48:1898.

64. Covington TR, Alexander VL. Drug use evaluation: the fundamentals. Indianapolis, IN: Eli Lilly & Co.; 1991.

65. Schaff RL, Schumock GT, Nadzam DM. Development of The Joint Commission's indicators for monitoring the medication use system. Hosp Pharm. 1991;26:326-9, 350.

66. Bernstein SJ, Hilborne LH. Clinical indicators: the road to quality care? Jt Comm J Qual Improv. 1993;19(11):501-9.

67. Tully MP, Cantrill JA. The validity of explicit indicators of prescribing appropriateness. Int J Qual Health Care. 2006;18:87-94.

68. Wallerstedt SM, Belfrage B, Fastbom J. Association between drug specific indicators of prescribing quality and quality of drug treatment: a validation study. Pharmacoepidemiol Drug Saf. 2015;24:906-14.

69. Clark TR, Gruber J, Sey M. Revisiting drug regimen review, part III: a systematic approach. Consult Pharm. 2003;18:656-66.

70. Knapp DA. Development of criteria for drug utilization review. Clin Pharmacol Ther. 1991;50(Pt 2):600-3.

71. Threshold vs. standards. QRC Advisor. 1988;5(2):5.

72. Makela EH, Davis SK, Piveral K, Miller WA, Pleasants RA, Gadsden RH Sr., Leman RB. Effect of data collection method on results of serum digoxin concentration audit. Am J Hosp Pharm. 1988;45:126-30.

73. Forrest GN, Van Schooneveld TC, Kullar R, Schulz LT, Duong P, Postelnick M. Use of electronic health records and clinical decision support systems for antimicrobial stewardship. Clin Infect Dis. 2014;59:S122-33.

74. What is an adequate sample? QRC Advisor. 1985;1(Aug):4-5.

75. Grasela TH, Walawander CA, Kennedy, Jolson HM. Capability of hospital computer systems in performing drug-use evaluations and adverse event monitoring. Am J Hosp Pharm. 1993;50:1889-95.

76. Zarowitz BJ, Petitta A, Mlynarek M, Touchette M, Peters M, Long P, Patel R. Bar-code technology applied to drug-use evaluation. Am J Hosp Pharm. 1993;50:935-9.

77. Burnakis TG. Facilitating drug-use evaluation with spreadsheet software. Am J Hosp Pharm. 1989;46:84-8.

78. Jha AK, Laguette J, Seger A, Bates DW. Can surveillance systems identify and avert adverse drug events? A prospective evaluation of a commercial application. J Am Med Inform Assoc. 2008;15:647-53.

79. Libby D, Grove C, Adams M. Collaborative use of informatics among hospitals to benchmark medication use processes. Jt Comm J Qual Improv. 1997;23:626-52.

80. Strykowski J, Hadsall R, Sawchyn B, VanSickle S, Niznick D. Bar-code assisted medication administration: a method for predicting repackaging resource needs. Am J Health Syst Pharm. 2013;70:154-60.

81. Soumerai SB, McLaughlin TJ, Avorn J. Improving drug prescribing in primary care: a critical analysis of the experimental literature. Milbank Q. 1989;67:268-317.

82. Avorn J, Soumeri SB, Taylor W. Reduction of incorrect antibiotic prescribing through a structured educational order form. Arch Intern Med. 1991;151:1825-32.

83. Kowalsky SF, Echols RM, Peck F. Preprinted order sheet to enhance antibiotic prescribing and surveillance. Am J Hosp Pharm. 1982;39:1528-9.

84. Pierson JF, Alexander MR, Kirking DM, Solomon DK. Physician's attitudes toward drug-use evaluation interventions. Am J Hosp Pharm. 1990;47:388-90.

85. Himmelberg CJ, Pleasants RA, Weber DJ, Kessler JM, Samsa GP, Spivey JM, Morris TL. Use of antimicrobial drugs in adults before and after removal of a restriction policy. Am J Hosp Pharm. 1991;48:1220-7.

86. Restino MS, Knodel LC. Drug information quality assurance program used to appraise students' performance. Am J Hosp Pharm. 1992;49(6):1425-9.

87. Wheeler-Usher DH, Hermann FF, Wanke LA. Problems encountered in using written criteria to assess drug information responses. Am J Hosp Pharm. 1990;47(4):795-7.

88. Moody ML. Revising a drug information center quality assurance program to conform to Joint Commission standards. Am J Hosp Pharm. 1990;47(4):792-4.

89. Smith CH, Sylvia LM. External quality assurance committee for drug information services. Am J Hosp Pharm. 1990;47(4):787-91.

90. Halbert MR, Kelly WN, Miller DE. Drug information centers: lack of generic equivalence. Drug Intell Clin Pharm. 1977;11:728-35.

91. Beard SL, Coley RM, Blunt JR. Assessing the accuracy of drug information responses from drug information centers. Ann Pharmacother. 1994;28(6):707-11.

92. Calis KA, Anderson DW, Auth DA, Mays DA, Turcasso NM, Meyer CC, Young LR. Quality of pharmacotherapy consultations provided by drug information centers in the United States. Pharmacotherapy. 2002;20:830-6.

93. Ghaibi S., Ipema H., Gabay M. ASHP guidelines on the pharmacist's role in providing drug information. Am J Health Syst Pharm. 2015;72:573-7.
94. Ogrinc G, Davies L, Goodman D, Batalden P, Davidoff F, Stevens D. SQUIRE 2.0 (Standards for QUality Improvement Reporting Excellence): revised publication guidelines from a detailed consensus process. BMJ Qual Saf. Published On-line First: [2015 Sept 14]. doi:10.1136/bmjqs-2015-004411. [cited 2016 Sep 2]. Available from: http://qualitysafety .bmj.com/content/early/2015/09/10/bmjqs-2015-004411.full

SUGGESTED READINGS

1. Warholak TL, Nau DP. Quality and safety in pharmacy practice. New York, NY: McGraw-Hill Medical; 2010.
2. Mainz J. Developing evidence-based clinical indicators: a state of the art methods primer. Int J Qual Health Care. 2003;15:Si5-Si11. Available from: https://m.intqhc.oxfordjournals. org/content/15/suppl_1/i5.full
3. An evaluation of the use of performance measures in health care. Technical Report, Rand Corporation. Santa Monica, CA. 2011. Available from: https://www.rand.org/pubs/technical_ reports/TR1148.html
4. Institute for Healthcare Improvement (IHI). How to improve. Available from: http://www .ihi.org/resources/Pages/HowtoImprove/default.aspx
5. Pharmacy Quality Measurement Resources. NCPA National Community Pharmacy Association. Available from: http://www.ncpanet.org/innovation-center/ownership/ pharmacy-quality-measurement-resources
6. PQA Performance Measures. PQA Pharmacy Quality Alliance. Available from: http:// pqaalliance.org/measures/default.asp
7. American Society of Health-System Pharmacists. ASHP statement on the health-system pharmacist's role in national health care quality initiatives. Am J Health-Syst Pharm. 2010; 67:578–9. Available from https://www.ashp.org/-/media/assets/policy-guidelines/ docs/statements-health-system-pharmacists-role-national-health-care-quality-initiatives .ashx?la=en

Chapter Seventeen

Medication Misadventures I: Adverse Drug Reactions

Kelly Besco

Learning Objectives

● *After completing this chapter, the reader will be able to*

- Define adverse drug reactions (ADRs).
- Discuss the impact of ADRs on health care systems and patients.
- Explain methods for determining causality and probability of an ADR.
- Identify specialty drug information resources that can be used to locate information related to ADRs.
- Classify ADRs based on type and severity.
- Use guidelines from national organizations to implement an ADR reporting program.
- Describe the use of technology in ADR monitoring and reporting.
- Explain when, where, and how to report an ADR to the U.S. Food and Drug Administration (FDA).
- Explain how to report adverse reactions related to dietary supplements and vaccines.

Key Concepts

❶ Adverse drug reaction (ADR) refers to any unexpected, unintended, undesired, or excessive response to a medicine.

❷ One of the first steps in establishing an ADR program is to define what each facility or organization categorizes as ADRs.

❸ Several algorithms have been published that try to incorporate information about an ADR into a more objective form.

❹ Communication is a critical component throughout the ADR monitoring process.

❺ Technology plays an important role in monitoring, identifying, and minimizing ADRs.

❻ ADR surveillance serves as a means to primarily provide early signals about possible problems with a medication.

Introduction

The terminology surrounding adverse drug reactions (ADRs) is often confusing. All adverse drug events (ADEs), ADRs, and medication errors fall under the umbrella of medication misadventures. Medication misadventure is a very broad term, referring to any iatrogenic hazard or incident associated with medications. An ADE is the next broadest term, and refers to any injury caused by a medicine. An ADE encompasses all ADRs, including allergic and idiosyncratic reactions, as well as medication errors that result in harm to a patient.[1-5] ADRs and medication errors are the most specific terms. ❶ *Adverse drug reaction refers to any unexpected, unintended, undesired, or excessive response to a medicine.* A medication error is any preventable event that has the potential to lead to inappropriate medication use or patient harm.[1] Figure 17-1 shows one way of graphically classifying these terms. Many of these concepts will be explored in greater depth elsewhere in this text as well as in Chapter 18 Medication Misadventures II: Medication and Patient Safety. The present chapter focuses on ADRs, highlighting the impact of ADRs, pertinent definitions and classifications, specialty drug information resources, ADR reporting systems, and future approaches to detecting and managing ADRs.

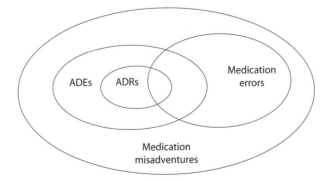

Figure 17–1. Relationship among medication misadventures, adverse drug events, medication errors, and adverse drug reactions. (Adapted from Bates DW, et al. Relationship between medication and errors and adverse drug events. J Gen Intern Med. 1995 Apr;10(4):199-205.)

Impact of Adverse Drug Reactions

All medications, including the inactive ingredients of a product, are capable of producing adverse reactions.[6] ADRs account for about 5% of all hospital admissions, cause patients to lose confidence in their health care providers, and lead to a significant increase in morbidity and mortality.[7] In 2014, there were nearly 50,000 deaths in the United States that were attributed to ADRs.[8]

ADRs have economic consequences as well. ADRs have been estimated to result in an annual cost of $30 billion in the United States.[9] These costs are attributable to the overall cost-of-illness generated by an ADR, including initial and prolonged hospitalization, loss of income from occupational absences, as well as utilization of new medication(s) for management of symptoms and conditions induced by the medication that initially caused the reaction. Direct hospital costs in the United States as a result of ADRs may be as high as $1.56 billion annually. After experiencing an ADR, patients spend an average of 8 to 12 days longer in the hospital, with potential to increase the cost of their hospitalization by $14,000 to $19,000.[9,10]

The incidence of ADRs for hospitalized patients has been reported to be as high as 16%.[10] Of course, ADRs do not affect hospitalized patients alone; however, there is limited data available regarding the incidence of ADRs that occur in the ambulatory care setting. It has been estimated that 4.5 million ambulatory visits each year in the United States are related to ADRs. These outpatient events typically result in visits to physician office practices.[11] Health care professionals agree that these estimates may be conservative because many ADRs go undetected, unreported, and untreated.[12] One systematic review of 37 studies concluded that the level of underreporting is likely to be in access of 90%.[13]

Although not all adverse reactions can be prevented, a large proportion of them can. The World Health Organization (WHO) estimates that at least 60% of ADRs are preventable. Preventable ADRs may be caused by such factors as the wrong diagnosis of a patient's condition, incorrect dosing or selection of a prescription medication, interactions with other drugs including dietary supplements, and patients who do not follow the instructions for taking a medication.[12] This highlights the need for health care practitioners and health care facilities to engage in the process of systematically preventing and responding to ADRs. WHO terms this **pharmacovigilance**, or the process of preventing and detecting adverse effects from medications.[14]

Several agencies and professional organizations across the United States have an active role in pharmacovigilance, and contribute efforts to minimize the occurrence and impact of ADRs. In addition to WHO, some of the key organizations include the FDA, The Joint Commission (TJC), and the American Society of Health-System Pharmacists (ASHP) (see Table 17-1). Despite the numerous organizations involved, pharmacovigilance depends heavily on individual health care practitioners, including pharmacists, physicians, and nurses, to take measures to minimize ADRs and report events. Practitioners

TABLE 17–1. ORGANIZATIONS INVOLVED IN PREVENTING ADVERSE DRUG EVENTS

Food and Drug Administration (FDA)	http://www.fda.gov
The Joint Commission (TJC)	http://www.jointcommission.org
World Health Organization (WHO)	http://www.who.int
Institute for Safe Medication Practices (ISMP)	http://www.ismp.org
The United States Pharmacopeial Convention (USP)	http://www.usp.org
American Society of Health-System Pharmacists (ASHP)	http://www.ashp.org
National Coordinating Council for Medication Error Reporting and Prevention (NCC MERP)	http://www.nccmerp.org
Agency for Healthcare Research and Quality (AHRQ)	http://www.ahrq.gov

need to understand the potential for ADRs and be prepared to recognize and prevent such occurrences in order to minimize adverse outcomes.

Pharmacists play a vital role in avoiding ADRs. One study published in Pharmacotherapy reviewed which inpatient-based, clinical pharmacy programs were associated with reduced ADR rates. Significant reductions occurred in hospitals offering pharmacist-obtained admission medication histories, drug protocol management, and ADR management programs. Facilities with these programs were found to have lower incidence of ADR rates as compared to hospitals without these services. Presence of these three services additionally translated to lower death rates, length of hospital stays, and inpatient drug charges. For example, hospitals without a pharmacist-led medication history service were found to have 86% increased likelihood of developing an ADR and $127,253 in additional Medicare patient charges.[15]

Definitions

After reading this chapter, the reader should be able to evaluate ADRs and, potentially, develop and implement an ADR surveillance program at their hospital, clinic, or community pharmacy. ❷ *One of the first steps in establishing an ADR program is to define what each facility or organization categorizes as ADRs.* There are many definitions for ADRs that have been described in the literature, including guidance from national and international organizations, as well as individual facilities and practitioners. Several of these definitions are presented below. Rather than getting bogged down in the differences between these many definitions, use this information for guidance when starting to evaluate ADRs and develop an ADR monitoring and reporting system. Remember that institutions, as well as clinicians, use different definitions depending on their practice needs.

WHO defines an ADR as "a response to a medicine which is noxious and unintended, and which occurs at doses normally used in man."[16] WHO additionally defines the term side effect, which is "any unintended effect of a pharmaceutical product occurring at doses normally used by a patient which is related to the pharmacological properties of the drug."[16] Note that, in clinical practice, side effect is a broad term that may be used synonymously with ADR, or may even refer to an ADE.

Defined by the FDA, an ADR is any "undesirable experience" associated with the use of a drug in a patient.[17] This definition is also fairly broad, and includes adverse events occurring from drug overdose as well as situations involving abuse. The FDA goes on to define an *unexpected* adverse reaction as one that is not listed in the current labeling for a medication as having been reported or associated with the use of the drug. This distinction is important, because unexpected ADRs are those that the FDA would like health care practitioners to report. Reporting ADRs to the FDA will be discussed later in this chapter. This definition focuses on reporting unusual, uncommon, or newly identified ADRs. Although common or expected ADRs are relevant and important, they do not provide the FDA with new or additional safety information. Unexpected drug reactions may be symptomatically or pathophysiologically related to an ADR listed in the current labeling, but may differ from the labeled ADR because of greater severity or specificity. For example, a medication may have abnormal liver function listed in its labeling as an adverse reaction. A health care practitioner should still report a case of hepatic necrosis following administration of the drug, because it represents an unexpected ADR of greater severity.[18]

Edwards and Aronson[19] propose another definition of an ADR: "An appreciably harmful or unpleasant reaction, resulting from an intervention related to the use of a medicinal product, which predicts hazard from future administration and warrants prevention or specific treatment, or alteration of the dosage regimen, or withdrawal of the product." This is a very practical definition for health care practitioners, because it highlights the need to take action in order to manage the effects of the adverse reaction.

Finally, Karch and Lasagna,[20] two prominent researchers in the area of ADRs, define a drug, an ADR, and a patient drug exposure as follows:

> "Drug: a chemical substance or product available for an intended diagnostic, prophylactic or therapeutic purpose.
>
> Adverse Drug Reaction: any response to a drug which is noxious and unintended and which occurs at doses used in man for prophylaxis, diagnosis or therapy, excluding therapeutic failures. (As stated by the WHO, this definition excludes intentional and accidental poisoning as well as drug abuse situations.)
>
> Patient–Drug Exposure: a single patient receiving at least one dose of a given drug."[20]

Many institutions use Karch and Lasagna's definition because it excludes accidental poisonings as well as problems with drugs of abuse.

Remember, these definitions are intended to provide guidance and food for thought; in daily practice, the differences between these descriptions may not be relevant or clinically meaningful. What is important is that individuals find or develop a definition of ADRs that works for the needs of their pharmacy, clinic, or hospital.

Causality and Probability of Adverse Drug Reactions

One of the challenges in defining and managing ADRs is determining causality. How can it be determined whether or not a drug caused a patient's adverse reaction? Cause and effect is difficult to prove in general, and ADRs are no exception. Many investigators have dealt with this problem by developing and publishing definitions, algorithms, and questionnaires that try to determine the probability of a reaction—that is, the likelihood that an ADR was caused by a particular drug or medication. There are over 30 different published methods for assessing ADR causality. They fall into three broad categories[21]:

1. **Expert judgment/Global introspection:** This method involves the individual assessment of the event by a health care practitioner, based on his or her clinical knowledge and experience without using any form of standardized tool.
2. **Algorithm:** This method uses specific questions to assign a weighted score that helps determine the probability of causality in a given reaction.
3. **Probabilistic:** This method uses Bayesian approaches and epidemiological data to calculate and estimate the probability of causality with advanced statistical methods.

To date, none of these attempts have been able to prove actual causality. These tools, however, are used to determine the probability that a particular drug caused an adverse event and will be described further below.

These algorithms and definitions use several important key concepts.[17,22] Dechallenge and rechallenge are often discussed. **Dechallenge** occurs when the drug is discontinued and the patient is then monitored to determine whether the ADR abates or decreases in intensity. **Rechallenge** occurs when the drug is discontinued and, after the ADR abates, the same drug is administered in an attempt to elicit the response again. Dechallenge and rechallenge are effective means for establishing a strong case that the drug was responsible for the ADR. A dechallenge is often essential in clinical practice, but a rechallenge may not be practical and may actually cause further harm to the patient. Nevertheless, a rechallenge may be clinically necessary if the medication the patient is allergic to is essential to sustain life (e.g., chemotherapy). Rechallenges are typically performed under medical supervision through use of a desensitization protocol. If successful, desensitization will allow a patient to tolerate exposure to a specific medication to which they are allergic. Desensitization protocols involve giving the medication to the patient in slowly increasing amounts, starting with small doses, and ending with the full dose prescribed by a physician. Unfortunately, the lasting effects of desensitization are somewhat uncertain. For medications that are taken on a daily basis, the body remembers and retains a state of desensitization; however, if more than 2 days pass between doses, desensitization often needs to be performed again prior to rechallenging the patient to the medication.[23]

Another important concept to consider is the temporal relationship between the drug and the event. Does the timeframe for development of the ADR make sense? Did the patient's exposure to the drug precede the suspected ADR? If there are previous reports of the ADR in the literature, do these reports describe a temporal relationship between the drug and the event? Case reports, specialty drug information resources, and package inserts can be helpful in noting if a drug has been known to cause a certain type of reaction in a certain timeframe in the past. Unfortunately, the literature is not likely to be helpful for rare or new ADRs, but this does not discount the fact that a reaction may have occurred.

Naranjo and colleagues[22] developed the following definitions to assist in determining the probability of a suspected ADR:

> "Definite ADR is a reaction that: (1) follows a reasonable temporal sequence from administration of the drug, or in which the drug level has been established in body fluids or tissue; (2) follows a known response pattern to the suspected drug; (3) is confirmed by dechallenge; and (4) could not be reasonably explained by the known characteristics of the patient's clinical state.
>
> Conditional ADR is a reaction that: (1) follows a reasonable temporal sequence from administration of the drug; (2) does not follow a known response pattern to the suspected drug; and (3) could not be reasonably explained by the known characteristics of the patient's clinical state.
>
> Doubtful ADR is any reaction that does not meet the criteria above."[22]

USING ALGORITHMS

❸ *Several algorithms have been published that try to incorporate information about an ADR into a more objective form.* As described above, these algorithms each use a set of specific questions to determine the likelihood that the drug was responsible for the reaction, and establish a rational and scientific approach to what previously required strictly clinical judgment. Although algorithms are helpful in offering a systematic approach to assessing the probability of ADRs, they can be very time-consuming and the results vary significantly according to the interpretation of multiple observers.

In 1979, Kramer and colleagues[24] published a questionnaire composed of 56 yes or no questions (See Appendix 17-1). This questionnaire includes sections about the patient's previous experience with the drug or related drugs, alternative etiologies, timing of events, drug concentrations, dechallenge, and rechallenge. Responses to each question are given a weighted value and these values are totaled. The total value then correlates to one of four categories: unlikely, possible, probable, or definite. One of the problems with the Kramer method (as well as other algorithms) is that clinicians can disagree on the weighted values because the user must make subjective judgments for some of the questions. Another problem inherent with this questionnaire is that an unexpected ADR may not score well because of lack of literature or previous experience with the ADR. If the reaction is not universally accepted or in the most recent edition of the Physicians' Desk Reference, the suspected reaction would score a zero in this section. This makes the method devised by Kramer and associates less useful for new medications and for unexpected or emergent ADRs. Overall, however, the questionnaire provides health care professionals with the opportunity to use a standardized tool. Hutchinson and colleagues[25] evaluated the reproducibility and validity of the Kramer questionnaire and concluded that, although the questionnaire was cumbersome to use, the method was superior to clinical judgment alone.

Naranjo and colleagues[22] developed an alternative algorithm in 1981 (See Appendix 17-2). This algorithm asks 10 questions involving the following areas: temporal relationship, the pattern of response, dechallenge or administration of an antagonist, rechallenge, alternative causes, placebo response, drug level in the body fluids or tissue, dose-response relationship, previous patient experience with the drug, and confirmation by any other objective evidence. Like the algorithm proposed by Kramer et al., the answer to each question is assigned a score. The score is then totaled and placed into a category from definite to doubtful. In the initial published report of this algorithm, Naranjo and colleagues tested the reproducibility and validity of the algorithm and found that their tool was a valid means of assessing ADRs. Today, the Naranjo algorithm is one of the most commonly used methods to assess ADR causality, and has been considered a gold standard for assessing ADR causality. Compared to the method devised by Kramer et al., the Naranjo tool is much quicker to administer. However, it is not without its faults. The tool emphasizes rechallenge and dechallenge, which may pose some problems in evaluating ADRs as described previously. The Naranjo algorithm also asks about a response to placebo, which is rarely (if ever) administered in clinical practice today.

In 1982, Jones published an algorithm that allows health care practitioners to answer a series of yes or no questions to determine the probability that an ADR occurred (See Appendix 17-3).[26] The Jones algorithm asks similar questions as those used in the methods described above, but uses a dichotomous key design. Like the Naranjo algorithm, the tool developed by Jones is shorter and quicker to complete than Kramer's questionnaire.

Unlike either Kramer or Naranjo's algorithms, the Jones method does not require summation of a score. Of note, the Jones algorithm was originally designed for use in a community health setting, illustrating that the assessment of ADRs is not limited to inpatient or institutional settings only.

All of the algorithms described above possess a certain degree of observer variability. However, each can be used to help determine whether an adverse event was precipitated by a certain drug or drug-drug combination. Michel and Knodel[27] compared the three algorithms by Kramer, Jones, and Naranjo. Their study found that the Naranjo algorithm was simpler and less time-consuming, and compared favorably to the 56 questions asked by Kramer. Although there was agreement between the Naranjo and Jones algorithms, the study found a higher correlation between the Naranjo algorithm and the Kramer questionnaire. The authors concluded that more data was needed to support the use of the algorithm developed by Jones and colleagues.

A modern approach to assessing the causality of ADRs has been developed by researchers at the University of Liverpool's Institute of Translational Medicine (See Appendix 17-4).[28] Their algorithm, the Liverpool ADR Causality Assessment Tool (CAT), has been proposed as an alternative to traditional methods, and aims to improve the inter-rater reliability of ADR assessment techniques. The Liverpool CAT includes a sequence of questions that allow a user to arrive at a decision as to if the presence of an ADR was definite, probable, possible, or unlikely. The tool was developed while the originators were undertaking an observational study of ADRs in children and encountered concerns with the sensitivity of the Naranjo scale to predict ADR likelihood.[28] While studies have yet to demonstrate if the Liverpool ADE CAT is superior to alternative algorithms, the originators believe the tool to be practical for assessing the probability of ADRs in a clinical setting and its use in observational studies regarding ADRs has continued to grow.

At this time, no algorithm for assessing the causality or probability of an ADR has been proven superior.[29] Therefore, it is reasonable to select a method based on factors such as availability, speed and ease of completing the tool, and clinician preference.

PROBABILISTIC METHODS

A Bayesian approach to assessing adverse reactions has been developed by Lane.[30] Using the Bayesian approach, relevant information is collected and a quantitative measure of the odds that a particular drug caused a particular event is calculated. The Bayesian approach has the potential to be an outstanding tool for predicting populations that may be at higher risk for ADRs; however, this method requires complex calculations, significant time investments to develop the model, and the involvement of a statistician.[31] Due to these requirements, the Bayesian approach is likely not practical for implementation in individual clinics or hospitals, but the WHO is using these methods to analyze data in their international drug monitoring network.[17]

In addition to the methods for assessing ADR causality and probability discussed above, there are also tools for assessing specific types of ADRs. For example, different methods exist for assessing drug-related liver toxicity.[32]

Case Study 17-1

A patient presents to the Emergency Department with the complaint of rapid heart rate. He has no prior medical history of cardiovascular disease, including arrhythmias (i.e., irregular heartbeat). While interviewing the patient, you learn that he is a bodybuilder and about four weeks ago started taking a dietary supplement called *XL Fit* to help him lose weight. He states that every time he takes the product, he feels like his heart is racing. The symptom lasts about three hours and then goes away. You research the product and find out that it contains high doses of caffeine and a stimulant called synephrine that is similar to ephedrine.

- *In this case, was there a dechallenge? If so, what happened when the suspected product was dechallenged?*
- *Was there a rechallenge? Is so, what happened?*
- *Was there a temporal relationship between taking this product and the reaction the patient experienced?*
- *Based on what you know about this product, is the reaction consistent with its known pharmacology?*
- *What is the likelihood of this product causing the reaction?*

SPECIALTY RESOURCES FOR ADVERSE DRUG REACTIONS

Methods used to assess the causality of ADRs, including the Kramer and Naranjo algorithm, rely in part on previous documentation of the reaction occurring in response to administration of the suspected drug. For common or well-known ADRs, the prescribing information (also called the package insert) and major drug information compendia can be useful. However, for other suspected ADRs, specialty resources may be necessary.

Chapter 3 introduces ADR specialty resources, including gold standards references Meyler's Side Effects of Drugs and Side Effects of Drugs Annual. This section briefly describes a few additional specialty resources that may be useful.

FDA's MedWatch program for voluntary reporting of ADRs is discussed later in this chapter and Chapter 18. The results of this program are disseminated through a special section of the FDA website dedicated to ADRs and other medication safety topics (http://www.fda.gov/Safety/Medwatch). This online reference contains the FDA's latest safety alerts and recalls as well as resources for health care professionals. The site also provides monthly summaries of changes to drug labeling that the FDA has made in response to reports from health care providers and others involved in pharmacovigilance.[33] Users can sign up to receive safety alerts by e-mail, or follow FDA MedWatch on Twitter using Internet-enabled mobile devices such as smartphones or tablet computers (http://www.twitter.com/FDAMedWatch). The database is also searchable using http://fdable.com.

Because the FDA's website can be difficult to navigate, it is perhaps best used for current hot topics or news items related to ADRs. The search function is rudimentary, and searching MedWatch for previous reports of a suspected ADR can be challenging. An alternative solution is VigiAccess™ (http://www.vigiaccess.org), the WHO's global database of adverse reaction reports. The database is a user-friendly web application that allows the public to access information about adverse reactions with medicines and vaccines that have been reported to the WHO Programme for International Drug Monitoring (WHO PIDM) by its more than 110 members, including FDA's MedWatch. Although the depth of information provided by VigiAccess™ is minimal, the site can be used to determine whether an adverse reaction has been previously reported in response to a particular drug.[34]

Published case reports can also be useful in assessing and evaluating ADRs (see Chapter 5 for more information on evaluating case reports). Reactions Weekly is a weekly publication that indexes and abstracts ADR case reports and ADR-related news from around the world (see also Chapter 3). Because it pulls information from biomedical journals, scientific meetings, and the WHO PIDM, Reactions Weekly can be useful for efficiently searching the available information related to a suspected ADR.[35] Clin-Alert is a similar publication that summarizes reports of adverse clinical events from more than 100 key research journals, although its focus is primarily on reports of drug-drug interactions (DDIs).[36]

Classification of Adverse Drug Reactions

Various definitions and terminology have been used to classify ADRs. As discussed above, algorithms such as those developed by Naranjo, Kramer, and Jones have used the definite, probable, possible, and unlikely categories to classify ADRs by their probability. Other classification systems rank ADRs by severity or by their mechanism. When developing an ADR monitoring program, these various systems can be used to determine probability (cause and effect) and severity of ADRs and help describe and quantify data. The data may help identify severity of reactions that are occurring and which medications cause the most severe reactions. Classification systems can also help health care practitioners organize and present data, and facilitate monitoring of ADR trends and potential causative agents. These trends can be used to change prescribing habits or to alert institutions and organizations to potential problems with medications.

CLASSIFYING BY SEVERITY

Karch and Lasagna[20] developed a method of classifying ADRs by severity, from minor to severe, as defined below:

- **Minor:** No antidote, therapy, or prolongation of hospitalization is required in response to the ADR.
- **Moderate:** The management of the ADR requires a change in drug therapy, specific treatment, or an increase in hospitalization by at least 1 day.
- **Severe:** The ADR is potentially life threatening, causing permanent damage or requiring intensive medical care.
- **Lethal:** The ADR directly or indirectly contributes to the death of the patient.

The FDA and WHO also use severity to classify ADRs. According to these organizations, an ADR is serious when it results in death, is life threatening, causes or prolongs hospitalization, causes a significant persistent disability, results in a congenital anomaly, or requires intervention to prevent permanent damage.[7,37]

CLASSIFYING BY MECHANISM

Karch and Lasagna[20] also described various mechanisms by which ADRs occur. These mechanisms are related to the pharmacologic or pharmacodynamic properties of drugs, and can be used to classify the type of reaction that occurs:

- **Idiosyncrasy:** an uncharacteristic response of a patient to a drug, usually not occurring on administration.
- **Hypersensitivity:** a reaction, not explained by the pharmacologic effects of the drug, caused by altered reactivity of the patient and generally considered to be an allergic manifestation.
- **Intolerance:** a characteristic pharmacologic effect of a drug produced by an unusually small dose, so that the usual dose tends to induce a massive overaction.

- **Drug interaction:** an unusual pharmacologic response that could not be explained by the action of a single drug, but was caused by two or more drugs.
- **Pharmacologic:** a known, inherent pharmacologic effect of a drug, directly related to dose.

Classifying the ADR by its mechanism may aid in identifying similar drugs that can be expected to cause a reaction, or may help explain patient-specific reactions to medications.

Implementing a Program

Well-designed programs that monitor and identify ADRs, as well as broadcast information to the medical community, are essential. A later section of this chapter will discuss the importance of reporting suspected ADRs to the FDA and other stakeholders. But before ADRs can be reported, a program for detecting and capturing these reactions must be implemented at a facility or institution.

Prior to implementing an ADR program, the health care facility must educate its staff on the importance and significance of the program. The pharmacy department is in an excellent position to provide this education because of its involvement in the pharmacy and therapeutics (P&T) committee, pharmacokinetic dosing, medication use evaluation (MUE), and drug distribution. The pharmacy department can be an excellent resource for developing an ADR program, as well as providing data about ADRs to the P&T committee and/or the institution's medication safety committee.

STEPS FOR IMPLEMENTING A PROGRAM

Accrediting bodies like the Centers for Medicare & Medicaid Services (CMS)[38] and TJC[39] require that hospitals and health care organizations have an ADR reporting program. These programs are generally a function of the P&T committee (or other medical staff committee) and the department of pharmacy. ASHP also encourages pharmacists and health care practitioners to take an active role in monitoring adverse events. ASHP has published very specific guidelines on ADR monitoring and reporting as part of its practice standards.[40] TJC and ASHP standards can be used as a basis for starting an ADR monitoring program. In addition to the standards, the pharmacy and medical literature are rich with examples of successful programs, some of which will be reviewed in this chapter.

Steps for implementing an ADR monitoring program include the following:

1. Develop definitions and classifications of ADRs that work for the institution. The definitions and classifications in this chapter provide a good starting point for discussion.

2. Assign responsibility for the ADR program within the pharmacy and throughout other key departments. A multidisciplinary approach is an essential factor. This will improve awareness of the monitoring program and increase ADR reporting at all levels of patient care.

3. Develop a program with approval from the pharmacy department, risk management, the medical staff and nursing departments, as well as other appropriate areas within the facility. Cooperation is essential in initiation of a successful program.

4. Promote awareness of the program. Newsletters, e-mails, in-services, grand rounds presentations, and other educational programs are opportunities to increase awareness and garner support for the program.

5. Promote awareness of ADRs and the importance of reporting such events in order to increase patient safety. Again, newsletters, e-mails, in-services, grand rounds presentations, and other educations programs can be utilized to increase awareness of specific ADRs.

6. Establish mechanisms for screening ADRs continuously. These mechanisms should include retrospective reviews and concurrent monitoring, as well as prospective planning for high-risk groups. It is worthwhile to educate pharmacists to check for ADRs when they see orders for certain indicator drugs that are often used in treating an ADR (see Table 17-2), orders to discontinue or hold drugs, and orders to decrease the dose or frequency of a drug.[41] Also, electronic screening methods to check for laboratory tests that are indicative of ADRs (e.g., drug levels, *Clostridium difficile* toxin assays, elevated serum potassium, low white blood cell counts) can be helpful.[42] Emergency box usage is another event that may trigger investigation by the pharmacist to determine if an ADR has occurred (e.g., use of epinephrine, diphenhydramine).[43] The previous examples highlight specific approaches to monitor for ADRs continuously. Additionally, retrospective review of indicator drug orders, laboratory tests, and/or emergency box usage may also bring to light previously unreported ADRs.

7. Develop internal forms or other mechanisms for data collection and reporting of ADRs. A quick Internet search will identify a number of ADR report forms used at specific institutions across the country. Many institutions use computer reporting, as well as hotline phone numbers.

8. Develop policies and procedures for handling ADR reports. Indicate who is responsible for sending them to the FDA and review current accrediting body

criteria, such as CMS Conditions of Participation (CoPs)[38] and TJC Medication Management standards,[39] to ensure that the framework of the developed program meets expectations of regulatory agencies that regulate and certify the organization.

9. Establish procedures for evaluating the causality and probability of ADRs, usually based on one of the classification systems previously discussed.

10. Routinely review ADRs for trends.

11. Develop preventive interventions. Examples of these include flagging patients who are at high risk of developing ADRs and identifying specific drugs which are likely to cause ADRs. Monitoring these patients and drugs more closely will help prevent or reduce the severity of possible ADRs.

12. Report all findings to P&T committee, medication safety committee, and/or other appropriate committee(s).

13. Develop strategies for decreasing the incidence of ADRs, depending on the opportunities presented by the ADRs reported. This vital step has often been ignored in the literature; however, for an ADR program to be part of the quality assurance process, it must be included wherever possible.

❹ *Communication is a critical component throughout the ADR monitoring process.* To ensure that the suspected drug is not administered again, and that patients receive necessary treatment and monitoring, each ADR should be documented thoroughly in the patient's medical record. However, this action alone is not sufficient, as the information is often poorly visible and may be difficult to access. ISMP recommends that ADRs be communicated to members of the patient's health care team in a standardized manner,

TABLE 17–2. ADR INDICATOR DRUGS

Antidiarrheal agents
Atropine (except preoperatively)
Dextrose 50% (IV push)
Diphenhydramine (except at bedtime)
Epinephrine (IV push)
Flumazenil
Naloxone
Potassium supplement (diuretic or digoxin patients)
Protamine
Sodium polystyrene sulfonate (patients on potassium sparing diuretics or ACE inhibitors)
Topical steroids
Vitamin K

such as documenting the reaction on a standardized order form, either in paper or electronic form, just as if prescribing drug therapy or ordering lab draws.[44] This increases visibility of the information and facilitates a timely response by all individuals involved in the patient's care. In addition, ASHP recommends that patients and their caregivers be notified when a suspected ADR has occurred.[40] Well-informed patients can help prevent ADRs from recurring in the future.[44]

The Role of Technology in Adverse Drug Reactions Surveillance

❺ *Technology plays an important role in monitoring, identifying, and minimizing ADRs.* Information systems are available that can identify and alert practitioners to potential ADRs and detect potential DDIs that may contribute to ADRs. These systems search patient records and medical data to find drug names, drug levels, or drug-lab interactions (sometimes called triggers) that frequently indicate an ADR has occurred.[45] See Chapter 26 for more information on this topic. Sophisticated systems may also search through International Classification of Diseases (ICD-10) codes, nursing notes, or outpatient medical records. For example, a medication profile that includes an angiotensin-converting enzyme (ACE) inhibitor and a note in the medical chart that mentions cough might trigger the ADR surveillance system. This information is then used to alert a pharmacist or prescriber who can investigate the suspected ADR and manage any adverse effects.[45]

INPATIENT ADVERSE DRUG REACTIONS SURVEILLANCE PROGRAMS

An exemplar program was developed at Brigham and Women's Hospital. This system was programmed to detect a combination of patient-specific factors and medications that may indicate a patient who has the potential to experience an ADR. For example, patients taking medications that required renal function-based dosing and who had elevated serum creatinine were flagged as patients at risk for development of an ADR. Various other screening rules were also programmed. When compared to traditional methods of identifying ADRs, this system detected more ADRs than spontaneous reports, but fewer than retrospective chart review. Interestingly, the errors detected by the computer system were different than those detected by chart review, indicating that a combination of multiple ADR detection systems may provide the best results. As expected, using the computer system saved work time, requiring five times fewer person-hours than the chart review method.[46] In another study, a similar ADE detection system identified potential ADEs in 64 of every 1,000 admissions. The prescribing physician did not recognize 44% of the ADEs detected by the system.[47]

Duke University Health System (DUHS) in Durham, North Carolina, developed a sustainable model for computerized ADR surveillance in hospitalized patients that monitors medical records and automatically identifies patients who may have experienced an ADR.[48] The system screens DUHS' electronic health record (EHR) platform for abnormal laboratory results, medication orders for antidotes, and drug-laboratory combinations to identify potential ADRs. Once one of the aforementioned triggers is identified, a notification is transmitted to a web-based queue that is reviewed by a pharmacist who can follow-up to determine if an actual adverse event has truly occurred. The pharmacist reviews the patient's EHR and discusses the findings with clinicians involved in patient's care. Over a 1-year period for Duke University Hospital pediatric inpatients, the surveillance system was able to detect 1,537 medication-related events for required investigation.[49]

AMBULATORY ADVERSE DRUG REACTIONS SURVEILLANCE PROGRAMS

Because hospitals are required by accrediting bodies to have an ADR reporting system, the use of technology for identifying, reporting, and minimizing ADRs is very common in the inpatient setting. Unfortunately, this is quite different from the ambulatory care setting. In general, the reporting of ADRs and other drug-related events has experienced minimal uptake in the primary care setting. Reasons for this include busy physician schedules, high cost of implementation, and complexity of outpatient prescribing practices. Because of this, the Agency for Healthcare Research and Quality (AHRQ) initiated a project to develop and test a reporting system for use in ambulatory clinics nationwide. Called the Medication Error and Adverse Drug Event Reporting System (MEADERS), it was designed with input from a group of experts in patient and medication safety in the primary care setting. An intuitive electronic system was developed that allowed health care professionals to report events using both simple data entry and open text boxes in order to capture the complete story regarding each medication error or ADE. MEADERS also includes the option of sending each report to the FDA's MedWatch program.[50] ADR reports are documented via entry into an Internet-based system or a stand-alone system using Microsoft® Access™. MEADERS also includes an Internet-based report viewing system that allows users to browse reports from ambulatory setting across the country using the MedMarx[SM] database, a registry of ADE reports from over 400 health care facilities. This provides capabilities for practitioners to compare their local or organizational reports to national data.[51] Initial field testing of MEADERS involved 24 practice sites who submitted a total of 507 reports during the pilot period. Of these reports, 70% involved medication errors and 27% described ADEs linked to medication therapy. While physicians maintained that time was the primary barrier to reporting medication errors and ADEs, the average time spent per report was just 4.3 minutes. In addition, only eight reports were electronically forwarded to the FDA's MedWatch program. Thus, the development team is aiming to adapt the nuances of the system to make reporting a seamless component of the normal workflow.[50]

AHRQ had previously concluded that the data supporting ADR monitoring and reporting programs in the outpatient setting was limited, but initiatives like MEADERS demonstrate that evidence is still emerging in this practice setting.[45] Traditionally, hospital-based pharmacists have been the health care professional to provide the greatest number of spontaneous ADR reports to the FDA.[52] However, community pharmacists are in a unique position to report on ADRs relating to nonprescription medications and dietary supplements. Community pharmacists can also report on reactions that patients are likely to detect themselves, such as ophthalmic and dermatological disorders. In fact, in countries such as the Netherlands, Japan, and Spain, the majority of ADR reports originate from community, rather than hospital, pharmacists.[52]

One of the finest examples concerning the use of information technology for ADR monitoring and reporting comes from the Department of Veterans Affairs (VA). The VA refined its methods for collecting and reporting patient-specific ADR information by developing two distinct, yet complementary, databases. The first involves patient-specific information related to ADRs. Health care providers within the VA system are responsible for entering ADR information into a specific part of the patients' electronic medical record, called the Adverse Reaction Tracking (ART) package. This locally entered ADR information is then automatically extracted to construct a national ART database. Since its inception, the ART database has received over 50,000 entries per month. The second database, the VA Adverse Drug Event Reporting System (VA ADERS), is external to the electronic medical record and requires providers to report detailed information related to specific, preselected ADRs. VA ADERS also allows for direct submission to the FDA's reporting programs MedWatch and the Vaccine Adverse Event Reporting System (VAERS), discussed later in this chapter. The impact of VA ADERS on ADR reporting is demonstrated by the number of reports generated compared to the VA's previous system (the legacy Adverse Drug Event System). In the five years prior to the implementation of the VA ADERS, only 21,000 ADR reports were generated. In the three years after the implementation of the VA ADERS, nearly 150,000 ADR reports were generated.[53]

ROLE OF DRUG INTERACTION SCREENING IN ADVERSE DRUG REACTIONS SURVEILLANCE

Because DDIs may comprise as many as 59% of ADRs, computer systems that detect clinically significant interactions are also important for reducing ADRs.[54] Over the past 20 years, the integration of drug information databases with clinical information has allowed for increased screening of DDIs upon medication dispensing. As pharmacists are entering orders into patient profiles, the integrated drug information database is checking for DDIs with all concurrent medications. While these clinical decision support systems are a good first-line of defense in monitoring for DDIs, studies have suggested the interaction tools often perform at a suboptimal level, either by misclassifying the severity of specific DDIs or failing to provide sufficient evidence to support the supposed interaction. Additionally, studies have shown that clinicians override the majority of alerts, ignoring potentially important safety warnings, and may develop alert fatigue if they receive drug interaction alerts too frequently.[55]

Waller[56] proposed a potentially significant advancement in the use of technology for reporting ADRs. With this system, information regarding ADRs would be automatically captured from the computers of health care professionals. When a trigger event occurred, such as the administration of a drug antidote, reports could be generated and sent to the FDA or other regulatory bodies without any action at all from the practitioner. This proposal, while not without its challenges for implementation, has the capability to greatly reduce the underreporting of ADRs.

Due to high costs and the time required to educate health care professionals on the changes, the health care industry has traditionally lagged behind other industries in the implementation of high-end technology information systems.[57] The 2009 passage of the American Recovery and Reinvestment Act (ARRA), also known as the stimulus package, included the Health Information Technology for Economic and Clinical Health Act (HITECH) that provided financial incentives for adopting EHRs and associated technologies. As of 2014, eligible health professionals (both inpatient and outpatient) had received over $20 billion to implement EHRs as a result of funding provided by HITECH with 75.5% of hospitals and 51% of office-based physicians adopting an EHR system.[57] As the level of adoption of technology continues to increase, there is opportunity to harness large quantities of data to transform the way ADRs are identified and minimized. However, published accomplishments of using data analytics from EHRs tools to improve ADR detection and prevention continues to be minimal.

Reporting Adverse Drug Reactions

❻ *ADR surveillance serves as a means to primarily provide early signals about possible problems with a medication.* Because preapproval studies typically involve a limited number of patients and populations, it is not possible to anticipate all potential side effects a medication may produce once it is made available to the general public. Therefore, it is necessary to establish mechanisms to identify effects of a medication that did not appear during preapproval studies. This monitoring process is referred to as **postmarketing surveillance**, or the process of continually monitoring and reviewing suspected adverse reactions associated with medications once they reach the market and are available to the public (see Chapter 22 for more about postmarketing surveillance). In order to detect an ADR that occurs once in every 10,000 patients exposed to the drug, at least 30,000 people would need to be treated with the medication.[12] Clinical trials that are required to approve a new drug may not enroll a sufficient number of patients, and often exclude special groups such as children, pregnant women, and the elderly. Due to the limited sample size and populations included in these trials, the FDA relies on postmarketing information to establish a better understanding of adverse events. In addition, the short duration of most clinical trials means that they will not detect ADRs with a delayed onset.[58] Pharmaceutical companies are required by the FDA to submit quarterly reports of all ADRs for the first three years that a drug is on the market, followed by annual reports thereafter, as part of the postmarketing surveillance system. However, the success of post-marketing surveillance is directly dependent on the active involvement of health care practitioners. Postmarketing ADR reports from health care providers have led to changes in prescribing habits, changes to drug labeling, and the withdrawal of various drugs from the market.

REPORTING ADVERSE DRUG REACTIONS TO THE FDA

With the passage of the Kefauver-Harris Amendment of 1962, the FDA was required to maintain a Spontaneous Reporting System (SRS). The structure of the SRS has changed over time. Today, all health care professionals and consumers can report ADRs and participate in the postmarketing surveillance process by submitting reports to the FDA's MedWatch. With MedWatch, the FDA receives reports via mailings, phone calls, faxes, and the Internet. From 2006 to 2014, the number of reports submitted annually through MedWatch grew from 470,261 to 1,289,133.[59]

The current MedWatch system allows health care providers to report suspected ADRs using FDA Form 3500 (See Appendix 17-5), which can be submitted by mail, fax, phone, or online.[60] The MedWatch form asks for information related to the suspected ADR, the patient's relevant medical history and medication regimen, and pertinent laboratory tests, although this information does not need to be complete in order for an ADR report to be submitted. From start to finish, the FDA estimates that it takes 36 minutes to complete a MedWatch form, including gathering the patient's data, reviewing the instructions, and submitting the report.

Once submitted through the MedWatch system, ADR reports are received by a unit of the FDA called the Central Triage Unit. The Central Triage Unit screens reports and forwards them to the appropriate FDA program within 24 hours of receipt. The report becomes part of a database used by the FDA to identify signals or warnings related to drug safety which require further study or regulatory action (see Pharmacovigilance section of this chapter). As a reminder, MedWatch is interested in capturing reports of serious ADRs, which the FDA defines as death, life-threatening events, hospitalization, disability, congenital anomaly, or requiring intervention to prevent permanent impairment or damage, as well as unexpected ADRs. The MedWatch program asks individuals to report an event even if they are not certain that the drug product was the cause.[61]

Barriers to Reporting Adverse Drug Reactions

The MedWatch program does not overcome the traditional lack of reporting seen with voluntary systems. It is important to recall that pharmaceutical manufacturers are required to report all adverse events to the FDA, whereas individual health care practitioners do so only voluntarily. Various explanations can account for the failure of practitioners to participate in the FDA program. Hoffman[61] elucidates several reasons that physicians do not voluntarily report ADRs, as follows:

'1. Failure to detect the reaction due to a low level of suspicion.
2. Fear of potential legal implications.
3. Lack of training about drug therapy.
4. Uncertainty about whether the drug causes the reaction.
5. Lack of clear responsibility for reporting.
6. Paperwork and time involved.
7. No financial incentive to report.
8. Unaware of reporting procedure or little understanding of it.
9. Lack of readily available reporting forms.
10. Desire to publish the report.
11. Fear that a useful drug will be removed from the market or given a bad name.
12. Complacency and lethargy.
13. Guilty feelings because of patient harm.
14. Reaction not worth reporting.'

In a systematic review of available evidence, Lopez-Gonzalez and colleagues[62] identified additional reasons why ADRs are underreported, including the beliefs that a single ADR report cannot meaningfully contribute to medical knowledge and that only safe drugs are allowed on the market. Another potential explanation for the lack of reporting is that medical record personnel, whose job might be to categorize and report data, are not familiar with ADRs and/or their method of documentation.[61]

Many of the reasons noted above also explain pharmacists' barriers to ADR reporting. A survey of Texas pharmacists investigated attitudes about voluntary reporting of serious ADEs in both community and hospital settings. While nearly 90% of respondents felt reporting could improve patient safety, 72.6% noted that the reporting process was time-consuming. Furthermore, 55.5% of respondents felt the reporting process disrupted their normal workflow. Some of the pharmacists in this survey also mentioned the reporting would increase the risk of malpractice, compromise relationships with physicians, and potentially break trust with their patients.[63] Ultimately, the benefit of increased patient safety should be enough to overcome the barriers to reporting faced by health care practitioners.

Reporting by Consumers

Historically, consumer reporting of adverse events has provided little data to MedWatch in comparison to the number of reports submitted by health care professionals. With the passage of the Food and Drug Administration Amendments Act (FDAAA) in 2007, however, consumer reports have been increasing. The FDAAA called for increased measures to assure the safety of marketed drugs. In an effort to increase consumer reporting of adverse events to the FDA, the act requires direct-to-consumer advertisements of prescription drugs to include the following statement: "You are encouraged to report negative side effects of prescription drugs to the FDA. Visit http://www.fda.gov/medwatch, or call 1-800-FDA-1088."[64]

In fact, in 2006, before the FDAAA was passed, consumers reported only 126,918 adverse event reports to MedWatch. In 2014, consumers were responsible for reporting 823,813 adverse event reports, bypassing the total provided by all health care providers that year.[65] While this trend is encouraging, there is still room for an increased rate of reporting by consumers. Efforts to educate the public on its role in ADR reporting could significantly impact public health.

Although consumers have the option of submitting ADR reports directly to the MedWatch program, FDA Form 3500 may be difficult for patients to navigate and complete. For example, they may not have ready access to their medical records, laboratory test results, and so on. Fortunately, a simplified, consumer-focused Form 3500B is available for patients to report ADRs to the FDA. A reporting mechanism is available for these individuals through the FDA's Consumer Complaint Coordinators. Available by telephone, these coordinators listen to consumer complaints, document the suspected problem, and follow up when needed. In the past, FDA has recalled nonprescription products after just two or three reports of serious problems were received through the Consumer Complaint Coordinators.[66]

DIETARY SUPPLEMENT ADVERSE DRUG REACTIONS REPORTING

Dietary supplements, including herbs, vitamins, minerals, and other so-called "nutraceuticals," can and do cause ADRs. Many of these products have powerful pharmacological effects and, therefore, can cause ADRs. The medical literature contains many case reports that describe ADRs related to dietary supplements. However, the exact incidence of ADRs with dietary supplements is not known. In one survey of 2,743 adults, 4% who took a dietary supplement reported an adverse event in the previous 12 months.[67]

Dietary supplements are regulated much differently than pharmaceuticals. The most striking difference is that these supplements can reach pharmacies and grocery store shelves without FDA approval and without any proof of safety or effectiveness. In the past, manufacturers of these products were not required to monitor safety of their products through postmarketing surveillance, nor were they required to share information about safety with the FDA. However, the Dietary Supplement and Nonprescription Drug Consumer Protection Act of 2006 changed this. This legislation now requires that any manufacturer, packager, or distributor of a dietary supplement whose name appears on a product label must collect and report ADR information related to their product(s). Manufacturers or marketers of dietary supplements who receive reports or information about severe adverse reactions related to their products are now required to share these reports with FDA.[68] Retailers who sell these products may report events upstream to the manufacturer, packer, or distributor.

An interesting case related to dietary supplements and ADRs involves the herb ephedra, also known as *ma huang*. This herb was marketed as a dietary supplement and promoted primarily for weight loss and enhancing athletic performance. It received lots of negative media attention when a Minnesota football player died of heat exhaustion during a training session. It turned out that the football player was using ephedra for weight loss. Over a period of several years, there were well over 100 reports to the FDA of life-threatening ADRs linked to ephedra, including heart attacks, strokes, seizures, and death. In March 2004, the FDA banned the sale of dietary supplements containing ephedra,[69] although this ban was lifted by a judge in 2010.[70] Still, the FDA could not prove that ephedra was the cause of these numerous ADRs. Because there were no reporting standards or requirements for manufacturers to collect data on their products' safety at this time, it would be unlikely that the FDA would ever have enough data to scientifically prove causality; they had to act based upon the best available evidence. The FDA's actions on ephedra will have long-lasting effects, and has ultimately set the precedent by which other cases against dietary supplements will be decided.

Currently, ADRs related to dietary supplements can be submitted by health care practitioners and consumers through the Department of Health and Human Services' Safety Reporting Portal. Previously, dietary supplement ADRs could be reported directly to FDA MedWatch program using the same approach that is used for prescription drugs. In 2014, FDA transitioned the reporting process to the Safety Reporting Portal to improve the efficiency and convenience of the reporting process.[71] There are also third-party systems for collecting adverse event data such as Natural MedWatch. Natural MedWatch (https://natural-database.therapeuticresearch.com/nd/adverseevent.aspx?s=ND&cs=naturalstandard)

allows consumers or health care professionals to complete an electronic form reporting an adverse event related to any dietary supplement. This system uses a database of around 90,000 commercially available dietary supplements that allows the user to select the specific commercial product used by the patient. Since many commercially available dietary supplements contain multiple ingredients, this system may improve the reliability of adverse reaction reporting for supplements. Natural MedWatch is integrated with the drug information resource Natural Medicines (https://naturaldatabase.therapeuticresearch.com/nd/adverseevent.aspx), which increases its accessibility for health care practitioners. Natural MedWatch asks similar questions to those on the FDA MedWatch Form 3500, and all reports submitted through this system are also simultaneously shared with the FDA.[72]

Just as with conventional drugs, reporting ADRs related to dietary supplements is voluntary for health care professionals. Practitioners and consumers have many options for reporting dietary supplement ADRs. As described above, they may submit them directly to the FDA via the Safety Reporting Portal, through a third-party system such as Natural MedWatch, or to the manufacturer or product distributor. Each of these avenues ultimately results in the information being provided to FDA for evaluation and analysis. Within the FDA, these reports are sent to the Center for Food Safety and Applied Nutrition (CFSAN), which maintains a special group charged with evaluating these adverse events. The CFSAN Adverse Event Reporting System (CAERS) allows for a more efficient evaluation of reports specifically related to dietary supplements.[73]

Despite the availability of this reporting infrastructure, the number of adverse events submitted by health professionals is minimal. From 2007 to 2010, an average of only 440 voluntary reports related to dietary supplement ADRs were submitted to FDA each year.[74] During the same time frame, about 790 per year were reported through mandatory mechanisms, such as manufacturer or distributor reporting. Most of these reports originate from consumers rather than health professionals.[73]

There may be a variety of reasons why few health professionals submit reports on dietary supplements to the FDA. Some of these may include:

- Patients often do not tell their providers about supplements use, or about the adverse effects they experience.
- Health professionals often do not ask about the use of dietary supplements.
- Consumers do not believe health professionals are able to answer questions about dietary supplements.
- Health professionals do not know where or how to submit reports of adverse reactions.
- There is a lack of information available to assess dietary supplement adverse reactions.

- Health care professionals may face a lack of time or support from management.
- Practitioners may have a fear of litigation.

ADRs related to dietary supplements can be assessed in much the same way as conventional drugs. However, there are some unique considerations. For example, when it comes to supplements, there is no such thing as generic equivalency. In other words, two supplement products made by different manufacturers cannot be considered equivalent. Different manufacturing practices and different extraction methods can dramatically change how a substance acts in the body, and this is especially true when it comes to herbal extracts. Because herbal extracts are made from plant material, variables such as extraction method, time of harvest, growing conditions, and so on can affect the chemical makeup of the extract. Therefore, two supplements containing Echinacea should not necessarily be considered equivalent. This may also mean that an ADR caused by one version of a supplement may not occur with another version.

VACCINE ADVERSE DRUG REACTIONS REPORTING

While MedWatch accepts adverse event reports for all FDA-regulated drugs, biologics, and medical devices, a separate process has been established for the reporting of adverse reactions related to vaccinations. The VAERS is a postmarketing surveillance program supported by the FDA and the Centers for Disease Control and Prevention (CDC). It was established after the passage of the National Childhood Vaccine Injury Act in 1986. This act requires health care providers to report specific adverse events that follow vaccination. These events include those listed by the vaccine manufacturer as a contraindication to subsequent doses of the vaccine, as well as certain other reactions defined by the FDA and CDC. A list of these reportable reactions is available on the VAERS website (http://vaers.hhs.gov).[75] Around 30,000 reports are submitted to VAERS annually. Of these, approximately 13% are considered serious.[76]

Similar to the MedWatch program, patients and practitioners can submit reports of adverse reactions to VAERS online, by fax, or by mail. Detailed instructions regarding this process are also available on the VAERS website.

_____ **Case Study 17–2**

A patient approaches you at the community pharmacy. She explains that she began taking a dietary supplement called *Kool Nights* about three weeks ago to help with insomnia. The patient awoke this morning with a rash over her face and torso. You research the product and find out that it contains kava kava, which is known to cause dermatologic side effects. After interviewing the patient and evaluating the available information, you decide that *Kool Nights* is causing the patient's rash.

- *As a health care professional, how can you report this suspected ADR to the FDA?*
- *Your patient decides she would like to take responsibility for reporting this ADR on her own. How can she accomplish this task?*

Future Approaches to Pharmacovigilance

The FDA has recognized that voluntary postmarketing evaluations of drug safety data alone are not sufficient to identify serious ADRs. High-profile adverse events related to drugs, such as rofecoxib (Vioxx®) and isotretinoin (Accutane®), are prime examples of the insufficiency of the voluntary reporting system. The FDA, working with private companies and academic researchers, has developed new methodologies to get early detection signals about safety issues with medications. These latest techniques include the development of additional pharmacovigilance methods as well as the improvement of the existing SRS. For example, the FDA is using data mining approaches for a more rapid identification of potential problems. Data mining is a statistical process that attempts to find a drug-associated event that appears more often in the ADR databases than would normally be expected to occur in the general population. When a higher-than-expected event occurs, this is referred to as signal detection. Statistics are used to identify these signals using both Bayesian and non-Bayesian methods. When an association is flagged in the system, the FDA then requires a clinical review involving experts to decide if any further action is needed for these events.[77] Although data mining and signal detection cannot determine a causal relationship between a drug and an adverse reaction, it is an efficient means of identifying ADRs that may warrant further investigation by the FDA.

With these new techniques, some hospitals have investigated pharmacovigilance methods for evaluating the safety profile of drugs at their institutions. The New York Presbyterian Hospital implemented a pharmacovigilance system that involved the EHR and used natural language computer processing. Various statistical techniques were used to establish associations between drugs and ADRs, as well as cutoff thresholds. In the hospital's feasibility study, seven drug classes were evaluated for novel adverse events. The researchers believed that the use of a comprehensive, unstructured data-monitoring program of EHRs was a feasible option for computerized pharmacovigilance at the local health-system level. This study demonstrates that data mining and signal detection, even at the local level, provide an effective mechanism for ADR reporting.[78]

The traditional randomized controlled clinical trial (RCT) is primarily designed to test the effectiveness of a drug or therapy, and is not usually powered to detect relevant safety information. With this in mind, it is easy to see why adverse reactions may go undetected in these trials. As discussed previously, it has been estimated that any ADR that occurs in few than 1 in 10,000 people will not be detected in most RCTs. Therefore, some experts have recommended the use of what is known as a large, simple trial (LST) to increase sample sizes and to monitor larger numbers of patients during clinical testing. LSTs have less stringent eligibility criteria than traditional RCTs, and subjects are typically studied for shorter periods of time. LST designs still use randomization techniques and continue to have important safety monitoring thresholds; they are not powered to determine efficacy. The larger sample sizes seen with the LST design provide more data for ADR monitoring methods like signal detection. In addition, the larger number of subjects increases the probability of picking up adverse events that are less common.[79] However, because LSTs are of relatively short duration, they do not overcome the challenge of detecting ADRs with a long latency.

Pharmacovigilance has traditionally relied on retrospective reports of ADRs, and relatively little information is available that helps health care professionals prospectively decide whether or not to use a drug in a particular patient. Pharmacogenomics may offer a solution for identifying characteristics and risk factors that predispose an individual to an ADR.[54] Genetic variations in enzymes that metabolize and eliminate drugs can lead to a patient's increased exposure to a medication, potentially increasing their risk for adverse effects.[80] Genome-wide association studies scan for genetic markers across the DNA of many individuals to find variations that may be associated with serious ADRs.[81,82] A list of over 150 pharmacogenomic associations that have been identified and validated is available from the FDA and is regularly updated with label warnings of new medications found to have genomic biomarkers.[83]

Conclusion

ADRs are a serious problem in the United States health care system, causing significant morbidity and mortality as well as costing billions of dollars annually. The problem is undeniably widespread, with the FDA receiving 1.2 million ADE reports in 2015, which was a 32.9% increase as compared to 2014 and nearly five times the total reports received in 2005.[84] Because of documented underreporting, these numbers represent only a small fraction of the ADRs occurring annually. Recognition of the problem is an important step in developing strategies to minimize the occurrence of ADRs. Reporting of these reactions by health care professionals is vital to gauging progress and directing the U.S.'s efforts in medication safety and patient care.

Health care practitioners play a vital role in developing, maintaining, and promoting ADR monitoring programs. Key steps in the development of these programs include identifying an institution-wide definition of ADRs, obtaining buy-in throughout the facility, establishing a mechanism to continuously screen for ADRs, and assigning responsibility for transmitting ADR reports. These programs provide valuable information about ADRs within the institution, as well as spontaneous reports of ADRs that can be forwarded to the FDA to aid in signal detection. ADR monitoring programs improve communication channels, generate additional education on adverse events, and positively impact patient care.

Technology is essential for monitoring, identifying, and minimizing ADRs, with most institutions and facilities utilizing computerized systems to screen for and alert practitioners to potential ADRs. The role of technology continues to expand as the FDA develops new approaches for signal detection and data mining. In addition, advances in pharmacogenetics may soon help practitioners proactively identify risk factors that predispose patients to an ADR, optimizing prescribing and medication management practices.

Despite the impact of ADRs and the tools available to assist in their management, ADRs remain underreported. Physicians and pharmacists report several barriers to reporting ADRs, including the time and hassle involved in reporting, as well as the belief that a single ADR report cannot contribute to medical knowledge to influence change in practice and regulations. ADR monitoring programs can only be successful if health care providers believe in their potential to improve patient safety and are willing to be active participants. Therefore, future efforts should focus on strategies for overcoming barriers to ADRs reporting in order to improve medication safety-related outcomes and improve patient care.

Self-Assessment Questions

1. Which of the following refers to an adverse drug reaction (ADR)?
   a. Any iatrogenic hazard or incident associated with a medication
   b. Any injury caused by a medication
   c. Any preventable event that leads to inappropriate medication use or patient harm
   d. Any unexpected, unintended, undesired, or excessive response to a medication
   e. Any reaction related to the intentional or unintentional overdose of a medication

2. Which of the following reactions is **NOT** an example of an ADR that the FDA would like health care professionals to report?
   a. A life threatening reaction to a drug
   b. An ADR that is not currently listed in the drug's labeling
   c. A reaction that is a more severe form of a previously reported ADR
   d. A common or expected side effect
   e. An ADR of which the exact cause is not known

3. The first step in establishing an adverse drug reaction program at a facility is to:
   a. Determine the institution's definition of an adverse drug reaction
   b. Decide who is responsible for reporting adverse reactions to the FDA
   c. Develop an ADR reporting hotline
   d. Identify drugs most likely to cause adverse reactions
   e. Report findings of the ADR program to the P&T committee

4. Which of the following factors is **NOT** used to determine adverse reaction causality?
   a. Dechallenge
   b. Rechallenge
   c. Temporal relationship
   d. Patient gender
   e. Known response pattern

5. Which of the following is the most commonly used algorithm for determining adverse reaction causality?
   a. Bayesian approach
   b. Kramer method
   c. Naranjo algorithm
   d. Larch algorithm
   e. Karch tool

6. Which of the following statements is/are **TRUE** regarding the Vaccine Adverse Event Reporting System (VAERS)?
   a. VAERS is a partnership between the FDA and the CDC.
   b. ADRs related to vaccine administration should be reported to VAERS instead of MedWatch.
   c. VAERS provides specific guidance on the kind of reactions that should be reported.
   d. Over 30,000 ADR reports are reported to VAERS annually.
   e. All of the above are true.

7. Which of the following best describes the role of technology in the management of ADRs?
   a. Technology can help identify and alert practitioners to potential ADRs.
   b. Technology eliminates the need for pharmacists to get involved in ADR management.
   c. Technology systems have not proven useful in the management of ADRs.
   d. Technology can only be used to report ADRs, not to aid in their detection.
   e. Technology has nearly eliminated fatalities due to ADRs.

8. Patients that experience an ADR typically encounter the following **EXCEPT**:
   a. Loss of income from occupational absences
   b. Initial or prolonged hospitalization
   c. Increased visits to their primary care physician
   d. Lower cost of hospitalization
   e. Use of new medications to manage symptoms induced by the ADR

9. Which of the following are resources that can be used to assess and evaluate ADRs?
   a. Clin-Alert
   b. Reactions Weekly
   c. Vigiaccess
   d. Meyler's Side Effects
   e. All of the above

10. Which of the following requires FDA to maintain a Spontaneous Reporting System for adverse events?
    a. Kefauver-Harris Amendment of 1962
    b. Dietary Supplement and Nonprescription Drug Consumer Protection Act of 2006
    c. Food and Drug Administration Amendments Act (FDAAA) of 2007
    d. American Recovery and Reinvestment Act (ARRA) of 2009
    e. The Health Information Technology for Economic and Clinical Health (HITECH) Act of 2009

11. Which of the following statements about ADRs associated with dietary supplements is **TRUE**?
    a. Manufacturers of dietary supplements are not required to share ADR reports they receive with the FDA.
    b. Only health care professionals can report dietary supplement ADRs to the Department of Health and Human Services' online Safety Reporting Portal.
    c. Dietary supplements are approved by the FDA and have a decreased chance of causing an ADR.

d. Patients often do not tell their health care provider about supplement use or the ADRs they experience from them.

e. The majority of dietary supplement ADR reports originate from health care providers.

12. Which of the following inpatient-based pharmacy programs have been proven to decrease ADR rates?
    a. Medication history service
    b. Drug protocol management
    c. ADR management programs
    d. a and b
    e. All of the above

13. Preventable ADRs may be caused by all of the following **EXCEPT**:
    a. Correct diagnosis
    b. Drug interactions
    c. Incorrect dosing
    d. Failure of patient to follow instructions for taking a medication
    e. All of the above

14. Using the classification of ADR severity developed by Karch and Lasagna, an event where an antidote was required to reverse the symptomatic effects of the event would be classified as:
    a. Minor
    b. Moderate
    c. Severe
    d. Lethal
    e. Administration of an antidote would not qualify as an ADR

15. Using the classification of ADR event type developed by Karch and Lasagna, an event where a patient developed an allergic rash subsequent to taking a medication would be labeled as:
    a. Idiosyncrasy
    b. Hypersensitivity
    c. Intolerance
    d. Drug interaction
    e. Pharmacologic

REFERENCES

1. American Society of Health-System Pharmacists. Suggested definitions and relationships among medication misadventures, medication errors, adverse drug events, and adverse drug reactions. Am J Health Syst Pharm. 1998;55:165-6.

2. Rich DS. A process for interpreting data on adverse drug events: determining optimal target levels. Clin Ther. 1998;20(Suppl C):C59-C71.

3. Rich DS. The Joint Commission's revised sentinel event policy on medication errors. Hosp Pharm. 1998;33:881-5.

4. Kohn LT, Corrigan JM, Donaldson MS, editors. Institute of medicine. To err is human: building a safer health system. Washington, DC: National Academy Press; 1999 Nov 1. p. 311.

5. White TJ, Arakelian A, Rho JP. Counting the costs of drug-related adverse events. PharmacoEconomics. 1999;15:445-8.

6. Wong YL. Adverse effect of pharmaceutical recipients in drug therapy. Ann Acad Med. 1993;22:99-102.

7. Kongkaew C, Noyce PR, Ashcroft DM. Hospital admissions with adverse drug reactions: a systematic review of prospective observational studies. Ann Pharmacother. 2008;42(7):1017-25.

8. Kochanek KD, Murphy SL, Xu J, Tejada-Vera B. Deaths: final data for 2014. Natl Vital Stat Rep. 2016 Jun 30;65(4):1-122.

9. Sultana J, Cutroneo P, Trifiro G. Clinical and economic burden of adverse drug reactions. J Pharmacol Pharmacother. 2013 Dec;4(Suppl 1):S73-S77.

10. Miguel A, Azevedo LF, Arajuo M, Pereira AC. Frequency of adverse drug reactions in hospitalized patients: a systematic review and meta-analysis. Pharmacoepidemiol Drug Saf. 2012;21(11):1139-54.

11. Sarkar U, Lopez A, Maselli JH, Gonzales R. Adverse drug events in U.S. adult ambulatory medical care. Health Serv Res. 2011 Oct;46(5):1517-33.

12. Fincham JE. An overview of adverse drug reactions. Am Pharm. 1991;NS31:435-41.

13. Hazell L, Shakir SA. Under-reporting of adverse drug reactions: a systematic review. Drug Saf. 2006;29(5):385-96.

14. World Health Organization. Medicines: safety of medicines—adverse drug reactions [Internet]. Geneva: World Health Organization; c2013. 2008 Oct [cited 2016 Aug 12]. Available from: http://www.wiredhealthresources.net/resources/NA/WHO-FS_Medicines SafetyAdverseReactions.pdf

15. Bond CA, Raehl CL. Clinical pharmacy services, pharmacy staffing, and adverse drug reactions in United States hospitals. Pharmacotherapy. 2006 Jun;26(6):735-47.

16. Lepakhin VK. Safety of medicines—a guide to detecting and reporting adverse drug reactions—why health professionals need to take action. Geneva: World Health Organization; 2002. p. 16.

17. U.S. Food and Drug Administration. An FDA guide to drug safety terms [Internet]. Silver Spring, MD: U.S. Food and Drug Administration. 2016 Aug 3 [cited 2016 Sept 6]. Available from: http://www.fda.gov/ForConsumers/ConsumerUpdates/ucm107970.htm

18. U.S. Food and Drug Administration. Code of Federal Regulations Title 21 [Internet]. Silver Spring, MD: U.S. Food and Drug Administration. 2015 Apr 1 [cited 2016 Sept 6]. Available from: http://www.accessdata.fda.gov/scripts/cdrh/cfdocs/cfcfr/cfrsearch.cfm?fr=312.32

19. Edwards R, Aronson JK. Adverse drug reactions: definitions, diagnosis, and management. Lancet. 2000;356:1255-9.

20. Karch FE, Lasagna L. Toward the operational identification of adverse drug reactions. Clin Pharmacol Ther. 1977;21:247-54.

21. Agbabiaka TB, Savovic J, Ernst E. Methods for causality assessment of adverse drug reactions: a systematic review. Drug Saf. 2008;31:21-37.

22. Naranjo CA, Busto U, Sellers EM, Sandor P, Ruiz I, Roberts EA, Janecek E, Domecq C, Greenblatt DJ. A method of estimating the probability of adverse drug reactions. Clin Pharmacol Ther. 1981;30:239-45.

23. Castells MC, Solensky R. Rapid drug desensitization for immediate hypersensitivity reactions. In: Adkinson NF, editor. UpToDate. [Internet]. Waltham, MA. UpToDate; 2017 [cited March 3, 2017]. Available from: www.uptodate.com

24. Kramer MS, Leventhal JM, Hutchinson TA, Feinstein AR. An algorithm for the operational assessment of adverse drug reactions: I. Background, description, and instructions for use. JAMA. 1979;242:623-32.

25. Hutchinson TA, Leventhal JM, Kramer MS, Karch FE, Lipman AG, Feinstein AR. An algorithm for the operational assessment of adverse drug reactions: II. Demonstration of reproducibility and validity. JAMA. 1979;242:633-8.

26. Jones JK. Adverse drug reactions in the community health setting: approaches to recognizing, counseling, and reporting. Fam Comm Health. 1982;5(2):58-67.

27. Michel DJ, Knodel LC. Comparison of three algorithms used to evaluate adverse drug reactions. Am J Hosp Pharm. 1986;43:1709-14.

28. Gallagher RM, Kirkham JJ, Mason JR, Bird KA, Williamson PR, Nunn AJ, Turner MA, Smyth RL, Pirmohamed M. Development and inter-rater reliability of the Liverpool Adverse Drug Reaction Causality Assessment Tool. PLoS ONE. 2011;6(12):e28096. doi:10.1371/journal.pone.0028096

29. Agababiaka TB, Savovic J, Ernst E. Methods for causality assessment of adverse drug reactions: a systematic review. Drug Saf. 2008;31(1):21-37.

30. Lane DA. The Bayesian approach to causality assessment: an introduction. Drug Info J. 1986;20:455-61.

31. Lactot KL, Naranjo CA. Comparison of the Bayesian approach and a simple algorithm for assessment of adverse drug events. Clin Pharmacol Ther. 1995;58:692-8.

32. Garcia-Cortes M, Stephens C, Fernandez-Castaner A, Andrade RJ, Spanish Group for the Study of Drug-Induced Liver Disease. Causality assessment methods in drug induced liver injury: strengths and weaknesses. J Hepatol. 2011;55(3):683-91.

33. U.S. Food and Drug Administration. Medical product safety information [Internet]. Silver Spring, MD: U.S. Food and Drug Administration. 2016 Aug 15 [cited 2016 Sept 6]. Available from: http://www.fda.gov/Safety/MedWatch/SafetyInformation/default.htm

34. VigiAccess. About [Internet]. [place unknown]: World Health Organization; [cited 2016 Sep 10]. Available from: http://www.vigiaccess.org/.

35. Springer—International Publisher Science, Technology, Medicine. Reactions Weekly: About this journal [Internet]. Berlin, DE: Springer Science+Business Media; c2016 [cited 2016 Sept 10]. Available from: http://www.springer.com/adis/journal/40278

36. SAGE Journals. Clin-Alert [Internet]. Thousand Oaks, CA: SAGE Journals; c2016 [cited 2016 Sept 10]. Available from: http://cla.sagepub.com/.

37. U.S. Food and Drug Administration. What is a serious adverse event? [Internet]. Silver Spring, MD: U.S. Food and Drug Administration. 2016 Feb 1 [cited 2016 Sept 10]. Available from: http://www.fda.gov/medwatch/report/desk/advevnt.htm

38. Centers for Medicare & Medicaid Services. Transmittal 72 Revised Appendix A: conditions of participation and interpretive guidelines for hospitals [Internet]. Baltimore, MD: Department of Health & Human Services and Centers for Medicare & Medicaid Services. 2011 Nov 18 [cited 2016 Sept 13]. Available from: https://www.cms.gov/Regulations-and-Guidance/Guidance/Transmittals/downloads/R72SOM.pdf

39. Joint Commission. Comprehensive Accreditation Manual for Hospitals (e-edition). Joint Commission Resources; c2016 [cited 2016 Sept 13]. Available from: https://e-dition.jcrinc.com/MainContent.aspx

40. ASHP guidelines on adverse drug reaction monitoring and reporting. Am J Health Syst Pharm. 1995 Feb 15;52(4):417-9.

41. Saltiel E, Johnson E, Shane R. A team approach to adverse drug reaction surveillance: success at a tertiary care hospital. Hosp Form. 1995 Apr;30(4):226-8, 231-2.

42. Classen DC, Pestotnik SL, Evans RS, Burke JP. Computerized surveillance of adverse drug events in hospitalized patients. Qual Saf Health Care. 2005 June;14:221-6.

43. American Society of Consultant Pharmacists. Guidelines [Internet]. Alexandria, VA; c2016. Guidelines for detecting and reporting adverse drug reactions in long-term care environments. 1997 Jul 17 [cited 2016 Sept 10]. Available from: http://www.ascp.com/resources/policy/upload/Gui97-ADRs.pdf

44. Institute for Safe Medication Practices. Acute Care Newsletters [Internet]. Horsham, PA; c2016. Adverse drug reactions: documentation is important but communication is critical. 2000 Sept 6 [cited 2016 Sept 10]. Available from: http://www.ismp.org/Newsletters/acutecare/articles/20000906.asp

45. AHRQ: Archive [Internet]. Rockville, MD; c2016. Making health care safer: a critical analysis of patient safety practices—evidence report/technology assessment, No. 43. 2001 Jul [cited 2016 Sept 10]. Available from: http://archive.ahrq.gov/clinic/ptsafety/.

46. Jha AK, Kuperman GJ, Teich JM, Leape L, Shea B, Rittenberg E, Burdick E, Seger DL, Vander Vliet M, Bates DW. Identifying adverse drug events: development of a computer-based monitor and comparison with chart review and stimulated voluntary report. J Am Med Inform Assoc. 1998 May-Jun;5(3):305-14.

47. Raschke RA, Gollihare B, Wunderlich TA, Guidry JR, Leibowitz AI, Peirce JC, Lemelson L, Heisler MA, Susong C. A computer alert system to prevent injury from adverse drug events. JAMA. 1998 Oct 28;280(15):1317-20.

48. Cozart H, Horvath MM, Long A, Whitehurst J, Eckstrand J, Ferranti J. Culture counts—sustainable inpatient computerized surveillance across Duke University Health System. Q Manage Health Care. 2010 Oct-Dec;19(4):1-10.

49. Ferranti J, Horvath MM, Cozart H, Whitehurst J, Eckstrand J. Reevaluating the safety profile of pediatrics: a comparison of computerized adverse drug event surveillance and voluntary reporting in the pediatric environment. Pediatrics. 2008 May;121(5):e1201-1207.

50. Hickner J, Zafar A, Kuo GM, Fagnan LJ, Forjuoh SN, Knox LM, Lynch JT, Stevens BK, Pace WD, Hamlin BN, Scherer H, Hudson BL, Oppenheimer CC, Tierney WM. Field test results of a new ambulatory care medication error and adverse drug event reporting system—MEADERS. Ann Fam Med. 2010 Nov-Dec;8(6):517-25.

51. Zafar A, Hickner J, Pace W, Tierney W. A medication error and adverse drug event reporting system for ambulatory care (MEADERS). AMIA Annu Symp Proc. 2008;6:839-43.

52. van Grootheest AC, de Jong-van den Berg LTW. The role of hospital and community pharmacists in pharmacovigilance. Res Soc Admin Pharm. 2005 Mar;1(1):126-33.

53. Emmendorfer T, Glassman PA, Moore V, Leadholm TC, Good CB, Cunningham F. Monitoring adverse drug reactions across a nationwide health care system using information technology. Am J Health Syst Pharm. 2012 Feb 15;69(4):321-8.

54. Davies E, Green C, Taylor S, Williamson P, Mottram D, Primohamed M. Adverse drug reactions in hospital in-patients: a prospective analysis of 3695 patient-episodes. PLoS ONE. 2009;4(2):e4439.

55. Issac T, Weissman JS, Davis RB, Massagli M, Cyrulik A, Sands DZ, Weingart SN.Overrides of medication alerts in ambulatory care. Arch Intern Med. 2009 Feb 9;169(3):305-11.

56. Waller P. Making the most of spontaneous adverse drug reaction reporting. Basic Clin Pharmacol Toxicol. 2006 Mar;98(3):320-3.

57. DesRoches CM, Painter MW, Jha AK. Health information technology in the United States, 2015: transition to a post-HITECH World. Robert Wood Johnson Foundation; 2015.

58. Harmark L, van Grootheest AC. Pharmacovigilance: methods, recent developments and future perspectives. Eur J Clin Pharmacol. 2008 Aug;64:743-52.

59. FDA: Drugs [Internet]. Silver Spring, MD. c2016. Reports received and reports entered into AERS by year. 2015 Nov 24 [cited 2016 Sept 10]. Available from: http://www.fda.gov/Drugs/GuidanceComplianceRegulatoryInformation/Surveillance/AdverseDrugEffects/ucm070434.htm

60. FDA: Safety [Internet]. Silver Spring, MD. c2016. Reporting by health professionals. 2016 Mar 25 [cited 2016 Sept 10]. Available from: http://www.fda.gov/Safety/MedWatch/HowToReport/ucm085568.htm

61. Hoffman RP. Adverse drug reaction reporting—problems and solutions. J Mich Pharm. 1989;27:400-3, 407-8.

62. Lopez-Gonzalez E, Herdeiro MT, Figueiras A. Determinants of under-reporting of adverse drug reactions: a systematic review. Drug Saf. 2009;32(1):19-31.

63. Gavaza P, Brown CM, Lawson KA, Rascati KL, Wilson JP, Steinhardt M. Influence of attitudes on pharmacists' intention to report serious adverse drug events to the Food and Drug Administration. Br J Clin Pharmacol. 2011 Jul;72(1):143-52.

64. Du DT, Goldsmith J, Aikin KJ, Encinosa WE, Nardinelli C. Despite 2007 law requiring FDA hotline to be included in print drug ads, reporting of adverse events by consumers still low. Health Aff. 2012 May;31(5):1022-9.

65. FDA: Drugs [Internet]. Silver Spring, MD. c2016. AERS reporting by healthcare providers and consumers by year. 2015 Nov 24 [cited 2016 Sept 10]. Available from: http://www.fda.gov/Drugs/GuidanceComplianceRegulatoryInformation/Surveillance/AdverseDrugEffects/ucm070456.htm

66. FDA: For consumers [Internet]. Silver Spring, MD; c2016. FDA 101: how to use the consumer complaint system and MedWatch. 2016 Sept 9 [cited 2016 Sept 10]. Available from: http://www.fda.gov/ForConsumers/ConsumerUpdates/ucm049087.htm

67. Timbo BB, Ross MP, McCarthy PV, Lin CT. Dietary supplements in a nationwide survey: prevalence of use and reports of adverse events. J Am Diet Assoc. 2006;106:1966-74.

68. U.S. Food and Drug Administration. Selected amendments to the FD&C Act: Dietary Supplement and Nonprescription Drug Consumer Protection Act [Internet]. Silver Spring, MD: U.S. Food and Drug Administration. 2006 Dec 22 [updated 2009 May 20; cited 2017 Sept 24]. Available from: https://www.fda.gov/RegulatoryInformation/LawsEnforcedbyFDA/SignificantAmendmentstotheFDCAct/ucm148035.htm

69. U.S. Government Printing Office. Federal Register Volume 69, Number 28 [Internet]. Washington, DC: U.S. Government Printing Office. 2004 Feb 11 [cited 2016 Sept 11]. Available from: http://www.gpo.gov/fdsys/pkg/FR-2004-02-11/html/04-2912.htm

70. American Botanical Council. Federal court overturns FDA ban on ephedra at low doses [Internet]. Austin, TX: American Botanical Council; c2016 [cited 2016 Sept 11]. Available from: http://cms.herbalgram.org/press/FDAephedra.html

71. U.S. Food and Drug Administration. FDA initiates new online reporting method for dietary supplement adverse events to facilitate reporting [Internet]. Silver Spring, MD: U.S. Food and Drug Administration. 2014 Jan 13 [cited 2016 Sept 11]. Available from: http://www.fda.gov/Food/NewsEvents/ConstituentUpdates/ucm381317.htm

72. Natural Medicines Comprehensive Database. Natural MedWatch: adverse event reporting form [Internet]. Stockton, CA: Therapeutic Research Center; c2016 [cited 2016 Sept 11]. Available from: https://naturaldatabase.therapeuticresearch.com/nd/adverseevent.aspx

73. Woo JJY. Adverse event monitoring and multivitamin-multimineral dietary supplements. Am J Clin Nutr. 2007;85:323S-324S.

74. Fabricant D. Dietary supplement update. Presented at: U.S. Food and Drug Administration; 2011 Jun 6; Silver Spring, MD.

75. Vaccine Adverse Event Reporting System. Information for healthcare professionals [Internet]. Rockville, MD: U.S. Department of Health and Human Services [cited 2016 Sept 11]. Available from: http://vaers.hhs.gov/professionals/index

76. Vaccine Adverse Event Reporting System. About the VAERS program [Internet]. Rockville, MD: U.S. Department of Health and Human Services. Vaccine Adverse Event Reporting System Web site [cited 2016 Sept 11]. Available from: http://vaers.hhs.gov/about/index

77. Van Manan RP, Fram D, DuMouchel W. Signal detection methodologies to support effective safety management. Drug Saf. 2007;6:451-64.

78. Want XY, Hripcsak G, Markatou M, Friedman C. Active computerized pharmacovigilance using natural language processing, statistics, and electronic health records: a feasibility study. J Am Med Inform Assoc. 2009;16:328-37.

79. Peto R, Collins R, Gray R. Large-scale randomized evidence: large, simple trials and overview of trials. J Clin Epidemiol. 1995;48:23-40.

80. National Human Genome Research Institute. Genome-wide association studies fact sheet [Internet]. Bethesda, MD: National Institutes of Health. 2015 Aug 15 [cited 2013 Aug 16]. Available from: http://www.genome.gov/20019523

81. Kacevska M, Ivanov M, Ingelman-Sundberg M. Perspectives on epigenetics and its relevance to adverse drug reactions. Clin Pharm Ther. 2011;89(6):902-7.

82. Daly AK. Using genome-wide association studies to identify genes important in serious adverse drug reactions. Ann Rev Pharmacol Toxicol. 2012;582:21-35.

83. U.S. Food and Drug Administration. Table of pharmacogenomic biomarkers in drug labeling [Internet]. Silver Spring, MD: U.S. Food and Drug Administration. 2016 Nov 7 [cited 2017 Mar 5]. Available from: https://www.fda.gov/drugs/scienceresearch/researchareas/pharmacogenetics/ucm083378.htm

84. Moore TJ, Cohen MR, Furberg CD, Mattison DR. Quarter watch annual report issue [Internet]. Horsham, PA: Institute for Safe Medication Practices. 2016 Jun [cited 2017 Mar 9]. Available from: http://www.ismp.org/QuarterWatch/pdfs/2015Q4.pdf

SUGGESTED READINGS

1. Harmark L, van Grootheest AC. Pharmacovigilance: methods, recent developments and future perspectives. Eur J Clin Pharmacol. 2008;64:743-52.

2. Lepakhin VK. Safety of medicines—a guide to detecting and reporting adverse drug reactions—why health professionals need to take action. Geneva: World Health Organization; 2002. Available from: http://apps.who.int/medicinedocs/en/d/Jh2992e/.

3. Naranjo CA, Busto U, Sellers EM, Sandor P, Ruiz I, Roberts EA, Janecek E, Domecq C, Greenblatt DJ. A method for estimating the probability of adverse drug reactions. Clin Pharmacol Ther. 1981;30:239-45.

Chapter Eighteen

Medication Misadventures II: Medication and Patient Safety

Kathryn A. Crea

Learning Objectives

● *After completing this chapter, the reader will be able to*

- Define and compare the terms medication errors, adverse drug events, and adverse drug reactions.
- Describe methods to identify medication errors and adverse drug events.
- Discuss the role of Patient Safety Organizations (PSOs) in health care.
- Assign an event severity rating to reported errors and events.
- Discuss two methods of analyzing medication errors and adverse drug events that are utilized to develop action plans for prevention of recurrence.
- Describe examples of skill-based, rule-based, and knowledge-based errors.
- Explain a systems approach to error.
- Compare a Just Culture with a culture of shame and blame.
- Determine strategies health care practitioners and health systems can implement to reduce medication errors.
- Reflect on the benefits of interprofessional education and training on quality and safety principles.

Key Concepts

❶ The terms medication error, adverse drug event, and adverse drug reaction are similar and often confused. They are interrelated, yet distinct occurrences.

❷ Several methods of identifying errors are recommended to gain a more global understanding of the risks and errors occurring within an organization.

3. Classification of errors by type is a common method to identify common themes and causes of events.

4. Thorough analysis of safety events through root cause analysis (RCA), failure mode and effects analysis (FMEA), or other methods is a key activity to support learning from errors in an effort to prevent recurrence.

5. Human beings (including health care professionals of all types) have a propensity to commit errors in all aspects of their lives. To err is human.

6. Understanding the three modes of human performance (skill based, rule based, and knowledge based) is very important to understanding errors and events, and in developing appropriate strategies to reduce the risks of recurrence.

7. Poorly designed health care systems and processes are a significant contributor to individual human error and subsequent patient harm.

8. A Just Culture is one in which discipline is applied in a consistent manner based on the intentions of the individual and the situation in which they were placed, not on the outcome.

9. All health professionals should be trained to deliver patient-centered care as members of an interdisciplinary team, emphasizing evidence-based practice, quality improvement approaches, and informatics.

10. There are many resources available that identify best practice error prevention strategies.

11. Researching, recognizing, and designing with human factors principles in mind is a great way to improve the safety of any process.

Introduction

Much attention has been focused on adverse outcomes in health care in the past 15 years. While pockets of research in medical errors were developing prior to 2000, the Institute of Medicine's report, To Err Is Human: Building a Safer Health System,[1] released in late 1999, served as a catalyst for additional research in the causes and methods to prevent adverse outcomes in health care. The mortality estimates documented in this report (an estimated 44,000 to 98,000 people die each year as a result of medical errors) were derived from two landmark studies.[1-3] The report notes that **medication errors** alone, whether occurring within or outside of the hospital, were estimated to account for over 7,000 deaths annually. The majority of literature to date has focused on work in the hospital setting, as it is, for the most part, a closed and controlled environment. Other settings are less well researched, although early studies of nursing homes and ambulatory settings have shown significant opportunities for improvement. It is clear that medication safety, and the broader category of patient safety, represents a serious concern for patients and health care providers.

While many health care professionals have roles in the medication use process, pharmacists play a pivotal role in ensuring the safe use of medication. Pharmacists' provision of accurate drug information and identification of potential medication-related adverse effects to diverse health care providers is of vital importance. Throughout the medication use process, there are many opportunities for unexpected adverse events, including errors in prescribing, dispensing, and administering medications, idiosyncratic reactions, and other adverse effects. These events can all be described as medication misadventures.[4] All health care providers need a sound understanding of the risks for error and the ability to identify the underlying causes of medication misadventures and be responsible for taking steps to prevent such occurrences and minimize adverse outcomes. This usually involves collaborative work with interprofessional health care team members to ensure optimal outcomes. Pharmacists in particular are well positioned to lead these efforts in reducing harm to patients.

Definitions: Medication Errors, Adverse Drug Events, and Adverse Drug Reactions

❶ *The terms medication error, adverse drug event, and adverse drug reaction are similar and often confused. They are interrelated, yet distinct occurrences.* The terminology surrounding medication misadventures is often confusing; there are many definitions that are very similar. The term medication misadventure is an overarching term which includes medication errors, **adverse drug events (ADEs), and adverse drug reactions (ADRs).** The American Society of Health-System Pharmacists[4] (ASHP) defines a **medication misadventure** as[5] an iatrogenic hazard or incident that

- is an inherent risk when medication therapy is indicated
- is created through either omission or commission by the administration of a medicine or medicines during which a patient may be harmed, with effects ranging from mild discomfort to fatality
- whose outcome may or may not be independent of the preexisting pathology or disease process
- may be attributable to error (human or system, or both), immunologic response, or idiosyncratic response
- is always unexpected or undesirable to the patient and the health professional

The National Coordinating Council for Medication Error Reporting and Prevention (NCCMERP), an organization composed of 24 national organizations and individual members, including the U.S. Food and Drug Administration (FDA), American

Medical Association (AMA), American Pharmacists Association (APhA), United States Pharmacopeial Convention (USP), and several others (See Table 18-1), has developed a detailed definition of what constitutes a medication error:

> "Any preventable event that may cause or lead to inappropriate medication use or patient harm while the medication is in the control of the health care professional, patient, or consumer. Such events may be related to professional practice, health care products, procedures, and systems, including prescribing; order communication; product labeling, packaging, and nomenclature; compounding; dispensing; distribution; administration; education; monitoring; and use."[6]

TABLE 18–1. NATIONAL COORDINATING COUNCIL FOR MEDICATION ERROR REPORTING AND PREVENTION MEMBER ORGANIZATIONS

Founding Members
American Association of Retired Persons (AARP)
American Hospital Association (AHA)
American Medical Association (AMA)
American Nurses Association (ANA)
American Pharmacists Association (APhA)
American Society of Health-System Pharmacists (ASHP)
Food and Drug Administration (US FDA)
Generic Pharmaceutical Association (GPhA)
The Joint Commission (TJC)
National Association of Boards of Pharmacy (NABP)
National Council of State Boards of Nursing (NCSBN)
Pharmaceutical Research and Manufacturers of America (PhRMA)
U.S. Pharmacopeial Convention (USP)
Regular Members
American Association of Homes and Services for the Aging (AAHSA)
American Society for Healthcare Risk Management (ASHRM)
American Society of Consultant Pharmacists (ASCP)
Department of Defense (DoD)
Department of Veterans Affairs (VA)
Institute for Healthcare Improvement (IHI)
Institute for Safe Medication Practices (ISMP)
National Alliance of State Pharmacy Associations (NASPA)
National Association of Chain Drug Stores (NACDS)
National Council on Patient Information and Education (NCPIE)
National Patient Safety Foundation (NPSF)

Key points related to medication errors include:

- medication errors are preventable
- medication errors can be caused by errors in the planning (deciding what to do—which drug and/or what dose) or execution stages (completing the task that was decided on—administering the drug to the wrong patient)
- medication errors include errors of omission (missed dose or appropriate medication not prescribed) or commission (wrong drug given)
- medication errors may or may not cause patient harm

Based on the NCC MERP definition, an error may occur as a result of not adequately counseling or educating a patient on proper use of medication. When, for example, a patient inappropriately uses a metered-dose inhaler for asthma and fails to receive the full amount of the medication, a medication error has occurred. The error may be secondary to a lack of education or may have occurred despite adequate counseling and education. Independent of the cause, based on the above definition, a medication error did occur.

Based on this definition, medication errors also occur when a prescriber prescribes the incorrect dose of a medication. Even if the prescriber is called by a pharmacist to clarify and change the order and the patient eventually receives an appropriately dosed medication, an error did occur in the process. An adverse outcome is not necessary to classify an event as a medication error.

An ADE involves harm to a patient. An ADE is defined as an injury from a medicine or lack of intended medicine.[7] An ADE refers to all ADRs, including allergic or idiosyncratic reactions, as well as medication errors that result in harm to a patient. It is estimated that 3% to 5% of medication errors result in harm to a patient and can also be classified as an ADE.

An ADR is defined by the World Health Organization (WHO) as "any response that is noxious, unintended, or undesired, which occurs at doses normally used in humans for prophylaxis, diagnosis, therapy of disease or modification of physiological function."[8]

The relationship between the terms is illustrated in Figure 17-1 (see previous chapter). While there are standard definitions for medication errors, there may be significant differences in the interpretation, reporting rates, and severity ranking between institutions. Common questions that arise are included in Table 18-2. For example, one institution may determine that an error has occurred when a dose is not received by a patient within 30 minutes of the scheduled time, where another may permit 60 minutes before or after the scheduled administration time. Some institutions may not report an inappropriately written prescription, if that error is caught by a clinician before the medication reaches the patient. Instead, a pharmacist or nurse may report it as a professional intervention. According to most definitions, this would count as an error. These variations make it very difficult to compare data from one institution to another. Therefore, it is best for an institution to use its own data to monitor improvement.

TABLE 18–2.   COMMON QUESTIONS THAT ARISE IN DEFINING MEDICATION ERRORS AND ADVERSE DRUG EVENTS

- Is it an error if it does not reach the patient?
- Is it an error if it does not cause harm?
- What constitutes minimal harm? Moderate? Severe?
- Is it an error or event if it is not clinically significant?
- Should pharmacist's interventions related to inappropriate orders by prescribers be documented and counted as prescribing errors?
- What is considered preventable?

The Impact of Errors on Patients and Health Care Systems

Patients depend on health care systems and health care professionals to help them stay healthy. As a result, patients frequently receive drug therapy with the notion that these medications will help them lead a healthier life. The initiation of drug therapy is the most common medical treatment received by patients.[9] In virtually all cases, patients and their health care providers understand that when medications are given, there are some known and some unknown risks. It is important that patients understand that they may experience unexpected drug-related morbidity and mortality which, although rare, may be significant.

Several landmark studies have identified the risk of medication errors and ADEs in varying populations and settings. The Harvard Medical Practice Study I was a landmark study that estimated that 3.7% of hospitalized patients experience adverse events.[2] The findings and extrapolated statistics from this study along with the Harvard Medical Practice Study II served as the grounds for the statement (from To Err Is Human) that approximately 44,000 to 98,000 people are killed by medical error every year. Specifically related to medication errors, Bates and associates[7] identified 6.5 ADEs per hospital admission. In the nursing home setting, Gurwitz and associates[10] identified 227 ADEs per 1,000 resident years. Gurwitz and associates[11] also studied the ambulatory patient population, finding 50.1 ADEs per 1,000 person-years. Interestingly, preventability of all

ADEs in these studies ranged from 27% to 51%, while the preventability of serious and life-threatening ADEs ranged from 42% to 72%, potentially indicating that improved processes and behaviors should be able to prevent serious harm events.

The economic impact of medication errors and ADEs is staggering and adds unnecessarily to the health care cost burden. Several important studies documented the economic burden of these events.[12-15] A landmark study in 1995 estimated that ADE-related costs were $76.6 billion annually in ambulatory patients alone.[12] Drug expenditures in ambulatory patients at that time were $80 billion per year. This means that for every $1 spent for a drug, almost $1 was also being spent due to a drug-related problem. These costs exceed the total cost of managing patients with diabetes or cardiovascular diseases.[13] A subsequent study demonstrated the cost of drug-related morbidity and mortality in the ambulatory setting exceeded $177 billion in 2000.[15]

While it was initially thought that medication misadventures were caused by individual health care practitioners, including pharmacists, physicians, and nurses, now it is clear that our health care systems and processes often are causative or contributing factors in the majority of errors and events. Efforts to decrease adverse outcomes will not be successful if these system and process-related issues are not addressed. Multiple agencies and professional organizations across the country are now contributing efforts to minimize these events (See Table 18-3), which will be discussed in the section Best Practices for Error Prevention.

TABLE 18–3. ORGANIZATIONS INVOLVED IN PREVENTING ADVERSE DRUG EVENTS

Organization	Website
Food and Drug Administration (FDA)	www.fda.gov
The Joint Commission (TJC)	www.jointcommission.org
World Health Organization (WHO)	www.who.int
Institute for Safe Medication Practices (ISMP)	www.ismp.org
The United States Pharmacopeial Convention (USP)	www.usp.org
American Society of Health-System Pharmacists (ASHP)	www.ashp.org
National Quality Forum (NQF)	www.qualityforum.org
Agency for Healthcare Research and Quality (AHRQ)	www.ahrq.gov
Patient Safety Network	www.psnet.ahrq.gov
Web M&M: Morbidity and Mortality Rounds on the web	www.psnet.ahrq.gov
Institute for Healthcare Improvement (IHI)	www.ihi.org
Health Resources and Services Administration (HRSA)	www.hrsa.gov
National Patient Safety Foundation (NPSF)	www.npsf.org
Centers for Medicaid and Medicare Services (CMS)	www.cms.hhs.gov
Centers for Disease Control and Prevention (CDC)	www.cdc.gov
The Leapfrog Group	www.leapfroggroup.org

Identification and Reporting of Medication Errors and Adverse Drug Events

❷ *Several methods of identifying errors are recommended to gain a more global understanding of the risks and errors occurring within an institution.* It is important that a systematic approach to the identification and assessment of errors and adverse events be utilized in order to identify trends and opportunities for improvement based on events occurring at a location. This should involve several methods, and include prospective and retrospective methods of identifying errors and risks when possible. Many methods of identifying errors in health care exist, including voluntary reporting, direct observation, chart review, trigger identification, and computerized monitoring. These methods are described further here.

1. A voluntary reporting system (paper, telephonic, or online) is the most common method of identification of errors and events. Many institutions include an anonymous option for those who do not feel comfortable providing their name and contact information. Anyone detecting or committing an error can report it without associating their name with the error. It is essentially risk free for the reporter and, therefore, it may increase the likelihood of having an error reported. While voluntary reporting is the least labor-intensive method, it only identifies approximately 1 out of 20 errors when compared to other identification methods.[16] Therefore it is important to include other methods of detection.

2. The direct-observation method uses trained observers to watch the real-time delivery of medications. Notes from the observations are compared with prescriber's orders to determine if an error has occurred. Results with this method are more valid and reliable than with self-reporting, but the impact of the observer on the subject being observed and interobserver agreement has been questioned.[17,18] This method is costly, time consuming, and limited to the identification of errors that occur during the administration phase of the medication use process. It typically samples a selected time period on a selected unit, limiting the extrapolation to other time periods or patient care areas. On the positive side, errors are often identified that may never be discovered through other methods as they may go unrecognized.

3. Chart review identification of medication errors and ADEs is very labor intensive and is not generally practical outside of the research environment. Various trained staff review charts looking for particular cues or data elements that signify an error or event has occurred. This method relies on practitioners to document these events when identified, which may lead to an underestimation of the true occurrence.

4. A modified version of manual chart review is the use of the **ADE Trigger Tool**. It is a tool that is promoted by the Institute for Healthcare Improvement (IHI). It is

an augmented chart review method that uses automated systems to identify alerts or triggers that have been shown to efficiently identify patients with potential ADEs.[19-27] The triggers are cues that a patient may have experienced an error and/or adverse event. Example triggers include the use of reversal agents (e.g., flumazenil, naloxone, phytonadione) or abnormal values for labs, such as partial thromboplastin time (PTT), international normalized ratio (INR), or a low blood glucose value. When these triggers are identified, it is suspected that the patient may have experienced a medication error. The patient's chart is reviewed for evidence of error and/or level of harm and data is collected and collated to determine potential common causes. For example, reviewing the charts of patients who experience hypoglycemia may reveal errors, such as incorrect insulin dosing while patients are receiving nothing by mouth in preparation for a surgical procedure. Upon review of patients requiring the use of naloxone, it may be discovered that the dosing for hydromorphone and morphine are often confused during the prescribing, administration, and monitoring phases leading to oversedation. The advantage to using this trigger method is that these types of events are rarely reported as errors. These tools have been used in several ways—as a long-term trend and measure of ADEs and/or in a more focused scope such as triggers related to known high-risk classes of medications.[28-30] Specific information on the use of this tool is available at http://www.ihi.org.

5. Classen[20,21] and Jha[19] developed methods to identify ADEs using an electronic medical record (EMR) with text searching tools and logic-based computer rules. In Classen's model, the text within the computer charting (e.g., lab, nurses notes, physician progress notes and orders) is searched for defined conditions or cues, such as heparin-induced thrombocytopenia (HIT). When identified, a pharmacist is alerted, reviews the patient record, and relays an appropriate recommendation to the prescribing physician. This serves as a real-time intervention to prevent or mitigate harm to the patient. This seems to be an optimal model, allowing concurrent review of potential harm and intervention to prevent further error or harm. Unfortunately, while more organizations are implementing an EMR, many are not capable of searching text or have not yet implemented this option.

The use of technology has presented new sources of data on potential errors. The increased use of automated distribution machines, smart pumps, computerized prescriber order entry (CPOE), and bar-coding technology provides rich databases. For example, every keystroke a nurse makes in programming a smart infusion pump is recorded. Once an error is identified, it is possible to download the data and review details about the error. The challenge is sorting through the massive volumes of information to derive common themes and strategies to decrease risk and optimize the technology.

The 1999 IOM report spotlighted a serious need to capture data that would help to reduce harm to patients. Congress subsequently passed The Patient Safety and Quality Improvement Act of 2005 (Patient Safety Act). The act authorized the creation of a nationwide network of **Patient Safety Organizations (PSOs)** to improve safety and quality through the collection and analysis of data on patient events.[31] The act provides a venue for institutions to report information related to errors and events with the goal of collating the information and learning the underlying risks across similar types of events.

The act provides confidentiality and privilege protection to organizations. The fear of legal action related to reported event information has prevented many organizations from voluntarily reporting errors and events to external agencies. The confidentiality protections assure that information about an error that is provided to the authorized PSO is kept confidential. The privilege protections limit or forbid the use of protected information in criminal, civil, and other proceedings. Specifically, the information will not be subject to subpoena, discovery, or disclosure to any federal, state, or local criminal, civil, or administrative proceeding. The information may not be used in a professional disciplinary hearing, nor be admitted as evidence.

One example, the Pennsylvania Patient Safety Reporting System, has been collating error data since 2004 and publishes regular advisories with the goal of improving health care delivery systems and educating providers about safe practices. For example, in December 2009,[32] the advisory reviewed errors with neuromuscular blocking agents. In a five-year span, 154 reports related to neuromuscular blocking agents were submitted. The advisory provides specific information related to the contributing factors (unsafe storage, look-alike drug names, similar packaging, and unlabeled syringes) that increase the risk for a fatal error. Specific risk reduction strategies are outlined. The same errors tend to recur in facilities across the United States. There was a series of errors in the administration of heparin to premature infants[33] that occurred at least three times in different states with similar causes. It is imperative that health care professionals commit to learn from others and critically self-assess the processes within their own institution to assure their process is as safe as possible. Being a learning organization is essential to prevent errors within an organization. A learning organization is one in which the leadership supports organizational learning, creating an environment where structured processes are developed to support this. Examples include communication of performance data to the staff level, formal training in performance improvement and problem solving at the unit or department level, and active engagement of staff in local problem solving. It is recommended that hospitals, ambulatory centers, and other organizations join a PSO and commit to forwarding data related to adverse outcomes, enabling the collation of larger quantities of data, which the PSO can analyze and feedback recommendations to member organizations. This enables local and broad scale learning from errors and events.

Classification of Error Types

❸ *Classification of errors by type is a common method to identify common themes and causes of events.* The most common way to classify errors is to identify them by type of error. For medications, this classification focuses on whether an error was related to dispensing, administering, prescribing, monitoring, or other reasons. There have been many taxonomies of errors developed by various groups, including the WHO, The Joint Commission (TJC), MEDMARX®, and others. The ASHP previously designated categories of medication errors are listed here.[34] These are similar to those outlined by NCC MERP.

- Prescribing error
- Omission error
- Wrong time error
- Unauthorized drug error
- Improper dose error
- Wrong dosage form error
- Wrong drug preparation error
- Wrong administration technique
- Deteriorated drug error
- Monitoring error
- Compliance error
- Other medication error

As a result of the development of PSOs, a common taxonomy and language was developed to enable health care providers to collect and submit standardized information related to safety events. These standard event reporting forms are called the Common Formats. The Common Formats define the standardized data elements associated with errors and events that are to be collected and reported to the PSO. The scope of Common Formats applies to all patient safety concerns including events reaching the patient (with or without harm), near-miss events that do not reach the patient, and unsafe conditions that have the potential to cause an error or event.[35] The Common Formats most recently updated (V1.2) by the Agency for Healthcare Research and Quality (AHRQ) are likely to become the standard for reporting. The following event types have been defined for medication errors:

- Incorrect patient—An incorrect patient error occurs when a medication is given to the wrong patient, usually caused by an error in patient identification and confirmation. Two identifiers should be used to identify the patient every time a patient is given a medication. Confirming patient identification is necessary whenever a pharmacist or physician writes or enters an order, or dispenses a medication in outpatient areas, or when a nurse administers a medication.

- Incorrect medication—This error occurs when a medication is administered that was not ordered for the patient. This may occur when a patient receives a medication intended for another patient, due to inadequate patient identification, or when a nurse obtains the incorrect medication for administration, perhaps from floor stock. Barcode scanning is designed to prevent these errors and others.

- **Incorrect dose** (subcategories of overdose, underdose, omitted dose, extra dose, and unknown)—An incorrect dose error can occur when a prescriber orders an inappropriate dose of a medication or when the dose administered is different than what was prescribed. An omission error occurs when a patient does not receive a scheduled dose of medication. This is considered to be the second most common error in the medication use process.[36]

- **Incorrect route of administration** (subcategories include the intended route and the actual route)—Some of the most harmful incorrect route errors have included administration of enteral tube feeding into an intravenous line or instillation of an IV medication intrathecally that is not designed to be given this route. One significant cause is the fact that these varying types of tubing fit together, which is considered a systems problem. In an effort to reduce the chance of this occurrence, tubing designed to fit only based on the intended use would be optimal (e.g., IV, enteral feeding, intrathecal, dialysis).

- Incorrect timing (too early, too late, unknown)—What constitutes a wrong time error may vary considerably among organizations. In general, this type of error occurs when a dose is not administered in accordance with a predetermined administration interval. Most organizations realize that it is often impossible to be totally accurate with the administration interval and typically allow 15 to 60 minutes outside that interval. Establishing a policy to indicate what constitutes an error in this category is needed for consistent reporting and data collection.

- Incorrect rate (too fast, too slow, unknown)—This category generally applies to intravenous infusions, but can also apply to an intravenous push medication if the drug is pushed too quickly or too slowly.

- Incorrect duration—The patient receives the medication for a shorter or longer time period than prescribed. For example, a patient is prescribed a one-time dose of a medication. The pharmacist must enter the order as "daily" so it will show up on the medication administration record (MAR) for the nurse to administer and chart; however, he or she must remember to place "one time" in the correct field so it only appears to the nurse once to administer. If the pharmacist forgets that last step (relying on memory is a poor error-prevention strategy), the medication will appear on the MAR for daily administration.

- Incorrect dosage form (e.g., extended release instead of immediate release)—A wrong dosage form error can occur when the prescriber makes an error or when a patient receives a dosage form different from that prescribed, assuming the appropriate dosage form was originally ordered.

- Incorrect strength or concentration—This is an error that can occur at several points in the medication use process, from prescribing to administration. The pharmacist may choose the wrong strength when entering the order, a pharmacy technician may select the wrong drug for dispensing, or a nurse may choose the wrong drug upon administration. The appropriate use of barcode administration of medications in the inpatient setting makes it harder to make these errors.

- Incorrect preparation (e.g., splitting tablets, compounding errors)—When medications require some type of preparation, such as reconstitution, this type of error may occur. These kinds of errors may also occur in the compounding of various intravenous admixtures and other products and can occur when nurses, pharmacists, or technicians are preparing medications.

- Expired or deteriorated product—This error occurs when a drug is administered that has expired or has deteriorated prematurely due to improper storage conditions.

- Medication that is a known allergen to the patient—These errors may occur due to lack of adequate interfaces between different computer or technology software programs, resulting in the appropriate information not being available to apprise the appropriate people.

- Medication known to be contraindicated for the patient such as a drug-drug interaction or drug-food interaction.

- Incorrect patient action (patient taking a dietary supplement that interacted with medication, whether or not he or she was told to avoid taking it)—This type of error occurs when patients use medications inappropriately. Proper patient education and follow-up may play a significant role in minimizing this type of error. This type of error may be a direct result of insufficient patient counseling from a pharmacist, a prescriber, or both. Important components in counseling include consideration of the level of health literacy of the patient and methods to gauge their understanding of their medication regimen and information provided. An adequate learning needs assessment may assist in effective counseling based on an individual patient's needs.

The second classification section of the medication Common Formats report asks at what stage the incorrect action was discovered (regardless of where or when the incorrect action originated) with the following choices:

- Purchasing
- Storing
- Prescribing
- Transcribing
- Preparing
- Dispensing
- Administering to patient (including verifying medication)
- Monitoring

Prescribing errors generally focus on inappropriate drug selection, dose, dosage form, or route of administration. Examples may include ordering duplicate therapies for a single indication, prescribing a dose that is too high or too low for a patient based on age or organ function, writing a prescription illegibly, prescribing an inappropriate dosage interval, or ordering a drug to which the patient is allergic.

In one study, the most common type of prescribing error (56.1%) was related to an inappropriate dose (either too high or too low).[9] The second most common prescribing error was related to prescribing an agent to which the patient was allergic (14.4%). Prescribing inappropriate dosage forms was the third most common error (11.2%). Other relatively common prescribing errors have included failing to monitor for side effects and serum drug levels, prescribing an inappropriate medication for a particular indication, and inappropriate duration of therapy.

Monitoring errors occur when patients are not monitored appropriately either before or after they have received a drug. For example, if a patient is placed on warfarin therapy and adequate blood tests (baseline and ongoing) are not performed to assess the patient's response, a monitoring error has occurred and has the potential to result in a life-threatening hemorrhage. TJC recognized this as a significant safety risk and developed a National Patient Safety Goal in 2015 in an effort to encourage organizations to improve and standardize this process.[37]

These types of medication errors are not mutually exclusive. Multiple types of errors may occur during a single administration of a drug and a single adverse patient outcome may be the result of more than one type of error.[34]

Additional information is gathered in the PSO reporting process. As the use of Common Formats grows, individual health care organizations will need to adopt these classifications, likely developing a standard taxonomy over time. Visit the PSO website for updated versions of the Common Formats at https://www.pso.ahrq.gov/common.

Classifying Patient Outcomes

Although the classification of errors or events frequently is based on type, most are also classified by the patient outcome related to the error or event. When an error occurs, there is not always an adverse outcome. It is important for institutions to monitor both the types of errors that occur and the outcomes associated with them. Most reporting systems request information regarding type and outcome of a medication error.

The NCC MERP developed a medication error index that serves to categorize errors based on the severity or outcome of the error. This index is divided into four main categories and nine subcategories as follows.[38] See the index for event classification and corresponding algorithm at http://www.nccmerp.org/types-medication-errors.

1. No error
   - **Category A:** Circumstances or events that have the capacity to cause error.
2. Error, no harm
   - **Category B:** An error occurred, but the medication did not reach the patient.
   - **Category C:** An error occurred that reached the patient, but did not cause the patient harm.
   - **Category D:** An error occurred that resulted in the need for increased patient monitoring, but caused no patient harm.
3. Error, harm
   - **Category E:** An error occurred that resulted in the need for treatment or intervention and caused temporary patient harm.
   - **Category F:** An error occurred that resulted in initial or prolonged hospitalization and caused temporary patient harm.
   - **Category G:** An error occurred that resulted in permanent patient harm.
   - **Category H:** An error occurred that resulted in a near-death event (e.g., anaphylaxis and cardiac arrest).
4. Error, death
   - **Category I:** An error occurred resulting in patient death.

Oftentimes, the initial staff member(s) reporting the error has an opportunity to indicate their interpretation of the level of harm to the patient. In follow-up, a medication safety pharmacist and the unit/department manager may investigate further details and assign a final severity classification based on the ultimate outcome to the patient.

Institutions may use information about outcomes to focus their error prevention efforts on the types of errors resulting in the most serious outcomes. It is important to remember that examining near-miss events (those that do not reach the patient) can be as valuable in preventing future errors as focusing on serious outcomes. These near-miss events are often clues to the underlying process issues that require attention before they cause harm to a patient.

National Reporting

Reporting of medication errors is important for every practitioner without regard to their practice setting. However, institutional internal reporting is often emphasized (above external reporting). Drug information specialists or medication safety officers are in an ideal position to encourage the importance of medication error and ADR reporting to all health professionals, especially when they are consulted to answer questions related to potential cases. In an effort to share institutional experiences and avoid the same errors being repeated at several institutions, national reporting systems for institutions have evolved.

- **MedWatch:** This program was developed by the FDA Medical Products Reporting Program for the purpose of monitoring problems with medical products. MedWatch monitors quality, performance, and safety of medical products, devices, and medications. This program contributes to surveillance of medication errors that may be associated with product labeling and names.[39] MedWatch collects reports about faulty products (e.g., improperly functioning devices). Significant reports may result in distribution of e-mail and safety alerts to health care professionals. These announcements can also be viewed on the Internet at http://www.fda.gov/Safety/MedWatch/default.htm. Health care professionals and consumers can report ADEs and product problems by completing a MedWatch 3500 form (found on the website) and mailing it to the FDA, by calling 1-800-FDA-1088, or reporting online at https://www.accessdata.fda.gov/scripts/medwatch/index.cfm?action=reporting.home.
- **ISMP Medication Errors Reporting Program (MERP):** This program provides a venue for voluntary medication error reporting to the Institute for Safe Medication Practices (ISMP). Reports can be submitted online at http://www.ismp.org/reporterrors.asp. ISMP is a federally certified PSO which collates errors and provides summary information across multiple cases in an effort to identify risk and support prevention strategies.
- **Subscription-based reporting systems:** One example of a subscription-based reporting system is Quantros, which took over the prior USP-MEDMARX® reporting system. This program, and others, is an anonymous, subscription-based,

voluntary reporting system that enables facilities to collect and report medication error, ADE, and ADR data. Subscribing organizations utilize the system to report and monitor organization-specific errors online, as well as compares their error rates with other subscribing organizations of similar type. These products differ from the ISMP MERP program in that they are fee-based services that enable comparison to data within the database.

Managing an Event Reporting System

TJC and ASHP standards can be used as a basis for starting an error reporting program. In addition to the standards, the pharmacy and medical literature contain abundant examples of successful programs. The following steps are a compilation of several of these references:

1. Develop and utilize standardized definitions and classifications for errors and events. The definitions and classifications in the literature and this chapter provide a good starting point for discussion. It is anticipated that the Common Formats developed in preparation for external reporting to PSOs will eventually become the standard.

2. Assign responsibility for the error review program within the pharmacy and throughout other key departments. A multidisciplinary approach is an essential factor. The program needs a leader and an advocate. It also needs the involvement of nursing, physicians, quality, and risk management departments in order to function as a collaborative team to work toward improved processes.

3. Develop forms or online methods for data collection and reporting (see #1 above). Other mechanisms for reporting (hotline phone numbers) may be used as well. Electronic reporting can often be designed such that medication errors are reviewed by a medication safety pharmacist to confirm severity of the event and gather additional information as needed in order to determine whether additional analysis is appropriate. It is important to develop internal processes to assure awareness of key staff and leaders while maintaining protection from discovery. Protections vary from state to state making it important to work with legal and risk management. This serves as the voluntary reporting component of the program.

4. Promote awareness of the program and the importance of reporting errors and adverse events. Provide feedback to reporters and individual units that discuss their errors as well as those of others, along with steps taken to prevent them. Providing feedback is very important to assure that those reporting feel that the

identified errors are reviewed and methods to prevent recurrence are developed and implemented.

5. Develop policies and procedures for determining which errors, events, and ADRs are reported to the FDA. The responsibility for this reporting should be defined and usually resides with someone in the pharmacy department.

6. Establish mechanisms for regular screening and identification of potential medication errors and ADEs to supplement voluntary reporting. These mechanisms should include retrospective reviews, concurrent monitoring, as well as prospective planning for high-risk groups. It is worthwhile to educate clinicians to check for potential events or reactions when they see orders for certain triggers that are often used to treat an error or event (See Table 18-4), orders to discontinue or hold drugs, and orders to decrease the dose or frequency of a drug.[19] Additionally, electronic screening methods to check for laboratory tests that are indicative of potential events (e.g., drug levels, *Clostridium difficile* toxin assays, elevated serum potassium, and low white blood cell counts) can be helpful.[21]

7. Routinely review medication errors, ADEs, and ADRs for trends. Report all findings to the pharmacy and therapeutics committee and other hospital or organization quality and safety committees. It is beneficial to present facility specific data, nationally reported errors of significance, as well as incorporate storytelling into various presentations. Oftentimes, telling a de-identified story that engages one's

TABLE 18–4. ADVERSE DRUG EVENT TRIGGERS

Medications	Conditions
Antidiarrheal agents	PTT > 100 seconds
Atropine (exclude preoperative use)	INR > 6
Dextrose 50% (IV push)	WBC < 3,000
Diphenhydramine (excluding orders for sleep)	Glucose < 50 mg/dL
Epinephrine (IV push)	Rising serum creatinine
Flumazenil	*Clostridium difficile*-positive stool
Naloxone	Digoxin level > 2 ng/mL
Droperidol	Lidocaine level > 5 mcg/mL
Sodium polystyrene sulfonate	Gentamicin/tobramycin peak > 10 mcg/mL or trough > 2 mcg/mL
Vitamin K	Amikacin peak > 35 mcg/mL or trough > 10 mcg/mL
	Vancomycin trough level > 26 mcg/mL
	Theophylline level > 20 mcg/mL
	Oversedation, lethargy, fall, rash
	Abrupt medication stop
	Transfer to higher level of care

emotions, followed by your own data specific to the event, engages clinicians in the efforts to work toward safer processes.

8. Develop strategies for decreasing the incidence of medication errors and adverse events utilizing the data collected through the various identification and reporting systems. Use caution in aggregating data by error types or other surface level classifications. The key is getting to the causes of the errors—not just the fact that the majority of errors are omitted doses. Why are the doses omitted? Is the automated dispensing cabinet filled at inappropriate intervals, is there not a clear and standardized process for delivering medications where they are easily located, or do the batteries on the computers-on-wheels drain too quickly and the doses just are not charted? Seek to discover why the doses are omitted, as these are the issues that need to be resolved.

9. Review national resources that identify errors in other organizations such as the ISMP, the FDA, and the USP. It is likely that your institution is experiencing risks similar to other institutions. Learn what risk reduction strategies are recommended, take a close look at your own processes, and implement additional risk reduction strategies where warranted. There is no need to repeat errors at every institution to learn what steps need to be taken for prevention.

Types of Safety Event Analysis

❹ *Thorough analysis of safety events through root cause analysis (RCA), failure mode and effects analysis (FMEA), or other methods is a key activity to support learning from errors in an effort to prevent recurrence.* Analysis of near-miss events (errors that do not reach the patient) and precursors (errors reaching the patient but causing little to no harm) can be very valuable learning experiences. These may be documented in various ways—through interventions or error-reporting systems. These are valuable when reviewed in aggregate to determine if there are common themes or causes that may warrant further investigation and process changes. It is important to remember that the causes of near misses or errors causing minimal harm are often the same errors that lead to serious harm. For example, a nurse administers a dose of cefazolin to the wrong patient. Fortunately, the patient was not allergic and there was no adverse outcome. If the same error occurs with a different drug (e.g., a high-risk drug, such as a paralytic agent), the outcome can be fatal. Precursor events (those causing little to no harm) can be an important learning experience.

Medication errors that are rated severity E through I, using the NCC MERP severity rating system, cause harm to patients, ranging from minor harm to death. Many facilities conduct an investigation on these events to better understand the causes.

● SENTINEL EVENTS AND ROOT CAUSE ANALYSIS

TJC is an accrediting body that is focused on continuously improving health care for the public by evaluating health care organizations (e.g., hospitals, home care organizations, nursing homes, ambulatory care providers, clinical laboratories). The goal of TJC is to ensure each organization meets designated standards for quality and safety. A sentinel event is defined by TJC as "an unexpected occurrence involving death or serious physical or psychological injury, or the risk thereof. Serious injury specifically includes loss of limb or function. The phrase 'or the risk thereof' includes any process variation for which a recurrence would carry a significant chance of a serious adverse outcome."[40] The expectation is that the organization will conduct a timely, thorough, and credible root cause analysis (RCA) in response to a sentinel event, develop and implement an action plan to reduce the risk of recurrence, and monitor the effectiveness of the plan and its implementation. An RCA can also be conducted on events other than sentinel events, such as when a trend of similar precursor or near-miss events is identified.

GOAL OF ROOT CAUSE ANALYSIS

The goal of the RCA is to investigate the event in such detail that the true root cause(s) of the event are identified. This requires that the team completes a thorough analysis that includes reviewing the human errors and processes that may contribute to the event. An action plan should be developed with the intent of preventing the recurrence with certainty. Risk reduction strategies such as reeducating the department, asking staff to be more careful, and developing or editing a policy and procedure have been the norm for years. It is now recognized that these are weak action plans that are not able to prevent recurrence without some change to the processes. The concepts of mistake-proofing, standardization, and forcing functions are important considerations in the development of risk reduction strategies. Taking an action that physically prevents something from happening is the most effective method of preventing an inadvertent action—such as requiring the foot to be placed on the brake before placing a car in reverse. Another example of a forcing function is when a computer program requires confirmation to delete a file—it prevents inadvertent deletion. An example of a fail-safe is when a garage door will not continue to close if any motion is detected that interferes with the operation of the door.

One of the key challenges in completing a quality RCA is adequate training and coordinating time for front-line staff and management team members (e.g., physicians, vice presidents) to attend the meetings. One strategy is to have predetermined times designated for team meeting use if and when an RCA is indicated. This ensures that those with busy schedules have adequate time allotted for this most vital activity. A second key in preventing recurrence is monitoring the action plan to ensure that it is implemented in a timely and effective fashion. Measures should be defined as part of the action plan and revisited to assess the implementation and effectiveness of the action plan. Lastly, it is important to the continued development of a safety culture to be transparent within the organization (and between organizations who are a part of a system) about the lessons learned from events. Information about the event and the action plan should be shared within the facility through structured meetings and communications—all the way to the staff level. The last thing anyone wants is to restructure processes in one area of a facility and not translate the lessons learned to other applicable areas of the facility.

FAILURE MODE AND EFFECTS ANALYSIS

While RCA is a retrospective process, the use of FMEA is a prospective process that is required annually by TJC. This type of analysis involves a team that takes an issue that has been identified as a potentially risky process and examines the ways in which the process or product might fail. An FMEA can be done prior to implementation of a new process or technology in an effort to increase the awareness of how the implementation might fail, before it occurs. This allows the implementation team to take adequate steps before the new product or process is introduced to avoid failures. In an FMEA, each step of the process is outlined, the team brainstorms all the ways in which the process could fail, and defines the effect of each potential failure to the end user (often the patient). An estimation (on a 10-point scale) is made of the likelihood of the failure, the severity of the potential failure, and the probability that the failure will be detected. A criticality index is calculated and those failure modes with the highest scores are prioritized as important steps for which barriers are developed. Generally, an action plan to reduce risk within the process is developed, implemented, and monitored.

Case Study 18-1

At your institution, there have been seven significant errors with Lantus® insulin in the past three months. Fortunately no serious harm occurred, however transfer to higher level of care and treatment was required for all seven cases. It has been determined that you will combine information from all of the known cases and conduct an aggregate RCA.

An aggregate RCA[41,42] provides intense scrutiny of the cases to determine what opportunities exist to decrease the rate of the extravasations.

- *What are the advantages and disadvantages of including multiple cases in the RCA process?*

To Err Is Human

As long as human beings are a key component of processes such as the medication use process, errors are inevitable. Therefore, there exists a need for redundancies and incorporation of human factors principles as key elements to more reliable processes, preventing errors from reaching the patient.

When (not if) humans make errors, there are several ways to approach the event. ❺ *Human beings (including health care professionals of all types) have a propensity to commit errors in all aspects of their lives. To err is human.* Being human, health care professionals of all types have a propensity to commit errors in every area of their personal and professional lives, including the medication use process. One approach to error management places emphasis on the individuals involved, which generally implies blame. This approach generally puts the blame on the last person touching the patient, and does not usually acknowledge other factors contributing to the error. As a result, people are urged to be more careful, pay more attention, and undergo remedial training. It also results in increased supervision and increased detail within policies and procedures. It is thought that if people are more vigilant, the number of errors will be reduced.[43] The other approach focuses on how the design of objects (e.g., smart pumps, drug names, labels for medications, connectors for IVs, and tube feedings), activities, and procedures (programming a pump that is infrequently used) contributes to the actions and behaviors of individuals. This approach believes that people come to work with good intentions, are skilled and experienced, but may be led to commit errors because of the way in which the design of the system shapes their behaviors.

According to Senders,[44] "An error is a psychological event with psychological causes...." Human error is inevitable; rather a fact of life. Most human error results in little to no consequence. It occurs regardless of occupation, although the consequences vary significantly depending on the specific occupation. Therefore an error in medicine can be fatal, as can an error in the airline industry.

To better understand why health care professionals commit errors, it is necessary to look at the cognitive processes that occur at the time of the error. Norman and Reason have written wonderful books reflecting philosophies of human error.[45-47] Humans will most likely commit errors at an unacceptable rate despite best efforts to understand and remedy the occurrence. With this in mind, it is necessary to develop systems of medication use that account for human error and have processes in place to identify and correct human error before medications reach patients.

THREE MODES OF HUMAN PERFORMANCE

⑥ *Understanding the three modes of human performance (skill based, rule based, and knowledge based) is very important to understanding errors and events, and in developing appropriate strategies to reduce the risks of recurrence.*

- **Skill-based human performance:** When in skill-based level of performance, humans are doing very routine tasks that are very practiced and automatic. People are very good at these tasks, as they do them all the time. In skill-based mode, a decision has been made on what the intended action is and the individuals are now in the process of executing a task. Activities such as eating or driving a car to work fit into this category. These are effortless and really unconscious activities that do not require much thought or attention. Skill-based errors are termed slips, lapses, or fumbles.[46] They are easily identified. Slips are usually associated with attention or perception failures and lapses generally involve memory failures.
  - When a person places the cereal in the refrigerator instead of the milk, this is an example of a slip. The task is something people do all the time successfully but for some reason they err. Perhaps he or she was briefly interrupted by children or the dog and unconsciously reached for the wrong container.
  - An example of a lapse might be when a person walks into a room only to say— "Now why did I come in here?".
  - If the milk is accidentally knocked over while in the process of putting it back into the refrigerator, a fumble has occurred.
- **Rule-based human performance:** Humans perform in rule-based mode when problem solving or making decisions. Perhaps there has been a change in the situation—like an exit is closed on the usual route to work and it is necessary to choose an alternate route. The person begins to problem solve, realizing that he or she has been in this situation before. People are trained to deal with many situations; perhaps by learning a policy or procedure. It is possible to determine which rule to apply to the situation encountered. This is called an if-then scenario—if this situation, then do this action. Several scenarios can occur:
  - A wrong rule may be chosen because one misperceives the situation and applies the wrong rule.
  - If one misapplies a rule, a rule-based error has occurred. It is possible to unconsciously pull the wrong pattern or rule from memory. Memory may be

biased for many reasons: overgeneralization, recent occurrences (causing one to choose the first answer that comes to mind—despite available evidence that would lead us to another conclusion), or other factors.

○ There is also intentional rule-based noncompliance (with defined policies and procedures) in which an individual chooses an action despite the knowledge that they should take a different action (e.g., a nurse administers a medication without checking the patient's arm band because he or she is sleeping soundly or the barcode reader is not conveniently located).[46]

• **Knowledge-based human performance:** The other decision-making type is knowledge-based mode. Knowledge-based errors occur when the individual is in a situation to which he or she has never been exposed, or has no preprogrammed rules to apply. The person has a lack of required knowledge to complete the task, or has possibly misinterpreted the problem. When in knowledge-based mode, people are much more likely to make an error than when in skill-based or rule-based mode. The best scenario is that the person recognizes that he or she is lacking the information needed and takes the time to consult with other sources (e.g., colleagues, texts, policies, literature) to determine the next course of action. Oftentimes, humans feel pressured to proceed in the face of uncertainty, because of perceived time constraints, to avoid acknowledging lack of knowledge to complete the task, or because of overconfidence. The worst-case scenario is that an individual does not realize he or she is in knowledge-based mode, has misinterpreted the situation, and proceeds without any question. "You don't know what you don't know" is a representative phrase in this situation.

CONFIRMATION BIAS

One very common type of human error is called confirmation bias. Confirmation bias refers to a type of selective thinking where individuals select what is familiar to them or what they expect to see, rather than what is actually there. A similar type of error is inattentional blindness. Inattentional blindness occurs when the person is so focused on performing the assigned task that he or she fails to see an error or change right in front of his or her eyes, which should have been plainly visible, and cannot explain the lapse. In many cases, people involved in the errors have been labeled as careless and negligent. It is human nature for people to associate items by certain characteristics, for example, color of vial, cap, or text. It is very important for the health care community to recognize the role that confirmation bias may play in medication errors and to work to develop systems with the understanding that this phenomenon exists and is part of natural human behavior. These types of accidents are common—even with intelligent, vigilant, and attentive people.[48] Attempts to combat these errors are difficult. Paying more attention is not effective. The use of barcoding has increasingly been used to avoid this phenomenon.

System Error

❼ *Poorly designed health care systems and processes are a significant contributor to individual human error and subsequent patient harm.* Interestingly enough, behind the majority of individual human errors, one or more system errors exist that contributed to the human error. Therefore, it is of utmost importance to recognize system errors and gaps when developing prevention strategies. Systems have common characteristics—these generally include technology, tools and machines, interfaces, processes, products, user interaction with the system, and people. The health care system has become, and continues to become, very complex. There are many layers and components to the health care system: individual practitioners, teams working together, policies and procedures (generally for each individual entity), regulations, devices and equipment, communications, leadership, and management. It would be optimal if all of the parts of the system were integrated and had seamless communication and coordination, but that is not the case. They are each managed separately and are likely to have their own culture, that is, common goals, values, beliefs, and behaviors. It is rare that each component of the system has similar cultures, even when speaking of departments or units within an organization, such as the patient-care areas of a hospital.[40] It is clear that the development and management of systems and processes has a direct link to the actions of individuals. According to TJC's analysis of multiple sentinel events,[49] ineffective communication contributes to a significant number of adverse outcomes (60% to 70%). Optimization of systems and processes is essential to optimization of health care safety. This section discusses system failures that contribute to error that must be identified and corrected to provide safe care.

LATENT FAILURE

A latent failure is a weakness that is usually unconsciously built into a system or, more commonly, develops over time. When making decisions about processes, it is not uncommon that the solution to one problem actually creates a problem in another part of the system (i.e., an unanticipated consequence). One example: if barcoding medication administration technology using computers on wheeled carts is purchased to prevent administration errors, yet there are not adequate outlets or batteries to keep the computer charged, nurses are faced with skipping the scanning step, finding another computer, or rebooting the computer. The latter two options delay the patient's medication—perhaps only 5 to 10 minutes. However, when a patient is in severe pain, the nurse has been placed in a situation where it seems better to give the medication in a timely fashion and then scan once a viable computer is found. These gaps are inevitable and usually lie relatively undetected. They may appear periodically in a near-miss event, where the error slips through several points, but is caught by one last stop-gap (a good catch). If organizations do not learn from the near misses, it is quite possible that eventually the same gaps will result in an adverse event.

UNDERSTANDING SYSTEM DESIGN

When an analysis, such as an RCA is undertaken, a thorough understanding of how the system is designed (what are the defined policies and procedures) and how it actually functions (include staff in the RCA or go to the location and observe the process) is very important. When designing an action plan, include more than just actions taken with individuals (e.g., peer review, disciplinary action). A good action plan should address the gaps that were found in the system with prevention strategies to prevent the identified causes. If during a code, nursing staff pulled the wrong drug from the crash cart and it was determined that not all crash carts had the same contents and the medication labels were not readily visible, the medications were combined with other supplies, and the contents were in different drawers depending on what unit the cart was found, blaming the staff for not reading the label will not effectively prevent the next person from having similar difficulties finding the correct medication. Address the system and process issues that contributed to the human error. Appropriate to the findings of the investigation, the action plan may include standardization of the carts, with the same drugs found in the same place regardless of cart location, placement of dosing charts in the cart to avoid calculation errors, positioning of pharmacists to pull and prepare medications, or other action to address the true causes of the error.

Case Study 18–2

A pharmacist is staffing the surgery satellite alone, entering postoperative orders for Sue Doe. She is interrupted by a nurse caring for a different postoperative patient Janie Snow from earlier in the day who has a question about her patient's orders. The pharmacist can only view one patient's profile at a time so she pulls up the computer profile to answer a question about Janie Snow. When the pharmacist returned to her original task of entering the orders for Sue Doe, she inadvertently entered them on the wrong patient. It was determined that there is a system that automatically links the scanned order page to the correct patient, but the current version of computer software does not support this process.

Discussion Question: Debate and discussion often ensues over whether it is possible to eliminate all errors, eliminate all harm events, or eliminate preventable harm events. Think about human nature and system design. Designate two groups to review the literature around this topic paying specific attention to human error science and system design science (mistake-proofing and similar topics). Then facilitate a discussion around the following questions:

- *Is it possible to eliminate all errors? What should be the goal? No errors? No events of harm? No preventable harm?*
- *What questions would you like to ask the pharmacist involved in the error as part of an interview?*
- *Would you classify this error as human-error only, system-error only, or a combination of both and why?*

A Just Culture—Not Shame and Blame

In some instances, reporting medication errors, particularly severe or life-threatening errors, have had adverse consequences for both individuals and the organizations involved. Health care professionals have lost their jobs or voluntarily resigned from their jobs and, at times, have left their profession. Consequently, health care professionals and health systems have been reluctant to open themselves up to adverse outcomes associated with reporting medication errors.[50] For example, in one hospital there were only 36 incident reports regarding medication errors over a yearlong reporting period. At the same institution, an observational study revealed that as many as 51,200 errors were likely to have actually occurred during that same reporting period.[51]

Hindsight bias often plays a role in the way people react to an error. Hindsight bias is the inclination to see events that have occurred as being more predictable than they were before the event took place. In other words, the person should have known that this would be the outcome. It is very easy to examine the information after the event and conclude that of course this bad outcome was going to occur. What investigators and facilitators do not have the benefit of is the vast number of exact circumstances and choices that the individual was facing, along with their thought processes that led them to their conclusions.

In Nevada, a pharmacy was fined two weeks' net profit for a dispensing error that resulted from understaffing.[49] A medical center in New Jersey was successfully sued for $12 million and fined by the state board of pharmacy after a medication error killed an infant.[52] In 1996, a medication error occurred in a hospital in Colorado that resulted in the death of a newborn infant. Three nurses involved in the infant's care were indicted on charges of criminally negligent homicide.[53] District attorneys in Colorado pressed criminal charges that could have resulted in three to five years imprisonment. A pharmacist in Ohio was indicted and jailed for a chemotherapy error resulting in the death of a young patient.[54] In these cases, there were underlying system concerns that likely contributed to the event. Without resolution of these system issues, a similar event may occur with a different clinician. These cases reiterate the need to identify root causes to prevent recurrence.

DEFINITION OF JUST CULTURE

Learning from errors, events, and near misses is vital to improvement. Despite the negative actions that have been taken against individuals and organizations in the past, the health care culture is evolving toward a culture of safety. Leaders are learning more about **Just Culture**. Just Culture is a culture in which discipline is applied in a consistent manner based on the intentions of the individual and the circumstances in which they were working—not the outcome. One must understand the circumstances (including poorly designed systems) in which errors occur before decisions related to discipline are made. If a system sets up one individual to fail, the next person in the same situation is also likely to fail in the same manner as the first. If the system is not specifically designed to avert likely human errors (no double check of a high-risk calculation, such as chemotherapy), human errors will continue to reach patients with significant potential for harm.

Action plans to prevent recurrence of an event should be designed according to the type of error(s) made. It does not make sense to retrain someone in a procedure if they are very skilled, were distracted by a colleague, and made a skill-based error. Similarly if a knowledge-based error is identified, working to decrease distractions and interruptions will have little impact on decreasing future repeat errors with the activity. When interviewing individuals involved in errors, be sure to ask them to describe what happened and what else was going on at the time, ask them to walk through their decision-making process, and find out why they think the event occurred. Be sure to understand the options presented to them at the time.

Recall those headlines again—Child Dies from Medication Error, Journalist Dies of Chemotherapy Error.... The rest of the story usually involves details about what happened (on the surface) and who was fired or reprimanded. What disciplinary action should be taken in these cases—if any? It depends on the circumstances entirely. It is important to have a good understanding of exactly what happened and the "whys" behind the decisions and actions taken. If an individual did not consciously make an unsafe decision, how does discipline help one learn from mistakes? Will not staff be less willing to report and discuss them without fear of retribution? Retraining, counseling, and discipline have been hallmark actions taken to prevent error and have failed to substantially improve patient care.

The culture of blame shifted in the 1990s in the health care industry when it was recognized that the punitive nature of discipline was not the best way to encourage staff to talk about risks and errors, and assist in the process of decreasing errors. The culture then shifted to a blame-free culture in an effort to promote reporting. This culture recognized that humans will err, that most unsafe acts are slips or lapses, and that weaknesses in systems and environments contribute significantly to errors in medicine.[55]

What was not recognized at the time was that a solely blame-free culture (also termed nonpunitive) failed to attend to those few who knowingly ignore designated safety procedures and those who are unreasonably reckless or negligent. This undermines those who work hard at providing safe care.

8 *A Just Culture is one in which discipline is applied in a consistent manner based on the intentions of the individual and the situation in which they were working—not the outcome.* A Just Culture is somewhere between the two extremes described above, with blaming individuals on one end, blame-free culture on the other end, and a Just Culture somewhere in the middle. It is unacceptable to discipline all errors regardless of their circumstances, and is just as unacceptable to be nonpunitive in the face of individuals who are intentionally ignoring safe operating principles.

The hard part is distinguishing between those who make a conscious decision to complete an unsafe action, despite knowledge that it is unsafe (i.e., at-risk behavior), and those who usually work in a safe manner and experienced a slip or lapse. The use of a substitution test has proven to be useful in these instances.[47] When dealing with a serious event and a person is implicated in an unsafe act, describe the scenario to several other individuals (at least three) of the same qualifications and experience (optimally, who are not aware of the actual incident) and ask them in the circumstances at the time, what decisions they would have made. If they would have made the same decision and completed the same actions, then blaming the individual is not likely appropriate as there is evidence that this issue has a larger scope. Another option is to observe individuals in the same situations, if possible, to determine how others behave in similar instances. This helps one determine whether the problem may lie with an individual, an expanded group (perhaps a unit or department), or is a more global problem. This also helps in the development of an action plan. There is no need to reeducate an entire department on a process, if there is only one individual that is in need of coaching.

The use of a series of questions helps determine the culpability and accountability of a person's actions and are taken from the Decision Tree for determining the Culpability of Unsafe Acts.[47] Appropriate discipline, when warranted, should be taken when unsafe behaviors are identified, regardless of the outcome.[56]

1. Were the actions as intended?
2. Was the person under the influence of unauthorized substances?
3. Did he or she knowingly violate a safe operating procedure? If so, was the procedure available, workable, intelligible, and correct? This gets at those procedures that staff feel make no sense and are not value-added in their workflow. Perhaps they have a point and there is a component of system-induced error.
4. Do they pass the substitution test described above? Would others have made the same decisions and, if so, less likely to be culpable? If not, were there deficiencies in training or experience?
5. Does the individual have a history of unsafe acts? If not, again less likely to be culpable.

The use of these questions should be used to assist in determining the level of culpability of an individual. The actions in the first few questions bear more culpability than those that occur in the last several questions. Therefore, disciplinary actions are more likely to be appropriate for those acts that are intended and/or undertaken while under the influence of unauthorized substances.

There are always a few outliers within any profession; those who intentionally do not follow the processes as designed, feeling that they are immune from human error and/or believing their process is better. There is a difference between unintentional human error, at-risk behavior, and reckless behavior. Intentionally unsafe behavior is identified by the first question and is generally dealt with through disciplinary action. At-risk behavior may be amenable to coaching about the reason for the process as designed and a request to commit to better choices.

Case Study 18–3

Patient Samuel Sneer received an overdose of a diltiazem drip and became hypotensive, requiring fluid boluses, but recovered without further effects. After further investigation, it was discovered that the nurse changed the diltiazem bag as it was nearly empty. The pump required the nurse to enter the concentration (drug in milligrams and then volume of fluid). Instead of entering the drug dose first, she mistakenly entered the fluid volume first. This is the way the concentration information appeared on the labeled bag, which was to what she was referring.

The nurse was under time pressure and was caring for more patients than the usually accepted ratio due to the flu epidemic. The pump has programmed minimum and maximum settings, and the rate was just over the maximum setting, meaning she received a warning about the error and overrode it. This is the first error identified for this nurse who has practiced here for over a year.

- *What system issues contributed to the error?*
- *Walk the error through the Just Culture algorithm to determine your reaction as manager of the unit (coaching, consoling, or disciplinary action).*
- *What potential system fixes can you identify?*

Risk Factors for Errors and Events

The ultimate purpose for defining, classifying, analyzing, and reporting medication errors is to enable individuals and organizations to implement better systems that prevent medication errors. The ASHP has identified a multitude of risk factors associated with the occurrence of medication errors as outlined below.[34]

- Shift work—switching from days to nights or vice versa
- Inexperienced or inadequately trained staff
- Medical services with special needs (e.g., pediatrics and oncology)
- Higher number of medications per patient
- Environmental factors such as high levels of noise, poor lighting, and frequent interruptions
- High workload for staff
- Poor communication among health care providers
- Dosage form—more errors with injectable drugs
- Drug category—more errors with certain classes of drugs (e.g., antibiotics)
- Type of drug distribution systems—unit dose system is associated with fewer errors; high levels of floor stock are associated with increased errors
- Improper drug storage
- Calculations—increased errors with increased complexity and frequency of amount of calculations required
- Poor handwriting
- Verbal orders

- Lack of effective policies and procedures
- Poorly functioning oversight committees

Personal and environmental factors are thought to interact to influence cognitive function that may lead to slips. There are several factors specific to the professional involved and their working environment that may contribute to their risk of committing an error. Grasha and O'Neill[57] have outlined some of the factors that may affect cognitive processes, resulting in lapses of performance.

1. **Excessive task demand:** Many clinicians attribute their errors to this situation, complaining that their workload is so heavy and they are overloaded with tasks, making it difficult to work error free. In one survey, 68% of pharmacists rated work overload as a major contributing factor to the committal of dispensing errors.[58] Most pharmacists and experts in medication errors agree that work overload may be the most significant factor contributing to medication errors. Reevaluation of the workload distribution, with an eye for streamlining processes, may be valuable. Developing a detailed map of all of the steps required to accomplish a task is one way to discover the complexity of a task. This is called **process mapping.**

2. **Personal characteristics:** Personal factors, such as age, sensory deficits, or state of health, may contribute to performance lapses. Personal levels of stress or fatigue may also have an impact. Someone who is bored at work may be more error prone.

3. **Extraorganizational factors:** Factors, such as similar product names or packaging from pharmaceutical companies, may have an extensive impact on the commission of errors with particular drugs. In one study, look-alike or sound-alike drugs were involved in 37% of medication errors.[59] As an example, this issue is currently being addressed for the sound-alike drugs celecoxib (Celebrex®), fosphenytoin (Cerebyx®), and citalopram (Celexa®). Complex insurance plans are also extraorganizational factors that may serve to complicate the medication use process and contribute to slips. The profession of pharmacy has been referred to as the most heavily regulated of all professions. Legal mandates for policing illegal prescriptions and other regulatory requirements are also good examples of extraorganizational factors.

4. **Work environment:** Poor working conditions may influence the rate of error committal. Poor illumination and high noise levels have been shown to affect the dispensing error rate in pharmacies.[60] Other factors in this category may include high ambient temperatures and frequent interruptions from the telephone or patients.

5. **Intraorganizational factors:** There is a significant emphasis on other factors besides the quality and safety of medication use within health care systems. Concerns related to finances, throughput, customer service, and quality of employee

work life are often competing priorities and major areas of focus in many institutions. Policies and procedures demanding high output or mandating long working hours may significantly affect cognition and the ability to prevent error occurrence.

6. **Interpersonal factors:** Conflicts among coworkers or with patients may distract professionals from the tasks at hand and contribute to error commission. General interruptions from people may also fall into this category.

Some factors that may contribute to cognitive lapses and the commission of medication errors may fall into more than one of these categories. Furthermore, factors from multiple categories may occur simultaneously to contribute to error commission.

Health care professionals have indicated that other factors may also contribute to medication errors. Some of those factors are as follows:

1. **Lack of effective communication:** This factor may also fall under interpersonal factors listed above. Failure to communicate effectively among fellow employees or among health care professionals has frequently been named as contributing to medical and medication errors. For example, an error may be more likely to occur if a pharmacist chooses not to clarify physician orders, or if the pharmacist does not communicate all of the pertinent information so the physician can make an informed decision. Poor physician handwriting and verbal orders are also significant contributing factors.[36]

2. **Failure to comply with policy:** This is a common factor in dispensing and administering drugs. In one survey, 42% to 46% of pharmacists said that failing to check drugs before dispensing was a significant factor in dispensing errors.[58] Noncompliance with policy has also been associated with drug administration errors and is the result of several factors: perceived burden of the task, perceived risk of a bad outcome, and the perceived risk of being observed. Often, nurses develop specific personal routines for administration of certain agents, which they perceive to be an improvement in the medication administration process, despite contrary policy.[36] It is important to understand the challenges that make work difficult. Assure that processes have been designed with safety in mind.

3. **Lack of knowledge:** This is a frequently cited factor in the committal of medication errors. Mistakes, rather than slips, are typically committed as a result of inadequate knowledge. Placing inexperienced recent graduates in positions where they cannot interact with more experienced practitioners may increase medication errors. Nonspecialists covering a service that is normally staffed by a specialist may also lead to errors.[60] Nurses with less exposure to pharmacology may be less likely to recognize potential inconsistencies in disease state and medication usage and doses, resulting in the possibility of increased medication errors reaching the patient.[36]

4. **Lack of patient counseling:** The last safety check prior to dispensing medication should be counseling the patient. Talking to the patient allows the pharmacist to correlate the medication and dose with the patient's condition and helps the pharmacist to detect any errors that may have occurred in the medication use process. In one study, 89% of errors committed in a community pharmacy were detected during patient counseling.[50] However, errors may occur not only from a lack of counseling, but also from providing incorrect information during patient counseling.[61] Providing incorrect information may also fall in the lack of knowledge category. One additional factor that plays a major part in understanding the patient is health care literacy. All professionals should assess the level of patient literacy to assure that appropriate language and teaching methods are used in their interactions with the patient.

The examples provided above are a partial list of contributory factors at the level of the health care practitioner. These factors influence the occurrence of slips or performance lapses and mistakes committed by individuals. They do not address failure of a system or failure of a safety net as a whole process. The medication use process involves multiple health care professionals, nonprofessional staff, patients, and multiple physical environments. To adequately address the causes of errors, failures in the system must be addressed. Although, it is important to address the problem of individuals committing errors (e.g., increasing training if a knowledge deficit was identified and enforcing policy), adequately developed safety systems should be in place to significantly minimize the number of errors reaching patients.

Health Professions Education

Most health care professionals are trained with the thought that individuals cannot make mistakes in health care; when dealing with patients, it is unacceptable to cause an error. Students, as well as practicing professionals (e.g., physicians, nurses, pharmacists, respiratory therapists) learn little about human factors thinking, systems design, quality improvement, and reliability. They do not learn that humans err in many ways. Thus, when they do make an error in practice, many either deny the fact or are jolted into the realization that they should be more careful and develop reliable habits. Many times, the realization that they have made an error causes physicians, pharmacists, nurses, and other professionals to avoid discussion about errors—with colleagues and patients. When an error or safety event is investigated and analyzed, individuals and/or professions may point fingers at the other, some may avoid telling the whole story, some do not realize the value of the process, and many do not recognize the contribution that processes and systems play in their own errors. Many of the Institute of Medicine reports on quality and safety have referenced the need for changes in health professions education. Pertinent quotes from "To Err is Human: Building a Safer Health System"[1] include:

> "Clinical training and education is a key mechanism for cultural change. Colleges of medicine, nursing, pharmacy, health care administration, and their related associations should build more instruction into their curriculum on patient safety and its relationship to quality improvement."
>
> "Many believe that initial exposure to patient safety should occur early in undergraduate and graduate training programs, as well as through continuing education."
>
> "The need for more opportunities for interdisciplinary training was also identified. Most care delivered today is done by teams of people, yet training often remains focused on individual responsibilities leaving practitioners inadequately prepared to enter complex settings."

Another report by the Institute of Medicine, "Crossing the Quality Chasm,"[62] identified health professions education as a priority.

Subsequently, a summit of over 150 interdisciplinary participants met in 2002 and developed recommendations for reaching this goal. The proceedings and recommendations from the summit are compiled in "Health Professions Education: A Bridge to Quality."[63] This committee developed the following vision statement:

❾ *"All health professionals should be educated to deliver patient-centered care as members of an interdisciplinary team, emphasizing evidence-based practice, quality improvement approaches, and informatics."*

The following strategies are outlined in the book:

- Develop and build consensus around a common language and core competencies.
- Integrate core competencies into oversight processes.
- Motivate and support leaders, and monitor progress of reform effort.
- Develop evidence-based curricula and teaching approaches.
- Develop faculty as teaching and learning experts.

The IHI has developed an interprofessional, international educational online community. The IHI Open School provides a mechanism by which students and their mentors in nursing, medicine, pharmacy, dentistry, health care administration, and other health care professions can interact and learn in an interdisciplinary fashion. There are online courses in quality and safety, basic and advanced certifications in quality improvement and patient safety, case studies, podcasts, videos, and feature articles. The IHI's Open School program[64] is one example where online modules on quality and safety can be completed either during professional education or as a part of continuing education and learning for practitioners. See http://www.ihi.org for additional information. This is a great start to providing the types of interdisciplinary learning that will be of great value to the health care community and patients.

Best Practices for Error Prevention

❿ *There are many resources that identify best practice error prevention strategies.* Listed here are various resources as well as strategies to assure medication use processes are as safe as they can be. Commit to be a learning organization by constantly reviewing local and national information and taking proactive steps to prevent error. Do not wait until it happens to you.

The Institute for Safe Medication Practices publishes a "Quarterly Action Agenda" that describes known risks and errors and describes recommendations for risk reduction strategy implementation. These can be found on the website at http://www.ismp.org.

The Institute for Healthcare Improvement has sponsored several campaigns (The 100,000 Lives Campaign and the 5 Million Lives Campaign) to save lives and protect patients from harm. At least half of the 12 recommended interventions within the two campaigns involve improving the safe use of medications. Pharmacists should be integrally involved in the institution team to assure successful interventions (See Table 18-5). In addition to these two campaigns, the IHI offers many programs, conferences, IMPACT network associations, best practice postings, the IHI Open School, and much more. Visit http://www.ihi.org for more information.

The Joint Commission's National Patient Safety Goals can serve as a guide to improving the safety of health care. Many of TJC's National Patient Safety Goals released each year are related to safe medication use and pharmacists should be involved in assuring that the facility meets these goals. They are divided into the type of health care provided—hospital, home care, ambulatory care, behavioral health care, etc. There are other goals aside from those listed, some of which indirectly relate to pharmacy. These goals change frequently. A partial list includes:

- Accurately and completely reconcile medications during transitions within and across organizations (inpatient to outpatient).
- Improve the effectiveness of communication between caregivers.
  - Write down and read back verbal orders (and critical test results)—TJC safety goal sets the expectation that for all verbal orders, the receiver of the order must write the order down on the order page and then read the transcribed order back to the practitioner, who then verifies that the order has been transcribed as intended.

TABLE 18–5. INTERVENTIONS RECOMMENDED BY THE INSTITUTE FOR HEALTHCARE IMPROVEMENT (IHI) TO SAVE LIVES AND REDUCE PATIENT INJURIES[65]

Strategies from the 100,000 Lives Campaign

- **Deploy rapid response teams**...at the first sign of patient decline
- **Deliver reliable, evidence-based care for acute myocardial infarction**...to prevent deaths from heart attack
- **Prevent adverse drug events (ADEs)**...by implementing medication reconciliation
- **Prevent central line infections**...by implementing a series of interdependent, scientifically grounded steps
- **Prevent surgical site infections**...by reliably delivering the correct perioperative antibiotics at the proper time
- **Prevent ventilator-associated pneumonia**...by implementing a series of interdependent, scientifically grounded steps

Strategies from the 5 Million Lives Campaign

- **Prevent harm from high-alert medications**...starting with a focus on anticoagulants, sedatives, narcotics, and insulin
- **Reduce surgical complications**...by reliably implementing all of the changes recommended by SCIP, the Surgical Care Improvement Project
- **Prevent pressure ulcers**...by reliably using science-based guidelines for their prevention
- **Reduce methicillin-resistant *Staphylococcus aureus* (MRSA) infection**...by reliably implementing scientifically proven infection control practices
- **Deliver reliable, evidence-based care for heart failure**...to avoid readmissions
- **Get boards on board**...by defining and spreading the best-known leveraged processes for hospital boards of directors, so that they can become far more effective in accelerating organizational progress toward safe care

This prevents transcription errors in which the receiver may have heard the order correctly and made an error in writing/entering the order after the conversation has ended and prevents errors in which the order was heard and transcribed incorrectly. This is also referred to as closed-loop communication in which the giver and recipient confirm that the information provided and received is accurate.
  ◦ Designate unapproved abbreviations and monitor their use.
- Implement a standardized approach to handoff communications, including an opportunity to ask and respond to questions.
- Improve the safety of using medications.
  ◦ Develop risk reduction strategies around look-alike and sound-alike medications such as the use of tall man letters to draw attention to differences in similar drug names such as DAUNOrubicin and DOXOrubicin.
  ◦ Label all medications, medication containers (e.g., syringes, medicine cups, basins), or other solutions on and off the sterile field.
- Reduce the likelihood of patient harm associated with the use of anticoagulant therapy.
  ◦ Includes an anticoagulation management program, approved protocols for initiation and maintenance, individualized care, appropriate baseline and ongoing lab monitoring.

○ Includes notification and involvement of the dietary department, patient education, use of infusion pumps for heparin, and evaluation of anticoagulation safety.
- Implement best practices for preventing surgical site infections. Timely administration of appropriately chosen antibiotics just prior to the surgical procedure is essential to preventing surgical site infections. Most preoperative antibiotics must be given within 1 hour prior to the incision time. There are many errors that may contribute to the development of infection at the surgical site: lack of timely access to the medication, incorrect medication selection, or administration of the drug too early. At one time, the preoperative antibiotic was administered on the patient care unit before transporting the patient to the operating room, however, there are often delays in getting the patient to the operating room.

● Consult TJC website for the most up-to-date standards (http://www.jointcommission. org/standards_information/npsgs.aspx).

● **The National Quality Forum's (NQF) Safe Practices for Better Healthcare** identifies 34 practices that have been demonstrated to be effective in reducing the occurrence of adverse events in health care. While two best practices have been identified within a chapter titled Improving Patient Safety Through Medication Management, many of the other Safe Practices involve medication use. The Safe Practices associated with this chapter are as follows:

- Medication reconciliation—Many adverse events are the result of patients presenting to an acute care facility such as a hospital, identifying a list of the medications that are taking at home, yet somewhere during the admission, transfer, or discharge process, these medications are inadvertently omitted or duplicate therapy occurs due to therapeutic substitution at discharge. The organization must develop a process to identify, reconcile (compare and confirm which medications are appropriate for the patient to take during the hospitalization or outpatient visit), and communicate an accurate patient medication list throughout the continuum of care (to other primary care and specialist providers).
- Pharmacist leadership structure—Pharmacy leaders should have an active role on the administrative leadership team that identifies their accountability for the performance of the medication management systems across the institution.

Other Safe Practices which relate to medication use include:

- Improving patient safety by creating and sustaining a culture of safety.
    ○ The elements of this safe practice include leadership structures and systems, culture measurement and intervention, teamwork training, and identification and mitigation of risks and hazards.

- Improving patient safety by facilitating information transfer and clear communication.
  - Elements of this chapter include communication of critical information, order read-back, safe adoption of CPOE, and avoiding unapproved abbreviations. Each organization must define a list of unapproved abbreviations, monitor the frequency of use, and develop strategies to reduce the use of these abbreviations. Several high-risk abbreviations have been identified (by ISMP and other organizations) such as MSO_4 and $MgSO_4$ which may be inadvertently misread and administered causing harm to patients and U (for units) which has been misinterpreted as a zero, causing 10-fold overdoses of insulin.
- Improving patient safety through prevention of health care-associated infections.
  - This chapter includes practices around aspiration and ventilator-associated pneumonia (VAP) prevention, surgical site infection prevention, multidrug-resistant organism prevention, hand hygiene, and influenza prevention through administration of appropriate vaccines to all qualified patients. Administration of appropriate antibiotic prophylaxis in a timely manner is a key prevention strategy for surgical site infections.
- Improving patient safety through condition and site-specific practices.
  - This grouping includes perioperative myocardial infarction and ischemia prevention, venous thromboembolism prevention, anticoagulation therapy, and contrast media-induced renal failure prevention.

Many of the practices involve medication use and pharmacy should be integrally involved in efforts to meet these goals. Visit the website for the latest version (http://www. qualityforum.org/Publications/2014/02/NQF_safe_practices_and_related_processes. aspx). These two resources combined create a great roadmap for working toward safer medication use systems.

Incorporate human factors principles into the design of processes. ⓫ *Researching, recognizing, and designing with human factors principles in mind is a great way to improve the safety of any process.* Human factors research is a developing type of research in health care, where other industries have developed strategies around human factors to successfully improve the safety (e.g., nuclear power, air travel). Some of the core principles of human factors design include the following:

- Simplify and standardize—A process that requires a policy and procedure of 20 pages is one that is much too complex.
- Reduce reliance on memory—The human mind can only hold a limited amount of things in short-term memory (four to seven items depending on what source is read). Therefore formulating other methods of prioritization or reminders is likely to be more effective than relying on recall of individuals.

- Use constraints and forcing functions—Mistake-proofing is the use of process or design features to prevent errors or the negative impact of errors. Mistake-proofing is also known as *poka-yoke* (pronounced *pokayokay*), Japanese slang for avoiding inadvertent errors.[66] One great example is the file cabinet. Tons of papers are stored in file cabinets. An example is when one file drawer, and then a second drawer, is opened, which may cause the entire cabinet falling over. If more than one file drawer is opened at a time, the center of gravity moves, causing the file cabinet to fall. Modern file cabinets are designed to avoid this type of injury, as opening one drawer locks the rest. The design forces correct behavior and only allows for proper use. It takes longer to file, but it prevents injury. Several approaches to mistake-proofing include mistake prevention, mistake detection, and reduction of the effect of user errors.
- Improve information access—Coordination and interfacing computer systems is a huge challenge, but is often the only way to assure that all information is available to those who need it.
- Decrease reliance on vigilance—Humans will err; therefore other mechanisms to prevent errors from reaching the patient are much more effective than asking people to be careful. They may be more vigilant for a brief time, and then revert back to previous habits.
- Increase feedback—Feedback (of actions taken and processes improved as a result of reported events) to reporters, end-users, and management staff is critical to the development of a safety culture. At times, staff report errors and never see any changes which is discouraging and results in staff less likely to report. If there is never any perceived action taken in response to the report, no review of the reports, no activity to improve the system, or no follow-up or feedback of information back to the reporter, the staff perceives that reporting the known risks they encounter is a waste of time, and they will stop reporting. Completing a report (especially if there is no harm to a patient) takes away time from the bedside or other critical activities.
- Reduce and/or improve the reliability of handoffs—Handoffs are one of the more common points for error. Oftentimes when contacting a physician, handing off a patient to another caregiver, or during a change of shift report, only portions of the patient's pertinent history are provided. The information provided is often variable, dependent on the person handing off the information, and other factors, such as time pressure. There are often gaps when critical information (e.g., allergies, code status, pending physician response to resolve medication-related questions) is not provided, leading to errors and omissions in care.
- A structured handoff process has been incorporated as a National Patient Safety Goal by TJC as a method of reducing the likelihood that important information is

not passed on to the next shift or the next caregiver. The use of SBAR as a communication tool during handoffs of patients or information is one method that has proven useful in reducing the errors introduced during the handoff of patients within or between institutions. SBAR stands for the following:

◦ Situation—Describe the current situation and reason for the call
◦ Background—Provide pertinent background information (e.g., history, current medications, labs, vital signs) to the situation
◦ Assessment—Provide your assessment of the situation
◦ Recommendation/Request—Provide your request or recommendation in succinct terms.

Other Principles of Error Management

- **Implement new technology and information systems—with caution.** There have been many advances in technology and information systems available within health care: barcoding technology, smart pumps, CPOE, automated dispensing and distribution technologies, and more. These all have the potential to provide great value, however, one should undertake the implementation of these new technologies carefully. The curse of the unintended consequence is often discovered during or after implementation. Unintended consequences may occur when a new technology is implemented and a new problem develops as a result of the technology. In some cases, an FMEA is used prior to new technology implementation to brainstorm what could go wrong and develop strategies and educational tools to prevent deviations from the desired outcome. Reviewing technology from a human factors perspective early in the process is recommended. For example, placing a computer on top of an automated distribution machine provides great access to information that nursing and pharmacy staff need during the retrieval or refilling of these machines. However, if the font is so small that no one can read it, this technology may actually cause more errors by selecting the wrong patient or wrong drug. It is always recommended that the end-user be involved in the selection process of these technologies, as they are the ones who interact with the products daily. They can identify potential issues very quickly.
- **Use quality improvement techniques to improve safety.** Develop metrics and monitor progress. While it is not necessary to conduct a randomized controlled trial with every intervention to improve safety, it is valuable to develop measures, gather baseline data, and remeasure to show improvement. The Plan-Do-Study-Act (PDSA) cycle is one structured method to lead teams through the improvement

process. This process involves a planning stage in which a problem statement and implementation strategy is developed based on gaps identified within a process (plan), the strategy is implemented (do), the results are analyzed (study), and any refinements are made to the plan (act). These cycles repeat until a reliable and efficient process is finalized. See Chapter 16 for additional information on this process. Rapid-cycle tests of change are great ways to avoid full blown implementation of a poorly designed process. Rapid-cycle testing involves identification of a new process to be considered or implemented followed by a very brief trial or pilot with just one patient, one physician's patients, or one unit. The learning from this short pilot will be used to edit the new method, allow time to try it again (often several times), gain the input and support of staff in the process, and provide valuable revisions before implementation. Once the cycles have ironed out all of the apparent problems, the process is rolled out on a broader basis.

- **Evaluate areas for environmental contributions to error.** There are numerous workplace factors that may contribute to performance lapses and medication errors. Low lighting, high levels of noise, high temperatures, and stressful work environments are examples. Distractions and interruptions as part of the workflow should also be evaluated and minimized.
- **Involve patients on committees such as the patient safety committee.** Place some thought into who might be chosen to join the team. Use an application process to identify the best people. Assure that a confidentiality agreement is signed. Choose someone who will listen to other perspectives, yet provide constructive feedback into how to think from a patient's perspective. It is amazing what changes can result when involving patients and/or family members. The team will alter their thinking and priorities, becoming more patient-centered.
- **Establish redundancies around high-risk processes and high-risk medication use.** As humans are susceptible to error, it is recommended that redundancy be a part of processes. This allows an error caused by a slip or lapse to be caught downstream before it reaches a patient. Independent double checks are recommended for high-risk processes and medications, such as for chemotherapy and neonatal parenteral nutrition. For maximal effectiveness, double checks should be limited to assure they are completed appropriately. It is recommended that double checks be limited to the following:[67]
  - Situations that involve high-alert medications, such as chemotherapy (including methotrexate), insulin, opiates, and anticoagulants.
  - Complex processes (compounding, calculating doses).
  - High-risk patient populations (children and adolescents, elderly or pregnant patients; patients with severe congestive heart failure; and patients with known renal impairment or liver disease).

TABLE 18–6. ORGANIZATIONS PROMOTING BEST PRACTICES IN PATIENT AND MEDICATION SAFETY

Agency for Healthcare Research and Quality	www.ahrq.gov
AHRQ Patient Safety Network	www.psnet.ahrq.gov
American Society of Health-System Pharmacists	www.ashp.org
Centers for Disease Control and Prevention	www.cdc.gov
Institute for Healthcare Improvement	www.ihi.org
Institute for Safe Medication Practices	www.ismp.org
Massachusetts Coalition for the Prevention of Medical Errors	www.macoalition.org
National Patient Safety Foundation	www.npsf.org
National Quality Forum	www.qualityforum.org
Patient Safety and Quality Healthcare	https://www.psqh.com/
The Joint Commission	www.jointcommission.org
The Joint Commission International	www.jointcommissioninternational.org
The Advisory Board	www.advisory.com
United States Pharmacopeia (USP)	www.usp.org
U.S. Food and Drug Administration (FDA)	www.fda.gov

The average number of errors missed on a check is about 5%. In studies using simulated cart-fills, 93% to 97% of these errors were identified with an independent double check. While these numbers seem small, they add up quickly with the number of medications dispensed daily. Be sure to define exactly what is meant by an independent double check. One person should do the calculations and document the results. Then a second person, without reviewing the work of the first person, should complete the same calculations and then compare the answers for consistency. This is important to avoid confirmation bias. Recall that confirmation bias is a natural tendency to see what we think we see. When glancing at an order to confirm it for another person who has just asked, "Do you think this order says warfarin?", the chance to be biased to see warfarin in the order greatly increases. If they had just asked what the order appeared to say, there is much less chance for this bias.

Table 18-6 identifies several websites that remain sources of updated safe practices and updated news related to safety risks and hazards.

Putting It All Together

Providing safe medication use is paramount to the safety of all patients. Diligent efforts to identify errors (utilizing several methods), understand human capability and propensity to commit errors in everyday life, analyze and determine the root causes and contributing factors, and devise systems that support humans and prevent expected errors are all a part of developing a culture of safety. Involving staff on the front line when reviewing safety events and developing action plans to prevent recurrence is important. It is important not only to the development of an appropriate action plan, but also to garner support and confidence that once errors are identified, leadership is committed to improving the processes in which staff have to work every day.

Case Study 18–4

A nurse caring for a birthing mother removed a bag of bupivacaine from the automated dispensing machine prior to the arrival of the anesthesiologist in order to have everything readily available when needed. The anesthesiology department had requested a preparation checklist with other supplies and the epidural. The same patient required prophylactic penicillin based on Group B streptococcus. Both bags of similar size were in the patient's room. The nurse administered what was thought to be the penicillin bag, but did not use the bar-coding system. The patient immediately decompensated and expired. It was discovered that the epidural bupivacaine was administered IV instead of the penicillin bag.

Upon further investigation, it was identified that the barcoding system had been implemented in the majority of the hospital, but was not fully implemented in the Labor and Delivery area due to several technologic and cultural issues.

- *What system or process issues can you identify?*
- *Read the related article cited below to identify additional information about the case. Lead a discussion related to system errors and their impact on health care professional's behaviors and the potential impact to patients.*

Smetzer J, Baker C, Byrne FD, Cohen MR. Shaping systems for better behavioral choices: lessons learned from a fatal medication error. Jt Comm J Qual Patient Saf. 2010 Apr;36(4):152-63.

- *Discuss challenges with implementation of new technology.*
- *Discuss challenges in culture and prioritization of safety principles.*
- *Discuss confirmation bias and look-alike packaging.*

Conclusion: Safety as a Priority

In 1998, the IOM formed the Quality of Healthcare in America Committee that was charged with developing a strategy to improve quality in health care. In their published report, "To Err is Human: Building a Safer Health System,"[1] the committee highlighted what was currently known about the extent of medical errors, what contributes to medical errors, and recommendations to minimize errors and improve the quality of health care in the United States. Many of the goals set forth in this report are becoming closer to reality. The many other reports by the IOM have provided additional detail and insight into what is necessary to optimize the safety of the health care system in the United States.

Medication misadventures continue to be a serious problem in the United States health care system, both in the hospital and the ambulatory care setting. Working to provide safe care is a journey or, rather, a marathon. Changing a culture is not something that is accomplished in a few years; it may take 10 or more years. Much of that is dependent on the leadership of executives and staff. Those with a passion for safety may need to help enlighten those in higher leadership positions. Learn from others. It is an important method of preventing errors from occurring within one's institution/facility. Take a close look at processes when reading a local or national headline about an error. There continues to be ongoing research aimed at increasing the safety and quality of health care. Health care will continue to be complex and require effective coordination and communication. Technology will continue to evolve. Safety truly needs to be a core value that is held by all. Teamwork and mutual respect are vital parts to success. Only through collaboration and a shared, dedicated commitment will patient safety truly become a reality.

Self-Assessment Questions

1. In an effort to improve handoffs and communication, SBAR is a recommended technique. What does SBAR stand for?
   a. Summary, Background, Assignment, and Review
   b. Summary, Briefing, Assessment, and Recollection
   c. Situation, Background, Assessment, and Recommendation/Request
   d. Situation, Briefing, Assessment, and Recommendation

2. Which of the following is **NOT** an advantage of the use of SBAR?
   a. Encourages the clinician to be prepared and succinct when contacting a provider with a concern
   b. Encourages the clinician to anticipate questions related to the patient's care prior to contacting a provider

c. May take longer to prepare for the conversation with the provider

d. Ultimately saves time with the provider due to appropriate preparation and succinct discussion

3. Congress passed the Patient Safety and Quality Improvement Act of 2005, from which Patient Safety Organizations (PSOs) were created. Which of the following is **NOT** a true statement?

a. This act provides two types of protections: confidentiality and privilege protections.

b. One of the goals of the PSOs is to collate and analyze data related to safety errors and events.

c. PSOs will forward information about facility-specific reported events to The Joint Commission and the media.

d. PSOs will require the use of Common Formats (standardized reporting and terminology) for reporting errors and events.

4. Patient A is given a low dose of regular insulin intended for Patient B. The patient became hypoglycemic and required two doses of D50W to reverse the effects, but did become symptomatic and did not require further treatment. Which of the following NCC MERP classification is most appropriate?

a. Category A

b. Category B

c. Category C

d. Category E

e. Category F

5. You are an experienced nurse who was asked to float to a surgical floor. Your patient has intentionally retained packing. You have been asked to change the packing and have never completed this task and are unaware of the requirements and documentation needs. You make a first attempt, but due to your uncertainty you decide (appropriately) to ask the charge nurse for assistance. Without help, what type of human error might you have made?

a. Skill-based error

b. Rule-based error

c. Knowledge-based error

d. Interruption-based error

6. A Just Culture exists when there is a punitive environment, where staff are disciplined based on errors, to assure events will not recur.

a. True

b. False

7. Which of the following methods utilizes observation of drug administration and comparison with physician orders in order to identify medication errors and is considered very time consuming, rarely used on an ongoing basis?
   a. ADE Trigger Tool
   b. Observation method
   c. Voluntary reporting method
   d. None of the above

8. Which of the following is a thorough and deliberate retrospective analysis of an error or event in an effort to design risk reduction strategies to prevent a recurrence?
   a. Root cause analysis (RCA)
   b. Interview people involved in previous errors
   c. Failure mode and effects analysis (FMEA)
   d. Trending of error and event reports

9. Which of the following strategies was **NOT** one recommended by the IHI 100,000 Lives Campaign?
   a. Prevent adverse drug events
   b. Prevent central line infections
   c. Prevent surgical site infections
   d. Develop a culture of safety

10. Which of the following statements are **TRUE**?
    a. All adverse drug events involve harm
    b. All medication errors cause harm
    c. There is no harm involved in an adverse drug reaction
    d. All of the above are true

11. Which of the following does **NOT** describe the vision statement related to interprofessional education around quality and patient safety—from "Crossing the Quality Chasm"?
    a. All health professional should learn about quality in their own undergraduate program.
    b. All health professionals should be taught to deliver patient-centered care as members of an interdisciplinary team.
    c. There should be emphasis on evidence-based practice and interdisciplinary teamwork within health profession education.
    d. Common language and core competencies should be developed and taught among health professional education programs.

12. Which is these strategies are generally the **LEAST** effective or less reliable than other strategies?
    a. Change a policy or procedure
    b. Re-educate everyone (especially when was an individual failure)
    c. Coach associate(s) to be more careful (vigilant)
    d. All of the above are examples of less reliable strategies

13. Which term refers to a type of selective thinking where individuals select out what is familiar to them or what they expect to see, rather than what is actually there?
    a. Hindsight bias
    b. Confirmation bias
    c. System failure
    d. Just Culture

14. A pharmacist is alone in the pharmacy, entering a physician order, when she receives a call about a patient. In order to answer the question, she must exit the current patient's profile to pull up another patient's profile. Once the question has been answered, she hangs up and proceeds to finish entering the order on the patient's profile (the wrong patient). Which error prevention strategy would most likely be the **LEAST** effective at preventing a recurrence of this error?
    a. Discipline the pharmacist and remind her to be more careful—do patient identification correctly on every order.
    b. Purchase (or develop) technology that automatically links a physician order to the patient's profile in the pharmacy system—a forcing function.
    c. Alter the practice such that there are minimal to no interruptions for pharmacists entering orders (route calls to one area and responsible staff, segregate order-entry staff to decrease interruptions).
    d. All of the above will be effective and prevent the recurrence.

15. Which of the following strategies do **NOT** promote safe medication use?
    a. Requesting a double check for a high-risk medication like insulin
    b. Writing down and repeating back a telephone order
    c. Using an IV syringe to administer an oral medication
    d. Using a leading zero in writing an order for a medication dose less than 1 mg

REFERENCES

1. Institute of Medicine. To err is human: building a safer health-system. Washington, DC: National Academy Press; 1999.
2. Brennan TA, Leape LL, Laird NM, Hebert L, Localio R, Lawthers AG, Newhouse JP, Weiler PC, Hiatt HH. Incidence of adverse events and negligence in hospitalized patients: results of the Harvard Medical Practice Study I. N Engl J Med. 1991;324:370-6.

3. Leape LL, Brennan TA, Laird NM, Lawthers AG, Localio AR, Barnes BA, Hebert L, Newhouse JP, Weiler PC, Hiatt H. The nature of adverse events in hospitalized patients: results of the Harvard Medical Practice Study II. N Engl J Med. 1991;324(6):377-84.

4. American Society of Health-System Pharmacists. Suggested definitions and relationships among medication misadventures, medication errors, adverse drug events, and adverse drug reactions. Am J Health Syst Pharm. 1998;55:165-6.

5. ASHP Report: suggested definitions and relationships among medication misadventures, medication errors, adverse drug events and adverse drug reactions. Am J Health Syst Pharm. 1998;55:165-6.

6. Joint Commission Resources. Medication use: a systems approach to reducing errors. Porche RA, editor. 2nd editor. Oak Brook, IL: JCR; 2008:16.

7. Bates DW, Cullen DJ, Laird N, Peterson LA, Small HD, Servi D, Laffel G, Sweitzer BJ, Shea BF, Hallisey R, Vander Vliet M, Nemeskal R, Leape LL, for the ADE Prevention Study Group. Incidence of adverse drug events and potential adverse drug events. JAMA. 1995;274:29-34.

8. Lamy PP. Adverse drug effects. Clin Geriatr Med. 1990;6:293-307.

9. Lesar TS, Lomaestro BM, Pohl H. Medication-prescribing errors in a teaching hospital: a 9-year experience. Arch Intern Med. 1997;157:1569-76.

10. Gurwitz JH, Field TS, Avorn J, McCormick D, Jain S, Eckler M, Benser M, Edmondson AC, Bates DW. Incidence and preventability of adverse drug events in nursing homes. Am J Med. 2000;109:87-94.

11. Gurwitz JH, Field TS, Harrold LR, Rothschild J, Debellis K, Seger AC, Cadoret C, Fish LS, Garber L, Kelleher M, Bates DW. Incidence and preventability of adverse drug events among older persons in the ambulatory setting. JAMA. 2003;289:1107-16.

12. White TJ, Arakelian A, Rho JP. Counting the costs of drug-related adverse events. PharmacoEconomics. 1999;15:445-58.

13. Johnson JA, Bootman JL. Drug-related morbidity and mortality. Arch Intern Med. 1995;155:1949-56.

14. Classen DC, Pestotnik SL, Evans S, Loyd JF, Burke JP. Adverse drug events in hospitalized patients. JAMA. 1997;277:301-6.

15. Ernst FR, Grizzle AJ. Drug-related morbidity and mortality: updating the cost-of-illness model. J Am Pharm Assoc. 2001;41:192-9.

16. Phillips MA. Voluntary reporting of medication errors. Am J Health Syst Pharm. 2002;59:2326-8.

17. Barker KN, Flynn EA, Pepper GA. Observation method of detecting medication errors. Am J Health Syst Pharm. 2002;59:2314-6.

18. Barker KN, Mikeal RI, Pearson RE, Illig NA, Morse ML. Medication errors in nursing homes and small hospitals. Am J Hosp Pharm. 1982;39:987-91.

19. Jha AK, Kuperman GJ, Teich JM, Leape L, Shea B, Rittenberg E, Burdick E, Seger DL, Vander Vliet M, Bates DW. Identifying adverse drug events: development of a computer-based monitor and comparison with chart review and stimulated voluntary reporting. J Am Med Inform Assoc. 1998;3:305-14.

20. Classen DC, Pestotnik SL, Evans RS, Burke JP. Description of a computerized adverse drug event monitor using a hospital information system. Hosp Pharm. 1992;27:774, 776-9, 783.

21. Classen DC, Pestotnik SL, Evans RS, Burke JP. Computerized surveillance of adverse drug events in hospital patients (published erratum appears in JAMA. 1992;267:1992). JAMA. 1991;266:2847-51.

22. AHRQ Evidence Report/Technology Assessment No. 43: making healthcare safer [Internet]. 2001 Jul 20 [cited 2017 Apr 4]. Available from: https://archive.ahrq.gov/clinic/ptsafety/pdf/ptsafety.pdf

23. VHA, Inc. Monitoring adverse drug events: finding the needles in the haystack. Vol. 9. Irving, TX: VHA; 2002. VHA 2002 Research Series.

24. Raschke RA, Gollihare B, Wunderlich TA, Guidry J, Leibowitz A, Peirce J, Lemelson L, Heisler MA, Susong C. A computer alert system to prevent injury from adverse drug events: development and evaluation in a community teaching hospital (published erratum appears in JAMA 1999;281:420J). JAMA. 1998;280:1317-20.

25. Bates DW, Evans RS, Murff H, Stetson PD, Pizziferri L, Hripcsak G. Detecting adverse events using information technology. J Am Med Inform Assoc. 2003;10:115-28.

26. Bates DW. Using information technology to screen for adverse drug events. Am J Health Syst Pharm. 2002;59:2317-9.

27. Schneider PJ. Using technology to enhance measurement of drug-use safety. Am J Health Syst Pharm. 2002;59:2330-2.

28. Rozich JD, Haraden CR, Resar RK. Adverse drug event trigger tool: a practical methodology for measuring medication related harm. Qual Saf Health Care. 2008;12:194-200.

29. Rozich JD, Resar RK. Medication safety: one organization's approach to the challenge. J Clin Outcomes Manage. 2001;8(10):27-34.

30. Crea KA, Sherrin TP, Morehead D, Snow R. Reducing adverse drug events involving high-risk medications in acute care. J Clin Outcomes Manage. 2004;11(10):640-6.

31. The Patient Safety Act and Quality Improvement Act of 2005. Public Law 109-41, 109th Congress, July 29, 2005.

32. Pennsylvania Patient Safety Authority. Vol 6(4), December 2009.

33. ISMP Newsletter. Heparin errors continue despite prior, high-profile fatal events [Internet]. 2008 Jul 17. Available from: http://www.ismp.org/newsletters/acutecare/articles/20080717.asp

34. American Society of Hospital Pharmacists. ASHP guidelines on preventing medication errors in hospitals. Am J Hosp Pharm. 1993;50:305-14.

35. Patient Safety Organization Privacy Protection Center (PSOPPC). Available from: https://www.psoppc.org/psoppc_web

36. Pepper GA. Errors in drug administration by nurses. Am J Health Syst Pharm. 1995 Feb 15;52(4):390-5.

37. Sipkoff M. Joint Commission sets anticoagulant therapy safety goal. Drug Topics-Hospital/Health-System Pharmacy [Internet]. 2007 Aug 20:[about 1 p.]. Available from: http://drugtopics.modernmedicine.com/drug-topics/news/clinical/hospitalhealth-system-pharmacy/joint-commission-sets-anticoagulant-therapy

38. Dunn EB, Wolfe JJ. Medication error classification and avoidance. Hosp Pharm. 1997;32:860-5.

39. Kessler DA, for the working group. Introducing MedWatch: a new approach to reporting medication and device adverse effects and product problems. JAMA. 1993:269(21):2765-8.

40. The Joint Commission Sentinel Event Policy and Procedure. Available from: http://www. jointcommission.org/sentinel_event_policy_and_procedures/.

41. Using aggregate root cause analysis to improve patient safety. Jt Comm J Qual Patient Saf. 2003 Aug;29(8):434-9.

42. Using aggregate root cause analysis to reduce falls. Jt Comm J Qual Patient Saf. 2005 Jan;31(1):21-31.

43. Bogner MS. Human error in medicine. Hillsdale, NJ: Lawrence Erlbaum Associates; 1994.

44. Senders JW. Theory and analysis of typical errors in a medical setting. Hosp Pharm. 1993;28:505-8.

45. Norman DA. The design of everyday things. New York, NY: Basic Book; 1988.

46. Reason J. Human error. Cambridge: Cambridge University Press; 1990.

47. Reason J. Managing the risks of organizational accidents. Burlington, VT: Ashgate; 1997.

48. ISMP Newsletter. Inattentional blindness: what captures your attention? Available from: www.ismp.org/newsletters/acutecare/articles/20090226.asp

49. The Joint Commission (TJC). Sentinel Events Statistics, March 31, 2007. Available from: http://www.jointcommission.org/sentinel_event_data_general/.

50. Abood RR. Errors in pharmacy practice. US Pharm. 1996;21:122-32.

51. Coleman IC. Medication errors: picking up the pieces. Drug Top. 1999;143:83-92.

52. Glut of medication errors focuses pharmacists on event reporting. Drug Util Rev. 1998:201-6.

53. Cohen MR. ISMP medication error report analysis: the mistake of blaming people and not the process. Hosp Pharm. 1997;32:1106-11.

54. ISMP Newsletter. An injustice has been done: jail time given to pharmacist who made an error. August 21, 2009. Available from: http://www.ismp.org/pressroom/injustice-jailtime-for-pharmacist.asp

55. ISMP Newsletter. Our long journey towards safety-minded just culture. Part I: where we've been. Available from: http://www.ismp.org/newsletters/acutecare/articles/20060907 .asp?

56. GAIN Working Group E, Flight Ops/ATC Ops Safety Information Sharing. A roadmap to a just culture: enhancing the safety environment. Available from: http://flightsafety.org/ files/just_culture.pdf

57. Grasha AF, O'Neill M. Cognitive processes in medication errors. US Pharm. 1996;21:96-109.

58. Ukens C. Breaking the trust: exclusive survey of dispensing errors. Drug Top. 1992;136:58-69.

59. DeMichele D. Preventing medication errors. US Pharm. 1995;20:69-75.

60. Davis NM. Lack of knowledge as a cause of medication errors. Hosp Pharm. 1997;32:16-25.

61. Fitzgerald WL, Wilson DB. Medication errors: lessons in law. Drug Top. 1998;142: 84-93.

62. Institute of Medicine. Crossing the quality chasm. Washington, DC: National Academy Press; 2001.

63. Institute of Medicine. Health professions education: a bridge to quality. Washington, DC: National Academy Press; 2003.

64. Institute for Healthcare Improvement—Open School. Available from: http://www.ihi.org/education/ihiopenschool/pages/default.aspx

65. Berwick DM, Calkins DR, McCannon CJ, Hackbarth AD. The 100,000 Lives Campaign: setting a goal and a deadline for improving health care quality. J Am Med Assoc. 2006 Jan;295(3):324-7.

66. Grout J. Mistake-proofing the design of health care processes. Rockville, MD, AHRQ Publication No. 07-0020, 2007.

67. Grissinger M. The virtues of independent double checks: they really are worth your time! P&T. 2006;31:9.

SUGGESTED READINGS

1. Gandhi TK, Weingart SN, Borus J, Seger A, Peterson J, Burdick E, Seger D, Shu K, Federico F, Leape L, Bates D. Adverse drug events in ambulatory care. N Engl J Med. 2003;348:1556-64.

2. Rozich JD, Haraden CR, Resar RK. Adverse drug event trigger tool: a practical methodology for measuring medication related harm. Qual Saf Health Care. 2008;12:194-200.

3. Jha AK, Kuperman GJ, Teich JM, Leape L, Shea B, Rittenberg E, Burdick E, Seger DL, Vander Vliet M, Bates DW. Identifying adverse drug events: development of a computer-based monitor and comparison with chart review and stimulated voluntary reporting. J Am Med Inform Assoc. 1998;3:305-14.

4. Howard R, Avery A, Bissell P. Causes of preventable drug-related hospital admissions: a qualitative study. Qual Saf Health Care. 2008;17:109-16.

5. Kale A, Keohane CA, Maviglia S, Gandhi TK, Poon EG. Adverse drug events caused by serious medication administration errors. BMJ Qual Saf. 2012;21:933-38.

6. Bagian JP, Gosbee J, Lee CZ, Williams L, McKnight SD, Mannos DM. The Veterans Affairs root cause analysis system in action. Jt Comm J Qual Improv. 2002;28:531-45.

7. Smetzer J, Baker C, Byrne FD, Cohen MR. Shaping systems for better behavioral choices: lessons learned from a fatal medication error. Jt Comm J Qual Patient Saf. 2010 Apr;36(4):152-63.

Chapter Nineteen

Policy, Procedure, and Guideline Development

Sabrina W. Cole • Gregory Heindel • Conor Hanrahan

Learning Objectives

After completing this chapter, the reader will be able to

- Differentiate between types of practice documents (e.g., policy, procedure).
- Assess various document management philosophies.
- Discuss the roles and responsibilities of individuals/groups involved in the practice document development and review process (e.g., document owner, stakeholders, consultants).
- Identify factors that influence document development (e.g., regulations, scope, review periods).
- Describe the systematic methodology to develop and revise practice documents.

Key Concepts

1. Documents should ultimately meet the need of employees who are responsible to adhere to the policy, procedure, or guideline that is intended to result in perpetual compliance and safe medication practices.

2. The first step to understanding the practice document development requirements is to evaluate the process for the organization.

3. Review periods for documents can vary depending on the organization (typically a biennial or triennial review) or defined by a regulatory agency.

4. The first step in developing practice documents is to identify the need for the document.

⑤ It is important to gather relevant data to the practice document topic.

⑥ Practice documents should be evidence based and reflect standard of care or best practice.

⑦ Ensure the format, ease of use, and reading level are appropriate for the intended audience and end users.

⑧ After composition, the draft document must then be disseminated for review and comments.

⑨ After approval, publication and education are essential to the success of any practice document.

⑩ The last step in the development and maintenance of practice documents is to ensure compliance with any changes.

Introduction

Health care professionals in health systems are often asked to develop **policies, procedures, and guidelines** that not only apply to their department, but pertain to other parts of the health system or even the system in its entirety. Given the breadth of knowledge that pharmacists possess regarding medication use, they are poised to contribute to development of **practice documents** affecting each aspect of the medication use cycle (e.g., prescribing, preparation, administration). These types of practice documents are appropriate for various reasons and are often created to establish a clinical best practice, ensure safe and reliable operational practices, and meet regulatory requirements. Further explanation of these various types and justifications for document development is included throughout this chapter.

Document development is unfamiliar to many clinicians. Literature available to help the health care professional on document development is limited and often directed toward more general application of evidence-based medicine and use of outcomes research in the medication use policy development process.[1-3] Selected resources are also available in the nursing literature.[4] Much of what the individual is exposed to in these areas is on-the-job training. This skill set should be taught early in the educational process for pharmacists, with a specific recommendation from the Center for the Advancement of Pharmacy Education to engage pharmacy students in the development of professional documents that are relevant to needs of various organizations, specifically formulary monographs and policy development.[5] This may be accomplished in the drug information curriculum. The information presented in this chapter is derived from the literature and other available resources and designed to assist with policy, procedure, and guideline development.[6]

Regulatory Considerations

Health care is a highly regulated field, with clinical and operational regulations from many organizations, including **The Joint Commission (TJC)**, state regulators, boards of pharmacy, the U.S. Food and Drug Administration (FDA), URAC®, and the Drug Enforcement Administration, among others. Hospitals and health systems often employ compliance programs to manage these regulations and ensure safe and appropriate practice in all areas of the organization. Health care professionals and leaders should be engaged in the understanding of regulatory requirements in addition to the level of detail and/or documentation that is expected to meet the requirements of these accrediting or regulatory bodies. As a result, clinicians often are responsible to develop, review, and revise practice documents on a routine basis. It is important to note that while practice documents should be compliant to all regulatory requirements, the ❶ *documents should ultimately meet the need of employees who are responsible to adhere to the policy, procedure, or guideline that is intended to result in perpetual compliance and safe medication practices.* Additional considerations to ensure regulatory compliance are detailed in the systematic approach to practice documents later in this chapter.

Practice Document Design and Organization

Practice document design and organization is institution- or organization-specific. Appendix 19-1 provides an example policy. ❷ *The first step to understanding the practice document development requirements is to evaluate the process for the organization.* While some organizations still manage practice documents, including policies and procedures, manually, some employ workflow software solutions for document management. There is not a standard approach to designing and organizing the documents themselves. It must be understood what the organizational standard is for requirements of each individual document in addition to the types of documents employed. For example, some organizations use policies and procedures, while others supplement policies and procedures with additional guidance documents, such as practice guidelines or protocols. Practice documents commonly include policies, procedures, and guidelines. Organizations generally adopt one of two standard works for document management. The combining of both policy statements and procedural steps in a single document is considered a unified approach. Alternatively, individual, but related, documents may be created, which includes development of a policy and a procedure in separate documents. Another option is the development of a manual to implement a policy. A benefit of this approach is the agile and timely process to update the manual, which is connected to a policy as a reference document.

Factors Influencing Practice Document Development

A step-wise approach to document development is presented in the following section. However, an understanding of factors that may influence the development of practice documents is warranted. To begin, it is necessary to look at the time frame in which these documents need to be approved and reapproved. Some documents need regular review. ❸ *Review periods for documents can vary depending on the organization (typically a biennial or triennial review) or defined by a regulatory agency* (e.g., URAC® requires a review of documents annually). Attention is required to ensure adequate time for all stakeholders to review and edit the documents prior to approval in the required review cycle. Documents should have a defined scope, which may include by facility, practice area, patient versus non-patient care areas, or other considerations. It is important to identify the scope statements for the organization and indicate the most appropriate statement for the document created. The subject matter of the document varies. Table 19-1 details common health system policy classifications.

As mentioned previously, document management may be automated or manual. Appropriate time should be allowed to follow the defined process. Some workflows for document review and approval collect feedback from all stakeholders concurrently. A sequential feedback and approval process may be beneficial if the organization has divided responsibilities among several groups. For example, if several groups or disciplines need to review the document, consider that the sequence of the review may be of importance. It would be prudent for those reviewing for clinical content to provide feedback prior to a group who reviews the final draft to ensure regulatory compliance. A sequential review process should eliminate the risk of duplicative work among stakeholders. Table 19-2 provides an example for a sequential review process. A continuous quality improvement process should be applied to practice document development. A thorough discussion on continuous quality improvement is found in Chapter 16.

There are several critical skills that are beneficial when overseeing document development and management. Attention to detail, strong written communication skills, and

TABLE 19−1. HEALTH SYSTEM POLICY SAMPLE CLASSIFICATIONS

Administrative: Policies that address organizational operations

Department specific: Policies that address an individual department or work area (e.g., pharmacy, nursing, laboratory, food and nutrition)

Human resources: Policies that address the work environment and employee rights

Patient care: Policies that affect patient care directly or indirectly and cross more than one department or work area

Procurement: Policies that address purchasing and inventory management

Safety policies and emergency operations plans

TABLE 19–2. SEQUENTIAL DOCUMENT REVIEW PROCESS EXAMPLE

1. Document owner identifies need for revision (e.g., scheduled review, new information)
2. Document owner identifies content experts and coordinates a review and update by these stakeholders
3. Document owner incorporates feedback and submits review document to pharmacy document coordinator (e.g., Drug Information Service) for review of content, format, consistency with other documents
4. Pharmacy document coordinator facilitates approval and publication of the revised document with the organizational department responsible for all practice documents (e.g., compliance department)

a system or population perspective to clinical care are needed. Pharmacists with additional training in drug information are often involved with policy development given their involvement with medication safety and formulary management.[7] Additionally, a pharmacist with a strong drug information skill set is an ideal candidate to participate in policy development since it requires thorough and accurate analysis of evidence-based medicine and quality improvement initiatives.

Systematic Method for Practice Document Development and Maintenance

Before undertaking the task of practice document development or maintenance, it is important to appreciate the approval process at an institution. The approving bodies, time needed for approval, and relevant stakeholders may vary greatly from one institution or practice document to the next. Fully understanding the process at an individual institution will help determine the timeline, urgency for review, and prioritization for development of different documents. While individual practice documents, institutions, and scenarios may require unique considerations, the overall approach will generally consist of many similar steps. Table 19-3 describes the systematic method for development and maintenance of practice documents. This framework may be followed for both new documents and revisions of existing documents. It is important to note that some aspects of this framework may need slight adjustment based upon culture, manpower, and stakeholders at different institutions. The necessary steps are described below.

STEP 1: IDENTIFY THE NEED

❹ *The first step in developing practice documents is to identify the need for the document.* A wide spectrum exists for the need of practice documents. Accrediting bodies (e.g., TJC, URAC®, American Society of Health-System Pharmacists [ASHP]) may require up-to-date

TABLE 19-3. SYSTEMATIC METHOD FOR PRACTICE DOCUMENT DEVELOPMENT AND MAINTENANCE

Before beginning: evaluate and understand institution-specific process

1. Identify need and determine purpose
2. Gather data
3. Research regulations, standard of care, best practices, and published evidence
4. Synthesize practice document and incorporate stakeholder input
5. Gain document approval
6. Publication and education
7. Continual evaluation of practice document compliance

practice documents. Internal groups, such as the human resources department, may require other departments to maintain specific practice documents to establish clear expectations within the workplace (e.g., paid time off, dress codes). Practice documents may also be utilized to limit the variability in a process through standardization (e.g., the patient identifiers used prior to dispensing a prescription, the appropriate steps to unit-dose packaging tablets). Established practice documents also enable managers to hold workers accountable to the clear standards for practice and, if needed, discipline violators of those standards. Finally, clinical guidelines and best practice recommendations (e.g., from the Institute for Safe Medication Practices [ISMP] or the Infectious Diseases Society of America [IDSA]) can be executed through practice document development, approval, and implementation.

STEP 2: GATHER RELEVANT DATA

Next, ❺ *it is important to gather relevant data to the practice document topic.* Internal data, such as medication error reports or TJC findings, may help inform decisions or identify gaps that the practice document should address. Data may also be helpful in defining the scope of the practice document and identifying the relevant institutions, departments, or practice areas. A search for other similar or related practice documents should also be completed to ensure the content is not duplicative or contradictory. For example, the institution-wide document describing paid time off requests may be adequate for a pharmacy department to adopt and a new document may not be required. Similarly, storage and temperature monitoring standards for medication refrigerators may be within pharmacy, nursing, and environmental department-specific documents. The defined expectations should, at minimum, not conflict and the need for duplicative documents certainly warrants discussion. Understanding the purpose and the need (or lack thereof) for a practice document in context of internal data is an important step to help prioritize work and direct research efforts in the next step.

STEP 3: FOLLOW BEST-PRACTICE RECOMMENDATIONS

Whenever possible, ❻ *practice documents should be evidence based and reflect standard of care or best practice.* The appropriate sources for information related to practice documents may vary depending on subject matter, but will likely include a combination of tertiary and primary literature. Clinical practice guidelines should be informed heavily by professional organizations' recommendations. For example, a clinical practice guideline on pulmonary arterial hypertension should consider the published recommendations from the American College of Chest Physicians. For more detailed information on evidence-based practice guidelines, see Chapter 8. Professional organization's position papers and other recommendations are also available for nonclinical topics and should be incorporated when relevant (e.g., ISMP List of High-Alert Medications in Acute Care Settings).[8] Regulatory guidelines and requirements should also be reviewed to ensure that the practice document meets appropriate accreditation and legal standards. Subject-matter experts should also be consulted to identify unpublished considerations. Lastly, a survey of other institutions may help identify solutions, safeguards, or overlooked considerations.

STEP 4: DRAFT THE DOCUMENT

After gathering all of the pertinent background information, recommendations, and literature, the information should be synthesized into a working draft. Most organizations or departments have specific templates that should be followed for each of the different types of practice documents. Depending on the complexity and content of the document, the document owner may individually draft the document, or the owner may assemble a work group to jointly develop the document. Regardless of the method, an evidence-based approach to the review of information and development of documents is preferred. ❼ *Ensure the format, ease of use, and reading level are appropriate for the intended audience and end users.* Relevant key words and links to supporting documents should also be incorporated. Educational efforts and tools addressing potential practice changes for affected individuals are also important to consider.

STEP 5: DISSEMINATE FOR REVIEW AND COMMENTS

❽ *After composition, the draft document must then be disseminated for review and comments.* Stakeholder and experts' review and input are probably most important at this stage of the systematic method, but would also be valuable in both previous steps and later steps, depending on the scenario. See Chapter 20 on project management for details on how to best identify appropriate stakeholders. Typically, the document owner will compile comments and make edits as needed. The finalized document should integrate an evidence-based practice with clinical and stakeholder expertise. It is important to acknowledge that this review, comment, and edit cycle may be repeated many times before the documents are ready to move on to the approval process.

STEP 6: RECEIVE APPROVAL

The approving bodies for practice documents will fluctuate immensely between different institutions, subject matters, and types of practice documents. Table 19-4 provides common types of practice documents, approval bodies, and relevant stakeholders. In general, departmental-specific documents may be reviewed by a process manager or relevant committee. Interdisciplinary and interdepartmental documents will often require approval through one or more interdisciplinary committees. The **pharmacy and therapeutics committee** (see Chapter 13) is probably the most common interdisciplinary body that regularly approves pharmacy-related documents. Regardless of the approving body, the approval

TABLE 19–4.   COMMON EXAMPLES OF PRACTICE DOCUMENTS, APPROVAL BODIES, AND IMPORTANT STAKEHOLDERS

Practice Document	Approval Bodies	Important Stakeholders
Medication Storage Policy	Pharmacy and therapeutics committee	Pharmacy operations managers Nurse unit managers Environmental services Infection control Legal/Risk management
Patient Identification Before Dispensing Medications Procedure	Legal/Risk management	Pharmacists Technicians Medication safety pharmacist Nurses Legal/Risk management
Antibiotic Desensitization Guideline	Pharmacy and therapeutics committee	Infectious disease specialists Allergy/Immunology specialist Infectious disease pharmacists IV pharmacists Nurses
Intravenous (IV) Batch Procedure	Pharmacy operations committee, IV room manager	IV pharmacists IV technicians
Central Venous Catheter Assessment Policy	Nurse practice council	Infection control Nurses Pharmacists Infectious disease specialists

of documents, the stakeholders included, and any relevant discussion points should always be recorded. This information is important not only to implementation and enforcement of the document, but a powerful reference tool during upcoming reviews of the document.

STEP 7: PUBLISH AND EDUCATE

❾ *After approval, publication and education are essential to the success of any practice document.* In general, the document should be readily accessible to end users as a point-of-care reference or guide. Some institutions provide printed copies within relevant areas, while others actively restrict the ability to print or save digital copies. Documents for an entire health system, institution, or department may also be stored in one physical or virtual location or may be spread into separate and secluded sections. Links within electronic health records and/or electronic formularies may also be considered. Each of these strategies presents different advantages and disadvantages with regard to the effort required to access documents, the ease of end users to find relevant documents, and the energy required to update all copies of a document. Nonetheless, robust education about document changes is crucial to successful adoption of new practice documents. The mode(s) of education and communication regarding practice documents should be carefully considered throughout the process.

STEP 8: MONITOR COMPLIANCE

❿ *The last step in the development and maintenance of practice documents is to ensure compliance with any changes.* This often overlooked step is arguably the most important. The value of a practice document lies in the intent and purpose (identified in step 1) and compliance audits represent an evaluation of the successful execution of that intent or purpose. A compliance audit ensures specific requirements of the policy or procedure were adopted into practice. Poor compliance may indicate the need for reevaluation of the stakeholder input, publication, or education process. Finally, document management strategies should be assessed by compliance with the established review periods and adjusted as indicated and a process should be implemented to ensure the change is successfully maintained.

Conclusion

Clinicians, with their expertise in pharmacotherapy, medication safety, operations, and formulary management are uniquely situated to be involved in and lead policy development. The tools that health care professionals use for these activities are gradually being introduced via the health care literature and professional societies. Pharmacists with additional training in drug information are often involved with policy development given their involvement with medication safety and formulary management. Additionally, a pharmacist with a strong drug information skill set is an ideal candidate to participate in policy development since it requires thorough and accurate analysis of evidence-based medicine and quality improvement initiatives. For more in-depth training, professional certificate programs or a Master of Business Administration (MBA) program may be of interest.

Case Study 19–1

As a clinical pharmacist at a large academic medical center, you participate in formulary management to support the efforts of the pharmacy department and the health system to provide safe, effective, and cost-effective medications for use within the system. Currently, pantoprazole, a proton pump inhibitor, is the formulary agent in this class. Nonformulary usage reports indicate significant dispensing of esomeprazole and lansoprazole as well. You are asked to develop an automatic therapeutic interchange policy for the health system to decrease the amount of nonformulary prescribing of these agents.

- *List the steps used to approach this assignment.*
- *Discuss the resources used when gathering background information.*
- *Explain the process to summarize the information collected for development of the policy.*
- *Define stakeholder and identify key stakeholders for this policy.*

Self-Assessment Questions

1. The following health system policies require a pharmacist's participation, **EXCEPT**:
   a. Herbal product use
   b. High-alert medications
   c. Medical resident supervision
   d. Electrolyte infusions
   e. Drug shortages

2. When gathering information for inclusion in a health system policy, what is the initial step?
   a. Conduct a literature search using CINAHL Information Systems
   b. Ask for a meeting with the director of pharmacy
   c. Contact colleagues who work at other health systems
   d. Gather background information including the justification of the policy
   e. Conduct a literature search using PubMed®

3. Which of the following provides specific guidance on a how to perform a given task?
   a. Policy
   b. Procedure
   c. Project description
   d. Purpose statement
   e. Project activities

4. Which of the following resources may be used to research the standard of care before engaging in writing a policy?
   a. Tertiary references
   b. Clinical treatment guidelines
   c. Primary literature
   d. Colleagues and coworkers
   e. All of the above

5. Which of the following is/are a type(s) of health system policy classification?
   a. Patient care
   b. Procurement
   c. Administrative
   d. Human resource
   e. All of the above

6. Additional resources to build a skill set in practice document development include:
   a. Professional pharmacy organization programs
   b. Business programs (e.g., MBA program)
   c. Tertiary references (e.g., textbooks)
   d. Agency for Healthcare Research and Quality (AHRQ)
   e. All of the above

7. Organizations follow a triennial review process for all practice documents, including policies and procedures.
   a. True
   b. False

8. Which of the following represents the correct sequence of the systematic approach for practice document development?
   a. Gather relevant data, identify the need, draft document, ensure compliance with the policy/procedure, provide education to end users
   b. Identify the need, gather relevant data, draft document, provide education to end users, ensure compliance with the policy/procedure
   c. Ensure compliance with the policy/procedure, identify the need, gather relevant data, draft document, provide education to end users
   d. Provide education to end users, identify the need, gather relevant data, draft document, ensure compliance with the policy/procedure
   e. Draft document, identify the need, gather relevant data, ensure compliance with the policy/procedure, provide education to end users

9. The following stakeholders would be **MOST** appropriate to involve in the policy development of antimicrobial stewardship within the organization:
   a. Pharmacist, infectious diseases physician, chief financial officer
   b. Infectious diseases physician, pharmacist, pharmacy and therapeutics committee chairperson
   c. Legal/Risk manager, infectious diseases physician, chief operating officer
   d. Environmental services, infection control, infectious diseases physician
   e. Quality officer, infectious diseases physician, pharmacist

10. Which of the following allows for the rapidly changing information and an agile approach to document management?
    a. Procedure
    b. Guideline
    c. Protocol
    d. Manual
    e. Policy

11. Guidelines are prescriptive in their direction.
    a. True
    b. False

12. Poor compliance with practice documents may indicate which of the following?
    a. Need for additional education
    b. Reevaluation of stakeholder input
    c. Reevaluation of the formatting and reading level
    d. Reevaluation of standard of care or best practice
    e. All of the above

13. Practice documents should always be in compliance with all related regulatory requirements.
    a. True
    b. False

14. A purpose statement of the policy is a step-by-step description of how the issue addressed in the policy should be managed.
    a. True
    b. False

REFERENCES

1. Gray T, Bertch K, Galt K, Gonyeau M, Karpiuk E, Oyen L, Sudekum MJ, Vermeulen LC. Guidelines for therapeutic interchange—2004. Pharmacotherapy. 2005;25(11):1666-80.
2. Vermeulen LC, Beis SJ, Cano SB. Applying outcomes research in improving the medication-use process. Am J Health Syst Pharm. 2000;57:2277-82.
3. Vermeulen LC, Rough SS, Thielke TS, Shane RR, Ivey MF, Woodward BW, Pierpaoli PG, Thomley SM, Borr CA, Zilz DA. Strategic approach for improving the medication-use process in health systems: the high-performance pharmacy practice framework. Am J Health Syst Pharm. 2007;64:1699-710.
4. Oman KS, Duran C, Fink R. Evidence-based policy and procedures: an algorithm for success. JONA. 2008;38(1):47-51.
5. Medina MS, Plaza CM, Stowe CD, Robinson ET, DeLander G, Beck DE, Melchert RB, Supernaw RB, Roche VF, Gleason BL, Strong MN, Bain A, Meyer GE, Dong BJ, Rochon J, Johnston P. Center for the Advancement of Pharmacy Education (CAPE) educational outcomes 2013. Am J Pharm Educ. 2013;77(8):article 162.
6. AHRQ: Agency for Healthcare Research and Quality [Internet]. Rockville, MD: US Department of Health & Human Services; [cited 2017 Apr 1]. Available from: https://www.ahrq.gov
7. Tyler LS, Cole SW, May JR, Millares M, Valentino MA, Vermeulen LC, Wilson AL. ASHP guidelines on the pharmacy and therapeutics committee and the formulary system. Am J Health Syst Pharm. 2008;65:1272-83.
8. ISMP: Institute for Safe Medication Practices [Internet]. Horsham, PA; [cited 2017 Mar 28]. Available from: https://www.ismp.org

20

Chapter Twenty

Project Management

Conor Hanrahan • Candice Burns Wood • Sabrina W. Cole

Learning Objectives

After completing this chapter, the reader will be able to

- Differentiate between a project, program, and portfolio.
- Assess the viability and value of projects.
- Describe the key components of a project charter, including scope, goals, success criteria, and stakeholders.
- Discuss tools used for planning projects, including a work breakdown structure, requirements matrix, risk management plan, communication management plan, and change management plan.
- Explain factors important for the successful execution of a project.
- List key activities to complete when closing a project.

Key Concepts

1. Understanding programs and portfolios is critical to successful project management.
2. Knowing the success criteria is critical because they provide a measurable way to define when the project is finished and the goal has been achieved.
3. Knowing the stakeholders involved is a key step because many times the success of the project depends on their buy-in and input.
4. It is extremely important to define the scope because it puts boundaries on the project and defines what the endpoint is.
5. After identifying tasks and the resources needed to accomplish those tasks, a project timeline can be developed.

Introduction

Health care today is perhaps more complex than it has ever been in history. Instead of the autonomous, physician-centric model of medicine practiced for decades, more organizations are recognizing the value of an interdisciplinary, patient-centric, and population-health approach. Furthermore, integrated health care delivery systems, as opposed to independently owned and disparate entities, are becoming the norm. Standardization and quality improvement processes are now core to many organizations wanting to reduce costs, improve safety, and increase their overall ability to care for patients. Government agencies are further propelling this transformation through changes in payment models and new regulations, adding another layer of complexity.

As a result, health care professionals are increasingly inundated with projects and responsibilities, often without being given more time or resources. Furthermore, most health care workers have historically not applied project management frameworks to these complex tasks. It is little surprise, therefore, that many projects in health care fail to succeed. Imagine, for instance, that a surgeon is about to perform a complex cardiac operation. However, instead of reading through the patient's chart, talking with the surgical team, prescheduling time in the operating room, and working through the step-by-step techniques needed to perform the operation, the physician decides to just begin the surgery without a plan. It should be clear that this patient's outcome would likely not be good, or at least that the surgery itself would not go smoothly. The same principle is also true with projects. Although a well thought out plan and systematic approach cannot guarantee success, it can certainly help increase the likelihood of success, improve productivity, reduce unnecessary stress and waste, and increase quality.

The practice of pharmacy is no exception. Drug Information specialists and other pharmacy specialties develop, manage, and execute projects every day—everything from policy and guideline development to sweeping standardization efforts and patient care initiatives. As such, strong project management skills are paramount to success. In many ways, project management can be thought of as an extension of the existing drug information skill set by helping work get done quicker and more efficiently, as well as ensuring that best practices are implemented correctly.

Thus, the goal of this chapter is to provide readers with a meaningful framework for managing projects (see Figure 20-1). While several tools and strategies will be discussed, it is important to recognize that the level of project planning rigor should be proportional to the project at hand. For instance, the effort that goes into planning a six-week long project should be much less than the planning needed for a two-year long endeavor. As such, it is incredibly important to balance the planning of the project in relation to its urgency and complexity.

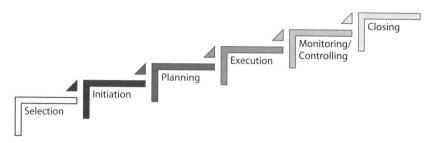

Figure 20–1. Overarching steps in project management.

Projects, Programs, and Portfolios

At a basic level, **projects** are finite endeavors with a distinct beginning and end. Projects are also considered to be progressively elaborate, meaning that at the beginning there is relatively little information or detail; however, as the project evolves, a greater level of detail and planning is achieved. In contrast, **operations** encompass more routine day-to-day activities, are not progressively elaborate, and do not have a finite beginning and end. For example, designing a new car would be considered a project, whereas the ongoing manufacturing of the car after it has been designed would be considered an operation. Another example related to health care could be that of intravenous medication compounding. Implementing a technical solution to ensure safe and accurate compounding would be considered a project, whereas the ongoing use of that technology to compound medications would be considered an operation.

Understanding the relationship between a project, program, and portfolio is also important (see Figure 20-2). At the highest level is a **portfolio**, which encompasses various plans to meet an overall strategic objective. Within a portfolio are **programs**, which involve a group of related projects that are managed in a coordinated way. Programs have their own goals and objectives that ultimately support the main strategic objective of the portfolio. For instance, the Pharmacy Services Department of a hospital might be considered a portfolio, while the subdivisions within Pharmacy

Figure 20–2. Relationship between projects, programs, and portfolios.

Services (e.g., hospital, community, specialty) would be considered programs. Each subdivision has their own goals and undertakes projects that support the overall Pharmacy Services strategy.

❶ *Understanding programs and portfolios is critical to successful project management.* Perhaps most importantly, a project that is aligned with portfolio and program goals will help ensure that the organization is achieving what it wants to accomplish. In such cases, it is also much easier to obtain project buy-off and approval. Alignment with organizational goals will also help in the prioritization of projects—especially in situations where there are many good ideas, but limited resources.

Selecting Projects

PROJECT VIABILITY AND VALUE

One of the most challenging aspects of project management can be that of selecting and prioritizing projects. As mentioned above, successful projects are often those that are aligned with organizational priorities and can add value when completed. Value can be provided in many different ways depending on the culture and objectives of the organization. Value might be demonstrated as the ability to execute on the organization's strategy and bring goals to fruition. It may also be shown in the ability to enable and bring forth change—particularly in rigid environments that lack the ability to change and adapt. Process improvement, or the idea that existing processes could become more efficient, safer, etc., is also a common way of providing value. Additionally, improved regulatory compliance and avoidance of legal risk are sometimes used as a value proposition. Lastly, and perhaps most commonly, value is demonstrated through financial means (e.g., saving money, increasing revenue, better reimbursement).

In all cases, the added value should be measurable and quantifiable. For instance, if the value of implementing a new compounding system is in saving patient lives, then one should be able to define how many lives are being harmed with current processes and how many lives the new technology might save. Ideally, an unbiased and evidence-based assessment should be done when determining value—especially with measures that are more malleable or harder to quantify. In addition to being quantifiable, it is important to ensure that the added value is meaningful and relevant in the eyes of those approving the project. This nuance is particularly helpful when multiple projects are competing for the same pool of limited resources. Those projects where the return-on-investment and the value proposition are high will often be prioritized above projects that show less value to the organization.

CREATING A BUSINESS CASE

Once the added value has been determined, it is often necessary to develop a compelling business case that can be presented to those approving the project. Without a cogent case or argument for the project, there may not be a convincing reason to move forward. While each organization may have their own requirements for a business case, it should typically include an overview of the current landscape or issue to be addressed, what will be accomplished, and a description of the value proposition. Details regarding business case development are beyond the scope of this chapter; however, several useful resources have been written on this topic if more information is desired.[1-3]

Initiating a Project

After a project has been selected, two key deliverables related to initiation can be developed: the **project charter** and the **stakeholder matrix**. The charter is a written document that serves as the guidepost for the project and helps outline the overall vision. Although project charters can vary, they typically contain several key elements including goals and success criteria, final deliverables, stakeholders, budgets, as well as any obvious assumptions, risks, and dependencies. An example of a project charter and its components is outlined in Appendix 20-1. The concept of the stakeholder matrix will be discussed more below.

GOALS, SUCCESS CRITERIA, AND DELIVERABLES

Project goals refer to the desired outcome of the project, whereas **success criteria** are quantifiable measures that define when the goal is accomplished. For example, if a goal is to regain a lost market segment of specialty pharmaceuticals, a success measure might be a 30% increase in sales. ❷ *Knowing the success criteria is critical because they provide a measurable way to define when the project is finished and the goal has been achieved.* Importantly, it should be noted that success criteria might be easier or harder to measure depending on the goal. A goal to improve the reliability of the compounding process, for instance, will have markedly different success criteria than a goal to reduce deaths associated from errors in compounding. Thus, a thoughtful and realistic approach is required when developing goals and success criteria. Lastly, a **deliverable** refers to the tangible component that will be produced as a result of the project in order to achieve the success criteria. For example, if a criterion for success is a 30% improvement in sales, a deliverable might include a real-time dashboard that tracks sales over time.

STAKEHOLDERS

The other key deliverable during project initiation involves the identification of stakeholders. A **stakeholder** refers to anyone (internal or external to the organization) involved in, interested in, or impacted by the project. For instance, stakeholders for a project to install a new robot for filling prescriptions in a community pharmacy might include the pharmacists and technicians who would use the robot, the pharmacy manager or director who has oversight of the pharmacy and budget, patients whose prescriptions will be filled by the machine, environmental or maintenance services who install the robot, as well as information technology specialists who must integrate the robot with existing pharmacy dispensing software. ❸ *Knowing the stakeholders involved is a key step because many times the success of the project depends on their buy-in and input.* Stakeholders can be identified in many ways. An impact analysis and/or benefits analysis could be conducted to help recognize people affected by the project. Similarly, evaluating past projects could provide insight regarding individuals who might be interested or involved in the current endeavor. Those with responsibility for project approval and budgeting are also likely going to be key stakeholders. Consultation with the project sponsor or senior leaders may also be helpful.

Stakeholder Matrix

Once the stakeholders have been identified, it is important to understand their needs and manage them appropriately. One way to do this is to develop a stakeholder matrix or registry, which outlines who they are, their involvement in the project, their expectations from the project, their interest in the project, and how to engage them (see Appendix 20-2). With regard to stakeholder interest level, it can vary considerably and can often be classified into one of five categories:

1. Unaware: refers to those who are not aware of the project or its impact.
2. Resistant: refers to those who are aware of the project, but resistant to the change.
3. Neutral: refers to those who are aware of the project, but have no interest.
4. Supportive: refers those who are aware and supportive with the project.
5. Leading: refers to those who are aware and actively engaged in the project.

Once the interest level of a stakeholder is known, it can be combined with their power/influence over the project to determine how they should be managed and engaged (see Figure 20-3). For instance, a stakeholder with low interest and low power would not require as much attention as someone with both high interest and high power. Such analyses are helpful to determine how often each stakeholder should receive communication about the project or how they should be strategically engaged (e.g., weekly e-mails, monthly in-person meetings).

Figure 20–3. Stakeholder power/interest grid.

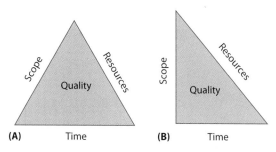

Figure 20–4. Influence of project constraints on quality. **(A)** Quality is a function of the project constraints (such as scope, available resources, and time), which are balanced in this figure. In Part **(B)**, however, notice that if the time constraint is decreased, either the resources needed increase or scope must decrease in order to maintain the same level of quality.

PROJECT CONSTRAINTS

In addition to analyzing stakeholders, it is also helpful to assess **project constraints**—namely scope, time, and available resources, with resources encompassing aspects such as funding, staff, available technology, etc. (see Figure 20-4). Knowing the constraints of the project and managing them effectively are critical to success and the ultimate outcome. For instance, if the staff resources that are needed to complete a project are limited, then either the time needed to complete the project must be increased or the scope must be decreased to compensate. Similarly, if the allotted timeline for the project is shortened, this means that either the scope must decrease or the available resources must increase to maintain quality.

ENVIRONMENTAL AND SWOT ANALYSES

Aside from the charter and stakeholder matrix, it is also generally important to understand the operating environment and all external aspects that may impact a potential project. As such, it may be useful to conduct a **PESTLE analysis**, which encompasses political, economic, social, technological, legal, and environmental factors that may influence the project (see Appendix 20-3).[4] The probability, severity, and potential response to the event can then be determined as a means to help mitigate risk. These analyses are helpful in projects related to the health care field. For instance, a wholesaler who wants to implement a new software program for shipping medications must be aware of regulatory requirements with the Drug Supply Chain and Security Act, which could alter the software and reporting needs.

Another common tool is a **SWOT analysis**, which evaluates strengths, weaknesses, opportunities, and threats. In particular, such analyses are helpful to capitalize on strengths and opportunities, while minimizing weaknesses and threats. For instance, a potential strength within an organization might be the high level of engagement from colleagues about the project, while a weakness that should be minimized may include a reduction in funding due to budget cuts. It should be noted that it is typically more useful and efficient to focus on minimizing threats and weaknesses, rather than improving them.

Planning a Project

After completing the assessments and components associated with project initiation, the next part of the project management process is to actually develop the project plan. This planning typically involves defining scope, identifying resources and deliverables, creating a timeline, and other various management plans, which are reviewed below.

SCOPE

Project **scope** refers to the amount of work to be done, as well as what the project will and will not entail. ❹ *It is extremely important to define the scope because it puts boundaries on the project and defines what the endpoint is* (recall that projects must have a clearly defined end). Without a clearly defined scope, it is nearly impossible to know when the project is considered to be finished. In fact, the project may continue to grow and encompass aspects not originally intended at the outset (a concept referred to as "scope creep"). A clear scope also helps to set expectations with those impacted by the project and helps in the determination of timeline and budget considerations.

WORK BREAKDOWN STRUCTURE AND PROJECT TIMELINE

One of the key elements used when planning a project is a **work breakdown structure (WBS)**. As the name implies, a WBS is essentially a large task list that encompasses all of the deliverables for the project (see Appendix 20-4). Each deliverable is then broken down into the other deliverables or inputs that are required for completion. For example, one major deliverable when building a new house is the exterior finishes. Exterior finishes can be further broken down to include shutters, driveway, mailbox, etc. Another example might be that of adding a new sterile compounding hood in a pharmacy clean room. A major deliverable would include a document detailing a modification to the pharmacy's workflow, which could be further broken down into the following inputs: a description of the current pharmacy workflow before the hood, the future state of the new workflow after installation of the hood, and a workflow gap analysis to identify potentially important issues or barriers. Doing so helps visualize and identify all of the tasks involved in a project and ensures that important deliverables are not missed.

Additionally, the WBS can also be used to elucidate the number resources needed. For instance, after completing the WBS for the new sterile compounding hood, it is estimated that 30 days worth of pharmacist effort is required. Knowing that only one pharmacist is available to work on this project, and that only a few hours per day of this pharmacist's time can be spent completing the work, it is possible to estimate the total time needed to complete the hood installation project. However, if the compounding hood has to be installed and functioning by a certain date, one could estimate the number of additional pharmacist resources needed to meet the project deadline.

❺ *After identifying tasks and the resources needed to accomplish those tasks, a* **project timeline** *can be developed.* A project timeline is useful for assigning a timeframe to each task and, ultimately, determining an overall project schedule. For example, installation of the driveway for the new house might be assigned to the pavers and require two days worth of work, while installation of the mailbox might be assigned to the general contractor and take three hours. Once all of the required times are known, a clearer understanding of the total project time can be elucidated. Another useful byproduct of a project timeline is the identification of dependencies between tasks and inputs. For instance, in the sterile compounding hood example, the gap analysis is dependent on the current and future workflow evaluation (i.e., it cannot be completed before those other actives are finished). However, in the new home example, installation of the exterior shutters is not dependent on installation of the mailbox (i.e., it can be completed either before or after).

Estimating how long a task will take can be challenging and highly nuanced. In general, it is helpful to think of time in terms of effort (the time actively involved in doing the work) and duration (the length of time it will actually take to complete). In the sterile compounding hood scenario, for example, the overall effort time to conduct the gap analysis might be two days; however, because the person responsible also has to attend meetings, care for patients during rounds, teach learners, etc., the total time in terms of duration might be 14 days. In many cases, it is not always clear exactly how long a task may take to complete. In these scenarios, it is often helpful to compare the activity to one that has already been completed. Alternatively, it may be useful to consider the best-case scenario

Figure 20–5. Gantt chart for a simple project using Microsoft Excel® software.

(the soonest it could be completed) and the worst-case scenario (the longest it might take), and then use an average. Achieving a balance will help avoid developing timelines that are either too aggressive or too lax. Regardless, it is important to be realistic about the time required and understand that people usually have other responsibilities and cannot dedicate all of their time to the project.

Gantt Chart

Once all of the dependencies and durations of the tasks are known, a **Gantt chart** can be created. Gantt charts are used to show a visual progression and overall timeline for the project (see Figure 20-5). Depending on the complexity of the project and the needs of the project owner, a Gantt chart can be quite intricate (including every task and associated dependencies) or more global (only including the major deliverables or milestones). These charts can often be developed using common software, such as Microsoft Excel®, although more nuanced charts may require dedicated project management software, such as Microsoft Project® (an in-depth discussion of project management software is beyond the scope of this chapter). Although not every project will need a Gantt chart, such visuals are often useful as a communication and tracking tool for stakeholders and leaders supporting the project.

Case Study 20–1

You are a clinical pharmacist practicing in an inpatient care unit of a large, academic medical center. As part of your job responsibilities, you periodically participate in formulary management activities designed to ensure that evidence-based, safe, and cost-effective medications are used within your facility. One of your assignments for this year is to evaluate the formulary status of tumor necrosis factor (TNF) inhibitor medications. Currently, your hospital uses infliximab (Remicade®) and adalimumab (Humira®) as the formulary-preferred products.

- *What other information would you want to know before starting this assignment or outlining a charter?*
- *Discuss potential success criteria and deliverables for this project.*
- *List potential stakeholder groups relevant to this project.*
- *Describe potential constraints for this project.*
- *Identify some important tasks that should be included in a work breakdown structure that informs the project timeline.*

OTHER COMPONENTS OF A PROJECT PLAN

Requirements Matrix

A **requirements matrix** is a tool used to align the requirements of a project with the goals in the charter. Defining the relationship between goals and requirements at the onset of the project clarifies scope and stakeholder expectations. Within the requirements matrix, each requirement is assigned a person responsible for its completion, a way to track whether or not it has been completed, and some type of quality assessment metric. Documenting and tracking these details helps ensure that the day-to-day activities are executed in a manner that supports the vision for the project. It is also a useful means of monitoring goal completion and can serve as the documentation used for closing the project (discussed further below).

Risk Management Plan

Risk can be thought of as uncertainty during a project that can impact the ability to meet overall goals. In a risk management plan, potential risks are identified and then analyzed in terms of the probability (or likelihood) of it occurring and impact it would have if it did occur. Impact is typically described using a continuum that includes no impact, minimal impact, moderate impact, severe impact, and project failure. Risks with both a high probability of occurrence and high impact require a thoughtful response plan. Although some types of risks are unavoidable, most can usually be mitigated or even avoided. For instance, one risk during the implementation of a new electronic health record system might be a hospital-wide power outage. Having identified this risk, a response plan that includes clear downtime procedures could be developed in order to mitigate the impact of any outages that occur.

Communication Management Plan

Another important aspect of the project plan involves communication. Having an up-front strategy for clear and regular communication with stakeholders helps to create transparency, avoid uncertainty, and maintain engagement. These plans are typically based on the results of the stakeholder matrix analysis conducted during the initiation phase. For instance, stakeholders who are highly interested and have a great amount of power over the project may require more frequent and detailed status reports, whereas someone with low interest and power may only want a brief monthly e-mail. When thinking about a communication plan it is also important to understand the organization's culture and how receptive it is to the change. Project implementation may not succeed unless people within the organization have had time to adjust and buy-in to the concept. Thus, the communication plan may also need to be designed to communicate benefits and advantages of the project to facilitate acceptance.

Change Management Plan

Change, whether expected or not, is likely to happen at some point during the course of a project. Without a well-defined change management process, the scope of the project may expand beyond the initial commitment. Such scope creep can lead to unanticipated delays in implementation, strained resources, budget overruns, unmet expectations, and failed projects. Thus, changes to the project should usually go through a formal and objective review process to fully understand the impact. Depending on the complexity of the project, formal approval or vetting through a change management advisory board may be needed.

Executing a Project

Once the project has been planned, it can then be executed. Following the previously defined strategy for the project will make the work more straightforward and increase the likelihood of accomplishing it successfully. Along the way, it is important to keep team members engaged and maximize their efforts. It is also important to track the planned work versus the work actually accomplished and communicate this information to relevant stakeholders. Not only does this help track if the project is on schedule, but it is also useful to estimate what additional resources are needed in the event work must be accelerated. For instance, knowing that only 30% of the planned work has been completed allows the project coordinator to estimate how much additional time or resources are needed to finish the project.

Monitoring and Controlling a Project

It is important to be able to navigate unanticipated obstacles that may occur during project execution. While most challenges can be prepared for ahead of time using tools such as a risk management plan, many projects fail because of unanticipated issues. As such, continuously evaluating and managing quality throughout the project is crucial. **Project quality** essentially refers to how good the end result or accomplishment will be. To achieve the highest quality, equal parts of time, scope, and resources are needed; however, quality might suffer if any of these three components are limited or not balanced appropriately. It may also be a measure of stakeholder expectations and how well the deliverables conform to their requirements.

Measuring quality is typically done through quality assurance and quality control mechanisms. **Quality assurance** refers to activities that ensure the value of the final product/deliverable itself, whereas **quality control** refers to activities that prevent deficiencies along the process. For example, quality control would include checks put in place during the sterile compounding process (e.g., routine use of isopropyl alcohol, garbing requirements). Quality assurance would include quarantining the final compounded product and conducting a sterility test. Usually it is best to strike a balance between prevention techniques and detection techniques; however, this choice will depend on the nature of the project. As alluded to above, it is also useful to conduct and document quality checks as the project goals or deliverables are completed. It is important to remember that it is the project coordinator's responsibility to keep the project plan up-to-date and stakeholders involved when quality issues my impact the project.

Closing a Project

After all of the work has been completed, several key steps should be taken to close the project. One of the most important activities is to ensure all of the predetermined requirements have been met and accepted by the project sponsor and key stakeholders. Recall that the success criteria developed during project initiation and the requirements matrix developed during project planning are useful tools in this endeavor. Additionally, it is very important to celebrate with the project team and evaluate lessons learned. Depending on the scope and nature of the project, a fun group lunch or social outing could be a great way to congratulate the team and show appreciation for their work. It also provides an opportunity for open discussion about how the project went—evaluating what went well and what could be done differently for next time. Such iterative learning and improvement is invaluable for future projects. Lastly, it is important to finish any project documentation (budgets, completed requirements matrix, etc.) and store it in a readily accessible place. Past project materials often serve as useful templates for the future and having them easily available can save time and work.

Conclusion

Projects are a part of daily life in today's health care environment. Knowing how to manage them appropriately is not only vital to personal success, but can also help improve project outcomes and quality; increase overall efficiency; reduce stress and uncertainty; and lower costs. Although several key concepts to project management were discussed throughout this chapter, it is important to remember that the rigor involved should be proportional to the project at hand. For example, smaller projects or those that need to be completed within a limited time frame may not benefit from a detailed WBS. Nevertheless, the critical components of effective project management should still be considered, including defining the scope, goals, and success criteria, developing a stakeholder matrix and risk mitigation strategy, and outlining a realistic timeline for the major tasks involved. Various project management programs, such as Microsoft Project®, can also be leveraged. Again, however, routine use of these tools is often unnecessary for the average health care professional who deals with projects. General workplace productivity software and resources are often sufficient (e.g., Microsoft Excel®, Microsoft Word®, white boards). The key is to use a routine, organized, and systematic process that can be followed from project selection through completion.

Self-Assessment Questions

1. Which one of the following best describes a project?
   a. Ongoing, day-to-day activities that support an organization
   b. A group of plans that support an overall strategic organizational objective
   c. A finite, progressively elaborate endeavor with a beginning and end
   d. An endeavor with a larger scope than either a program or portfolio
   e. None of the above

2. Which one of the following is used to define/identify when a project is complete?
   a. Deliverables
   b. Success criteria
   c. Work breakdown structure (WBS)
   d. Scope
   e. Constraints

3. Which of the following considerations is important when determining the value proposition of a project?
   a. Measurable and quantifiable
   b. Aligned with the priorities of the organization
   c. Related to financial incentives or profits
   d. Both a and b
   e. All of the above

Please use the following case for questions 4 through 6

A pharmacist wants to conduct a project to standardize how concentrated 23.4% normal saline is stored and dispensed within a hospital. After discussing the project with leadership the pharmacist decides to develop a project charter.

4. Which one of the following individuals would **NOT** be considered a stakeholder for this project?
   a. Nurse manager in the neuro intensive care unit
   b. Inpatient pharmacy operations manager
   c. Medication safety officer for the hospital
   d. Physician chair of intensive medicine for the hospital
   e. Radiology technician in the medical intensive care unit

5. Individuals classified as which of the following in a stakeholder matrix should receive the most attention?
   a. Low interest, high power
   b. High interest, high power
   c. Low interest, low power
   d. High interest, low power
   e. All stakeholders should receive equal attention

6. Which of the following might be considered a constraint of this project?
   a. A completion deadline of two weeks from the start of the project
   b. Limited space in the automated dispensing cabinets in the patient care units
   c. Only one staff member in the neuro intensive care unit is available to help

d. Both a and b

e. All of the above

7. A SWOT analysis is often used to identify ways to capitalize on strengths and opportunities, while minimizing weaknesses and threats to a project.

a. True

b. False

8. Which one of the following is used to put boundaries on the project?

a. Deliverables

b. Success criteria

c. Work breakdown structure (WBS)

d. Scope

e. Constraints

9. Which one of the following is used to organize and identify the tasks needed to accomplish major project deliverables?

a. Deliverables

b. Success criteria

c. Work breakdown structure (WBS)

d. Scope

e. Constraints

10. _____ is a useful tool for visualizing the progression and timeline of a project.

a. Gantt chart

b. Work breakdown structure (WBS)

c. PESTLE analysis

d. SWOT analysis

e. Charter

11. Which of the following correctly outlines the progression of a project?

a. Selection, initiation, planning, execution, monitoring, closing

b. Initiation, selection, planning, execution, monitoring, closing

c. Selection, planning, initiation, execution, monitoring, closing

d. Selection, initiation, planning, monitoring, execution, closing

12. When monitoring and controlling a project, which of the following is the most important?

a. Review the Gantt chart and work breakdown structure daily

b. Conduct regular SWOT and PESTLE analyses

c. Continually assess and manage the quality of the project

d. Routinely update the project charter

e. Document daily status reports for leadership

13. Project quality is dependent on which of the following?
    a. Time
    b. Resources
    c. Scope
    d. Both a and b
    e. All of the above

14. A debrief with team members should be conducted after closing a project in order to learn and improve.
    a. True
    b. False

15. Smaller projects, or projects with short timelines, should still use a detailed work breakdown structure, charter, change management strategy, and all other components of a project plan.
    a. True
    b. False

REFERENCES

1. Schumock GT, Stubbings J. How to develop a business plan for pharmacy services. 2nd rev. ed. Lenexa, KS: American College of Clinical Pharmacy; 2013.
2. Sahlman WA. How to write a great business plan. Harv Bus Rev. 1997 Jul-Aug;75(4):98-108.
3. Chishold-Burns MA, Vaillancourt AM, Shepherd M, editors. Pharmacy management, leadership, marketing, and finance. Burlington, MA: Jones & Bartlett Learning, LLC; 2014.
4. What is PESTLE analysis? A tool for business analysis [Internet]. Newark, DE: Weberience LLC; [cited 2017 Apr 3]. Available from: http://pestleanalysis.com/what-is-pestle-analysis/.

SUGGESTED READINGS

1. Kerzner H. Project management: a systems approach to planning, scheduling, and controlling. 11th rev. ed. Hoboken, NJ: Wiley; 2013.
2. Project Management Institute homepage [Internet]. Newtown Square, PA: Project Management Institute; [cited 2016 Sept 22]. Available from: http://www.pmi.org
3. Project Management Institute. A guide to the project management body of knowledge (PMBOK®). 5th rev. ed. Newtown Square, PA: Project Management Institute, Inc.; 2013.
4. Schwalbe K, Furlong D. Healthcare project management. Minneapolis, MN: Schwalbe Publishing; 2013.

Chapter Twenty-One

Investigational Drugs

Bambi Grilley

Learning Objectives

After completing this chapter, the reader will be able to

- List the major legislative acts that led to the current system of drug evaluation, approval, and regulation used in the United States.
- List the steps in the drug approval process.
- List the components of an investigational new drug (IND) application.
- Recognize the difference between a commercial IND, treatment IND, an emergency use IND, and an individual investigator IND.
- Define orphan drug status and list the advantages of classifying a drug as an orphan drug.
- List all of the requirements (as specified by the Office of Human Research Protections [OHRP]) for an Institutional Review Board (IRB).
- Prepare appropriate protocol assessments for use by the IRB or other review committees when they evaluate new human subject protocols.
- Describe the type of support that is necessary for clinical research, including (but not limited to):
  a. ordering drug supplies for ongoing clinical trials;
  b. maintaining drug accountability records as required by the Food and Drug Administration (FDA);
  c. preparing drug and protocol data sheets for use by health care personnel in the hospital;
  d. preparing pharmacy budgets for sponsored clinical research;
  e. aiding investigators in designing and conducting clinical trials in their institution;
  f. assisting investigators in initiating and conducting clinical trials (including emergency use INDs).

Key Concepts

1 The Food and Drug Administration (FDA) is the federal agency that decides which drugs, biologics, and medical devices are safe and efficacious, determinations upon which the agency decides if a product can be marketed in the United States.

2 In addition to review by the FDA, research protocols are also reviewed for ethical appropriateness by IRBs.

3 The drug approval process in the United States is standardized by FDA review. It consists of preclinical testing and Phase I through IV of clinical testing.

4 The investigational new drug (IND) application is the application by the study sponsor to the FDA to begin clinical trials in humans.

5 The IND should be amended as necessary. The four types of documents used to amend the IND include:

    a. Protocol amendments

    b. Information amendments

    c. IND safety reports

    d. IND annual reports

6 After sufficient evidence is obtained regarding the drug's safety and effectiveness, the sponsor will submit a new drug application/biologics licensing application to the FDA requesting approval of the agent for marketing.

7 The FDA allows the manufacturer to charge for an investigational drug under certain conditions.

8 An orphan drug is one that is used for the treatment of a rare disease, affecting fewer than 200,000 people in the United States, or one that will not generate enough revenue to justify the cost of research and development.

9 Drug accountability records are mandated by law. They can be computerized or in paper form. Necessary components include:

    a. Transaction date

    b. Transaction type

    c. The receiving party (for patient dispensing this should include patient initials/identifying number)

    d. The dose/number of units dispensed/received

    e. The lot number dispensed/received

    f. The initials of the person who performed the transaction

Introduction

It is now estimated that approximately $2.6 billion is spent to get a new drug product to market in the United States.[1] Although there is some controversy surrounding these estimates, there is no doubt that the costs of drug development continue to escalate.[2] Currently the Pharmaceutical Research and Manufacturers of America (PhRMA) database is tracking 3,500 new compounds in development in the United States with more than $58.8 billion invested in research and development (R&D) in 2015.[3] This should be compared to 45 novel drugs approved by the Food and Drug Administration (FDA) in 2015.[4] ❶ *The FDA is the federal agency that decides which drugs, biologics, and medical devices are safe and efficacious, determinations upon which the agency decides if a product can be marketed in the United States.* In fact, the FDA monitors the manufacture, import, transport, storage, and sale of 25% of all goods purchased in the United States annually.[5] The centers of the FDA involved in regulating drugs, biologics, and medical devices used in humans are as follows:

- Center for Biologics Evaluation and Research (CBER)
- Center for Drug Evaluation and Research (CDER)
- Center for Devices and Radiological Health (CDRH)[6]

Since this book only includes drug-related information, this chapter will concentrate only on the regulations associated with CBER and CDER.

Since 1940, more than 10,000 new drug applications (NDAs) have been approved in the United States.[7] It is very important that the clinical trials upon which the FDA will base their decisions be both scientifically accurate and complete. Health care professionals can play an important role in ensuring that the clinical trials conducted at their institutions meet the goals set forth by the study sponsor, the local investigator, and ultimately the FDA.

Currently, most research conducted on investigational drugs is performed in medical schools, hospitals, and organizations specifically designed to conduct clinical research trials. In some institutions, a pharmacist will be hired specifically to handle investigational drugs. More frequently, however, this role falls to other health care providers. To successfully manage investigational drugs, this individual or team of individuals must be a bookkeeper, inventory control manager, and, most importantly, an information disseminator. Before proceeding, it is necessary to define a number of terms that will be used in this chapter.

Definitions

- **Biologics license application (BLA):** A BLA is a submission that contains specific information on the manufacturing processes, chemistry, pharmacology, clinical pharmacology, and the medical effects of the biologic product. It is a request for permission to introduce, or deliver for introduction, a biologic product into interstate commerce.[8]
- **Clinical investigation:** Any experiment in which a drug is administered or dispensed to one or more human subjects. An experiment is any use of a drug (except for the use of a marketed drug) in the course of medical practice. Although there are many other definitions, this is the FDA's definition and would seem the appropriate one to use, given the nature of this topic. Please note that the FDA does not regulate the practice of medicine and prescribers are (as far as the agency is concerned) free to use any marketed drug for off-label use.[9]
- **Commercial IND:** An IND for which the sponsor (see below) is usually either a corporate entity or one of the institutes of the National Institutes of Health (NIH). In addition, CDER may designate other INDs as commercial, if it is clear that the sponsor intends the product to be commercialized at a later date.[10]
- **Control group:** The group of test animals or humans that receive a placebo (a dosage that does not contain active medicine) or active (a dosage that does contain active medicine) treatment. For most preclinical and clinical trials, the FDA will require that this group receives placebo (commonly referred to as the placebo control). However, some studies may have an active control, which generally consists of an available (standard of care) treatment modality. An active control may, with the concurrence of the FDA, be used in studies where it would be considered unethical to use a placebo. A historical control is one in which a group of previous patients is compared to a matched set of patients receiving the new therapy. A historical control might be used in cases where the disease is consistently fatal (i.e., acquired immunodeficiency syndrome [AIDS]). (Refer to Chapter 4 for additional information on control groups.)[11]
- **Contract research organization (CRO):** An individual or organization that assumes one or more of the obligations of the sponsor through an independent contractual agreement.[9]
- **Drug master file (DMF):** A submission to the FDA that may be used to provide confidential, detailed information about facilities, processes, or articles used in the manufacturing, processing, packaging, and storing of one or more human drugs.[12]
- **Drug product:** The final dosage form prepared from the drug substance.[8]
- **Drug substance:** An active ingredient that is intended to furnish pharmacological activity or other direct effect in the diagnosis, cure, mitigation, treatment, or

prevention of disease or to affect the structure or any function of the human body.[13]

- **Food and Drug Administration (FDA):** The agency of the U.S. government that is responsible for ensuring the safety and efficacy of all drugs on the market in the United States.[9]

- **Good clinical practice (GCP):** A standard for the design, conduct, monitoring, analyses, and reporting of clinical trials that provides assurance that the results are credible and accurate, and that the rights of study subjects are protected.[14]

- **Institutional Review Board (IRB)/Institutional Ethics Committee (IEC):** A committee of reviewers that is responsible for ensuring the protection of the rights, safety, and well-being of human subjects involved in a clinical investigation.[9]

- **Investigational new drug:** A drug, antibiotic, or biologic that is used in a clinical investigation. The label of an investigational drug must bear the statement: "Caution: New Drug—Limited by Federal (or U.S.) law to investigational use."[9]

- **Investigational new drug (IND) application:** A submission to the FDA containing chemical information, preclinical data, and a detailed description of the planned clinical trials. Thirty days after submission of this document to the FDA by the sponsor, clinical trials may be initiated in humans, unless the FDA places a clinical hold. When the FDA allows the studies to proceed, this document allows unapproved drugs to be shipped in interstate commerce.[15]

- **Investigator:** The individual responsible for initiating the clinical trial at the study site. This individual must treat the patients, assure that the protocol is followed, evaluate responses and adverse reactions, assure proper conduct of the study, and solve problems as they arise.[9]

- **New drug application (NDA):** The application to the FDA requesting approval to market a new drug for human use. The NDA contains data supporting the safety and efficacy of the drug for its intended use.[16]

- **New molecular entity (NME):** A compound that can be patented and has not been previously marketed in the United States in any form.[4]

- **Regulatory project manager (RPM):** This will be the sponsor's (see below) primary FDA contact person. Each application that is submitted is assigned an RPM. Contact information for the RPM is provided in the letter sent to the applicant acknowledging receipt of the application. If the RPM is changed during the course of the review, the applicant is notified by the new RPM.[17]

- **Sponsor:** An organization (or individual) who takes responsibility for and initiates a clinical investigation. The sponsor may be an individual or pharmaceutical company, government agency, academic institution, private organization, or other organization.[9]

- **Sponsor-investigator:** An individual who both initiates and conducts a clinical investigation (i.e., submits the IND and directly supervises administration of the drug as well as other investigator responsibilities).[9]
- **Subject:** An individual who participates in a clinical investigation (either as the recipient of the investigational drug or as a member of the control group).[9]

History of Drug Development Regulation in the United States

For more than a century after the Declaration of Independence, drug products were not regulated in the United States. Available drugs were often ineffective, but some were addictive, toxic, or even lethal. During this same period, physicians were not licensed and nearly anyone could practice medicine. The public was, for the most part, responsible for using common sense when evaluating which products they would use.

The evolution of drug regulations in this country is a study in human tragedy. Crises have instigated the development of many of the laws regulating drug development, preparation, and distribution.

The first federal law developed to deal with drug quality and safety was the Import Drug Act of 1848. This law was passed after it was discovered that American troops involved in the Mexican War had been supplied with substandard imported drugs. The act provided for the inspection, detention, and destruction or reexport of imported drug shipments that failed to meet prescribed standards.

The Pure Food and Drugs Act was passed in 1906. This law required that drugs not be mislabeled or adulterated, and stated that they must meet recognized standards for strength and purity. Mislabeling in this context only referred to the identity or composition of drugs (not false therapeutic claims). False therapeutic claims were prohibited with the passing of the Sherley Amendment in 1912.

In 1937, the drug sulfanilamide was released. This drug showed promise as an anti-infective agent and was prepared as an oral liquid. The vehicle used for this preparation was diethylene glycol (a sweet-tasting solvent similar to ethylene glycol, which was used as an automobile antifreeze). A total of 107 people died after taking this preparation. Within one year of this tragedy, the Food, Drug, and Cosmetic Act of 1938 was enacted. This law required that the safety of drugs, when used in accordance with the labeled instructions, be proven through testing before they could be marketed. It was in this law that the submission of an NDA to the FDA was first described. The NDA was required to list the drug's intended uses and provide scientific evidence that the drug was safe.

If after 60 days the FDA had not responded to the manufacturer regarding the NDA, the manufacturer was free to proceed with marketing of the product.

In 1951, the Durham-Humphrey Amendment was passed. This law divided pharmaceuticals into two distinct classes:

1. Over-the-counter (OTC) medications that could be safely self-administered.
2. Prescription (℞) medications that had potentially dangerous side effects and therefore required expert medical supervision.

This law required the following statement be added to the labels for all prescription medications: "Caution: Federal Law prohibits dispensing without a prescription."

In 1962, another drug tragedy occurred that resulted in additional regulations. In that year, an inordinate number of pregnant women in Western Europe gave birth to children with severe deformities. These deformities were related to the use of the drug thalidomide. Although U.S. consumers were not directly affected by this tragedy, because thalidomide had not been released in the U.S. market, it was a compelling reason for the legislature to develop stronger laws regarding the testing of new drug products. The Kefauver-Harris Drug Amendment was passed the same year. This law specified that the manufacturer had to demonstrate proof of efficacy, as well as safety, prior to marketing any new drug. Additionally, this law required that drug manufacturers operate in conformity with Current Good Manufacturing Practices (CGMP). Finally, it stated that the FDA had to formally approve an NDA before the drug could be marketed.[18]

There are numerous other laws and regulations that affect drug products in the United States, but those mentioned above provide the legal foundation for the current regulation of drug products in the United States. Based on these laws, the FDA has assumed a large role in assessing the safety and efficacy of drug products prior to their distribution in the United States.

EVOLUTION OF THE FDA'S DRUG APPROVAL PROCESS

❶ *The FDA decides which drugs, biologics, and medical devices are safe and efficacious and therefore can be marketed in the United States.* The goal of the FDA is to provide American consumers with safe and effective drugs, biologics, and devices.[5] Extensive debate regarding the need to reform the FDA has been ongoing in the United States for years. Critics of the FDA have long claimed that the approval process for drugs in the United States is too costly and time consuming.[19,20] Interestingly however, data shows that the FDA leads the world in the first introduction of new active substances and that the majority of novel therapeutic agents are approved in the United States first. Additionally, approval times in the United States are on average two months faster than in the European Union (E.U.) and

Canada.[21] Nevertheless, over the past two decades, the FDA and the federal government have initiated many reforms and initiatives designed to address these criticisms. Included in these reform acts are the Prescription Drug User Fee Act of 1992 (PDUFA), which was reauthorized in 1997 and reauthorized every 5 years with the most recent reauthorization occurring in 2012, and the Food and Drug Administration Modernization Act of 1997 (FDAMA). PDUFA redefined the time frames for NDA reviews and established revenues to fund the increased demands created by the new time frames.[22] The FDAMA, which reauthorized PDUFA in 1997, was much broader in scope and impacted not only the drug approval process, but also other aspects of the practices of pharmacy and medicine.[23] The Food and Drug Administration Amendments Act (FDAAA), which was signed into law in 2007, further expanded PDUFA to provide the FDA with additional resources to conduct timely and comprehensive reviews of new drugs in the United States.[24] Most recently, the Food and Drug Administration Safety and Innovation Act of 2012 (FDASIA) signed into law on July 9, 2012, not only reauthorized PDUFA, it also gave the FDA a new product designation known as the "breakthrough therapy" designation, that will be discussed in more detail later in this chapter.[25]

Aside from looking at review times, the FDA has also been concerned about the increasing difficulty in drug and biologic development. To attempt to address this issue, the FDA launched a new initiative in March 2004 called the Critical Path Initiative. The Critical Path Initiative is the FDA's attempt to facilitate modernization of the sciences and improve regulatory decision making. The FDA has been working with the public, the pharmaceutical industry, other regulatory agencies, and academia to identify projects that they feel are most likely to help the drug development process from test tube to bedside.[26]

More recently, as a result of FDASIA, the FDA has increased their focus on patient engagement.[25] A notable example of this initiative is a patient advocacy-initiated draft guidance submitted to the FDA to help accelerate development and review of potential therapies for Duchenne muscular dystrophy. A major point of emphasis was that the parents of children affected by Duchenne muscular dystrophy were willing to accept a higher risk profile for potential therapies even in evaluation of products that may improve patient quality of life without prolonging life.[27,28]

Finally, the FDA has undertaken many information technology initiatives to facilitate the regulatory review process. Included in these initiatives is the development of systems allowing for electronic submission, management, and review of regulatory information.[29] In fact, the FDA has mandated that all NDA, BLA, ANDA, and DMFs must be in the eCTD format by May 2017 while all commercial INDs must be in eCTD format by May 2018.[30]

Overall, the goal of the initiatives is to review priority drugs in 6 months and standard drugs within 10 months.[31] Other attempts by the FDA to increase availability of investigational drugs to patients will be discussed later in this chapter.

TRANSPARENCY AND HARMONIZATION OF DRUG DEVELOPMENT

First initiated in response to components of FDAMA, the NIH developed a web-based system that offers information about ongoing clinical trials for a wide range of diseases and conditions. The system allows potential study subjects to search for studies for particular diseases and identify treatment centers that offer enrollment into those studies. Requirements for postings have become more stringent over the past five years. Most recently, in 2007 FDAAA required more types of trials to be registered, additional trial registration information, and submission of summary results including adverse events for certain trials. The site is available at http://clinicaltrials.gov. Study sponsors are required to verify that the study is posted on the ClinicalTrials.gov website as part of the IND submission process through submission of a Form 3674.[32,33]

Increasingly, pharmaceutical companies are involved in global drug development. Historically, the regulatory requirements for drug approval varied from country to country, resulting in a significant amount of time and money being spent to receive multiple approvals. For this reason, the International Conference on Harmonization (ICH) has brought together officials from Europe, the United States, and Japan to develop common guidelines for ensuring the quality, safety, and efficacy of drugs. The FDA has been very involved in the development of the ICH guidelines. The ultimate goal of these guidelines is to provide pharmaceutical firms a method to ensure simultaneous submission and rapid regulatory approval in the world's major markets. This would minimize duplication of effort, improve efficiency, and increase the quality and consistency of medical treatments available to patients worldwide.[34]

For gene therapy products, submission to the NIH Office of Scientific Policy is required with a potential selection for review by the Recombinant DNA Activities Committee.[35] Review and approval by the local Institutional Biosafety Committee(s) is required. These submissions and reviews are in addition to review and approval by the FDA and IRB (discussed below). The review process for gene therapy products is a separate topic that will not be further addressed in this chapter. Individuals interested in regulatory requirements of gene therapy products can refer to other references such as the book chapter entitled Regulations Governing Clinical Trials in Gene Therapy included in the book Cancer Gene Therapy by Viral and Non-viral Vectors.[36]

PROTECTION OF HUMAN SUBJECTS

❷ *In addition to the regulatory review of investigational drugs by the FDA, research protocols are also reviewed for ethical appropriateness by IRBs.* The formalized process for protecting human subjects began with the Nuremberg Code. This code was used to judge the human experimentation conducted by the Nazis around the middle of the twentieth century. The Nuremberg Code states that "the voluntary consent of the human subjects is absolutely essential." The code goes on to specify that the subject must have the capacity to consent, must be free from coercion, and must comprehend the risks and benefits involved in the research.[37] The Declaration of Helsinki reemphasized the above points and distinguished between therapeutic and nontherapeutic research. This document was first developed in 1964 and has been revised multiple times, most recently in 2013.[38]

The NIH, as part of the Department of Health and Human Services (DHHS), used these two documents to develop its own policies for the Protection of Human Subjects in 1966. These policies were raised to regulatory status in 1974 and established the IRB as a mechanism through which human subjects would be protected. The Belmont Report, released in 1978, further delineates the basic ethical principles underlying medical research on human subjects.[39] Title 45 Part 46 of the Code of Federal Regulations (CFR), which was released in 1981, was designed to make uniform the protection of human subjects in all federal agencies.[40] Title 21 Part 50 (approved in 1980) of the CFR sets forth guidelines for appropriate informed consent and Title 21 Part 56 (approved in 1981) of the CFR sets forth guidelines for the IRB.[41,42] Copies of these regulations can be obtained on the Internet at http://www.ecfr.gov.

These two documents are used by the FDA and the DHHS to evaluate the ethical conduct of clinical trials in the United States. Further information regarding the role of the IRB will be presented later in this chapter.

The Drug Approval Process

6 *The drug approval process in the United States is standardized by FDA review. It consists of preclinical testing and Phase I through IV of clinical testing.* The first step in the drug approval process is preclinical testing. This testing is conducted either *in vitro* or in animals. Before filing an IND, the sponsor must have developed a pharmacologic profile of the drug, determined its acute and subacute toxicity, and have sufficient information regarding chronic toxicity to support the drug's use in humans.[43]

INVESTIGATIONAL NEW DRUG APPLICATION

After the preclinical testing is completed, the sponsor will file an IND with the FDA. **4** *The IND is the application by the study sponsor to the FDA to begin clinical trials in humans.* Most often, the sponsor is a pharmaceutical company, but occasionally an individual investigator will file an IND and serve as a sponsor-investigator. An investigator IND is submitted when a physician plans to use an approved drug for a new indication (i.e., one that is outside the package labeling) or on occasion, for an unapproved product or for an NME. The IND requirements for the sponsor-investigator are the same as those for any other sponsor. For that reason, no differentiation will be made in the following discussion of the drug approval process.

An IND is not required if the drug to be studied is marketed in the United States and all of the following requirements are met:

1. The study is not to be reported to the FDA in support of a new indication.
2. The study does not involve a different dose, route, or patient population that increases the risk to patients.
3. IRB approval and informed consent are secured.
4. The study will not be used to promote the drug's effectiveness for a new indication.

The FDA has developed a guidance document specifically to assist in determining whether or not an IND is required. However, in situations where it is unclear whether an IND is required or not, a call to the FDA is the best way to determine the appropriate way to proceed.[44]

In recent years, there have been several therapeutic products developed that depend on the use of an *in vitro* companion diagnostic device (or test) for its safe and effective use. It is important to note that in this situation, the *in vitro* device should be approved or cleared concurrently by FDA for the use indicated in the therapeutic **product labeling**. To be clear, this might require the study of the diagnostic device under an **investigational device exemption (IDE)** while the therapeutic product is being studied under an IND. If the diagnostic device and therapeutic product are to be studied together to support their respective approvals (or clearance in the case of a device) both products can be studied in the same investigational study if the study has been developed and conducted in a manner that meets both IND and IDE regulations.[45] One other interesting issue related to devices is the use of a mobile app (i.e., a software application on a mobile platform such as an iPhone or Android) for the diagnosis of disease, or the cure, mitigation, treatment or prevention of disease or to affect the structure of function of the body. In these situations, the mobile app can be considered to be a medical device subject to IDE regulations.[46] IDE regulations and components will not be further discussed in this chapter; however, the applicable regulations can be found in 21CFR812 and the FDA has extensive guidance regarding these products and their development.

Contents of IND

An IND application needs to contain the following information:

1. **Cover sheet:** Form 1571 (available at the FDA website under Forms, see Appendix 1). This form identifies the sponsor, documents that the sponsor agrees

to follow appropriate regulations, and identifies any involved CRO. This is a legal document.

2. **Table of contents**

3. **Introductory statement:** States the name, structure, pharmacologic class, dosage form, and all active ingredients in the investigational drug; the objectives and planned duration of the investigation should be stated here.

4. **General investigational plan:** Describes the rationale, indications, and general approach for evaluating the drug, the types of trials to be conducted, the projected number of patients that will be treated, and any potential safety concerns; the purpose of this section is to give FDA reviewers a general overview of the plan to study the drug.

5. **Investigator's brochure:** An information packet containing all available information on the drug including its formula, pharmacologic and toxicologic effects, pharmacokinetics, and any information regarding the safety and risks associated with the drug. It is important that this brochure be kept current and comprehensive; therefore, it should be amended as necessary. The investigator's brochure may be used by the investigator or other health care professionals as a reference during the conduct of the research study.

6. **Clinical protocol**
   - *Objectives and purpose:* A description of the purpose of the trial (a typical Phase I objective would be to determine the maximum tolerated dose of the investigational drug, whereas a typical Phase III objective would be to compare the safety and efficacy of the investigational drug to placebo or standard therapy).
   - *Investigator data:* Provides qualifications and demographic data of the investigators involved in the clinical trial (may be presented on Form 1572 [available at the FDA website under Forms, see Appendix 2]).
   - *Patient selection:* Describes the characteristics of patients that are eligible for enrollment in the trial and states factors that would exclude the patient.
   - *Study design:* Describes how the study will be completed; if the study is to be randomized, this will be described here with a description of the alternate therapy.
   - *Dose determination:* Describes the dose (with possible adjustments) and route of administration of the investigational drug; if retreatment or maintenance therapy of patients is allowed, it will be detailed in this section.
   - *Observations:* Describes how the objectives stated earlier in the protocol are to be assessed.
   - *Clinical procedures:* Describes all laboratory tests or clinical procedures that will be used to monitor the effects of the drug in the patient; the collection of this data is intended to minimize the risk to the patients.

- *IRB approval for protocol:* Documentation of this approval is not required as part of the IND application process; however, Form 1571 does state that an IRB will review and approve each study in the proposed clinical investigation before allowing initiation of those studies.

7. **Chemistry, manufacturing, and control data**
   - *Drug substance:* Describes the drug substance including its name, biological, physical, and chemical characteristics; the address of the manufacturer; the method of synthesis or preparation; and the analytical methods used to assure purity, identity, and the substance's stability.
   - *Drug product:* Describes the drug product including all of its components; the address of the manufacturer; the analytical methods used to ensure identity, quality, purity, and strength of the product; and the product's stability.
   - *Composition, manufacture, and control of any placebo used in the trial:* The FDA does not require that the placebo be identical to the investigational drug; however, it wants to ensure that the lack of similarity does not jeopardize the trial.
   - *Labeling:* Copies of all labels and labeling used for the drug substance or product, and packages as it will be provided to each investigator. Labels in this context meaning the information affixed to product and used to identify the contents while labeling in this context relates to product information including prescribing information.
   - *Environmental assessment:* Presents a claim for categorical exclusion from the requirement for an environmental assessment (a statement that the amount of waste expected to reach the environment may reasonably be expected to be nontoxic).

8. **Pharmacology and toxicology data**
   - *Pharmacology and drug disposition:* Describes the pharmacology, mechanism of action, absorption, distribution, metabolism, and excretion of the drug in animals and *in vitro*.
   - *Toxicology:* Describes the toxicology in animals and *in vitro*.
   - A statement that all nonclinical laboratories involved in the research adhered to Good Laboratory Practice (GLP) regulations.

9. **Previous human experience:** Summary of human experiences, which includes data from the United States and, where applicable, foreign markets. Known safety and efficacy data should be presented (especially if the drug was withdrawn from foreign markets for reasons of safety or efficacy).

10. **Additional information**: Other information that would help the reviewer evaluate the proposed clinical trial should be included here. For example, if a drug has the potential for abuse, data on the drug's dependence and abuse potential should be discussed in this section.[43]

The letter of authorization (LOA) to cross reference a DMF, IND application, or NDA (referred to in item 9 on page 1 of Form 1571) is required when the investigational product (or some component of the investigational product) being used in the research is being supplied by a manufacturer other than the study sponsor. The original holder of the IND/NDA/DMF prepares the LOA. An LOA is frequently required when two companies are working together toward development of a product.[47]

Finally, proof of compliance with the requirements of ClinicalTrials.gov through submission of Form 3674 (available at the FDA website under Forms, http://www.fda.gov/AboutFDA/ReportsManualsForms/Forms/default.htm) is required as part of the IND.[32]

Amendment of IND

● ❺ *The IND should be amended as necessary.* There are four types of documents that may be used to amend the IND. They are as follows:

1. **Protocol amendments:** Submitted when a sponsor wants to change a previously submitted protocol or add a new study protocol to an existing IND.[48]
2. **Information amendments:** Submitted when information becomes available that would not be presented using a protocol amendment, IND safety report, or annual report (e.g., new chemistry data).[49]
3. **IND safety reports:** Reports clinical and animal adverse reactions; reporting requirements depend on the nature, severity, and frequency of the experience. The following definitions are used to help evaluate adverse reactions.
   - *Suspected adverse reaction:* An adverse reaction for which there is evidence to suggest a causal relationship between the drug and the adverse event.
   - *Serious adverse event or serious suspected adverse reaction:* An event that results in any of the following outcomes: death, a life-threatening adverse drug experience, inpatient hospitalization or prolongation of existing hospitalization, a persistent or significant disability/incapacity, or a congenital anomaly/birth defect. Important medical events that may not result in death, be life threatening, or require hospitalization may be considered a serious adverse drug experience when, based on appropriate medical judgment, they may jeopardize the patient or subject and may require medical or surgical intervention to prevent one of the outcomes listed in this definition.
   - *Unexpected adverse event or unexpected suspected adverse reaction:* An adverse reaction that is not listed in the current labeling for the drug product. This includes events that may be symptomatically and pathophysiologically related to an event listed in the labeling, but differs from the event because of greater severity or specificity.

For serious and unexpected, fatal, or life threatening suspected adverse reactions, the sponsor is required to notify the FDA by telephone or fax within seven calendar days after the sponsor receives the information. The sponsor must also submit a written report within 15 calendar days. For clinical and nonclinical adverse reactions that are both serious and unexpected, the sponsor must notify the FDA in writing within 15 calendar days. The written reports should describe the current adverse event and identify all previously filed safety reports concerning similar adverse events. The written report may be submitted as a narrative or as Form 3500A (available at http://www.fda.gov/safety/medwatch/howtoreport/downloadforms/default.htm).[50,51]

4. **Annual reports**: Submitted within 60 days of the annual effective date of an IND; it should describe the progress of the investigation including information on the individual studies, summary information of the IND (summary of adverse experiences, IND safety reports, preclinical studies completed in the last year), relevant developments in foreign markets, and changes in the investigator's brochure.[52]

Each submission to a specific IND is required to be numbered sequentially (starting with 000). A total of three sets (the original and two copies) of all submissions to an IND file (whether a new IND or revisions to an existing IND) are sent to the FDA.[43]

Once submitted to the FDA, the IND will be forwarded to the appropriate review division based on the therapeutic category of the product. Examples of the different divisions include oncology products, hematology products, anti-infective products, and medical imaging products. Following submission, the IND and clinical trial will be assigned to a review team that includes:

- The project manager,
- A chemistry, manufacturing, and controls (CMC) reviewer,
- A nonclinical pharmacology/toxicology reviewer,
- A clinical reviewer, and
- Other reviewers as needed (e.g., statisticians, epidemiologists, site inspectors, patient representatives).[17]

The FDA has 30 days after receipt of an IND to respond to the sponsor. The sponsor may begin clinical trials if there is no response from the FDA within 30 days.[53] The FDA delays initiation of a new study or discontinues an ongoing study by issuing a clinical hold. Clinical holds are most often used when the FDA identifies an issue (through initial review or through later submissions) that the agency feels poses a significant risk to the subjects. After this issue has been satisfactorily resolved, the clinical hold can be removed and the investigations can be initiated or resumed.[54]

PHASES OF CLINICAL TRIALS

❸ *There are four phases of clinical trials.* Clinical studies generally begin cautiously. As experience with the agent grows, the dose and duration of exposure to the agent may also increase. The number of patients treated at each phase of study and the duration of the studies can vary significantly depending on statistical considerations, the prevalence of patients affected by the disease, and the importance of the new drug. However, some general guidelines regarding the four phases of clinical testing are presented below.

Phase I

A Phase I trial is the first use of the agent in humans. As such, these studies are usually initiated with cautious (low) doses and in a small numbers of subjects. Doses may be increased as safety is established. A Phase I study will usually treat 20 to 80 patients and last an average of six months to one year. The purpose of a Phase I trial is to determine the safety and toxicity of the agent. Frequently these trials include a pharmacokinetic portion. These trials assist in identifying the preferred route of administration and a safe dosage range. When possible, these trials are initiated in normal, healthy volunteers. This allows for evaluation of the effect of the drug on a subject who does not have any preexisting conditions. In situations in which this is not practical, such as oncology drugs, in which the drug itself can be highly toxic, these drugs are usually reserved for patients who have exhausted all conventional options.

Phase II

A Phase II trial is one in which the drug is used in a small number of subjects who suffer from the disease or condition that the drug is proposed to treat. The purpose of a Phase II trial is to evaluate the efficacy of the agent. Data from the Phase I trial, *in vitro* testing, and animal testing may be used to identify which group of patients is most likely to benefit from therapy with this agent. Phase II trials usually treat between 100 and 200 patients and will average about two years in duration. Following Phase II trials study sponsors will frequently assess these preliminary results and predicted marketability of the product prior to initiating the larger and more expensive Phase III trials.

Phase III

Phase III trials build on the experience gained during the Phase II trials. The purpose of a Phase III study is to further define the efficacy and safety of the agent. Frequently, in Phase III studies, the new agent is compared to current therapy. These trials are usually multicenter studies, generally treat from several hundred to 3,000 patients, and usually last about three years. Usually, some of the Phase III trials will be considered pivotal studies and will serve as the basis for the NDA/BLA for a medicinal product's marketing approval.[55]

One interesting scientific advance in the area of drug development has been the impact of pharmacogenomics (PGx) on the field. PGx is the study of variations of DNA and RNA characteristics as related to drug response including effectiveness and adverse effects. As such, PGx can contribute to evaluation of interindividual differences in the response to drugs. The FDA is encouraging study sponsors to include PGx in early stage studies to assist in areas such as identifying populations that should receive a lower or higher dose of a drug; identify potential responder populations; and identify groups at risk of serious adverse effects. An important prerequisite to using PGx in drug development is collection and storage of DNA samples from all clinical trials. Ideally, sample collection should be collected at the time of study enrollment or at baseline in order to avoid bias related to subjects who do not complete the study. At the time of drug approval, information gained from PGx studies would be included in the product labeling to inform prescribers of the impact of a certain genotype or phenotype relative to response or adverse events. Similar approaches should be considered for proteomic (scientific analysis of proteins) and metabolomic evaluations (scientific analysis of the chemical processes involving metabolites).[56]

Case Study 21-1

Company CaCure (not a real company) has developed a drug called ALLCure. The product is approved as an intravenous product used to treat severe headaches. Dr. Smith has conducted preclinical laboratory work that indicates that when given intrahepatically, the product can cause shrinkage of liver metastases.

Dr. Smith wants to try to use this ALLCure in 10 patients with cancer that is metastatic to the liver and see if the results hold true in humans.

- *Does Dr. Smith or ALLCure need approval from the FDA to transition this work into patients?*

NEW DRUG APPLICATION

❻ *After Phase III trials have been completed, the sponsor will submit an NDA/BLA to the FDA requesting approval of the medicinal product for marketing.* The FDA requires the completion of two well-designed, controlled clinical trials prior to submission to the FDA.

However, the sponsor will include information gathered from all of the clinical trials to show that the medicinal product is safe and effective and to describe the pharmacology and pharmacokinetics of the drug. The NDA/BLA will include all preclinical data, clinical data, manufacturing methods, product quality assurance, relevant foreign clinical testing (or marketing experience), and all published reports of experience with the medicinal agent (whether sponsored by the company or not). A proposed package insert will be supplied as well.[57]

Review of NDA

The NDA/BLA will be distributed to the same FDA review division assigned while the product was under IND status. As noted, these divisions are based on the therapeutic group of the medicinal agent. The same reviewer may be assigned to review the IND and the NDA/BLA.[17]

The speed at which the NDA will be processed is to some extent determined by the classification the drug receives during its initial review. Each agent is rated with a number-letter designation that evaluates two separate aspects of the agent. The number portion of the rating is associated with the uniqueness of the drug product (ranging from 1 for an NME to 7 for a drug that has already been marketed, but without an approved NDA/BLA—see Table 14-1). The letter portion of the rating is associated with the therapeutic potential of the medicinal agent. The P (priority review) designation is given to drugs that represent a therapeutic advance with respect to available therapy, whereas an S (standard review) is given to drugs that have little or no therapeutic gain over previously available drugs—see Table 14-2. BLA prioritization is slightly simplified but similar.[58]

During the review process, the FDA may utilize one of its prescription drug advisory committees to help review the NDA. These committees are composed of experts who provide the agency with independent, nonbinding advice and recommendations regarding the NDA. Currently the FDA has 50 advisory committees many of which are composed of various panels. Examples of such committees include the antiviral drugs advisory committee and the oncologic drug advisory committee.[58,59] Within 180 days of receipt of an NDA, the FDA will review the application and send the applicant an approval letter or a complete response letter.[60] When an approval letter is sent, the drug is considered approved as of the date of the letter.[61] A complete response letter is issued to let the sponsor know that the review period for the drug is complete, but that the application is not yet ready for approval. It will describe specific deficiencies and when possible, identify recommended actions that the sponsor might take to address those deficiencies. In response to the complete response letter, the sponsor amends the NDA, withdraws the NDA, or requests a hearing with the FDA to clarify whether grounds exist for denying approval of the application.[62]

Expanded Access to Investigational Drugs for Treatment Use

As mentioned previously in this chapter, the FDA has been under considerable criticism relative to the time taken for drug review. They have implemented many initiatives to address these criticisms. The most recent initiative implemented by the FDA is referred to as "Expanded Access to Investigational Drugs for Treatment Use." The expanded access rule clarifies existing regulations and adds new types of expanded access for treatment use. Specifically, the rule allows for investigational drugs to be used for treatment use in patients with serious or life-threatening diseases where there is no other comparable or satisfactory alternative therapy. The FDA defines immediately life-threatening conditions as those where death is likely to occur within a matter of months or in which premature death is likely without early treatment. Serious conditions are defined as those associated with morbidity that has substantial impact on day-to-day functioning.[63] The rules specify different requirements for expanded access for individual patients in emergencies; intermediate-size patient populations; and larger populations under a treatment protocol or treatment IND.[64]

The FDA must determine that in addition to the patient having a serious or immediately life-threatening disease for which there is no satisfactory alternative therapy, the potential patient benefit must outweigh the risk and that the requested used will not interfere with clinical investigations that could support marketing approval of the expanded access use. In all cases, an expanded access submission to the FDA is required. The submission may be a new IND or a protocol amendment to an existing IND (see the above explanation). Except as justified by emergency-use guidelines further discussed below, all other regulations governing new INDs and protocol amendment including regulations regarding study initiation, adverse reaction reporting, and annual reports is identical to that described for standard INDs and described elsewhere in this chapter.[65]

For individual patients, submission requirements must include information adequate for the FDA to determine that the risk to the person from the investigational drug is not greater than the probable risk from the disease and that the patient cannot obtain the drug under another type of IND. Treatment is generally limited to a single course of therapy for a specified duration unless FDA expressly authorizes multiple courses or chronic therapy. In this type of submission, the FDA does allow for emergency procedures if the patient must be treated before a written submission can be made. In that situation, the FDA may authorize the emergency use by telephone. The sponsor must agree to submit an expanded access submission within 15 business days of the FDA's authorization of the use.[66] In addition, although the FDA must authorize emergency use of a test article (investigational drug), prospective IRB approval is not required.[67]

For intermediate patient populations, there must be sufficient evidence that the drug is safe at the dose and duration proposed for treatment, and that there is at least preliminary clinical evidence of effectiveness of the drug. The sponsor must also indicate whether the drug is being developed and define the patient population. If the drug is being studied in a clinical trial, the sponsor must explain why the expanded access patient population cannot be enrolled in the clinical trial and under what circumstances the sponsor would conduct a clinical trial in those patients.[68]

The treatment IND, or treatment protocol, is a way the FDA has allowed for increased accessibility of experimental drugs for widespread treatment use. The drug must be investigated in a clinical trial under an IND designed to support a marketing application for the expanded access use, or if all clinical trials have been completed, the sponsor must be actively pursuing marketing approval of the drug for the expanded access use. When the expanded access use is for an immediately life-threatening disease, the available scientific evidence (usually clinical data from Phase II or Phase III trials) must provide reasonable assurance that the drug may be effective for the expanded access use and would not expose patients to significant risk.[69]

Cost of Using Investigational Drugs

❼ *The FDA allows for the manufacturer to charge for an investigational drug under certain conditions.* The sponsor must obtain prior written authorization from FDA to charge for an investigational drug. In order to charge for an investigational drug, the sponsor must provide evidence that the drug has a potential clinical benefit that would provide a significant advantage over available products, demonstrate that the data to be obtained from the clinical trial would be essential to establishing that the drug is effective or safe, and demonstrate that the clinical trial could not be conducted without charging because the cost of the drug is extraordinary to the sponsor. The sponsor may only charge recovery costs for direct cost attributable to making the investigational drug, including raw materials, labor, nonreusable supplies, and equipment used to manufacture the drug or costs to acquire the drug from another manufacturer or to ship and handle the drug. In addition, for expanded access studies for intermediate-size patient populations or treatment IND/protocols a sponsor may recover the cost of monitoring the expanded access IND or protocol, complying with IND reporting requirements, and other administrative costs directly associated with the expanded access IND.[70-72]

Expedited Review for New Drugs

The FDA has also attempted to expedite the review process for new drugs in several ways:

1. **Priority review:** CDER determines a drug will potentially provide a significant advance in medical care and sets a target to review the drug within six months instead of the standard 10 months.
2. **Fast Track review:** CDER determines that a drug can treat unmet medical needs. Fast Track speeds new drug reviews, for instance, by increasing the level of communication FDA allocates to developers and by enabling developers to use a

rolling review process such that CDER can review portions of an application ahead of the submission of the full application.

3. **Accelerated Approval program:** Allows for early approval of a drug for serious or life-threatening illness that offers a benefit over current treatments. This approval is based on a surrogate endpoint (e.g., a laboratory measure) or other clinical measure that FDA considers reasonably likely to predict clinical benefit. After this approval, the drug must undergo additional testing to confirm the benefit.

4. **Breakthrough Therapy:** Allows for expedited development and review of drugs which are intended to treat serious conditions and which may demonstrate a substantial improvement over available therapy.[73]

PHASE IV: POSTMARKETING SURVEILLANCE

After the drug has been approved, postmarketing studies may be initiated. They are conducted for the approved indication, but may evaluate different doses, the effects of extended therapy, or the drug's safety in patient populations that were not represented in premarketing clinical trials. **❸❶** *The final phase of clinical studies is referred to as Phase IV trials.* These Phase IV trials may be requested by the FDA or they may be initiated by the sponsor in an attempt to gather more data on the safety and efficacy of the drug or to identify a competitive advantage of the drug over other available therapies.

Risk Evaluation and Mitigation Strategies (REMS)

In some situations, the FDA may actually approve a product with restrictions limiting the facilities or physicians where the product may be used, or limiting the patient population to only those who have demonstrated certain performance on specified medical procedures.[74,75] Specifically, the FDA has started to utilize REMS when they determine that safety measures are needed beyond the labeling to ensure that a drug's benefits outweigh its risks. REMS can be required before or after a drug is approved. REMS are developed by drug sponsors; however, the FDA reviews and approves them. Factors that are considered in determining the need for an REMS include:

- The size of the population likely to use the drug
- The seriousness of the disease
- Expected benefits
- Expected duration of treatment
- Seriousness of adverse events (known or potential)
- Whether the drug is an NME[50]

The REMS may include the following components: a medication guide (or patient package insert), a communication plan (for providing key information to health care providers), Elements to Assure Safe Use (ETASU), and an implementation system. Sample ETASU components include required training or certifications for health care providers, limitations on health care settings where the drug can be infused, specific laboratory results, monitoring of drug use by the patient, and enrollment of the patient on a registry. The REMS must be assessed for adequacy at least by 18 months, 3 years, and 7 years after approval.[76]

Case Study 21–2

CaCure (refer to Case Study 21-1) decided to help develop ALLCure for this indication. They successfully submitted an IND and have now completed not only Phase I and Phase II studies, but have completed two positive Phase III studies in patients with metastatic disease to the liver. The company can now apply for an NDA for this new application. Unfortunately, during the studies they became aware that some patients developed cirrhosis months or even years after treatment.

- *Assuming that the cirrhosis is related to this new route of administration, what would be an important component of the submission to the FDA as they seek licensing approval?*
- *What will be appropriate components of the REMS?*

The Orphan Drug Act

Outside of the drug development process described above, the FDA has developed an incentive program to encourage manufacturers to develop products with limited potential profit. This incentive program is known as The Orphan Drug Act and it was passed in 1983. This act provides incentives for manufacturers to develop orphan drugs. ❽ *An orphan drug is one used for the treatment of a rare disease, affecting fewer than 200,000 people in the United States, or one that will not generate enough revenue to justify the cost of research and development.* There are more than 6,000 rare diseases impacting more than 25 million Americans. The Orphan Drug Act is administered by the FDA's Office of Orphan Products Development. The orphan drug designation provides the following incentives:

- **Tax incentives:** The sponsor is eligible to receive a tax credit for up to 50% of money spent on R&D of an orphan drug.
- **Waive filing fees:** The sponsor is eligible to file for a waiver from the application fee associated with the review of an NDA.

- • **Protocol assistance:** If a sponsor can show that a drug will be used for a rare disease, the FDA will provide assistance with developing the preclinical and clinical plans for the product.
- • **Grants and contracts:** The FDA budget may allot money for grants and contracts to be used in developing orphan drugs. On average the annual budget for orphan drug grants is $14 million and 10 to 15 applications are funded per year for development of orphan drugs.[77] Phase I clinical trials are eligible for up to $250,000 per year for three years while Phase II to III clinical trials may receive up to $500,000 per year for four years.[78]
- • **Marketing exclusivity:** The first sponsor to obtain marketing approval for a designated orphan drug is allowed seven years of marketing exclusivity for that indication, but identical versions of the same product marketed by another manufacturer may be approved for other indications.

The Orphan Drug Act does not provide advantages for the drug approval process. Sponsors seeking approval for drugs that will be designated as orphan drugs must still provide the same safety and efficacy data as all other drugs evaluated by the FDA. Exceptions to the rules governing the number of patients that should be treated in the clinical trials may be made based on the scarcity of patients with the condition. Additionally, because in many cases there are no alternative therapies for the disease, the drug may be given a high review priority during the NDA process.[79,80]

Having discussed the federal infrastructure under which clinical research is conducted, now the approvals that need to be obtained locally before research in human subjects can be initiated will be discussed.

Institutional Review Board/Institutional Ethics Committee

The IRB/IEC is a committee formed to review proposed clinical trials and the progress of such studies to ensure that the rights and welfare of human subjects are protected. In the United States the standard designation for this type of committee is the IRB. The IRB must contain at least one member who has specialized in a scientific area (usually this will be a physician) and at least one board member who has a specialty in a nonscientific area such as law, ethics, or religion. Additionally, the IRB must contain at least one individual who is not affiliated with the institution where the research is being conducted. Membership of the IRB varies between institutions. Common members of IRBs include physicians, pharmacists, nurses, lawyers, clergy, and laypeople. The IRB is also responsible for ensuring that the proposed clinical trial is not in conflict with the institution's research policies or philosophy. The IRB and the study sponsor will have little, if any, direct contact. The primary investigator (PI) generally acts as the liaison between these two parties.

REVIEW OF A CLINICAL RESEARCH PROTOCOL

The IRB should evaluate the research proposal to ensure that the following requirements are met:

- The risks to subjects are minimal.
- The expected risk/anticipated benefit ratio must be reasonable.
- Equitable subject selection is used.
- Informed consent must be received from each participant (or his or her legally authorized representative).
- Informed consent must be documented in writing.
- Data must be monitored to ensure subject safety.
- Patient confidentiality must be maintained.
- If appropriate, additional safeguards against coercion must be included in studies that include vulnerable subjects (children, prisoners, pregnant women, mentally disabled people, or economically or educationally disadvantaged persons).

A notable exception to the requirements for written informed consent, as described above, has been provided for research done in emergency circumstances involving human subjects who cannot give informed consent because of their emerging, life-threatening medical condition (for which available treatments are unproven or unsatisfactory), and where the intervention must be administered before informed consent from the subject's legally authorized representative is feasible. In these situations, the exception from informed consent requirements may proceed only after the sponsor has received prior written permission from the FDA (via IND approval) and from the IRB. In this type of research, both community consultation and public disclosure must be provided for the protocol.[81]

RESPONSIBILITIES OF IRB COMMITTEES

The IRB must, at a minimum, perform annual reviews of all ongoing clinical trials and evaluate adverse experiences to ensure that the criteria listed above continue to be met.[82,83]

The IRB must maintain documentation of all IRB activities including copies of all research proposals reviewed, minutes of IRB meetings, records of continuing review activities, copies of all correspondence between the IRB and the investigators, a list of IRB members, written procedures of the IRB, and statements of significant new findings provided to subjects. This documentation and records that pertain to research should be retained for three years after the research is completed.[84,85]

Some institutions divide their review of proposed clinical research into two separate processes. One of these is the review of the protocol for scientific worth (scientific review), and the other is the review of the protocol for ethical considerations (IRB review). For many years the role of the IRB and the effectiveness of the informed consent process have been questioned.[86,87] Federal officials and regulatory agencies continue to contemplate reform of the process to better meet the goals of providing study subjects with information from which they can make an educated decision regarding whether or not they wish to participate in a clinical trial. Information regarding the role the pharmacist can assume in both IRB and scientific reviews of protocols will be presented later in the chapter.

In some institutions, the IRB is also responsible for evaluating research misconduct. Research misconduct means fabrication, falsification, or plagiarism in proposing, performing, or reviewing research, or in reporting research results.[88] Research misconduct is an issue of increasing concern to study sponsors, institutions, and the government as the pressure on investigators and their associates to produce results has increased. In most institutions as the emphasis on identifying and handling research misconduct has increased, the institutions have developed separate review processes and policies to deal with the issue.

IRBs also get involved in evaluating conflict of interest (CofI). As with research misconduct, evaluation and control of CofI is a shared responsibility for the institution, the IRB, and the investigator (and staff). Of specific concern to the IRB is whether or not financial interests may impact the protection of human subjects. The IRB should identify a mechanism for reporting such CofI, develop a mechanism for managing or eliminating such CofI, and as deemed necessary require that such conflicts be provided to potential study subjects as part of the informed consent process.[89]

Training of investigators and staff in human subject protections, GCP, and CofI is an institutional responsibility that is sometimes enforced by the IRB. Many institutions use the Collaborative Institutional Training Initiative (CITI) to provide and track such training of investigators and staff.[90]

Case Study 21-3

The FDA has mandated that before ALLCure (refer to Case Study 21-1) can be approved, further clinical trials will be required to determine the mechanism of action of developing cirrhosis and if there are clinical or genetic factors that can define the at-risk population. The lawyers at CaCure do not want the cirrhosis information provided in the consent form as the relationship between the toxicity and the drug is not yet definitely proven.

- *What is a likely IRB determination?*
- *What special issues need to be considered if children are to be included in this study to further define the risk of cirrhosis?*
- *What is required if a child reaches their legal age of majority (as defined by state law) while enrolled in this study?*

Next the role of health care professionals in clinical research will be discussed.

Role of the Health Care Professional

The health care professional can play a vital role in the clinical research process by

- being the PI on a study,
- reporting adverse events,
- preparing the IND,
- serving on the IRB and, where applicable, on the Scientific Review Committee,
- providing financial evaluations of investigational protocols,
- disseminating information regarding both the protocol and the investigational drug to other health care personnel,
- maintaining drug accountability records,
- ordering, maintaining and, when necessary, returning drug supplies for ongoing clinical trials,
- randomizing and, when necessary, blinding drug supplies for a clinical trial.

GETTING INVOLVED IN CLINICAL RESEARCH

The health care professional can serve as the PI on clinical research studies. The type of study for which an individual can serve as a PI varies based on their expertise and experience. Common types of studies for which nonphysicians serve as PIs include pharmacoeconomic, pharmacology/pharmacokinetic, quality of life, and other nontherapeutic and minimal risk. For some of these trials, an IRB may insist that a physician be a coinvestigator.

The health care professional can assist the investigator by reporting clinical trial adverse reactions to the FDA. A discussion of the types of adverse reactions and the applicable reporting requirements was presented in the section of this chapter referred to as the drug approval process. Further information about the concept of adverse drug reaction reporting, including identification and classification of adverse events, can be found in the adverse drug reaction section of Chapter 17.

The health care professional can assist in preparing the IND by following the guidelines presented earlier in this chapter. Equally important, the health care professional can assist in writing the protocol. One issue that should be considered when writing a protocol is the issue of potential drug shortages of commercially available products. As discussed in Chapter 15 of this book, drug shortages are an increasingly common problem in the United States. In the context of clinical trials if a drug that is included in a protocol is unavailable for any portion of the study the impact on study conduct and outcome evaluations can be significant. In such a situation the following options are available:

1. Temporary or permanent study hold/termination
2. Drug substitution

If drug substitution is selected, there are two possible options to consider including a specific drug (as specified by the sponsor) or allowing for drug substitution by individual investigators without specification by the sponsor. While the second option may allow for better personalized clinical decision making, it is likely to yield study outcomes that are difficult to interpret. In any event, the decision about how to proceed at the time of a drug shortage will be driven by the length of time the drug is anticipated to be in short supply, the role (pivotal or not) of the drug in the study and study questions, and the rapidity at which drug substitutions need to be made. In general, drug substitutions will need to be made in the body of the protocol as an amendment; however, for a drug with therapeutic purposes where the suspected time of drug shortage may be prolonged, the treatment may need to be altered prior to approval of the amendment. This type of rapid modification of treatment is allowed for in situations where the subjects are considered to be at immediate risk of harm.[19,43] More generally, the impact of drug shortages on protocols can be avoided by only specifying drugs that are critical to study outcomes, allowing for institutional preferences in drug selection, and referencing institutional treatment standard operating procedures (SOPs) rather than specific drugs.

Preferably, health care professionals are voting members of the IRB and as such may have some control over clinical trials initiated at the institution. More important, however, is the role they may have in the scientific review of the protocol, whether this occurs as part of the scientific review board review or as part of the IRB review. When reviewing a protocol for scientific purposes, they should help verify that the information in the protocol is complete and that it is logistically possible for the protocol to be conducted as presented. In addition, the health care professional should confirm that any potential toxicities specified in the protocol are detailed for the patient in the informed consent of the protocol.

Some roles are more specific to the training of the health care professional. Following is a description of the role of the pharmacist in clinical research.

ROLE OF THE PHARMACIST

Reviewing the Research Protocol

The pharmacist should verify that the protocol or associated documents such as the investigator's brochure contain the following information:

1. The name and synonyms of the study agent,
2. The chemical structure of the study agent,
3. The mechanism of action of the study agent,
4. The dosage range of the study agent (with appropriate rationale),
5. Animal toxicologic and pharmacologic information (when available, any known human toxicologic and pharmacologic information should also be presented),
6. How the agent will be supplied (dosage form and size),
7. The preparation guidelines for the agent (including stability and compatibility information when appropriate),
8. The storage requirements of the agent (both before and, when appropriate, after preparation), and
9. The route of administration (and, if applicable, the rate of administration).

The pharmacist should also review the protocol for other potential problems (such as incompatibilities and inappropriate infusion devices). Frequently, nurses do not have an opportunity to review protocols prior to initiation and it falls to the pharmacist to ensure that the drug can be given as specified in the protocol. The pharmacist can review the protocol for clinical and scientific issues appropriate to his or her knowledge level and experience. Those pharmacists with research experience or a strong clinical background may, and probably should, comment on the study design or scientific merit of a particular protocol.

Managing Drug Costs

With the central role of financial considerations in today's research environment, pharmacists can also provide valuable insight into the costs associated with clinical research. Traditionally, the study sponsors would provide the investigational drug free of charge to the hospital (and to the patient) and the patient (or the third-party payer) would be responsible for paying for all other charges associated with therapy. These charges could include hospitalization charges, laboratory tests, and examinations to name a few. Some third-party payers are reluctant to pay for such charges unless they can be considered to be standard of care. Effective in September 2000, Medicare began to cover the costs of qualifying clinical trials (QCTs) inclusive of items and services that are generally available to Medicare recipients excluding only the investigational agent, evaluations being done only for research purposes, and other items and services customarily provided by research sponsors.[91] Hospitals and other health care institutions and providers are increasingly using the QCT determination system to evaluate the costs and financial risks of the research protocol. Many (but not all) insurers will agree to cover similar costs for subjects not enrolled on research studies. However, uninsured, underinsured and patients whose insurance will not accept the QCT assessment are left in a financially risk situation. This financial risk is ultimately shared by the health care provider and the institution. This leaves the patient, and subsequently the health care institution, in a financially risky situation. Developing cost assessments and QCT evaluations can assist the investigator, the institution, and the review boards with important information regarding the potential cost of the research allowing all parties to make a more educated decision regarding appropriation of resources for research purposes (sample economic analysis form can be found in Appendix 3). When preparing an economic review of a protocol, important aspects to consider include:

1. Can the therapy be converted from inpatient to outpatient?
2. Can the method of infusion or the infusion device be changed to one that is more cost effective?
3. Does the treatment plan call for administration of compatible medications that could be mixed in the same container?
4. Is the supportive care adequate and not excessive (this is especially important with high-cost drugs such as antiemetics and growth factors)?

More recently, some sponsors have started to implement programs for cost recovery for investigational drugs. As discussed in Key Concept 7, the sponsor applies to and receives approval from the FDA for a specific dollar amount that can be charged. FDA approval of this charge must be in place before cost recovery can begin.[66,70,71,72] The institution will need to have procedures in place for billing properly for investigational drugs.

Disseminating Research Information

Following approval of the research project, the pharmacist can assist in disseminating information regarding both the protocol and the investigational agent by preparing data sheets that may be used by pharmacy and nursing personnel (and in some situations by physicians who may be unfamiliar with the research). This information can be distributed using various methods including paper, web-based systems, and the electronic medical record. The investigational agent data sheet should include the following elements:

- Agent name (synonyms)
- Therapeutic classification
- Pharmaceutical data
- Stability and storage data
- Dose preparation guidelines (where applicable)
- Usual dosage range
- Route of administration
- Known side effects and toxicities
- Mechanism of action
- Status (phase of study)
- Date effective (and dates of revision)
- References

The protocol data sheet should include the following elements:

- Protocol number (as assigned by the institution)
- Protocol title
- Agent name(s) (synonym[s])
- Protocol description
  1. Objectives
  2. Study design
     a. Registration requirements
     b. Primary location of patients
     c. Type of study
  3. Treatment course (including retreatment criteria)
- Availability
  1. Supplier
  2. Status
  3. How supplied
- Storage, stability, and compatibility
  1. Intact drug
  2. Prepared drug (for injectables this should include both reconstitution and dilution guidelines)
- Dosage range
- Dose preparation guidelines
- Administration guidelines
- Special notes

- PI
- Key study staff including the research nurse

The PI and study sponsor should approve both the drug data sheet and the protocol data sheet before dissemination. This will help eliminate any potential errors and may reduce the liability the pharmacist assumes in preparing and distributing these documents.

Securing Drug Supplies for Research

The pharmacist can assume primary responsibility for ordering and maintaining adequate drug supplies for conducting the clinical trial. All investigational drugs should be stored in a locked area, preferably a pharmacy. Usually, ordering can be done via telephone; however, sometimes study sponsors require written drug orders. If the drug under investigation is a controlled substance, a written order will definitely be required. Shipment and receipt of the drug can vary from one day to several weeks (or sometimes months for very specialized drug products). The individual responsible for ordering drug must be sufficiently knowledgeable regarding the rate of patient enrollment in the protocol and subsequent drug usage to ensure that the institution does not run out of drug. The same individual(s) should also assume responsibility for returning unused drug supplies at the completion of the study. The sponsor may authorize on-site destruction of unused supplies provided this will not increase the risk to humans (or provide a risk to the environment). Many study sponsors will attempt to have the site save and return all used drug supplies as well. This is not an FDA requirement and for safety and space reasons should be discouraged.

Maintaining Drug Accountability Records

Related to the activities above, the same individuals (or team) should assume responsibility for maintaining drug accountability records. ❾ *Maintenance of such records is required by law.* Again, it is preferable to have this handled by a pharmacist. These records can be maintained manually or on a computer. The records must document all drug shipments, returns, and dispensing to patients. *At a minimum*, these records should document:

- The date of the transaction,
- The type of the transaction,
- The recipient of the transaction (if this is a drug dispensing, the patient initials and an identifying number are required),
- The number of units being used or received (or patient dispensing this should include the actual dose the patient will receive),
- The lot number of the drug (if multiple lot numbers were used, each one should be documented), and
- The initials of the individual who performed the transaction.

An audit trail is required. The National Cancer Institute (NCI) has prepared a sample drug accountability form that may be used as a guide (see Appendix 4).

Computer systems that will maintain drug accountability records are available commercially. Both personal computer (PC) based and web-based systems exist. Some of these systems will also provide drug labels, drug and protocol information, summaries of investigational drug dispensing (useful in the preparation of productivity reports), and even monthly billing summaries to be used for posting charges to the study budget. Examples of such systems include IDEA© being marketed by DDOTS, Inc.[92] and Velos Investigational Drug System.[93] Obviously, the development of a personalized system that meets the specific needs of the institution or pharmacy is another possibility; however, this can be costly, laborious, and time consuming. If a personalized system is developed, it is important to remember that the system must be able to maintain the integrity of the records and that a clear audit trail needs to be maintained. Ultimately, the decision to computerize drug accountability records and the selection of which system to use is one that should be made only after evaluating the needs of the institution/pharmacy and the available budget.[93-95]

Drug accountability records and drug supplies may be inspected at any time by the sponsor. The frequency of these inspections may vary according to the wishes of the sponsor. They may be monthly, quarterly, or annually. The FDA also has the right to inspect these records. The investigational drug pharmacist should play a key role in providing drug accountability information to either the FDA or the sponsor during an audit. If proper records are not being maintained, the sponsor or the FDA may discontinue the investigator's participation in the clinical investigation.

After the clinical trial is complete, records must be maintained at the study site for the following time periods:

- Two years after approval of the NDA *or*
- Two years after the FDA received notification that the investigation was discontinued.[96]

Randomizing and Blinding Interventions

The pharmacist should also assume primary responsibility for randomizing and, where appropriate, blinding clinical trials. These two activities assist the sponsor in reducing or eliminating the bias of the clinical trial (see Chapter 4). A randomized study is one in which patients are randomly assigned (similar to flipping a coin) to different therapies. More details regarding the statistical basis for randomized studies is included in Chapter 6 of this book. Usually the assignment is done using a computer-generated randomization list; however, a manual list may be used as well. The randomization groups may include a number of different therapy options (e.g., a study may have four different treatment arms with an equal number of patients assigned to each arm). The number of patients assigned to the different groups may vary as well (e.g., a study may have two different treatment regimens where patients will be assigned in a 2:1 ratio to the first treatment option). The investigator should not be aware which arm the patient has been assigned to before randomization. Therefore, the involvement of a third party (such as the pharmacist) is important. A blinded study is one in which, after the patient has been randomized, the drug is masked so that at least one of the involved parties (e.g., physician, nurse, patient, pharmacist) is not aware of what the patient is to receive. In a single-blind study, the only individual who is not aware of what the patient is receiving is the patient him or herself. In a double-blind study, the nurse, physician, and patient are all unaware of what the patient is receiving. The role of a pharmacist in a double-blind study is crucial and sloppy work in this area destroys a clinical investigation. A triple-blind study is one in which the drug arrives at the pharmacy already blinded. In this scenario, the patient, nurse, physician, and pharmacist are not aware of what drug the patient is to receive. Although this may seem simpler than a double-blind study, it is equally difficult because each patient has his or her own supply of medication and it is important that the supplies be dispensed appropriately. In a triple-blind study, the sponsor supplies the investigator with a mechanism for removing the blind from the patient (in case of emergency). It is critical that the pharmacist keep the master list. The protocol should state who has access to the master list and under what conditions this access should occur. If the FDA discovers that the investigator had access to this list, the study will be considered invalid.

Seeking Reimbursement for Services

Pharmacists should be willing and able to request reimbursement for the services they provide. Funds for these services are usually negotiated directly with the study sponsor before initiation of the protocol. The majority of pharmacies charge a base fee for each protocol initiated at the institution (these fees generally range from $1,000 to $2,000 per protocol). This base fee may be fixed or it may vary based on the size of the patient population, the complexity of the protocol, or the number of doses to be prepared. Some institutions also charge an annual renewal fee for ongoing clinical trials (ranging from $500 to $1,500). Most pharmacies will charge a separate fee for randomizing and blinding a clinical trial. This fee can be a one-time (per study) fee or it can be a per patient fee. Some hospitals also charge dispensing fees per dose or per the amount of time required to prepare a dose. These fees can range from about $15 for oral doses to $50 for more complicated products such as intravenous chemotherapy. Pharmacies can also charge a monthly fee for drug storage and inventory. This fee varies based on the amount of space and type of storage (freezer, room temperature, or refrigerator) required. The pharmacist can also charge a professional fee for services that exceed the standard services provided for in the base fee. Examples of pharmacy-specific additional services include special compounding, ordering and handling controlled substances, and completing sponsor-specific drug accountability records. These services are usually charged using an hourly rate.[97] More generally clinical research services that should be considered when developing a study budget include charges for regulatory submission preparation, coordination of protocol-driven care, monitoring of patients, and completion of case report forms.

Conclusion

Assisting in the implementation and conduct of clinical trials can be a satisfying role for the health care professional. Clinical trials that utilize drugs, biologics, and devices in the United States are largely controlled by the FDA and by local IRBs. A thorough understanding of the regulations governing those entities is extremely helpful when conducting clinical trials. The health care professional can use that knowledge to help investigators develop clinical trials, obtain and maintain proper approvals for those clinical trials, and assist in the conduct of clinical trials. Related to the conduct of clinical trials, health care professionals (and specifically pharmacists) are frequently involved in obtaining, storing, and dispensing the agents being utilized in the clinical trial. In addition, the health care professional (and specifically pharmacists) can be quite involved in providing protocol and drug information to the investigators, other study personnel, and equally importantly to the study subjects. Health care professionals can and should play an integral role in the conduct of clinical trials at their institution.

Self-Assessment Questions

1. What is the primary role of the FDA related to drugs, biologics, and medical devices in the United States?
   a. Evaluating the safety and efficacy of the products
   b. Determining that the rights and welfare and human subjects are protected
   c. Evaluating of prescribing trends of physicians among similar products
   d. Determining the price of the products

2. What is the primary purpose of IRB review of research?
   a. Evaluating the safety and efficacy of products used in an investigational protocol

    b. Determining that the rights and welfare and human subjects are protected

    c. Evaluating the risk benefit ratio of an investigational protocol

    d. Determining that the consent form is written at an appropriate reading level

3. The drug approval process in the United States as codified by the FDA includes:

    a. Phase I to V testing

    b. Postmarketing usage evaluations

    c. IND/NDA (BLA) submissions

    d. Cost recovery evaluations

4. A treatment IND:

    a. Is any IND that includes a product with therapeutic intent

    b. Allows for treatment of patients even when consent cannot be obtained

    c. Is part of Fast Track review

    d. Allows for increase accessibility of the product for widespread use

5. IND safety reports:

    a. Are submitted annually to describe the progress of the investigation

    b. Should be submitted if a manufacturing change may impact product safety

    c. When there is proof that an adverse event is related to the product

    d. Should be submitted for new safety data obtained from humans or animals

6. What would be an appropriate example of an REMS and the associated requirements to mitigate those risks?

    a. Liver damage—counseling patients on signs of liver failure

    b. Serious infection—sending patients home with antibiotics

    c. Severe birth defects—requiring a negative pregnancy test prior to dispensing each dose of medication

    d. Leukemia—meeting with an oncologist prior to initiating treatment

7. An Orphan Drug designation:

    a. Can be given to any product affecting less than 500,000 people worldwide

    b. Provides funding to all manufacturers of products used to treat rare diseases

    c. Encourages the development of products with limited potential profit

    d. Allows approval of products with limited safety and efficacy data

8. A manufacturer can charge for an investigational product:

    a. If it is part of a QCT

    b. When they demonstrate that the cost of the drug is extraordinary

    c. When Phase III protocols are initiated

    d. If it is part of a treatment IND

9. What does an NDA/BLA allow a sponsor to do?
   a. Market the product
   b. Charge for the product
   c. Advertise for the product
   d. Name the product

10. Who is the sponsor's primary contact at the FDA?
    a. Medical reviewer
    b. Pharmacology/Toxicology reviewer
    c. Regulatory project manager
    d. CMC reviewer

11. What was the most recent reform act intended to improve FDA inclusive of attempts to speed drug evaluation timeframes?
    a. Kefauver-Harris Drug Amendment
    b. FDAAA
    c. FDASIA
    d. PDUFA

12. Protocols using gene transfer products are uniquely submitted to the:
    a. FDA
    b. NIH/OSP
    c. IRB
    d. Scientific Review Committees

13. The drug data sheet should include the following elements:
    a. Dose preparation guidelines
    b. Principal investigator name
    c. Indications for use
    d. The lot numbers of the product to be dispensed

14. The protocol data sheet should include the following elements:
    a. The proposed label to be used
    b. Dose administration guidelines
    c. The lot numbers of the product to be dispensed
    d. Eligibility criteria for subjects enrolled on the protocol

15. The FDA regulates:
    a. Illegal drugs of abuse
    b. Practice of medicine
    c. Advertising for prescription drugs
    d. Reimbursement for drugs and devices

REFERENCES

1. DiMasi JA, Grabowski HG, Hansen RW. Innovation in the pharmaceutical industry: new estimates of R&D costs. JHE. 2016 May;47:20-33.
2. Carroll A. $2.6 billion to develop a drug? New estimate makes questionable assumptions. The New York Times [Internet]. 2014 Nov 18 [cited 2016 Sept]:[4 p.]. Available from: http://www.nytimes.com/2014/11/19/upshot/calculating-the-real-costs-of-developing-a-new-drug.html?_r=0
3. Ubi S. PhRMA member companies invested $58.8 billion in R&D in 2015. PhRMA [Internet]. 2016 May 16 [cited 2016 Sept]:[8 p.]. Available from: http://catalyst.phrma.org/phrma-member-companies-invested-58.8-billion-in-rd-in-2015
4. Food and Drug Administration [Internet]. Novel drug approvals for 2015. Updated through 2016 Apr [cited 2016 Sept]:[20 p.]. Available from: http://www.fda.gov/downloads/drugs/developmentapprovalprocess/druginnovation/ucm485053.pdf
5. Food and Drug Administration [Internet]. Advancing regulatory science at the FDA. 2011 Aug [cited 2016 Sept]:[38 p.]. Available from: http://www.fda.gov/downloads/sciencere search/specialtopics/regulatoryscience/ucm268225.pdf
6. Food and Drug Administration [Internet]. FDA organization chart. Updated through 2016 Jul [cited 2016 Sept]:[2 p.]. Available from: http://www.fda.gov/aboutfda/centers offices/organizationcharts/ucm393155.htm
7. Food and Drug Administration [Internet]. Summary of NDA approvals & receipts, 1938 to the present. Updated 2013 Jan [cited 2016 Sept]:[3 p.]. Available from: http://www.fda.gov/aboutfda/whatwedo/history/productregulation/summaryofndaapprovalsreceipts 1938tothepresent/default.htm
8. Food and Drug Administration [Internet]. Drugs@FDA glossary of terms. Updated through 2012 Feb [cited 2016 Sept]:[3 p.]. Available from: http://www.fda.gov/drugs/informationondrugs/ucm079436.htm
9. United States Federal Government Code of Federal Regulations. 21CFR312.3. Updated 2016 Apr 1.
10. CDER; Food and Drug Administration [Internet]. MAPP 6030.1: IND process and review procedures. Updated 1998 May 1 [cited 2016 Sept]:[12 p.]. Available from: http://www.fda.gov/downloads/aboutfda/centersoffices/officeofmedicalproductsandtobacco/cder/manualofpoliciesprocedures/ucm082022.pdf
11. International Conference on Harmonization (ICH) [Internet]. Guidance for Industry: E10 choice of control group and related issues in clinical trials. 2000 June [cited 2016 Sept]:[29 p.]. Available from: http://www.ich.org/fileadmin/Public_Web_Site/ICH_Products/Guidelines/Efficacy/E10/Step4/E10_Guideline.pdf
12. United States Federal Government Code of Federal Regulations. 21CFR314.420. Updated 2016 Apr 1.
13. United States Federal Government Code of Federal Regulations. 21CFR314.3. Updated 2016 Apr 1.
14. International Conference for Harmonization (ICH) [Internet]. E6 guideline for good clinical practice: glossary. 1996 Apr [cited 2016 Sept]:[4 p.]. Available from: http://ichgcp.net/1-glossary

15. United States Federal Government Code of Federal Regulations. 21CFR312.20. Updated 2016 Apr 1.

16. United States Federal Government Code of Federal Regulations. 21CFR314. Updated 2016 Apr 1.

17. Yager JA, Kallgren DL. Roles of regulatory project managers in the U.S. Food and Drug Administration's Center for Drug Evaluation and Research. Drug Inf J. 2000;34:289-93.

18. Meadows M. Promoting safe and effective drugs for 100 years. FDA Consum [Internet]. Last updated 2009 June [cited 2016 Sept]:[9 p.]. Available from: http://www.fda.gov/aboutfda/whatwedo/history/productregulation/promotingsafeandeffectivedrugsfor100years/default.htm

19. Bruderle TP. Reforming the Food and Drug Administration: legislative solution or self-improvement: Am J Health Syst Pharm. 1996;53:2083-90.

20. Reichert J. A guide to drug discovery: trends in development and approval times for new therapeutics in the Unites States. Nat Rev Drug Discov. 2003 Sept;2(9):695-702.

21. Downing NS, Aminawung JA, Shah ND, Braunstein JB, Krumholz HM, Ross JS. Regulatory review of novel therapeutics—comparison of three regulatory agencies. NEJM [Internet]. 2012 June [cited 2016 Sept]:[5 p.]. Available from: http://www.nejm.org/doi/full/10.1056/NEJMsa1200223#t=articleBackground

22. Food and Drug Administration [Internet]. Prescription Drug User Fee Act (PDUFA). Last updated 2016 Aug [cited 2016 Sept]. Available from: http://www.fda.gov/forindustry/userfees/prescriptiondruguserfee/default.htm

23. Food and Drug Administration [Internet]. Food and Drug Administration Modernization Act of 1997. Updated 2013 Nov [cited 2016 Sept]. Available from: https://www.fda.gov/RegulatoryInformation/LawsEnforcedbyFDA/SignificantAmendmentstotheFDCAct/FDAMA/default.htm

24. Food and Drug Administration [Internet]. Food and Drug Administration Amendments Act of 2007. Updated 2011 Dec 2 [cited 2016 Sept]. Available from: https://www.fda.gov/RegulatoryInformation/LawsEnforcedbyFDA/SignificantAmendmentstotheFDCAct/FoodandDrugAdministrationAmendmentsActof2007/default.htm

25. Food and Drug Administration [Internet]. Food and Drug Administration Safety and Innovation Act (FDASIA). Updated 2015 Oct [cited 2016 Sept]. Available from: https://www.fda.gov/RegulatoryInformation/LawsEnforcedbyFDA/SignificantamendmentstotheFDCAct/FDASIA/default.htm#stakeholder

26. Food and Drug Administration [Internet]. Critical path initiative. Updated 2016 Jan [cited 2016 Sept]. Available from: http://www.fda.gov/ScienceResearch/SpecialTopics/CriticalPathInitiative/ucm076689.htm

27. CDER; Food and Drug Administration [Internet]. Duchenne muscular dystrophy and related dystrophinopathies: developing drugs for treatment: Guidance for Industry. 2015 Jun [cited 2016 Sept]. Available from: http://www.fda.gov/downloads/drugs/guidancecomplianceregulatoryinformation/guidances/UCM450229.pdf

28. FDA draft guidance on Duchenne. EndDuchenne.org [Internet]. 2014 Jun [cited 2016 Sept]. Available from: http://www.parentprojectmd.org/site/PageServer?pagename=Advocate_fdaguidance

29. Food and Drug Administration [Internet]. Electronic regulatory submissions and review. Updated 2016 Aug [cited 2016 Sept]. Available from: http://www.fda.gov/Drugs/DevelopmentApprovalProcess/FormsSubmissionRequirements/ElectronicSubmissions/default.htm

30. Food and Drug Administration [Internet]. Electronic Common Technical Document (eCTD). Updated 2016 Aug [cited 2016 Sept]. Available from: http://www.fda.gov/Drugs/DevelopmentApprovalProcess/FormsSubmissionRequirements/ElectronicSubmissions/ucm153574.htm

31. Woodcock J. FDA user fee agreements: strengthening FDA and the medical products industry for the benefit of patients [Internet]. Presented to: Committee on Health, Education, Labor and Pensions United States Senate; 2012 Mar [cited 2016 Sept]. Available from: http://www.fda.gov/NewsEvents/Testimony/ucm297390.htm

32. Food and Drug Administration [Internet]. FDA's role: ClinicalTrials.gov information. 2013 Nov [cited 2016 Sept]. Available from: http://www.fda.gov/scienceresearch/specialtopics/runningclinicaltrials/fdasroleclinicaltrials.govinformation/default.htm

33. ClinicalTrials.gov [Internet]. History, policies, and law. Last reviewed 2016 Mar [cited 2016 Sept]. Available from: https://clinicaltrials.gov/ct2/about-site/history

34. International Conference on Harmonization [Internet]. History of ICH. Updated 2000 [cited 2016 Sept]. Available from: http://www.ich.org/about/history.html

35. NIH OSP [Internet]. Appendix M: points to consider in the design and submission of protocols for the transfer of recombinant or synthetic nucleic acid molecules into one or more human research participants (points to consider). Available from: https://osp.od.nih.gov/wp-content/uploads/2013/06/NIH_Guidelines.pdf

36. Grilley BJ. Regulations governing clinical trials in gene therapy. In: Brenner M, Hung M, editors. Cancer gene therapy by viral and non-viral vectors. John Wiley & Sons, Inc., Hoboken, New Jersey; 2014:131-49.

37. Office of NIH History [Internet]. The Nuremberg Code. Trials of war criminals before the Nuremberg Military Tribunals under Control Council Law. 1949 [cited 2016 Sept]. Available from: https://history.nih.gov/research/downloads/nuremberg.pdf

38. The World Medical Association [Internet]. Declaration of Helsinki. Updated 2013 Oct [cited 2016 Sept]. Available from: https://www.wma.net/policies-post/wma-declaration-of-helsinki-ethical-principles-for-medical-research-involving-human-subjects/.

39. The Belmont Report: ethical principles and guidelines for the protection of human subjects of research [Internet]. 1979 Apr 18 [cited 2016 Sept]. Available from: http://www.hhs.gov/ohrp/regulations-and-policy/belmont-report/index.html

40. United States Federal Government Code of Federal Regulations. 45CFR46. Updated 2015 Oct.

41. United States Federal Government Code of Federal Regulations. 21CFR50. Updated 2016 Apr.

42. United States Federal Government Code of Federal Regulations. 21CFR56. Updated 2016 Apr.

43. United States Federal Government Code of Federal Regulations. 21CFR312.23. Updated 2016 Apr.

44. CDER/CBER; Food and Drug Administration [Internet]. Guidance for Industry: Investigational New Drug Applications (INDs)—determining whether human research studies can be conducted without an IND. 2013 Sept [cited 2016 Sept]. Available from: http://www.fda.gov/downloads/drugs/guidancecomplianceregulatoryinformation/guidances/ucm229175.pdf

45. CDER/CBER/CDRH; Food and Drug Administration [Internet]. Guidance for Industry and Food and Drug Administration staff: in vitro companion diagnostic devices. 2014 Aug [cited 2016 Sept]. Available from: http://www.fda.gov/downloads/medicaldevices/deviceregulationandguidance/guidancedocuments/ucm262327.pdf

46. CBER/CDRH; Food and Drug Administration [Internet]. Guidance for Industry and Food and Drug Administration staff: mobile medical applications. 2015 Feb [cited 2016 Sept]. Available from: http://www.fda.gov/downloads/medicaldevices/deviceregulationandguidance/guidancedocuments/ucm263366.pdf

47. CDER; Food and Drug Administration [Internet]. Guideline for drug master files. Updated 2015 Nov [cited 2016 Sept]. Available from: http://www.fda.gov/Drugs/DevelopmentApprovalProcess/FormsSubmissionRequirements/DrugMasterFilesDMFs/ucm073164.htm

48. United States Federal Government Code of Federal Regulations. 21CFR312.30. Updated 2016 Apr.

49. United States Federal Government Code of Federal Regulations. 21CFR312.31. Updated 2016 Apr.

50. United States Federal Government Code of Federal Regulations. 21CFR312.32. Updated 2016 Apr.

51. CDER/CBER; Food and Drug Administration [Internet]. Guidance for Industry and investigators: safety reporting requirements for INDs and BA/BE studies. 2012 Dec [cited 2016 Sept]. Available from: http://www.fda.gov/downloads/Drugs/GuidanceComplianceRegulatoryInformation/Guidances/UCM227351.pdf

52. United States Federal Government Code of Federal Regulations. 21CFR312.33. Updated 2016 Apr.

53. United States Federal Government Code of Federal Regulations. 21CFR312.40. Updated 2016 Apr.

54. United States Federal Government Code of Federal Regulations. 21CFR312.42. Updated 2016 Apr.

55. Food and Drug Administration [Internet]. The FDA's drug review process: ensuring drugs are safe and effective. Updated 2014 Nov [cited 2016 Sept]. Available from: http://www.fda.gov/Drugs/ResourcesForYou/Consumers/ucm143534.htm

56. CDER/CBER/CDRH; Food and Drug Administration [Internet]. Clinical pharmacogenomics: premarket evaluation in early-phase clinical studies and recommendations for labeling. 2013 Jan [cited 2016 Sept]. Available from: http://www.fda.gov/downloads/Drugs/GuidanceComplianceRegulatoryInformation/Guidances/UCM337169.pdf

57. United States Federal Government Code of Federal Regulations. 21CFR314.50. Updated 2016 Apr.

58. Food and Drug Administration [Internet]. Drug development and review definitions. 2015 Aug [cited 2016 Sept]. Available from: http://www.fda.gov/Drugs/Development ApprovalProcess/HowDrugsareDevelopedandApproved/ApprovalApplications/ InvestigationalNewDrugINDApplication/ucm176522.htm

59. Food and Drug Administration. 21CFR14: public hearing before a public advisory committee. Updated 2016 Apr.

60. United States Federal Government Code of Federal Regulations. 21CFR314.100. Updated 2016 Apr.

61. United States Federal Government Code of Federal Regulations. 21CFR314.105. Updated 2016 Apr.

62. United States Federal Government Code of Federal Regulations. 21CFR314.110. Updated 2016 Apr.

63. United States Federal Government Code of Federal Regulations. 21CFR312.300. Updated 2016 Apr.

64. CDER/CBER; Food and Drug Administration. Expanded access to investigational drugs for treatment use—questions and answers. 2016 Jun [cited 2016 Sept]. Available from: http://www.fda.gov/downloads/drugs/guidancecomplianceregulatoryinformation/ guidances/ucm351261.pdf

65. United States Federal Government Code of Federal Regulations. 21CFR312.305. Updated 2016 Apr.

66. United States Federal Government Code of Federal Regulations. 21CFR312.310. Updated 2016 Apr.

67. United States Federal Government Code of Federal Regulations. 21CFR56.104. Updated 2016 Apr.

68. United States Federal Government Code of Federal Regulations. 21CFR312.315. Updated 2016 Apr.

69. United States Federal Government Code of Federal Regulations. 21CFR312.320. Updated 2016 Apr.

70. CDER/CBER; Food and Drug Administration [Internet]. Charging for investigational drugs under an IND—questions and answers. 2016 Jun [cited 2016 Sept]. Available from: http://www.fda.gov/downloads/drugs/guidancecomplianceregulatoryinformation/ guidances/ucm351264.pdf

71. United States Federal Government Code of Federal Regulations. 21CFR312.7. Updated 2016 Apr.

72. United States Federal Government Code of Federal Regulations. 21CFR312.8. Updated 2016 Apr.

73. CDER/CBER; Food and Drug Administration [Internet]. Expedited programs for serious conditions—drugs and biologics. 2014 May [cited 2016 Sept]. Available from: http:// www.fda.gov/downloads/drugs/guidancecomplianceregulatoryinformation/guidances/ ucm358301.pdf

74. Food and Drug Administration [Internet]. Phase IV commitment category. 2014 Dec [cited 2016 Sept]. Available from: http://www.fda.gov/drugs/developmentapprovalprocess/

formssubmissionrequirements/electronicsubmissions/datastandardsmanualmono
graphs/ucm071716.htm

75. United States Federal Government Code of Federal Regulations. 21CFR314.520. Updated 2016.

76. Food and Drug Administration [Internet]. FDA basics webinar: a brief overview of risk evaluation and mitigation strategies (REMS). Updated 2016 Sept [cited 2016 Sept]. Available from: http://www.fda.gov/AboutFDA/Transparency/Basics/ucm325201.htm

77. Food and Drug Administration [Internet]. Information on the Orphan Products Natural History Grants Program. 2016 Feb [cited 2016 Sept]. Available from: https://www.fda.gov/ForIndustry/DevelopingProductsforRareDiseasesConditions/OrphanProductsNaturalHistoryGrantsProgram/ucm487336.htm

78. Food and Drug Administration [Internet]. FAQ concerning the Orphan Products Natural History Grants Program. 2016 Apr [cited 2016 Sept]. Available from: https://www.fda.gov/ForIndustry/DevelopingProductsforRareDiseasesConditions/OrphanProductsNaturalHistoryGrantsProgram/ucm487385.htm

79. United States Federal Government Code of Federal Regulations. 21CFR316. Updated 2016 Apr.

80. Food and Drug Administration [Internet]. Developing products for rare diseases and conditions. 2016 Mar [cited 2016 Sept]. Available from: http://www.fda.gov/forindustry/developingproductsforrarediseasesconditions/default.htm

81. United States Federal Government Code of Federal Regulations. 21CFR50.24. Updated 2016 Apr.

82. United States Federal Government Code of Federal Regulations. 45CFR46.108. Updated 2015 Oct.

83. United States Federal Government Code of Federal Regulations. 21CFR56.109. Updated 2016 Apr.

84. United States Federal Government Code of Federal Regulations. 21CFR56.115. Updated 2016 Apr.

85. United States Federal Government Code of Federal Regulations. 45CFR46.115. Updated 2015 Oct.

86. Laurence DJ. The therapeutic misconception: not just for patients. J Can Chiropr Assoc. [Internet]. 2008 Aug [cited 2016 Sept]. Available from: http://www.ncbi.nlm.nih.gov/pmc/articles/PMC2528258/.

87. Hochhauser M. "Therapeutic misconception" and "recruiting doublespeak" in the informed consent process. IRB Ethics Hum Res. 2002 Jan-Feb;24(1):240-1.

88. Office of Research Integrity [Internet]. Research misconduct. [cited 2016 Sept]. Available from: http://ori.hhs.gov/research-misconduct-0

89. Department of Health and Human Services [Internet]. Financial conflict of interest: HHS guidance. 2004 May [cited 2016 Sept]. Available from: http://www.hhs.gov/ohrp/regulations-and-policy/guidance/financial-conflict-of-interest/#

90. Collaborative Institutional Training Initiative (CITI) Program [Internet]. [cited 2016 Sept]. Available from: https://www.citiprogram.org/rcrpage.asp

91. Medicare Coverage~Clinical Trials: final national coverage decision [Internet]. [cited 2016 Sept]. Available from: https://www.cms.gov/medicare/coverage/clinicaltrialpolicies/downloads/finalnationalcoverage.pdf

92. DDOTS, Inc. [Internet]. [cited 2016 Sept]. Available from: http://www.ddots.com

93. Velos Investigational Drug System. [cited 2016 Sept]. Available from: http://ids.velos.com

94. Burnham NL, Elcombe SA, Skorlinski CR, Kosanke L, Kovach JS. Computer program for handling investigational oncology drugs. Am J Hosp Pharm. 1989;46:1821-4.

95. Grilley BJ, Trissel LA, Bluml BM. Design and implementation of an electronic investigational drug accountability system. Am J Hosp Pharm. 1991;48:2816.

96. United States Federal Government Code of Federal Regulations. 21CFR312.57. Updated 2016 Apr.

97. Veteran's Medical Research Foundation Pharmacy Service [Internet]. [cited 2016 Sept]. Available from: http://www.vmrf.org/researchcenters/pharmacy-service/pharmacy.html

SUGGESTED READINGS

1. NIH/Office of Science Policy (OSP). Available from: http://osp.od.nih.gov/office-biotechnology-activities/.

2. FDA. Available from: http://www.fda.gov/.

3. FDA forms. Available from: http://www.fda.gov/opacom/morechoices/fdaforms/fda forms.html/.

4. Code of Federal Regulations. Available from: http://www.ecfr.gov

5. FDA Dockets Management page. Available from: http://www.fda.gov/ohrms/dockets/default.htm

6. ICH. Available from: www.ich.org

7. NIH/OHRP. Available from: http://www.hhs.gov/ohrp/.

8. CenterWatch. Available from: http://centerwatch.com/.

Chapter Twenty-Two

Pharmaceutical Industry and Regulatory Affairs

Bhavini T. Parikh

Learning Objectives

● *After completing this chapter, the reader will be able to*

- Design an organization chart for a pharmaceutical company.
- Discuss opportunities for health care professionals (HPs) within the pharmaceutical industry.
- Describe how HPs are regulated in pharmaceutical industry.
- Determine acceptable interactions between pharmaceutical companies and practitioners.
- List the components of a standard response and personalized letter.
- Explain the importance of collecting adverse event information.
- Identify pharmaceutical industry-associated organizations.
- Recommend methods for communicating safety information to consumers.
- Describe the role of the Division of Drug Information (DDI) at the Food and Drug Administration (FDA).
- List the main differences between the DDI and a typical drug information center.
- Illustrate the different types of drug information services provided by the FDA.
- Identify factors that guide selection of a specific FDA-sponsored resource or website.
- Discuss student and professional opportunities within the FDA.

Key Concepts

❶ Pharmaceutical companies' scientific or medical departments are staffed with highly trained health care professionals (HPs) working in a multitude of specialized fields.

❷ Medical information specialists respond to inquiries, provide training, and draft materials for a variety of internal and external audiences.

❸ Pharmaceutical companies are regulated both externally by the FDA and internally by standard operation procedures (SOPs).

❹ The FDA's draft Guidance for Industry "Responding to Unsolicited Requests for Off-Label Information About Prescription Drugs and Medical Devices" describes the FDA's current thinking about how manufacturers and distributors of prescription human drug products can respond to unsolicited requests for information about unapproved indications (off-label information) related to their FDA-approved or cleared products.

❺ Unsolicited requests are those initiated by persons or entities that are completely independent of the relevant firm.

❻ The FDA considers requests for off-label information that are prompted in any way by a manufacturer or its representatives to be solicited.

❼ Interactions between pharmaceutical companies and HPs are defined, but not regulated, by a code of conduct established by the Pharmaceutical Research and Manufacturers of America (PhRMA) through the revised version of the *Code on Interactions with Health Care Professionals*.

❽ Clinical response letters, also known as standard responses, are written correspondence that are internally reviewed and contain content in response to an unsolicited request for medical information.

❾ Patient variability, clinician experience, and previously unaddressed questions require personalized responses that cannot be fulfilled with a standard response letter.

❿ Adverse drug experiences, or adverse events, are required to be reported to the FDA by pharmaceutical companies.

⓫ The mission of the FDA is to protect "the public health by assuring the safety, efficacy, and security of human and veterinary drugs, biological products, medical devices, our nation's food supply, cosmetics, and products that emit radiation."

⓬ Timely communication of important drug safety information provides HPs, patients, consumers, and other interested persons with access to the most current information concerning the potential risks and benefits of a marketed drug, helping them to make more informed treatment choices.

⓭ The FDA uses various tools and methods to communicate drug safety information to the public.

⑭ The mission of the Division of Drug Information (DDI) is to optimize the Center for Drug Evaluation and Research's (CDER) educational and communication efforts to the global community. DDI supports the FDA's mission to promote and protect public health.

⑮ DDI has built effective internal and external interactions to provide timely, accurate, and useful information through both traditional and social media channels.

⑯ In addition to dedicated Drug Safety Communication (DSC) channels, DDI has several proactive and innovative tools to communicate information about human drug products to the public.

⑰ The FDA offers many opportunities for health professional students. One of the most popular programs is the FDA Pharmacy Student Experiential Program. Student opportunities are also available within the United States Public Health Service (USPHS) Commissioned Corps.

Introduction

There are many roles available to health care professionals (HPs) within the pharmaceutical industry and regulatory agencies focused on public health. In the industry, these roles span medical education, publications, marketing, medical information, regulatory affairs, and more. In public health agencies, the roles are usually separate functions supporting the organizational mission statement and generally pertain to protecting the health of all citizens and providing essential human services, especially for those who are least able to help themselves. Job titles and descriptions may vary slightly from company to company or agency to agency, but the importance of HPs within each area is constant across organizations.

Throughout this chapter, the reader will become familiar with the organization of a pharmaceutical company, professional mentoring relationships, pharmaceutical industry's regulated interactions with outside HPs, fulfillment of a medical information request (MIR) and responses to unsolicited inquiries, the many roles and career paths available to HPs in industry, and the importance and requirements of adverse event (AE) reporting and **postmarketing surveillance**. Information surrounding the role of medical information within a regulatory agency, specifically the U.S. Food and Drug Administration (FDA), will then be presented. At the end, the reader should have a general knowledge of the roles and responsibilities of HPs employed in the pharmaceutical industry and FDA, the expectations that HPs may have when receiving medical information from a pharmaceutical company or regulatory agency, and how to pursue opportunities and careers within the pharmaceutical industry or a regulatory agency with a public health mission.

Opportunities for Health Professionals within Industry

❶ *Pharmaceutical companies' scientific or medical departments are staffed with highly*
● *trained HPs working in a multitude of specialized fields* (see Figure 22-1).[1] The following
section will highlight specific opportunities within the pharmaceutical industry for HPs.

CONSUMER RESPONSE CENTER

● Customer response center representatives are the first-line response team for unsolicited requests* for medical information. HPs in this setting are well trained for customer
response center representative positions, as many have direct patient care experience
from previous roles, including nurses, pharmacists, nurse practitioners, physician assistants, etc. HPs in customer response center are faced with a variety of responsibilities
as the first-line of communication with patients and providers. Responsibilities include
capturing AEs that are reported and triaging nonmedical and MIRs. Customer response
center HPs are provided with a variety of tools, including but not limited to product labeling (or package inserts), response letters, question & answer (Q&A) documents, and
clinical topic overviews, typically drafted by peers in the medical information department
to assist in answering unsolicited requests for product information. A guidance document
published by the FDA, regarding responding to unsolicited requests*, also offers industry
the FDA's current thinking on this topic.[2] Customer response center staff uses product
labeling, response letters, and literature searches to assist them in responding to MIRs.
HPs serving in this capacity must have excellent verbal communication skills and are
highly trained in effectively searching for information. Some MIRs may require additional
research or analysis resulting in the customer response center HPs escalating the inquiry

Figure 22–1. Organization of pharmaceutical companies medical department.[1]

---

* Unsolicited requests must be created by the requestor, free from prompting by the pharmaceutical
company or its representatives.

to a medical information specialist for further investigation. Medical information specialists have a variety of education and training, including health professionals (e.g., pharmacists, nurses) and other scientific degrees (PhD). The skills required for this position include literature evaluation, communication of scientific information, medical writing ability, and knowledge of disease states and medications.

MEDICAL INFORMATION

❷ *Medical information specialists respond to inquiries, provide training, and draft materials for a variety of internal and external audiences.* Medical information specialists are HPs who respond to unsolicited MIRs, write and update response letters, conduct scientific analysis of medical literature topics, review promotional materials, develop Academy of Managed Care Pharmacy (AMCP)-formatted dossiers for formulary consideration, and train company staff (e.g., sales force, peers, account managers [see Figure 22-2]).[3,4]

Medical information specialists also respond to MIRs that are escalated to them by customer response center representatives. Escalation, or the transfer of MIRs, occurs frequently when the customer response center representatives do not have the resources and expertise necessary to formulate a response. Frequently, escalations involve questions about off-label use of a medication in question. This will be discussed later in the section entitled Regulation of Health Professionals in Industry. Medical information specialists may have access to additional resources, such as comprehensive reports from

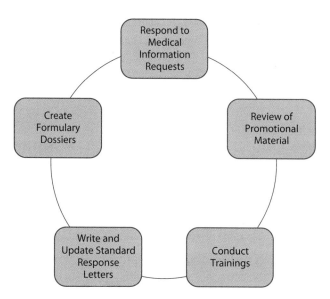

Figure 22–2. Responsibilities of medical information specialists.[1,2]

clinical trials, information provided to study investigators, marketing materials, posters and abstracts, and contacts in other departments, which makes them invaluable resources for analyzing and synthesizing information.

MEDICAL SCIENCE LIAISONS

Medical science liaisons (MSLs) originated as a highly specialized customer response center representative and have varying responsibilities (Table 22-1). An MSL supports, and is supported by, the scientific affairs and medical information team. MSLs have a close working relationship with **key opinion leaders** and are expected to engage in clinical conversations ranging from broad clinical guidelines to patient-specific care.[5] MSLs are expected to attend national meetings and to provide comprehensive clinical presentations. These individuals engage in scientific exchange with experts, support clinical trial development and enrollment, and serve as the liaison between the key opinion leaders and company to develop externally sponsored research. MSLs may focus on one product or therapeutic area, so there may be overlapping MSLs working for the same company in one location, supporting different products and specialty areas, or vice versa, there may be one MSL in a remote location responsible for multiple products and therapeutic areas.

MANAGED MARKETS

Managed market specialists are known in some companies as field-based outcomes liaisons or FBOLs. This position is similar to that of an MSL, except the focus of FBOLs may be to demonstrate the value of a product to managed care organizations (e.g., accountable care organizations), pharmacy benefit managers (PBMs), or other HPs in similar decision-making roles through the generation of outcomes data. Outcomes data typically provides studies focused on identifying, measuring, and evaluating the end result of a

TABLE 22–1. RESPONSIBILITIES OF MEDICAL SCIENCE LIAISONS[3,5]

Building and maintaining relationships with key opinion leaders
Recruiting interested investigators for clinical trial research
Supporting advisory boards
Assisting with company projects
Providing peer-to-peer exchange of information
Presenting at meetings with formulary decision makers
Conducting training sessions for branded product speakers, medical residents, and/or sales representatives
Performing and overseeing clinical trial and health outcomes research
Providing continuing education and branded product presentations

health care service or treatment. For example, a company that is marketing an antiplatelet medication might request their FBOLs demonstrate to customers the value of the product through quality-life years gained or may request the FBOLs create a risk stratification tool (e.g., stratification of risk for patients with cardiovascular disease) to assist clinicians in determining appropriate therapy options for their patients.

OUTCOMES RESEARCH

Health economics and outcomes research (HEOR) compares a product's effectiveness to other interventions, evaluates the efficacy of a product or services, and assesses the cost efficiency compared to incremental benefit. These studies may be retrospective or prospective and utilize electronic medical records (EMR), data collected from physicians, and patient-reported outcomes to provide real-world evidence. Studies can assess drug utilization, medication adherence and compliance, quality of life, patient-reported outcomes, burden of illness, and health care utilization and costs. The HEOR department can work with key experts in a certain field, including academicians, to generate new evidence. For example, clinical studies published in the literature may have insufficient data or inconsistent conclusions regarding cost and resource utilization (e.g., physician office visits, pharmacy claims, hospitalizations) for a specific disease state. To address this lack of information, individuals in HEOR design a study using a national claims database, which contains data from thousands of individuals with the same private insurance. These researchers conduct a retrospective analysis that provides information on the burden of the specific disease state on the health care industry and areas that may require improvement. Data generated from the HEOR department supports the conversations driven by liaisons in the managed markets field-based positions.

MEDICAL EDUCATION

HPs in medical education evaluate funding requests for continuing medical education (CME), continuing education (CE), and other programs submitted by qualified organizations. Grants are reviewed by medical education to ensure the program outlined in the grant addresses specific needs of clinicians in clinical practice and is consistent with the company's educational goals and objectives for a specific therapeutic area.[1] Additionally, the pharmaceutical industry collaborates with CE companies to provide education to various HPs. These programs may include various topics, such as disease state, changes to clinical practice, and medication therapy management. CE programs must meet standards set by the corresponding accrediting body for the audience (e.g., Accreditation Council for Continuing Medical Education [ACCME]) and should follow guidance documents published by regulatory bodies (e.g., FDA).[6,7]

MEDICAL AFFAIRS

Medical affairs HPs have strategic oversight of marketed products, and typically manage Phase IV clinical trial programs. They may also be involved with preclinical studies through Phase IV or postmarketing studies. These HPs are primarily conducting research on marketed pharmaceuticals in areas of high therapeutic demands or information need. Medical affairs HPs play a key role in shaping the direction of future clinical development including where to focus resources on specific disease states, what drug candidates to support in human clinical studies, and what marketed drugs to develop with new indications or to study through the investigator-initiated study process. In addition, medical affairs staff is involved in a variety of tasks with peers in medical information, marketing, and with key opinion leaders in the field. These tasks include reviewing promotional and marketing materials, supporting Phase IV clinical trial sites and maintaining communication with trial investigators, reviewing product labeling, formulary dossiers, training materials for promotional and education purposes, and developing and presenting original research in the form of posters, abstracts, and manuscripts. Medical affairs HPs are responsible for reviewing these materials for accuracy of medical information and to ensure that the final products (e.g., promotional materials, package inserts) are unbiased, fair balanced, and not misleading.[1]

MARKETING

HPs in the marketing department of a pharmaceutical company are responsible for developing the branded messages for a product. The tag lines and main selling points seen in journal advertisements, on web pages, and on printed materials are created by the marketing department. It is important for HPs in marketing to understand the clinical practice environment of their peers, so they can provide useful, valuable tools and materials. Marketing drafts a plethora of promotional materials such as journal and television advertisements to functional educational tools such as dose conversion guides. These materials are then reviewed by peers in medical information and medical affairs, and other internal business partners in regulatory and legal.[1] Direct-to-consumer advertising (DTCA) is a source of information for patients and caregivers, which is allowed in a limited number of countries (e.g., the United States, New Zealand) and is regulated by various government agencies. DTCA can impact multiple factors, including patient education and awareness of treatments and enhanced discussion between physician and patient. However, DTCA may also be associated with medication utilization, health care costs, and misinformation.

PUBLICATIONS

The team of HPs in the publications department has the important task of ensuring the appropriate information reaches the appropriate audience. The publication process includes planning the dissemination of preclinical studies, clinical trials, and review articles for therapeutic areas of interest and company-sponsored studies through scientific channels. For example, a company coming to market with a new antihypertensive medication would want its publications department to create a plan that would publish trial data (preclinical through *post hoc* and review data) concurrently with major meetings of prescribers treating hypertension. The publications department ensures that reprints of posters, abstracts, and manuscripts are readily available for dissemination to HPs in the field. HPs in this department are also responsible for reviewing the final content of publications and drafting comments if necessary, often through a partnered review process with medical affairs and medical information, to make certain accurate information is available for practitioners in clinical practice.[1]

REGULATORY AFFAIRS

Many HPs work within the regulatory affairs role, which combines the clinical expertise of an HP with regulatory knowledge. The responsibilities of individuals in regulatory affairs are to interact with regulatory governing bodies, including FDA, develop strategies for submission documents (e.g., new drug applications [NDAs], investigational new drug [IND] applications), and prepares product labeling. Regulatory interactions within FDA include contacts with various offices, including, the Office of New Drugs, Office of Drug Evaluation, among others. The regulatory affairs department also understands and interprets the changes in the regulatory environment to the company's standard procedures. Personnel in regulatory affairs work closely with the development of a drug and ensure that the company adheres to regulatory requirements.

OPPORTUNITIES WITHIN THE PHARMACEUTICAL INDUSTRY

There are several opportunities for both current and future HPs within the pharmaceutical industry.

FOR THE STUDENT

There are many opportunities for HP students in training to gain exposure to the roles and responsibilities within the pharmaceutical industry. Many pharmaceutical companies offer internships in various departments, which allow students to learn the skills required for these positions, network with industry professionals, and understand the work environment. Additionally, many companies host students in different health professions during advanced rotational experiences. Some companies allow their HPs to visit school campuses to share and promote their upcoming internship opportunities.

FOR THE GRADUATE

Many postgraduate opportunities are available upon completion of school and training. This includes postdoctoral fellowships which are structured for graduates to gain in-depth knowledge of the industry, advances professional development, and allows HPs to utilize their clinical knowledge to help patients and providers better manage their health. Pharmaceutical industry fellowships vary in curriculum, structure, and objectives. Fellowships can be focused in one specific department or multiple departments in a rotational fashion (e.g., medical information, regulatory affairs, medical education). Many programs offer rotational opportunities within regulatory agencies or partner with an agency for a more regulatory focused experience. Additionally, some programs include academic opportunities, such as serving as a preceptor to students, working within a clinical environment and providing direct patient care, researching and publishing articles or conference posters, or teaching in a didactic nature and obtaining a teaching certificate. Upon completion of the fellowship, individuals have a wide breadth and depth of experience that allows them to successfully contribute to the pharmaceutical industry.

FOR THE PROFESSIONAL

The various roles in the pharmaceutical industry allow HPs to incorporate their expertise and experience to complex medical conditions and corporate environment. HPs have the ability to interpret scientific literature and guidelines, understand the nuances of complex health care systems and formulary plans, and provide advice regarding patient therapy management, all which influence strategic decisions made about a drug product. HPs are able to utilize their clinical skills to collaborate with other professionals in an effort to develop new medications to bring to patients.

As outlined in this section, HPs have many varied opportunities within the industry. Each of the functions described previously abide by a set of rules and regulations. Understanding and complying with these rules and regulations help ensure the success of industry-employed HPs.

Regulation of Health Professionals in Industry

❸ *Pharmaceutical companies are regulated both externally by FDA and internally by standard operating procedures (SOPs).*[8,9] To help internal staff to understand the regulations governing their department's duties and to establish an efficient methodological approach to the business, SOPs are developed internally by the company.[3,9] While practitioners in clinical practice may not be governed by the same regulations as industry, having a basic understanding of company's regulations will help align the external clinicians' expectations with what can be provided by internal industry HPs.

STANDARD OPERATING PROCEDURES

SOPs provide additional guidance to employees, supplementing regulations from federal and state government agencies. SOPs allow a company to digest federal regulations, making them applicable to employees and their everyday job functions.[3,9] The pharmaceutical industry employs HPs and lawyers in regulatory affairs to ensure SOPs are up-to-date and provide employees proper guidance for complying with all applicable regulations. Examples of SOPs include the process to respond to unsolicited requests and the development of standard response letters.

CODE OF FEDERAL REGULATIONS

The Code of Federal Regulations (CFR) Title 21 regulates the U.S. pharmaceutical industry throughout the life cycle of a product, from before the investigational new drug application (pre-IND) through Phase IV clinical trials, including postmarketing data collection.[6,7,10,11] HPs working for a U.S. pharmaceutical company must achieve a thorough understanding of these regulations to ensure compliance with the regulations that pertain to their daily duties.

FDA GUIDANCE DOCUMENTS

FDA guidance documents represent the FDA's current thinking on a topic. Guidance documents do not create or confer any rights for or on any person and do not operate to bind the FDA or the public. Guidance documents are very useful because they expand upon the regulations. ❹ *FDA's draft Guidance for Industry "Responding to Unsolicited Requests for Off-Label Information About Prescription Drugs and Medical Devices" describes the FDA's current thinking about how manufacturers and distributors of prescription human drug products can respond to unsolicited requests for information about unapproved indications (off-label information) related to their FDA-approved or cleared products.* An important portion of this guidance document for pharmaceutical companies is the discussion of unsolicited requests that are encountered through emerging electronic media. First though, several important definitions are provided with examples.

UNSOLICITED REQUESTS

❺ *Unsolicited requests are those initiated by persons or entities that are completely independent of the relevant firm.* The requestors may include many HPs, health care organizations, members of the academic community, and formulary committees, as well as consumers such as patients and caregivers. Requests that are prompted in any way by a manufacturer or its representatives are not unsolicited requests.

FDA has long taken the position that firms can respond to unsolicited requests for information about FDA-regulated medical products by providing truthful, balanced, non-misleading, and non-promotional scientific or medical information that is responsive to the specific request, even if responding to the request requires a firm to provide information on unapproved indications or conditions of use.[2]

Two Types of Unsolicited Requests

Nonpublic unsolicited requests: A nonpublic unsolicited request is an unsolicited request that is directed privately to a firm using a one-on-one communication approach. For example, an individual calls or e-mails the medical information staff at a firm seeking information about an off-label use. In this case, neither the request nor the response would be visible to the public.

Public unsolicited requests: A public unsolicited request is an unsolicited request made in a public form, whether directed to a firm specifically or to a forum at large. For example, during a live presentation, an individual asks a question, directed to a firm's representative but heard by other attendees, regarding off-label use of a specific product. This request is a public request. Similarly, a response by the firm that is conveyed to the same audience as the original question would be considered a public response. Another example is if an individual posts a question about off-label use of a specific product on a firm-controlled website (or a third-party discussion forum) that is visible to a broad audience. The request could be directed to a firm specifically or posed to users of a discussion forum at large. This request is a public online request. Similarly, a response by the firm that is visible to the same audience as the original question would be considered a public online response.

SOLICITED REQUESTS

❻ *The FDA considers requests for off-label information that are prompted in any way by a manufacturer or its representatives to be solicited.* Such solicited requests may be considered evidence of a firm's intent that a drug be used for an unlabeled indication. For example, if a firm announces results of a study via a microblogging service (e.g., Twitter) and suggests that an off-label use of its product is safe and effective, any comments and requests received as a result of the original message about the off-label use would be considered solicited requests (Case Study 22-1).

Case Study 22-1

■ DRUG A

DRUG A® is an FDA-approved medication for the treatment of moderate to severe hiccups, manufactured by the pharmaceutical company Amazing Drugs LP. Since initial approval of DRUG A®, their first approved medication, the company is planning to file a supplemental new drug application (sNDA) for the indication of uncontrollable laughter. Amazing Drugs LP employs HPs in various functions, including regulatory affairs, medical affairs, and marketing to ensure the successful launch of DRUG A®. However, since they are relatively a small company and this is their first sNDA, they require additional employees. A priority review (a drug product with priority status is reviewed faster than one with standard status) was granted for DRUG A®, with an expected approval action in 6 months following sNDA filing.

- *What internal documents should Amazing Drugs LP prepare so their employees are aware of the regulations governing their job functions?*
- *What external regulations should Amazing Drugs LP include in education for their staff?*
- *Discuss the job responsibilities in the current departments at Amazing Drugs LP.*
- *What are some other departments Amazing Drugs LP should consider developing in the future? What are some of the job responsibilities of these departments?*

The Code on Interactions with Health Care Professionals

HPs within the pharmaceutical industry hold themselves to a high standard when it comes to providing accurate, concise, and timely information. ❼*Interactions between pharmaceutical companies and HPs are defined, but not regulated, by a code of conduct established by the Pharmaceutical Research and Manufacturers of America (PhRMA). This is done through the revised version of the Code on Interactions with Health Care Professionals.*[10] The prior edition from 2002 addressed primarily drug products being marketed and activities prior to the launch of a medication. The updated version released in January 2009 includes more specific guidance regarding the interactions between pharmaceutical industry representatives and HPs. The goal of these regulations is to provide transparency to HPs and patients alike as to the motives and channels through which pharmaceutical industry conducts business with external customers and business partners[10,11] (Case Study 22-2).

Case Study 22–2

Use information from Case Study 22-1

- *What department(s) would review grants for educational programming for DRUG A®?*
- *What department(s) may be involved in approving marketing materials for DRUG A®?*
- *What department(s) may be involved in engaging in scientific exchange with external HPs who specialize in uncontrollable laughter?*

Fulfillment of MIRs

HPs and patients may contact a pharmaceutical company with questions regarding a medication when an answer is not readily available. A typical process for responding to these questions is described in Figure 22-3.

RESPONSE LETTERS

❽ *Clinical response letters, also known as standard responses, are written correspondence that are internally reviewed and contain content in response to unsolicited requests for medical information.* The use of evidence-based medicine in response letters allows consumers and HPs to be confident that they are receiving fair-balanced, unbiased, and not misleading information.[11] Response letters are usually created according to a template for consistency (see Table 22-2) and drafted in anticipation of, or in response to, frequently asked questions.[12] Solvay Pharmaceuticals determined that prior to the launch of a product, response letters took 4 to 8 hours each to create. The time spent by Solvay's staff to

Figure 22–3. Medical information request receipt and fulfillment process.

TABLE 22–2. COMPONENTS OF A STANDARD RESPONSE LETTER[11,12]

Opening
Indication(s)
Disclaimer
Body
Closing
Adverse Event Reporting
Signature and Contact Information
Enclosure(s)
References

create a response letter following launch of its product significantly increased, taking 4 to 7 days to create. This was directly related to the increased workload and the continuous arrival of new MIRs.[13] Once a product is available on the market, the number and complexity of MIRs are likely to increase. This increases HPs' total workload and therefore increases the time it takes to complete individual tasks, such as creating response letters. Because of this, the time to create a response letter and respond to an MIR may differ from Solvay's initial estimate.

Pharmaceutical companies' response letters are created from source documents in response to frequently asked questions and are peer-reviewed internally.[14,15] Standard response letters developed by companies may be either proactive or reactive. For example, if the evening news reports that STRIPES® causes yellow stripes to appear on patients' skin, the company that makes STRIPES® should react immediately by developing a response letter to address questions from HPs and patients on this AE (i.e., reactive). In another example, a company launching Drug A, a drug with a similar mechanism of action to STRIPES®, may wish to proactively develop a response letter in anticipation that the likelihood of experiencing yellow stripes with Drug A will be frequently asked, based on the report of this reaction with STRIPES®. Using the example above, the company that manufacturers Drug A may need more than 1 day to prepare a complete, concise response and, thus, in the meantime may tell customers that they are currently researching the issue in question. When this short response is provided, the requestor should expect a complete response to be delivered in a timely manner (see Appendix 22-1 for an example of a response letter).

UNIQUE RESPONSES FOR NON-FREQUENTLY ASKED QUESTIONS

❾ *Patient variability, clinician experience, and previously unaddressed questions require personalized responses that cannot be fulfilled with a standard response letter.* HPs in the customer response center and medical information department then use their literature search and evaluation skills to determine if relevant information has been published or is available through internal company data (also known as data on file) that addresses the inquiry.[15] If no information is found, the requestor is contacted with the results and a statement that the company cannot provide any information. If relevant publications are found, a response is drafted that includes the citations or reprints (when copyright allows) of the information and this is provided to the requestor along with a verbal conversation (if possible) to discuss the findings and applicability to the requestor's situation.[14] An internal peer review is conducted in order to ensure the accuracy of the information provided and that the response adequately answers the original inquiry. Requestors expect their inquiry to be addressed in a timely manner and often prefer a verbal answer, allowing for a peer-to-peer discussion and the option to request written information.[15] All MIRs are valuable and provide timely information to the company regarding the current state of the product in clinical practice. MIRs are typically compiled and analyzed periodically to identify trends and patterns. These trends are published internally in the form of periodic reports; this may signal to a company that a response letter is needed on a particular topic that is reported frequently, identify new educational gaps, or lead to the development of new product formulations. Periodic reports may alternatively signal to a company that previous "hot topics" or frequently asked questions, are no longer of interest to practitioners in clinical practice, often times identifying new areas of interest that practitioners need to have addressed (Case Study 22-3).

Case Study 22–3

DRUG A® receives approval for the indication of uncontrollable laughter and HPs have quickly adopted the medication into their practice. Since approval, Amazing Drugs LP has received multiple MIRs from HPs who are interested in using DRUG A® for off-label uses and learning the scientific literature that supports its indication. To adequately answer these inquiries, Amazing Drugs LP has expanded the number of HPs working in multiple departments within the medical department. Many companies are investigating similar compounds and one has successfully completed Phase III studies. This company has developed the product STRIPES® for the treatment of uncontrollable laughter, and received approval by the European Medicines Agency (EMA) for use in Europe. The NDA was recently submitted to FDA, and it is suspected that STRIPES® will have a **Risk Evaluation and Mitigation Strategy** (REMS) (see description later in the chapter) and restricted distribution program approved by FDA along with the drug because it is well-known to occasionally cause yellow stripes to appear on the skin.

- *What should Amazing Drugs LP do to prepare for inquiries regarding product comparisons to STRIPES® and other investigational compounds?*
- *What questions should Amazing Drugs LP anticipate receiving due to their similar indication to STRIPES®?*

AE Reporting

FDA approval of a medication does not denote complete safety of the product. It is important to keep in mind that any medicine capable of curing or treating a disease may also have the potential for serious AEs. An adverse drug experience is defined by the CFR Title 21, Section 314.80—Postmarketing reporting of adverse drug experiences, as, "Any adverse event associated with the use of a drug in humans, whether or not considered drug related, including the following: an adverse event occurring in the course of the use of a drug product in professional practice; an adverse event occurring from drug overdose whether accidental or intentional; an adverse event occurring from drug abuse; an adverse event occurring from drug withdrawal; and any failure of expected pharmacological action."[16] ⑩ *Adverse drug experiences, or AEs, are required to be reported to the FDA by pharmaceutical companies.* It is the charge of the pharmaceutical company to monitor these risks once the drug is on the market, also known as the postmarketing phase of the drug's life cycle.[16,17]

Pharmaceutical companies obtain information regarding AEs in a variety of ways including postmarketing trials, publications, customer calls, physician reports, social media sites, blogs, and in some cases, even by being in close proximity to a personal conversation. The reporting process may vary from company to company so long as the information required by FDA is reported with each AE through completion of FDA Form 3500A. FDA Form 3500A differs from voluntary FDA Form 3500 and Form 3500B which are intended for HPs and consumers, respectively. FDA Form 3500A requests such information as patient demographics, medication identifiers, and a description of the AE.[17] Further information on reporting adverse effects may be found in Chapter 17 (Case Study 22-4).

Case Study 22–4

Use information from previous case.

The company that manufactures DRUG A® begins receiving reports of patients noting yellow stripes on their skin.

- *How must Amazing Drugs LP document patient reports of yellow stripes?*
- *Does Amazing Drugs LP need to send the reports of yellow stripes to any additional agency or organization?*

Staying Connected with Pharmaceutical Industry

Pharmaceutical companies are dynamic entities that are constantly evolving. In today's media, it is possible to keep up-to-date with new information from industry including drug approvals, publications and presentations, as well as safety alerts and labeling changes. The Drug Information Association (DIA) and other industry-associated organizations (see Table 22-3) are resources for pharmaceutical company information. HPs in clinical practice should familiarize themselves with these reliable sources for industry news so that they can share current industry information with their patients and other clinicians.

Anatomy of DHHS and FDA

The Department of Health and Human Services (DHHS) is the U.S. government's principal agency for protecting the health of all Americans and providing essential human services, especially for those who are least able to help themselves. DHHS is headed by the Secretary who is the chief managing officer for the DHHS family of agencies,

TABLE 22-3. PHARMACEUTICAL INDUSTRY ORGANIZATIONS

Organization	Website
American Association of Pharmaceutical Scientists (AAPS)	https://www.aaps.org/default.aspx
Association of Clinical Research Professionals (ACRP)	http://www.acrpnet.org/default.aspx
Drug Information Association (DIA)	http://www.diaglobal.org/en.aspx
Generic Pharmaceutical Association (GPhA)	http://www.gphaonline.org/
Health Industry Representatives Association (HIRA)	http://www.hira.org
Industry Pharmacists Organization (IPhO)	http://www.industrypharmacist.org
Institute for Safe Medication Practices (ISMP)	http://www.ismp.org/
National Association of Pharmaceutical Sales Representatives (NAPSRx®)	http://www.napsronline.org/
Pharmaceutical Research and Manufacturers of America (PhRMA)	http://www.phrma.org/
Regulatory Affairs Professionals Society (RAPS)	http://www.raps.org/

including various operating divisions, regional offices, and the Office of the Secretary.[18,19] Table 22-4 describes each agency and office and provides the mission statement for each. This illustrates how DHHS programmatic areas each have their own goals and objectives. The composition of each agency or office under DHHS varies. Ultimately, a common theme can be applied to these agencies. DHHS creates agencies to address specific

TABLE 22–4. LIST OF HEALTH AND HUMAN SERVICES AGENCIES AND OFFICES

Agency or Office	Purpose
Office of the Secretary (OS)	"To help provide the building blocks that Americans need to live healthy, successful lives"
Administration for Children and Families (ACF)	"...to provide family assistance (welfare), child support, child care, Head Start, child welfare, and other programs relating to children and families."
Administration on Aging (AoA)	"...to develop a comprehensive, coordinated and cost-effective system of home and community-based services that helps elderly individuals maintain their health and independence in their homes and communities."
Agency for Healthcare Research and Quality (AHRQ)	"...to improve the quality, safety, efficiency, and effectiveness of health care for all Americans. Information from AHRQ's research helps people make more informed decisions and improve the quality of health care services."
Agency for Toxic Substances and Disease (ATSDR)	"... serves the public by using the best science, taking responsive public health actions, and providing trusted health information to prevent harmful exposures and diseases related to toxic substances."
Centers for Disease Control and Prevention (CDC)	"...serves as the national focus for developing and applying disease prevention and control, environmental health, and health promotion and health education activities designed to improve the health of the people of the United States."
Centers for Medicare and Medicaid Services (CMS)	"... to ensure effective, up-to-date health care coverage and to promote quality care for beneficiaries."
Food and Drug Administration (FDA)	...to protect "the public health by assuring the safety, efficacy, and security of human and veterinary drugs, biological products, medical devices, our nation's food supply, cosmetics, and products that emit radiation."
Health Resources and Services Administration (HRSA)	"... to improve health and achieve health equity through access to quality services, a skilled health workforce and innovative programs."
Indian Health Service (IHS)	"...to raise the physical, mental, social, and spiritual health of American Indians and Alaska Natives to the highest level."
National Institutes of Health (NIH)	"...to seek fundamental knowledge about the nature and behavior of living systems and the application of that knowledge to enhance health, lengthen life, and reduce the burdens of illness and disability."
Office of Inspector General (OIG)	"...to protect the integrity of Department of Health and Human Services (HHS) programs, as well as the health and welfare of the beneficiaries of those programs."
Substance Abuse and Mental Health Services Administration (SAMHSA)	"...to reduce the impact of substance abuse and mental illness on America's communities."

areas of public health. Each organization is further divided into groups depending on the roles and responsibilities assigned to the agency. These agencies are further divided into centers supporting the role assigned to the agencies. In the United States, there is a center or office available to provide some regulatory guidance on most, if not all, areas of public health. One of such agencies is FDA.

MISSION OF FDA

⓫ *The mission of the FDA is to protect "the public health by assuring the safety, efficacy, and security of human and veterinary drugs, biological products, medical devices, our nation's food supply, cosmetics, and products that emit radiation."*[20] The FDA consists of nine Centers and Offices. Figure 22-4 shows the FDA's organization chart. The Center for Drug Evaluation and Research (CDER) is of particular interest to pharmacists and other HPs because of the Center's responsibility for ensuring that drug products are of high quality, and are safe and effective for their intended use.[21] CDER provides the public with access to accurate, science-based information needed to evaluate the risks and benefits of human drugs and strives to provide easily retrievable information about human drugs through the FDA website, www.fda.gov.

SAFETY COMMUNICATION BY FDA

⓬ *Timely communication of important drug safety information provides HPs, patients, consumers, and other interested persons with access to the most current information concerning the potential risks and benefits of a marketed drug, helping them to make more informed treatment choices.*[22] The FDA's safety assessment of medicines does not diminish after drugs are approved for marketing.[23] Although the premarket phase of study is very intensive, much work still remains to monitor approved drugs over time. Once a drug is approved and marketed, the FDA often gains additional information as the drug is used and studied in broader and more diverse populations. Such information helps provide a better picture of a drug's benefits, risks, and enables FDA to give HPs and patients the latest information on potential or newly identified risks, and strengthens FDA's ability to safeguard patients against unacceptable risks.

SAFETY COMMUNICATION TOOLS

The FDA has created effective and ongoing relationships with a wide array of trade and professional associations, patient advocacy and consumer groups, safety organizations, media, and other entities. When drug safety issues arise, FDA contacts these groups and works with them to communicate the safety issue to their constituencies.[23,24] ⓭ *FDA uses*

FOOD AND DRUG ADMINISTRATION

Figure 22–4. Organization of centers and offices within FDA. July 2016. FDA = Food and Drug Administration: This figure represents an overview of how FDA is organized. Every Center and Office at FDA has their own organization chart. (Source: http://www.fda.gov/AboutFDA/CentersOffices/OrganizationCharts/ucm393155.htm)

various tools and methods to communicate drug safety information to the public. Important tools used in this effort include, but are not limited to, FDA-approved prescribing information (i.e., drug labeling) and a postmarket communication tool called a *Drug Safety Communication* (DSC), along with other important tools and methods used to communicate drug safety information to the public and HPs.

LABELING UPDATES

The drug labeling, or written material that accompanies drug products, is the most complete single source of information on the drug. A change to the drug label may have tangible benefit in expanding the education of risks, benefits, and optimal usage of marketed drugs.

Over time, new information often emerges about a product, such as side effects, dosing, warnings (boxed warning), drug interactions, and new indications.

This new information is added by the manufacturer to the drug's label so consumers and HPs have all the information necessary for safe and effective use of the drug. All changes to a drug's label must be approved by FDA. The manufacturer sends proposed changes to FDA for review and revision if necessary.

Risk Evaluation and Mitigation Strategies

The creation of **Risk Evaluation and Mitigation Strategies** (REMS) is one of the many methods of communicating safety information to patients and practitioners beyond the traditional labeling.[24,25] REMS were enacted on September 27, 2007 as part of the FDA Amendments Act (FDAAA). An REMS provides information regarding the risks ("above the average risks") of a specific medication in an effort to ensure that the benefits will outweigh the risks for a potential patient, mitigating the likelihood of a negative outcome with the product's use. Following the enactment of FDAAA, FDA may request a manufacturer to develop REMS programs for a particular drug as part of the NDA process. An REMS may also be submitted voluntarily by the manufacturer as part of the NDA prior to receiving a request from FDA. Finally, FDA may request an REMS after a drug receives approval. When determining the need for an REMS, multiple factors are considered including, severity of disease, population intended to use the drug, expected benefits, duration of therapy, and seriousness of known or potential AEs. General REMS program requirements are outlined by FDA, subject to FDA's approval, and enforceable through penalties.[25]

Prior to the codification of REMS, **risk minimization action plans (RiskMAPs)** were established. RiskMAPs are safety plans that are designed to achieve prespecified goals and objectives[24] to minimize known safety risks of a medication while concomitantly

TABLE 22–5.   OTHER METHODS OF COMMUNICATING SAFETY INFORMATION TO CONSUMERS[26,27,28]

Medication Guides	Medication Guides may be required: • If patient labeling could mitigate serious adverse events • If the product has serious adverse events relative to benefits that may cause patients to reconsider their use of the product • If patient adherence can seriously alter the drug's effectiveness
Patient package inserts (PPIs)	PPIs may be required if FDA believes the package insert will help mitigate a serious risk. Usually a Medication Guide or PPI exists for a product, not both.
Communication plan	A communication plan may be requested in which a company submits their plan to educate practitioners about their strategy for minimizing risk/maintaining benefit as outlined in their REMS.
Elements to Assure Safe Use (ETASU)	In certain cases, if these previously described measures are not sufficient to mitigate the risks associated with the medication, additional ETASU may be implemented. ETASU include specific goals to minimize serious risk. If an REMS program includes ETASU, the REMS must also include a specific implementation plan, and education for the patient to be able to monitor and evaluate the risks of the medication and to recommend improvements to the ETASU.

maintaining the benefits. RiskMAPs can employ one or more tools to achieve its set goals and objectives (see Table 22-5 for more detail). Some drug and biological products that were previously approved and/or licensed with RiskMAPs are now deemed to have an REMS.[25]

Medication Guides and Patient Package Inserts

Medication Guides and patient package inserts (PPI) are other examples of safety measures required by FDA prior to 2007. Medication Guides are paper handouts issued with certain prescription medications to address safety concerns specific to that drug or drug class in an effort to reduce AEs.[26] All Medication Guides are subject to the requirements of 21 CFR 208, which means that the Medication Guide must be provided directly to the patient or their agent by HPs when the drug product is dispensed, unless an exemption applies. Alternatively, PPIs are required to be issued with oral contraceptive products to satisfy the requirement that patients using these products are fully informed of all the potential risks and benefits.[27] Manufacturers of oral contraceptives may request informal guidance from FDA to help them create a PPI.

Drug Safety Communications

A DSC is a specific tool used by FDA to communicate to the public important information about safety issues, including emerging safety information, about marketed drugs.[28] DSCs are standardized electronic communications posted on the FDA website. Written as clearly as possible, DSCs are targeted to both HPs and patients. DSCs generally communicate the following information:

- A summary of the safety issue and the nature of the risk being communicated
- The established benefit or benefits of the drug being discussed
- Recommended actions for HPs and patients, when appropriate
- A summary of the data reviewed or being reviewed by FDA

The DSC is the FDA's primary safety communication tool for important postmarket drug safety issues. In the past, safety communications were issued by FDA in a variety of formats. They were issued under different titles and targeted to different audiences. Safety communications have been issued under the titles *Early Communications about Ongoing Safety Reviews, Public Health Advisory, Patient Information Sheet, Healthcare Professional Sheet*, and *Alerts on Patient Information and Healthcare Professional Sheets*. In early 2010, FDA began using a single communication tool—the *Drug Safety Communication*.

It is important to note that while a DSC communicates important safety issues about marketed drugs, it is not a crisis communication document. If a drug product is defective or tainted, or poses some other form of immediate danger, FDA uses other communication tools, such as *Public Health Alerts*, press releases, stakeholder calls, and media briefings, to inform the public rapidly (Case Studies 22-5 and 22-6).

Case Study 22–5

DRUG A® and STRIPES® are found to have a high incidence of causing yellow stripes on the skin. FDA believes this AE warrants additional communication to patients regarding safety information.

- *What are some examples of ways safety information is communicated to patients?*

Case Study 22–6

The manufacturer of SPOTS®, a drug with a similar mechanism of action to DRUG A and STRIPES®, is preparing its NDA for submission to FDA for approval to market their product for the treatment of uncontrollable laughter.

- *What might SPOTS® manufacturer want to submit voluntarily with its NDA package given the known risks associated with DRUG A® and STRIPES®?*

ADVISORY COMMITTEES

Advisory committees play an important role in regulatory activities by providing expert advice and opinions that are independent of the FDA. The advisory committee meeting process allows FDA access to advice from public stakeholders, such as patient advocacy groups, HPs, patients, and caregivers. Topics can include the approval of a drug product, premarket approval of medical devices, trial design specifications, or policy issues. The advisory committee, after hearing from multiple sources, provides recommendations to FDA. Although recommendations are provided, the FDA makes final decisions on these matters.

Division of Drug Information

The focal point at FDA for public inquiries related to human drugs is the Division of Drug Information (DDI). **⓮** *The mission of DDI is to optimize CDER's educational and communication efforts to its global community. DDI supports the FDA's mission to promote and protect public health.*[29] DDI is staffed with a team of HPs. They provide expert advice and guidance on a broad range of CDER activities. This requires DDI's staff to have an extensive knowledge of human drug products and the regulations guiding drug development and marketing. The role of DDI is unique from hospital and academic-based drug information centers because it serves the general public domestically and internationally through direct contact via phone, letter, and e-mail. DDI also works internally to support the Center by collaborating with experts throughout the Center to effectively communicate important and emerging topics.

The division has several unique characteristics that differentiate it from a more traditional drug information center. First, DDI has a unique visitor (customer) make up. Visitors include U.S. and international regulated industry, consumers, HPs, insurance companies, academia, law enforcement, attorneys, and other government agencies. The majority of requests received from U.S. visitors are from consumers, followed by industry and HPs. Industry and small businesses make up most of international requests.

It is not uncommon for DDI to prepare responses for a wide variety of requestors. The preponderance of the information used by DDI to answer drug information queries comes directly from FDA's website. DDI's staff is comprised of highly trained experts in drug information and retrieval. In fact, DDI's drug information specialists are able to answer most inquiries without further consult by using their knowledge of FDA's available public resources. Sometimes, an inquiry cannot be addressed using readily available information. In that case, DDI staff work with subject matter experts across the Center to find information suitable to answer the inquiry.

DDI SERVES THE CENTER AND PUBLIC HEALTH

Drug information services provided by DDI fit generally into one of three categories: correspondence, dissemination, and other (Table 22-6). Correspondence represents a majority of direct contact provided by DDI. In an average month, DDI responds to 1,300 e-mails, 4,000 telephone calls, and over 60 letters. The most common inquiries are related to regulatory issues, such as the drug review and approval process. Many times the same question will be asked in a different way by a different requestor. For example, a consumer might call FDA asking for more information about a DSC. The same question might be addressed by an HP wanting to know the impact on clinical practice and possible labeling changes.

FDA DRUG INFORMATION RESOURCES

⓯ *DDI has built effective internal and external interactions to provide timely, accurate, and useful information through both traditional and social media channels.* Table 22-7 lists commonly used FDA websites and the intended purpose of each page. In order to select the most appropriate FDA-sponsored resource/website, practitioners should have a basic understanding of what websites are available and what information is provided. Table 22-7 provides a brief overview of these websites. Practitioners are strongly encouraged to visit and explore these websites to become familiar with what is offered.

⓰ *In addition to dedicated DSC channels, DDI has several proactive and innovative tools to communicate information about human drug products to the public.* Information is disseminated through DDI's listservs, RSS feeds, CDERLearn Continuing Education (CE) programs, videos, Twitter, and audio podcasts. All of these examples represent new ways to promote the safe and effective use of human drug products.

CDER SMALL BUSINESS & INDUSTRY ASSISTANCE

Most DI centers would not have a component that serves industry, which is a unique characteristic of this federal DI center. DDI is the home of CDER's Small Business & Industry Assistance (SBIA) program and interacts with regulated industry by assisting domestic and international industry seeking timely and accurate information relating to

TABLE 22–6.   DRUG INFORMATION SERVICES PROVIDED BY DDI

Correspondence
- Phone calls
  - Drug Information 1-855-543-DRUG (3784)
  - MedWatch Adverse Event Reporting (1-800-FDA-1088)
  - CDER Small Business & Industry Assistance (1-866-405-5367)
- E-mails
  - Drug Information and MedWatch (DrugInfo@fda.hhs.gov)
  - CDER Small Business Assistance (CDERSBIA@fda.hhs.gov)
  - GDUFA (AskGDUFA@fda.hhs.gov)
  - GADIS (GADIS@fda.hhs.gov)
- Mail

Division of Drug Information (CDER) or CDER SBIA

Office of Communications

10001 New Hampshire Avenue

Hillandale Building, 4th Floor

Silver Spring, MD 20993

Dissemination
- DDI website
- Listservs: DDI, CDER Small Business Assistance, GADIS
- Twitter @FDA_Drug_Info
- Publications, posters, presentations
- Exhibits
- Student webinars
- CDERLearn
- CDER small business workshops and webinars
- CDER Trade Press

Other
- Imprint identification
- International visitations
- FDA Pharmacy Student Experiential Program
- Regulatory Pharmaceutical Fellowship
- Global Alliance of Drug Information Specialists

development and regulation of human drug products. Small business outreach activities include a series of online webinars and live workshops held around the United States. Inquiries are received, triaged to subject matter experts if necessary, and responses are coordinated from the CDERSBIA@fda.hhs.gov e-mail account. Additional key elements of the industry assistance program are monthly webinars and CDERLearn CE programs. These are methods by which FDA educates specific audiences about the safe use of medicine, the drug regulatory process, the vital role HPs play to assist FDA in fulfilling its

TABLE 22–7.   FDA-SPONSORED DRUG INFORMATION LINKS

Website	Purpose
www.fda.gov/aboutddi	Division of Drug Information (DDI) home page
	Provides background, mission, and purpose of DDI
	Also maintains several helpful links for finding information relating to:
	• Student and fellowship opportunities
	• Small Business & Industry Assistance
	• CE programs, webinars, trainings, audio podcasts, videos, Twitter, and listserv
	• Drug identification
www.fda.gov/drugs	CDER home page
	DDI's first resource for responding to questions from the public and where most questions pertaining to regulations can be answered.
	Site maintains sections dedicated to the following topics:
	• Drug approvals and databases
	• Drug safety and availability
	• Drug development and approval process
	• Guidances, compliance, and regulatory information
	• Drug science and research
	• Consumer, health professional, and industry resources
	• Recalls and alerts
	• Approvals and clearances
http://www.fda.gov/Drugs/ DrugSafety/PostmarketDrug SafetyInformationforPatientsand Providers/ucm111085.htm	Index to drug-specific information
	This page provides a list of drugs that have been the subject of postmarketing drug safety communication efforts.
http://www.fda.gov/AboutFDA/ ContactFDA/StayInformed/ GetEmailUpdates/default.htm	E-mail updates home page
	This page allows users to sign up for the FDA e-mail alert service that distributes important FDA news and information as it is available.
www.fda.gov/drugsatfda	Drugs@FDA home page
	Searchable FDA database containing official information about FDA-approved brand and generic drugs and therapeutic biological products. This database also contains:
	• Labels for approved drug products
	• Consumer information for drugs approved after 1998
	• Approval history for drug products (including FDA review documents)
www.fda.gov/cder/ob	Orange Book: approved drug products with therapeutic equivalence evaluations home page
	Free electronic access to the approved drug products with therapeutic equivalence evaluations list
	Can search by active ingredient, proprietary name, patent, applicant holder, or application number

continued

TABLE 22–7. FDA-SPONSORED DRUG INFORMATION LINKS (*CONTINUED*)

Website	Purpose
www.fda.gov/cder/ndc	National Drug Code Directory home page
	Searchable list of universal product identifier for human drugs. OLD and NEW NDC directories available, background page provides overview of differences between the two databases.
http://www.fda.gov/Training/ForHealthProfessionals/default.htm	CDERLearn home page
	Web page for CDER-sponsored educational tutorials, some of which have CE credit available
www.fda.gov/MedWatch	MedWatch home page
	Home page for FDA's safety information and adverse event reporting program. Contains a searchable list of safety labeling changes and updated safety information. Also, it contains links to online and downloadable forms to report serious problems to FDA.
http://www.fda.gov/DrugSafetyPodcasts	Drug Safety Podcasts home page
	Podcasts broadcast in conjunction with the release of new Drug Safety Communication. Also available on iTunes under drug safety podcasts.
www.fda.gov/DrugInfoRounds	FDA Drug Info Rounds
	Series of training videos for practicing clinical and community pharmacists. Also available on YouTube.
www.fda.gov/smallbusinessdrugs	CDER's Small Business & Industry Assistance
	Interacts with regulated industry by assisting regulated domestic and international small pharmaceutical business seeking timely and accurate information relating to development and regulation of human drug products. Information about outreach activities including workshops and webinars available.
www.fda.gov/gadis	Global Alliance of Drug Information Specialists: a partnership among pharmacists for the advancement of public health
	GADIS provides a network among drug information pharmacists and the FDA to support collaborative strategies on critical trends and transformations for addressing FDA regulatory actions.

duties, and many other important issues with the added benefit of CE credit for pharmacists, physicians, and nurses, many of whom work in industry.

CDER TRADE PRESS

An additional team within DDI, the CDER Trade Press team, provides members of the trade press with accurate and timely information regarding CDER policies, programs, and initiatives. In addition to facilitating interactions between trade press and FDA subject matter experts, CDER Trade Press also alerts FDA leadership and staff to relevant FDA coverage in the trade media. Relationships with members of the trade press are fostered, and maintained by this unique team of practitioners. The CDER Trade Press team provides general and ongoing assistance to FDA's Field Office Public Affairs Specialists (PASs).

SOCIAL MEDIA OUTREACH

● DDI uses social media to reach audiences that prefer to receive the latest drug information in a variety of media formats. DDI tweets the latest drug information and may be followed on Twitter @FDA_Drug_Info. FDA Drug Info Rounds is a series of training videos for practicing clinical and community pharmacists written and casted by DDI pharmacists. These videos may be viewed on FDA's website and on YouTube. Audio podcasts are broadcast in conjunction with the release of each new DSC. If interested, a person may find and subscribe to FDA's Drug Safety Podcasts on iTunes and FDA's website RSS feed.

GLOBAL ALLIANCE OF DRUG INFORMATION SPECIALISTS (GADIS)

● DDI networks with fellow drug information specialists around the world through the GADIS. GADIS advances public health by promoting partnerships among drug information pharmacists in academia, hospitals, and federal government. GADIS establishes a community among DI specialists to support collaborative strategies, a forum for the exchange of evidence-based best practices, and an opportunity to gain insights and feedback from peers to support collaborative strategies on critical trends and transformations for addressing FDA regulatory actions. GADIS offers online webinars with speakers from within the FDA, and external experts on topics such as the implementation of REMS programs (Case Study 22-7).

Case Study 22–7—Topical Antimicrobial
Drug Products

In December 2013, the FDA issued a proposed rule requesting manufacturers to submit information and data to demonstrate the safety of long-term daily use of these products and that they are more effective than soap and water in preventing illness and the spread of infections. Some of these products could pose health risks, including bacterial resistance and hormonal effects. Manufacturers did not provide the necessary information to demonstrate safety and effectiveness for 19 active ingredients included in the tentative final monograph (TFM). For these ingredients, no data or insufficient information was submitted to the FDA. In September 2016, FDA announced a final rule to amend the

1994 TFM for over-the-counter (OTC) antiseptic drug products (59 FR 31402) as part of the ongoing review of OTC drug products. This rule established that as of September 6, 2017 the marketing of OTC consumer antiseptic wash products containing certain active ingredients, including triclosan and triclocarban, have to stop. Many consumers contacted DDI with questions and concerns regarding the discontinuation of these antiseptic wash products.

- *Since the rules stated that production had to stop by September 6, 2017, a pharmacist wanted to know if she can still stock these antibacterial products in the OTC section of the pharmacy until she runs out. Can she do this? What information can you find on FDA's website to support your answer?*
- *A pharmacist wants to know if this rule applies to antibacterial products in the hospital? Does the pharmacy need to discard of all antibacterial products in the hospital that is used by various HPs?*
- *A patient was complaining that regular hand soap and water does not work for them. What do you tell them? What alternatives can you offer the patient?*
- *An advocacy group comprised of patients who regularly used soap containing triclosan to prevent illness sent hundreds of e-mails to FDA regarding the issue. What type of response does FDA have regarding the safety and effectiveness of these medications? What authority does FDA have over the regulation of OTC products?*
- *A manufacturer of an OTC antibacterial soap product containing chloroxylenol sends a letter to FDA requesting that they be allowed to continue marketing of this product. How does the final rule apply to this specific ingredient? What can you tell them?*

Opportunities within the FDA

There are several opportunities for both current and future HPs within the FDA.

FOR THE STUDENT

⑰ *The FDA offers many opportunities for health professional students. One of the most popular programs is the FDA Pharmacy Student Experiential Program.*[30] *Student opportunities are also available within the United States Public Health Service (USPHS) Commissioned Corps.*[31] The experiential program provides an opportunity for students to gain experience working in various divisions within the FDA. Depending on where the student is placed, he or she will have the chance to learn about the FDA's multidisciplinary processes for addressing public health issues involving drugs, biologics, or medical devices. Pharmacy students who complete the FDA Pharmacy Student Experiential Program gain unique experience in regulatory affairs that proves beneficial to their future careers.

The Commissioned Corps created the Commissioned Corps Officer Student Training and Extern Program (COSTEP) for students studying in the health professions field. There are two programs, the Junior COSTEP and Senior COSTEP. Students in selected health fields can apply to the Junior COSTEP program if they have completed at least 1 to 2 years of their professional program. The Junior COSTEP program takes place during school breaks and most assignments last anywhere from 1 to 4 months. There is no obligation to commit or work for the Commissioned Corps after graduation as this opportunity is focused on allowing students to experience the program before joining. One major benefit for those students enrolled in the COSTEP programs is the diverse opportunities available after completion of the program. Some have gone on to provide clinical services in the Indian Health Service, work in labs at the National Institutes of Health, provide care to patients in the Bureau of Prisons, or join agencies within FDA or Centers for Disease Control and Prevention, just to name a few. For those students who wish to find out more information or apply, they are encouraged to visit the U.S. Public Service website at http://www.usphs.gov/student/.

FOR THE PHARMACY GRADUATE

Postgraduate opportunities for students are also available with the FDA. Many fellowship programs offer rotational opportunities within regulatory agencies, which provide individuals an internal insight into the regulatory environment. One opportunity is the Regulatory Pharmaceutical Fellowship.[32] The purpose of this fellowship is to develop candidates with advanced experience in the medical and regulatory aspects of drug information dissemination, drug safety, or drug marketing and advertising. The program exposes fellows to three areas of regulatory pharmaceutical experience: FDA, academia, and pharmaceutical industry.

Only a few of the potential opportunities for health professional students are described in this chapter. There are several opportunities for students interested in regulatory affairs beyond what is described here, and students are encouraged to research and contact those programs directly for further information.

FOR THE PROFESSIONAL

Due to new legislation, CDER has an ongoing need to recruit qualified HPs in order to carry on the mission of the FDA. HPs have several opportunities to serve either as civil service or join the U.S. Commissioned Corps. Physicians are needed to help evaluate submitted clinical trial data of new drugs for safety and efficacy. Pharmacists are needed for a variety of duties including reviewing, evaluating, and recommending approval (or non-approval) of new and generic drugs. Scientists evaluate the technical portions of applications such as INDs and NDAs. Mathematical statisticians and computer specialists are hired for statistical and technical support of human drug product reviews. Consumer safety officers are vital to managing and monitoring regulatory teams in certain divisions. The consumer safety officer is sometimes referred to as a project manager or division liaison and often these roles are filled with biologists, chemists, pharmacists, nurses, physicians, engineers, and others. The team of HPs working at the FDA is diverse and so are the opportunities to help fulfill the mission of assuring the quality, safety, and efficacy of drugs available to the American public.

Conclusion

Pharmaceutical companies and regulatory agencies provide many services to and have many opportunities for HPs. Pharmaceutical companies' scientific or medical departments are filled with highly trained HPs working in a variety of specialized fields in order to provide medical information and support for various brands marketed by the company. Efforts are currently ongoing to make the pharmaceutical industry more transparent in the way they conduct the business of drug development and product marketing. Regulatory agencies are also focusing on ways to be more transparent, and monitor and improve the communication of the benefit/risk equation to the general public. The DDI offers traditional and social media channels to those seeking regulatory drug information. Most pharmaceutical companies have detailed and structured processes for responding to clinician's questions. DDI uses effective internal and external interactions to provide timely, accurate, and useful responses to individual inquiries. An informed HP is a professional who is aware of the valuable information available from industry and FDA, can effectively communicate safety and risk information, and dedicates their career to positively impacting public health.

Self-Assessment Questions

1. Which of the following is *NOT* a department within the medical department of a company that employs HPs?
   a. Regulatory Affairs
   b. Publications
   c. Market Research

d. Medical Information

e. Outcomes Research

2. What resources can a customer service representative in the pharmaceutical industry utilize to respond to customer inquiries?

a. Standard response letter

b. Study publication

c. Competitor package insert

d. Online drug information website

e. Social media websites

3. What can studies created by the Outcomes Research department evaluate?

a. Health care utilization

b. Patient adherence and compliance

c. Efficacy of product

d. a and b

e. b and c

4. Which of the following departments may be involved in approving a standard response letter?

a. Medical Publications

b. Marketing

c. Medical Information

d. Metrics

e. Marketing

5. HPs are regulated in industry in which of the following ways?

a. Externally by Food and Drug Administration

b. Externally by Food and Drug Administration Amendments Act

c. Internally by standard operating procedures

d. Externally by the Code of Federal Regulations

e. All of the above

6. Identify which interaction between pharmaceutical industry and HPs is unacceptable according to PhRMA's *Code on Interactions with Health Care Professionals*.

a. An industry representative stops by a clinician's office to invite them to an upcoming industry-sponsored continuing medical education event.

b. An industry representative makes an appointment with a practitioner to discuss a newly approved indication for BESTDRUGEVER®.

c. An industry representative answers an on-label question asked by a health professional with the prescribing information.

d. An industry representative refers a health professional to contact their medical information department when asked about an off-label use.

e. An industry representative drops off tickets to a local sports game to a health professional's office.

7. What is the purpose of FDA mandating pharmaceutical industry collect adverse event information?

a. FDA wants to ensure pharmaceutical industry captures all postmarketing AEs.

b. FDA wants to ensure pharmaceutical industry professionals are busy at their desks.

c. FDA wants to ensure pharmaceutical industry is burdened by AE paperwork.

d. FDA wants to ensure pharmaceutical industry captures all bad doctors causing AEs.

e. FDA wants to ensure pharmaceutical industry is overloaded with phone calls.

8. Which of the following is NOT a responsibility of medical science liaisons within the pharmaceutical industry?

a. Support medical affairs by providing insight into therapeutic area

b. Engage in scientific exchange with key opinion leaders

c. Draft standard response letters and AMCP dossiers

d. Support clinical trial development and enrollment

e. Aid in the development of externally sponsored research

9. Identify which of the following is an organization associated with the pharmaceutical industry.

a. American Pharmaceutical Association

b. Drug Information Association

c. American Medical Association

d. Parenteral Drug Association

10. The role of the Division of Drug Information (DDI) at Food and Drug Administration (FDA) is best described by which of the following?

a. CDER is the last option for unanswered general inquiries regarding regulations and human drug products.

b. The division exists as a traditional drug information center responding to calls and questions from the general consumer.

c. CDER is the focal point for public inquiries regarding food and tobacco products.

d. The Division supports the FDA's mission to promote and protect public health by building effective internal and external interactions to provide timely, accurate, and useful information through both traditional and social media channels.

e. b and d only.

11. Which of the following is NOT a tool used by FDA to communicate drug safety information?
    a. Drug Safety Communication
    b. Standard response letters
    c. Medication Guide
    d. Risk Evaluation and Mitigation Strategies
    e. Product labeling

12. A pharmaceutical industry Customer Service Representative speaks to a patient regarding the proper way to take her medication. What would be the best resource for the representative to use to answer this question?
    a. Package insert
    b. Medication Guide
    c. Drug Safety Communication
    d. a and b
    e. b and c

13. An international manufacturer e-mails DDI with questions regarding the regulatory pathway for marketing an all-natural toothpaste in the United States. When DDI responds, this activity would best be categorized by which of the following?
    a. Correspondence of information by FDA
    b. Dissemination of information by FDA
    c. Development of a standard response
    d. Reactive responses by FDA
    e. Other

14. A pharmacist contacts DDI and asks if they can assist in identifying the exclusivity for a specific medication. Which website would be the best place to refer the requestor for this information?
    a. CDER home page
    b. Federal Register
    c. Electronic Orange Book
    d. National Drug Code Directory online
    e. CDER Small Business & Industry Assistance home page

15. Which of the following is NOT a student opportunity within the FDA?
    a. Junior COSTEP Program
    b. Senior COSTEP Program
    c. FDA Pharmacy Student Experiential Program
    d. FDA/CDER Academic Collaboration Program
    e. Commissioned Corps Officer Student Training and Extern Program

REFERENCES

1. Cadogan AA, Fung SM. The changing roles of medical communications professionals: evolution of the core curriculum. Drug Inf J. 2009 Nov;43(6):673-84.

2. U.S. Food and Drug Administration [Internet]. Silver Spring, MD: U.S. Department of Health and Human Services; c2011. FDA guidance for industry: responding to unsolicited requests for off-label information about prescription drugs and medical devices. Draft Guidance; [cited 2016 Aug 25]; [15 screens]. Available from: http://www.fda.gov/down loads/Drugs/GuidanceComplianceRegulatoryInformation/Guidances/UCM285145.pdf

3. Soares SC, March C. Metrics implementation in an industry-based medical information department and comparison to metrics tracked within other industry-based medical information departments. Drug Inf J. 2008 Mar;42(2):175-82.

4. Academy of Managed Care Pharmacy (AMCP) [Internet]. Alexandria, VA: Academy of Managed Care Pharmacy; c2016. The AMCP format for formulary submissions Version 4.0; 2016 April [cited 2016 Aug 26]; [about 62 screens]. Available from: http://www.amcp .org/FormatV4/

5. Marrone CM, Bass JL, Klinger CJ. Survey of medical liaison practices across the pharmaceutical industry. Drug Inf J. 2007 Jul;41(4):457-70.

6. Department of Health and Human Services (U.S.). FDA guidance for industry: industry-supported scientific and educational activities. Final rules. Fed Regist. 1997 Nov;62 (232):64093.

7. ACCME standards for commercial support: standards to ensure the independence of CME activities. Chicago, IL: Accreditation Council for Continuing Medical Education (U.S.); 2007:3.

8. Electronic records; electronic signatures, 21 C.F.R. Sect. 11 (2009).

9. Gough J, Hamrell M. Standard operating procedures (SOPs): how companies can determine which documents they must put in place. Drug Inf J. 2010 Jan;44(1):49-54.

10. PhRMA: Progress. Research. Hope [Internet]. Washington, DC: Pharmaceutical Researchers and Manufacturers of America; c2008. Code on interactions with healthcare professionals; 2009 Jan [cited 2016 Aug 26]; [about 36 screens]. Available from: http:// www.phrma.org/sites/default/files/pdf/phrma_marketing_code_2008.pdf

11. Bryant PJ, Steinberg MJ, Marrone CM. A practical approach to evidence-based medicine for the medical communications professional. Drug Inf J. 2009 Nov;43(6):663-72.

12. Gazo A, Wyble C, Schiappacasse H, Petses J, Toscano M, El-Toukhy N, Fierro L. Mega mergers: a systematic approach to the integration of two medical information departments. Drug Inf J. 2008 Mar;42(2):183-91.

13. Donald T, Marsh C, Ashworth L. An assessment of preparation methods and personnel requirements in a medical information department during product launch. Drug Inf J. 2007 Mar;41(2):241-49.

14. Black P, March C, Ashworth L. Assessment of customer satisfaction with verbal responses provided by a pharmaceutical company's third-party medical information call center. Drug Inf J. 2009 May;43(3):263-71.

15. Fett R, Bruns K, Lischka-Wittmann S. Results of a qualitative market research study evaluating the quality of medical letters. Drug Inf J. 2009 Nov;43(6):697-703.

16. U.S. Food and Drug Administration [Internet]. Silver Spring, MD: U.S. Department of Health and Human Services; c2010. FDA guidance for industry: format and content of proposed risk evaluation and mitigation strategies (REMS): REMS assessments, and proposed REMS modifications. Draft Guidance; [cited 2016 Aug 23]; [39 screens]. Available from: http://www.fda.gov/downloads/Drugs/GuidanceComplianceRegulatoryInformation/Guidances/UCM184128.pdf

17. U.S. Food and Drug Administration [Internet]. Silver Spring, MD: U.S. Department of Health and Human Services; c2010. MedWatch Form FDA 3500A; [cited 2016 Aug 24]; [2 screens]. Available from: http://www.fda.gov/downloads/AboutFDA/Reports ManualsForms/Forms/UCM048334.pdf

18. U.S. Department of Health and Human Services [Internet]. Washington, DC: U.S. Department of Health and Human Services; c2015. About HHS; [cited 2016 Aug 26]; [about 1 screen]. Available from: http://www.hhs.gov/about/

19. U.S. Department of Health and Human Services [Internet]. Washington, DC: U.S. Department of Health and Human Services; c2015. About HHS; [cited 2016 Aug 26]; [about 1 screen]. Available from: http://www.hhs.gov/about/index.html

20. U.S. Food and Drug Administration [Internet]. Silver Spring, MD: U.S. Department of Health and Human Services; c2015. What we do; 2015 Dec 7 [cited 2016 Aug 23]; [about 1 screen]. Available from: http://www.fda.gov/AboutFDA/WhatWeDo/default.htm

21. U.S. Food and Drug Administration [Internet]. Silver Spring, MD: U.S. Department of Health and Human Services; c2011. A conversation about the FDA and drug regulation with Janet Woodcock, M.D., Deputy FDA Commissioner for Operations; [cited 2016 Aug 23]; [3 screens]. Available from: http://www.fda.gov/Drugs/ResourcesForYou/Consumers/ucm143467.htm

22. U.S. Food and Drug Administration [Internet]. Silver Spring, MD: U.S. Department of Health and Human Services; c2012. FDA guidance: drug safety information—FDA's communication to the public; [cited 2016 Aug 23]; [17 screens]. Available from: http://www.fda.gov/downloads/Drugs/GuidanceComplianceRegulatoryInformation/Guidances/UCM295217.pdf

23. U.S. Food and Drug Administration [Internet]. Silver Spring, MD: U.S. Department of Health and Human Services; c2016. FDA basics: how does FDA monitor safety after drugs are approved and marketed?; [cited 2016 Aug 23]; [1 screen]. Available from: http://www.fda.gov/AboutFDA/Transparency/Basics/ucm305058.htm

24. U.S. Food and Drug Administration [Internet]. Silver Spring, MD: U.S. Department of Health and Human Services; c2010. FDA guidance for industry: development and use of risk minimization action plans; [cited 2016 Aug 24]; [27 screens]. Available from: http://www.fda.gov/downloads/RegulatoryInformation/Guidances/UCM126830.pdf

25. Federal Register [Internet]. Silver Spring, MD: U.S. Department of Health and Human Services; c2008. [Docket no. FDA-2008-N-0174] Identification of drug biological products deemed to have risk evaluation and mitigation strategies for purposes of the Food and Drug Administration Amendments Act of 2007; [cited 2016 Sept 1]; [2 screens]. Available from: http://www.fda.gov/OHRMS/DOCKETS/98fr/E8-6201.pdf

26. U.S. Food and Drug Administration [Internet]. Silver Spring, MD: U.S. Department of Health and Human Services; c2016. Medication guides; [cited 2016 Aug 25]; [1 screen]. Available from: http://www.fda.gov/Drugs/DrugSafety/UCM085729

27. U.S. Food and Drug Administration [Internet]. Silver Spring, MD: U.S. Department of Health and Human Services; c2011. FDA guidance for industry: medication guides—distribution requirements and inclusion in risk evaluation and mitigation strategies (REMS); [cited 2016 Sept 1]; [12 screens]. Available from: http://www.fda.gov/down loads/Drugs/GuidanceComplianceRegulatoryInformation/Guidances/ucm244570.pdf

28. U.S. Food and Drug Administration [Internet]. Silver Spring, MD: U.S. Department of Health and Human Services; c2012. FDA guidance: drug safety information—FDA's communication to the public; [cited 2016 Aug 26]; [17 screens]. Available from: http://www .fda.gov/downloads/Drugs/GuidanceComplianceRegulatoryInformation/Guidances/ UCM295217.pdf

29. U.S. Food and Drug Administration [Internet]. Silver Spring, MD: U.S. Department of Health and Human Services; c2016. Division of Drug Information; 2016 Feb 16 [cited 2016 Aug 28]; [about 3 screens]. Available from: http://www.fda.gov/AboutFDA/ CentersOffices/OfficeofMedicalProductsandTobacco/CDER/ucm082585

30. U.S. Food and Drug Administration [Internet]. Silver Spring, MD: U.S. Department of Health and Human Services; c2010. FDA Pharmacy Student Experiential Program; 2016 Sept 19 [cited 2010 May 3]; [about 3 screens]. Available from: http://www.fda .gov/AboutFDA/WorkingatFDA/FellowshipInternshipGraduateFacultyPrograms/ PharmacyStudentExperientialProgramCDER/default.htm

31. U.S. Public Health Service Commissioned Corps [Internet]. Rockville, MD: U.S. Department of Health and Human Services; c2010. Student opportunities; 2014 Feb 3 [cited 2016 Aug 28]; [about 4 screens]. Available from: http://www.usphs.gov/student/

32. U.S. Food and Drug Administration [Internet]. Silver Spring, MD: U.S. Department of Health and Human Services; c2016. Regulatory Pharmaceutical Fellowship; 2016 Feb 11 [cited 2016 Aug 28]; [about 2 screens]. Available from: http://www.fda.gov/AboutFDA/ CentersOffices/OfficeofMedicalProductsandTobacco/CDER/ucm162733.htm

SUGGESTED READINGS

1. Drug Safety Communications. Available from: http://www.fda.gov/Drugs/DrugSafety/ ucm199082.htm

2. Guidance "Drug Safety Information—FDA's Communication to the Public". Available from: http://www.fda.gov/downloads/Drugs/GuidanceComplianceRegulatoryInformation/ Guidances/UCM295217.pdf

3. Guidance for Industry "Expanded Access to Investigational Drugs for Treatment Use— Questions and Answers". Available from: http://www.fda.gov/downloads/Drugs/ GuidanceComplianceRegulatoryInformation/Guidances/UCM351261.pdf

23

Chapter Twenty-Three

Assessing Drug Promotions

Robert D. Beckett • Genevieve Lynn Ness

Learning Objectives

After completing this chapter, the reader will be able to

- Define drug promotions.
- List recommendations by the World Health Organization (WHO) for appropriate drug promotions.
- Describe the role of the U.S. Food and Drug Administration (FDA) Office of Prescription Drug Promotion (OPDP).
- Determine whether a piece of direct-to-consumer advertising (DTCA) has been cited in FDA warning letters to companies.
- Describe the allowed content for a specific type of DTCA.
- Evaluate a given piece of DTCA based on FDA and Pharmaceutical Research and Manufacturers of America (PhRMA) guidelines.
- Report a drug promotion concern using the Bad Ad program.
- Evaluate the appropriateness of a piece of drug promotion designed for a health care professional.
- List systematic and individual strategies that may be used to combat proliferation of misinformation in drug promotions.
- Identify logical fallacies used in drug promotion, when given an interaction with a pharmaceutical industry representative.
- Describe the goals and design of academic detailing programs.
- Describe the clinical, economic, and humanistic effects of academic detailing.

Key Concepts

❶ Drug promotion is defined by the World Health Organization (WHO) as material or information provided by drug manufacturers with the ultimate goal of increasing prescribing or purchasing of medications.

❷ The FDA currently recognizes and outlines appropriate content for three types of direct to consumer advertising (DTCA): help-seeking ads, reminder ads, and product claim ads.

❸ The following information should be considered when validating appropriateness of DTCA: (1) balance of risk and benefit information and inclusion of a brief summary of the risks listed in the labeling, (2) a statement encouraging patients to seek information from their physician, and (3) references to other sources to find the full prescribing information.

❹ Drug promotion to health care professionals makes up the majority of drug promotions activity in terms of financial expenditure on the part of pharmaceutical industry; this information can be effective in eliciting changes in prescribing behavior.

❺ All health care professionals, including pharmacists, should arm themselves using strategies of information mastery and vigilance for potentially flawed reasoning when interacting with pharmaceutical sales representatives.

❻ Health care professionals are encouraged to report drug promotion violations to the FDA's Bad Ad program.

❼ Academic detailing programs, often led by pharmacists, are designed to combat pharmaceutical industry detailing by providing evidence-based information in the form of one-on-one or small-group interactions between a clinician and prescribers.

Introduction

❶ *Drug promotion is defined by the World Health Organization (WHO) as material or information provided by drug manufacturers with the ultimate goal of increasing prescribing or purchasing of medications.* Each year, the pharmaceutical industry spends billions of dollars advertising their medications to the public and to health care professionals.[1-11] In 2014, Johnson and Johnson, Novartis, and Pfizer spent $17.5, $14.6, and $11.4 billion on marketing their products, respectively.[12] The channels that companies use for advertising include medical journals, newspapers, radio, television, magazines, websites, social media, search engine marketing, distributed promotional materials, billboards, direct mailings, medication samples, and sales representatives.[2,7,9,13-15] In addition, a report assessing drug advertising submissions to the FDA by pharmaceutical companies from 2001 to 2014 found that there were three times more non-Internet advertisements targeting health care professionals than consumers.[16]

Health care professionals and consumers may not recognize the impact that drug promotion can have on individual behavior.[7] The literature has reported increased prescribing patterns, rapid implementation of new medications, and an increase in inappropriate prescribing among physicians who utilize promotional materials to obtain drug information.[7] The effect of medication promotion on overall public health remains uncertain. The WHO suggests clinical trials be conducted to assess the correlation of drug promotion with inappropriate prescribing and the occurrence of adverse events, to identify the public health outcomes of drug promotion.[7] For these reasons, health care professionals must be prepared to critically interpret and evaluate verbal and written drug promotions. In particular, pharmacists play an important role as an interpreter of drug advertisements to their patients. The following section describes the full scope of drug promotion according to the WHO.

Ethical Criteria for Medicinal Drug Promotion

In 1988, the WHO published criteria for the ethical promotion of medications.[17] The guidelines state the promotion of drugs should comply with the national standards established by the country where the drugs are being promoted. These guidelines apply to both domestic and exported drug products. Overall, information presented for the purposes of promotion should be balanced, accurate, and current. Advertisements targeted specifically to health care professionals should follow the approved product labeling and all writing should be clear and readable.[17]

HEALTH CARE PROFESSIONALS

A scientific summary is required when product claims are made within an advertisement directed at health care professionals. These advertisements should include generic name, brand name, amount of active ingredient per dosage form, other ingredients that can lead to allergies or adverse effects, indications, dosage form, adverse reactions, warnings and precautions, contraindications, drug interactions, additional notable interactions, manufacturer/distributor name and address, and scientific literature references. Detailed information about the scientific properties of a medication should be made available to health care professionals as appropriate.

CONSUMERS

The WHO criteria also provides information about direct-to-consumer advertising (DTCA).[17] According to WHO, DTCA should assist consumers in making decisions about nonprescription medications; however, the use of DTCA for prescription medications is not recommended. Scientific evidence must support all factual information provided. DTCA should not use fearful language or tactics, but use only information available in the approved labeling, including the following: generic name, brand name, indications, major warnings and precautions, contraindications, and the manufacturer/distributor name and address.

PHARMACEUTICAL REPRESENTATIVES

The WHO also outlines guidelines for pharmaceutical representatives.[17] These personnel should be properly trained and retain adequate technical and medical knowledge. The information presented should only discuss the material from the approved labeling. The pharmaceutical industry is responsible for the statements made by their sales representatives and the salary of those representatives should not be influenced by the number of prescriptions written for the product they are promoting. The WHO recognizes that free samples of prescription medications can be given to prescribers in small quantities upon request.

The WHO guidelines outline the proper features of drug promotion that are required to produce beneficial and accurate materials. These criteria provide the basis of drug promotion regulations and evaluative strategies that will be discussed in more detail later in this chapter.

Direct-to-Consumer Advertising (DTCA)

DEFINITION OF DTCA

The U.S. FDA defines DTCA as any advertisement created by a pharmaceutical company to promote products to a general audience.[15] The goal of such advertising is to encourage patients to discuss a medication with their prescriber, ultimately leading to a prescription.[11]

DTCA has increased steadily over the last few years. In a report of FDA drug advertising submissions, advertisements directed toward consumers increased from 6,870 in 2001 to 15,993 in 2009.[16] However, this number did decrease in 2014 to 15,186.[16]

There are many methods that pharmaceutical companies use to present DTCA to patients. The three most well-known are (1) print, through magazines or newspapers, (2) broadcast through television, and (3) electronic, in online banners, videos, search engine ads, and websites.[18] The Pharmaceutical Research and Manufacturers of America (PhRMA) defines direct-to-consumer print advertisements as "space that is bought by a company in newspaper or magazine publications targeted to patients or consumers, or a direct mail communication paid for and disseminated by a company to patients or consumers, for the purpose of presenting information about one or more of the company's medicines."[19] The PhRMA also defines direct-to-consumer television advertisements as, "portion of television air time on broadcast or cable television that is bought by a company for the purpose of presenting information about one or more of the company's medicines."[19] The most common form of DTCA submitted to the FDA in 2014 was Internet materials (12,136 submissions).[16] The increase in the use of the Internet for DTCA may be due to the fact that this type of advertising can focus on specific patient populations, exposes a larger number of consumers to medications, and is more cost effective than television or print advertisements.[18] Pharmaceutical companies have also increased their presence on social media. In a study assessing 15 pharmaceutical companies, 14 had links to social media sites on their websites with Twitter being the most common (93%, 14/15).[20] Facebook followed behind with 66% of the companies linking to this social media site.[20]

EFFECTS OF DTCA ON PRESCRIPTIONS

DTCA has been known to increase prescription drug profit for the pharmaceutical industry.[21] Specifically, for each dollar spent on DTCA, the company makes about $4.20 in sales.[11,21] A study assessing the promotion of aromatase inhibitors found that, for every million dollars spent on DTCA, new prescriptions for the products increased by 0.15% after 3 months.[22] One study, assessing data from 1992 to 1997, found that 32 extra diagnoses and 41 additional prescriptions for *statin* medications were prescribed for every $1,000 spent on DTCA.[6] In 2002, the U.S. General Accounting Office (GAO) projected that 8 million Americans requested and received prescriptions due to DTCA each year.[6] A study in 2009 found that there were an additional 1 million physician visits and 397,025 additional irritable bowel syndrome (IBS) diagnoses after the promotion of tegaserod (Zelnorm®).[21] In addition, 1,796 prescriptions were written for every 1 million dollars spent on tegaserod DTCA (95% confidence interval [CI] 1,041 to 2,529).[6,21] A study assessing the DTCA of Advair®, Singulair®, Symbicort®, and Asmanex® found that the average rate of doses dispensed per 100,000 patients increased from 392,000 in 2005 to 483,000 in 2009 per designated marketed area.[23] Additionally, for every additional advertisement to which the household was exposed, a 2% higher rate of prescriptions was dispensed after adjusting for designated-marketed-area characteristics.[23]

COSTS OF DTCA

Based on these reports, it is not surprising that, between 1996 and 2005, spending on DTCA increased from $985 million to about $4 billion.[2-4] DTCA spending peaked at $5.4 billion in 2006; however, spending had decreased to $4.8 billion, $4.3 billion, and $3.83 billion in 2007, 2010, and 2013, respectively.[2,8-10,24] These spending decreases could be due to loss of patent on highly advertised medications, fewer products being brought to the market, an increase in consumer doubt, and budget cuts due to the recession.[2] Since then, DTCA has made a comeback with an increase in spending to $4.53 billion in 2014.[24] From January 2007 to March 2011, the highest DTCA marketed products were atorvastatin (Lipitor®, $917.70 million), duloxetine (Cymbalta®, $820.50 million), and fluticasone/ salmeterol (Advair®, $766.3 million).[6] Recently, it was reported that Pfizer spent the most on prescription drug advertisements compared with other pharmaceutical companies in 2014 ($1.4 billion).[24] Specifically, Pfizer spent $221 million on Eliquis®, $232 million on Viagra®, and $246 million on Lyrica®.[24]

Today, most of the DTCA spending is allotted for television advertisements which results in the average American watching about 16 hours of televised drug advertisements per year.[6,9,25] However, one study reported that the average household exposure to televised DTCA peaked in 2007 with 195.3 ads monthly and had since steadily decreased to 111.1 monthly in 2011.[26] Interestingly, smoking cessation products, impotence medications, and antidepressant television ads have the highest changing-channel rates among viewing audiences.[2] The ads that retain most of the television audience through commercials include overactive bladder treatments and osteoporosis medications.[2]

TYPES OF DTCA

❷ *The FDA currently recognizes and outlines appropriate content for three types of DTCA: help-seeking advertisements, reminder advertisements, and product claim advertisements.* The following describes each of these types of advertisements in detail, including evaluative criteria.[15]

- **Help-seeking advertisements** do not recommend a particular medication but provide information about a disease state or condition.[6,9,15,21,27] The advertisement can describe particular symptoms, point patients to discuss their symptoms with their physician, and offer a phone number for more information about the disease state.[27,28] These advertisements are regulated by the Federal Trade Commission (FTC) since a specific drug product is not mentioned.[27,28] In a study assessing pharmaceutical companies' use of social media for DTCA, help-seeking ads were found to be the most common form of DTCA (40%, 301/740).[20] These were found mostly on YouTube and Twitter as opposed to Facebook.

- **Reminder advertisements** do not describe the indication of a medication but do present the brand name.[6,9,15,21,29] These particular advertisements are created with the assumption that patients are already familiar with the drug's indication.[27] Risk information is not included in these advertisements and therefore, reminder advertisements of drugs with boxed warnings are illegal.[6,9,27,30] Any information or even implied information (through images or text) about a product's benefits or risks are not permitted in reminder advertisements.[27] For example, a medication for osteoporosis would not have an image of bones in the reminder advertisement as this implies the product's indication.[27]

- **Product claim advertisements** require more detail and should contain the drug name, the indication, as well as a balance between the risks and benefits associated with the product.[6,9,15,21,27,29] Specifically, printed product claim advertisements should include a brief summary that provides details about all of the risk information listed in the FDA-approved labeling.[9,27] Printed advertisements must also include a reference to the FDA MedWatch program (http://www.fda.gov/Safety/MedWatch/) for patients to report side effects to the medication.[27] Product claim advertisements that are broadcasted either by television, radio, or phone are not required to include the brief summary of risk information.[2,15,27] Instead, television advertisements are required to contain a **major statement** of the main risks associated with the product, which can be presented verbally.[8,9,27,29,31] In addition, when broadcast advertisements do not include all risk information listed in the labeling, the advertisement is expected to provide resources that patients can consult to obtain the full prescribing information.[27] For example, the advertisement can refer a patient to consult with their health care professional, call a toll-free number, visit the product website, or refer to a printed advertisement that contains information that is more detailed.[15,27,31] This is known as the adequate provision requirement.[3,9,27] Information DTCAs are not required to include is listed in Table 23-1.[32]

TABLE 23–1. INFORMATION NOT REQUIRED FOR INCLUSION IN DTCA[32]

Cost information
Generic availability
Availability of similar drugs that have the same indication with less adverse effects
Whether lifestyle changes could help the condition (this is only required if it is listed in the prescribing information for the product)
Incidence of the disease that the medication treats
Mechanism of action:
Onset of action (if the product states that it works quickly it must define the meaning of quickly)
How many people have experienced benefit from the drug

Tone and themes of DTCA can vary.[29,31] Many advertisements portray patients after successfully taking the product (i.e., healthy patients); similarly, advertisements tend to portray the product as a facilitator of healthy or recreational activities.[29] Most advertisements rely on emotional, rather than logical appeals; these emotional appeals could be positive, negative, or both. One study performed content analysis to describe major themes present in advertisements and found that promotion, prevention, individualism, collectivism, cheerfulness, quiescence, dejection, agitation, fear, and affection were all prevalent.[31]

DTCA LEGISLATION

Currently, among developed countries, DTCA is only permitted in the United States and New Zealand.[6,9,15,21,29] DTCA is currently banned in Canada; however, in the mid-1990s and early 2000s, Health Canada permitted the dissemination of unbranded "help-seeking" advertisements and branded prescription "reminder advisements" to consumers.[33] New Zealand relies on self-regulation of DTCA by the pharmaceutical companies; however, in the United States, the FDA is responsible for overseeing DTCA.[6]

● FDA's Oversight on DTCA

The FDA's authority over prescription drug advertising targeted to health care professionals was established in 1962 by the Kefauver-Harris Amendment.[3,9,34] Shortly after, in 1969, the FDA released regulations requiring drug advertisements to (1) be accurate and not misleading, (2) contain a brief summary of indications, adverse effects, warnings, and contraindications, (3) be **fair balanced**, and (4) include only factual information about the product's advertised uses.[7,9,31,35,36] At this time, television advertisements were also required to contain the brief summary, which made these ads too lengthy for broadcast.[2]

The FDA first allowed companies to promote their products directly to consumers in 1985.[3,9,10] In 1997, the FDA released a draft guidance stating that television advertisements no longer required the brief summary; however, the guidance did require a **major statement** of the main safety risks and referral to a source for detailed information about the product.[1,2,8,9,15,31] This guidance was finalized in 1999.[3,9] In addition, printed product claim advertisements were required to include the entire prescribing information prior to the release of 2004 regulations stating that only a simplified brief summary is required.[9] However, patient mailings, brochures, and other drug company materials that promote a drug product are still required to include the full FDA-approved prescribing information if any such materials mention the benefits of the medication.[27] In 2007, the Food and Drug Administration Amendments Act (FDAAA) required the MedWatch reporting statement to be added to all printed advertisements, which states: "You are encouraged to report negative side effects of prescription drugs to the FDA. Visit MedWatch, or call

1-800-FDA-1088."[27,37] Today, prescription drug advertising regulations can be found in title 21, volume 4, part 202 of the Code of Federal Regulations (CFR).[36]

Enforcement of the DTCA Legislation

To ensure that DTCAs are following FDA guidelines and to protect consumers from false information, the FDA maintains a surveillance and enforcement program through their Office of Prescription Drug Promotion (OPDP) division.[15] It is important to remember that FDA has the authority only over DTCA for prescription medications.[32] DTCA for nonprescription medications and help-seeking ads are regulated by the FTC.[27,28,32] In addition, the FDA does not require pharmaceutical companies to submit DTCA prior to its distribution or being aired.[32] However, the FDA does require advertisements to be submitted for review as soon as they are released to the public.[6,11,32]

If the FDA discovers that a DTCA is not in compliance with the set of laws in place, warning letters can be issued to the pharmaceutical company, requesting the removal of the advertisement and to address the material that violates the law.[11,32] These letters are publically available on the FDA's Warning Letters website.[32,38] If the advertisement has created a severe threat on public health, the FDA can also request the company to correct the advertisement and publish or broadcast the corrected version.[32] In rare cases, the FDA may bring criminal charges against the company in court and seize the company's drug supply.[32] The FDA does not have authority to levy fines on pharmaceutical companies for DTCA violations.[11]

There has been a decrease in the number of DTCA regulatory actions by the FDA.[9] Critics say that this could be the result of decreased FDA supervision or, in contrast, could be due to better compliance with DTCA laws.[9] Another added factor is that all warning letters must be reviewed and approved by the FDA's Office of Chief Counsel, which was mandated by the Secretary of Health and Human Services (HHS) in 2002.[9] This action alone may have resulted in a decline in the number of promotional-related warning letters issued between 2001 and 2002, which were 68 and 28, respectively.[9] In addition, the FDA has limited staff to review DTCA.[9] Fewer than six FDA employees were assigned to review greater than 15,000 brochures and DTCA in 2006.[9] Since then, the OPDP staff has increased to accommodate the growing number of advertisements to review.

Monitoring Online Promotion

There is still a need for FDA guidelines in regards to online promotion of prescription medications.[9] After warning letters issued from the FDA in 2009 stating that online search engine results need to include risk information since both the drug name and indication are mentioned, the pharmaceutical companies now only include either the name of the drug or the indication in search engine links.[9] A study assessing 73 FDA notices of violations and warning letters for online DTCA from 2004 to 2014 found that 47.9% were in reference to advertisements on drug websites, 24.7% for links on search engines and banner ads, 21.9% for videos, 2.7% for e-mails, and 2.7% for social media widgets.[18] The main violation reported in the warning letters for these online DTCA was omission or minimization of risk (32.4%).[18] Strategies that pharmaceutical companies have used to promote their products on social media include "one clicks," which provide risk information "one click away," and human interest stories with branded medication information excluded, which do not fall under FDA DTCA regulation.[39]

Since studies have reported a lack of consumer awareness of the FDA role in DTCA oversight, it is vital for health care professionals to monitor and evaluate DTCA.[6,9]

PhRMA'S GUIDING PRINCIPLES FOR DTCA

With the increasing role of DTCA in health care, the PhRMA established guiding principles for DTCA of prescription medications.[19] These principles are voluntary, but do serve as guidance for pharmaceutical companies to create accurate, educational, and encouraging DTCAs that follow FDA regulations.[19] See Table 23-2 for an overview of the PhRMA principles. A commitment to follow the PhRMA guiding principles and completion of an annual certification entitles the company to be identifiable as a signatory company and be recognized by PhRMA online.[19]

SUPPORT FOR DTCA

Supporters of DTCA believe these advertisements serve a public health need.[6,15,19] Through DTCA, patients become educated about different disease states, which can assist them in making better treatment decisions and create more knowledgeable patients in the health care environment.[1,6,9,10,19,35,40] A related point is that DTCA can help improve the quality of patient-professional interactions and help patients identify meaningful questions to ask of their health care providers, as well as improve adherence to prescribed treatment.[6,9,15,19] DTCA provides patients with information about treatment options available early on, which can result in lower health care costs.[9] Similarly, DTCA may also increase appropriate care for underdiagnosed diseases.[1,6,9,15,19] It has been asserted that health care costs can be saved if medication therapy is started sooner because of DTCA for a disease that could eventually lead to surgery if not treated.[9] However, there is limited data to support this claim.[9] Supporters mention that DTCA can lower drug prices due to increased competition between products.[9] DTCA also has been credited with reducing the stigma of certain diseases making them acceptable for discussion (e.g., psychiatric disorders).[6,9,10,15,41] In addition, a 2015 study credited depression-related DTCA for assisting patients in remembering to take their depression medication, which can result in an increase in medication adherence.[42]

TABLE 23–2.   PhRMA GUIDING PRINCIPLES FOR DTCA[19]

1. DTCAs should follow all FDA standards including the absence of off-label promotion.
2. The company should obtain insight from patients and health care professionals to identify what educational information should be included in DTCA.
3. Prescription medications should be clearly identified as such in the DTCAs.
4. The ad should encourage patients to discuss the risks and benefits of the advertised medication with their prescriber.
5. Health care professionals should be educated about new prescription medications prior to the release of DTCA in order to be able to accurately respond to patient questions.
6. Once unknown safety risks about an advertised product are discovered, companies should edit or remove DTCA while continuing collaboration with the FDA.
7. All new DTCAs should be submitted to the FDA prior to public release. DTCAs that have been significantly changed including additional indications, new patient populations, additional safety information, or new outcome claims should also be submitted to the FDA. If companies would like to obtain FDA comments, they should submit a feedback request with the DTCA. Timelines for review are 30 days for priority review and greater than 30 days for non-priority.
8. All printed DTCA should contain the FDA's MedWatch number or website to report adverse events. Television DTCA should point patients to print advertisements with the FDA's MedWatch information and/or present the organization's toll-free number.
9. The ad should clearly identify the use of actors as health care professionals and disclose any financial compensation if actual health care professionals are utilized.
10. If a celebrity advocate is used in the DTCA, the claims made by the celebrity should reflect their factual views and experiences while taking the medication.
11. When applicable, the DTCA should also highlight alternatives to treat the condition being advertised such as diet and lifestyle changes.
12. Television DTCA that discuss a particular product should present the major risks and the approved indications.
13. Medication benefit and risk information should be balanced including information about boxed warnings (presented in plain language). Television DTCA should point patients to where they can obtain additional information about product risks and benefits.
14. The disease state should be presented seriously and reverently throughout the DTCA.
15. DTCA that may be inappropriate for children should not be aired or published in mediums where children could witness the advertisement.
16. Information about the disease and health awareness should be presented in DTCA.
17. Patient assistance programs for the uninsured and underinsured population should be mentioned in DTCA when applicable.

OPPOSITION TO DTCA

In contrast, many who oppose DTCA express its potential threat to public health.[15] DTCAs could contain inaccurate or misleading information in addition to inadequate information about adverse effects and risks.[1,15]

Imbalance Between Benefits and Risks

Sixty-five percent of physicians reported that patients tend to underestimate the risks and overemphasize the benefits of a drug, mostly after viewing a television advertisement.[11] A study analyzing television drug advertisements found that patients remembered the benefits of a drug more easily than the risks.[11] This may be due to the dominance of visual messages over audio when presented jointly and the fact that much of the safety information is presented verbally in television advertisements.[9] Patients may also overemphasize a product's benefits because DTCA is known to exaggerate the happiness achieved with a medication.[9] A study assessing social media advertising found that drug product claim posts mentioned only benefits (44.8%, 216/482) more often than both risks and benefits (28%, 135/482) and risks alone (27.2%, 131/482).[20]

Opponents of DTCA state that FDA regulations are too lenient because the pharmaceutical companies are only held responsible for the information presented in DTCA if there is a violation.[9] As a result, some advertisements include inappropriate information. For example, in 1996, only 65% of DTCA in newspaper and magazines were reported to be fair balanced.[7] Unfortunately, consumers will remember the information presented in an ad even if there are violations.[9] The PhRMA has released DTCA guidelines that suggest companies should submit DTCA to the FDA for review prior to distribution; however, these guidelines are optional and unenforceable.[9]

The content of DTCA is usually not written in lay person language (i.e., an eighth grade reading level) making it challenging for consumers to understand the content.[9] Along these lines the use of words, such as usually, mild, and may, to describe safety information may lead to consumer confusion about the exact meaning of these terms.[9]

Statistical Inaccuracy

There have also been multiple reports of statistical exaggeration of product benefits in advertisements.[43] Particularly, in DTCA, one study reported that only 2 of 67 advertisements found in U.S. magazines presented results of the clinical trials assessing the promoted drug versus placebo as absolute rates of clinical outcomes, which is considered the appropriate way to represent data. Other advertisements only presented data in the form of relative risk reduction (RRR); absolute risk reduction (ARR) was not included (see Chapter 4 for further information about RRR and ARR). Some provided references to clinical studies but did not provide any data from the studies in the advertisements. One additional advertisement claimed that the promoted drug provided a clinical cure compared with competitors but did not explain exactly what was defined as a clinical cure. In a study assessing 16 advertisements, only 1 ad provided frequency of adverse effect, using quantitative methods, 2 presented using comparative language, and the majority used a qualitative approach.[43] Prevalence of the disease state that the product is treating is also rarely reported in advertisements. In a study from 2004, only 3 of 31 advertisements provided information on disease prevalence.[43]

Potential for Inappropriate Prescribing

Due to DTCA, there has been an increase in patients requesting advertised medications during their provider visits.[7] This can lead to the undermining of health care professional authority and hinder the provider-patient relationships.[3,6,9,10] This has been reported in the literature by 30% of patients and 39% of physicians who participated in a national survey.[9] In particular, if a physician refuses to prescribe a medication that the patient is requesting, the patient is more likely to switch physicians.[9] This pressure on prescribers from patients can increase the risk of inappropriate prescribing.[3,4,6,9,10,15] An FDA study reported about 50% of physicians felt some pressure to prescribe a particular medication after a patient reported seeing a DTCA for the product.[11,35] One study found that during physician visits, 40% of patients requested a medication that they saw on a DTCA and about 50% of the requests were granted by the prescriber.[9] However, a study conducted in 2006 reported that, of the patients who requested a medication due to a DTCA, only about 2% to 7% received a prescription for the product in the end.[9] It has been reported that patients may try to fit the type of patient that is presented in the DTCA, which can also lead to inappropriate prescribing, diagnosis, and ultimately unnecessary side effects.[6,9] A study found that about half of physicians, participating in a focus-group discussion, presumed that patients diagnosed themselves accurately based on DTCA.[6] This increase in unnecessary prescribing can lead to an increase in prescription drug spending.[8]

The added time for providers and patients to discuss DTCA during scheduled appointments could take away from other important aspects of the appointment and lead to negative patient outcomes.[10] DTCA can lead to unnecessary physician visits and make patients believe that they have a particular disease.[1,8,9] For example, critics blame DTCA for converting menopause from a normal life process into an insufficient hormone disease.[9]

Increased Health Care Costs

In addition, use of DTCA to advertise me-too drugs can increase health care costs since many patients will request the brand name drug when there may be inexpensive generic options available.[4,9,15] A study found that patients were more likely to switch from lansoprazole to omeprazole in areas that were more exposed to DTCA since omeprazole was advertised via DTCA and lansoprazole was not.[6] The expense of DTCA may also drive up the consumer costs for the product as pharmaceutical companies increase prices to compensate for advertising costs.[5] For example, one study found that the cost of clopidogrel increased by $0.40 (12%) per unit after the launch of the DTCA campaign.[5,6] In a study assessing television DTCA, the high-cost medications had longer air time for the ads (60 seconds) compared with medium-cost medications (47.9 seconds).[1] Due to concerns regarding the increasing cost of medications, the American Medical Association (AMA) called for a ban on DTCA in November 2015.[44] The AMA criticized these ads for causing the increased demand for novel and expensive treatment options when generic alternatives were available.[44]

Insufficient Safety Data with DTCA

Critics mention that the safety information required in the DTCA could cause patients to have concerns about the safety of a medication and may lead to issues with patient compliance.[9] However, most of the time, DTCA is released to the public before the majority of the safety information is collected (i.e., postmarketing surveillance).[9] For example, rofecoxib (Vioxx®), which was one of the most promoted medications in the United States ($100 million/year spent on promotion), was not discovered to cause myocardial infarction (80,000 to 140,000 cases) or stroke until after the DTCA campaign.[6,9] This additional safety information led to its voluntary recall in 2004.[6,9] Another example of a highly marketed product whose side effects were not fully discovered until after DTCA was tegaserod (Zelnorm®), which was later withdrawn from the market due to increased risk of cardiovascular-related adverse effects.[21,45]

For the many reasons described above, information included in DTCA, in addition to advertisements intended for health care professionals, should be closely scrutinized for errors, promotional violations, and other misleading information.

SUGGESTIONS FOR IMPROVEMENT

Suggestions for the improvement of DTCA have been reported in the literature. One suggestion would eliminate the need for DTCA altogether; a group of representatives from industry, government, and academia would be tasked to create public service announcements discussing appropriate treatment for conditions that are known to cause morbidity or mortality, have effective and safe treatments available, and are identified as being undertreated and underdiagnosed.[8,9] This solution has not been implemented at this time. The U.S. Institute of Medicine (IOM) proposed enforcing a 2-year delay from the time a drug product is released to launching DTCA.[6,9] This can ensure that adequate time has passed for postmarketing data to be collected and allow physicians to become educated about the product.[9] However, in 2011, the U.S. Congressional Budget Office stated that the benefits of providing information about new medications outweighed the risks and, therefore, the proposal was not supported.[6] To have the FDA review all DTCA before being released to the public is another recommendation.[9] However, this would only be achievable assuming additional user fees were paid to the FDA by pharmaceutical industry. There was a proposal for such a program in 2008, but it was not funded by

Congress and, therefore, could not be enforced by the FDA. Another suggestion involves the use of a television control device which would give the patient or consumer the option to watch TV with or without DTCA.[46]

There have also been debates about the most appropriate DTCA format.[47] A study assessing consumer preferences found that more patients preferred the drug-facts-box format which is similar to the nonprescription labeling.[47] In addition, more patients were able to recall risk information when presented in this matter. Other suggestions include listing adverse effects on drug advertisements in bullet form from the highest to the lowest possibility of occurring.[10] In August 2015, the FDA proposed new changes to print DTCA, which would include a new "consumer brief summary" that would include "the most important risk information" that can easily be comprehended by patients.[48,49]

Requiring quantitative data in the DTCAs, as well as mentioning if a generic alternative is available for the product, have also been described as possible solutions.[9] The latter suggestion may not be well accepted by the pharmaceutical industry but has been suggested in the literature. Another study suggested requirements to include specific information about the population at risk for the condition being advertised, describing **nonpharmacologic treatment**, and discuss the effectiveness of other therapies in the ads.[29]

In order to increase transparency, there has been a suggestion to have the following information reported on an online, publically available database: (1) monetary amount spent on the DTCA, (2) type of DTCA, (3) marketing channel, (4) language, (5) demographic location in which the DTCA is presented, (6) time when the DTCA will be available, (7) type of product being marketed, (8) therapeutic category of product, (9) disease that the medication treats, and (10) branded name of product.[50] With the solutions, suggestions, and continued evolvement, the hope for future DTCAs will be a greater emphasis on using medications appropriately, sustained use of medications, and medication adherence.[2]

EVALUATING DTCA

❸ *The following information should be considered when validating appropriateness of DTCA: (1) balance of risk and benefit information and inclusion of a brief summary of the risks listed in the labeling, (2) a statement encouraging patients to seek information from their physician, and (3) references to other sources to find the full prescribing information.*

In general, DTCA must present only accurate statements, maintain a balance of risk versus benefit information throughout, align with the information presented in the FDA-approved labeling, and only present content that is supported by robust evidence.[19,51] Common violations found in advertisements include (1) omitting or softening risk, (2) overstating effectiveness, and (3) misleading drug comparisons.[52] When evaluating DTCA, consider using the process outlined in Table 23-3[53] (Case Study 23-1).

TABLE 23–3. ISSUES TO CONSIDER WHEN EVALUATING DTCA[43,53]

Issues for health care professionals and patients to consider:

- Identify what condition or disease state the advertised product treats.
- Determine the reasoning behind why the patient believes that they have the advertised condition.
- Decide if the patient would be considered an appropriate candidate for the drug based on the information.
- Recognize if the patient is permitted to take the medication with their current comorbidities.
- Identify if the patient is taking any other medications that could interact with the advertised medication.
- Determine which adverse effects that may concern the patient.
- Decide if the drug could be affected by certain foods, dietary supplements, vitamins, or alcohol.
- Pinpoint any other medications (including generic products) that could treat the patient's current condition.
- Determine if other medications to treat this condition have different or less serious side effects.
- Identify if diet and exercise could help the patient with their condition.
- Locate additional information about the disease state and the drug described in the advertisement.

Additional issues for health care professionals to consider:

- Determine if absolute risk reduction (ARR) or number needed to treat (NNT) was used to present results (e.g., "Three out of five patients benefit from Drug X").
- Assess the appropriateness of the use of confidence intervals.
- Identify if statistical power has been adequately explained in the advertisement if referenced.
- Determine if the referenced literature is from the main journal in which the data were published and not from a supplement or symposia.
- Evaluate the appropriateness of presented graphs and tables.
- Recognize if claims are being supported by emotional reports rather than numerical data.

Case Study 23–1

While using a common commercial search engine, you identify a reminder advertisement regarding asthma. Since this advertisement is visible to many members of the public, you decide to evaluate if it is appropriate.

- *What information should the help-seeking advertisement include?*
- *What information should the help-seeking advertisement not include?*

The FDA also provides information for patients and health care professionals on how to determine if an advertisement is false or misleading based on the type.[54] FDA

TABLE 23–4. FDA GUIDANCE FOR EVALUATING SPECIFIC TYPES OF ADVERTISEMENTS[28,30,37]

A product claim ad should:

- Identify the product's brand and generic name.
- State the product's FDA-approved indication (all claims made in the ad must be backed by clinical experience or evidence).
- Include a statement that the product is only available by prescription.
- Contain balanced amounts of drug's risk and benefit information.
- Clearly state that the product is intended for adults or children (this includes the use of pictures, such as children being featured for pediatric medications).
- Include the FDA MedWatch statement about reporting serious adverse effects to the FDA.
- Contain a brief summary of the product's risks listed in the FDA-approved labeling.
- Encourage patients to ask their physician about the medication, signifying that the patient cannot make the decision to prescribe.
- Include references to other resources to obtain detailed product information including a website or toll-free telephone number.

A reminder ad should:

- Include a product's brand and generic name.
- Not list the product's indication.

A help-seeking ad should:

- Include appropriate images of individuals who may be experiencing the discussed symptoms, but not include images of drug products.
- List possible symptoms but does not mention a treatment for these symptoms.
- Encourage patients to discuss their symptoms and seek medical advice from their prescriber.
- Provide company information and references to a telephone number or website for more information.

guidance for evaluating specific types of advertisements is provided in Table 23-4. The FDA encourages patients to report promotional violations to OPDP by calling 301-796-1200 or mailing a written complaint directly to the division.[32,55] Health care professionals are encouraged to report promotional violations using the Bad Ad program described below.

Promotions to Health care Professionals

❹ *Drug promotion to health care professionals makes up the majority of drug promotions activity in terms of financial expenditure on the part of pharmaceutical industry; this information can be effective in eliciting changes in prescribing behavior.* The following sections describe the scope and response to this issue.

DETAILING

Marketing of prescription medications differs from typical consumer products in that one individual—the prescriber—directly controls, to a large extent, purchasing decisions on behalf of the ultimate patient.[56] For this reason, in addition to the very high expenditures of pharmaceutical industry on DTCA, even greater financial resources are dedicated to promotions made directly to health care professionals, or **detailing**. In 2010, an estimated $27.7 billion was spent in pharmaceutical promotions: $4.4 billion (16%) on DTCA and $23.3 billion (84%) on promotions to providers. Of the $23.3 billion directed toward professionals, $13.9 billion was spent on samples, $5.3 billion on office visits, and $2.8 billion on conferences and meetings.[57] Similarly, in an assessment of the promotional pieces submitted to FDA, there were 58,142 professional pieces compared with 27,322 pieces intended for patients (i.e., DTCA).[16] Detailing, like any type of marketing, combines use of scientific knowledge, logic, and reason with appeals to emotions through techniques such as slogans and use of wishful thinking.[56] Detailing may be defined as a one-on-one or group interaction in which a pharmaceutical industry representative, who might or might not have a clinical background, provides drug information and marketing materials to a prescriber or health care professional.[56,58] The most commonly provided types of non-Internet materials include direct mailings, exhibits, sales aids, and presentation slides.[16] These activities could involve provision of product samples and continuing education. At its core, detailing is designed to produce a change in prescribing behavior. The extraordinary expenditures on detailing and related activities, as well as cases of illegal and unsupported drug promotion to health care professionals, suggest that critically assessing the information delivered in these interactions is of vital importance.

LEGAL ISSUES

The same criteria described earlier for DTCA also apply to formal advertisements intended for health care professionals and information promotions such as detailing.[59] Briefly, the information provided must provide fair balance in addressing safety risks and efficacy benefits, describe factual information, and not be misleading. Additionally, information must be consistent with the FDA-approved product labeling (i.e., the package insert), including indications for which the medication may be used.[60] Off-label information may be provided in scientific exchanges and at the request of a health care professional but not in the context of promotion. The legality of off-label promotion is an often-debated First Amendment issue.[60,61] Pharmaceutical companies are allowed to provide off-label information in response to an unsolicited request from a health care professional, may provide peer-reviewed articles, clinical practice guidelines, and reference books that discuss off-label information, and may support continuing education that addresses off-label uses.[62]

However, recent cases suggest that FDA may be willing to allow pharmaceutical companies to provide non-misleading, truthful off-label promotion; at the time of writing, FDA has committed to update its guidance to industry regarding communication practices, including off-label promotion.

FDA advertising rules also apply to industry-sponsored education programs that are, in actuality, promotional activities.[59] For a program to be considered independent and non-promotional (and, thus, qualify as continuing education), the program must be conducted by a third party who controls the educational content. Additionally, all relevant financial relationships must be disclosed. PhRMA members adhere to voluntary standards that prohibit direct speaker honorariums, entertainment (e.g., sporting-event tickets), gifts, and noneducational practice-related items (e.g., coffee mugs, pens) at continuing education events and during detailing.[63] All programs must be conducted through an independent continuing-education provider.

PROMOTION EFFECTIVENESS

The majority of scientific literature assessing health care professionals' interactions with pharmaceutical industry centers around medical students, physicians, and nurse practitioners, and finds success on the part of industry in achieving their desired changes in attitudes and behaviors.[4,64–73] Little information is available regarding promotions targeted toward pharmacists. Two studies have attempted to quantify exposure to pharmaceutical promotion during medical training, with high proportions of medical students (mean of one gift or exposure per week) and residents (median of one personal representative meeting and 10 marketing lunches per year) reporting attending sponsored events.[64,65] Similar studies have not been repeated since the PhRMA Code on Interactions with Health Care Professionals took effect in 2009; however, in 2013, it was found that approximately 62% of medical students had been exposed to drug promotions even prior to medical school.[74]

Studies vary in the degree to which medical residents and students value industry-sponsored information; however, survey responders generally perceive that they do not feel prepared to manage these types of interactions, but that drug promotions would not influence their prescribing habits. One survey of nurse practitioners found that this group does not prefer to receive drug information from pharmaceutical industry sources, but also found that approximately 36% have been offered paybacks in return for changes to prescribing habits.[66] Limited research describes which prescribers are more likely to meet with pharmaceutical industry representatives. One cross-sectional study found that factors of higher prescription volume (coefficient beta [CB] 0.286), rural practice (CB 0.069), and specialization in primary care (CB 0.132) were positively associated with this risk, and having a restrictive policy for representative interactions (CB −0.327), practice setting size (CB −0.95), and academic affiliation (CB −0.082) were inversely associated with this risk.[67]

Several studies have assessed effects of detailing and related activities on prescribing patterns. Two studies found increased prescribing and loyalty to brand-name prescription medications when physicians were exposed to detailing.[4,21] Similar results have been found in a study assessing effectiveness of industry-sponsored continuing education for physicians,[68] although it should be noted that it was conducted prior to publication of current industry guidelines.[63] One systematic review noted that 17 of 29 assessed articles found increased prescribing of a target medication as a result of one-on-one detailing; the remaining studies found no difference in practice.[69] Similarly, five out of eight articles assessing effectiveness of sponsored education events found the expected changes in practice (i.e., increased prescribing of the target medication). In the inpatient setting, one study found that physicians who request a medication to be added to formulary are more likely to have accepted payment from industry to attend or lead symposia or to have personally met with industry representatives from the company producing the medication.[70] Use of coupons and samples have also been suggested to have significant impact on prescribing habits in theoretical models and experimental studies.[71–73]

COMBATTING MISINFORMATION

❺ *All health care professionals, including pharmacists, should arm themselves using strategies of information mastery and vigilance for potentially flawed reasoning when interacting with pharmaceutical sales representatives.* Systematic and individual strategies for combatting potential misinformation provided by pharmaceutical industry are discussed in the following sections.

Both approaches are needed to ensure that undesired effects of drug promotions to health care professionals are minimized. This need is illustrated by several cases in which the pharmaceutical industry was fined for inappropriate promotion to health care professionals, including cases brought against the manufacturers of olanzapine (Zyprexa®), gabapentin (Neurontin®), and valdecoxib (Bextra®) for off-label promotion and/or lack of fair balance.[75]

A number of systematic strategies are active or have been proposed to decrease the potentially significant effect of promotions on prescribers and pharmacists at local, institutional, and national levels. Several of these strategies are described below.

- **Academic detailing**: Research has demonstrated the value of structured one-on-one visits between traveling clinicians, or academic detailers, and prescribers in terms of evidence-based prescribing habits and increased use of generic medications.[58] Applications of academic detailing are described later in the chapter.

- Conflict of interest policies: Conflict of interest policies have been used in residency programs, colleges of medicine, and health systems in order to decrease the effect of pharmaceutical promotions.[76,77] Many health systems have very specific policies regarding the allowed interactions with industry representatives. The policy may even be that such meetings are prohibited.
- Education: Several studies have assessed effectiveness of educational sessions focusing on pharmaceutical industry interactions with medical students and residents.[78-80] Study participants have generally expressed improved knowledge of the pharmaceutical industry and a greater ability to critically assess promotions, and identified potential behaviors they will change as a result of the program (e.g., stop seeing industry representatives).
- National initiatives: In the United States, OPDP is responsible for review of submitted promotional materials, monitoring at professional meetings for inappropriate promotion, and review of Internet sites related to prescription medications.[81]
- Representative tracking: Health systems often use industry credentialing programs to enforce institutional policies regarding content, frequency, and length of meetings between clinicians and industry representatives.[82] These programs allow health systems administrators to know when representatives are on campus and with whom they are meeting.

Additionally, several professional organizations provide guidelines regarding information provided by the pharmaceutical industry. The American Society of Health-System Pharmacists (ASHP) guides members that a third party should control educational content of all industry-sponsored continuing education.[83] Similarly, the AMA recommends physicians select continuing education that is accredited and fair balanced. Promotional continuing education should be clearly denoted as such.[84] Both organizations counsel members to limit interactions with pharmaceutical industry to professional, scientific exchange of information and to avoid situations in which professional judgment is at risk and impropriety may be perceived.[83,84]

Even in the presence of systematic approaches to preventing misinformation in drug promotions, the need for health care professionals to critically evaluate specific information provided in drug promotions is clear. Considering the volume of medical information emerging every day, the task of analyzing, retaining, and synthesizing this information can be monumental.[85] For this reason, health care professionals must develop skills and confidence in searching the medical literature and practicing evidence-based medicine (i.e., information mastery) using both patient-specific and general approaches (i.e., top down versus bottom up, see Chapter 8). It is recommended that health care professionals preferentially use tertiary drug information resources that are either FDA-approved (i.e., the prescribing information) or prepared and published by unbiased sources

TABLE 23–5. EXAMPLE LOGICAL FALLACIES USED IN PHARMACEUTICAL PROMOTION[56]

Fallacy	Description	Example
Appeal to authority	Appeal to knowledge of a known expert with or without conferring with that expert	"I just spoke with the Head of Surgery who says he used Drug X in nearly every case."
Appeal to pity	Appeal to the inner desire to "do good" without focusing on evidence	"Patients whom my other prescribers work with have benefited so much from Drug X. It's really been life-changing for them."
Bandwagon effect	Appeal to popularity with or without confirming if that popularity is true or false	"All the other tertiary medical centers in the city have added Drug X to their formulary."
Red herring	Including extraneous, irrelevant details in an argument	"In clinical studies, Drug X had a lower rate of headache (2%) compared with Drug Y (3%)."

TABLE 23–6. RECOMMENDED PRACTICES FOR INTERACTIONS WITH PHARMACEUTICAL INDUSTRY[84]

- Conduct visits politely and professionally.
- Determine the content of meetings ahead of time.
- Clearly communicate expectations for content and duration of meetings with the representative.
- Prepare for meetings using unbiased tertiary resources and review of primary literature.
- Come prepared with specific questions in mind.
- Use active listening skills.
- Use critical thinking to catch potential errors in reasoning.

(e.g., *AHFS® Drug Information*, Micromedex 2.0). If health care professionals do meet with pharmaceutical industry representatives or use other promotional materials, they should be prepared to rigorously assess pharmaceutical promotions in the same way they would any tertiary resource (see Chapter 3). Additionally, health care professionals should evaluate any print pharmaceutical promotions distributed by industry representatives using strategies similar to DTCA, outlined in Tables 23-2, 23-3, and 23-4.

Many pharmaceutical industry representatives use flawed logic in order to persuade prescribers and pharmacists that their product is the ideal choice for their patients.[56] Errors in reasoning can introduce self-doubt on the part of the health care professional and increase likelihood of a behavior change. It is important to identify when arguments are logical and when they are irrational. In particular, pharmacists who manage pharmacy and therapeutics committee initiatives should be vigilant in their awareness of flawed logic and misleading messages. One of the best methods for combating logical fallacies is reviewing relevant information prior to interacting with an industry representative. See Table 23-5 for examples of misleading strategies that industry representatives might use. See Table 23-6 for general recommendations for interacting with pharmaceutical industry representatives (Case Study 23-2).

Case Study 23-2

As part of your work with the pharmacy and therapeutics committee at an academic, tertiary care hospital, you are asked to conduct monthly meetings with pharmaceutical industry representatives. Your goal for these meetings is to stay up-to-date on competitive pricing information.

- *What systems should you ensure are in place prior to scheduling such visits?*
- *What strategies should you use to prepare for visits once you know which representatives will be attending?*
- *What strategies can you use to remain objective during the visits?*

REPORTING INAPPROPRIATE ADVERTISEMENTS

❻ *Health care professionals are encouraged to report advertising violations to the FDA's Bad Ad program.* All health care professionals have a responsibility to report inappropriate drug promotions using the process described below.

Health care professionals, particularly prescribers, are also targets of drug promotion in the form of print advertisements in medical journals.[86,87] One study found that approximately 16% of the pages in one oncology journal were devoted to drug promotion.[86] Advertisements appearing in medical journals are subject to the same standards as other print advertisements discussed earlier in the chapter, as well as ideally be in compliance with a journal's advertising policy. Advertising policies should be robust and available to the reader. Advertisements in these journals should be assessed using the same methods described for DTCA.

The FDA's Bad Ad Program encourages prescribers to report misinforming or incorrect prescription drug advertising and promotion to FDA.[51,55] This assists OPDP in identifying and ceasing such advertisements.[51] Advertisements for products such as dietary supplements, medical devices, and nonprescription drugs should not be reported through the Bad Ad Program since OPDP does not regulate the promotion of these products. In the past, OPDP obtained information about prescription drug promotion violations through complaints and comments about medication promotion, medical conference observations, review of company submitted promotional materials, and Internet searches.[55] Due to the inability of FDA employees to be present at all dinner programs, promotional speaker events, and prescribers' offices, the FDA seeks the help of health care professionals to report promotional violations through this program.[55]

If an ad is found to be in violation, the FDA can take enforcement action or continue to monitor additional advertisement activities.[51] Advertising methods that are assessed and can be reported through the Bad Ad Program include information presented in printed or written drug promotional materials or by sales representatives, presentations by program speakers, as well as advertisements on radio or television.[51,55]

Common violations identified in drug advertisements include (1) inadequate risk information including downplaying potential risks, (2) exaggeration of benefits, (3) off-label or unapproved information, and (4) false or deceiving comparisons with other medications.[51]

Comments to the FDA through the Bad Ad program can be submitted anonymously; once received, they are analyzed by a member of the OPDP team.[51] FDA accepts comments from health care professionals via e-mail BadAd@FDA.gov or by phone 855-RX-BADAD (855-792-2323) (Case Study 23-3).

Case Study 23–3

You have been asked to attend a dinner program sponsored by the pharmaceutical industry. The main goal for you attending the program is to learn about a new product to treat rheumatoid arthritis.

- *How do you interpret the information being presented at the program?*
- *What are the common violations that can occur in this setting?*
- *How do you report a violation to the FDA?*

ACADEMIC DETAILING

❼*Academic detailing programs, often led by pharmacists, are designed to combat pharmaceutical industry detailing by providing evidence-based information in the form of one-on-one or small-group interactions between a clinician and prescribers.* The following sections address the design, effectiveness, and roles for pharmacists in academic detailing.

Definition

Academic detailing, also known as counter-detailing, prescriber outreach, and prescriber support and education, is a proactive approach developed to combat proliferation of potentially biased information provided by pharmaceutical sales representatives in prescriber workplaces.[58,88,89] The goal of academic detailing is to provide objective, scientific evidence to prescribers in order to improve patient outcomes. While originally focused on increasing use of generic medications when the practice emerged in the 1980s, today's

TABLE 23-7. CORE FUNCTIONS OF AN ACADEMIC DETAILING PROGRAM[58,89,90]

- Identify a target therapeutic issue based on local trends (e.g., demographics, endemic disease states, prescriber preference, prescribing patterns).
- Identify a target prescriber population based on specific criteria (e.g., level of experience, prescribing patterns).
- Synthesize the available evidence using strategies discussed in Chapters 2 and 8.
- Provide the synthesized evidence in an engaging small-group or one-on-one format using a concise message that can be easily implemented into practice.
- Monitor program using identified metrics related to scope (e.g., quantity and quality of visits) and effectiveness (e.g., generic versus brand prescribing, therapeutic area-specific issues).
- Develop relationships with prescribers by increasing communication and face time.

academic detailing programs have expanded clinical roles including promotion of evidence-based medicine and dissemination of comparative effectiveness research. Although most commonly associated with outpatient settings, academic detailing programs have also been reported in inpatient and long-term care practices.[90,91] Pharmaceutical and academic detailing are similar in that both are designed to change prescribing behavior.[58,88,89,92]

Designing Academic Detailing Program

The core process of an academic detailing program is outlined in Table 23-7.[89,90] At its heart is a one-on-one, face-to-face interaction between a traveling health care professional (e.g., physician, pharmacist, nurse) and a prescriber.[58,88,89,92] The academic detailer may also have a concurrent academic or clinical appointment.[88,89] While the original format for these interactions was inspired by the success of pharmaceutical detailing, a key difference is that academic detailing is intended to focus purely on evidence-based information without a promotional perspective.[58,88,89,92] Individuals providing academic detailing should have knowledge of clinical and information sciences as well as experience in providing direct patient care.[88] Interactions between the detailer and prescriber should be nonjudgmental, empathetic, and professional. Although there are examples of peer academic detailing, where fellow prescribers lead the initiative and provide the information,[93,94] most programs are led by or largely rely on pharmacists.

The most accepted goal of academic detailing is promotion of rational prescribing and increasing transparency by providing scientific information regarding medication efficacy, safety, and effectiveness.[58,88,89] One somewhat controversial aspect of academic detailing is whether improving cost-savings-related outcomes should also be a core function of these initiatives.[88] Programs are occasionally accused of allowing pursuit of cost savings to supersede promotion of evidence-based medicine. While simply encouraging use of generic medications in place of branded product is a generally accepted aim, therapeutic substitution of a different medication in the same class is a more divisive issue. Differences in philosophy may vary depending on the organization sponsoring the program; for-profit, third-party, and government organizations may be more likely than academic groups to acknowledge a cost-savings goal.[58,88,89,92]

Examples of Academic Detailing Program

For-profit, nonprofit, government, and academic organizations are all known to sponsor academic detailing programs.[58,88–92,95,96] Many of the most successful programs are collaborations among multiple groups. Large-scale academic detailing has been conducted by several Canadian provinces and at a national level in Australia; several states in the United States are considering or have developed programs modeled after the success of programs in these countries (where large-scale academic detailing has a much longer history).[88,89] One of the most well-known academic detailing programs in the United States is the Independent Drug Information Service (iDiS), a division of the Pennsylvania Department of Aging's Pharmaceutical Contract for the Elderly (PACE) program.[95] This program spends approximately $600 million annually to provide medication to over 300,000 elderly patients who are ineligible for Medicaid.[88,95] PACE reports that cost savings generated from improving prescribing of common chronic medications (e.g., antihypertensives, anti-inflammatories) more than cover the costs of this program.[88,89] The content for iDiS visits is developed by an independent group of physicians, the National Resource Center for Academic Detailing (NaRCAD), located at Harvard Medical School and Brigham and Women's Hospital, and then provided by 10 academic detailers in approximately 1,000 physician visits annually.

Another example of an American academic detailing collaboration is the South Carolina Medicaid Academic Detailing Program (SCORxE), a collaboration of the South Carolina Department of Health and Human Services and the South Carolina College of Pharmacy.[88,96] This program focuses on providing pharmacist-led academic detailing with prescribers who provide care for rural and urban Medicaid patients, primarily on mental health topics.[97] The programming is provided by full-time pharmacists across 18 counties, with support from the Medical University of South Carolina Drug Information Center.

Nationally, leadership in the area of academic detailing comes from NaRCAD, an Agency for Healthcare Research and Quality (AHRQ)-supported initiative.[58,98] NaRCAD collaborates with states and private organizations to determine their specific needs in an academic detailing program, based on local medication use.[88,89,99] Additionally, the service translates important comparative effectiveness research into usable tools, conducts education on academic detailing best practices and implementation, and helps organizations develop an assessment plan for their programs.[58,99] A final key role of NaRCAD is enlarging the network of organizations providing academic detailing in order to encourage information exchange (Case Study 23-4).

Case Study 23–4

As part of your work in a large health system with a network of physician-office clinics, you are asked to develop an academic detailing program designed to improve safety, efficacy, and cost effectiveness of prescribing in an area of psychiatry.

- *How would you go about determining on which class of medications or disease state to focus?*
- *How would you develop your clinical materials? With which external organizations could you partner?*
- *Would you take a one-on-one or group approach to academic detailing? Discuss why you selected the strategy you did.*
- *What metrics could you assess to determine the effectiveness of your program?*

Effectiveness of Academic Detailing

While theoretical and observational data suggest huge potential for improvement in clinical and economic outcomes from academic detailing programs,[100,101] results from prospective, interventional studies assessing effectiveness of academic detailing programs have been mixed.[88,89,91,102–107] The nationwide academic detailing program in Australia has demonstrated significant cost effectiveness; however, less public information is available regarding tangible cost savings of such programs in the United States.[101] One analysis suggests that academic detailing provided by a pharmacist to small groups of physicians would result in average annual net savings of approximately $1,000,000 per 10,000 physicians. From a clinical perspective, some individual programs have demonstrated both improved prescribing practices in addition to some cost savings in areas such as control of vasodilator use, adherence to hypertension clinical practice guidelines, statin prescribing, smoking cessation, oral diabetic selection, reducing inappropriate antibiotic prescribing, and evidence-based treatment of gastrointestinal reflux disease (GERD) and related disorders.[102–104,108–112] Another study found improved prescribing practices regarding use of antipsychotics in long-term care.[91] Conversely, some studies have had only marginal clinical and economic results.[105,106]

Most published studies of academic detailing have limited generalizability due to conduct in a specific HMOs or institution, and interventions performed by a low number of individuals; however, these same limitations could signal good internal validity of individual programs and customizing based on local need, a key principle of academic detailing.[91,102–112] Another concern regarding effectiveness of academic detailing is that the resources dedicated to these programs are much less than the resources dedicated toward pharmaceutical detailing on the part of industry.[88,89,100] Meta-analyses of academic detailing studies found a consistent, small-to-moderate benefit in terms of changes in targeted practice behavior, but did not assess pharmacoeconomic outcomes.[113,114]

Pharmacist's Role in Academic Detailing

With their strong academic background in drug information and drug literature evaluation, pharmacists can be ideally positioned to engage in academic detailing.[58,88,89] Indeed, many of the academic detailing programs described in clinical literature and the media are centered around a team of pharmacists.[88–90,92,102,106,107] Pharmacists with postgraduate training in drug information may be particularly well-equipped for these types of positions as a result of their special skills in drug information service management, evidence-based medicine, and communications.[115] Pharmacists seeking to engage in academic detailing should critically assess local demographics and prescribing patterns in order to identify a specific detailing target, network and collaborate with established programs through organizations such as NaRCAD and local key stakeholders, and strive to build strong interpersonal relationships with target prescribers. Finally, as with any novel clinical service, identifying and monitoring key metrics is vital to justify direct and indirect costs of the program. Considering the mixed results of published studies and their remote time of publication, pharmacists participating in academic detailing are encouraged to share more current effectiveness information.

Conclusion

Drug promotion, including DTCA and promotion to health care professionals, represents significant expenditure on the part of pharmaceutical industry. The controversial issues surrounding DTCA and off-label promotion, in particular, continue to raise concerns about the benefits and harms of providing this type of information to patients. Detailing and direct advertisement to health care professionals continues to be an effective method of promotion. FDA calls on health care professionals to play a key role in reporting drug-promotions violations related to advertising, detailing, and continuing education. As drug-promotional methods evolve, pharmacists will continue to serve both health care professionals and the public as a valuable source in deciphering and evaluating materials distributed by pharmaceutical industry. Academic detailing may be one avenue for drug information specialists and health care professionals to combat the influence of drug promotions on prescribing.

Self-Assessment Questions

1. Which of the following is considered the goal of drug promotion?
   a. Developing a better physician-patient relationship
   b. Increasing the prescribing or purchasing of medications
   c. Increasing medication compliance among patients
   d. Informing patients about generic alternatives

2. World Health Organization (WHO) does NOT recommend the use of DTCA for which of the following product types:
   a. Prescription drugs
   b. Nonprescription drugs
   c. Vitamins and minerals
   d. Herbal products

3. The Kefauver-Harris Amendment:
   a. Required the MedWatch reporting statement to be included on printed ads
   b. Eliminated the requirement for the brief summary on television ads
   c. Gave the FDA authority over prescription drug advertising
   d. Required printed ads to include the entire prescribing information

4. Help-seeking ads are regulated by which government agency?
   a. FTC
   b. FDA
   c. DEA
   d. USP

5. What types of advertisements are illegal for medications with boxed warnings?
   a. Help-seeking
   b. Reminder
   c. Product claim
   d. Academic detailing

6. Which of the following components of product claim ads are required by FDA regulations?
   a. Fair-balanced risks and benefits
   b. Mechanism of action
   c. Cost information
   d. Onset of action

7. The PhRMA Guiding Principles for DTCA are voluntary and are **NOT** enforced by the FDA.
   a. True
   b. False

8. According to the PhRMA Guiding Principles for DTCA which of the follow ads are NOT acceptable?
   a. A printed advertisement for a cholesterol medication that includes information about the patient assistance program sponsored by the company.
   b. A television commercial portraying a child playing outside for a medication for a pediatric allergy medication.
   c. An advertisement for an obesity medication that mentions diet and exercise as adjunctive therapy.
   d. A television advertisement for an erectile dysfunction medication being aired during Saturday morning cartoons.

9. If a DTCA violates FDA advertising regulations, the FDA has the authority to:
   a. Ban the company from producing DTCA
   b. Issue warning letters to the company
   c. Levy fines against the company
   d. The FDA does not have the authority to take action against the company

10. Due to concerns about the increasing cost of medications, the American Medical Association (AMA) called for which of the following actions in 2015?
    a. Tighter regulation of DTCA by the FDA
    b. The development of a public access database
    c. A ban on DTCA in the United States
    d. The implementation of a pricing cap for drugs

11. A pharmaceutical representative is permitted to provide off-label information regarding use of prescription medications when responding to an unsolicited request from a health care professional.
    a. True
    b. False

12. All of the following are proposed means to combat potential for biased information discussed in pharmaceutical detailing EXCEPT:
    a. Academic detailing to prescribers based on identified issues
    b. Developing conflict of interest policies outlining permitted interactions
    c. Education to physicians-in-training regarding information mastery
    d. Requiring detailing to be performed by a health care professional

13. The red herring logical fallacy refers to:
   a. Bandwagon effect
   b. Making the discussion personal
   c. Providing distracting, unrelated detail
   d. Referencing local content experts

14. Academic detailing programs ideally are designed to:
   a. Decrease use of brand medications
   b. Promote evidence-based prescribing
   c. Provide cost savings to third-party payers
   d. Punish low-performing physicians

15. Academic detailing programs in the United States have been shown to:
   a. Achieve the desired change in prescribing behavior
   b. Achieve national improvements in economic outcomes
   c. Decrease the rate of evidence-based prescribing
   d. Have similar success to pharmaceutical detailing

REFERENCES

1. Brownfield ED, Bernhardt JM, Phan JL, Williams MV, Parker RM. Direct-to-consumer drug advertisements on network television: an exploration of quantity, frequency, and placement. J Health Commun. 2004;9(6):491-7.
2. Bulik B. Pharmaceutical marketing. Chicago, IL: Ad Age; 2011 [updated Oct 17; cited 2016 Sept 27]. Available from: http://gaia.adage.com/images/bin/pdf/WPpharmmarketing_revise.pdf
3. Greene JA, Herzberg D. Hidden in plain sight marketing prescription drugs to consumers in the twentieth century. Am J Public Health. 2010;100(5):793-803. doi:10.2105/AJPH.2009.181255.
4. Hansen RA, Chen S-Y, Gaynes BN, Maciejewski ML. Relationship of pharmaceutical promotion to antidepressant switching and adherence: a retrospective cohort study. Psychiatr Serv. 2010;61(12):1232-8. doi:10.1176/appi.ps.61.12.1232.
5. Law MR, Soumerai SB, Adams AS, Majumdar SR. Costs and consequences of direct-to-consumer advertising for clopidogrel in Medicaid. Arch Intern Med. 2009;169(21):1969-74. doi:10.1001/archinternmed.2009.320.
6. Mintzes B. Advertising of prescription-only medicines to the public: does evidence of benefit counterbalance harm? Annu Rev Pub Health. 2012;33:259-77. doi:10.1146/annurev-publhealth-031811-124540.
7. Norris P HA, Lexchin J, Mansfield P. Drug promotion—what we know, what we have yet to learn—reviews of materials in the WHO/HAI database on drug promotion—EDM Research Series No. 032. World Health Organization and Health Action International;

2005 [cited 2016 Sept 27]. Available from: http://apps.who.int/medicinedocs/pdf/s8109e/s8109e.pdf

8. Ross JS, Kravitz RL. Direct-to-consumer television advertising: time to turn off the tube? J Gen Intern Med. 2013;28(7):862-4. doi:10.1007/s11606-013-2424-2. PubMed PMID: 23539285.

9. Ventola CL. Direct-to-consumer pharmaceutical advertising: therapeutic or toxic? PT. 2011;36(10):669-84.

10. Womack CA. Ethical and epistemic issues in direct-to-consumer drug advertising: where is patient agency? Med Health Care Philos. 2013;16(2):275-80. doi:10.1007/s11019-012-9386-8.

11. Vastag B. FDA considers tightening regulations for direct-to-consumer advertising. J Natl Cancer Inst. 2005;97(24):1806-7.

12. Pharmaceutical marketing. Washington, DC: DrugWatch.com; [updated 2015 Aug 25]. Available from: https://www.drugwatch.com/featured/big-pharma-marketing/

13. Othman N, Vitry A, Roughead EE. Quality of pharmaceutical advertisements in medical journals: a systematic review. PLoS ONE. 2009;4(7):e6350-e. doi:10.1371/journal.pone.0006350.

14. Palmer E. Top 10 drug advertising spends—q1 2012. Fierce Pharma; 2012 [updated Aug 9; cited 2016 Sept 27]. Available from: http://www.fiercepharma.com/special-reports/top-10-drug-advertising-spends-q1-2012

15. Keeping watch over direct-to-consumer ads. Silver Spring, MD: U.S. Food and Drug Administration; 2010 [cited 2016 Sept 27]. Available from: http://www.fda.gov/downloads/ForConsumers/ConsumerUpdates/ucm107180.pdf

16. Sullivan HW, Aikin KJ, Chung-Davies E, Wade M. Prescription drug promotion from 2001-2014: data from the U.S. Food and drug administration. PLoS ONE. 2016;11(5):e0155035. doi:10.1371/journal.pone.0155035.

17. Ethical criteria for medicinal drug promotion. Geneva: World Health Organization; 1988 [cited 2016 Sept 27]. Available from: http://apps.who.int/medicinedocs/documents/whozip08e/whozip08e.pdf

18. Kim H. Trouble spots in online direct-to-consumer prescription drug promotion: a content analysis of FDA warning letters. Int J Health Policy Manag. 2015;4(12):813-21. doi:10.15171/ijhpm.2015.157.

19. PhRMA guiding principles direct to consumer advertisements about prescription medicines. Washington, DC: Pharmaceutical Research and Manufacturers of America (PhRMA); [updated 200 Dec; cited 2016 Sept 27]. Available from: http://www.phrma.org/sites/default/files/pdf/phrmaguidingprinciplesdec08final.pdf

20. Tyrawski J, DeAndrea DC. Pharmaceutical companies and their drugs on social media: a content analysis of drug information on popular social media sites. J Med Internet Res. 2015;17(6):e130. doi:10.2196/jmir.4357.

21. Dorn SD, Farley JF, Hansen RA, Shah ND, Sandler RS. Direct-to-consumer and physician promotion of tegaserod correlated with physician visits, diagnoses, and prescriptions. Gastroenterology. 2009;137(2):518. doi:10.1053/j.gastro.2009.05.005.

22. Abel GA, Chen K, Taback N, Hassett MJ, Schrag D, Weeks JC. Impact of oncology-related direct-to-consumer advertising. Cancer. 2013;119(5):1065-72.

23. Daubresse M, Hutfless S, Kim Y, Kornfield R, Qato DM, Huang J, Miller K, Emery SL, Alexander GC. Effect of direct-to-consumer advertising on asthma medication sales and health-care use. Am J Respir Crit Care Med. 2015;192(1):40-6. doi:10.1164/rccm.201409-1585OC.

23: Daubresse M, Hutfless S, Kim Y, Kornfield R, Qato DM, Huang J, Miller K, Emery SL, Alexander GC

24. Staton T. Pharma's ad spend vaults to $4.5b, with big spender Pfizer leading the way. FiercePharma. 2015.

25. Mackey TK, Cuomo RE, Liang BA. The rise of digital direct-to-consumer advertising? Comparison of direct-to-consumer advertising expenditure trends from publicly available data sources and global policy implications. BMC Health Serv Res. 2015;15:236. doi:10.1186/s12913-015-0885-1.

26. Kornfield R, Alexander GC, Qato DM, Kim Y, Hirsch JD, Emery SL. Trends in exposure to televised prescription drug advertising, 2003-2011. Am J Prev Med. 2015;48(5):575-9. doi:10.1016/j.amepre.2014.12.001.

27. Basics of drug ads. Silver Spring, MD: U.S. Food and Drug Administration; [updated 2012 Sept 13; cited 2016 Sept 27]. Available from: http://www.fda.gov/Drugs/ResourcesForYou/Consumers/PrescriptionDrugAdvertising/ucm072077.htm

28. Correct help-seeking ad. Silver Spring, MD: U.S. Food and Drug Administration; [updated 2012 Sept 13; cited 2016 Sept 27]. Available from: http://www.fda.gov/Drugs/ResourcesForYou/Consumers/PrescriptionDrugAdvertising/ucm082288.htm

29. Frosch DL, Krueger PM, Hornik RC, Cronholm PF, Barg FK. Creating demand for prescription drugs: a content analysis of television direct-to-consumer advertising. Ann Fam Med. 2007;5(1):6-13.

30. Reminder ad (correct). Silver Spring, MD: U.S. Food and Drug Administration; [updated 2012 Sept 13; cited 2016 Sept 27]. Available from: http://www.fda.gov/Drugs/ResourcesForYou/Consumers/PrescriptionDrugAdvertising/ucm083573.htm

31. Sumpradit N, Ascione FJ, Bagozzi RP. A cross-media content analysis of motivational themes in direct-to-consumer prescription drug advertising. Clin Ther. 2004;26(1):135-54.

32. Prescription drug advertising: questions and answers. Silver Spring, MD: U.S. Food and Drug Administration; [updated 2012 Sept 13; cited 2016 Sept 27]. Available from: https://www.fda.gov/Drugs/ResourcesForYou/Consumers/PrescriptionDrugAdvertising/ucm076768.htm

33. Lexchin J, Mintzes B. A compromise too far: a review of Canadian cases of direct-to-consumer advertising regulation. Int J Risk Saf Med. 2014;26(4):213-25. doi:10.3233/JRS-140635.

34. Kefauver-Harris amendments. Silver Spring, MD: U.S. Food and Drug Administration; [updated 2013 Apr 11; cited 2016 Sept 27]. Available from: http://www.fda.gov/ForConsumers/ConsumerUpdates/ucm322856.htm

35. The impact of direct-to-consumer advertising. Silver Spring, MD: U.S. Food and Drug Administration; [updated 2013 Apr 12; cited 2016 Sept 27]. Available from: http://www.fda.gov/Drugs/ResourcesForYou/Consumers/ucm143562.htm

36. CFR—Code of Federal Regulations Title 21: Part 202—prescription drug advertising. Silver Spring, MD: U.S. Food and Drug Administration; [updated 2012 Apr 1; cited 2016 Sept 27]. Available from: http://www.accessdata.fda.gov/scripts/cdrh/cfdocs/cfCFR/CFRSearch.cfm?fr=202.1

37. Product claim ad (correct). Silver Spring, MD: U.S. Food and Drug Administration; [2012 updated Sept 13; cited 2016 Sept 28]. Available from: http://www.fda.gov/Drugs/ResourcesForYou/Consumers/PrescriptionDrugAdvertising/ucm082284.htm

38. Warning letters and notice of violation letters to pharmaceutical companies. Silver Spring, MD: U.S. Food and Drug Administration; [2012 updated Jan 25; cited 2016 Sept 28]. Available from: http://www.fda.gov/Drugs/GuidanceComplianceRegulatoryInformation/EnforcementActivitiesbyFDA/WarningLettersandNoticeofViolationLetterstoPharmaceuticalCompanies/default.htm

39. Yang YT, Chen B. Legal considerations for social media marketing by pharmaceutical industry. Food Drug Law J. 2014;69(1):39.

40. Tan ASL. Potential spillover educational effects of cancer-related direct-to-consumer advertising on cancer patients' increased information seeking behaviors: results from a cohort study. J Cancer Educ. 2014;29(2):258-65. doi:10.1007/s13187-013-0588-4.

41. Corrigan PW, Kosyluk KA, Fokuo JK, Park JH. How does direct to consumer advertising affect the stigma of mental illness? Community Ment Health J. 2014;50(7):792-9. doi:10.1007/s10597-014-9698-7.

42. Bhutada NS, Rollins BL. Disease-specific direct-to-consumer advertising for reminding consumers to take medications. J Am Pharm Assoc. 2015;55(4):434-7. doi:10.1331/JAPhA.2015.14234.

43. Lexchin J. Statistics in drug advertising: what they reveal is suggestive what they hide is vital. Int J Clin Pract. 2010;64(8):1015-8. doi:10.1111/j.1742-1241.2010.02398.x.

44. AMA calls for ban on direct to consumer advertising of prescription drugs and medical devices. American Medical Association; 2015 [cited 2016 Jun 29]. Available from: http://www.ama-assn.org/ama/pub/news/news/2015/2015-11-17-ban-consumer-prescription-drug-advertising.page

45. Public health advisory: tegaserod maleate (marketed as zelnorm). Silver Spring, MD: U.S. Food and Drug Administration; [2013 updated Aug 19; cited 2016 Sept 28]. Available from: http://www.fda.gov/Drugs/DrugSafety/PostmarketDrugSafetyInformationforPatientsandProviders/ucm051284.htm

46. Guessous I, Dash C. Direct to consumer advertising: the case for greater consumer control. J Gen Intern Med. 2015;30(4):392-4. doi:10.1007/s11606-015-3187-8.

47. Aikin KJ, O'Donoghue AC, Swasy JL, Sullivan HW. Randomized trial of risk information formats in direct-to-consumer prescription drug advertisements. Med Decis Making. 2011;31(6):E23-33. doi:10.1177/0272989X11413289.

48. Greene JA, Watkins ES. The vernacular of risk—rethinking direct-to-consumer advertising of pharmaceuticals. N Engl J Med. 2015;373(12):1087-9. doi:10.1056/NEJMp1507924.

49. Brief summary and adequate directions for use: disclosing risk information in consumer-directed print advertisements and promotional labeling for prescription drugs: Guidance for Industry. Revised 2nd ed. Rockville, MD: U.S. Food and Drug Administration; 2015.

50. Mackey TK, Liang BA. It's time to shine the light on direct-to-consumer advertising. Ann Fam Med. 2015;13(1):82-5. doi:10.1370/afm.1711.

51. Reporting misleading Rx drug promotion. Silver Spring, MD: U.S. Food and Drug Administration; [cited 2016 Sept 28]. Available from: http://www.fda.gov/downloads/Drugs/GuidanceComplianceRegulatoryInformation/Surveillance/PrescriptionDrugAdvertisingandPromotionalLabeling/UCM209847.pdf

52. Truthful prescription drug advertising and promotion. Silver Spring, MD: U.S. Food and Drug Administration; [updated 2015 Oct 20; cited 2016 Jun 19]. Available from: http://www.fda.gov/Drugs/GuidanceComplianceRegulatoryInformation/Surveillance/DrugMarketingAdvertisingandCommunications/ucm209384.htm

53. Prescription drug advertising: questions to ask yourself. Silver Spring, MD: U.S. Food and Drug Administration; [updated 2015 Jun 19; cited 2016 Sept 28]. Available from: http://www.fda.gov/Drugs/ResourcesForYou/Consumers/PrescriptionDrugAdvertising/ucm071915.htm

54. Prescription drug advertising. Silver Spring, MD: U.S. Food and Drug Administration; [updated 2015 Jun 19; cited 2016 Sept 28]. Available from: http://www.fda.gov/Drugs/ResourcesForYou/Consumers/PrescriptionDrugAdvertising/default.htm

55. Bad Ad program. FDA aims to keep drug promotion truthful. Silver Spring, MD: U.S. Food and Drug Administration; [updated 2015 Oct 20; cited 2016 Sept]. Available from: http://www.fda.gov/Drugs/GuidanceComplianceRegulatoryInformation/Surveillance/DrugMarketingAdvertisingandCommunications/ucm209384.htm

56. Shaughnessy AF, Slawson DC, Bennett JH. Separating the wheat from the chaff: identifying fallacies in pharmaceutical promotion. J Gen Intern Med. 1994;9(10):563-8.

57. Kornfield R, Donohue J, Berndt ER, Alexander GC. Promotion of prescription drugs to consumers and providers, 2001-2010. PLoS ONE. 2013;8(3):e55504. doi:10.1371/journal.pone.0055504.

58. Detailing NaRCAD. About academic detailing. Boston, MA: Brigham and Women's Hospital and Harvard Medical School, Department of Medicine, Division of Pharmacoepidemiology and Pharmacoeconomics; [cited 2017 Mar 15]. Available from: https://www.narcad.org/about.html

59. Abood R. Pharmacy practice and the law. 7th ed. Burlington, MA: Jones & Bartlett Learning; 2014.

60. Greenwood K. The ban on "off-label" pharmaceutical promotion: constitutionally permissible prophylaxis against false or misleading commercial speech? Am J Law Med. 2011;37(2-3):278-98.

61. Kesselheim AS, Avorn J. Pharmaceutical promotion to physicians and first amendment rights. N Engl J Med. 2008;358(16):1727-32. doi:10.1056/NEJMsb0708920.

62. Richardson E. Off-label drug promotion. Health Aff. June 30, 2016; Health Policy Briefs.

63. Code on interactions with health care professionals. Washington, DC: Pharmaceutical Research and Manufacturers of America; [cited 2016 Sept 20]. Available from: http://www.phrma.org/code-on-interactions-with-healthcare-professionals

64. Sierles FS, Brodkey AC, Cleary LM, McCurdy FA, Mintz M, Frank J, Lynn DJ, Chao J, Morgenstern BZ, Shore W, Woodard JL. Medical students' exposure to and attitudes about drug company interactions: a national survey. JAMA. 2005;294(9):1034-42.

65. Hodges B. Interactions with the pharmaceutical industry: experiences and attitudes of psychiatry residents, interns and clerks. CMAJ. 1995;153(5):553-9.

66. Clauson KA, Khanfar NM, Polen HH, Gibson F. Nurse prescribers' interactions with and perceptions of pharmaceutical sales representatives. J Clin Nurs. 2009;18(2):228-33. doi:10.1111/j.1365-2702.2008.02536.x.

67. Alkhateeb FM, Khanfar NM, Clauson KA. Characteristics of physicians who frequently see pharmaceutical sales representatives. J Hosp Mark Public Relations. 2009;19(1):2-14. doi:10.1080/15390940802581374.

68. Bowman MA, Pearle DL. Changes in drug prescribing patterns related to commercial company funding of continuing medical education. J Contin Educ Health Prof. 1988;8(1):13-20.

69. Spurling GK, Mansfield PR, Montgomery BD, Lexchin J, Doust J, Othman N, Vitry A. Information from pharmaceutical companies and the quality, quantity, and cost of physicians' prescribing: a systematic review. PLoS Med. 2010;7(10):e1000352. doi:10.1371/journal.pmed.1000352.

70. Chren MM, Landefeld CS. Physicians' behavior and their interactions with drug companies. A controlled study of physicians who requested additions to a hospital drug formulary. JAMA. 1994;271(9):684-9.

71. Mackey TK, Yagi N, Liang BA. Prescription drug coupons: evolution and need for regulation in direct-to-consumer advertising. Res Social Adm Pharm. 2014;10(3):588-94. doi:10.1016/j.sapharm.2013.08.002.

72. Hurley MP, Stafford RS, Lane AT. Characterizing the relationship between free drug samples and prescription patterns for acne vulgaris and rosacea. JAMA Dermatol. 2014;150(5):487-93. doi:10.1001/jamadermatol.2013.9715.

73. Daugherty JB, Maciejewski ML, Farley JF. The impact of manufacturer coupon use in the statin market. J Manag Care Pharm. 2013;19(9):765-72.

74. Hodges LE, Arora VM, Humphrey HJ, Reddy ST. Premedical students' exposure to the pharmaceutical industry's marketing practices. Acad Med. 2013;88(2):265-8. doi:10.1097/ACM.0b013e31827bfbce.

75. Lexchin J. Models for financing the regulation of pharmaceutical promotion. Global Health. 2012;8:24. doi:10.1186/1744-8603-8-24.

76. Epstein AJ, Busch SH, Busch AB, Asch DA, Barry CL. Does exposure to conflict of interest policies in psychiatry residency affect antidepressant prescribing? Med Care. 2013;51(2):199-203. doi:10.1097/MLR.0b013e318277eb19.

77. Grande D, Frosch DL, Perkins AW, Kahn BE. Effect of exposure to small pharmaceutical promotional items on treatment preferences. Arch Intern Med. 2009;169(9):887-93. doi:10.1001/archinternmed.2009.64.

78. Fugh-Berman AJ, Scialli AR, Bell AM. Why lunch matters: assessing physicians' perceptions about industry relationships. J Contin Educ Health Prof. 2010;30(3):197-204. doi:10.1002/chp.20081.

79. Shankar PR, Singh KK, Piryani RM. Knowledge, attitude and skills before and after a module on pharmaceutical promotion in a Nepalese medical school. BMC Res Notes. 2012;5:8. doi:10.1186/1756-0500-5-8.

80. Shankar PR, Singh KK, Piryani RM. Student feedback about the skeptic doctor, a module on pharmaceutical promotion. J Educ Eval Health Prof. 2011;8:11. doi:10.3352/jeehp.2011.8.11.

81. Office of Prescription Drug Promotion. Silver Spring, MD: U.S. Food and Drug Administration; [updated 2011 Oct 17; cited 2013 Apr 29]. Available from: http://www.fda.gov/Drugs/GuidanceComplianceRegulatoryInformation/Surveillance/DrugMarketing AdvertisingandCommunications/default.htm

82. About Reptrax. Flower Mound, TX: IntelliCentrics, Inc.; [cited 2013 Apr 29]. Available from: https://www.reptrax.com/about/reptrax

83. ASHP guidelines on pharmacists' relationships with industry. Bethesda, MD: American Society of Health-Systems Pharmacists, ASHP Council on Legal and Public Affairs; 1992 [updated 2001]. Available from: https://www.ashp.org/-/media/assets/policy-guidelines/docs/guidelines-pharmacists-relationships-industry.ashx.

84. AMA's Code of Medical Ethics: 9.2.6 continuing medical education. Chicago, IL: American Medical Association, Council Ethical and Judicial Affairs; 1993 [updated 1996; cited 2013 Apr 29]. Available from: https://www.ama-assn.org/sites/default/files/media-browser/code-of-medical-ethics-chapter-9.pdf.

85. Slawson DC, Shaughnessy AF, Bennett JH. Becoming a medical information master: feeling good about not knowing everything. J Fam Pract. 1994;38(5):505-14.

86. Yonemori K, Hirakawa A, Ando M, Hirata T, Yunokawa M, Shimizu C, Tamura K, Fujiwara Y. Content analysis of oncology-related pharmaceutical advertising in a peer-reviewed medical journal. PLoS ONE. 2012;7(8):e44393. doi:10.1371/journal.pone.0044393.

87. Kesselheim AS. Covert pharmaceutical promotion in free medical journals. CMAJ. 2011;183(5):534-5. doi:10.1503/cmaj.110156.

88. Academic detailing: a review of the literature and states' approaches. Baltimore, MD: The Hilltop Institute; [updated 2009 Jan 18; cited 2013 Apr 29]. Available from: http://www.hilltopinstitute.org/publication_view.cfm?pubID=270&st=tbl_Publications

89. Reck J. A template for establishing and administering prescriber support and education programs: a collaborative, service based approach for achieving maximum impact. 2008 [cited 2013 Apr 26]. Available from: http://www.policychoices.org/reports.shtml

90. Levinson W, Dunn PM. Counter-detailing. JAMA. 1984;251(16):2084.

91. Avorn J, Soumerai SB, Everitt DE, Ross-Degnan D, Beers MH, Sherman D, Salem-Schatz SR, Fields D. A randomized trial of a program to reduce the use of psychoactive drugs in nursing homes. N Engl J Med. 1992;327(3):168-73.

92. Greg M. Confessions of a pharmacy counter-detailer. Drug Topics; [updated 2011 Apr 15; cited 2013 May 23]. Available from: http://drugtopics.modernmedicine.com/drug-topics/news/modernmedicine/modern-medicine-now/confessions-pharmacy-counter-detailer

93. Grover ML, Nordrum JT, Mookadam M, Engle RL, Moats CC, Noble BN. Addressing antibiotic use for acute respiratory tract infections in an academic family medicine practice. Am J Med Qual. 2013;28(6):485-91. doi:10.1177/1062860613476133.

94. Rognstad S, Brekke M, Fetveit A, Dalen I, Straand J. Prescription peer academic detailing to reduce inappropriate prescribing for older patients: a cluster randomised controlled trial. Br J Gen Pract. 2013;63(613):e554-e62.

95. PACE, PACENET, and PACE Plus Medicare. Harrisburg, PA: Pennsylvania Department of Aging; [cited 2013 Apr 26]. Available from: http://www.aging.state.pa.us/portal/server .pt/community/pace_and_affordable_medications/

96. What is SCORxE? Columbia, SC: South Carolina College of Pharmacy, SCORxE; [cited 2017 Mar 15]. Available from: https://sccp.sc.edu/scorxe

97. Wisniewski CS, Robert S, Ball S. Collaboration between a drug information center and an academic detailing program. Am J Health Syst Pharm. 2014;71(2):128-33. doi:10.2146/ ajhp130225. PubMed PMID: 24375605.

98. National Resource Center for Academic Detailing. About us. Boston, MA: Brigham and Women's Hospital and Harvard Medical School, Department of Medicine, Division of Pharmacoepidemiology and Pharmacoeconomics; [cited 2013 Apr 26]. Available from: http://www.narcad.org/about

99. National Resource Center for Academic Detailing. Our services. Boston, MA: Brigham and Women's Hospital and Harvard Medical School, Department of Medicine, Division of Pharmacoepidemiology and Pharmacoeconomics; [cited 2017 Mar 15]. Available from: https://www.narcad.org/training-series.html

100. Cost effectiveness of prescriber education ("academic detailing") programs. Boston, MA: Pew Prescription Project; [updated 2008 Mar 12; cited 2013 Apr 26]. Available from: http://www.communitycatalyst.org/

101. Soumerai SB, Avorn J. Economic and policy analysis of university-based drug "detailing". Med Care. 1986;24(4):313-31.

102. Avorn J, Soumerai SB. Improving drug-therapy decisions through educational outreach. A randomized controlled trial of academically based "detailing". N Engl J Med. 1983;308(24):1457-63.

103. Simon SR, Rodriguez HP, Majumdar SR, Kleinman K, Warner C, Salem-Schatz S, Miroshnik I, Soumerai SB, Prosser LA. Economic analysis of a randomized trial of academic detailing interventions to improve use of antihypertensive medications. J Clin Hypertens. 2007;9(1):15-20.

104. Ofman JJ, Segal R, Russell WL, Cook DJ, Sandhu M, Maue SK, Lowenstein EH, Pourfarzib R, Blanchette E, Ellrodt G, Weingarten SR. A randomized trial of an acid-peptic disease management program in a managed care environment. Am J Manag Care. 2003;9(6):425-33.

105. Franzini L, Boom J, Nelson C. Cost-effectiveness analysis of a practice-based immunization education intervention. Ambul Pediatr. 2007;7(2):167-75.

106. Farris KB, Kirking DM, Shimp LA, Opdycke RAC. Design and results of a group counter-detailing DUR educational program. Pharm Res. 1996;13(10):1445-52.

107. Wall GC, Smith HL, Craig SR, Yost WJ. Structured pharmaceutical representative interactions and counterdetailing sessions as components of medical resident education. J Pharm Pract. 2013;26(2):151-6. doi:10.1177/0897190012465988.

108. Clyne B, Smith SM, Hughes CM, Boland F, Bradley MC, Cooper JA, Fahey T; OPTI-SCRIPT study team. Effectiveness of a multifaceted intervention for potentially inappropriate prescribing in older patients in primary care: a cluster-randomized controlled trial (opti-script study). Ann Fam Med. 2015;13(6):545-53. doi:10.1370/afm.1838.

109. Vinnard C, Linkin DR, Localio AR, Leonard CE, Teal VL, Fishman NO, Hennessy S. Effectiveness of interventions in reducing antibiotic use for upper respiratory infections in ambulatory care practices. Popul Health Manag. 2013;16(1):22-7. doi:10.1089/pop.2012.0025.

110. Ho K, Nguyen A, Jarvis-Selinger S, Novak Lauscher H, Cressman C, Zibrik L. Technology-enabled academic detailing: computer-mediated education between pharmacists and physicians for evidence-based prescribing. Int J Med Inform. 2013;82(9):762-71. doi:10.1016/j.ijmedinf.2013.04.011.

111. Jin M, Gagnon A, Levine M, Thabane L, Rodriguez C, Dolovich L. Patient-specific academic detailing for smoking cessation: feasibility study. Can Fam Physician. 2014;60(1):e16-23.

112. Lowrie R, Lloyd SM, McConnachie A, Morrison J. A cluster randomised controlled trial of a pharmacist-led collaborative intervention to improve statin prescribing and attainment of cholesterol targets in primary care. PLoS ONE. 2014;9(11):e113370. doi:10.1371/journal.pone.0113370.

113. O'Brien MA, Rogers S, Jamtvedt G, Oxman AD, Odgaard-Jensen J, Kristoffersen DT, Forsetlund L, Bainbridge D, Freemantle N, Davis DA, Haynes RB, Harvey EL. Educational outreach visits: effects on professional practice and health care outcomes. Cochrane Database Syst Rev. 2007;(4):CD000409.

114. Chhina HK, Bhole VM, Goldsmith C, Hall W, Kaczorowski J, Lacaille D. Effectiveness of academic detailing to optimize medication prescribing behaviour of family physicians. J Pharm Pharm Sci. 2013;16(4):511-29.

115. American Society of Health-System Pharmacists. Educational outcomes, goals, and objectives for a drug information PGY2 pharmacy residency. Bethesda, MD; 2008 [cited 2017 Mar 15]. Available from: https://www.ashp.org/-/media/assets/professional-development/residencies/docs/pgy2-drug-information.ashx?la=en&hash=32836B4FCF65E23774CDD25C6947374C652D0F90.

Chapter Twenty-Four

Drug Information in Ambulatory Care

Suzanne M. Surowiec

Learning Objectives

After completing this chapter, the reader will be able to

- Describe the importance of drug information provided by the health care professional in the ambulatory care setting.
- Discuss the importance of access to up-to-date formulary information in the provision of care in the ambulatory setting.
- Identify sources with links to full-text evidence-based practice guidelines.
- Describe desired characteristics of drug information resources specific to the ambulatory care environment.
- Describe reputable drug information resources geared toward the health care professional that are also useful in providing drug information to patients.
- List ways that practitioners may address concerns regarding access to information.
- Discuss the importance of providing drug information regarding disposal of unused, unwanted, or expired medications.
- Identify appropriate resources to obtain immunization information.
- Identify resources providing quality assurance indicators for optimal provision of ambulatory care.

Key Concepts

❶ The clinician in the ambulatory care setting routinely utilizes multiple drug information skills on a daily basis to not only provide drug information to patients and other health care providers, but to function competently and efficiently within this practice setting.

❷ The ambulatory care practitioner is the individual with the greatest opportunity to fill the role of medication information provider and interpreter to the lay public.

❸ Knowledge of formulary status of medications is only one part of the prescription decision-making process. Whenever they exist, evidence-based clinical practice guidelines should guide prescriptive decision making.

❹ Ambulatory care practitioners have the responsibility to remain up-to-date regarding current practice guidelines.

❺ Increasingly more medical literature, including tertiary references, is being provided in the electronic or Internet-based format, and such references are attractive to utilize in ambulatory care for multiple reasons.

❻ Ambulatory care clinicians bear a responsibility to educate patients on the proper disposal of unused and unwanted medications and should therefore be aware of pertinent sites for information.

❼ While ambulatory care clinicians (in particular, pharmacists) typically recommend and/or dispense most medications, immunizations are medications that are _administered_ in the ambulatory care setting. Those practitioners immunizing in this setting have the obligation to not only provide these services safely, but to serve as immediate sources of information (i.e., drug information) regarding the medications they are administering.

❽ Health care professionals involved in providing patient care in the ambulatory care setting should familiarize themselves with the pertinent, established quality measures.

Introduction

This chapter covers a long list of drug information topics and skills specific to the ambulatory care setting, although not every clinician will use all of these skills on a daily basis. ❶ _The clinician in the ambulatory care setting routinely utilizes multiple drug information skills on a daily basis to not only provide drug information to patients and other health care providers, but to function competently and efficiently within this practice setting._

The ambulatory care practitioner is required to use a variety of drug information skills and resources during routine encounters with patients to provide information at a personalized and appropriate level. Before doing so, the practitioner must know where to look for appropriate information, and how to interpret and practically apply this information to a specific patient or population.

It is commonly recognized that patients are technologically savvy and utilize the Internet and news media to provide self-care in the outpatient setting. The quality of the medical and drug information that patients obtain themselves varies widely, depending on the source (see Chapters 4 and 5 for drug literature evaluation); however, even when quality information is obtained by a patient or family member, someone with clinical expertise and drug information training is necessary to explain medical information and to provide guidance in the decision-making process.

Moreover, with increasing numbers of team-based patient care models, such as the **patient-centered medical home** (PCMH), in existence across the country, the provision of accurate, comprehensive drug information in the ambulatory setting is growing exponentially. Thus, it is crucial to (a) research appropriate medical treatment, especially of chronic conditions, (b) bridge the gap between data provided from health information technology and how to most effectively use this data to treat patients on an individual and on a population-based basis, and (c) educate patients on their treatment.

This chapter will discuss the resources and skills commonly needed by the ambulatory care practitioner to provide appropriate drug information. Topics covered will include (a) commonly used references for prescription formularies and for obtaining evidence-based guidelines, (b) desired characteristics of drug information resources and examples of those particularly useful to the ambulatory care clinician, (c) information resources pertinent to the current trends in ambulatory care, such as the proper disposal of unused, unwanted, or expired medications, (d) preventive health information (specifically regarding immunizations), and (e) quality assurance measures in ambulatory care.

Ambulatory care encompasses a variety of settings. For example, an ambulatory care practitioner may be a clinician who practices in a community pharmacy (including persons in medication-dispensing roles), a clinic or physician's office, an outpatient setting of an institutional care facility, or someone who provides onsite services within an employer-provided wellness and disease management program. As such, the case scenarios within this chapter include examples where the practitioner is in a medication-dispensing role as well as where the practitioner is in a non-dispensing role.

Providing Drug Information in the Ambulatory Care Setting

"I CAN JUST GOOGLE® IT MYSELF"

Given the name of a medication, the average layperson may well be able to Google® the name of the drug, and would very likely find general information regarding its use and side effects. Blogs regarding the experiences of other people taking that medication may also be easily found, as well as anecdotal comments about the drug and the condition being treated, including outdated information. The average patient is, in fact, able to access a plethora of information via websites and blogs; however, the reliability, accuracy, and timeliness of this information can vary widely, as discussed in Chapter 3. While some of these sources of drug information may be reputable, they are impersonal and can only offer general information to the reader. Such sites typically advise patients to talk with their practitioner for specific personal questions. For example, clinicians usually have experience with other patients using a particular medication; practitioners can speak to the fact that an adverse effect may be listed online, but the patients they have encountered have never experienced said side effect. In contrast, these practitioners may be able to justify an adverse effect being caused from a medication that the patient did not correlate to that specific drug. As one can see, Google® cannot always provide such patient-specific information as well as the clinical judgment needed for optimal medical care.

WHAT SHOULD THE PUBLIC (OR OTHER HEALTH CARE PROVIDERS) KNOW ABOUT UTILIZING CLINICIANS TRAINED IN DRUG INFORMATION VERSUS PERFORMING THEIR OWN SEARCHES?

In today's environment, with direct-to-consumer advertising (see Chapter 23) and increasing numbers of nonprescription medications that were formerly available only by prescription, the decision to use a medication is not made solely by prescribers but also by patients themselves. It is evident that all decision makers need guidance. Who guides these decision makers?

Health care providers fill an important role in the provision, interpretation, perspective on clinical application, and perhaps most importantly, providing patient-specific application of drug information that is often targeted toward the layperson by the media. While there is an ever-increasing trend toward patient empowerment, self-care, and self-education, the lay public is often unaware that the health care provider has access not only to the same websites as the patient, but also to professional literature and databases (see Chapter 3) that expand and often provide critical analysis of the information the public accesses. The layperson is unable to access or interpret such information. Depending on their clinical training, even certain health care providers may also lack knowledge regarding available resources and how to best interpret health information data, making it necessary to improve clinical training in this area, where necessary.

❷ *The ambulatory care practitioner is the individual with the greatest opportunity to fill the role of medication information provider and interpreter to the lay public.*

Although in some cases individuals may be able to personally access secondary or even primary literature, interpreting this information and putting it into context with their personal health conditions as well as with current evidence-based guidelines (see Chapter 8) requires a health care professional trained in drug information. Interpreting and evaluating primary literature (see Chapters 4 and 5) as well as locating and interpreting evidence-based guidelines are skills that require training and practice. Pharmacists are the health care professionals with the greatest amount of time devoted to this in their professional training. As such, this profession bears the responsibility to educate both the public and fellow health care providers. Examples of this type of education in the ambulatory setting may include:

- ensuring that biased sources such as pharmaceutical representatives are not the main source of new product education for prescribers
- leading or facilitating discussions with prescribers regarding newly published studies, meta-analyses, and clinical guidelines, with emphasis on understanding limitations of these publications and how they apply specifically to those prescribers' patient populations
- researching and answering drug information questions (which may or may not be patient-specific)
- writing newsletters regarding topics pertinent in the media or in the condition-specific clinic(s) in which the pharmacist works
- "debunking" misperceptions that may arise from direct-to-consumer-advertising regarding exaggerated efficacy or risk associated with treatments
- providing basic statistical training, including terms such as relative risk versus actual risk of treatments, and how to determine them (see Chapter 6).

In addition, in order to provide patient-specific drug information, complete medication profiles must be obtained, and this often involves communication between not only outpatient/ambulatory care clinics, but with one or more pharmacies to get the full picture regarding all pertinent medical conditions and medications (medication reconciliation).

In today's busy society, the case for the pharmacist (and subsequent pharmacist-provided drug information) needs to be concise and to the point. Until that case is made to the public and other payers for health care, including both employers and legislators, so that pharmacists can get provider status and be reimbursed for ambulatory care services, it is likely that pharmaceuticals will continue to have the unintended effect of increasing, rather than decreasing morbidity and mortality, and contributing to rising health care expenditures in at least some patients. To further assist in decreasing morbidity and mortality, pharmacists are actively pursuing provider status to be able to improve quality of life and health outcomes of patients. Studies and practice-based experiences have shown that when pharmacists are involved as members of the health care team, patient outcomes improve and health care costs are reduced.[1]

The following section discusses resources integral to the provision of drug information in ambulatory care.

Drug Information Responsibilities in Ambulatory Care

Integral drug information-related responsibilities of the ambulatory care clinician are many. Several key responsibilities include but are not limited to:

- assisting prescribers and consumers to find the most cost-effective and safe drug to treat a given condition,
- ensuring a prescribed medication is appropriate and follows current treatment guidelines,
- ensuring a patient's understanding of the appropriate use of their medications,
- guiding others regarding the proper disposal of unused or unwanted medications,
- delivering preventive health information, and
- incorporating quality assurance indicators into daily practice.

Practitioners who may not be the initial prescribers of medications (e.g., those who work under consult or collaborative practice agreements or who work with supervisory physicians or collaborating physicians) must be familiar with this information. Regardless of the location in which a clinician practices, and regardless of health care provider degree (e.g., Doctor of Pharmacy, Bachelor of Science in Pharmacy, Physician Assistant, Certified Registered Nurse Practitioner), sound recommendations regarding modifications in drug therapy, drug therapy renewal, and initial drug therapy recommendations all hinge upon a solid understanding of drug formularies, appropriate practice guidelines, and drug information database considerations.

DRUG FORMULARY INFORMATION

A major key to assisting prescribers and consumers in finding the most cost-effective treatment is familiarity with drug **formularies**. Whether a clinician is prescribing or filling a prescription order, formulary restrictions influence **medication usage patterns**. With a prescription insurance plan, a formulary is typically a list of medications that are approved to be paid for or provided at a discounted rate by the plan. It is important to note that even if a medication is not included on a formulary (i.e., is considered "non-formulary"), or is not listed as a preferred option by the payer for a patient's prescription drugs, the prescriber is *not* bound to this when deciding whether to prescribe the medication, and nothing prohibits the pharmacist from filling an appropriate medication for a patient, *regardless* of its formulary status.

Additionally, there are some medications that, while on formulary, may require prior authorization from the insurance company before it will be paid for. That does not mean it cannot be dispensed—it only means that if the patient wants the insurance company to pay for the medication, additional information must be provided in advance regarding the medical need. The pharmacist plays an integral role in working with the prescriber on a patient's behalf to obtain an insurance company's authorization to fill a prescription for such a medication.

What formulary status ultimately affects is the amount the patient will personally pay for a medication, and thus the patient's adherence to therapy. Several useful resources exist to assist in determining formulary restrictions and then making decisions as to risks versus benefits of abiding by these restrictions.

Centers for Medicaid and Medicare Services (CMS)

The CMS is a government agency within the U.S. Department of Health and Human Services that is responsible for the administration of the U.S. Medicare and Medicaid services, through which medical and prescription benefits are derived for select components of the populations, *traditionally* for the poor, elderly, and disabled. Historically, private insurances have modeled reimbursement structures for medical and medicine-related costs after the CMS model. The Affordable Care Act has resulted in increasing numbers of persons who in the past were either uninsured or underinsured (without adequate prescription insurance to cover medical-related costs) to now being insured through either Medicaid or other government-mandated programs, although it is uncertain whether even further changes are coming. In other words, the landscape of prescription coverage has changed in recent years, and many patients' prescription constraints have shifted from those related to personal finance to those related to formulary restrictions.

In addition, it remains a fact that the largest proportion of the population taking prescription medications are already Medicare recipients. These persons' drug coverage is provided through a component of Medicare called Medicare Part D. Through this program, various insurances provide government-funded prescription coverage for Medicare recipients. Each insurance company has a different formulary or list of drugs that are provided at a reduced price to Medicare recipients. As such, understanding formularies and their restrictions as well as the ability to access Medicare drug plan (i.e., Medicare Part D) formulary information is paramount.

Although many patients may select their own Medicare drug provider and plan, others often look to a health care professional to assist them in this decision. Drug plan selection is done largely online and is based on a patient's prescription profile as well as geographic location. A pharmacist is an ideal person to assist with this process as this is the provider likely to be most familiar with various drug classes listed on drug plan formularies as well as acceptable over-the-counter and generic alternatives to specific medications. Information to guide selection is available at http://www.medicare.gov and clicking on the link to "Find health and drug plans," https://www.medicare.gov/find-a-plan/questions/home.aspx. Users choose their state of residence, by entering their zip code, and enter their prescription drug profile (i.e., the list of prescriptions the patient takes). The program will then provide a list of Medicare Part D plans that include some or all of the medications the patient takes, as well as information regarding the status of each medication in a particular plan, and the number of pharmacies that participate with a plan in a given state. Users, including prescribers, can also download complete formularies, as well as appeals and exceptions forms. These are forms that may be completed, usually by the prescriber, on behalf of the patient asking for consideration of payment for a drug due to extenuative circumstances or a situation specific to that patient. This website can be used by patients alone or may be used by a provider on behalf of the patient. Additionally, it is useful for the provider needing to complete necessary forms for patients requiring a medication not covered on their formulary plan. Finally, although not required to prescribe for medications on a patient's specific drug plan, providers may use the site to determine if a drug will be paid for, and if not, if there are acceptable therapeutic alternatives that will be covered.

An additional method for obtaining formulary information via the Internet is by typing the name of the prescription insurance provider + formulary + the calendar year you desire (e.g., 2018) in the Internet search engine (e.g., Google®, Bing™). Most prescription providers will have webpages that include (1) a full formulary guide, (2) a list of covered medications listed by drug name or by drug class, (3) **medication tier status** in which participants are subject to varying levels of co-payment options for a given medication depending on its formulary status, (4) links to suggested alternatives to a medication if it is not covered, and (5) links for forms necessary for prior approval, appeals, and exceptions. An advantage to using these websites is immediate access to information and necessary forms. Each insurance provider, however, will have a different webpage design and there is often not consistency as to where the user will find such information.

Electronic Prescribing Platforms

Electronic prescribing (e-prescribing) is a prescriber's ability to electronically send an accurate, error free, and understandable prescription directly to a pharmacy from the point of care, which is an important element in improving the quality of patient care.[2] Clinicians with prescribing privileges should note that e-prescribing platforms provide drug and formulary information at the point of care. In a 2008 study conducted by the Agency for Healthcare Research and Quality (AHRQ) and published in the Archives of Internal Medicine, prescribers utilizing e-prescribing platforms with **formulary decision supports** (FDS) were significantly more likely to prescribe tier 1 medications, with resulting significant potential cost savings.[3] Chang and associates[4] evaluated over 21,000 prescriptions for just over 1 year, and reported in 2010 that generic drug use was 6% higher, formulary drug use was 3% higher, and cost savings for the payer and prescription drug member was over 17% higher for those prescriptions electronically prescribed. It is important to note that electronic prescribing has now become a mandate to avoid penalty fees from CMS for Medicare patients, so the majority of health care practitioners should have access to an electronic prescribing platform in their practice. While this feature can be beneficial, it is not always accurate; insurance information for medical coverage is oftentimes included in the electronic medical record, but prescription coverage/insurance can be missing.

Some pharmacy apps/databases also contain formulary information. See the section entitled "A Review of Selected Drug Information Resources for the Ambulatory Care Clinician" for further details.

❸ *Knowledge of formulary status of medications is only one part of the prescription decision-making process. Whenever they exist, evidence-based clinical practice guidelines should guide prescriptive decision making.*

CURRENT PRACTICE GUIDELINE INFORMATION

It is beyond the scope of this chapter to discuss in depth the development and the interpretation of evidence-based clinical practice guideline recommendations (see Chapter 8). It is important to note, however, that ❹ *ambulatory care practitioners have the responsibility to remain up-to-date regarding current practice guidelines.* No individual can be expected to know the current treatment guidelines for every condition; however, clinicians can and should be expected to be able to retrieve this information quickly and efficiently. The following sections outline several sources for such retrieval.

Open-Access Databases

Typically, government-sponsored organizations such as Centers for Disease Control and Prevention (CDC), National Heart, Lung, and Blood Institute (NHLBI), and National Cancer Institute (NCI) publish clinical practice guidelines on their websites for free. Some of these guidelines are also available in mobile applications (apps), which may be most useful to ambulatory care practitioners. The CDC website includes free mobile apps (compatible with Apple® and Android®) for a variety of medical conditions, available at http://www.cdc.gov/mobile/mobileapp.html.

Clinicians searching for current practice guidelines may also wish to visit the National Guideline Clearinghouse (NGC) at http://guidelines.gov. This compilation of evidence-based clinical practice guidelines is a project of the AHRQ, Silverchair, and ECRI Institute. The NGC includes links to full-text current treatment guidelines, guidelines in process, as well as archived guidelines. Side-by-side comparison of two or more treatment guidelines for a given condition is also available. Users may search this site by disease/condition, by treatment/intervention, or by organization.[5] If Internet or Wi-Fi access (depending on practice location) is not readily available, users can download guidelines, often at no cost, in HTML format to their personal handheld devices for quick reference.

Clinicians in this situation may wish to consider downloading treatment guidelines that they most commonly refer to in their particular practice, checking regularly for updates. The NCG website also provides links to the websites of various guideline developers (e.g., American Academy of Dermatology, American Academy of Family Physicians) for those which have mobile-device-friendly formats of their guidelines.

- Health Services Technology Assessment Texts (HSTAT) (http://www.ncbi.nlm.nih .gov/books/NBK16710/) via the National Library of Medicine is a useful source for locating several evidence-based summaries and reports.

- The Turning Research Into Practice (TRIP) database (http://www.tripdatabase.com) and PubMed® (https://www.ncbi.nlm.nih.gov/pubmed/) are great resource for locating pertinent and current practice guidelines; they allow the user to establish (for free) a user account, and the viewer can filter searches to include review articles (which may include clinical practice guidelines). However, the guidelines may or may not be accessible in full text, depending on the specific subscription that the practitioner's institution has. Those that do not provide full-text article links provide full citations.[6]

Professional Associations' Websites

- Many health professions organizations publish links to current, pertinent practice guidelines in full text on their websites. For example, American Diabetes Association (ADA) guidelines, the current American College of Cardiology/American Heart Association (ACC/AHA) guidelines on the treatment of blood cholesterol to reduce atherosclerotic cardiovascular risk in adults, and the current Joint National Committee (JNC) guidelines for the treatment of hypertension are available on the websites without any subscription. Clinicians who may work primarily with a specialized population may wish to tailor the organizations' websites and downloads to those pertinent to their area of practice. The American Society of Health-Systems Pharmacists (ASHP) also provides links to their Best Practice policies and treatment guidelines (https://www.ashp.org/Pharmacy-Practice/ Resource-Centers). The American Pharmacists Association (APhA) also provides links from its website to select practice guidelines (http://www.pharmacist.com).

Subscription-Based Databases

- MEDLINE® (which is partially available via PubMed), EMBASE, and the Cochrane Database of Systematic Reviews indexing systems are excellent resources for retrieving clinical practice guidelines; however, they require subscriptions and familiarity with the search techniques in order to yield optimal results. The reader should refer to Chapters 3 and 8 for a more detailed description of each of these, as well as other databases that may be utilized when searching for clinical practice guidelines. Of note, the most effective search term may be *practice guideline* in the publication type field of various search pages. An additional useful search term may be *treatment guideline*.

Case Study 24-1

Dr. Miller, an internal medicine physician that works with you, the clinical ambulatory care pharmacist, approaches you with a drug information question. "Can you help me? I am trying to find updated guidelines for the treatment of psoriasis for one of my patients. I don't treat this condition very often, so I want to know what my drug therapy options are?"

• *Where would you direct Dr. Miller to look to obtain current treatment guidelines?*

DESIRED CHARACTERISTICS OF DRUG INFORMATION RESOURCES IN THE AMBULATORY SETTING

❺ *Increasingly more medical literature, including tertiary references, is being provided in the electronic or Internet-based format, and such databases are attractive to utilize in ambulatory care for multiple reasons.*

- **Easy access:** Electronic databases are easily accessible, which is of utmost importance, as ambulatory care may take place in clinics or pharmacies that are part of the same health system, but located in multiple locations.
- **Frequent update:** Electronic databases tend to be updated more easily and frequently, with new drug updates and pertinent changes in patient and disease management versus print copies of drug information that may outdate quickly.
- **Efficient retrieval:** Electronic drug information databases are more quickly and easily searched for specific topics pertinent to a given patient, and often utilize hyperlinks or search functions.
- **Appropriate level of information:** Recall that, as reviewed in Chapter 3, regardless of the format (electronic versus print), patient education materials should contain language that is directed either toward the patient, parent, or caregiver, and be written at an appropriate reading level. It is recommended that databases specify the reading level of patient education material.

Examples of particularly useful databases are provided below.

A REVIEW OF SELECTED DRUG INFORMATION RESOURCES FOR THE AMBULATORY CARE CLINICIAN

The following is a brief overview of selected resources that (a) are available electronically and as apps for Apple® and Android® devices, (b) are primarily geared toward the health care professional and are also particularly useful to the ambulatory care practitioner, (c) provide in-depth drug and alternative product monographs, and (d) provide useful patient-oriented material. More detailed information on these resources can be found in Chapter 3.

Clinical Pharmacology®

Available as an online subscription through Elsevier Gold Standard, http://www.clinical pharmacology.com, this database includes MedCounselor® Consumer Drug Information Sheets that are available in both English and Spanish, and includes the date of last revision of any given patient education sheet. MedCounselor® Sheets are available via hyperlinks from drug monographs or by searching by drug product under a patient education tab within the site. This product includes patient education materials written at a 6th to 8th grade reading level regarding prescription, nonprescription, and some herbal medications.

In addition to this information geared toward the consumer, this database also includes clinical calculators, manufacturer contact information, normal laboratory reference values, drug class overviews, clinical comparison reports, and convenience charts (e.g., meds that should not be split, meds that interact with grapefruit juice). Information on complementary and alternative medicine (CAM) is also found in this database. This may be of particular value in the ambulatory setting as these patients are most likely to be concurrently taking or inquiring about CAM in addition to their prescription medications.

Drug Facts and Comparisons®

Available through Wolters Kluwer, http://www.factsandcomparisons.com, the electronic version of this database, http://online.factsandcomparisons.com, utilizes MedFacts Patient Information®, which provides customizable patient information in both English and Spanish for over 4,000 brand and generic drugs, and includes some herbal medication patient education materials. The reading level is written at the 8th grade level or below, with the date of last issue clearly provided on each education sheet.

In addition, the ambulatory care clinician can find within this database: clinical calculators, comparative data tables and comparative efficacy tables within drug classes, a "don't crush/chew" list of medications, a drug identifier tool, drug interactions tool, immunization schedules, and even information regarding patient assistance programs for those patients experiencing difficulty affording their medication(s). Additional information on medication use during pregnancy and lactation, natural medicines, and toxicology treatment guidelines (e.g., for overdose treatment or for reversal of effects of medications) is also available within this database.

● Epocrates®

Many clinicians may be familiar with Epocrates®, Inc. software programs (http://www.epocrates.com/). Epocrates®, Inc. markets programs with a variety of content areas including calculations, continuing medical education, diagnostics, a medical dictionary, disease state information, drugs, drug identification, medical news, and tables. These content areas are bundled into various data packages, some of which are free. All Epocrates® programs, including those that are available at no cost, include both national and regional formulary information, including Medicare Part D. Users can access formulary status and restrictions for over 3,300 brand and generic medications. Users of these programs select the formulary or formularies they desire to include in their searches. Epocrates®, Inc. updates formulary information at least once per week.[7]

Epocrates® accounts may be established on the Internet, but for those practitioners who work with limited Internet access, these programs are downloadable to handheld electronic devices (e.g., tablets and smartphones). This program may prove to be a practical solution for providers who require timely formulary information and who operate without full Internet access.

● Lexicomp® Online

Available as an online subscription through Wolters Kluwer, http://www.wolterskluwercdi.com/lexicomp-online/, Lexicomp® Online incorporates an Internet-based platform to provide not only the electronic version of information found in Lexicomp's Drug Information Handbook, but, depending on the subscription purchased, may also include information from AHFS® Drug Information reference and prescription drug plans including information regarding pricing, formulary status, and prior authorization status. Of particular interest to the ambulatory clinician, this resource includes links within drug monographs to Patient Education Modules (PEM).

PEM delivers patient-specific education regarding a particular medication, disease, condition, or procedure. Condition and procedure information is available in either English or Spanish, with medication leaflets available in up to 19 different languages. PEM are also available for select natural products. Patient information is written at a 5th to 7th grade reading level, and may be personalized and printed for distribution to the patient.[8] The practitioner specifies whether a PEM is for an adult or pediatric patient, with pediatric information written toward the parent or caregiver.

● Micromedex® Healthcare Series' Detailed Drug Information for the Consumer™

Available as an online subscription through Truven Health Analytics, www.micromedex.com, the Micromedex Patient Connect Suite® includes educational resources written at a 3rd to 7th grade reading level in up to 15 languages that may be delivered in multiple media formats (e.g., written, video, interactive tools, and more). This suite of resources is intended for use by not only retail and hospital pharmacists, physicians, and nurses, but also patient education program coordinators.[9]

Separate tabs contain information within this database regarding drug interactions, drug identification, calculators, and toxicology/drug effect reversal. The toxicology section may be of particular interest to clinicians in an ambulatory setting who work with high-risk medications such as anticoagulants (e.g., warfarin) or insulin products.

CareNotes™ System

Also available via a subscription by Truven Health Analytics, http://www.micromedex.com, the CareNotes® System enables the clinician to provide customizable patient education documents (in 15 different languages, confirmed to be written at a 6th to 8th grade reading level in English and Spanish). These documents may address general health condition information, pre-procedure or pre-surgical information, and information regarding inpatient and discharge care for patients, laboratory test information, and a section titled DrugNotes, which includes patient-directed drug information for both prescription and nonprescription medications.[13]

In addition, of use to the ambulatory care provider in particular, this database includes drug identification, toxicology management, drug comparison tables, clinical calculators, and even pricing and manufacturing information in medical *devices* and select diagnostic equipment (e.g., blood glucose monitors).

Medscape®

Medscape®, www.medscape.com, provides a very comprehensive set of tools to assist clinicians in practice. This database contains a drug reference, drug interaction checker, medical calculators, disease and condition reference, procedure reference, as well as formulary information. There are almost 2,000 insurance plans, covering all 50 states, included to assist with comparison of tier drug status for patients. Furthermore, Medscape® also includes medical news, continuing education to support professional development for medical providers, and links to the MEDLINE® database to review journal articles and clinical evidence.

Natural Medicines®, Pharmacist's Letter®, and Prescriber's Letter®

All published by Therapeutic Research Center, subscriptions to each of these publications are available electronically, may be downloaded to electronic handheld devices, and may be of great value, especially in the ambulatory care setting.

Natural Medicines®

Natural Medicines® (https://naturalmedicines.therapeuticresearch.com) (subscription required), provides evidence-based information regarding complementary, alternative, integrative medicine, and natural medicines. The database, which combined former Natural Standard® with Natural Medicines Comprehensive Database®, provides full monographs with evidence-based ratings, safety ratings, and interaction ratings based on currently available literature. Natural Medicines® includes a useful natural product/drug interaction checker, and patient handouts written in both English and Spanish.[10]

Of use to the ambulatory clinician, enabling frank discussion of the risk versus benefit of complementary or natural medicines is an "efficacy" rating, which rates each natural medication on the likelihood of its being effective for a given condition, coined the NMBER™ (Natural Medicines Brand Evidence-based Rating). Information regarding perioperative use of natural medications is also available.

Pharmacist's Letter® and Prescriber's Letter®

Pharmacist's Letter® (http://pharmacistsletter.com) and Prescriber's Letter® (http://prescribersletter.com) (subscription required), provide detailed information regarding traditional prescription and nonprescription medication, including full monographs with evidence-based ratings, safety rating, and interactions based on currently available literature. The main difference between these two databases is the target audience. These publications cover new developments in drug therapy and trends in pharmacy practice, concise updates, and advice regarding current therapeutic issues with links to a detail document with a more in-depth explanation of the topic. These publications also include very useful comprehensive disease-, medication-, and practice-related charts. For example, ambulatory care clinicians may find comparison charts for statins, insulin products, injectable anticoagulants, anticipated availability of first-time generics, etc. Links for treatment guidelines for a variety of commonly treated conditions are also available (e.g., cardiology, diabetes, gastroenterological conditions, asthma, COPD). A "Rumor vs. Truth" section may also be of use for quick reference when fielding questions from the public on misstated facts or exaggerated efficacy claims in the media, for example.

● ACCESS CONSIDERATIONS

Because of increasing amounts of current drug information available exclusively online, or for which online access provides regularly updated information not otherwise available, it is strongly recommended that all providers of drug information and direct patient care have access to Internet-based information in order to ethically, accurately, and competently perform their responsibilities. Health care providers and employers should ensure that this is available to those providing medical information to others.

Practitioners may also note that by partnering with colleges of pharmacy or medicine to provide experiential education to students, they may expand their access to drug information databases to which the college subscribes, depending on subscription limitations.

PATIENT EDUCATION

The preceding sections (e.g., practice guidelines, desired characteristics of databases, and other drug information resources) address the role of the ambulatory care provider in researching appropriate medical treatment and using this data to treat patients on an individual basis. This section focuses on yet another important aspect to ambulatory drug information: educating patients on the appropriate use of their medications. Certainly documents generated from the databases outlined above, manufacturer-provided patient information leaflets, and direct patient counseling at the pharmacy all serve to educate patients on intended use(s), cautions, possible side effects, and required monitoring for each medication, but this is not enough. Ambulatory care clinicians fill an important role in educating patients regarding the proper *administration* of certain medications (e.g., insulin, inhalers, injectable anticoagulants), the *management* of adverse reactions (e.g., hypoglycemia, bleeding), and dosing adjustments that may be required such as during perioperative periods or during periods of illness. While most of this information may be found within the individual drug information databases (e.g., how to reverse the effects of hypoglycemia caused by excess insulin or how to reverse the effects of warfarin), it is not always included in patient education materials, and must be **taught to the patient.** Additionally, for those medications that require specific administration technique, providing patients with written instructions is not enough.

Hands-on demonstration and teach-back communication is vital to ensuring medications are used optimally. Manufacturers of drug products that require special administration typically provide patient handouts for this purpose. The CDC website, http://www.cdc.gov, also has useful videos as well as tutorial sheets (e.g., asthma inhaler use, how to check blood glucose), which may be modified or used "as-is." Finally, for the condition of interest, there are often topic-specific patient education materials available from a national website for the disorder being treated. For example, http://www.diabetes.org includes links for recognizing and treating hypoglycemia, for testing blood glucose, and for "sick-day" management. Information obtained from any of these places, however, must be explained, tailored to the patient and the situation, and even demonstrated (e.g., glucose monitor, insulin pen) for the patient; ambulatory clinicians fill an important role in the provision of this type of drug information.

Case Study 24–2

Consider the following scenario:

Claire Collins, PharmD, is working in an outpatient anticoagulation clinic at a local physician's office, when PP, a Hispanic man in his mid-60s who takes warfarin for atrial fibrillation stops by to report a new medication and to confirm it is "okay" to take with his warfarin. PP states that "I'm always nervous about taking any new medication! I just filled the prescription and it was really expensive—they told me it "wasn't on formulary," whatever that means." After some discussion, Dr. Collins discovers that PP has been experiencing arthritis pain for the last month and saw his family doctor today who prescribed him celecoxib.

- *In addition to asking Dr. Collins to check for a drug interaction between warfarin and celecoxib, what drug information questions has PP either requested or implied he needs to know?*
- *How might Dr. Collins begin to answer each of these questions?*

The patient (PP) requires the ambulatory care pharmacist to assist with several drug information queries. Before leaving the clinic, PP now asks for any information available (in addition to the leaflet stapled to the prescription bag he picked up at the pharmacy) regarding his new prescription. PP further requests that, if possible, he would like information in Spanish, as it is easier for him to read health-related information in his first language.

- *What resource database(s) could Dr. Collins refer to with patient information written at an appropriate level? Are there databases that are useful for traditional drug information geared toward the health care professional and that also have information geared toward patient education?*
- *Do any of these databases provide patient information in multiple languages?*

PATIENT DISPOSAL OF UNUSED MEDICATIONS

Near the end of 2014, the Drug Enforcement Administration (DEA) approved allowing community pharmacies to voluntarily take part in drug take-back programs; this allows pharmacies to collect and appropriately dispose of unused medications from patients. This ruling affords patients the option of mailing their unused medications or placing them in pharmacy-maintained collection containers at a pharmacy. These containers can also be found at several local law enforcement agencies.[11] Health care providers can also take the next step and provide drug information to the inquirer regarding the safe and appropriate disposal of medications.

More often than in any other setting, ambulatory care practitioners are asked about disposal of unused or unwanted medications. While there are no specific laws regarding *personal* disposal of medications by patients, disposal of unused or unwanted pharmaceuticals (both prescription and nonprescription) is becoming an emerging and complex environmental issue. In a 2006 survey published in the Journal of the American Board of Family Medicine, of 301 patients surveyed at an outpatient pharmacy, 50% reported storing unused or expired medications and another 50% report they have flushed such medications. Less than 20% of respondents reported having been counseled by a health care provider about the appropriate means of medication disposal.[12] Drug information is often considered the provision of information to patients or health care providers about safe and appropriate use of medications, but it also includes serving as a resource for information about the proper storage and disposal of medications when they are not in use. ❻ *Ambulatory care clinicians bear a responsibility to educate patients on the proper disposal of unused and unwanted medications and should therefore be aware of pertinent sites for finding this information.*

The FDA, http://www.fda.gov, provides consumer health information regarding the disposal of unused medicines and has worked with the White House Office of National Drug Control Policy (ONDCP) to develop consumer guidance regarding this topic. Documents developed by these organizations are available online at the FDA and the ONDCP website.[13,14]

In addition, disposal information for some, but not all, medications may be found on DailyMed, http://dailymed.nlm.nih.gov/dailymed/about.cfm, by searching within monographs in one or more of the following fields: Information for Patients and Caregivers, Patient Information, Patient Counseling Information, Safety and Handling Instructions, or Medication Guide.

Additional useful online resources with information on the safe disposal of medications include those of the Pharmacist's Letter®, http://www.pharmacistsletter.com, and the Institute for Safe Medical Practice (ISMP), http://www.ismp.org. Finally, the Community Medical Foundation for Patient Safety, http://www.comofcom.com/, has developed a very useful document, the National Directory of Drug Take-Back and Disposal Programs.[15] Local and state drug take-back initiative sites may be listed on a case-by-case basis online; however, one site attempts to centralize drug take-back information on a national basis. The Product Stewardship Institute (PSI) addresses appropriate disposal of multiple types of products, including pharmaceuticals, and visitors to the PSI website may research take-back efforts and activities on a state-by-state basis.[16]

There are a select few medications for which flushing *is* the FDA-recommended method of disposal. For these medications, the sentiment of FDA officials is that in order to best protect persons and animals that could inappropriately use these medications, prompt flushing of unused or unwanted medication is the preferred method of disposal.[17] The drugs are listed in Table 24-1.

TABLE 24–1. MEDICATIONS FOR WHICH FLUSHING REMAINS THE FDA-RECOMMENDED METHOD OF DISPOSAL

Medicine	Active Ingredient
Abstral, tablets (sublingual)	Fentanyl
Actiq, oral transmucosal lozenge*	Fentanyl citrate
Avinza, capsule (extended release)	Morphine sulfate
Belbuca, soluble film (buccal)	Buprenorphine hydrochloride
Buprenorphine hydrochloride, tablets (sublingual)*	Buprenorphine hydrochloride
Buprenorphine hydrochloride; Naloxone hydrochloride, tablets (sublingual)*	Buprenorphine hydrochloride; Naloxone hydrochloride
Butrans, transdermal patch system	Buprenorphine
Daytrana, transdermal patch system	Methylphenidate
Demerol, tablets*	Meperidine hydrochloride
Demerol, oral solution*	Meperidine hydrochloride
Diastat/Diastat AcuDial, rectal gel	Diazepam
Dilaudid, tablets*	Hydromorphone hydrochloride
Dilaudid, oral liquid*	Hydromorphone hydrochloride
Dolophine hydrochloride, tablets*	Methadone hydrochloride
Duragesic, patch (extended release)*	Fentanyl
Embeda, capsules (extended release)	Morphine sulfate; Naltrexone hydrochloride
Exalgo, tablets (extended release)	Hydromorphone hydrochloride
Fentora, tablets (buccal)	Fentanyl citrate
Hysingla ER, tablets (extended release)	Hydrocodone bitartrate
Kadian, capsules (extended release)	Morphine sulfate
Methadone hydrochloride, oral solution*	Methadone hydrochloride
Methadose, tablets*	Methadone hydrochloride
Morphabond, tablets (extended release)	Morphine sulfate
Morphine sulfate, tablets (immediate release)*	Morphine sulfate
Morphine sulfate, oral solution*	Morphine sulfate
MS Contin, tablets (extended release)*	Morphine sulfate
Nucynta ER, tablets (extended release)	Tapentadol
Onsolis, soluble film (buccal)	Fentanyl citrate
Opana, tablets (immediate release)	Oxymorphone hydrochloride
Opana ER, tablets (extended release)	Oxymorphone hydrochloride
Oxecta, tablets (immediate release)	Oxycodone hydrochloride
Oxycodone hydrochloride, capsules	Oxycodone hydrochloride
Oxycodone hydrochloride, oral solution	Oxycodone hydrochloride
Oxycontin, tablets (extended release)*	Oxycodone hydrochloride
Percocet, tablets*	Acetaminophen; Oxycodone hydrochloride

continued

TABLE 24–1. MEDICATIONS FOR WHICH FLUSHING REMAINS THE FDA-RECOMMENDED METHOD OF DISPOSAL *(CONTINUED)*

Medicine	Active Ingredient
Percodan, tablets*	Aspirin; Oxycodone hydrochloride
Suboxone, film (sublingual)	Buprenorphine hydrochloride; Naloxone hydrochloride
Targiniq ER, tablets (extended release)	Oxycodone hydrochloride; Naloxone hydrochloride
Xartemis XR, tablets	Oxycodone hydrochloride; Acetaminophen
Xtampza ER, capsules (extended release)	Oxycodone
Xyrem, oral solution	Sodium oxybate
Zohydro ER, capsules (extended release)	Hydrocodone bitartrate
Zubsolv, tablets (sublingual)	Buprenorphine hydrochloride; Naloxone hydrochloride

*These medications have a generic version or are only available as a generic. Updated April 2016.

Case Study 24–3

Abby P., who works in a diabetes and cardiology clinic, is approached by the widow of a former patient. The man is carrying a grocery bag which appears to be full of prescription bottles, insulin pens, and vials. "Can you take these, and perhaps donate or give them to someone who could use them? My wife passed away last month, and I probably have hundreds of dollars' worth of medication in this bag! If you can't use them, can you tell me where I should take them?"

- *Where can unused, unwanted, or expired medications be taken?*
- *If a patient wishes to dispose of medications, are there any associated legal requirements or guidelines?*

DRUG REPOSITORY PROGRAMS

Drug repository programs, which allow nursing homes, long-term care pharmacies, and wholesalers to donate unused medication for redistribution to those patients who meet prespecified criteria, may exist in certain states. While patients understandably may be reluctant to throw away their personal unused or unwanted medications, these medications, once dispensed and in patients' homes, are not eligible for donation to drug repository programs, as these drugs have left the custody and controlled environment of a pharmacy or institution. Practitioners should refer to their respective state's Board of Pharmacy website for information regarding drug repository programs.

PROVIDING IMMUNIZATION INFORMATION

Formerly provided primarily in the traditional clinician's office or in county or city health departments, immunizations are increasingly being delivered by pharmacists and other health care providers in ambulatory care settings, including pharmacies and retail grocery stores. ❼ *While ambulatory care clinicians (in particular, pharmacists) typically recommend and/or dispense most medications, immunizations are medications that are administered in the ambulatory care setting. Those practitioners immunizing in this setting have the obligation to not only provide these services safely, but to serve as immediate sources of information (i.e., drug information) regarding the medications they are administering.*

Sources of Immunization Information

Centers for Disease Control and Prevention

While multiple texts exist regarding immunization and vaccine-preventable disease, the U.S. Department of Health and Human Services CDC website, http://www.cdc.gov, provides the most comprehensive, regularly updated information regarding immunizations. Links are available from the CDC webpage titled Vaccines and Immunizations, http://www.cdc.gov/vaccines, for both the health care provider and for patients that provide up-to-date information regarding vaccine-preventable disease, as well as safety, adverse events, administration schedule, and dosing recommendations for immunizations. Also available from this site are vaccine information statements (VISs), which must be distributed with their respective immunizations.

Epidemiology and Prevention of Vaccine-Preventable Disease

The textbook, commonly referred to as the Pink Book, is published annually by the Public Health Foundation.[18] It provides health care providers such as physicians, nurses, nurse practitioners, physician assistants, and pharmacists comprehensive information regarding vaccine-preventable diseases. The textbook is available for purchase in print; however, PDFs of each chapter are available fully formatted for download from the CDC website. While this text does not provide vaccine-specific information, it provides detailed information regarding respective vaccine-preventable disease, including epidemiology, prevalence, and prevention recommendations.

Immunization Training for the Pharmacist

The prerequisites for pharmacists to administer immunizations vary from state to state, and pharmacists are advised to refer to their state's laws and confer with their state board of pharmacy regarding specific questions; however, in each state that allows for pharmacist-administered vaccines, a training program approved by the state pharmacy board is required. The most widely recognized training program, Pharmacy-Based

Immunization Delivery, is offered nationally by the APhA (http://www.pharmacist.com). Other programs do exist that may be recognized nationally or within specific states only. Pharmacists may wish to inquire with their specific state board of pharmacy regarding recognized and approved training programs. Regardless of the training program initially utilized, it is expected that pharmacists, as well as all other providers of health care, maintain and document appropriate continuing education for the immunizations and the associated drug information they deliver.

QUALITY ASSURANCE CONSIDERATIONS IN AMBULATORY CARE

Quality assurance is one of the key responsibilities of ambulatory care practitioners. While institutions that are under the umbrella of a health care facility generally consider the standards set forth by The Joint Commission as a primary source of quality assurance guidelines, several other organizations provide quality assurance guidelines that may be applied to a variety of care settings.

Via a variety of initiatives, including the **Accountable Care Organizations** (ACOs) model, CMS has specified 33 required **quality measures** that are evaluated to determine payment structure for patient care networks, which are inclusive of ambulatory care settings. The quality measures themselves are standards set forth that evaluate efficiency (or resource use), structure, process, intermediate outcome, long-term outcome, and patient centeredness (which includes patient reports of satisfaction).[19] CMS has also contracted with Florida Medical Quality Assurance, Inc. (FMQAI) in a project particularly pertinent to quality assurance in the ambulatory care setting. The project, Medication Measure Special Innovation Project, is tasked with maintaining the current 33 quality measures and expanding them to include new measures focused on medication-related patient safety (e.g., detecting/preventing medication errors, adverse drug reactions). The project specifically includes a portfolio of six National Quality Forum (NQF)-endorsed measures for the ambulatory care setting, including measures related to patient adherence to specific medication classes, adherence to regular monitoring for warfarin (both routine and when on antibiotics), and adherence of patients with schizophrenia to antipsychotic therapy.

❽ *Health care professionals involved in providing patient care in the ambulatory care setting should familiarize themselves with the pertinent, established quality measures.*

Assuring patient safety is a crucial component of quality care and the ISMP is an important resource for health care providers in any setting. The ISMP publishes four distinct newsletters, each geared toward practitioners in a different health care setting. The ISMP Medication Safety Alert! Community/Ambulatory Care edition is targeted toward pharmacists, pharmacy technicians, nurses, physicians, and other community health professionals. This newsletter is sent monthly as an e-mail, and provides up-to-date information about medication-related errors, adverse drug reactions, and their implications for community practice sites. Finally, the newsletter includes recommendations on how to improve medication safety within the community setting (http://www.ismp.org/Newsletters/default .asp). A subscription to this newsletter is recommended for all ambulatory care providers (ISMP Medication Safety Alert! Community/Ambulatory Care edition). More information regarding ISMP as well as its newsletters can be found at http://www.ismp.org.[20]

Finally, the tracking, reporting, and prevention of not only medication errors, but of "near misses," is paramount to assuring quality in any health care setting, including ambulatory care. ISMP and the National Coordinating Council for Medication Error Reporting and Prevention (NCC MERP) are two organizations dedicated to this task. The reader should refer to Chapter 18 for a complete discussion on organizations and programs devoted to assuring quality by reporting and prevention of medication errors.

The APhA website http://www.pharmacist.com has a Patient Safety and Quality Assurance page that provides links to AHRQ, ISMP, the National Patient Safety Foundation (NPSF), the United States Pharmacopeia (USP) Medication Errors Reporting Form, and the PSPC Collaborative.

Case Study 24-4

Paul, a recent graduate from a college of pharmacy, is working in a private practice ambulatory care clinic where he provides medication recommendations to prescribers and counsels patients regarding disease state management. The manager of the clinic approaches Paul and asks him to become involved in measuring quality assurance indicators for all health care providers in the clinic, including patient satisfaction with the care that has been provided.

- *What type of quality assurance indicators/metrics are utilized by outside organizations?*
- *Is patient satisfaction with care a recognized quality indicator?*
- *Are there published guidelines for quality indicators in ambulatory care?*

Conclusion

As health professionals committed to optimal patient care, the provision of drug information goes far beyond providing patient information leaflets with medications. Application of drug information is performed routinely in the ambulatory care setting in a variety of manners, and it is in this setting that the clinician pulls it all together and takes the most important step—imparting this information not only to patients and their caregivers, but to other health care providers in an understandable, personalized, and practical format that will serve to improve health care.

Self-Assessment Questions

1. **ALL** of the following statements support the need for the skilled provision of drug information in ambulatory care **except:**
   a. There is not a consistent level of drug information education in the curricula of various health care professions.
   b. There is a lack of drug information freely available to the public.
   c. The ambulatory care clinician is able to access databases that may not be available to the public.
   d. A significant number of emergency room visits and hospital admissions each year are attributed to pharmaceuticals.

2. Which of the following best describes the drug information responsibilities of an ambulatory care clinician?
   a. Assisting prescribers and patients find the most cost-effective drug therapy for a given condition
   b. Ensuring a prescribed medication is appropriate and follows current treatment guidelines
   c. Ensuring a patient's understanding of the appropriate use of his/her medications
   d. Guiding individuals regarding the proper disposal of unused or unwanted medications
   e. All of the above

3. Which of the following statements is **TRUE** regarding prescription formularies?
   a. Prescription insurance providers often require cardholder identification information in order to gain full access to formulary information.
   b. Clinician use of electronic prescribing has not been shown to affect the likelihood of prescribing tier 1 medications.
   c. Software programs such as Lexicomp® and Epocrates® include formulary information that can be downloaded to a handheld electronic device.
   d. Medicare Part D participants cannot perform side-by-side comparisons of prescription plans that are available to them and that cover some or all of their medications.

4. Which of the following medication tiers will result in the lowest patient responsibility for payment?
   a. Tier 1 medication
   b. Tier 2 medication
   c. Tier 3 medication
   d. Not covered

5. Evidence-based clinical practice guidelines:
   a. Are used solely by practitioners who develop formularies.
   b. Are accessible without a fee only to practitioners who are members of the organization that developed a given set of guidelines.
   c. Are typically too large to download to most handheld devices.
   d. Are freely available in full text from a variety of government and public Internet sites.

6. A physician would like to know which sources he can utilize to find current practice guidelines for his patient with diabetes. All of the following are appropriate to recommend **EXCEPT**:
   a. National Guideline Clearinghouse (NGC)
   b. American Diabetes Association
   c. Institute for Safe Medical Practice (ISMP)
   d. Centers for Disease Control and Prevention (CDC)

7. Which of the following supports the desirability of electronic drug information resources in the ambulatory setting?
   a. Ambulatory care may be provided in multiple sites by the same organization.
   b. Updates to information are more readily performed.
   c. Electronic databases are conducive to faster and more efficient searches.
   d. More than one of the above.
   e. All of the above.

8. A patient brings to her wellness appointment a variety of herbal supplements that she wants to know more about prior to taking. She requests information about the supplements' efficacy as well as safety. Which of the following databases would **BEST** assist the ambulatory practitioner in answering this patient's inquiries?
   a. Clinical Pharmacology®
   b. Drug Facts and Comparisons®
   c. Natural Medicines®
   d. Micromedex®
   e. Prescriber's Letter®

9. The Pharmacist's Letter® website provides all of the following **EXCEPT**:
   a. Comparison tables for drug classes
   b. Links to medication error reporting databases
   c. Developments in drug therapy
   d. Downloadable documents for handheld devices

10. Which of the following are potential options to increase access to drug information when resources are limited?
   a. Encourage employers to ensure Internet access is available to all those providing medical information to others
   b. Consider partnering resources with a local college of medicine or pharmacy
   c. Utilize the services of a drug information center
   d. All of the above

11. All of the following are recommended by the Food and Drug Administration (FDA) as inappropriate in the disposal of unwanted medications **EXCEPT**:
   a. Flushing unused liquid medications
   b. Mixing medications with cat litter
   c. Burning with other trash
   d. Using a community dumpster

12. Which of the following statements is **FALSE** regarding immunizations?
   a. They are not considered medications
   b. They may be administered by pharmacists
   c. They must be accompanied by a vaccine information statement (VIS) upon administration
   d. They are becoming increasingly available in a variety of community settings including grocery stores and pharmacies

13. Which of the following organizations utilizes reports which include quality indicators as rated by consumers of health care?
   a. Institute for Safe Medical Practice (ISMP)
   b. Centers for Medicare and Medicaid Services (CMS)
   c. Patient Safety Clinical Pharmacy Services (PSPC)
   d. Food and Drug Administration (FDA)

14. Which of the following organizations provides recent drug-related news, drug approvals, recalls and safety warnings, therapeutic equivalency codes, and MedWatch adverse event reporting data?
   a. Centers for Disease Control and Prevention (CDC)
   b. Food and Drug Administration (FDA)

    c. Medscape

    d. White House Office of National Drug Control Policy (ONDCP)

15. Team-based health care delivery led by a physician or other primary care provider and includes multiple other types of providers including pharmacists to optimize patient outcomes is called:

    a. Patient Centered Medical Home (PCMH)

    b. Accountable Care Organization (ACO)

    c. Agency for Healthcare Research and Quality (AHRQ)

    d. Electronic Health Record (EHR)

REFERENCES

1. Provider status: what pharmacists need to know now. American Pharmacists Association. 2013 Aug [cited 2017 Jan 30]. Available from: http://www.pharmacist.com/provider-status-what-pharmacists-need-know-now

2. Centers for Medicare and Medicaid Services. E-prescribing; [updated 2014 Feb 26; cited 2016 Aug 9]. Available from: https://www.cms.gov/Medicare/E-Health/Eprescribing/index.html?redirect=/eprescribing/.

3. Fischer MA, Vogeli C, Stedman M, Ferris T, Brookhart A, Weissman JS. Effect of electronic prescribing with formulary decision support on medication use and cost. Arch Intern Med. 2008;168(22):2433-9.

4. Chang C, Nguyen N, Smith A, Huynh D. Electronic prescribing increases generic and formulary drug use; [updated 2010 Jun 7; cited 2016 Aug 10]. Available from: http://www.physicianspractice.com/articles/electronic-prescribing-increases-generic-and-formulary-drug-use

5. Agency for Healthcare Research and Quality. National Guideline Clearinghouse (NGC) [Internet]. Rockville, MD: Agency for Healthcare Research and Quality; [cited 2017 Feb 11]. Available from: https://www.guidelines.gov/.

6. National Center for Biotechnology Information, U.S. National Library of Medicine, National Institutes of Health. PubMed.gov; [cited 2016 Jul 1]. Available from: http://www.ncbi.nlm.nih.gov/pubmed/.

7. Epocrates®. San Mateo, CA: Epocrates, Inc. 2011 [cited 2016 Jul 1]. Available from: http://www.epocrates.com./products/comparison_table.html

8. Lexicomp ONLINE User Guide. Hudson, OH: Lexicomp™, Inc.; [cited 2016 Jul 1]. Available from: http://online.lexi.com

9. Micromedex Consumer Health Information™. Ann Arbor, MI: Truven Health Analytics Inc.; [cited 2016 Jul 1]. Available from: http://www.truvenhealth.com/your_healthcare_focus/hospital_patient_care_decisions/consumer_engagement.aspx

10. Natural Medicines. Somerville, MA: Therapeutic Research Center; [cited 2016 Jul 1]. Available from: https://naturalmedicines.therapeuticresearch.com/.

11. DEA: Pharmacies can voluntarily participate in take-back programs. American Pharmacists Association; [updated 2014 Oct 1; cited 2017 Jan 30]. Available from: http://www.pharmacist.com/dea-pharmacies-can-voluntarily-participate-take-back-programs

12. Seehusen D, Edwards J. Patient practices and beliefs concerning disposal of medications. J Am Board Fam Med. 2006;19(6):542-7.

13. FDA Consumer Health Information. How to dispose of unused medications; [updated 2013 Dec; cited 2016 Jul 1]. Available from: http://www.fda.gov/downloads/Drugs/ResourcesForYou/Consumers/BuyingUsingMedicineSafely/UnderstandingOver-the-CounterMedicines/ucm107163.pdf

14. Disposal of unused medications: what you should know; [cited 2016 Jul 1]. Available from: http://www.fda.gov/Drugs/ResourcesForYou/Consumers/BuyingUsingMedicineSafely/EnsuringSafeUseofMedicine/SafeDisposalofMedicines/ucm186187.htm

15. Communities now has a resource to get rid of unused and expired medicines from home. News Release; [updated 2011 Sept 16; cited 2016 Jul 1]. Available from: http://www.comofcom.com/News%20Release_National%20Directory%20091611.pdf

16. Product Stewardship Institute. The drug take-back network; [cited 2016 Jul 1]. Available from: http://www.productstewardship.us/page/GoToGuide

17. Medicines recommended for disposal by flushing; [updated 2016 Apr; cited 2016 Jul 1]. Available from: http://www.fda.gov/downloads/Drugs/ResourcesForYou/Consumers/BuyingUsingMedicineSafely/EnsuringSafeUseofMedicine/SafeDisposalofMedicines/UCM337803.pdf

18. Centers for Disease Control and Prevention. Epidemiology and prevention of vaccine-preventable diseases [Internet]. Hamborsky J, Kroger A, Wolfe S, editors. 13th ed. Washington, DC: Public Health Foundation; 2015 [cited 2016 Oct 16]. Available from: http://www.cdc.gov/vaccines/pubs/pinkbook/index.html

19. Centers for Medicaid and Medicare Services. Quality measures and performance standards; [updated 2015 Mar 2; cited 2016 Jul 1]. Available from: http://www.cms.gov/Medicare/Medicare-Fee-for-Service-Payment/sharedsavingsprogram/Quality_Measures_Standards.html

20. ISMP Medication Safety Alert®! Newsletters. Institute for Safe Medical Practice; [cited 2016 Jul 1]. Available from: http://www.ismp.org/Newsletters/default.asp

SUGGESTED READING

1. Centers for Medicare and Medicaid Services. Accountable Care Organizations (ACO); [updated 2015 Jan 6; cited 2016 Jul 1]. Available from: http://www.cms.gov/Medicare/Medicare-Fee-for-Service-Payment/ACO/index.html

Chapter Twenty-Five

Drug Information and Contemporary Community Pharmacy Practice

Morgan L. Sperry • Heather A. Pace

Learning Objectives

After completing this chapter, the reader will be able to

- Discuss limitations of the current approaches pharmacists use to deliver drug information to their patients.
- Compare and contrast patient education and consumer health information (CHI) as drug information sources for patients.
- Define social networking and describe how patients use this tool as a drug information source.
- Discuss mobile health information technology and its impact on how consumers are obtaining information.
- Describe the model for drug information services delivered by pharmacists.
- Design three strategies using electronic media to assist patients in receiving and applying high-quality drug information.
- List 13 characteristics of a high-quality health literate Internet site.
- Define participatory medicine and describe how this model changes the dynamic of the patient and the health care professional.

Key Concepts

❶ The trend for patients to obtain their health information from sources disconnected from health care professionals is not going away and it has shifted relationships between patients and their traditional touchstones in health care, namely physicians, nurses, and pharmacists.

❷ Answering drug information questions is a routine part of a pharmacist's day, but it is too often a passive process that hinges upon the patient's initiative to ask the important questions regarding their health.

❸ Patient education delivers written or verbal drug information through a planned activity initiated by a health care provider. The goal is to change patient behavior, improve adherence, and ultimately improve health.

❹ Consumer health information (CHI) is actively sought by the patient in response to their need for more information about their health. Importantly, CHI is not individualized for a specific patient.

❺ Social media sites allow patients to create content and share information about their health on the Internet.

❻ Wisdom of crowds is a belief that when patients share information about their common conditions through social networking, their collective wisdom is more beneficial than the expert opinion of just one individual.

❼ The use of mobile technology to obtain CHI has experienced a sharp increase within the last few years and continues to skyrocket.

❽ Pharmacists should discuss with their patients why they remain an important source of drug information. Patients should be encouraged not to see CHI as a replacement for actual interaction with a health care provider, but as an extension of care and a way to improve communication.

❾ Patients often have difficulty finding accurate information in response to their specific health concerns on the Internet.

❿ Once patients identify or are given quality health information, they still may face barriers in being able to use it to improve their health.

⓫ The term participatory medicine is a recent movement for a new model of cooperative health care. In this model, patients no longer play a passive part when it comes to their health care but an active role alongside the health care provider. Patients are seen as a valuable health care resource and providers are encouraged to view them as equal partners.

Introduction

Pharmacists' roles and responsibilities continue to evolve in response to changing pharmacy practice acts and a dynamic health care environment. One constant is the pharmacist's key function as a provider of quality, evidence-based drug information. However, pharmacists are not the only source of drug information. Use of the Internet, including social networking sites, and mobile technology has made information from sources other than health care professionals exponentially more accessible. The move toward patient-centered care and consumerism increases the desire for patients to be in control of their health care and be an active part of the decision-making process. ❶ *The trend for patients to obtain their health information from sources disconnected from health care professionals is not going away and it has shifted relationships between patients and their traditional touchstones in health care, namely physicians, nurses, and pharmacists.*[1] Recent surveys suggest 72% of Internet users went online to search for some type of health or wellness information within the past year. In fact, one-third of adults in the United States report going online to self-diagnose their illnesses. This group of people is often referred to as "online diagnosers."[2] The pharmacist's role as drug information expert may also be changing in the eyes of the patient. The clinician still remains a central health information resource for a majority of patients, but the role that friends, family, and peers are playing both offline and online is ever expanding.[3]

Pharmacy practice is moving away from its emphasis on the hands-on drug distribution model toward an emphasis on system management and patient care services.[4,5] It is important for pharmacists to enhance patient care services because of significant expenditures seen with unresolved drug-related problems. Nonadherence to medication therapy was estimated to cost $105 billion annually in direct and indirect costs by the IMS Institute for Healthcare Informatics.[6,7] A key strategy to improve adherence is to improve patients' understanding of their disease and its management, and includes individual needs in the treatment planning. Both strategies require individualized care that is not available from the Internet and other information sources. Pharmacists can remain a valuable drug information source for patients because they are one of the most accessible health care practitioners. Pharmacists can help patients customize information they find on the Internet and from other sources such as social media and mobile health applications. Project Destiny was an initiative introduced in 2008 that encouraged pharmacists to "embrace community pharmacy health care beyond dispensing." Now a historical document, Project Destiny paved the way for improved medication therapy management (MTM) services otherwise known as MTM today. Within the MTM model, a pharmacist's role is not just narrowed to providing health care services related to medications but providing comprehensive health care that optimizes patient outcomes and can contribute to the overall lowering of health care costs.[8] MTM services performed by pharmacists might include performing patient assessment, comprehensive medication reviews, developing a medication treatment plan, monitoring efficacy and safety of medication therapy, emphasizing the importance of medication adherence through patient empowerment and education, and communicating MTM services to prescribers in order to sustain comprehensive patient care. In addition, pharmacists must step up and add drug information services beyond what a patient can find on their own, as well as demand for these services. Pharmacists are well positioned to address these drug information needs as they are medication experts and trusted professionals. In this MTM model, patients should view pharmacists as a key medication advisor. For example, patients will often see results from clinical research on the news or through the Internet. They may not understand how these results relate directly to them and may reconsider continuing their medication. Pharmacists, with their understanding of both the literature and the patient's medical history, can help the patient understand whether these new findings are relevant to their individual situation.

According to a recent survey, 94% of patients selected a specific pharmacy based on location and convenience. When price is not a factor, accuracy and trust provided by the pharmacists were cited as a reason for going to a pharmacy only 9% and 4% of the time, respectively. These results further support the need to develop consumer demand for patient care services.[9] The purpose of this chapter is to shed light on how increased patient demand for autonomy and responsibility over their own health care and use of information sources beyond health professionals impacts pharmacy. Additionally, new models for pharmacists delivering drug information will be addressed.

Pharmacists as Drug Information Providers

Pharmacists are ideally advantaged to provide health information to their patients regarding medications and disease states because of the variety of health care settings they are placed within. Whether it is a long-term care facility, an ambulatory care clinic, a patient's hospital room, or the local pharmacy, pharmacists have the most access and ability to be a patient's primary drug information provider.

In the community setting, pharmacists are required by Omnibus Budget Reconciliation Act of 1990 (OBRA 90) to deliver patient counseling when they dispense a Medicaid prescription.[10] Individual states can and sometimes do mandate that counseling be extended to all patients, irrespective of their insurance. Some pharmacists are very diligent in providing important information to their patients when they pick up a prescription, while others only give information if specifically asked. Patients may be asked by pharmacy staff to electronically sign to decline counseling without being asked whether they want it or not. Some patients do not even know what they are signing. ❷ *Answering drug information questions is a routine part of a pharmacist's day, but it is too often a passive process that hinges upon the patient's initiative to ask the important questions regarding their health.* A variety of reasons make patients reluctant to use their pharmacist as a primary health information resource. Although the most accessible health care professional to patients, pharmacists often may appear too busy and unavailable within the sometimes hectic pharmacy. Technicians or cashiers may be the only staff who speaks directly to the patient. Simply asking whether or not a patient has questions is the wrong way to initiate counseling. Patients may not be sure what they need to know in the first place, or feel embarrassed to admit their lack of knowledge. In some cases, patients are unaware they should be asking questions. Some simply do not understand the impact of pharmacotherapy to their long-term health and well-being and are not invested in learning about the appropriate medication use.

Patient leaflets are just one example why patients may not seek out their pharmacist as a primary health information resource. Instead of direct patient communication, patient leaflets are commonly stapled to the prescription as a substitute for actual patient education. Additionally, many of these leaflets do not adhere to the qualities of good health literacy, making them hard for patients to use as a source of health information. In fact, research has shown that the majority of patients do not even bother reading through the leaflet due to the complex language, small typeface, narrow spacing, and poor design.[11] Additional information on the importance of good health literacy will be discussed later in the chapter.

Some pharmacies have developed websites to direct patients to quality drug information and offer an additional path for patients to ask questions. Many large chain pharmacies and mail-order pharmacies have begun to post answers to the most frequently asked drug information questions for their consumers on their websites and some allow for even more interaction online by giving patients the opportunity to ask their questions to a pharmacist. In addition, these websites also provide general information regarding medications in the form of patient leaflets. It is important to note that while these pharmacies are headed in the right direction in terms of giving patients more readily available access to quality health information online, these websites still have many limitations. Patients enrolled in disease state management and MTM programs require the pharmacist to be engaged in focused and directed patient education as part of a comprehensive treatment plan; something that cannot be done by passive answering of questions or interfacing with a website alone.

Opportunities to provide quality health information to patients also exist for pharmacists working in many other settings. From counseling that occurs during a clinic visit to discharge counseling done at the end of a hospital stay, pharmacists should have face-time with patients in order to ensure the patients understand how to best manage their medications and disease state(s) going forward. Pharmacists also play an important role within the emerging movement toward more effective transitions of care for patients. Moving patients around between various health care settings as their condition and care needs change is often a barrier to providing quality health information. The Joint Commission names ineffective patient education as one of the root causes for why breakdown occurs during the transition of care process. Patients and caregivers often are given conflicting recommendations, complex medication regimens, and confusing instructions on how to follow-up with their care. This is an area where pharmacists can provide an extremely beneficial service within the transitions of care multidisciplinary team.[12]

Patient Sources of Drug Information

The practice of drug information continues to evolve along with the profession. Drug information can be as simple as obtaining information from references, or an interactive experience between a specific patient and the pharmacist.[13] Drug information can be as active as counseling a patient on all of his or her medications and disease states or as passive as a pharmacy technician dispensing a medication leaflet with a prescription. Regardless of how drug information is delivered, patients are in need of a more connected experience when receiving drug information, not only from health care professionals, but from peers.

PATIENT EDUCATION VERSUS CONSUMER HEALTH INFORMATION

Patient education and **consumer health information (CHI)** are two distinct ways patients get information about medications, although the two may merge when pharmacists truly engage their patients. ❸ *Patient education delivers written or verbal drug information through a planned activity initiated by a health care provider. The goal is to change patient behavior, improve adherence, and ultimately improve health.*[14] Pharmacist-driven patient education formats include brief counseling when a patient picks up their medication, more comprehensive education as a part of MTM, point-of-care testing (e.g., blood glucose or cholesterol testing), and health screenings. Patient education can be delivered face-to-face or through a variety of technologies, including the telephone, e-mail, and webcams. The key is that pharmacists interact with individual patients to customize the information to their specific situation.

❹ *CHI is actively sought by the patient in response to their need for more informa-tion about their health. Importantly, CHI is not individualized for a specific patient.* Unlike patient education which is initiated by the pharmacist, CHI is completely patient-driven and has evolved out of the patient's need to be their own advocate. CHI has long been available to patients, but the Internet along with social media and mobile applications accelerated both the access to and the volume of information; the choices are endless for patients seeking their own information. In 2013, at least 60% of U.S. adults had looked online for health information within the past year.[15] For either patient education or CHI to be of any value to the patient, it is crucial that information presented to the patient be of high quality and strength. Controlling quality during a patient education encounter is easier because the health care professional filters information distributed to patients. In contrast, the quality and reliability of CHI are variable.[16] CHI may be of excellent quality and beneficial to the patient, or it may be of high quality but dangerous because it lacks relevance to their situation, be incomplete, or simply be wrong. Table 25-1 lists examples of popular CHI sites.

TABLE 25–1. EXAMPLES OF CONSUMER HEALTH INFORMATION AND SOCIAL MEDIA SITES[17–23]

Consumer Health Platform	Description
Angie's List® (http://www.angieslist.com)	Website tailored to help consumers find high-quality unbiased reviews and recommendations on a variety of services including contractors, service companies, home repair, and health care providers. Allows patients to seek perspectives and opinions from fellow patients who have previously seen certain health care providers in their area. Angie's List maintains that both patient members and health care providers benefit from feedback given. Consumers may choose from several different membership options which include monthly and annual payment plans.
Consumer Reports® (http://www.consumerreportshealth.org)	Requiring a monthly or annual subscription, this online resource provides patients with information and unbiased ratings on topics such as healthy living, conditions and treatments, physicians, insurance companies, natural health, and prescription drugs. Health expert blogs are also provided for subscribers on an array of health topics. The Best Buy Drugs feature of this website was created in 2004 to help patients compare brand prescription drugs against generics and provide consumers with the best medicine to treat their disease state for their money.
Healthfinder (http://www.healthfinder.gov)	A site operated by the Department of Health and Human Services that serves as a gateway to consumer information. The major goal of this site is to improve consumer access to health information via government agencies, their partner organizations, and other trustworthy sources that serve the public interest.

continued

TABLE 25–1. EXAMPLES OF CONSUMER HEALTH INFORMATION AND SOCIAL MEDIA SITES[17–23] *(CONTINUED)*

Consumer Health Platform	Description
Microsoft® HealthVault (http://www.healthvault.com)	Offers patients a way to store their personal or family's health information all in one location. Patients are then given the option to make their health information accessible to personal health care providers. HealthVault works with physicians, pharmacies, insurance providers, hospitals, and employers to ensure ease of adding information electronically to the HealthVault record. The site is also compatible with certain health devices such as blood pressure monitors and heart rate monitors allowing patients to upload important health data and readings straight to their HealthVault. The goal of this website is to provide the consumer with a more complete picture of their overall health and give them an opportunity to make the best informed decision.
PatientsLikeMe® (http://www.patientslikeme.com)	Privately funded social media site that was founded in 2004 with the intent of positively impacting patients diagnosed with life-changing diseases. This site primarily focuses on neurological, neuroendocrine, psychiatric, and immune conditions and is geared toward developing a new system of health care created by patients for patients. Through an online community of physicians, organizations, and patients, patients are encouraged to share information about their disease states, treatments, and overall experiences. The hope is that through this online platform patients will feel more connected to others going through similar circumstances as well as empowered and in more control of their disease state.
Everyday Health® (http://www.everydayhealth.com)	Consumer-centric health company founded to empower and encourage patients to put themselves at the center of their health care. Claims to be a site for comprehensive health and medical information. Free to consumers, the site gears information toward the person they consider the family's chief medical officer (CMO), women, or other caregivers. Blogs, forums, and online communities are available so patients can talk to people just like them.
WebMD® (http://www.webmd.com)	Health website allowing patients to obtain their health information via a variety of different ways. Health information is available on a wealth of different topics such as drugs and treatments, disease states, and prevention. Online communities for patients seeking support or desiring to share their experiences are also set up in the form of blogs, video, and message boards. Additionally patients have access to slide shows, newsletters, FDA consumer updates, symptom checkers, drug identifiers, and ask the expert feature. WebMD has established an Independent Medical Review Board to ensure all health information made available to the public is accurate and timely.

SOCIAL MEDIA

Patients have long used friends, family, coworkers, and support groups as sources of medical information. The Internet adds to these traditional sources through **social media** as described in Table 25-2.[1] **⑤** *Social media sites allow patients to create content and share*

TABLE 25-2. SOCIAL MEDIA DEFINITIONS AND PLATFORMS USED TO OBTAIN HEALTH INFORMATION[1]

Social Media	Definition	Platform Examples	URLs
Wikis	Allows user editing and adding of content via a collaborative website	Wikipedia Flu Wiki	http://www.wikipedia.org http://flu.wikia.com/wiki/Flu_Wiki
Social networks	A website where those with special interests in common can connect and share with one another	Angie's List® PatientsLikeMe® Everyday Health® Facebook Twitter	http://www.angieslist.com http://www.patientslikeme.com http://www.everydayhealth.com http://www.facebook.com http://www.twitter.com
Blogs	An online diary; one can log their personal thoughts on various topics and post to a web page	WebMD® Mayo Clinic	http://www.webmd.com http://www.mayoclinic.com/health/blogs/BlogIndex
Online forums	Thoughts and ideas are shared and open discussion takes place via various mediums such as a website, newspaper, or radio	Everyday Health® Google Health Yahoo! Groups	http://www.everydayhealth.com http://groups.google.com http://groups.yahoo.com
Video-sharing	A medium where information, ideas, and opinions can be shared via videos accessible to many	YouTube	http://www.youtube.com

information about their health on the Internet. Through the power of social media, the Internet goes beyond being merely a search engine and a source of information to a platform to create, share, and collaborate in developing new knowledge. Social networking is the phenomenon of online communities in which people share interests and/or activities with one another and has become an essential part of why patients are flocking to these sites. With the number of U.S. adults using social media climbing from 8% to 72% since 2005, it is clear this trend is not going anywhere.[24] With respect to CHI, patients no longer just read about their health information online, but can have an active role in controlling content, creating new information, and sharing their experiences with others. This is often described as peer-to-peer health care. Patients realize that health care professionals provide a wealth of information but believe the wealth of information they can obtain from their peers with similar illnesses can be a significant supplement.[25] For example, PatientsLikeMe® (http://www.patientslikeme.com/) is a privately funded company with the purpose of creating a community of patients with neurological, neuroendocrine, psychiatric, and immune conditions. Site content is posted by actual patients and includes anything from treatments they have tried, what works and what does not work for them, and what side effects they experience. Discussions often include the quality of the care delivered by their providers.

❻ *Wisdom of crowds is a belief that when patients share information about their common conditions through social networking, their collective wisdom is more beneficial than the expert opinion of just one individual.* Patients do not completely resist the advice of health professionals, but are just not as willing to rely on a single expert opinion for their information.[1] Health information received via social media is greatly valued by many consumers, especially the "net generation" as described by Don Tapscott in Grown Up Digital.[26] This "net generation," made up of consumers born in the early 1980s or after, has grown up online and prefers to engage and collaborate via technology. Extremely used to the digital world, they often trust a search engine on the Internet to provide answers or an online peer review over an expert. Opinions, stories, successes and failures, treatment options, and adverse effects are just some of what this "net generation" of patients share on social media. This feeling of camaraderie and support obtained via networks is something patients feel they cannot attain from most health care professionals. Some patients may even have reservations when it comes to trusting their health care professional. According to the Edelman Trust Barometer, people are inclined more than ever to trust social media as a source for information.[27] In fact, almost one in five adult Internet users state they have gone online to connect with other people who have health conditions similar to themselves.[25] The concern with social media is that posts made by patients are a reflection of their unique experience and may be incorrect or inappropriate for another individual. It is imperative patients keep in mind that the information retrieved from peers should be used only to supplement the information provided by practitioners and that the Internet does not replace health care professionals.[28] Information found on social media can often lack quality and reliability, and be unreferenced and incomplete. As practitioners, evidence-based medicine minimizes the importance of anecdotal reports where social media tends to affirm them, combining several different patient experiences into collective medical knowledge.[24] Most social media outlets that give consumers the ability to post opinions, recommendations, and health information state that they are not a substitute for advice of a qualified health professional. While the provision of these disclaimers can be a sign of a quality site, unfortunately, they are not always posted in the most visible place for many consumers on these websites, nor do consumers often heed these disclaimers' warning.

Social media also creates an additional opportunity for health care professionals to connect with their patients. Four out of 10 consumers report that health information found via social media influences the way they approach their health.[29] This means that health care professionals have a duty to be a part of that discussion. By creating educational content as well as providing health information via social media platforms, health care professionals are able to reach a much larger audience all the while correcting misinformation and providing accurate information. Many physicians are already using social media to bolster patient health care education. By tweeting, making blog posts, recording videos, and participating in disease-specific discussions focused on patient education, some health care professionals are doing all they can to ensure evidence-based health information is getting to patients rather than inaccurate data that can be found on the Internet.[24] Patients appreciate interacting with their health care professionals online and a majority say they trust social media posts and activity by health care professionals over any other group.[28] In fact, recent studies have shown that social media interventions made by health care professionals affect patients in a variety of different ways such as weight loss, smoking cessation, reducing risky sexual behaviors, and increasing physical activity.[24]

Case Study 25–1

You are the only pharmacist on duty at a local community pharmacy. You are short staffed, the phone is ringing, and you have 50+ prescriptions yet to verify. You are doing your best to make the wait as short as possible. In the midst of all this, one of your regular patients comes up to the counter and announces that she will no longer be taking her anticonvulsant medication. She describes how lately she has been feeling strange and feels fairly certain it is due to the carbamazepine. She then explains to you how she has recently gone online to find more information about the specific medication she is taking. "You wouldn't believe all the good information that is out there," she says, "I was able to talk to other patients and they were so helpful!" She then goes on to talk about the many patient testimonials she read telling her to discontinue her medication.

The patient seems adamant that she is going to stop taking her medication. As a pharmacist, this concerns you. The pharmacy technician calls you to resume verifying prescriptions because the pharmacy is quickly getting out of control.

- *Do you take the time to counsel this patient or do you get back to filling prescriptions before patients start complaining about the wait time?*
- *If you decide to counsel this patient, how would you educate her on the appropriate use of online resources to find health information?*
- *After counseling your patient, she still is determined to stop her carbamazepine. What is the most important advice you can give her at this point?*

MOBILE HEALTH

❼ *The use of mobile technology to obtain CHI has experienced a sharp increase within the last few years and continues to skyrocket.*

Smartphones have made obtaining health information online or via mobile software applications (also referred to as apps) that much easier. In 2015, a total of 64% of U.S. adults owned a smartphone, 62% of which had accessed health information with their smartphone within the past year. Among 18- to 29-year-olds, 75% of them had gone online with their smartphone to look up a health condition.[30] With nearly two-thirds of Americans owning a smartphone, retrieving health information is literally as simple as the touch of a fingertip. Fifty-eight percent of smartphone owners report downloading at least one mobile **health application** to their phone, with exercise, weight, pregnancy, and diet apps being among the most popular.[31] The market revenue for mobile health apps is projected to grow to $26 billion worldwide or more towards the end of this decade. According to IMS Institute for Healthcare Informatics, there are currently more than 165,000 mobile health apps available through the Apple iTunes and Android app stores.[32] Consumers who download these health applications may have a high trust in the accuracy of the information they provide.[30] It is clear smartphone use is here to stay which means that U.S. adults are not only going on the Internet to find health information, but are also tracking and managing their own health data. This mobile health era is yet another facet of technology that health care professionals must adapt to and understand to better serve their patients. Table 25-3 introduces just a few of the smartphone apps of which health care professionals should be aware.

The idea that health care professionals could start medically prescribing health apps for their patients is a concept that has gained momentum because many of them do not just track health data, but function as a mechanism for patients to manage various disease states. For example, WellDoc® is one of the first health care companies to gain Food and Drug Administration (FDA) approval for their smartphone health app as a medical device. This device gathers data on meals, carbohydrates, blood sugar levels, insulin doses, exercise, and medication about specific patients. The application, BlueStar®, then advises the patient on how to treat episodes of low blood sugar. It can also send medical data and clinical recommendations to the health care provider. The IMS Institute for Health Care Informatics found that one-third of physicians have prescribed mobile health apps to patients. Thirty-day adherence rates were 10% higher for apps prescribed by a physician compared to if a patient had downloaded the app on their own. Adherence rates were 30% higher for fitness apps.[31] The number of health apps being developed to function as medical devices are increasing and more are entering the market on a daily basis. This trend has created a need for guidelines regarding the regulation required for health apps and clarification of the role of the FDA in the approval process. Currently, developers of health care apps are providing a laundry list of disclaimers to accompany their product to avoid FDA clearance and the requirement of medical device application.[46] Criteria for what

TABLE 25–3. EXAMPLES OF FREE MOBILE HEALTH AND FITNESS APPLICATIONS[33–45]

Health and Fitness Applications	Description	Smartphone Availability	Fee
First Aid	This app provides immediate first aid information to help with a variety of common emergencies. It is available through the American Red Cross.	iPhone, iPad, and Android	Free
GlucoseBuddy	An application designed for diabetic users who can monitor blood glucose levels, record when they take medication, and track food intake and physical activity.	iPhone, iPod touch, and iPad	Free
iTriage®	iTriage was created by two emergency room physicians that wanted to help users more easily determine what medical condition they might have and where the best place to go for treatment is located.	iPhone and Android	Free
Lose It!	Users looking to lose weight download this app in order to set daily calorie goals, track physical activity, find new exercises, and search for new health-conscious recipes. Progress reports are also available for the consumer as well as the ability to share accomplishments via social media.	iPhone and iPad	Free
MapMyRun	This app not only tracks the runners' exact path but also records other aspects of a workout like speed, distance, pace, and calories burned. The runner can also share their run data via social media. Versions also exist for walking, hiking, biking, and triathlons.	iPhone, Android, iPad, and Windows	Free—lite version Paid—full version
MyFitnessPal	A popular app that gives users the ability to track their daily activity and food intake. Another feature making this a unique download is the searchable food database providing nutritional information on over 2 million items. The app even comes with a bar code scanner so users can easily upload nutritional data anywhere. Users can also get support from friends with similar health goals and track each other's progress.	iPhone, iPod touch, iPad, Blackberry, Android, and Windows	Free
MyPlate	A calorie tracker app developed by LiveStrong.com that gives users access to largest database of nutritional information on food and restaurant items. It provides personalized daily calorie and water intake goals as well as allows the user to update others of their progress via social media.	iPhone, Android, iPad, Blackberry, and Windows	Free—lite version Paid—full version

continued

TABLE 25–3. EXAMPLES OF FREE MOBILE HEALTH AND FITNESS APPLICATIONS[33–45] *(CONTINUED)*

Health and Fitness Applications	Description	Smartphone Availability	Fee
My Pregnancy & Baby Today	An app developed by Baby Center that is trusted by more than 300 million women. It provides expert advice and tips to help moms navigate through every day of pregnancy and baby's first year.	iPhone, iPad, and Android	Free
MyQuitCoach	This app put out by Livestrong.com helps smokers quit the habit gradually or right away. Users trying to quit can track their progress and will receive motivational tips and inspirational messages to help them remain strong.	iPhone, iPod touch, iPad	Free—lite version Paid—full version
RunKeeper	Developed for the runner, this app tracks the progress of a workout and the global positioning system (GPS) lets users know where they are running, how fast they are going, and how many calories they have burned. Similar to MapMyRun, this app allows users to share statistics via social media. Other versions track activities like walking and cycling.	iPhone, iPod touch, iPad, Windows, and Android	Free
TravWell	Brought to you by the Centers for Disease Control and Prevention (CDC), this app provides assistance to travelers who are looking for guidance on how to prepare for travel internationally. Some features include destination-specific vaccine recommendations, packing lists, emergency services phone numbers, as well as travel tips for a safe and healthy vacation.	iPhone, iPod touch, iPad, and Android	Free
WebMD®	Few users are unfamiliar with WebMD and all it has to offer. This mobile app provides much of the same information found online such as popular symptom checker. It also provides first aid information that is available without a wireless connection in emergency instances where Internet access is unavailable. WebMD Pain Coach and WebMD Baby are also available.	iPhone, iPad, and Android	Free
ZocDoc	An application developed to provide users a way to peruse reviews of local doctors and dentists while also conveniently booking appointments.	iPhone, iPod touch, iPad, Android, and Blackberry	Free

TABLE 25–4. AREAS OF EVALUATION FOR CONSUMER MOBILE HEALTH APPLICATIONS[48]

Areas of Evaluation	Questions to Consider
Credibility of app	Are credentials of app suitable?
	Are authors/publishers clearly listed?
	Are there advertisements?
	Is the organization that developed the app reputable?
	Are there disclaimers of content?
Accuracy of information	Is it peer reviewed?
	Is the information current and/or frequently updated?
	Are recent and reputable guidelines used to support recommendations made?
	Are references cited?
Evidence-based medicine	Are recommendations evidence based?
	Do recommendations target a specific audience or are they general in nature?
	Are opinion statements clearly marked?
	Are users directed to a health care professional before making changes to health care routine?
Ease-of-use	Does the app fit to the screen?
	Is the set-up of the app well designed and organized?
	Is the app easily navigated?
	Does the app have a search function?
	Is there a main menu that helps clearly lay content out?
Health literacy	Is medical jargon used easy for the lay reader to understand?
	Is font and set-up of app easy to read?
	Does app gear information for the consumer?

the FDA considers a mobile medical app that they need to regulate versus which apps they will exercise discretion with can be found at http://www.fda.gov/MedicalDevices/DigitalHealth/MobileMedicalApplications/default.htm.[47]

With health care shifting into this era of health information exchange, the role of the practitioner must also evolve and transform. As with health information found on the Internet, the lack of efficacy and safety information for most mobile health applications means health care professionals have a duty to warn patients to proceed with caution. This is an area where pharmacists especially can make an important impact. Sifting through the plethora of mobile health apps can be overwhelming for patients and health care professionals, but there are several platforms available that rate, evaluate, and certify mobile health apps. For example, the IMS Institute for Healthcare Informatics launched AppScore in 2013. It evaluates mobile health apps and includes physician input and patient feedback into their ratings. Various alternative mobile health rating tools include SocialWellth®, iMedical Apps, and iGetBetter. Considerations for evaluation of mobile health apps are presented in Table 25-4.

You are providing discharge counseling to a patient after a short hospital stay for a minor surgery. He brings up the fact that four or five months ago, he downloaded the most amazing app for his smartphone that allows him to more easily manage his diabetes. He shares that the app does things like track his blood glucose levels, food intake, and physical activity. The app also adjusts his insulin dose based on his specific data. He swears by the app and is convinced his diabetes is better controlled and that he has never felt better. He also states that he suffers from fewer hypoglycemic episodes than he previously used to experience. You are unfamiliar with the app he is talking about.

- *What initial follow-up questions do you have for this patient?*
- *What guidance do you have for this patient navigating the mobile health arena?*

During the patient's next office visit with his primary care provider, he is sure to mention the diabetes app that he has been using, following his discussion with you (refer to Case Study 25-2). The provider is unsure what process he should be using to evaluate this app for his patient. He has contacted and asked for you to provide some guidelines to help him evaluate this app as well as other apps that his patients are using to manage various disease states.

- *What suggestions do you have to help the physician in evaluating mobile health apps?*

A New Model of Drug Information

According to a 2014 Pew Research Center report, even with the explosion of online and mobile CHI opportunities, a majority of people still turn to a health care professional before using the Internet to find information. For the meantime, it appears patients still view the Internet's role as supplemental and are looking at health care professionals to guide them in their search.[49] However, this trend is shifting and pharmacists should anticipate patients may likely seek health information before talking to their health care provider.

This can be a dangerous practice as many patients are ill equipped to find and understand all the information they need to address their health care situation. Pharmacists have an option to either ignore the fact that patients can seek health information elsewhere, or embrace the opportunity to collaborate with their patients as they seek and use information to improve their health and quality of life. As part of the screening process, pharmacists should ask their patients where they get health information and what their preferred method is to obtain such information. Inquiring about a patient's degree of access and use of online health information should become as routine as gathering vital signs at an office visit. The answer to these simple questions can open the door to more specific education about how the patient can obtain useful, quality health information. Pharmacists must be aware of the wide range of CHI sources and how and why their patients use them. ❽ *Pharmacists should discuss with their patients why they remain an important source of drug information. Patients can be encouraged not to see CHI as a replacement for actual interaction with a health care provider, but as an extension of care and a way to improve communication.* Pharmacists can direct patients to quality CHI sites tailored to their situation and teach them how to seek information from the web. This skill is important as three out of four patients report just using a general search engine to seek out health information online versus a more specific site that specializes in health information. In addition, one-third of patients report using the Internet as a diagnostic tool.[15] Pharmacists may consider developing a list of online resources that have their seal of approval as providing high-quality information. Pharmacist recommended websites can be shared in a variety of different ways ranging from pamphlets, bulletin boards, social media, and space provided on the pharmacy website. Such a service is something relatively easy and quick to do and goes a long way to helping patients avoid low-quality or risky information. When providing resources, it is imperative they are monitored and updated on a consistent basis; otherwise, potential exists for these same resources to become yet another avenue that low-quality CHI reaches patients. Patients will also need tips on how to navigate the range of information sources as well as how to decide what information is relevant to their individual situation. Not only does this include aiding the navigation of health information found on the web, but also in other resources, such as brochures and patient leaflets given out with prescriptions. The success of a website in delivering meaningful information is heavily reliant upon the consumers' ability to identify, interpret, and apply information that is relevant to their situation. If the patient does not understand their health condition, they may use the wrong information for their situation, even if it is of good quality. A study in the Journal of the American Medical Informatics Association gave patients a scenario describing angina symptoms, but not the actual diagnosis. They used MedlinePlus® to find information on the condition. The authors found that searches yielded information leading patients to draw incorrect conclusions 70% of the time. The authors concluded that patients and/or family and friends of patients searching the web for information without a diagnosis most likely are confronted with a wealth of information and are unable to sift through what is relevant versus irrelevant.[50]

❾ *Patients often have difficulty finding accurate information in response to their specific health concerns on the Internet.*

Additionally, pharmacists may offer classes to teach patients how to use CHI to their advantage. Patients can be taught about the Health On the Net Foundation (HON). This nonprofit, nongovernmental organization's mission is to assess and stringently review those Internet sites out there offering health information. Sites passing inspection receive HON certification and are given the HON symbol to place on a visible area of their website for patients to see, giving assurance the website provides reliable and appropriate information. Unfortunately, as the number of health Internet sites increase, there are more and more places patients will find their health information and many may not have the HON seal of approval. The National Institutes of Health (NIH) has also developed a website for both consumers and health care professionals to better determine quality of health information found online. This information can be found at https://nccih.nih.gov/health/webresources.[51-53] Furthermore, patients can be referred to the National Library of Medicine's tutorial through MedlinePlus®. It is specifically dedicated to giving patients instruction on how to evaluate health information they find on the web and is located at http://www.nlm.nih.gov/medlineplus/webeval/webeval.html.[54] Moreover, pharmacists can function as rumor control for misinformation on the Internet, mainstream media, or from family and friends.

EVALUATING THE QUALITY OF HEALTH INTERNET WEBSITES

Questions have been raised about current standards for evaluating the quality of health and medical information on the Internet; many health care professionals feel proxy measures for evaluating the quality of such websites are less than ideal. One study suggests that even sites certified with the HON code may be questionable with little correlation between certification and accuracy or completeness of information.[16] Table 25-5 is an example of the aforementioned current standards in health Internet evaluation.

Much focus is put on structural design of a website, who the site sponsor is (e.g., government, nonprofit, academic institution), and whether or not the site lists its sources, but little emphasis is placed on actual content made available to consumers. When actual health information content has been reviewed in terms of a specific disease state across many different websites, website sponsorship has been a very poor predictor of quality.[55] In fact, most health information available on the Internet is not monitored for quality or accuracy. According to the Federal Trade Commission (FTC), health care professionals review only about 50% of the health and medical content on websites.[56] This suggests there is no real efficient and effective method in place to evaluate the quality of health

TABLE 25–5. EXAMPLE OF CURRENT STANDARDS USED TO EVALUATE THE QUALITY OF HEALTH INFORMATION ON THE INTERNET[49]

Considerations when Determining Whether or Not Health Information on the Internet Is Reliable
Who is responsible for the website? Does the website provide this information? Is the sponsor a government agency, a medical school, or a reliable health-related organization?
Is the only purpose of the website to provide information or is the website trying to sell something?
If the website inquires about personal information, does it offer a reason why and give an explanation about what it will do with that information once collected?
Is health information provided on the website backed up with evidence? Are there references to support recommendations being made, etc.?
Does the website give the source of their health information? If so, is that source credible? Does the website provide explanation about whether or not health information is reviewed and by whom?
Is health information provided in an unbiased and objective manner? Is material written in a way that would be understandable to most patients no matter their health literacy level?
Does health information on the website get updated regularly? Is material provided current?
Does health information on the website seem reasonable and credible overall?
Does the information provided by the site allow visitors to contact website owners with feedback, problems, and questions?

information online. The only real way is for the pharmacist to individually review each website or mobile application and evaluate health information content provided before they recommend them to patients. Sites devoted to a particular disease state tend to be much more complete and more accurate than sites that attempt to cover multiple health topics, but there are still no guarantees. The World Health Organization (WHO) is currently attempting to address the problem by requesting that the Internet Corporation for Assigned Names and Numbers create a domain suffix that would only be used when health information found on a website was validated. The WHO's goal is to have content on every website with this new domain suffix be rigorously monitored for quality and compliance. Additionally, any website with this domain address would be prioritized as the top result when using any search engine to research a health-related question.[24] Complete regulation of all health content on the Internet is improbable, but health care providers can attempt to help patients by selecting and evaluating a handful of sites to recommend for patients.[53]

HEALTH LITERACY—FINAL KEY TO THE PATIENT'S SUCCESSFUL USE OF INFORMATION

❿ *Once patients identify or are given quality health information, they still may face barriers in being able to use it to improve their health.* **Health literacy** is the capability of patients to read or hear health information, understand it, and then act upon health information, which is a subset of literacy, which is the capability of patients to read and understand.[57] The Institute of Medicine estimates that nearly 90 million adults lack the ability to use the U.S. health system sufficiently due to their poor literacy skills. Patients with poor health literacy may have trouble recognizing when health information is needed, identifying or obtaining access to health information resources, determining the quality of health information resources or acknowledging that quality is even a problem, and even more so analyzing and understanding information found.[58] Studies show a strong correlation with adults who report having poor health as also having the most limited literacy, numeracy, and health literacy skills. Health literacy even affects those patients who otherwise have no problems with normal literacy issues in their daily life. As a result of health literacy issues being unfamiliar to most people, many patients find themselves struggling with unfamiliarity of medical terms and how their bodies work, being unable to accurately judge risk versus benefit for their particular health situation, complicated treatment plans to follow, as well as being scared and confused when diagnosed with a serious condition.[59]

Pharmacists must consider a patient's health literacy when they provide information and education to their patients. Studies show that most health-related materials whether on the web or given out in the pharmacy surpass most U.S. adults' average reading ability.[56] Table 25-6 describes the qualities of health literate websites and can be used as a screen for pharmacists as they identify websites for their patients. Visit the Agency for Healthcare Research and Quality at http://www.ahrq.gov/professionals/quality-patient-safety/quality-resources/tools/literacy-toolkit/tool3a/index.html for additional detail about health literacy standards and the role health care professionals can play in helping their patients.

PARTICIPATORY MEDICINE

⓫ *The term* **participatory** *medicine is a recent movement for a new model of cooperative health care.* In this model, patients no longer play a passive part when it comes to their health care but an active role alongside the health care provider. Patients are seen

TABLE 25–6. GUIDELINES FOR HIGH-QUALITY HEALTH LITERATE INTERNET SITES[60]

• Designed for old hardware and software	• Link clearly defined
• Simple home page	• Printer-friendly option
• Information prioritized	• Audio option
• Minimal text per screen	• Site map easy to find
• Navigation simple and consistent	• Contact information easy to find
• Searching simplified	• Content uses other principles of health literacy
• Scrolling need minimized	

as a valuable health care resource and providers are encouraged to view them as equal partners. By fostering a sense of patient/provider engagement and patient education and empowerment, the Society for Participatory Medicine hopes to improve health outcomes along with increasing patient satisfaction among other things. Studies show that nearly 90% of patients believe that working with their health care professional as a partner will help them to enhance their overall health situation. Participatory medicine is a concept that is definitely not new to patients. They have sought to be a part of the decision-making process when it comes to their health for quite some time. It is evident now more than ever that patients desire to equip themselves with the proper tools to be a valued part of the conversation regarding their health situation. Seeking health information online is a large way patients feel invested and with health care in the midst of a technology revolution in which the availability of health information is accelerating at an extraordinary rate, it is important that health care professionals do everything they can to ensure patients are accessing accurate and quality information. The U.S. Department of Health and Human Services even recognizes the importance of where health care professionals are going in terms of health communication and health information technology for patients. Through HealthyPeople 2020 (https://www.healthypeople.gov/) it is their mission to deliver health information to patients that is accurate, targeted, and tailored for the individual as well as to increase health literacy skills and step up health communication efforts online. This includes having a more active role in disease state self-management tools that can be accessed via mobile devices which is just another avenue patients are flocking to, to take an active part in their health. According to a survey done by the Society for Participatory Medicine, 84% of patients think sharing health data they have tracked themselves with their health care professionals between visits would greatly help them to better manage their health. It was also found that 76% would use a monitoring device to track personal clinical data with 81% of those patients saying that they would be more likely to use the device if their health care professional recommended it.

Participatory medicine encompasses both the patient and the health care professional, asking both to work together in making the best possible health care decision for the patient. From asking more useful questions of physicians and other health care providers to more effectively managing conditions and participating in their own treatment, participatory medicine may help patients have more control over their lives in terms of their health.

PHARMACISTS' PAYMENT FOR PROGRESSIVE HEALTH SERVICES

In order for pharmacists to evolve into progressive drug information practitioners, a sustainable business model that includes reimbursement must be designed. The need for reimbursement is key in light of declining revenues from the dispensing operation.

MTM is reimbursable through Medicare Part D and according to MTM program requirements optimum therapeutic outcomes must be ensured for patients through improved medication use and adverse event risk reduction.[61] Effective patient education can play a big role in helping MTM participants meet these specified requirements. Pharmacists should include the strategies described in this chapter in their MTM patient education approaches to begin to get reimbursed for these services. Additionally, some patients are willing to pay directly for care that they cannot receive from other sources.

Conclusion

A vast amount of choices exist for both patients and health care professionals when it comes to obtaining and using health information. It is vital that health care professionals be positioned to be an integral part of patients' approach to gaining an understanding of their health. Especially for pharmacists, as traditional roles change, new opportunities to get involved in managing patients' health care are presenting themselves. A lot is at stake if health care professionals do not move toward these new roles as someone else will step in and take over this responsibility. It has been the responsibility of health care professionals, especially pharmacists, for decades to educate and provide patients with quality drug information. In the end, it is up to health care professionals to design this new role and demonstrate value to the patient so that they continue to be used as a key ally in providing patient care.

Self-Assessment Questions

1. Which of the following are limitations a pharmacist faces when delivering drug information to their patients?
   a. Lack of readability of most patient leaflets given with prescription
   b. Pharmacists appear too busy and unavailable
   c. Counseling has become a passive process where patient education is only given if requested
   d. Pharmacists lack of understanding in regards to patient's desire to take control of their own health
   e. All of the above

2. Patient education is best described by the following:
   a. Delivered by health care professional verbally only
   b. Occurs with the pickup of new prescriptions only

    c. Unplanned activity
    d. b and c only
    e. None of the above

3. Consumer health information (CHI) is **BEST** described by the following:
    a. Tailored to a patient's specific situation
    b. Actively sought by patients
    c. Created in response to patients need for more information about their health
    d. b and c only
    e. None of the above

4. Which of the following site(s) is considered a consumer health information or social media site?
    a. WebMD®
    b. PatientsLikeMe®
    c. Everyday Health®
    d. b and c only
    e. All of the above

5. Through social media sites patients share a wealth of personal information regarding their disease states and conditions. Examples of personal information shared includes all of the following **EXCEPT**:
    a. Treatment successes
    b. Treatment failures
    c. Adverse effects
    d. Opinions
    e. None of the above

6. All of the following are reasons why some patients prefer the collective wisdom of a group over the advice of an expert individual **EXCEPT** for:
    a. Patients are provided with a feeling of camaraderie and support
    b. Patients may not trust their health care professional
    c. Patients are more inclined to trust a person like them
    d. Patients are not as willing to rely on a single expert for their information
    e. None of the above

7. Which of the following is **NOT** a useful strategy for pharmacists to employ when helping patients to empower themselves and effectively use consumer health information (CHI)?
    a. Ask patients where else they get health information besides their health care professional
    b. Encourage patients to quit seeking information online regardless of the source

    c. Become familiar with the range of CHI resources available

    d. Develop a list of smartphone health applications that are pharmacist-recommended

    e. Discuss with patients why pharmacists still remain an important DI source

8. Which of the following are questions to ask when evaluating consumer mobile health applications?

    a. Is the organization that developed the app reputable?

    b. Are recommendations evidence based?

    c. Is medical jargon used easy for the lay reader to understand?

    d. a and b only

    e. All of the above

9. Which of the following questions are considered standard for evaluating the quality of a consumer health information site?

    a. If the website inquires about personal information, does it offer a reason why and give an explanation about what it will do with that information once collected?

    b. Does health information on the website get updated regularly?

    c. Does the website require you to sign in with a username and password in order to access health information?

    d. a and b only

    e. All of the above

10. Which mobile health and fitness application provides its users with daily tips and expert advice on what to expect during pregnancy?

    a. MyPlate

    b. My Pregnancy & Baby Today

    c. MyFitnessPal

    d. iTriage®

    e. ZocDoc

11. The Centers for Disease Control and Prevention developed which of the following mobile health and fitness application(s)?

    a. MyPlate

    b. First Aid

    c. TravWell

    d. b and c only

    e. All of the above

12. Which mobile health and fitness application provides its users with direction on how to handle the most common first aid emergencies?
    a. MyPlate
    b. MyQuitCoach
    c. MyFitnessPal
    d. First Aid
    e. GlucoseBuddy

13. Which type of social media is **BEST** defined as "an online diary where one can log their personal thoughts on various topics and post to a web page"?
    a. Wiki
    b. Blog
    c. Social network
    d. b and c only
    e. None of the above

14. Which of the following are issues patients with poor health literacy may face?
    a. Trouble recognizing when health information is needed
    b. Trouble identifying or getting a hold of health information resources
    c. Trouble analyzing and understanding information found
    d. a and b only
    e. All of the above

15. Which of the following terms **BEST** describes a new model of cooperative health care where patients no longer play a passive part when it comes to their health but an active role alongside their health care provider?
    a. Participatory medicine
    b. Social media
    c. Medication therapy management
    d. a and c only
    e. None of the above

REFERENCES

1. California HealthCare Foundation [Internet]. Oakland, CA: California HealthCare Foundation; c2009. The wisdom of patients: health care meets online social media; 2008 Apr [cited 2009 Nov 10]. Available from: http://www.chcf.org/.
2. Fox S, Duggan M. Health Online 2013 [Internet]. Washington, DC: Pew Research Center; 2013 Jan [cited 2016 Sept 8]:[1 p.]. Available from: http://www.pewinternet .org/2013/01/15/health-online-2013/.

3. Fox S, Duggan M. Part Two: sources of health information [Internet]. Washington, DC: Pew Research Center; 2013 Nov [cited 2016 Sept 8]:[6 p.]. Available from: http://www.pewinternet.org/2013/11/26/part-two-sources-of-health-information/.

4. National Community Pharmacists Association [Internet]. American Pharmacists Association, National Association of Chain Drug Stores, National Community Pharmacists Association. Project Destiny executive summary; 2008 Feb [cited 2013 Jul 14]:[5 p.]. Available from: http://www.ncpanet.org/pdf/projectdestinyexecsummary.pdf

5. National Alliance of State Pharmacy Associations [Internet]. Joint Commission of Pharmacy Practitioners. Executive summary: an action plan for implementation of the JCPP future vision of pharmacy practice; 2007 Nov [updated 2008 Jan]:[86 p.].

6. IMS Institute for Healthcare Informatics [Internet]. Parsippany, NJ: Avoidable costs in U.S. healthcare: the $200 billion opportunity from using medicines more responsibly; 2013 Jun [cited 2016 Sept 8]. Available from: http://www.imshealth.com/en/thought-leadership/ims-institute/reports/avoidable-costs

7. Bullman R. Recognizing the full benefits of medication [Internet]. New York, NY: Media Planet; 2011 Mar [cited 2012 Dec 20]:[10 p.]. Available from: http://www.talkaboutrx.org/assocdocs/TASK/531/MedicationNonAdherenceFINALREPORT.pdf

8. Anderson S. Pharmacy outlook 2016. Arlington, VA: National Association of Chain Drug Stores; 2016.

9. Eder R. How consumers choose a primary pharmacy [Internet]; [updated 2012 16 Apr; cited 2012 Dec 20]. Available from: http://www.drugstorenews.com/article/how-consumers-choose-primary-pharmacy

10. Omnibus Budget Reconciliation Act of 1990, Pub. L. 101-508, 104 Stat.1388 (Nov 5, 1990).

11. Consumer reports [Internet]. Yonkers, NY: Can you read this drug label; 2011 Jun [cited 2016 Sept 8]. Available from: http://www.consumerreports.org/cro/2011/06/can-you-read-this-drug-label/index.htm

12. The Joint Commission. Transitions of care: the need for a more effective approach to continuing patient care. Joint Commission Center for Transforming Healthcare. 2012:1-8.

13. Malone PM, Kier KL, Stanovich JE, Malone MJ. Drug information: a guide for pharmacists. 5th ed. New York, NY: McGraw-Hill; 2014.

14. Massengale L. Resources for quality health information online. Proceedings of the 119th Annual Meeting of the American Association of Colleges of Pharmacy. 2008 July 19-23; Chicago, IL.

15. Fox S, Duggan M. Information triage [Internet]. Washington, DC: Pew Research Center; 2013 Jan [cited 2016 Sept 8]:[11 p.]. Available from: http://www.pewinternet.org/2013/01/15/information-triage/.

16. Felkey BG, Fox BI, Thrower MR. Health care informatics: a skills-based resource. Washington, DC: American Pharmacists Association; 2006.

17. Angie's List. [Internet]. Indianapolis, IN: Angie's List; c1995-2012 [cited 2012 Dec 12]. Available from: http://www.angieslist.com

18. Consumer Reports Health [Internet]; c2004-2012 [cited 2012 Dec 12]. Available from: http://www.consumerreportshealth.org

19. Healthfinder [Internet]; c2012 [cited 2012 Dec 18]. Available from: http://www.healthfinder.gov

20. Microsoft HealthVault [Internet]; c2013 [cited 2013 Jun 12]. Available from: https://www.healthvault.com/us/en

21. PatientsLikeMe [Internet]; c2005-2012 [cited 2012 Dec 12]. Available from: http://www.patientslikeme.com

22. Everyday Health Group, LLC [Internet]; c2012 [cited 2012 Dec 12]. Available from: http://www.everydayhealth.com

23. WebMD [Internet]; c2005-2012 [cited 2012 Dec 12]. Available from: http://www.webmd.com

24. Ventola CL. Social media and health care professionals: benefits, risks, and best practices. Pharm Therapeut. 2014;39(7):491-9.

25. Fox S, Duggan M. Peer-to-peer health care [Internet]. Washington, DC: Pew Research Center; 2013 Jan [cited 2016 Sept 8]:[5 p.]. Available from: http://www.pewinternet.org/2013/01/15/peer-to-peer-health-care/.

26. Tapscott D. Grown up digital: how the net generation is changing your world. New York, NY: McGraw-Hill; 2009.

27. Edelman. 2012 Edelman Trust Barometer Executive Summary [Internet]. 2012 [cited 2017 Aug 11]. Available from: https://www.scribd.com/document/79026497/2012-Edelman-Trust-Barometer-Executive-Summary

28. Fox S. Medicine 2.0: peer-to-peer healthcare [Internet]. Washington, DC: Pew Research Center's Internet & American Life Project; 2011 Sept [cited 2017 Feb 28]:[10 p.]. Available from: http://www.pewinternet.org/2011/09/18/medicine-2-0-peer-to-peer-healthcare/.

29. 24 Outstanding statistics on how social media has impacted health care [Internet]. Physician Referral Management and EConsult Software—referral MD. 2015 [cited 2016 Sept 9]. Available from: https://getreferralmd.com/2013/09/healthcare-social-media-statistics/.

30. Smith A. U.S. smartphone use in 2015 [Internet]. Washington, DC: Pew Research Center; 2015 Apr [cited 2016 Sept 9]. Available from: http://www.pewinternet.org/2015/04/01/us-smartphone-use-in-2015/.

31. 58% of smartphone owners download, use mobile health apps [Internet]. mHealthIntelligence. 2015 [cited 2016 Sept 9]. Available from: http://mhealthintelligence.com/news/58-of-smartphone-owners-download-use-mobile-health-apps

32. Terry K. Number of health apps soars, but use does not always follow [Internet]. Medscape log in [cited 2016 Sept 9]. Available from: http://www.medscape.com/viewarticle/851226

33. First Aid [Internet]; c2016 [cited 2016 Sept 9]. Available from: http://www.redcross.org/get-help/prepare-for-emergencies/mobile-apps

34. GlucoseBuddy [Internet]; c2011-2012 [cited 2012 Dec 18]. Available from: http://www.mlanet.org/page/top-health-websites

35. iTriage [Internet]; c2008-2012 [cited 2012 Dec 18]. Available from: https://www.itriagehealth.com

36. Lose It! [Internet]; c2008-2012 [cited 2012 Dec 12]. Available from: http://www.loseit .com/.

37. MapMyRun [Internet]; c2005-2012 [cited 2012 Dec 18]. Available from: http://www .mapmyrun.com

38. MyFitnessPal [Internet]; c2005-2012 [cited 2012 Dec 18]. Available from: http://www .myfitnesspal.com

39. MyPlate [Internet]; c2011-2012 [cited 2012 Dec 18]. Available from: http://www .livestrong.com/calorie-counter-mobile/.

40. My Pregnancy & Baby Center [Internet]; c1997-2016 [cited 2016 Sept 9]. Available from: http://www.babycenter.com/mobile-apps

41. MyQuitCoach [Internet]; c2012 [cited 2012 Dec 18]. Available from: http://www .livestrong.com/quit-smoking-app/.

42. RunKeeper [Internet]; c2012 [cited 2012 Dec 18]. Available from: http://runkeeper .com/.

43. TravWell [Internet]; c2014 [cited 2016 Sep 9]. Available from: http://wwwnc.cdc.gov/ travel/page/apps-about

44. WebMD [Internet]; c2005-2012 [cited 2012 Dec 18] Available from: http://www.webmd .com/mobile

45. ZocDoc [Internet]; c2012 [cited 2012 Dec 18]. Available from: http://www.zocdoc.com/

46. Brustein J. Coming next: using and app as prescribed. New York Times (New York ed.). 2012 Aug 20:Sect. B:1.

47. Mobile medical applications [Internet]. Mobile medical applications; [cited 2016 Sept 9]. Available from: http://www.fda.gov/medicaldevices/digitalhealth/mobilemedicalapplica- tions/default.htm

48. Pope A, Bryant P, Pace H, Sperry M. Evaluation and ranking of consumer health and drug information smart phone applications. Poster session presented at: American Society of Health System Pharmacists Midyear Meeting; 2011 Dec 4-8; New Orleans, LA.

49. Fox S. The social life of health information [Internet]. Washington, DC: Pew Research Center's Internet & American Life Project; 2011 May [cited 2012 Dec 20]:[19 p.]. Available from: http://pewinternet.org/Reports/2011/Social-Life-of-Health-Info.aspx

50. Keselman A, Browne AC, Kaufman DR. Consumer health information seeking as hypoth- esis testing. J Am Med Inform Assoc. 2008;15(4):484-95.

51. Finding and evaluating online resources | NCCIH [Internet]. U.S. National Library of Medicine; [cited 2016 Sept 9]. Available from: https://nccih.nih.gov/health/webresources

52. U.S. Food and Drug Administration [Internet]. Silver Spring, MD: U.S. Health and Human Services. How to evaluate health information on the internet: information for consumers; 2010 Mar 9 [cited 2013 Jun 28]. Available from: http://www.fda.gov/Drugs/ ResourcesForYou/Consumers/BuyingUsingMedicineSafely/BuyingMedicinesOverthe Internet/ucm202863.htm#resources

53. Agency for Healthcare Research and Quality [Internet]. Rockville, MD: U.S. Health and Human Services. Assessing the Quality of Internet Health Information; 1999 Jun [cited 2013 Jun 28]. Available from: http://www.ahrq.gov/research/data/infoqual.html

54. Medline Plus [Internet]. Bethesda, MD: National Library of Medicine. 2007. Evaluating Internet health information: a tutorial from the National Library of Medicine; [cited 2009 Jan 12]. Available from: http://www.nlm.nih.gov/medlineplus/webeval/webeval.html

55. Center for Information Therapy [Internet]. Bethesda, MD: Center for Information Therapy, Inc. Seidman J, Steinwachs D, Rubin HR. The mysterious maze of the World Wide Web: what makes Internet health information high quality; 2004 Jul 6 [cited 2009 Jan 13]. Available from: http://www.ixcenter.org/publications/documents/e0035.pdf

56. Fox S, Rainie L. The online healthcare revolution: how the web helps Americans take better care of themselves [Internet]. Washington, DC: Pew Research Center's Internet and American Life Project; 2000 Nov [cited 2012 Dec 20]:[19 p.]. Available from: http://www.pewinternet.org/Reports/2000/The-Online-Health-Care-Revolution.aspx

57. Kutner M, Greenberg E, Jin Y, Paulsen C. The health literacy of America's adults: results from the 2003 National Assessment of Adult Literacy. Washington, DC: National Center for Education Statistics; 2003. Report No. NCES 2006-483. Supported by the U.S. Department of Education.

58. Nielsen-Bohlman L, Panzer AM, Kindig DA, eds. Health literacy: a prescription to end confusion. Board on Neuroscience and Behavioral Health, Committee on Health Literacy, Institute of Medicine. Washington, DC: National Academy of Sciences; 2004.

59. Understanding literacy and numeracy [Internet]. Centers for Disease Control and Prevention; 2015 [cited 2016 Sept 9]. Available from: http://www.cdc.gov/healthliteracy/learn/understandingliteracy.html

60. Agency for Healthcare Research and Quality. Accessible health information technology (IT) for populations with limited literacy: a guide for developers and purchasers of health IT. 2007 Oct [cited 2013 Jan 15]. Available from: http://healthit.ahrq.gov/sites/default/files/docs/page/LiteracyGuide_0.pdf

61. Centers for Medicare and Medicaid Service [Internet]. Baltimore, MD: Requirements for medication therapy management programs; 2013 Apr 10 [cited 2013 Jun 28]. Available from: http://www.cms.gov/Medicare/Prescription-Drug-Coverage/PrescriptionDrug CovContra/MTM.html

SUGGESTED READINGS

1. Agency for Healthcare Research and Quality (AHRQ). Health literacy: hidden barriers and practical strategies. Available from: http://www.ahrq.gov/professionals/quality-patient-safety/quality-resources/tools/literacy-toolkit/tool3a/index.html

2. Consumer and Patient Health Information Section (CAPHIS). Available from: http://www.mlanet.org/page/top-health-websites

3. iMedicalApps. Available from: http://www.imedicalapps.com/#

4. MedlinePlus®. Evaluating health information. Available from: http://www.nlm.nih.gov/medlineplus/evaluatinghealthinformation.html

5. MedlinePlus®. Guide to healthy web surfing. Available from: http://www.nlm.nih.gov/medlineplus/healthywebsurfing.html

6. National Institutes of Health. Finding and evaluating online resources. Available from: https://nccih.nih.gov/health/webresources

7. National Institutes of Health. Mobile (mHealth) health information and resources. Available from: http://www.fic.nih.gov/ResearchTopics/Pages/MobileHealth.aspx

8. Participatory Medicine. Available from: http://participatorymedicine.org/.

9. VUCA Health. Available from: www.vucahealth.com

Chapter Twenty-Six

Pharmacy Informatics: Enabling Safe and Efficacious Medication Use

Joshua C. Hollingsworth • Brent I. Fox

Learning Objectives

After completing this chapter, the reader will be able to

- List the activities that occur at each step of the medication use process.
- Define pharmacy informatics and other core informatics terms.
- Discuss the role of pharmacy informatics at each step of the medication use process.
- Describe challenges with implementing computerized provider order entry (CPOE).
- Describe the components of an e-prescribing system.
- Describe the role of the three primary components of a clinical decision support system (CDSS).
- Describe limitations of health information technology (HIT) that is used during the order verification step of the medication use process.
- Compare and contrast the health information technology used during dispensing in acute care and community pharmacy settings.
- Define the role of bar code medication administration.
- Describe the role of the three primary components of a clinical surveillance system.
- Describe the changing role of the patient in the U.S. health care system.
- Explain the importance of interoperability to the future of the U.S. health care system, including the role of the U.S. government.
- Describe the goal and structure of *Meaningful Use*.
- Compare and contrast privacy, security, and confidentiality as they relate to protected health information.

Key Concepts

① The medication use process is a system of interconnected parts that work together to achieve the common goal of safe and effective medication therapy.

② All pharmacists are affected by the electronic information systems that make up pharmacy informatics in virtually every aspect of practice.

③ The two broad categories of information used in pharmacy informatics, as well as other clinical informatics domains, are patient-specific information and knowledge-based information.

④ The vision of health care is becoming more patient-centered.

⑤ The current health care system is decentralized and fragmented. Because of this, significant communication gaps exist when multiple health care institutions provide care for the same patient. Substantial evidence suggests that more effective communication would improve patient care and reduce medical errors, such as adverse drug events (ADEs).

⑥ The desired result of interoperable systems and electronic health records (EHRs) is to readily provide all health practitioners in all locations, including the pharmacy, with access to information about a patient's care, as needed.

⑦ In order to increase adoption and Meaningful Use of EHRs by providers and hospitals, the Centers for Medicare and Medicaid Services (CMS) developed a monetary incentive program; the Meaningful Use program incentivizes hospitals and physicians to use EHRs to achieve specific outcomes, which may be process-oriented or patient-oriented. The goals of the Meaningful Use program are to (1) improve quality, safety, and efficiency, (2) engage patients and their families, (3) improve care coordination, as well as public and population health, and (4) maintain privacy and security of protected health information (PHI).

Introduction

Health care practitioners of today have a multitude of responsibilities within their scope of practice. For pharmacists, whether verifying and filling prescriptions, compounding medications, advising patients on proper medication use, or collaborating with other practitioners in the care of patients, the core responsibility lies on the safe and effective use of medication therapy. Clinicians aim to maximize patient safety while minimizing medication misadventures, such as medication errors and adverse drug events (ADEs), which are covered in Chapters 17 and 18. Given the sheer amount of information involved and available to take care of patients today, this focus on the safety and efficacy of medication use can only be reasonably obtained via clinicians' effective management of the information and related information systems involved in support of the medication use process. Health care providers, regardless of discipline and practice setting, must be able to input, access, share, evaluate, and utilize information in these systems to support their efforts in patient care.

Medication Use Process

❶ *The medication use process is a system of interconnected parts that work together to achieve the common goal of safe and effective medication therapy.* The interconnected parts include the people, systems, procedures, and policies that manage medications and related information in patient care. It should be noted here that Chapter 16 further covers a portion of the medication use process, specifically in the context of quality improvement. The medication use process is cyclical in nature and begins with the **prescribing** stage (Figure 26-1). In this stage, the practitioner assesses whether medication therapy

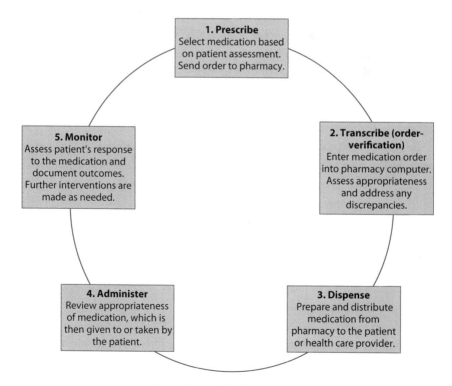

Figure 26–1.   Medication use process.

is warranted and, if so, orders therapy accordingly. The health information technology (HIT) utilized at the prescribing stage includes computerized provider order entry (CPOE), electronic prescribing (e-prescribing), and clinical decision support systems (CDSS), including various medication references.

In the next stage of the medication use process, the **order-verification or transcribing** stage, the ordered medication enters the pharmacy computer system, a pharmacist assesses the appropriateness of the order, and any issues or discrepancies are addressed. HIT tools used at the order-verification stage include CPOE and e-prescribing. Various drug information references, often electronic in nature, may be used and may be built into the systems (e.g., drug interaction screening systems).

Next is the **dispensing** stage. Here, the medication is prepared and distributed from the pharmacy, either directly to the patient or to a health care provider such as a nurse. There are many HIT tools utilized in the dispensing stage, including bar code verification, automated dispensing cabinets (ADCs), syringe fillers, total parenteral nutrition (TPN) compounders, and other robotics.

Following the dispensing stage is the **administration** stage in which the medication is reviewed for appropriateness and then given to, or taken by, the patient. Health care providers, caregivers, the patient, and the patient's family may be involved in the administration stage, depending on the setting. HIT tools used here may include point-of-care bar coding, electronic medication administration records (eMARs), and intelligent infusion (smart) pumps. Additionally, adherence monitoring technologies like medication event monitoring systems (MEMS) can be used to track patient medication usage by capturing each time when a medication is self-administered. To do so, MEMS utilize computer chips embedded in specialized medication bottle caps. The computer chip records each time the cap is removed, which serves as an indicator that the medication was taken by the patient. The final stage in the medication use process is **monitoring**. At the monitoring stage, the patient's response to the medication therapy is assessed, outcomes are documented, and interventions are made as necessary. HIT tools used here include ADE surveillance, antibiotic/drug surveillance, and rules engines. The following is a brief description of some of the HIT tools mentioned above in alphabetical order[1]:

- **Adverse drug event (ADE) monitoring**: Computer programs that use electronic data and predetermined rules to identify when an ADE may have occurred or is about to occur to a patient within a health care setting. This is separate from such programs as MedWatch (see Chapter 17) which is used to report adverse effects to the U.S. Food and Drug Administration (FDA).
- **Automated dispensing cabinets (ADCs)**: Automated devices with a range of functions. Core capabilities include medication storage and retrieval for administration to patients, especially in patient care areas, as well as audit trails of cabinet

access. Other functions can include medication charging and automated inventory management.

- **Bar code verification:** The use of bar code scanning to ensure that the correct drug, strength, and dosage form were dispensed in the drug selection process and to ensure that the six rights of medication administration (i.e., right patient, right drug, right dose, right route, right time, right documentation) are followed at the point of care.

- **Clinical decision support systems (CDSS):** Computer programs that augment clinical decision making by combining referential information with patient-specific information to prevent negative actions and update providers of patient status.

- **Computerized provider order entry (CPOE):** A process allowing medical provider instructions to be electronically entered for the treatment of patients who are under a provider's care.

- **Electronic medication administration record (eMAR):** An electronic version of the traditional medication administration record. It supports patient safety by incorporating clinical decision support and bar coded medication administration. It also enables real-time documentation and billing of medication administration.

- **Electronic prescribing (e-prescribing):** The electronic process in which a prescription is initially entered in an electronic format and then verified and processed in an electronic format, resulting in a labeled medication product, supportive documentation, and an updated, sharable patient electronic medication profile.

- **Intelligent infusion (smart) pumps:** Infusion pumps containing software designed to help eliminate pump programming errors through the use of standardized drug databases and dosing parameters.

- **Rules engines:** Computer programs, similar to ADE monitoring systems, with built-in logic rules designed to aid in monitoring specific aspects of patient care. For example, a rule developed in an attempt to prevent hypoglycemia in patients receiving insulin may require documentation of the patient's meal being delivered prior to the patient receiving mealtime insulin.

Pharmacy Informatics

The term informatics simply refers to the use of computers to manage data and information. *Informatics exists at the intersection of people, information, and technology.*[2] Pharmacy informatics refers to a form of clinical informatics that is applied to the discipline of pharmacy. More specifically, **pharmacy informatics** focuses on the use of information, information systems, and automation technology to ensure safe and effective medication usage.

❷ *All pharmacists are affected by the electronic information systems that make up pharmacy informatics in virtually every aspect of practice.* For example, patient records, medication administration and usage information, insurance information, as well as laboratory tests and results are just a few of the categories of information that are managed in electronic environments.

❸ *The two broad categories of information used in pharmacy informatics, as well as other clinical informatics domains, are patient-specific information and knowledge-based information.*[3] Patient-specific information, which is created and applied in the process of caring for individual patients, includes medication and medical histories, laboratory tests results, radiology interpretations, immunization histories, physical assessments, and other information that is unique to the specific patient. Today, this information is generated and housed in health care facilities, such as pharmacies, hospitals, and clinics. Consumer health informatics, a rapidly growing field, has created an environment in which patients themselves are also generating and managing health-related information in addition to and outside of these traditional settings. Aspects of consumer health informatics can include Internet-based direct-to-consumer advertising (see Chapter 23) and research activities.

Knowledge–based information, on the other hand, forms the scientific basis of health care and includes referential information (about medications, procedures, disease states, etc.), clinical practice guidelines, as well as many other domains of health and medical knowledge.[3] All health care providers make patient care decisions based on a combination of patient-specific and knowledge-based information, a process that can often be a real challenge. Informatics addresses this challenge by using information technology (IT) to manage information, and the medication use process is the context in which pharmacists work to promote safe and effective medication therapy. The following sections describe the role of pharmacists, pharmacy informatics, and other HIT in the medication use process.

Order Entry (Prescribing Stage)

In the 1999 report, *To Err Is Human: Building a Safer Health System*, the Institute of Medicine (IOM) estimated that 44,000 to 98,000 deaths occur each year in U.S. hospitals due to medical errors. A study published in 2016 by researchers at Johns Hopkins Medicine indicates that this number is likely much higher, estimating that 210,000 to 400,000 deaths due to medical error occur each year among U.S. hospital patients. This makes medical errors the third leading cause of death in the United States, behind heart disease and cancer.[4] ADEs undoubtedly make a significant contribution here. Chapters 17 and 18 provide a closer examination of ADEs and the larger topic of medication misadventures; brief statistics are provided here. Nineteen percent of the ADEs were deemed to be due to medication errors, by far the largest category of adverse events noted in the IOM report. The causes of errors and patient injury related to order entry identified in the report included illegible handwritten reports, manual order entry, and the use of nonstandard abbreviations.[5] Further, a study by Bates and associates,[6] which looked at more than 4,000 hospital admissions over a 6-month period, found that errors resulting in preventable ADEs occur most often (i.e., 56% of cases) at the prescribing stage of the medication use process. This same study judged 28% of ADEs as preventable. As such, it is imperative that pharmacists identify and prevent ADEs at this early stage in the medication use process. The three HIT tools that can aid in doing so include CPOE, e-prescribing, and CDSS.

COMPUTERIZED PROVIDER ORDER ENTRY

CPOE, described earlier, is the process allowing medical provider instructions to be entered electronically for the treatment of patients under a provider's care. Orders entered via a CPOE system are communicated to the medical staff and appropriate departments over a computer network. CPOE eliminates illegible handwriting, decreases medical errors as well as the delay in order completion, improves patient care, and is therefore an important component in health care information systems.[7,8] Although features of a CPOE system may vary, ideal features are described here:

- Provider orders should be standardized across the organization (see Chapter 13) but may also be individualized based on the provider or the provider's specialty through the use of order sets. Orders should be communicated to all departments and health care providers involved in the patient's care.
- Patient-centered decision support, including display of the patient's medical history, current test results, and evidence-based guidelines to support treatment options, should be readily available.
- CPOE systems must support clinical workflows through algorithms that provide clear, concise, and actionable advice and warnings. The order entry process should be simple and allow efficient use by new or infrequent users.
- Access must be secure, and a permanent record of access needs to be created with an electronic signature (i.e., any legally recognized means of indicating that a person accepts the contents of an electronic message).
- The CPOE system should be portable, accepting and managing orders from all departments through various devices, including desktop and laptop computers, smartphones, and tablets.

- Data should be collected for training, planning, and analysis of patient safety events as part of ongoing quality initiatives.
- Diagnoses should be linked to orders at the time of order entry to support drug-condition checking, improve documentation, and support appropriate charges.
- Like all HIT systems, appropriate backup and downtime procedures should be established and routinized.

Despite having the ability to decrease ADEs, CPOE also potentially introduces new types of errors.[9] Inexperienced providers and staff using CPOE may actually cause slower order entry and person-to-person communication, especially at first. Alerts and warnings that appear too frequently may lead to **alert fatigue**, a situation in which a provider ignores or overrides CDSS messages without giving them appropriate consideration, due to their sheer volume. Many other types of errors can occur, serving as a strong reminder that all health care providers share responsibility to ensure safe use of CPOE and other HIT systems. As such, implementation of CPOE in a complex medical environment can take years and requires ongoing design changes to adequately fit unique care settings.

Given these issues, as well as providers' resistance to change and the costs involved, adoption of this technology by providers and hospitals in the United States was slow for many years. However, use of CPOE has increased dramatically as more hospitals become aware of the financial benefits of CPOE and as hospitals comply with **Meaningful Use** criteria (see Key Concept 7 and below). A study by RAND Health found that the U.S. health care system could save $70 billion or more annually, reduce ADEs, and improve the quality of care if CPOE and other HIT were widely adopted.[10] Similarly, a 2013 study reported the findings of a systematic review, generating a pooled estimate of the effects of CPOE implementation on medication errors. The study concluded that CPOE implementation decreases the likelihood of a medication error by 48%. Based on CPOE adoption in hospitals at the time, this translates into over 17 million medication errors averted in the United States in 1 year.[11]

Challenges with CPOE Implementation

Despite these clear benefits, there are barriers that must be overcome for wide adoption to be realized. In 2004, Poon and colleagues[12] published a report identifying and addressing these barriers. First is provider and organization resistance to change and CPOE adoption. Reasons cited for this resistance vary and include perceptions that paper methods are faster or more efficient and that implementation attempts would be costly and unsuccessful. The authors of the report identified four key areas on which to focus to overcome resistance. Strong hospital leadership is a necessary factor of implementation of CPOE. Physician champions (i.e., well-respected physicians) should be identified and involved. Workflow concerns should be addressed and users should be reassured throughout the implementation process. And lastly, organizational expertise, being those providers who are more comfortable with IT or who have had experience with CPOE, should be leveraged.

The second major barrier identified is the high cost of CPOE implementation and lack of capital. Strategies identified to overcome high costs include realigning the hospital's priorities to focus on patient safety, leveraging external influences such as published literature to increase awareness about patient safety, and measuring CPOE's impact on hospital efficiency. The last major barrier identified was selection of a specific CPOE product from the many options available. As such, the report's authors concluded that the product or company selected should be (1) committed to the CPOE market, (2) willing and able to adapt products to specific hospital/health system workflows, (3) able to provide tools that help evaluate product functionality, and (4) able to provide information and references for other CPOE systems implemented by the company.

ELECTRONIC PRESCRIBING

Although many definitions exist, e-prescribing is commonly defined as ambulatory CPOE. A more precise definition would be a prescription entered by a prescriber directly into an electronic format using agreed-upon standards that is securely transmitted to the pharmacy that the patient chooses. Faxes and printed prescriptions are not e-prescriptions. One of the primary early challenges to nationwide e-prescribing was a network on which to transfer the prescriptions. Surescripts® provides the connection network and verification between prescribers, insurance providers, and pharmacies. The National Council for Prescription Drug Programs (NCPDP), which is accredited by the American National Standards Institute, provides the standards for provider identification and telecommunication of pharmacy claims in this process.[13]

Components of e-Prescribing

Aside from the prescriber, Surescripts®, and the pharmacy, there are many other components that make up an e-prescribing system. These components include:

- computer software
- the hardware needed to run the software
- the organizations that support transmission and sharing of data
- data standardization
- authorization of payment
- communications to the pharmacy
- the processing of prescriptions within the pharmacy.

The e-prescribing software should provide functionality to support accurate, efficient, and safe entry and transmission of prescriptions. The U.S. government provides incentives to health care providers who implement e-prescribing and EHRs that meet certain minimal requirements in their functionalities. Such functionality includes:

- generating a complete medication list
- supporting prescription ordering, printing, and electronic transmission
- including alerts for unsafe conditions (e.g., allergies)
- providing information on lower cost, therapeutic alternatives
- providing information on formulary and patient eligibility based on the patient's drug plan.[14]

The overall functionality of the e-prescribing software depends on the management of multiple databases.

- **A drug database** is necessary and should include decision support functions, such as therapeutic categories, drug-drug and drug-disease interactions, dose range checking, and allergy warnings.
- **A pharmacy database**, which supports selection of and communication with the patient's specific pharmacy, is needed.
- **A user database**, consisting of a list of prescribers and other users along with their authority to prescribe, Drug Enforcement Administration (DEA) number, and other identifiers, is also needed.
- **A patient database**, listing patients and all pertinent patient information to support e-prescribing functions, must be included and managed.
- Other necessary databases include medication insurance plans/formularies and medication profile information for individual patients.

Depending on the functionality of the e-prescribing software, additional clinical information may also be available, such as laboratory results, patient problems and diagnoses, and information from prior visits.

Workflow in e-Prescribing

To fully comprehend the functionality of an e-prescribing system, an understanding of prescribing workflow is necessary. The first step is patient registration and eligibility verification, which generally occurs prior to or at the time the patient arrives for an appointment. Here, the patient's insurance coverage and address are verified, and the patient is put on a readily available selection list within the e-prescribing system for prescribers. The patient's medication history and prescription eligibility, which are generally retrieved from Surescripts®, are assessed next.

Following this is the medication entry step. Since prescription entry can vary greatly between and within practices, the e-prescribing system should support quickly transitioning between patients, data gathering, and ordering. Portable devices and the ability to quickly log into an immobile device (e.g., desktop computer) are needed to support this type of workflow. Although not yet addressed by federal regulations, delegating the task of medication entry to support staff introduces the potential for errors as reading and translating written prescriptions are often involved in this approach. The next step in the prescribing workflow is prescriber selection of the pharmacy to which the prescriptions should be sent. A common error at this stage is selection of the wrong pharmacy from the searchable database. Once the pharmacy is selected, the prescription is transmitted to the pharmacy using standard NCPDP SCRIPT interface transactions.

One area that has great potential for improvement with e-prescribing is the renewal authorization process (i.e., authorization by the prescriber for additional refills). Prior to e-prescribing, renewal authorization required multiple telephone calls and was highly interruptive. Now, pharmacies can initiate electronic renewal requests which can be electronically processed and returned by the prescriber.

e-Prescribing of Controlled Substances

Federal law now allows electronic prescriptions (e-prescriptions) for controlled substances. However, both the prescriber's and the receiving pharmacy's e-prescription systems must first be verified by a DEA-approved third-party organization prior to their use. These systems are also subject to audit to ensure compliance with regulations. Although federal law began allowing controlled substances to be prescribed electronically in June 2010, adoption was slow.[15] It was not until September 2015 that all 50 U.S. states allowed the e-prescribing of controlled substances (Schedules II to V), with Vermont being the last state to fully adopt this practice. Like many other states, Vermont authorized e-prescribing of Schedule III to IV drugs prior to allowing e-prescribing of Schedule II drugs.[16,17] As a direct result of these state and federal legislative changes, e-prescribing of controlled substances has increased rapidly from 1,535 electronic prescriptions for controlled substances in 2012 to 4 million in the first half of 2015 alone.[18] Nationwide e-prescribing of controlled substances is expected to greatly decrease prescription fraud and abuse. In fact, progress in terms of allowing e-prescribing of controlled substances is closely linked with states' efforts to combat the current prescription drug abuse epidemic in the United States.[19] Moving beyond simply allowing e-prescribing, New York now has a mandate requiring practitioners to electronically prescribe both controlled and noncontrolled substances. There are however exceptions to the state mandate, which went into effect in March 2016.[20]

CLINICAL DECISION SUPPORT SYSTEMS

According to the American Medical Association (AMA), clinical decision support (CDS) is described as "providing clinicians, patients or individuals with knowledge and person-specific or population information, intelligently filtered or presented at appropriate times, to foster better health processes, better individual patient care, and better population health."[21] CDSS are the computing systems that provide CDS. The three basic components of a CDSS include (1) an inference engine, (2) a knowledge base, and (3) a communication mechanism. The inference engine, also known as the reasoning engine, forms the brain of the CDSS, working to link patient-specific information with information in the knowledge base. It evaluates the available information and determines what to present to the user. The knowledge base is composed of varied clinical knowledge, such as treatment guidelines, diagnoses, and drug-drug or drug-disease interactions. The communication mechanism allows entry of patient information and is responsible for communicating relevant information back to the clinician. A CDSS that checks a patient's age and immunization history against vaccination guidelines and then presents recommendations to a provider serves as a useful example.

CDS can be generated in a variety of forms, including alerts, reminders, information displays, CPOE, electronic templates, and guidelines. CDSS have been employed in many clinical care domains and can support a wide range of complex decisions at various stages in the patient care process. In terms of preventive care, CDSS can provide reminders for vaccinations, cancer screenings, cardiovascular risk reduction, and other preventive measures. A study by Shea and associates[22] found a 77% increase in the use of preventive practices when computer reminders were used. There are several CDSS that have been designed to help clinicians diagnose based on the signs and symptoms exhibited by a patient. These systems have the potential to reduce diagnostic errors and should be linked with an EHR to achieve their full potential.[23] CDSS are used to provide evidence-based treatment at the point of care, often drawing upon evidence-based guidelines, which are covered in Chapter 8.

Medication Decision Support

Medication decision support is a large portion of the knowledge base for any CDSS. Basic support in this area includes drug-allergy checking, basic dosing guidance, formulary decision support, duplicate therapy checking, and drug-drug interaction (DDI) checking. In the case of formulary decision support, CDSS can prompt prescribers of the preferred medications (according to the hospital's or insurer's formulary) at the point in time in which they are selecting from available medications. This allows prescribers to implement agreed-upon formularies (see Chapter 13) within their practice settings with minimal disruption. More advanced decision support may include dosing suggestions for geriatric patients or patients with renal insufficiency, guidance for medication-related laboratory testing, drug-disease and drug-lab interaction checking, and drug-pregnancy contraindication checking. CDSS are also used for follow-up or corollary orders as well as adverse event monitoring. In fact, a study by Overhage et al.[24] showed a 25% improvement in corollary orders (orders that are routine under certain situations, such as a stool softener when a patient is receiving a narcotic) with the use of CDSS. The main benefits of CDSS use include the ability to decrease ADEs, costs, and length of patient stay as well as improve clinical workflow, provide useful information at the point of care, draw attention to possible drug interactions, and provide reminders of warranted follow-up interventions.

CDSS also have their limitations. For instance, developing and maintaining a comprehensive knowledge base is time consuming and resource intensive. CDSS need to communicate with other clinical information systems, such as EHRs, CPOE systems, and pharmacy systems. Additionally, excessive alerting can lead to alert fatigue and clinicians ignoring the warnings (Case Study 26-1).

Case Study 26–1

While on a pharmacy informatics rotation, you as a pharmacy student attend rounds with medical students to gain insight into the use of HIT from a physician's standpoint. After the physician leading rounds illustrates the use of the hospital's CPOE and CDS systems, she mentions the challenges that the hospital faced when implementing their CPOE system. The discussion then turns to the potential problems, limitations, and benefits of CPOE and CDS systems. Since the physician knows that you are on a pharmacy informatics rotation, she asks for your input.

- *What is the difference between CPOE and e-prescribing systems?*
- *What are the challenges with CPOE implementation?*
- *What is a CDS system and what role does it play in CPOE and e-prescribing systems?*
- *What are the potential problems, limitations, and benefits of these two systems to users?*

Order Verification (Transcribing Stage)

Order verification occurs when prescribed medications are transferred, either manually or electronically, to the pharmacy. Once received, pharmacists must interpret the medication order and make an assessment in regards to any drug-related problems. The goal of this process is to transform the order into a dispensable form that can be safely and correctly interpreted at the administration step. Pharmacists may use CDSS, pharmacy computer systems, and evidence-based medicine tools at this stage to perform their cognitive and administrative functions.

Pharmacists have traditionally relied upon CDSS within the pharmacy information system to support safe and efficacious decision making regarding the filling of prescriptions. Although the use of CDSS at the prescribing stage helps improve the quality of orders received by the pharmacy, problems still exist with orders originating from CPOE systems and e-prescriptions. For instance, CPOE systems, while reducing certain errors, have been found to increase other types of errors. A study by Koppel and associates[9] found that a widely used CPOE system actually facilitated 22 types of medication error risks, including pharmacy inventory displays being mistaken for dosage guidelines, fragmented CPOE displays that prevent full view of a patient's medications, and inflexible ordering formats that result in wrong orders. As such, pharmacists must remain diligent in their review of orders prior to dispensing.

One of the main aspects of support provided by pharmacy CDSS software is information pertaining to DDIs. This information is meant to augment and increase pharmacists' ability to detect clinically significant interactions. However, a study by Saverno and associates, which analyzed the ability of pharmacy information systems and associated CDS to detect DDIs at 64 Arizona pharmacies, indicated that many pharmacy CDSS perform suboptimally in terms of identifying well-known, clinically relevant interactions. Specifically, only 28% of the participating pharmacies accurately identified the interactions and non-interactions involved in the study's fictitious patient medication orders.[25] This further reiterates the point that pharmacists must remain diligent when reviewing orders to be dispensed.

Dispensing

Medications are prepared and distributed to patients in the dispensing stage of the medication use process. The actual activities involved at this step vary depending on the setting: inpatient (institutional, acute care) versus outpatient care (community). However, there are many similarities shared between the two settings, including acquiring medications from a supplier, stocking medications based on needs, and safely and accurately preparing and dispensing medications based on the verified order. Further, there are many HIT tools utilized at the dispensing stage in both settings. That said, the two settings also have their differences when it comes to dispensing and the HIT tools used in the process.

ACUTE CARE PHARMACY SETTING

Many aspects related to dispensing from an acute care pharmacy (i.e., institutional pharmacy) can be automated by HIT. All automated systems utilized must be able to

(1) uniquely identify managed products, (2) receive and interpret medication orders, (3) perform appropriate dose calculations as needed, and (4) report transactions to other automated systems for billing or other purposes.

For this to occur, all prescription medication packaging must be marked with an assigned, 10-digit National Drug Code (NDC), a requirement by the FDA. All NDCs consist of three parts: a labeler code, a drug code, and a package code in one of the following configurations: 4-4-2, 5-4-1, or 5-3-2, representing labeler-drug-package. The labeler code is assigned by the FDA and identifies the vendor responsible for the final packaging of the drug. The drug code, which is assigned by the vendor, identifies the drug form and strength of the product. Lastly, the package code, also assigned by the vendor, identifies the packaging level type and size (e.g., unit, box, case, etc.). It should be noted that, due to a Health Insurance Portability and Accountability Act (HIPAA) standard, 10-digit NDCs must be converted into an 11-digit format in a 5-4-2 configuration for billing purposes.[26,27] The FDA maintains a central repository of NDCs. However, although manufacturers are required to report NDCs to the FDA, approval is not required. For automation to work properly, the pharmacy and related automated systems must maintain a current and accurate list of known NDCs. Compounded preparations, on the other hand, require their own unique bar codes produced by the pharmacy.[1]

Carousel cabinets, ADCs, robotic cart filling systems, and sterile compounding devices are some of the other prominent HIT tools used in automated drug distribution systems in acute care pharmacies. Carousel cabinets (e.g., MedCarousel®) contain shelves that are attached to a carousel, which rotates shelves for medication selection. Benefits of carousel cabinets include the freeing up of floor space, reduced walking associated with drug distribution, and more accurate accounting of inventory.

ADCs are similar to carousels, except they do not use rotating shelves. ADCs, which may be located either in the pharmacy or on patient-care units, maintain inventory and audit trails as well as perform charging functions (e.g., Pyxis®). Access to inventory contained in ADCs requires the user to log in, maintaining an audit trail of receiving and dispensing activity. ADCs can be configured with a variety of different drawers so that specified users may only have access to certain drawers or even specific drawer sections. Despite being able to limit access in this way, none of the drawers control the amount of product removed, which can be seen as a limitation. In some situations, like emergencies, override functions are permitted.[1] Despite the obvious benefit of override access, this practice has also been associated with medication errors, such as obtaining the wrong strength of medication and obtaining a medication after it has been discontinued.[28,29]

While not as common as ADCs, robotic cart filling systems are commonly found in hospital settings as well (e.g., Tug®). They utilize bar coding to locate, obtain, package, and deliver medications to a specified location (e.g., pediatric nursing unit).

This is done by filling unit-dose carts and most often requires significant repackaging efforts because the medications must be in containers that can be manipulated by the device.

The preparation of sterile products for administration can also be automated. The FDA classifies the devices that automate sterile dose preparations as pharmacy compounding devices.[30] TPN compounders are an example of this type of device. TPN compounders first compute a TPN formulation based on clinical requirements, and then drive a machine to deliver the correct ingredients in the correct amounts and sequence. Chemotherapy preparations which include hazardous medications to pharmacy personnel can also be compounded by an automated system (e.g., APOTECA).

COMMUNITY PHARMACY SETTING

Pharmacy Information Management System

In the community pharmacy, pharmacy information management systems (PIMS) serve as the core piece of HIT that supports pharmacy operations, managing all data associated with prescriptions, patients, and prescribers. They contain key databases, such as drug files, DEA and national provider identifier numbers, physician contact information, prescription pricing tables, third-party plan details, and patient profiles. The PIMS software and related databases commonly reside on a server in the pharmacy, but they may be located on a central server, allowing access from multiple sites. In the **software as a service (SaaS)** or **application service provider (ASP)** options, both the data and software are hosted off-site. PIMS may also have integrated workflow systems with multiple workstations assigned specific tasks (e.g., intake, processing, and verifying of prescriptions). For instance, faxed and paper prescriptions are scanned during intake, making the then digitized prescription available at the filling and verification steps. (Note: this is not an e-prescription.) The goal of digitization is to reduce the amount of paper handled and provide a faster way to file, index, share, and search for information. Bar code scanning is also an integral component of this workflow, which allows the tracking of every prescription through the filling queue. Such workflow systems provide efficiency and are usually found in high-volume pharmacies.[1]

Other HIT utilized in the community pharmacy setting includes automated counting systems and robotics, interactive voice response (IVR) systems (i.e., the automated menu that a caller is prompted through using the phone number pad), e-prescribing, and electronic signature capture. Refill requests are commonly routed into the PIMS filling queue via IVR, which guides patients in entering in their refill information. This practice reduces the number of phone calls that must be made and handled by pharmacy staff and also gives patients the ability to submit refills after hours. The Internet is also being utilized for patient-entered refill requests to the same effect. Further, IVR systems, along with text messaging, are being utilized to automate outbound contact with patients, such as prescription pick-up reminders and other informative messages. Another method by which new or refill prescriptions can enter the PIMS queue is via e-prescribing. E-prescribing is a feature of almost every PIMS, most of which route prescriptions through the Surescripts® network.[1]

Bar Coded Verification System

Through the use of counting systems or robotic dispensing systems, the majority of a community pharmacy's prescription volume can be automated. Counting systems include countertop devices and stand-alone cabinets while robotic dispensing fills and labels vials. Bar codes are used in the dispensing process to match (1) the medication with the prescription (avoiding an incorrect medication selection) and (2) the patient with the prescription (avoiding an incorrect patient selection) as entered in the computer system. This use of bar codes allows multiple checks as an additional layer of safety.[1] Further, bar codes on will-call bags are scanned when bags are hung. This information is updated in the pharmacy computer system for quick retrieval when the patient arrives, using light to identify the hanging bag in some instances.

Administration

Depending on the setting, medications may be administered by a health care provider, such as a physician, nurse, or pharmacist, by a caregiver, or by the patient themselves. Three important HIT tools being used in hospital settings at this stage of the medication use process are bar code medication administration (BCMA) systems, eMARs, and intelligent infusion devices ("smart pumps"). BCMA systems are used typically by nurses at the point of care to ensure that the six rights of medication administration are followed. While use of these systems has been increasing steadily, there is a major issue that hinders implementation. While most products used in the inpatient care setting have bar codes, there are some products (e.g., unit-dose packets) that still require pharmacy to create and attach the bar code, which is labor-intensive. Also, products that are compounded for local use, such as intravenous antibiotics, need special bar codes that are not supported by the basic linear bar coding format. Two-dimensional bar codes can at least partly solve this issue.

Alongside BCMA systems, the use of eMARs replaces paper records used by nurses to document medication administration. eMARs decrease the potential for errors by eliminating the need to handwrite changes in medications and allowing a medication change to be updated in real time in the patient's medical record.[1] They also automatically document the time at which medications are administered (i.e., scanned). This is especially important for evaluating the timing of administration of critical medications (e.g., antimicrobials).

Whereas BCMA commonly covers the administration of oral and topical dosage forms, intelligent infusion devices are increasingly being deployed in institutional settings to increase the safety of intravenous medication administration. Smart pumps, as they are commonly called, include drug libraries that contain standardized concentrations of drugs used in the institution, agreed-upon maximum and minimum dosing limits for continuous and bolus doses, and rate and volume limits. The development and refinement of the standardized information (e.g., libraries, dosing limits, etc.) found in smart pumps is an important opportunity for pharmacists to leverage their drug information expertise to support institutional-wide decisions that impact direct patient care. Additional benefits of the incorporation of standardized information in smart pumps include: (1) a double check of programming when nursing staff prepares a medication for administration, (2) soft and hard stops that can temporarily pause or suspend administration, and (3) an electronic audit trail.

A closed-loop medication administration system allows individuals responsible for a patient's care to have access to the same information at the same time. Being fully electronic, these systems collate data from CPOE, BCMA, smart pumps, EMRs, and other sources across the continuum of care at all steps of the medication use process via seamless documentation. Closed-loop medication administration systems allow health care providers access to nearly all activities related to a patient's care in real time, with decision support incorporated as needed. The primary focus of these systems is patient safety, and they have been shown to significantly reduce medication errors.

Monitoring

Clinicians' monitoring activities vary greatly depending on their work setting and available resources. No matter the setting however, monitoring activities should result in clinical interventions, when necessary. A clinical intervention is the act of interceding with the intent of modifying the medication use process. The broad categories of monitoring activities, and therefore clinical interventions, performed by health care providers include activities that promote safety, activities that promote quality, and activities that promote efficiency and cost-effectiveness. For instance, a pharmacist may intercept a medication ordered for which the patient has an allergy, or a pharmacist may identify a less expensive, therapeutic alternative to the prescribed medication in order to decrease costs for the patient.[1]

In the hospital setting, clinical surveillance systems are at the core of monitoring efforts. These systems exist as stand-alone applications and as components of integrated systems. Clinical surveillance refers to active surveillance or watchful waiting that includes a collection and analysis of patient-specific information that is then used to drive decisions. These systems are most often used by pharmacy to monitor information from the pharmacy system (i.e., medication lists), laboratory results, and patient demographics from the admission/discharge/transfer system. Rules are built to identify potential problems. Rules can be built locally or included with other information systems components. Often, pharmacy or others charged with medication safety will assume responsibility for rule construction and investigation. For example, a rule may monitor all patients for orders of naloxone, which is used to treat opioid overdose. Another rule may monitor for all patients receiving ranitidine, whose platelet count has decreased to less than 50% of the previous value, suggesting an occurrence of rare thrombocytopenia. Patients meeting these predefined rules are presented to pharmacy staff for follow-up and evaluation.

Once a need is established and a clinical intervention has taken place, the intervention must be well documented. The purpose of clinical intervention documentation is multifaceted. One primary purpose is to demonstrate the cost and quality impact of programs, such as clinical pharmacy services. Documenting clinical interventions can also be used for staff performance improvement as well as quality improvement activities. Documentation gives insight into what clinical staff members are doing, and therefore allows constructive feedback to be provided. Similarly, clinical intervention documentation can be utilized to improve workflow.

There are certain basic elements that a good documentation system should have.

- It should be easy to use and fit into the existing workflow as much as possible.
- It should allow for quick documentation that includes sufficient details. Specifically, the system should have the capability to add or modify interventions, manage drug and prescriber databases, and mirror the organization's security policies.
- All documentation should be searchable.
- The system should provide a complete record of all clinical activities.

Ideally, all practitioners providing care to the same patient would document all monitoring and intervention activities in a shared record. The record would then be accessible by all other providers who are also caring for that particular patient. In fact, a primary objective of the Pharmacy HIT Collaborative, a multi-organizational group focused on the role of pharmacists in the emerging electronic health record (EHR) landscape, is to ensure that this is the case for the patient care efforts of pharmacists.[31] Reporting, which is the critical output of the documentation system, should be quick and easy. It should allow real-time selection and inclusion of any combination of documented fields in the system[1] (Case Study 26-2).

Case Study 26-2

You are still on your pharmacy informatics rotation, and after your discussion on the potential problems/limitations of CPOE and e-prescribing systems from the physician's standpoint, the medical students with whom you are rounding ask you how pharmacists interface with CPOE and e-prescribing systems. The physician then illustrates the use of the hospital's BCMA system. The medical students inquire as to the purpose of the BCMA system. They also ask if HIT is used to actively monitor patients. Again, the physician leading rounds asks for your input.

1. *How do pharmacists interface with CPOE and e-prescribing systems?*
2. *What is a BCMA system and what is its purpose?*
3. *What HIT is used to actively monitor patients and how does it do so?*

PRESCRIPTION DRUG MONITORING PROGRAMS (PDMPS)

Monitoring of prescription narcotics, especially opioids, has become increasingly important in recent years. In fact, more than 40 people die per day due to use of prescribed opioids in the United States, more than heroin and cocaine combined.[32] PDMPs are central databases of statewide prescribing and dispensing records for controlled drugs and other drugs with high potential for abuse.[33] At the time of publication, all states except Missouri maintained a PDMP.

There are several PDMP vendors who develop and maintain the majority of states' databases. Access and reporting privileges and requirements vary among states. While the typical pharmacist may not have hands-on experience with the technical aspects of their state's PDMP, because of their access to PDMPs and to patients, pharmacists have an important role in curbing misuse of prescription medications. It is up to the pharmacist to review and act on the data found in their PDMP in those situations where concerns of abuse exist (Case Study 26-3).

Case Study 26–3

You are a student pharmacist completing an inpatient pharmacy administration rotation. Through your rotation experiences, you have observed and interacted with a variety of health information technologies and automation used to manage medications within the institution. Your preceptor gives you the following assignment.

- *What is the medication use process, and what health technologies are used at each stage of the medication use process to ensure safe and efficacious medication therapy?*

The Future: Informatics in the U.S. Health Care System

❹ *The vision of health care is becoming more patient-centered.* Health care is transitioning from industrial age medicine—which places focus on professional care and is segmented and also highly expensive—to a new approach, alternatively described as information age health care, which encourages lower cost individual care, getting friends and family involved, and using self-help networks as first-line approaches.[34] This transformation has been given the label, participatory care, in that the new approach involves patients as highly active, decision-making members of their own care team. **Health 2.0**, being the utilization of health care-related tools provided by Web 2.0, is the web-oriented extension of this new participatory care approach. Web 2.0 simply refers to those applications of the Internet that are interactive and social, allowing for collaboration and interactivity among patients, caregivers, and providers. Facebook (https://www.facebook.com/) is probably the most prominent example of Web 2.0. Facebook, as is well known, is a social networking portal that allows users to interact and share pictures, videos, and links, among other things. Patientslikeme (http://www.patientslikeme.com/), being a Health 2.0 social networking portal, is similar to Facebook except that it focuses on allowing people with the same medical condition to communicate with each other about health-related issues.

Other Web 2.0 and Health 2.0 resources include blogs, wiki sites, Twitter (https://twitter.com/), and **personal health records (PHRs)**. With a blog, anyone can post his or her thoughts on literally any topic at a particular site on the Internet as a blog entry. Readers can then leave related comments directly below the published material. Wiki sites allow the publication of monographs via group participation, and the published material can be updated at any time. The most well-known example of a wiki site is Wikipedia, "the free encyclopedia that anyone can edit."[35] As for Health 2.0, RxWiki (http://www .rxwiki.com/) is a wiki site that provides patients with drug monographs compiled by pharmacists. Twitter is a Web 2.0 service with the sole focus being the ability to send short messages to groups. Twitter users can follow one or more members as well as be followed by members who want to keep up with the insights of those they find interesting. Examples of pharmacy applications for this kind of resource include promoting medication adherence, promoting health behaviors, and producing warnings for patients. One of the best ways to learn about Health 2.0 resources (including primary literature, for example) is to search for "Health 2.0 journal" in your preferred search engine.

PHRs are Health 2.0 applications that provide the patient an increased opportunity to participate in the collection, maintenance, and sharing of their personal health-related information through a web-based environment. All the information is patient-maintained, and PHRs should be designed as a lifelong resource for the patient's health information. PHRs are ideally kept in a web-accessible, electronic format that is secure and private but also universally available to providers treating the patient. Further, the ability to move information from a patient's EHR, which is maintained by a health care organization, to the patient's PHR increases patient involvement in their own health care. Along with this ability, patients should also have the ability to annotate the information coming in from their providers or EHR. It should be noted here that the PHR does not and is not meant to replace the legal record of any provider.[36] In order for PHRs to be interoperable and share data with other systems as described, standards of data communication must be established and utilized. Current agreed upon standards include Continuity of Care Record (CCR) and Extensible Markup Language (XML). Strong levels of data encryption and passwords are also required. Although still evolving, there are dozens of PHRs available today. Two examples include Microsoft's HealthVault (https://www.healthvault.com) and AHIMA's MyPHR (http://www.myphr.com).

INTERNET OF THINGS

The *Internet of Things (IoT)* refers to the development of the Internet such that everyday physical objects or devices will be connected, enabling them to share information and communicate intelligently with other devices. This has been enabled by the increasing availability of broadband Internet, decreasing technology costs, and an increasing number of devices with built-in sensors and Wi-Fi capabilities. The possibilities in terms of the types of devices that could take part in the IoT are endless. Current examples range from light bulbs to children's toys to toothbrushes. Although the IoT is currently still in its infancy, IoT-enabling technology is rapidly maturing. Over the next decade, more than 250 billion devices are expected to connect to the Internet.

There are many current and potential use cases for the IoT in health care that may be of benefit to both patients and providers. Currently, mHealth applications and related devices allow patients to capture their personal biometric data, which can then be automatically or manually shared with health care providers. In hospitals, sensors can be used for indoor mapping, allowing visitors to use their smartphones to easily navigate to desired locations within the institution. In the same setting, IoT technology can be used to keep track of medical devices, personnel, and patients.[37] In the outpatient setting, application of IoT devices allows providers to monitor patients around-the-clock and in real time, whether present or remote.[38] Given these and many more potential uses of IoT in the field, health care is seen by some as one of the most promising applications of the IoT. According to a 2015 report, the health care IoT market is expected to reach $117 billion by 2020.[39] Along the way, standardization of data formats and optimization of transmission protocols are needed in order to maximize interoperability and minimize data-transfer costs.[38,40] Further, bounded latency and reliability are absolute requirements when being applied to emergency situations. Lastly, privacy, authentication, and integrity are requisites when dealing with protected health information[40] (Case Study 26-4).

Case Study 26–4

Your preceptor approaches you one morning and tells you about a new committee within the hospital that she has been asked to chair. The committee's role is to explore the emerging Health 2.0 domain and identify potential ways that the hospital can become involved. The committee is also interested in how the hospital can incorporate the IoT in ways that may benefit visitors, patients, and personnel. Knowing that you are a tech-savvy person, your preceptor asks you to help conduct some of the initial research into the Health 2.0 domain and potential uses of the IoT. You are given the following assignment.

- *What are the primary journals that address the Health 2.0 domain?*
- *Suggest a few ways the hospital can use popular Web 2.0 tools for Health 2.0 efforts.*
- *Suggest a few ways the hospital can use IoT applications and devices.*

THE EXPANDING ROLE OF DATA

Related to the IoT, two terms of increasing importance in today's health care space are *Big Data* and *Little Data*. Big Data has been defined as what organizations or businesses know about people (i.e., their customers and/or constituents), while Little Data is what people know about themselves.[41] Big Data are customarily captured through activities in the normal course of business and are often stored in large data repositories for analysis, which then drives decision making. In health care, for example, data are generated in the process of care and are increasingly being stored in EHRs and administrative claims databases. Through the use of extremely powerful software and hardware, these data can be analyzed to identify patterns and trends that can inform activities, such as clinical operations, research and development, and public health policies.[42]

Alternatively, Little Data are generated and maintained by individuals through their normal daily routines, including activities and experiences like shopping preferences, social networks, how we spend our time, and where we spend our money.[41] From a health and wellness point of view, several obvious examples of Little Data have permeated popular culture. Wearable devices that monitor physical activity and sleep patterns are continuously creating data that the individual can use as a guide in making decisions to improve overall health. Smartphone apps that enable routine recording of meals help individuals identify necessary changes to improve their dietary patterns.

An important difference between Big and Little Data is the owner: organizations own Big Data while the individual owns Little Data.[41] In the ideal future scenario, organizations and individuals will be able to leverage both types of data to optimize decision making. For example, Big Data describing the impact of a sedentary lifestyle among a specific subset of the population (e.g., women over 50 who primarily sit at a desk during the work day) will be informative to a specific member of said subset of the population. Using the Little Data that she has generated through a physical activity monitor, the individual will identify not only the outcomes of her lifestyle among similar individuals (using Big Data), but she will also be able to identify the impact of changing her lifestyle on our outcomes.

INTEROPERABLE ELECTRONIC HEALTH RECORDS

❺ *The current health care system is decentralized and fragmented. Because of this, significant communication gaps exist when multiple health care institutions provide care for the same patient. Substantial evidence suggests that more effective communication would improve patient care and reduce medical errors, such as ADEs.*[5,43] Beyond the clinical improvements, there are also major financial benefits to be had. It was projected in 2005 that greater health information exchange and interoperability could save the U.S. health care system $77.8 billion annually.[44] **Interoperability** is the ability of disparate computer systems to exchange information in a manner that allows the information to be used meaningfully.[45] **❻** *The desired result of interoperable systems and EHRs is to readily provide all health practitioners in all locations, including the pharmacy, with access to information about a patient's care, as* *needed.* As such, new health information systems (HIS) should focus on ensuring effective communication of data between and within institutions, which includes a focus on data transfer across applications, devices, and geographical locations. Communication standards are necessary to achieve this desired level of meaningful data exchange.

CURRENT STANDARDS

Several health care standards exist today. For instance, the NCPDP developed an e-prescribing standard, NCPDP SCRIPT, for the transmission of prescription information, along with relevant medical history information, electronically between prescribers, pharmacies, and payers. Mentioned previously, NDCs, created by manufacturers and the FDA, with whom they are registered, are used as a standard way to signify the drug manufacturer, the drug formulation, and the packaging type. RxNorm, produced by the National Library of Medicine (NLM), is a standard for supporting semantic interoperability between pharmacy systems and drug terminologies by providing a standardized naming system for generic and branded drugs.[46] Unified Medical Language System (UMLS), also maintained by the NLM, enables interoperability between computer systems, such as EHRs, by providing a set of files and software that bring together many medical vocabularies and standards.[47] Contained within the UMLS is the Logical Observation Identifiers Names and Codes (LOINC) terminology for laboratory test results and procedures. Another important medical terminology version also contained within UMLS is the Systematized Nomenclature of Medicine-Clinical Terms (SNOMED CT). SNOMED CT maps to diagnosis and billing codes known as the International Classification of Disease-tenth revision (ICD-10). Further, Current Procedural Terminology (CPT®) codes, produced by the AMA, provide medical nomenclature used to report medical procedures and services performed under private and public health insurance plans.[48]

THE GOVERNMENT'S ROLE IN INTEROPERABILITY

Technical standards are one piece of the interoperability puzzle. Other challenges include finding an organization or group to lead the charge through associated business, administrative, and financial considerations. The U.S. government has been leading these efforts, beginning in 2004 when President George W. Bush targeted computerizing health records in his State of the Union address. That same year, President Bush established the Office of the National Coordinator for Health Information Technology (ONC) within the Office of the Secretary of Health and Human Services (HHS).[49] The two major initial goals of the ONC were widespread adoption of EHRs by 2014 and the creation and implementation of an interoperable health information infrastructure.

❼ *In order to increase adoption and Meaningful Use of EHRs by providers and hospitals, CMS developed a monetary incentive program. The Meaningful Use program incentivizes hospitals and physicians to use EHRs to achieve specific outcomes, which may be process oriented or patient oriented. The goals of the Meaningful Use program are to (1) improve quality, safety, and efficiency, (2) engage patients and their families, (3) improve care coordination, as well as public and population health, and (4) maintain privacy and security of protected health information (PHI). For example, 60% of medication orders should be entered electronically or >50% of patients should have electronic access to their medical information within 36 hours after discharge.* It is hoped that the adoption of and compliance with Meaningful Use will result in better clinical outcomes, improved population health, increased health care transparency and efficiency, more robust data for research, and the empowerment of individuals and patients.[50]

Stages of Meaningful Use

Further, there are specific objectives, broken down into three stages, set by CMS that eligible providers and hospitals must achieve to qualify for the incentive program. Stage 1 began in 2011 and focused on providers capturing patient data and sharing that data with either the patient or other health care providers. Initiated in 2014, Stage 2 focused on advanced clinical processes, requiring that a specified number of core and menu objectives be met. Specifically, all of the 15 core objectives must be met, which include items such as the use of CPOE and e-prescribing, maintaining active drug and allergy lists, checking for drug-drug and drug-allergy interactions, implementation of CDS, and protection of electronic health information. As for the 10 menu objectives, which include items such as submitting electronic data to immunization registries, drug formulary checking, electronic access to health information for patients, and patient-specific education resources, 5 must be met.[51] Stage 3, began in 2016 and focuses specifically on improved patient outcomes.

EHR adoption has increased steadily since 2010. An estimated 75% of U.S. hospitals had at least a basic EHR in 2014. This was true of only 59% of hospitals in 2013. Further, core Stage 2 Meaningful Use criteria were met by just over 40% of U.S. hospitals in 2014. In 2013, these criteria were met by only 5.8% of hospitals. As of March 2016, over 90% of hospitals eligible for the Meaningful Use program have met Meaningful Use criteria.[52,53]

Despite this progress, the projected health and savings benefits of interoperable health IT systems have not been fully realized. This is due to many factors, including slower than expected adoption, adoption of systems that are neither interoperable nor easy to use, and failure to redesign health care approaches to take full advantage of health IT.[54]

Related challenges reported by hospitals include costs related to implementation and ongoing use, lack of support from physicians, and the complexity involved in meeting the Meaningful Use criteria.[52]

When practice sites already have computerized management systems (e.g., to capture patient information, schedule appointments, perform billing tasks, etc.), as most sites do, choosing an EHR or other health IT to implement can be difficult. These sites can choose to either integrate their existing management system with the EHR or adopt a completely new, integrated system. With the former approach, often referred to as a "best-of-breeds" system, the EHR is selected based on its inherent qualities. Often times, especially when the software applications are obtained from different vendors, interfaces must be built for them to exchange data. Integrated databases, on the other hand, share the same database, eliminating the need to build interfaces. Integrated systems also offer the convenience of having a single point of contact for technical support. However, the "best-of-breeds" approach is not without its advantages. It allows sites to keep their current, familiar software in place. This, combined with being able to choose an EHR based on its own merits, can make the choice between this approach and an integrated system a difficult one (Case Study 26-5).

Case Study 26–5

You are wrapping up your rotation, and your preceptor comes to you with a final assignment. She has been tasked with representing the Pharmacy Department on the committee that is overseeing the implementation of EHRs in the institution. She knows very little about EHRs and asks the following questions to get started.

1. *What are EHRs and how do they differ from PHRs?*
2. *What group or organization is overseeing EHR implementation?*
3. *Which governmental group is directing the Meaningful Use program?*
4. *Briefly describe the stages of Meaningful Use.*
5. *What are some known barriers to EHR implementation?*

SECURITY, PRIVACY, AND CONFIDENTIALITY OF PROTECTED HEALTH INFORMATION

As interoperability advances and more patient data is shared across providers and organizations, the issues of security, privacy, and confidentiality of protected health information

● inevitability arise. **Protected health information (PHI)** includes any information that can be used to identify a person, including information about medical conditions, payment for care, or actual care delivered.[1] Privacy refers to being free from unauthorized intrusions and the protection of PHI. In health care organizations, privacy is accomplished through policies that determine how and what information is gathered, stored, and used, and how patients are involved in the process. Security here refers to restricting access to patient health data to everyone except those with authorized access. This is accomplished through the use of electronic tools, such as login identifications and password protection. Confidentiality here refers to the provider-client privilege that, under most circumstances, any health-related information communicated between a provider and a patient is private. PHI can be in any form (e.g., written, oral, electronic), and examples include patient name, address, Social Security number, e-mail address, or any other part of a medical record that could be used to identify a patient.[1]

Health care providers need to be aware of the existing and emerging regulations that apply to the security, privacy, and confidentiality of PHI. For instance, the Health Breach Notification Rule, passed into law in 2009, requires that covered entities provide notice to patients following a breach in security. Also, the Patient Safety and Quality Improvement Act of 2005 (Patient Safety Act) establishes a framework that allows providers to voluntarily and confidentially report patient safety events to Patient Safety Organizations for aggregation and analysis purposes.[55]

HEALTH INSURANCE PORTABILITY AND ACCOUNTABILITY ACT (HIPAA)

Another major piece of legislation with which health care providers need to be intimately familiar is the HIPAA, passed into law in 1996. The main component of concern here is the HIPAA Privacy Rule, which establishes how medical information, should be handled. The major goal of the Privacy Rule is to ensure proper protection of individuals' health information while also allowing the flow of health information needed to provide high-quality health care. As such, the law defines PHI, describes how health care organizations can use and disclose PHI, and outlines the requirements of health organizations to protect PHI from inappropriate disclosure and misuse. For instance, the Privacy Rule specifies that PHI can be transmitted and used for treatment, payment, and operations (TPO) processes (i.e., general health care operational use).

As it is not intended to prevent providers from meaningfully discussing the treatment of their patients, the rule specifies that some incidental disclosures of PHI are permitted. That said, reasonable safeguards, such as speaking in a low voice, not discussing patient care in the presence of others, and closing patient charts after use, should be used to limit such incidental disclosures. There are also certain disclosures, permitted by law, which may be made to governmental agencies for such purposes as law enforcement, research, workers' compensation, and organ donation. Further, the HIPAA Privacy Rule requires that health care organizations notify patients of their rights when receiving care and also provides them with a process to exercise those rights. Also, patients should be given the opportunity to agree or object to disclosures of their PHI while under the care of a health care organization.[1,56]

There is also the HIPAA Security Rule that covers electronic PHI (ePHI). ePHI is simply PHI stored in electronic form. Health care organizations are required by the Security Rule to ensure the integrity, confidentiality, and availability of all ePHI created, received, maintained, or transmitted by the organization. As such, most all organizations have fax, Internet, and e-mail policies that outline appropriate use in order to protect ePHI.[57]

Conclusion

Pharmacy informatics is the scientific discipline found at the intersection of people, data, and technology systems. It is governed by business, technical, and regulatory standards to ensure optimal use of patient-specific and knowledge-based information. Health care providers rely on informatics to support all of their activities associated with the medication use process. As the United States advances efforts toward EHR, health care providers will continue to see a growing role of informatics in their practice, regardless of the setting.

Self-Assessment Questions

1. Which of the following represents the correct order of the medication use process?
   a. Monitoring, prescribing, order verification, administration, follow-up
   b. Prescribing, order verification, dispensing, administration, monitoring
   c. Order verification, dispensing, administration, monitoring, documentation
   d. Assessment, prescribing, order verification, administration, monitoring
   e. None of the above

2. Pharmacy informatics includes:
   a. People
   b. Information
   c. Technology
   d. a and b
   e. a, b, and c

3. The two primary types of information used in pharmacy informatics include:
   a. Patient-specific and clinical expertise
   b. Clinical expertise and knowledge-based
   c. Patient-specific and knowledge-based
   d. Referential and guidelines
   e. None of the above

4. The primary similarity between CPOE and e-prescriptions is they:
   a. Are easy to implement because they do not disrupt workflow
   b. Both address the dispensing stage of the medication use process
   c. Eliminate illegible prescriptions
   d. Eliminate all errors related to prescribing
   e. c and d

5. Which of the following provides the communication network for e-prescriptions?
   a. Clinical decision support systems
   b. Big Data
   c. Health 2.0
   d. Prescription drug monitoring programs
   e. Surescripts®

6. The three components of clinical decision support systems include:
   a. CPOE system, transmission network, transmission standards
   b. Knowledge base, e-prescription network, transmission standards
   c. Communication mechanism, knowledge base, CPOE system
   d. Inference engine, knowledge base, communication mechanism
   e. None of the above

7. The main benefits of CDSS include the ability to decrease:
   a. ADEs
   b. Costs
   c. Length of stay
   d. All of the above
   e. a and b

8. Prescriptions created electronically (by CPOE and e-prescribing) have already undergone clinical review by CDSS when they reach the pharmacists for order verification. Research suggests that:
   a. These prescriptions are ready for dispensing, requiring no additional review
   b. Problems still exist with prescriptions created electronically

   c. Pharmacists must remain diligent when reviewing all prescription orders

   d. Physicians do not rely on the information presented to them by CDSS

   e. b and c

9. Which of the following is true concerning NDCs?
   a. There is no single repository of NDCs
   b. The FDA assigns the first segment of the NDC
   c. NDCs are too long for some automation to read
   d. All NDCs are in the 5-4-2 format
   e. All of the above

10. Dispensing automation commonly found in hospitals include:
    a. Carousel cabinets
    b. Automated dispensing cabinets
    c. Robotic cart filling systems
    d. Sterile compounding devices
    e. All of the above

11. Which of the following is an example of a Big Data resource?
    a. Electronic health records
    b. Individuals' digital food log
    c. A hospital's Facebook page
    d. Personal health records
    e. b and d

12. Which of the following is an example of a Little Data resource?
    a. Electronic health records
    b. Individuals' digital food log
    c. A hospital's Facebook page
    d. Personal health records
    e. b and d

13. Which of the following is a potential application of the Internet of Things in the hospital setting?
    a. Automated tracking of the physical location of medical devices
    b. Use of stationary interactive digital kiosks to provide information to visitors
    c. Computer programs that are used to augment physicians' clinical decisions
    d. Use of electronic medication administration records
    e. Use of bar code verification during medication administration

14. The increase in regulation that allows for e-prescribing is closely linked to which of the following?
   a. Efforts to decrease in health care costs
   b. Efforts to increase in Meaningful Use
   c. Efforts to decrease prescription drug abuse and fraud
   d. Efforts to decrease errors in the medication use process
   e. Efforts to decrease the carbon footprint of the health care system

15. Which of the following is the primary purpose of prescription drug monitoring programs?
   a. Decrease health care costs
   b. Increase Meaningful Use
   c. Decrease prescription drug abuse and fraud
   d. Decrease errors in the medication use process
   e. None of the above

REFERENCES

1. Fox BI, Thrower MR, Felkey BG. Building core competencies in pharmacy informatics. Washington, DC: American Pharmacists Association; 2010.
2. Hersh W. A stimulus to define informatics and health information technology. BMC Med Inform Decis Mak. 2009;9(1):24.
3. Hersh W. Medical informatics—improving health care through information. JAMA. 2002;288:1955-8.
4. Makary MA, Daniel M. Medical error—the third leading cause of death in the US. BMJ. 2016;353:i2139.
5. Kohn LT, Corrigan JM, Donaldson MS. To err is human: building a safer health system. Washington, DC: National Academies of Science; 2000:1-5.
6. Bates DW, Cullen DJ, Laird N, Petersen LA, Small SD, Servi D, Laffel G, Sweitzer BJ, Shea BF, Hallisey R, Vander Vliet M. Incidence of adverse drug events and potential adverse drug events: implications for prevention. JAMA. 1995;274(1):29-34.
7. Kaushal R, Shojania KG, Bates DW. Effects of computerized physician order entry and clinical decision support systems on medication safety: a systematic review. Arch Intern Med. 2003;163(12);1409-16.
8. Bates DW, Leape LL, Cullen DJ, Laird N, Petersen LA, Teich JM, Burdick E, Hickey M, Kleefield S, Shea B, Vander Vliet M. Effect of computerized physician order entry and a team intervention on prevention of serious medication errors. JAMA. 1998;280(5):1311-6.
9. Koppel R, Metlay JP, Cohen A, Abaluck B, Localdo AR, Kimmel SE, Strom BL. Role of computerized physician order entry systems in facilitating medication errors. JAMA. 2005;293(10):1197-1203.

10. Hillestad R, Bigelow JH. Health Information Technology. Can HIT lower costs and improve quality? [Internet]. Santa Monica, CA: RAND Corporation; 2005 [cited 2016 Sept 16]. Available from: http://www.rand.org/pubs/research_briefs/RB9136.html

11. Radley DC, Wasserman MR, Olsho LE, Shoemaker SJ, Spranca MD, Bradshaw B. Reduction in medication errors in hospitals due to adoption of computerized provider order entry systems. J Am Med Inform Assoc. 2013;20(3):470-6.

12. Poon EG, Blumenthal D, Jaggi T, Honour MM, Bates DW, Kahshal R. Overcoming barriers to adopting and implementing computerized physician order entry systems in U.S. hospitals. Health Aff. 2004;23(4):184-90.

13. National Council for Prescription Drug Programs [Internet]. Scottsdale, AZ: National Council for Prescription Drug Programs; About Us; [cited 2016 Sept 16]; [about 1 screen]. Available from: https://www.ncpdp.org/About-Us

14. Centers for Medicare and Medicaid Services [Internet]. Baltimore, MD: Centers for Medicare and Medicaid Services; Electronic Prescribing (eRx) Incentive Program; 2013 May 28 [cited 2016 Sept 16]; [about 3 screens]. Available from: http://www.cms.hhs.gov/ERxIncentive

15. U.S. Department of Justice Drug Enforcement Administration, Office of Diversion Control [Internet]. Springfield, VA: Drug Enforcement Administration; Electronic Prescribing for Controlled Substances (EPCS); [cited 2016 Sept 16]; [about 2 screens]. Available from: http://www.deadiversion.usdoj.gov/ecomm/e_rx/index.html

16. Bonner L. Controlled substance e-prescribing now legal in all 50 states [Internet]. Washington, DC: Pharmacy Today; 2016 Jan [cited 2016 Jul 1]:[1 p.]. Available from: http://www.pharmacytoday.org/article/S1042-0991(15)00020-1/pdf

17. Administrative rules of the Board of Pharmacy [Internet]. Montpelier, VT: Vermont Board of Pharmacy; 2015 Jul 8 [cited 2016 Aug 4]:[89 p.]. Available from: https://www.sec.state.vt.us//media/690234/6-RX-Rules-2015-Final-Proposed-LCAR-Annotated-June-24-2015.pdf

18. E-prescribing of controlled substances now legal nationwide [Internet]. Alexandria, VA: Surescripts; 2015 Aug 28 [cited 2016 Aug 9]:[1 p.]. Available from: http://surescripts.com/news-center/press-releases/!content/e-prescribing-of-controlled-substances-now-legal-nationwide

19. With EPCS legal nationwide, there is still work to do [Internet]. Alexandria, VA: Surescripts; 2015 Aug 28 [cited 2016 Aug 9]:[1 p.]. Available from: http://surescripts.com/news-center/blog/!content/posts/2015/08/28/with-epcs-legal-nationwide-there-is-still-work-to-do

20. Electronic prescribing [Internet]. Albany, NY: New York State Department of Public Health; 2016 Apr [cited 2016 Sept 19]:[2 p.]. Available from: http://www.health.ny.gov/professionals/narcotic/electronic_prescribing/

21. Osheroff JA, Teich JM, Middleton B, Steen EB, Wright A, Detmer DE. A roadmap for national action on clinical decision support. J Am Med Inform Assoc. 2007;14(2):141-5.

22. Shea S, DuMouchel W, Bahamonde L. A meta-analysis of 16 randomized controlled trials to evaluate computer-based clinical reminder systems for preventive care in the ambulatory setting. J Am Med Inform Assoc. 1996;3(6):399-409.

23. Berner ES. Clinical decision support systems: theory and practice. 2nd ed. New York, NY: Springer; 2007.

24. Overhage JM, Tierney WM, Zhou XH, McDonald CJ. A randomized trial of "corollary orders" to prevent errors of omission. J Am Med Inform Assoc. 1997;4(5):364-75.

25. Saverno KR, Hines LE, Warholak TL, Grizzle AJ, Babits L, Clark C, Taylor AM, Malone DC. Ability of pharmacy clinical decision-support software to alert users about clinically important drug—drug interactions. Journal of the American Medical Informatics Association. 2010;18(1):32-7.

26. National Drug Code database background information [Internet]. Rockville, MD: U.S. Department of Health and Human Services, Food and Drug Administration. 2012 Jun 6 [cited 2016 Aug 4]:[4 p.]. Available from: http://www.fda.gov/Drugs/DevelopmentApprovalProcess/UCM070829

27. National Drug Code (NDC) conversion table [Internet]. Baltimore, MD: Department of Health and Mental Hygiene; [cited 2016 Aug 4]:[1 p.]. Available from: http://phpa.dhmh.maryland.gov/OIDEOR/IMMUN/Shared%20Documents/Handout%203%20-%20NDC%20conversion%20to%2011%20digits.pdf

28. Oren E, Griffiths LP, Guglielmo BJ. Characteristics of antimicrobial overrides associated with automated dispensing machines. Am J Health Syst Pharm. 2002;59(15):1445-8.

29. Kester K, Baxter J, Freudenthal K. Errors associated with medications removed from automated dispensing machines using override function. Hosp Pharm. 2006;41: 535-7.

30. Class II special controls guidance document: pharmacy compounding systems; final guidance for industry and FDA [Internet]. Rockville, MD: U.S. Department of Health and Human Services, Food and Drug Administration, Centers for Devices and Radiological Health. 2001 Mar 12 [cited 2016 Sept 16]:[9 p.]. Available from: http://www.fda.gov/downloads/medicaldevices/deviceregulationandguidance/guidancedocuments/ucm073589.pdf

31. Pharmacy Health Information Technology Collaborative home page [Internet]. Alexandria, VA: Pharmacy Health Information Technology Collaborative; c2011 [cited 2016 Aug 30]. Available from: http://www.pharmacyhit.org/

32. Injury prevention and control: opioid overuse [Internet]. Atlanta, GA: Centers for Disease Control and Prevention, National Center for Injury Prevention and Control, Division of Unintentional Injury Prevention. 2016 Sept 8 [cited 2016 Sept 16]:[1 p.]. Available from: http://www.cdc.gov/drugoverdose/index.html

33. Prescription drug monitoring programs (PDMPs) [Internet]. Atlanta, GA: Centers for Disease Control and Prevention, National Center for Injury Prevention and Control, Division of Unintentional Injury Prevention. 2016 Mar 23 [cited 2016 Jul 20]:[1 p.]. Available from: http://www.cdc.gov/drugoverdose/pdmp/

34. Smith R. Information technology and consumerism will transform health care worldwide. BMJ. 1997;314:1495.

35. Wikipedia: the free encyclopedia [Internet]. Wikipedia; [cited 2016 Sept 16]. Available from: http://en.wikipedia.org/wiki/Main_Page

36. AHIMA e-HIM Personal Health Record Work Group. The role of the personal health record in the EHR. J AHIMA. 2005;76(7):64A-D.

37. A guide to healthcare IoT possibilities and obstacles [Internet]. Atlanta, GA: TechTarget; [cited 2016 Sept 16]:[5 p.]. Available from: http://searchhealthit.techtarget.com/ essentialguide/A-guide-to-healthcare-IoT-possibilities-and-obstacles

38. Paschou M, Sakkopoulos E, Sourla E, Tsakalidis A. Health Internet of Things: metrics and methods for efficient data transfer [Internet]. Amsterdam, The Netherlands: Simulation Modelling Practice and Theory; 2013 May [cited 2016 Jul 27]:[14 p.]. Available from: http://www.sciencedirect.com/science/article/pii/S1569190X12001232?np=y

39. MarketResearch.com: IoT deployments in healthcare to reach $117 billion by 2020, says new Mind Commerce Report [Internet]. Albuquerque, NM: PR Newswire; 2015 Apr 22 [cited 2016 Jul 30]:[1 p.]. Available from: http://www.prnewswire.com/news-releases/ marketresearchcom-iot-deployments-in-healthcare-to-reach-117-billion-by-2020-says-new-mind-commerce-report-300070129.html

40. Bui N, Zorzo M. Health care applications: a solution based on the Internet of Things. Proceedings of the 4th International Symposium on Applied Sciences in Biomedical and Communication Technologies. 2011; Barcelona, Spain. Article 131.

41. Bonchek M. Little data makes big data more powerful [Internet]. Boston, MA: Harvard Business Review; 2013 May 3 [cited 2016 Aug 31]:[5 p.]. Available from: https://hbr .org/2013/05/little-data-makes-big-data-mor%20accessed%20August%2031

42. Raghupathi W, Raghupathi V. Big data analytics in healthcare: promise and potential. Health Inf Sci Syst. 2014:2:3.

43. eHealth Initiative. Migrating toward Meaningful Use: the state of health information exchange. Washington, DC: eHealth Initiative; 2009 Aug.

44. Walker J, Pan E, Johnston D, Adler-Milstein J. The value of health care information exchange and interoperability. Health affairs. 2005.

45. The National Alliance for Health Information Technology report to the Office of the National Coordinator for Health Information Technology on defining key health information technology terms [Internet]. Department of Health and Human Services; 2008 Apr 28 [cited 2016 Aug 1]:[40 p.]. Available from: http://cdm16064.contentdm.oclc.org/cdm/ singleitem/collection/p266901coll4/id/2086/rec/10

46. U.S. National Library of Medicine [Internet]. Bethesda, MD: U.S. National Library of Medicine; 1993 Oct 10 [updated 2013 Jul 3]. RxNorm Overview; 2005 May 5 [updated 2013 Mar 5; cited 2012 Dec 29]; [about 14 screens]. Available from: https://www.nlm.nih.gov/ research/umls/rxnorm/overview.html

47. U.S. National Library of Medicine [Internet]. Bethesda, MD: U.S. National Library of Medicine; 1993 Oct 10 [updated 2013 Jul 3]. UMLS Quick Start Guide; 2011 Mar 30 [updated 2012 Jul 27; cited 2012 Dec 29]; [about 2 screens]. Available from: http://www .nlm.nih.gov/research/umls/quickstart.html

48. American Medical Association [Internet]. Chicago, IL: American Medical Association; c1995-2013. About CPT®; [cited 2012 Dec 29]; [about 1 screen]. Available from: http:// www.ama-assn.org/ama/pub/physician-resources/solutions-managing-your-practice/ coding-billing-insurance/cpt/about-cpt.page

49. Bush GW. Executive Order 13335—incentives for the use of health information technology and establishing the position of the National Health Information Technology Coordinator [Internet]. Washington, DC: Federal Register; 2004 Apr 27 [cited 2012 Dec 29]:[3 p.]. Available from: http://www.gpo.gov/fdsys/pkg/FR-2004-04-30/pdf/04-10024.pdf

50. HealthIT.gov [Internet]. Washington, DC: The Office of the National Coordinator for Health Information Technology; Meaningful Use definitions and objectives; [cited 2012 Dec 29]; [about 1 screen]. Available from: http://www.healthit.gov/providers-professionals/meaningful-use-definition-objectives

51. An Introduction to the Medicaid EHR Incentive Program for Eligible Professionals [Internet]. Baltimore, MD: Centers for Medicare and Medicaid Services; [cited 2012 Dec 29]:[94 p.]. Available from: http://www.cms.gov/Regulations-and-Guidance/Legislation/EHRIncentivePrograms/Downloads/EHR_Medicaid_Guide_Remediated_2012.pdf

52. Adler-Milstein J, DesRoches CM, Kralovec P, Foster G, Worzala C, Charles D, Searcy T, Jha AK. Electronic health record adoption in US hospitals: progress continues, but challenges persist. Health Affairs. 2015;34(12):2174-80.

53. Quick Stats [Internet]. Washington, DC: The Office of the National Coordinator for Health Information Technology; 2015 May 31 [cited 2016 Sept 19]. Available from: http://dashboard.healthit.gov/quickstats/quickstats.php

54. Kellermann AL, Jones SS. What it will take to achieve the as-yet-unfulfilled promises of health information technology. Health Aff. 2013;32(1):63-8.

55. Summary of selected federal laws and regulations addressing confidentiality, privacy and security [Internet]. Washington, DC: The Office of the National Coordinator for Health Information Technology; 2010 Feb 18 [cited 2012 Dec 29]:[12 p.]. Available from: http://www.healthit.gov/sites/default/files/federal_privacy_laws_table_2_26_10_final_0.pdf

56. Summary of the HIPAA Privacy Rule [Internet]. Washington, DC: U.S. Department of Health and Human Services; 2003 May [cited 2012 Dec 29]:[25 p.]. Available from: https://www.hhs.gov/hipaa/for-professionals/privacy/laws-regulations/

57. HIPAA administrative simplification [Internet]. Washington, DC: U.S. Department of Health and Human Services; 2013 Mar [cited 2016 Aug 5]:[101 p.]. Available from: https://www.hhs.gov/sites/default/files/hipaa-simplification-201303.pdf

SUGGESTED READINGS

1. Fox BI, Thrower MR, Felkey BG. Building core competencies in pharmacy informatics. Washington, DC: American Pharmacists Association; 2010.

2. The Office of the National Coordinator for Health Information Technology [Internet]. Washington, DC: U.S. Department of Health and Human Services; [updated 2011 Feb 18; cited 2012 Dec 12]. Available from: https://www.healthit.gov/

3. Journal of the American Medical Informatics Association. Available from: http://jamia.bmj.com/

4. Friedman C. A 'Fundamental theorem' of biomedical informatics. JAMIA. 2009;16:169-70.

5. Pew Internet and American Life Project. Available from: http://www.pewinternet.org/

6. American Society of Health-System Pharmacists. Technology-enabled practice: a vision statement by the ASHP Section of Pharmacy Informatics and Technology. Am J Health Syst Pharm. 2009;66:1573-77.

7. Journal of Medical Internet Research. Available from: http://www.jmir.org

8. Journal of Participatory Medicine. Available from: http://www.jopm.org

9. Journal of Biomedical Informatics. Available from: http://www.sciencedirect.com/science/journal/15320464

10. Pharmacy Informatics. Available from: http://www.pharmacy-informatics.com

11. Dumitru D. The pharmacy informatics primer. Bethesda, MD: American Society of Health-System Pharmacists; 2009.

Chapter Twenty-Seven

Drug Information Education and Training

Michelle W. McCarthy

Learning Objectives

● *After completing this chapter, the reader will be able to*

- Determine fundamental drug information skills for all pharmacy students.
- Identify settings in which student's drug information skills can be developed and refined.
- Define the recommended training path for drug information specialists.
- Describe job responsibilities of contemporary drug information specialists.
- Formulate a strategy by which interested candidates can learn about available drug information residencies and fellowships.

Key Concepts

❶ Information retrieval, evaluation, and application skills represent a significant component of the core skill set each pharmacist must possess.

❷ Drug information skills are core concepts that must be incorporated in pharmacy curricula.

❸ The majority of foundational skill development should occur prior to student participation in advanced pharmacy practice experiences (APPEs).

❹ Drug information rotations may occur in institutional and nontraditional settings (e.g., pharmaceutical industry, managed care, group purchasing organization), a reflection of the expanding role of drug information in contemporary pharmacy practice.

❺ Pharmacy residency training standards include core drug information retrieval and evaluation skills for both postgraduate year one (PGY1) and postgraduate year two (PGY2) programs.

❻ Consistent with the profession-wide model for specialist training, the preferred training model for a drug information specialist is a PGY1 residency program, followed by completion of a PGY2 residency in drug information.

❼ The American Society of Health-System Pharmacists (ASHP), the organization charged with accrediting pharmacy residency programs, has developed outcomes, goals, and objectives that must be incorporated into ASHP-accredited PGY2 drug information residency programs.

❽ PGY2 programs in drug information are not limited to health systems, as programs exist in academic, industrial, and managed care settings.

❾ Fellowship programs build research skills beyond those provided during residency training programs.

Introduction

❶ *Information retrieval, evaluation, and application skills represent a significant component of the core skill set each pharmacist must possess.* To meet the profession's broader needs, the scope of drug information practice has evolved beyond a focus on literature retrieval, evaluation, and application to specific organizational needs and patient care situations such as therapeutic policy management, oversight of safe medication practices including information systems, and promotion of health and wellness. Combined with other practice responsibilities that have traditionally been linked to the practice of drug information (e.g., medication use policy), developing and maintaining practitioners with expertise in such activities is critically important.[1-3] This chapter will focus on key drug information education and training needs for all pharmacists, as well as for those practitioners specializing in drug information practice.

Drug Information in Pharmacy Curriculum

❷ *Drug information skills are core concepts that must be incorporated in pharmacy curricula.* Pharmacy curricula must be designed to prepare graduates in the knowledge, skills, abilities, behaviors, and attitudes necessary to apply the foundational sciences to the provision of patient-centered care.[2] The expectation of the Accreditation Council for Pharmacy Education (ACPE) accreditation standards is that students will develop the comprehensive knowledge base to be "practice and team-ready" and be able to retain, recall, build upon, and apply knowledge to deliver quality patient care in a variety of entry-level practice settings.[3] Educational outcomes of contemporary professional degree programs include four broad domains that are foundational knowledge, essentials for practice and care, approach to patient care, and personal and professional development, and 15 subdomains. Table 27-1 lists the educational outcomes, domains, subdomains, and example learning objectives that correlate to drug information practice.[2]

TABLE 27–1. CENTER FOR ADVANCEMENT OF PHARMACY EDUCATION (CAPE) EDUCATIONAL OUTCOMES (2013)[2]

Select learning objectives that correlate with drug information knowledge and skills

Domain 1: Foundational Knowledge

Subdomain 1.1 Learner: Develop, integrate, and apply knowledge from the foundational sciences (i.e., pharmaceutical, social/behavioral/administrative, and clinical sciences) to evaluate the scientific literature, explain drug action, solve therapeutic problems, and advance population health and patient-centered care.

Example learning objectives:

- 1.1.5 Critically analyze scientific literature related to drugs and disease to enhance clinical decision making.
- 1.1.6 Identify and critically analyze emerging theories, information, and technologies that may impact patient-centered and population-based care.

Domain 2: Essentials for Practice and Care

Subdomain 2.2 Medication use systems management: Manage patient health care needs using human, financial, technological, and physical resources to optimize the safety and efficacy of medication use systems.

Example learning objectives:

- 2.2.2 Describe the role of the pharmacist in impacting the safety and efficacy of each component of a typical medication use system (i.e., procurement, storage, prescribing, transcription, dispensing, administration, monitoring, and documentation).
- 2.2.3 Utilize technology to optimize the medication use system.
- 2.2.6 Apply standards, guidelines, best practices, and established processes related to safe and effective medication use.
- 2.2.7 Utilize continuous quality improvement techniques in the medication use process.

Domain 3: Approach to Practice and Care

Subdomain 3 Communication: Effectively communicate verbally and nonverbally when interacting with an individual, group, or organization.

Example learning objectives:

- 3.6.8 Develop professional documents pertinent to organizational needs (e.g., monographs, policy documents).

DRUG INFORMATION IN DIDACTIC CURRICULUM

The accreditation standards for professional degree programs identify required didactic elements for Doctor of Pharmacy (PharmD) curricula. The required didactic elements are written as broad learning outcomes to provide the comprehensive knowledge base required for entry-level practice. The goal of the latest ACPE standard is to ensure that critical areas of learning are included in pharmacy curricula; however, individual programs have the flexibility to determine how lessons are structured and delivered. The required didactic content that aligns with traditional and contemporary drug information skills are as follows[3]:

- Biostatistics (see Chapter 6)
- Health care systems
- Pharmacoeconomics (see Chapter 7)
- Pharmacy law and regulatory affairs (see Chapters 10 and 22)
- Practice management
- Professional communication (see Chapter 12)
- Research design (see Chapter 4)
- Health informatics (see Chapter 26)
- Health information retrieval and evaluation (see Chapters 2, 4, and 5)
- Natural products and alternative and complementary therapies
- Medication dispensing, distribution, and administration
- Patient safety (see Chapters 17 and 18)

The American College of Clinical Pharmacy (ACCP) Drug Information (DI) Practice and Research Network (PRN) published an opinion paper to ensure that drug information education and practice is designed to meet the needs of the changing health care environment. This paper recommended core-specific drug information concepts that should be formally taught and evaluated in all colleges of pharmacy (see Table 27-2).[4] Other topic areas closely aligned with drug information practice include alternative medicine, adverse drug event (medication misadventure) surveillance, drug shortage management and mitigation, safety monitoring during clinical trials, Risk Evaluation Mitigation Strategies (REMS), and managing investigational drug services.

A number of pedagogical approaches may be used to build drug information associated skills in the didactic setting. A 2012 survey conducted by the ACCP DI PRN summarized the methods by which colleges of pharmacy include drug information, literature evaluation, and biostatistics content into the curricula. Survey responses represented 50% of the pharmacy schools listed in the American Association of Colleges of Pharmacy (AACP) online directory. Instructional methodology used included didactic lectures, small group learning, Internet-based learning, and other formats. Survey respondents indicated

TABLE 27–2. ESSENTIAL DRUG INFORMATION CONCEPTS FOR PROFESSIONAL DEGREE CURRICULA[4]

- Applying medical information to specific patient situations
- Counterdetailing and appropriately interacting with the pharmaceutical industry
- Creating effective and efficient literature searching strategies
- Critically evaluating marketing and promotional materials and advertisements
- Critically evaluating medical literature
- Describing the process of drug regulation in the United States
- Distinguishing statistical versus clinical significance
- Discerning and communicating appropriate health information for patient education
- Evaluating drug use policies and procedures
- Identifying, evaluating, and utilizing key print (text) sources of medical information
- Identifying, managing, reporting, and preventing adverse drug events
- Incorporating principles and practices of evidence-based medicine (EBM) into pharmaceutical care
- Locating and critically evaluating medical information on the Internet
- Preparing, presenting, and participating in journal clubs
- Providing verbal and written responses to drug information requests
- Summarizing basic biostatistics and research design methods
- Understanding the creation, maintenance, and management of a drug formulary
- Using electronic medical information databases and other technologically enhanced references and resources in an effective and efficient manner to advance pharmaceutical care

using online course management programs, audience response systems, YouTube, online blogs, tweets, and wikis to teach drug information, literature evaluation, and biostatistics content.[5] The availability of instructional technologies and focus on active-learning components in the professional program provide many opportunities for instructors to engage learners through incorporation of practical, practice-oriented scenarios.

More recently, another survey of school of pharmacy faculty evaluated how and when medical literature evaluation skills were taught within the curriculum. The survey found that medical literature evaluation is a major topic taught in pharmacy schools. The most common response was that medical literature evaluation was taught in a stand-alone course (49% of respondents), and this course was placed within the second professional year (43%). However, teaching medical literature evaluation was also embedded within a drug information course for 37% and taught through laboratory-based courses for 11%.[6]

DRUG INFORMATION IN EXPERIENTIAL EDUCATION

❸ *The majority of foundational skill development should occur prior to student participation in advanced pharmacy practice experiences (APPEs).* Integration of practice-related

TABLE 27–3. ACPE GUIDANCE FOR PRE-APPE CORE COMPETENCIES[7]

Ability Statement:
Assess information needs of patients and health providers and apply knowledge of study design and literature analysis and retrieval to provide accurate, evidence-based drug information.

Example performance competencies
- Collect accurate and comprehensive drug information from appropriate sources to make informed, evidence-based, patient-specific, or population-based decisions
- Recognize the type of content that is available in general (tertiary), secondary, and primary information sources
- Collect, summarize, analyze, and apply information from the biomedical literature to patient-specific or population-based health needs
- Demonstrate utilization of drug information resources
- Describe the type of content in commonly used drug and medical information resources
- Collect and interpret accurate drug information from appropriate sources to make informed, evidence-based decisions
- Use effective written, visual, verbal, and nonverbal communication skills to accurately respond to drug information questions

activities in the introductory pharmacy practice experiences (IPPEs) are also important activities supported by the ACPE. Table 27-3 provides core competencies that pharmacy students must possess prior to APPE experiences.[2,7] Students in their final year of the professional curriculum would benefit greatly from a practice experience devoted to drug information practice. Having the opportunity to complete drug information-specific activities (e.g., responding to drug information requests, medication use evaluation, formulary class review or monograph, evaluation of adverse drug events) following completion of didactic coursework provides students even greater opportunities to apply pharmacotherapeutic, pharmacokinetic, legal, and ethical principles to their approach to providing drug information. Drug information historically was a required learning experience for each PharmD student. The growth in the number of colleges of pharmacy and pharmacy student population and reductions in the number of formal drug information centers has resulted in an inadequate number of teaching sites to support completion of required drug information APPEs for every student.[8] While some colleges have developed their own formalized centers, others provide only elective drug information APPEs.[1,8] ❹ *Drug information rotations may occur in institutional and nontraditional settings (e.g., pharmaceutical industry, managed care, group purchasing organization), a reflection of the expanding role of drug information in contemporary pharmacy practice.*

The new ACPE standard guidance document includes APPE activities to foster student drug information skill development (see Table 27-4).[7] Students require adequate

TABLE 27–4. DRUG INFORMATION ACTIVITIES INCLUDED IN APPE CURRICULA[3]

- Delivering evidence-based care through the retrieval, evaluation, and application of findings from the scientific and clinical literature
- Participating in the health system's formulary process
- Participating in the management of medication use systems and applying the systems approach to medication safety
- Conducting a drug utilization review
- Participating in the management of the use of investigational drug products
- Participating in therapeutic protocol development
- Performing prospective and retrospective financial and clinical outcomes analyses to support formulary recommendations and therapeutic guideline development

supervision and oversight to ensure the quality of service they provide, as well as to provide them valuable feedback to subsequently improve their performance. Sites often realize that incorporation of students into the practice site may expand the capacity of services provided, including responding to more drug information requests, preparing analyses of drug policy issues for consideration by the pharmacy and therapeutics committee, and conducting medication use evaluations or adverse drug reaction surveillance. Other advanced practice experiences beyond those labeled as drug information (e.g., pharmacy management, informatics, medication safety) also provide opportunities that are beneficial to building skills in drug information.

Postgraduate Training in Drug Information

Drug information skills are a core skill set for all pharmacists, regardless of their practice setting, area of therapeutic focus, or declared area of specialty. ❺ *Pharmacy residency training standards include core drug information retrieval and evaluation skills for both postgraduate year one (PGY1) and postgraduate year two (PGY2) programs.*[9,10] As early as 1966, the need for pharmacists with specialized skills in drug information was documented.[11] The focus of PharmD degree programs has evolved to the current model of postgraduate training, specifically through residency programs, to train drug information specialists. ❻ *Consistent with the profession-wide model for specialist training, the preferred training model for a drug information specialist is a PGY1 residency program, followed by completion of a PGY2 residency in drug information.* This training model is also supported by drug information specialist members of ACCP.[2]

SHORTAGE OF TRAINED DRUG INFORMATION SPECIALISTS

Although there is long-standing recognition regarding the importance of advanced training, one survey identified that 40% of drug information pharmacists have completed such training and the remaining 60% developed skill in their position responsibilities through on-the-job training.[12] This may reflect an imbalance in pharmacists with advanced training and available job openings. A relative lack of popularity or desirability of the specialty to students and new trainees, or pressures on employers to fill positions with applicants who lack the desired formal training may have contributed to this imbalance; no formal assessment of these or other factors has been conducted. One theory for the decreasing numbers of available PGY2 drug information residency programs is the misconception regarding the activities of drug information residents and specialists. Drug information has evolved from merely providing responses to drug information queries to serving as organizational leaders in medication use policy and safety.[13,14] The number of available positions for individuals with advanced training in drug information often exceeds the number of candidates who have completed advanced training. This imbalance is cause for concern and may result in a shortage of qualified candidates to meet the drug information needs of the changing health care environment.[2,13]

A 2006 survey of U.S. pharmacists with presumed drug information practices was conducted to determine the perceptions regarding drug information practice and training.[12] The survey was sent to members of the ACCP DI PRN, participants of a drug information practice listserv, and pharmacists employed by drug information centers; because of this methodology, the sample may not reflect all pharmacists with drug information responsibilities. The most common job responsibilities of those surveyed were instructing pharmacy students and staff (64%), maintaining formal drug information center operations (63%), responding to drug information queries (59%), conducting original research (53%), providing pharmacy and therapeutics committee support (46%), providing medication safety support (41.3%), publishing pharmacy-related newsletters (38%), and developing medication use policy (35%). Respondents generally felt prepared to undertake their responsibilities in relation to the extent of postgraduate training they received. However, areas in which pharmacists felt less prepared included information systems support (41%), pharmacoeconomic evaluations (32%), and clinical outcomes research (19%). Approximately 80% of those who had completed postgraduate training felt adequately prepared overall for their job roles. Preparing for practice changes and innovations is a focus of residency training and perhaps was reflected in the greater sense of preparedness reported by residency-trained pharmacists.[12] A 2011 survey of pharmacy residents and fellows identified that a new motivator of pharmacy students to pursue residency and fellowship training is that these additional training programs are prerequisites for certain jobs.[15]

ACCREDITATION STANDARDS FOR POSTGRADUATE TRAINING IN DRUG INFORMATION

❼ *The American Society of Health-System Pharmacists (ASHP), the organization charged with accrediting pharmacy residency programs, has developed outcomes/competency areas, goals, and objectives that are required to be included in ASHP-accredited PGY2 residency programs.*[9] In 2015, ASHP approved a new PGY2 Accreditation Standard where outcomes were replaced by competency areas.[16] ASHP is systematically working with practice experts to update each PGY2 programs' required and elective competency areas, goals, and objectives.[17] The available PGY2 drug information outcomes, goals, and objectives were written in 2007 and therefore lack correlation with the ASHP's 2015 PGY2 Accreditation Standard and contemporary practice. Until updated, the 2007 PGY2 drug information required outcomes, goals, and objectives that are to be incorporated into ASHP-accredited residency programs. These outcomes are to:

- demonstrate excellence in the provision of education, training, and evidence-based information for health care professionals and health care professionals in training
- contribute to the management of the organization's medication use policies processes
- exercise leadership and practice management skills
- conduct drug information practice related projects
- contribute to the management of the organization's budget.

There are additional outcomes suggested for those residencies conducted in formal drug information centers and hospitals or health systems.[9] The purpose of PGY2 residency programs is to "build on Doctor of Pharmacy (PharmD) education and PGY1 pharmacy residency programs to contribute to the development of clinical pharmacists in specialized areas of practice. PGY2 residencies provide residents with opportunities to function independently as practitioners by conceptualizing and integrating accumulated experience and knowledge and incorporating both into the provision of patient care that improves medication therapy. Residents who successfully complete an accredited PGY2 pharmacy residency should possess competencies that qualify them for clinical pharmacist and/or faculty positions and position them to be eligible for attainment of board certification in the specialized practice area (when board certification for the practice area exists)."[16] As noted in the 2006 survey, contemporary drug information specialists should be prepared to utilize technology and advance population-based approaches (e.g., data mining, pharmacoepidemiology, pharmacovigilance) to support a safe and effective medication use process.[12] These tools and approaches may include information-systems support, clinical outcomes research, pharmacoeconomic evaluations, and other such techniques that are also consistent with the Institute of Medicine's (IOM) focus on evidence-based medicine, technology, and quality assurance as core competencies for health care practitioners.[18]

OPPORTUNITIES FOR POSTGRADUATE RESIDENTS

❽ *PGY2 programs in drug information are not limited to health systems, as programs exist in academic, industrial, and managed care settings.* The ASHP required outcomes, goals, and objectives of PGY2 drug information residency programs provide opportunity for development of an advanced skill set that can be applied to many practice settings. Residency graduates who are actively engaged in the practice environment of their training program and then become employed in the same type of practice environment should be well equipped to effectively contribute to the drug information needs of their new organization, and the time to effectively transition from resident to independent practitioner may be shortened. For example, a graduate of an ASHP-accredited PGY2 drug information residency in an academic medical center would likely be a highly desirable candidate for drug information specialist positions within other hospitals and health systems. However, the skills afforded by advanced drug information training in any setting are transferable and beneficial to other settings since having a greater understanding of the operations of an alternate setting may improve decision making in the new environment. For example, training in pharmaceutical industry can better inform a pharmacist of the Food and Drug Administration (FDA) regulations and internal policies that may shape the manner in which a manufacturer can provide information about an investigational drug or suspected adverse effects of a marketed drug.

POSTGRADUATE FELLOWSHIP IN DRUG INFORMATION

❾ *Fellowship programs build research skills beyond those provided during residency training programs.* These fellowships have focus on a number of subspecialty areas including evidence-based practice, medical communications, medication use policy, medication safety, pharmacoepidemiology, and pharmacoeconomics. As with therapeutic specialties, fellowship training in drug information should focus on expanding the fellow's research abilities. There are no accreditation standards for fellowship programs, so their structure, duration, and delivery are guided by the program director.[19] Given the growing complexity and cost of health care, the need for practice-focused researchers has grown more vital. Drug information fellowships that focus on research skills in pharmacoepidemiology, pharmacoeconomics, and comparative effectiveness, or the role of informatics to support a safe and effective medication use system, would be well suited to fill this need.[2,12,15]

PURSUING SPECIALTY TRAINING

• Identifying potential residency or fellowship programs that may meet an individual's training needs should begin with a search of available training directories such as the ASHP online residency directory and the ACCP Directory of Residencies and Fellowships.[19,20] Different factors may be important to individual applicants as they evaluate available programs. Beyond traditional drug information activities like responding to queries and providing formulary management, factors that may be important to individual candidates include the ability to gain experience working with students or PGY1 residents, performing contract work, extensive opportunities to manage drug policy across a health system, and intensive training in medical writing. Regardless of the special features or characteristics, there should be opportunities that will prepare the individual for the type of practice envisioned for him or herself. In addition to being prepared for a position as a drug information specialist, graduates of PGY2 drug information residencies may pursue positions in medication safety (see Chapters 17 and 18), regulatory/quality pharmacists (see Chapter 22), drug policy (see Chapter 19), and medical writing (see Chapter 12). Settings in which positions may be available include hospitals and health systems, managed care organizations, government organizations, pharma-
• ceutical industry, and academia. A directory of accredited or accreditation-pending residency programs can easily be accessed from the ASHP Online Residency Directory (https://accred.ashp.org/aps/pages/directory/residencyProgramSearch .aspx).[20] In addition to employment (e.g., salary, benefits) and contact (e.g., program director) information, each program's listing includes a description of the practice site, key program features, application information, and a hyperlink to the program's website. More detailed information such as schedules, learning experience descriptions, and accomplishments of program graduates may be found on the
• websites of the individual programs. Residency programs, including those that are not accredited, may also be identified through a review of the Directory of Residencies, Fellowships, and Graduate Programs hosted on the ACCP website (http://www.accp. com/resandfel/).[19] This directory is also the primary catalog of possible fellowship options. Fellowship programs may be identified by searching drug information as well as the heading of the research focus (e.g., pharmacoeconomics, pharmacoepidemiology, outcomes research, medication safety). The program listings also provide descriptions of secondary specialty, which include evidence-based medicine or practice, medical communications, and medication use policy. These secondary specialty descriptions may continue to evolve as programs morph to meet the demands of the changing health care environment.

Conclusion

All pharmacists, regardless of practice setting, require drug information skills in order to provide evidence-based patient-centered care and appropriately support other health care professionals. Equipping pharmacists with those skills begins in professional degree programs, continues into residency training, and may extend into fellowship programs. Additionally, pharmacists may continue to expand drug information skill development throughout their careers by involvement in continuing professional development and on-the-job training. Each of these important elements of education and training should continue to evolve to meet contemporary practice and research needs and to prepare future practitioners to be "practice and team ready" to provide innovative services grounded in principles of evidence-based medicine.

Case Study 27–1

You have been hired as a drug information faculty member in a new school of pharmacy. You and your colleagues are evaluating how you will incorporate drug information skills into the curricula to ensure graduates are practice and team ready by providing evidence-based drug information to patients and other members of the health care team.

- *What methods may be used for incorporating drug information into the curricula?*
- *What structures can be used for teaching literature evaluation and when might this be taught?*

Case Study 27–2

A PharmD student has expressed interest in pursuing a career in drug information. The individual is seeking information about various practice settings and responsibilities. As the faculty advisor for the student, you have volunteered to identify shadowing opportunities for various drug information positions.

- *What positions may individuals with expertise in drug information hold?*
- *In what settings may these individuals practice?*
- *What advice regarding postgraduate training would you recommend for this student?*

Self-Assessment Questions

1. During your college's review of its professional degree program, a committee member recommends to eliminate a course entitled "Drug Information Skill Development." When asked to justify the recommendation, the faculty member replies, "The accreditation standards don't require a drug information course." What is a factual response to the statement?
   a. The standards *do not* prescribe specific concepts that must be taught in professional degree curricula
   b. The standards *do* require the inclusion of concepts generally categorized as drug information, in addition to related concepts
   c. Drug information concepts *are* required to be taught only during advanced pharmacy practice experiences (APPEs)
   d. All of the above
   e. None of the above

2. Although ACPE does not require pharmacy school graduates to have completed a drug information course or rotation, which of the following educational subdomains correlate with drug information knowledge and skills:
   a. Manage patient health care needs using human, financial, technological, and physical resources to optimize the safety and efficacy of medication use systems
   b. Develop, integrate, and apply knowledge from foundational sciences to evaluate the scientific literature, explain drug action, solve therapeutic problems, and advance population health and patient-centered care
   c. Effectively communicate verbally and nonverbally when interacting with an individual, group, or organization
   d. All of the above
   e. None of the above

3. Which specific drug information concept is **NOT** recommended by ACCP to be formally taught and evaluated in all colleges of pharmacy?
   a. Creating drug policies and procedures
   b. Critically evaluating medical literature
   c. Understanding the creation, maintenance, and management of a drug formulary
   d. Preparing, presenting, and participating in journal clubs

4. In which activity can you engage pharmacy students enrolled in a drug information course to demonstrate the broad applicability of drug information skills, using an example from the popular media?
    a. Critiquing the accuracy of a local television news reporter's segment about a newly approved prescription drug
    b. Crafting a letter to the editor describing the role pharmacists play in preventing medication errors, in response to an article about the national impact of medication errors published in the local newspaper
    c. Evaluating a front-page article from the New York Times regarding a recently published drug study
    d. All of the above
    e. None of the above

5. The college of pharmacy in which you work is unable to provide drug information APPEs in a traditional drug information setting. Which alternate APPE settings also provide opportunities to build drug information skills?
    a. Pharmacy management/administration
    b. Pharmacy informatics
    c. Medication safety
    d. All of the above
    e. None of the above

6. Which unique educational methods have been used to teach drug information concepts to pharmacy students?
    a. Small group hands-on assignments
    b. Online blogs, tweets, and wikis
    c. Audience response systems
    d. All of the above
    e. None of the above

7. The preferred credentials for a drug information specialist practicing in a hospital/health system/school of pharmacy are:
    a. Pharmacy degree
    b. Pharmacy degree + postgraduate year one pharmacy residency
    c. Pharmacy degree + pharmacoeconomics fellowship
    d. All of the above
    e. None of the above

8. What role(s) can postgraduate year two (PGY2) drug information residents play in the education of health care professionals and heath care professionals in training?
    a. Provide an in-service to nurses regarding a new medication
    b. Provide classroom instruction about literature evaluation skills to doctor of pharmacy students

  c. Prepare a newsletter article summarizing recently released therapeutic guidelines for distribution throughout the organization
  d. All of the above
  e. None of the above

9. What activities support the required outcomes, goals, and objectives of ASHP-accredited PGY2 drug information residencies?
  a. Develop therapeutic guidelines for high-cost agents used within an organization
  b. Peer review a paper submitted for publication
  c. Complete a pharmacoeconomic analysis to support a medication use policy or process
  d. All of the above
  e. None of the above

10. What types of positions may individuals completing an ASHP-accredited PGY2 drug information residency pursue?
  a. Drug information specialist in hospital/health system
  b. Editor at medical communications company
  c. Medication safety pharmacist
  d. All of the above
  e. None of the above

11. Drug information and associated fellowships may be desired by individuals interested in the following:
  a. Extensive research-related activities
  b. Pharmacoeconomics
  c. Pharmacoepidemiology
  d. All of the above
  e. None of the above

12. Where would you be able to find the employment paths graduates of PGY2 drug information residencies have pursued over the last 5 years?
  a. The individual training program's website
  b. The ACCP Online Residency Directory
  c. The ASHP Online Residency Directory
  d. All of the above
  e. None of the above

13. What job responsibilities are performed by contemporary drug information specialists:
   a. Supporting pharmacy and therapeutics committees
   b. Educating health care providers and health care providers in training on medication therapy
   c. Ensuring safe and effective use of medications through the use of technology
   d. Developing medication use policies
   e. All of the above

14. In what settings are drug information residencies and fellowships conducted:
   a. Hospitals/health systems
   b. Schools of pharmacy
   c. Pharmaceutical industry
   d. Managed care organizations
   e. All of the above

15. Which of the following statements is correct:
   a. Drug information APPEs are required for all pharmacy school graduates.
   b. Drug information practice has evolved from merely responding to drug information queries to serving as organizational leaders in medication use safety.
   c. AACP recommends drug information skills be taught only in didactic lectures.
   d. ASHP is the only organization that accredits drug information residency and fellowship programs.

REFERENCES

1. Wang F, Troutman WG, Seo T, Peak A. Rosenberg JM. Drug information education in doctor of pharmacy programs. Am J Pharm Educ. 2006;70:1-7.
2. Medina MS, Plaza CM, Stowe CD, Robinson ET, DeLander G, Beck DE, Melchert RB, Supernaw RB, Roche VF, Gleason BL, Strong MN, Bain A, Meyer GE, Don BJ, Rochon J, Johnston P. Report of the 2012-13 Academic Affairs Standing Committee: revising the Center for the Advancement of Pharmacy Education (CAPE) Educational Outcomes 2013. Am J Pharm Educ. 2013;77(8):Article 162.
3. Accreditation Council for Pharmaceutical Education. Accreditation standards and key elements for the professional program in pharmacy leading to the Doctor of Pharmacy degree. Chicago, IL: 2015 [cited 2016 Jul 22]. Available from: https://www.acpe-accredit .org/pdf/Standards2016FINAL.pdf
4. Bernknopf AC, Karpinski JP, McKeever AL, Peak AS, Smith KM, Smith WD, Timpe EM, Ward KE. Drug information: from education to practice. Pharmacotherapy. 2009 Mar;29(3):331-46.
5. Phillips JA, Gabay MP, Ficzere C, Ward KE. Curriculum and instructional methods for drug information, literature evaluation, and biostatistics: survey of US pharmacy schools. Ann Pharmacother. 2012;46:793-801.

6. O'Sullivan TA, Phillips J, Demaris K. Medical literature evaluation education at US Schools of Pharmacy. Am J Pharm Ed. 2016;80(1):Article 5.

7. Accreditation Council for Pharmacy Education. Guidance for the accreditation standards and key elements for the professional program in pharmacy leading to the Doctor of Pharmacy degree. Chicago, IL: 2015 [cited 2016 Aug 31]. Available from: https://www.acpe-accredit.org/pdf/GuidanceforStandards2016FINAL.pdf

8. Cole SW, Berensen NM. Comparison of drug information practice curriculum components in US colleges of pharmacy. Am J Pharm Educ. 2005;69:240-4.

9. American Society of Health-System Pharmacists. Educational outcomes, goals, and objectives for postgraduate year two (PGY2) pharmacy residencies in drug information; [cited 2017 Aug 23]. Available from: https://new.ashp.org/-/media/assets/professional-development/residencies/docs/pgy2-drug-information.ashx?la=en

10. American Society of Health-System Pharmacists. Required competency areas, goals, and objectives for postgraduate year one (PGY1) pharmacy residencies; [cited 2017 Aug 23]. Available from: https://www.ashp.org/-/media/assets/professional-development/residencies/docs/required-competency-areas-goals-objectives

11. Walton CA. Education and training of the drug information specialist. Drug Intell. 1967;1:132-7.

12. Gettig JP, Jordan JK, Sheehan AH. A survey of current perceptions of drug information practice and training. Hosp Pharm. 2009;44:325-31.

13. Vanscoy GJ, Gajewski LK, Tyler LS, Gora-Harper ML, Grant KL, May JR. The future of medication information practice: a consensus. Ann Pharmacother. 1996;30:876-81.

14. Ghaibi S, Ipema H, Gabay M. ASHP guidelines on the pharmacist's role in providing drug information. Am J Health Syst Pharm. 2015; 72:573-7.

15. McCarthy BC, Weber LM. Update on factors motivating pharmacy students to pursue residency and fellowship training. Am J Health Syst Pharm. 2013;70:1397-403.

16. American Society of Health-System Pharmacists. ASHP accreditation standard for postgraduate year two (PGY2) pharmacy residencies; [cited 2016 Jul 28]. Available from: https://www.ashp.org/-/media/assets/professional-development/residencies/docs/pgy2-residency-accreditation-standard-June2017.ashx?la=en&hash=FA375984733CEA67F705CB327A635777515EE65E

17. American Society of Health-System Pharmacists. Accreditation Services Division. PGY2 goals and objectives revision update. The Communiqué. 2016;19(1):5.

18. Institute of Medicine: executive summary. In: Greiner AC, Knebel E, editors. Health professions education: a bridge to quality. Washington, DC: National Academy Press; 2003:1-18.

19. American College of Clinical Pharmacy Directory of Residencies, Fellowships and Graduate Programs [Internet]. Lenexa, KS: American College of Clinical Pharmacy; c2016 [cited 2016 Aug 25]. Available from: https://www.accp.com/resandfel/

20. American Society of Health-System Pharmacists Online Residency Directory [Internet]. Bethesda, MD: American Society of Health-System Pharmacists; c2016 [cited 2016 Aug 25]. Available from: https://accred.ashp.org/aps/pages/directory/residencyProgramSearch.aspx

SUGGESTED READINGS

1. Bernknopf AC, Karpinski JP, McKeever AL, Peak AS, Smith KM, Smith WD, Timpe EM, Ward KE Drug information: from education to practice. Pharmacotherapy. 2009 Mar;29(3):331-46.

2. Cole SW, Berensen NM. Comparison of drug information practice curriculum components in U.S. colleges of pharmacy. Am J Pharm Educ. 2005;69:240-4.

3. Phillips JA, Gabay MP, Ficzere C, Ward KE. Curriculum and instructional methods for drug information, literature evaluation, and biostatistics: survey of US pharmacy schools. Ann Pharmacother. 2012; 46:793-801.

4. Gettig JP, Jordan JK, Sheehan AH. A survey of current perceptions of drug information practice and training. Hosp Pharm. 2009;44:325-31.

5. American Society of Health-System Pharmacists. Educational outcomes, goals, and objectives for postgraduate year two (PGY2) pharmacy residencies in drug information; [cited 2017 Aug 23]. Available from: https://new.ashp.org/-/media/assets/professional-development/residencies/docs/pgy2-drug-information.ashx?la=en

Appendices

Appendix 2–1

Example of Drug Information Consult Documentation Form

<table>
<tr>
<td>
☐ Completed (Review Pending)
☐ Reviewed
☐ Communicated
</td>
<td align="center">
DRUG CONSULTATION REQUEST FORM
DRUG INFORMATION SERVICE
NATIONAL INSTITUTES OF HEALTH
</td>
<td>
LOG# _____
Final QA Check _____
</td>
</tr>
</table>

REQUESTER INFORMATION

Date Received _____   Time Received _____ AM / PM *(circle one)*

Name _____   Phone# _____   FAX# _____

Pager# _____   e-mail _____

INTERNAL:	EXTERNAL:	AFFILIATION CATEGORY:
☐ MD ☐ DDS	☐ Pharmacist	☐ Institute _____
☐ RN	☐ Physician	☐ Clinic _____
☐ Pharmacist	☐ General Public	☐ Pt Care Unit _____
☐ Other Professional _____	☐ Other Healthcare Professional _____	☐ Other _____
☐ NIH Patient	☐ Other Professional/Organization _____	
☐ Other _____		

HOW RECEIVED: ☐ Phone ☐ Voice Mail ☐ E-Mail ☐ Mail ☐ FAX ☐ In Person ☐ Referred by :_____

PRIORITY: ☐ Urgent ☐ High Priority ☐ Routine ☐ Low Priority

ORIGINAL QUESTION / REQUEST

CLEAR STATEMENT(S) OF ACTUAL DRUG INFORMATION NEED

PERTINENT PATIENT DATA / BACKGROUND INFORMATION

Name _____   Pt Care Unit/Clinic _____   ☐ Inpatient ☐ Outpatient

Age _____ Race _____ ☐ Male ☐ Female   Height _____ cm _____ ft _____ in   Weight _____ lb _____ kg

Primary Diagnosis _____   Allergies/Intolerances _____

End-Organ Function _____   Special Circumstances _____

CC:

HPI:

PMH:

FH:

SH:

ROS:

Meds:

PE:

Labs:

Diagnostics:

Problem List:

LOG# _____

CLASSIFICATION(S) OF REQUEST

☐ Administration (Routes/Methods)
☐ Adverse Effects/Intolerances
☐ Allergy/Cross Reactivity
☐ Alternative Medicine
☐ Biotechnology/Gene Therapy
☐ Clinical Nutrition/Metabolic Support
☐ Compatibility/Stability/Storage
☐ Contraindications/Precautions
☐ Cost/Pharmacoeconomics
☐ Dose/Schedule
☐ Drug Delivery Devices/Systems/Forms
☐ Drug Interactions (Drug-Drug, Drug-Food)
☐ Drug of choice/Therapeutic Alternatives/Therapeutic Use
☐ Drug Standards/Legal/Regulatory
☐ Drug Use in Special Populations
  (Effects of Age, Organ System Function, Disease,
  Extracorporeal Circulation, etc.)
☐ Excipients/Compounding/Formulations

☐ Investigational Products (Pre–Clinical and Clinical)
☐ Lab Test Interferences (Drug-Lab Interactions)
☐ Monitoring Parameters
☐ Nonprescription Products
☐ Patient Information/Education
☐ Pharmacokinetics (LADME/TDM)
☐ Pharmacology/Mechanisms/Pharmacodynamics
☐ Physicochemical Properties
☐ Poisoning/Toxicology (Environmental/Occupational Exposure,
  Mutagenicity, Carcinogenicity)
☐ Pregnancy/Lactation/Teratogenicity/Fertility
☐ Product Availability/Status
☐ Product Identification (Tablet/Capsule)
☐ Product Identification (Generic, Brand, Orphan,
  Foreign, Chemical Substances, Discontinued Products, etc.)
☐ Product Information
☐ Study Design/Protocol Development/Research Support
☐ Other _____

REQUEST CATEGORY

☐ Patient Care   ☐ Research   ☐ Other _____

RESPONSE (Referenced)

REFERENCES (Numbered)

TRACKING / FOLLOW-UP

Request Received By_____   Reviewed By_____
Response Formulated By_____   Response Communicated By_____
                                          Time Required to Answer_____

☐ Documents/Literature Provided   ☐ Verbal Response   ☐ E-Mail   ☐ Written Response/Consult

OUTCOME / FOLLOW-UP

*U.S. GPO: 1998-445-295/89216

2—2

Appendix 2–2

Standard Questions for Obtaining Background Information from Requestors

Regardless of the type or classification of the question, the following information should be obtained:

1. The requestor's name.
2. The requestor's location and/or contact information.
3. The requestor's affiliation (institution or practice), if a health care professional.
4. The requestor's frame of reference (i.e., title, profession/occupation, rank).
5. The resources the requestor has already consulted.
6. If the request is patient-specific or academic.
7. The patient's diagnosis and other medications.
8. The urgency of the request (negotiate time of response).

The following questions should be asked when appropriate for specific requests*.

Availability of Dosage Forms

1. What is the dosage form desired?
2. What administration routes are feasible with this patient?
3. Is this patient alert and oriented?
4. Does the patient have a water or sodium restriction?
5. What other special factors regarding drug administration should be considered?

Identification of Product

1. What is the generic or trade name of the product?
2. Who is the manufacturer? What is the country of origin?
3. What is the suspected use of this product?
4. Under what circumstances was this product found? Who found the product?
5. What is the dosage form, color markings, size, etc.?
6. What was your source of information? Was it reliable?

General Product Information

1. Why is there a particular concern for this product?
2. Is written patient information required?

3. What type of information do you need?

4. Is this for an inpatient, outpatient, or private patient?

Foreign Drug Identification

1. What is the drug's generic name, trade, manufacturer, and/or country of origin?

2. What is the dosage form, markings, color, strength, or size?

3. What is the suspected use of the drug? How often is the patient taking it? What is the patient's response to the drug? Is the patient male or female?

4. If the medication was found, what were the circumstances/conditions at the time of discovery?

5. Is the patient just visiting, or are they planning on staying?

Investigational Drug Information

1. Why do you need this information? Is the patient in need of the drug or currently enrolled in a protocol?

2. If a drug is to be identified, what is the dosage form, markings, color, strength, or size of the product?

3. Why was the patient receiving the drug? What is the response when the patient was on the drug? What are the patient's pathological conditions?

4. If a drug is desired what approved or accepted therapies have been tried? Was therapy maximized before discontinued?

Method and Rate of Administration

1. What dosage form or preparation is being used (if multiple salts available)?

2. What is the dose ordered? Is the drug a one-time dose or standing orders?

3. What is the clinical status of the patient? For example, could the patient tolerate a fluid push of XX mL? Is the patient fluid or sodium restricted? Does the patient have CHF or edema?

4. What possible delivery routes are available?

5. What other medications is the patient receiving currently? Are any by the same route?

Incompatibility and Stability

1. What are the routes for the patient's medications?

2. What are the doses, concentrations, and volumes for all pertinent medications?

3. What are the infusion times/rates expected or desired?

4. What is the base solution or diluent used?

5. Was the product stored and handled appropriately, based on requirements?

6. When was the product compounded/prepared?

Drug Interactions

1. What event(s) suggest that an interaction occurred? Please describe.

2. For the drugs in question, what are the doses, volumes, concentrations, rate of administration, administration schedules, and length of therapies?

3. What is the temporal relationship between the drugs in question?
4. Has the patient received this combination or a similar combination in the past?
5. Other than the drugs in question, what other drugs is the patient receiving currently? When were these started?

Drug-Laboratory Test Interference

1. What event(s) suggest an interaction occurred? Please describe.
2. For the drug in question, what is the dose, volume, concentration, rate of administration, administration schedule, and length of therapy?
3. What is the temporal relationship between drug administration and laboratory test sampling?
4. What other drugs is the patient receiving?
5. Has clinical chemistry (or the appropriate laboratory) been contacted? Are they aware of any known interference similar to this event?
6. Was this one isolated test or a trend in results?

Pharmacokinetics

1. Which product (e.g., drug, dose, brand) is being used?
2. What are the dose and route of the drug?
3. What are the patient's age, sex, height, and weight?
4. What are the diseases being treated and the severity of the illness?
5. What is the patient's hepatic and renal functions?
6. What other medications is the patient receiving?
7. What physiologic conditions exist (e.g., pneumonia, severe burns, or obesity)?
8. What are the patient's dietary and ethanol habits?

Therapeutic Levels

1. Is the patient currently receiving the drug? Have samples already been drawn? At what time?
2. What is the disease or underlying pathology being treated? If infectious in nature, what is the organism suspected/cultured?
3. If not stated in the question, what was the source of the sample (blood, urine, saliva; venous or arterial blood)?
4. What was the timing of the samples relative to drug administration? Over what period of time was the drug administered and by what route?
5. What were the previous concentrations for this patient? Was the patient receiving the same dose then?
6. How long has the patient received the drug? Is the patient at steady state?

Therapy Evaluation/Drug of Choice

1. What medications, including doses and routes of administration, is the patient receiving?
2. What are the patient's pathology(ies) and disease(s) severity?
3. What are the patient's specifics: age, weight, height, gender, organ function/dysfunction?

4. Has the patient received the drug previously? Was response similar?
5. Has the patient been adherent?
6. What alternative therapies has the patient received? Was therapy maximized for each of these before discontinuation? What other therapies are being considered?
7. What monitoring parameters have been followed (serum concentrations/levels, clinical status, other clinical lab results, objective measurements, and subjective assessment).

Dosage Recommendations

1. What disease is being treated? What is the extent/severity of the illness?
2. What are the medications (all) being prescribed? Has the patient been adherent?
3. Does the patient have any insufficiency of the renal, hepatic, or cardiac system?
4. For drugs with renal elimination, what are the serum creatinine/creatinine clearance, blood urea nitrogen (BUN), and/or during output? Is the patient receiving peritoneal dialysis or hemodialysis?
5. For drugs with hepatic elimination, what are the liver function tests (LFTs), bilirubin (direct and indirect), and/or albumin?
6. For drugs with serum level monitoring utility, characterize the most recent levels per timing relative to dose and results.
7. Are these lab values recent? Is the patient's condition stable?
8. Does this patient have a known factor that could affect drug metabolism (ethnic background or acetylator status)?

Adverse Events

1. What is the name, dosage, and route for all drugs currently and recently prescribed?
2. What are the patient specifics (age, sex, height, weight, organ dysfunction, and indication for drug use)?
3. What is the temporal relationship with the drug?
4. Has the patient experienced this adverse relationship (or a similar event) with this drug (or similar agent) previously?
5. Was the suspected drug ever administered before? Why was it discontinued then?
6. What were the events/findings that characterize this adverse drug reaction (include onset and duration)?
7. Has any intervention been initiated at this time?
8. Does the patient have any food intolerance?
9. Is there a family history for this ADR and/or drug allergy?

Toxicology Information

1. What is your name, relationship to the patient, and telephone number?
2. What are the patient specifics (age, sex, height, weight, organ dysfunction, and indication for drug use)?
3. Is this a suspected ingestion or exposure?

4. What is the product suspected to have been ingested? What is the strength of the product and the possible quantity ingested (e.g., how much was in the bottle)?
5. How long ago did the ingestion occur?
6. How much is on the patient or surrounding area?
7. How much was removed from the patient's hands and mouth? Was the ingestion in the same room where the product was stored?
8. What has been done for the patient already? Has the Poison Control Center or emergency department been called?
9. Do you have Syrup of Ipecac available (only if recommended by a poison control center)? Do you know how to give it properly?
10. What is the patient's condition (sensorium, heart rate, respiratory rate, temperature, skin color/turgor, pupils, sweating/salvation, etc.)?
11. Does the patient have any known illnesses?

Teratogenicity/Drugs in Pregnancy

1. What is the drug the patient received and what was the dose? What was the duration of therapy?
2. Is the patient pregnant or planning to become pregnant?
3. When during pregnancy was the exposure (trimester or weeks)?
4. What are the patient specifics (age, height, weight, sex)?
5. Was the patient adherent?
6. For what indication was the drug being prescribed?

Drugs in Breast Milk/Lactation

1. What is the drug the patient received and what was the dose? What was the duration of therapy?
2. How long has the infant been breast-feeding?
3. Has the infant ever received non-maternal nutrition? Is bottle feeding a plausible alternative?
4. What is the frequency of the breast feeds? What is the milk volume?
5. How old is the infant?
6. Does the mother have hepatic or renal insufficiency?
7. What was the indication for prescribing the drug? Was this initial or alternate therapy?
8. Has the mother breast-fed previously while on the drug?

*Specific questions for only selected types of requests presented; other specific questions would be appropriate for other types of requests.

Appendix 3–1

Performing a PubMed Search

PubMed Search

PubMed is a database which is maintained by the National Library of Medicine and is available to the public at no charge. This database is available online at http://www.ncbi.nlm.nih.gov/PubMed. The information indexed by PubMed includes MEDLINE, OLDMEDLINE (articles from the 1950s to the mid-1960s), as well as citations for additional life science journals.

This database is especially helpful when looking for off-label uses of medications. For example, if a prescriber contacts you asking for information about the efficacy of fluoxetine in treatment of anorexia nervosa, it may be appropriate to seek information from the primary literature. A PubMed search might be a good place to start this search. When performing a search using PubMed one can begin with just a key word, for example, fluoxetine. As Figure 1 shows, just using the term fluoxetine yields in 10,310 results. The results can be narrowed by entering a second key word, such as anorexia nervosa, and combining the two terms with the Boolean operator AND.

While the addition of a second search term (see Figure 2) did narrow the results, there are still 88 results that match these two terms. At this time it may be wise to explore the limit options provided by the database. Limits allow the user to restrict the number of results returned for a search. Some databases allow searches to be limited by a variety of factors, including language of publication, year of publication, type of article (e.g., human study, review, case report) or by type of journal where publication is found. Since the requestor is seeking efficacy data it is appropriate to limit these search results to just clinical trials.

By limiting the results to only human clinical trials published in English, 23 citations of possible interest have been identified (Figure 3). It is now necessary to look at the abstracts for these citations (Figure 4) and determine if these are helpful to provide a response to the query. By clicking on the blue hyperlink an abstract is displayed, this abstract summarizes the information in the article, as well as providing complete citation information for that specific article. If the publisher's website offers full text of an article, a link is provided at the top of the page to the journal website. Some journals charge a fee for access to the full-text article while others do not. Those journals not charging for an article are clearly marked as "free full text." You can then select that icon and go directly to a full-text PDF or html of the desired article.

One additional helpful feature offered by PubMed is the "Related citations" link. The database will first identify the key words or Medical Subject Headings (MeSH) associated with the article selected and then identify secondary words and terms. The database will then compare these terms (both primary and secondary terms) with other articles indexed in PubMed to determine which other articles include similarly ranked terms and therefore might be of interest.

The best way to effectively search this database is by experience. However, PubMed offers a tutorial to gain additional experience in how to most effectively conduct literature searches. This interactive tutorial session is available at http://www.nlm.nih.gov/bsd/disted/pubmedtutorial/.

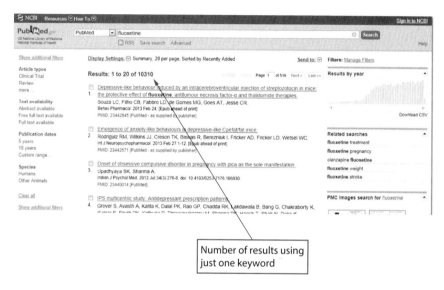

Figure 1. Key word search.

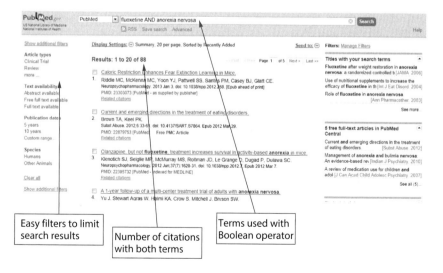

Figure 2. Multiple key word search.

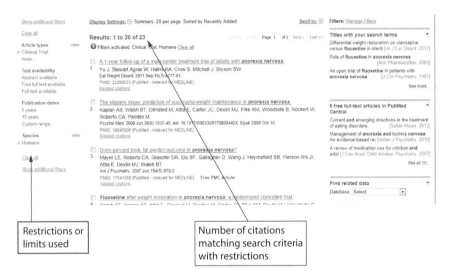

Figure 3. Results of search with restrictions.

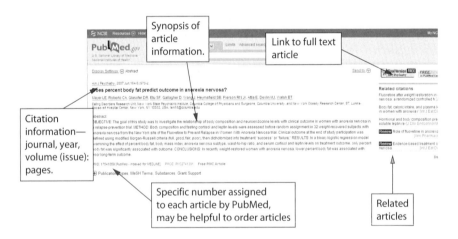

Figure 4. PubMed abstract.

Appendix 3–2

Selected Primary Literatures Sources

Journal Title	Publisher	ISSN	Areas Covered
American Journal of Health-System Pharmacy: AJHP	American Society of Health-System Pharmacy	1079-2082	Clinical and managerial areas of pharmacy practice in health systems
American Journal of Pharmacy Education	American Association of Colleges of Pharmacy	0002-9459	Scholarship and advancement of pharmacy education
Annals of Internal Medicine	American College of Physicians	0003-4819	Internal medicine, including management of disease states
Annals of Pharmacotherapy	Harvey Whitney Books Company	1060-0280	Safe, effective, and economical use of drugs
Antimicrobial Agents and Chemotherapy	American Society for Microbiology	0066-4804	Information regarding the use of antimicrobial agents
Archives of Internal Medicine	American Medical Association	0003-9926	Focus on the diagnosis and treatment of disease states
BMJ (British Medical Journal)	BMJ Publishing Group	0959-8138 (print) 1756-1833 (online)	A wide range of primary and tertiary papers regarding human health and include a suite of journals focusing on specialty care
Chest	American College of Chest Physicians	0012-3692 (print) 1931-3543 (online)	A wide range of research papers related to pulmonary and respiratory conditions, critical care, imaging, and cardiovascular diseases
Circulation	American Heart Association	0009-7322 (print) 1524-4539 (online)	Topics related to cardiovascular and cerebrovascular research, including clinical practice guidelines

continued

Journal Title	Publisher	ISSN	Areas Covered
Clinical Pharmacokinetics	Adis International Limited	0312-5963	Focus on pharmacokinetic and pharmacodynamic properties of drugs
Clinical Pharmacology and Therapeutics	Mosby Year Book Incorporated	0009-9236	The effect of drugs on the human body
Drug Information Journal	Drug Information Association	0092-8615	Technology related to disseminating drug information
Drug Topics	Thomson Healthcare	0012-6616	Focus on issues impacting community pharmacy and on new drug therapies
Drugs	Adis International Limited	0012-6667	Pharmacotherapeutic aspects of both new and established drugs
Formulary	Advanstar Communications Incorporated	1082-801X	Contemporary issues in drug policy management and pharmacotherapy
Hospital Pharmacy	Facts & Comparisons Incorporated	0018-5787	Issues related to pharmacy in institutional settings
JAMA (the Journal of the American Medical Association)	American Medical Association	0098-7484	New research and review information that impacts health care
Journal of Cardiovascular Pharmacology	Lippincott Williams & Wilkins	0160-2446	New information about the treatment of cardiovascular disease.
The Journal of Clinical Pharmacology	Lippincott Williams & Wilkins	0091-2700	Clinical information about the safety, tolerability, efficacy, therapeutic use, and toxicology of drugs
Journal of Pharmaceutical Sciences	Wiley	0022-3549	Application of physical and analytical chemistry to pharmaceutical sciences
Journal of Pharmacology and Experimental Therapeutics	American Society for Experimental Pharmacology and Therapeutics	0022-3565	Covers interaction between chemicals and biological systems as well as metabolism, distribution and toxicology
Journal of Pharmacy and Pharmacology	Pharmaceutical Press	0022-3573	Addresses a variety of practice areas including drug delivery systems, biomaterials and polymers, and implications of human genome on drug therapies
Journal of the American Pharmacists Association	American Pharmacists Association	1544-3191	News, information, and research in the area of pharmacotherapeutic management

continued

Journal Title	Publisher	ISSN	Areas Covered
Mayo Clinic Proceedings	Elsevier	0025-6196	A variety of articles related to health research, policy, and meeting reports as well as clinical practice recommendations
Medical Letter on Drugs and Therapeutics	Medical Letter, Inc.	0025-732X	Provides information on new drug therapies and drugs of choice for disease management
New England Journal of Medicine	Massachusetts Medical Society	0028-646X	Results of recent research considered important to the practice of medicine
Pharmaceutical Research	Plenum Press	0724-8741	Emphasis on drug delivery, drug formulation, pharmacokinetics, pharmacodynamics, and drug disposition
PharmacoEconomics	Adis International Limited	1170-7690	Information regarding the economical use of drug therapies
Pharmacological Reviews	American Society of Pharmacology and Experimental Therapeutics	0031-6997	Current topics of interest including cellular pharmacology, drug metabolism and disposition, renal pharmacology, and neuropharmacology
Pharmacotherapy	IOS Press	0277-0008	Published by American College of Clinical pharmacy and focused on original research in clinical practice
Pharmacy Times	Romaine Pierson Publishing Incorporated	0003-0627	Focus on new drug therapies and patient counseling as it relates to community pharmacy
PLoS ONE	PLOS	1932-6203	First multidisciplinary open access journal, covering a diverse topics of primary research and systematic reviews
The Lancet	Elsevier	0140-6736	New topics and research related to human health and include a suite of journals that focus on specialty areas of health care
Therapeutic Drug Monitoring	Lippincott Williams & Wilkins	0163-4356	Fosters exchange of knowledge between fields of pharmacology, pathology, toxicology, and analytical
U.S. Pharmacist	Jobson Publishing Corporation	0148-4818	Information regarding the practice of community pharmacy

Appendix 4–1

Drug Literature Assessment Questions for Clinical Trials

OVERALL ASSESSMENT

- Was the article published in a reputable, peer-reviewed journal?
- Are the investigator's training/education/practice sties adequate for the study objective?
- Can the funding source bias the study?

TITLE/ABSTRACT

- Was the title unbiased?
- Did the abstract contain information not found within the study?
- Did the abstract provide a clear over view of the purpose, methods, results, and conclusions of the study?

INTRODUCTION

- Did the authors provide sufficient background information to demonstrate the rationale for the study?
- Were the study objectives clearly identified?
- What were the major null hypothesis and alternate hypothesis?

METHODS

- Was an appropriate study design used to answer the question?
- Were reasonable inclusion/exclusion criteria presented to represent an appropriate patient population?
- Was a selection bias present?
- Was subject recruitment described? If so, how were subjects recruited? Was the method appropriate?
- Was IRB approval obtained?
- Was subject informed consent obtained?
- Were the intervention and control regimens appropriate?

- What type of blinding was used? Was this type appropriate?
- Was randomization included? If so, what type was used? Was this appropriate?
- Who generated the allocation sequence, enrolled participants, and assigned participants to groups? Was this appropriate?
- Which ancillary treatments were permitted? Would they have affected the outcome?
- Was a run-in period included? How does this affect the results?
- Did the investigators measure compliance? How was compliance measured? Was compliance adequate?
- Was the primary endpoint appropriate for the study objective?
- Were secondary endpoints measured? If so, were they adequate for what was being studied?
- Were planned subgroup analyses planned? If so, were they appropriate?
- Was the method used to measure the primary endpoint appropriate?
- What type of data best describes the primary endpoint?
- Were data collected appropriately?
- What number of patients was needed for the primary endpoint to detect a difference between groups (power analysis)? Was the necessary sample size calculated? Were there enough patients enrolled to reach this endpoint?
- What were the alpha (α) and beta (β) values? Were these appropriate?
- Were the statistical tests used appropriate?

RESULTS

- Were the numbers of patients screened, enrolled, administered treatment, completing, and withdrawing from the study reported? Were reasons for subject discontinuations reported? Were withdrawals handled appropriately?
- Was the trial adequately powered?
- Were the subject demographics between groups similar at baseline? If not, were the differences likely to have an effect on the outcome data?
- Were data presented clearly?
- Were the results adjusted to take into account confounding variables?
- Was intention-to-treat analysis used? Was this appropriate?
- Were estimated effect size, p-values, and confidence intervals reported?
- Were the results statistically significant? Clinically different?
- Was the null hypothesis accepted or rejected?
- Can the trial results be extrapolated to the population?
- Based on the results, could a Type I or Type II error have occurred?
- Are subgroup analysis presented? Are these appropriate?
- Was ancillary therapy included? Did this affect the study results?
- Were therapy adverse effects included?

CONCLUSIONS/DISCUSSION

- Did the information appear biased, and did the trial results support the conclusions?
- Were trial limitations described?
- Did the investigators explain unexpected results?
- Are the results able to be extrapolated to the population?
- Were the study results clinically meaningful?

REFERENCES

- Were the references listed well represented (e.g., current, well-representing the literature)?
- Is a comprehensive list of published articles related to the trial objective presented?

Appendix 5–1

Beyond the Basics: Questions to Consider for Critique of Primary Literature

RANDOMIZED CONTROLLED TRIAL

- Refer to Chapter 4: Drug Literature Evaluation I: Controlled Clinical Trial Evaluation

PHARMACO ECONOMIC ANALYSIS

- Refer to Chapter 7: Pharmacoeconomics

NON-INFERIORITY TRIAL

- Is the reference drug's efficacy established using adequate historical data and/or addition of a placebo arm?
- Are the participants and outcome measures for the non-inferiority similar compared to previous studies that confirmed the efficacy of the reference drug (e.g., constancy assumption)?
- Is the method used to determine the non-inferiority (NI) margin predetermined before the study, both clinically and statistically sound, and the reasoning clearly stated in the article?
- Was a per-protocol analysis used? If so, did they also perform an intention-to-treat analysis?
- Was the sample size modified as the study progressed? If so, was a clear explanation of how the blinded information was handled and by what method these modifications were determined also provided?
- Was this study an attempt to rescue a failed superiority trial?

N-OF-1 TRIAL

- Was assignment of active and control treatment to study periods randomized?
- Was the study blinded?
- Were multiple observation periods used?
- Were study endpoints clearly defined?
- Was the washout period between study periods adequate?

ADAPTIVE CLINICAL TRIAL (ACT)

- Are the methodologies used to make adaptive changes in the trial adequately described?
- What logistical issues exist and have they been adequately addressed?
- Are the adaptive changes based on evidence and good clinical judgment?
- Did extensive adaptation to the protocol occur during the study?
- To what extent is intrusion of bias noted?
- Who has access to the information created from interim analyses?
- If the study was stopped early, is the totality of evidence adequate?

STABILITY STUDY

- Were study methodologies and test conditions clearly defined?
- Were validated assays used?
- Were assays validated using time-zero measurements and an adequate number of test samples taken?

BIOEQUIVALENCY STUDY

- Did the protocol define the characteristics of the subjects?
- Were confounding factors (e.g., smoking, alcohol use) identified and controlled?
- Was a crossover design used?
- Was the study randomized and blinded?

PROGRAMMATIC RESEARCH

- Were one of two options used for subject comparison: (1) comparison of subjects to those not using the program or service, (2) comparison of subjects before or after initiation of the program or service?
- Was the program or service clearly defined?
- Did the authors specify from whose perspective (e.g., patient, provider, physician, third-party payer) the study was undertaken?
- If costs were analyzed, were all costs associated with provision of the program or service included in the analysis, including personnel, inflationary changes, and cost savings had the intervention not occurred?
- Were clinically important outcome parameters used to assess effectiveness of the program or service?

COHORT STUDY

- Was the research question clearly stated?
- Were inclusion and exclusion criteria described in detail?
- Were exposed and unexposed subjects similar in terms of demographic characteristics and susceptibility to disease states?
- Was selection bias obviously present?

- Were confounding factors obviously present?
- Were the same efforts to measure outcomes made in each group?
- Were 95% confidence intervals calculated?
- Were follow-up rates the same for the exposed and unexposed groups?

CASE-CONTROL STUDY

- Was predisposition of disease similar in cases and controls except for exposure to the risk factor?
- Were cases and controls matched?
- Was exposure to the risk factor similar to that which would occur in the general population?
- Did cases and controls undergo similar diagnostic evaluations?
- Were investigators who assessed patients or collected data blinded to the status of the subject as a case or control?
- Did the investigators compare cases with several different control groups?
- Were 95% confidence intervals calculated?

CROSS-SECTIONAL STUDY

- Did investigators ensure accuracy in data collection?
- If a survey or questionnaire was used, was it validated?
- Were the inclusion and exclusion criteria clearly defined and stated?
- Was selection of cases clearly described?

CASE STUDY, CASE REPORT, OR CASE SERIES

- Did the authors recognize the preliminary nature of the results (i.e., recommendations for clinical application of the results should be guarded)?

SURVEY STUDY

- Was the survey instrument valid and reliable? Was a pretest or pilot test conducted on the survey instrument?
- Was the sample size large enough to detect a difference between groups?
- Was the survey objective and carefully planned?
- Were data quantifiable?
- Was the sample representative of the target population?
- Was response rate high enough to reflect results that would be expected of the target population?
- Did the investigators determine whether nonresponders differed from responders?

POSTMARKETING SURVEILLANCE STUDY

- Was a large enough sample studied to reflect current uses of and side effects associated with the new drug therapy?
- Were appropriate methods used to measure clearly defined endpoints?

NARRATIVE (NONSYSTEMATIC) REVIEWS—QUALITATIVE

- Was an extensive search for available studies undertaken?
- Did the authors use a variety of resources to identify studies for inclusion in the review article?
- Was the review article focused on a clearly defined population?
- Did the studies included in the review article use valid research methods?
- Did the author examine reasons for differences in study results and conclusions?
- Were outcomes of the studies clinically important?
- Did the author consider benefits and risks of the drug therapy?

SYSTEMATIC REVIEWS—QUALITATIVE

- Did the authors clearly define the research question?
- Was the review article focused on a clearly defined patient population?
- Was an extensive search for available studies undertaken?
- Did the authors consider using results from both published and unpublished studies in the analysis?
- Did the authors clearly define criteria for study inclusion in the analysis?
- Did the authors list studies that were included in and excluded from the analysis?
- Did the authors provide details concerning methodologies of studies used in the analysis?
  - Were included studies addressing the same clinical question(s)?
  - Did all included studies use appropriate doses, regimens, and routes of administrations for both treatments and comparators?
  - Were all included studies of appropriate duration?
- Were those who selected studies for inclusion in the analysis blinded to the names of the original authors, place of publication of the study, and final study results?

META-ANALYSIS—QUANTITATIVE

- Did the authors clearly define the research question?
- Was the review article focused on a clearly defined patient population?
- Was an extensive search for available studies undertaken?
- Did the authors consider using results from both published and unpublished studies in the analysis?
- Did the authors clearly define criteria for study inclusion in the analysis?
- Did the authors list studies that were included in and excluded from the analysis?
- Did the authors include gray literature in the analysis?
- Did the authors provide details concerning methodologies of studies used in the analysis?
  - Were included studies addressing the same clinical question(s)?
  - Did all included studies use appropriate doses, regimens, and routes of administrations for both treatments and comparators?
  - Were all included studies of appropriate duration?
- Was a funnel plot provided to determine if publication bias was potentially present?
- Were tests of homogeneity performed and results reported?

- Were those who selected studies for inclusion in the analysis blinded to the names of the original authors, place of publication of the study, and final study results?
- Were appropriate statistical tests used and the probability of Type I and Type II errors considered?
- Were 95% confidence intervals calculated?
- Were results presented in a forest plot?

PRACTICE GUIDELINES

- Is there an explicit description of the procedures used to identify, select, and combine evidence?
- Are the recommendations valid?
- Are the guidelines regularly reviewed and updated to incorporate new evidence as it becomes available?
- Was the guideline peer reviewed?
- Can the recommendations be generalized to a larger population?
- Was the source of funding for the development of the guideline provided and could it bias the conclusions?
- If another group of experts were to independently develop a guideline on the same clinical situation, would the recommendations be the same (are the recommendations reliable)?

QUALITY-OF-LIFE STUDIES

- Are HR-QOL instruments validated?
- If a series of HR-QOL measurements are used, does this result in a valid HR-QOL battery?
- Are HR-QOL instruments sensitive to changes in the patients' status as the trial progresses?
- Are important aspects of patients' lives measured, as determined by patients themselves?
- Is timing of HR-QOL measurements to answer the research questions appropriately related to anticipated timing of the clinical effects?
- Were sequences of HR-QOL assessments conducted in the same order for all patients?
- Was mode of data collection (self-report versus trained interviewer) appropriate for type of questions being asked?
  - If mode of data collection was a trained interviewer, could the interview location lead to biased answers?
- Were response rates to questionnaires reported?
- Is there missing data?
  - If missing data exist, is there a specific pattern that suggests author manipulation providing desired results (missing data could have countered author's hypothesis)?
- If a multicenter trial, did all sites evaluate HR-QOL?
- Is the QOL instrument valid for examining the specific disease in question?
- Are both positive and negative findings reported?
- Are adverse drug events and HR-QOL measurements considered separately?
- Is impact of treatment effects included with HR-QOL measurements?
- Is there evidence that culturally defined factors may have impacted patient HR-QOL measurements and/or the assessment of these measurements?

- Does there appear to be a bias on the part of the study researchers?
- Were general measures of QOL evaluated?

DIETARY SUPPLEMENT MEDICAL LITERATURE

- Which plant part was utilized?
- Was a standardized botanical extract utilized?
- Was the study product standardization appropriate?
- Was a specific plant species or specific salt form utilized?
- Was the study dose appropriate?
- Was trial length appropriate to perceive treatment effects or differences?
- Was sample size sufficient to detect a difference between groups if one exists?

Appendix 8–1

Grade Evidence Profile: Antibiotics for Children with Acute Otitis Media

Quality Assessment | | | | | | **Summary of Findings** | | | | |

Number of studies (Design)	Limitations	Inconsistency	Indirectness	Imprecision	Publication bias	Number of patients		Relative risk (95% CI)	Absolute risk		Quality
						Placebo	Antibiotics		Control risk[a]	Risk difference (95% CI)	
Pain at 24 hours											
5 (RCT)	No serious limitations	No serious inconsistency	No serious indirectness	No serious imprecision	Undetected	241/605	223/624	RR 0.9 (0.78–1.04)	367/1,000	Not significant	⊕⊕⊕⊕ High
Pain at 2–7 days											
10 (RCT)	No serious limitations	No serious inconsistency	No serious indirectness	No serious imprecision	Undetected	303/1,366	228/1,425	RR 0.72 (0.62–0.83)	257/1,000	72 fewer per 1,000 (44–98)	⊕⊕⊕⊕ High
Hearing, inferred from the surrogate outcome abnormal tympanometry—1 month											
4 (RCT)	No serious limitations	No serious inconsistency	Serious indirectness (because of indirectness of outcome)	No serious imprecision	Undetected	168/460	153/467	RR 0.89 (0.75–1.07)	350/1,000	Not significant	⊕⊕⊕o Moderate
Hearing, inferred from the surrogate outcome abnormal tympanometry—3 months											
3 (RCT)	No serious limitations	No serious inconsistency (because of indirectness of outcome)	Serious indirectness	No serious imprecision	Undetected	96/398	96/410	RR 0.97 (0.76–1.24)	234/1,000	Not significant	⊕⊕⊕o Moderate
Vomiting, diarrhea, or rash											
5 (RCT)	No serious limitations	Serious inconsistency (because of inconsistency in absolute effects)	No serious indirectness	No serious imprecision	Undetected	83/711	110/690	RR 1.38 (1.09–1.76)	113/1,000	43 more per 1,000 (10–86)	⊕⊕⊕o Moderate

[a] The control rate is based on the median control group risk across studies.

GRADE = Grading of Recommendations Assessment, Development, and Evaluation; RCT = randomized controlled trials; CI = confidence interval; RR = risk ratio.

Reproduced from Journal of Clinical Epidemiology, Vol 64, Gordon Guyatt, Andrew D. Oxman, Elie A Akl, Regina Kunz, Gunn Vist, et al. GRADE guidelines: Introduction GRADE evidence profiles and summary of findings tables. p. 383–394, Copyright 2011, with permission from Elsevier.

Appendix 11-1

Code of Ethics for Pharmacists[1]

Pharmacists are health professionals who assist individuals in making the best use of medications. This Code, prepared and supported by pharmacists, is intended to state publicly the principles that form the fundamental basis of the roles and responsibilities of pharmacists. These principles, based on moral obligations and virtues, are established to guide pharmacists in relationships with patients, health professionals, and society.

I. A pharmacist respects the covenantal relationship between the patient and pharmacist.

Considering the patient-pharmacist relationship as a covenant means that a pharmacist has moral obligations in response to the gift of trust received from society. In return for this gift, a pharmacist promises to help individuals achieve optimum benefit from their medications, to be committed to their welfare, and to maintain their trust.

II. A pharmacist promotes the good of every patient in a caring, compassionate, and confidential manner.

A pharmacist places concern for the well-being of the patient at the center of professional practice. In doing so, a pharmacist considers needs stated by the patient as well as those defined by health science. A pharmacist is dedicated to protecting the dignity of the patient. With a caring attitude and a compassionate spirit, a pharmacist focuses on serving the patient in a private and confidential manner.

III. A pharmacist respects the autonomy and dignity of each patient.

A pharmacist promotes the right of self-determination and recognizes individual self-worth by encouraging patients to participate in decisions about their health. A pharmacist communicates with patients in terms that are understandable. In all cases, a pharmacist respects personal and cultural differences among patients.

IV. A pharmacist acts with honesty and integrity in professional relationships.

A pharmacist has a duty to tell the truth and to act with conviction of conscience. A pharmacist avoids discriminatory practices, behavior or work conditions that impair professional judgment, and actions that compromise dedication to the best interests of patients.

V. A pharmacist maintains professional competence.

A pharmacist has a duty to maintain knowledge and abilities as new medications, devices, and technologies become available and as health information advances.

VI. A pharmacist respects the values and abilities of colleagues and other health professionals.

When appropriate, a pharmacist asks for the consultation of colleagues or other health professionals or refers the patient. A pharmacist acknowledges that colleagues and other health professionals may differ in the beliefs and values they apply to the care of the patient.

VII. A pharmacist serves individual, community, and societal needs.

The primary obligation of a pharmacist is to individual patients. However, the obligations of a pharmacist may at times extend beyond the individual to the community and society. In these situations, the pharmacist recognizes the responsibilities that accompany these obligations and acts accordingly.

VIII. A pharmacist seeks justice in the distribution of health resources.

When health resources are allocated, a pharmacist is fair and equitable, balancing the needs of patients and society.

Adopted by the membership of the American Pharmacists Association, October 27, 1994.

REFERENCE

1. American Pharmacists Association. Code of ethics 1994 [updated 1994 Oct 27; 2010 Mar 26]. Available from: http://www.pharmacist.com/code-ethics

Appendix 12–1

Question Example

DRUG INFORMATICS CENTER

St. Anywhere Hospital

Name of Inquirer:	Dr. Meghan J. Malone	Date: XX/XX/XX
Address	2184 Fall St. Seneca Falls, NY 13148	Time Received: XX:XX am/pm
		Time Required: 5 hours
		Nature of Request: Therapeutics
Telephone Number:	(315)555-1212	Type of Inquirer: Pharmacist

QUESTION

A young, adult male patient recently arrived from Japan and presented to the physician with sparse medical records indicating he is suffering from tsutsugamushi disease. Because of the language difficulties, little is known about the patient, other than he is taking drug X for the illness. Physical exam reveals a patient in some discomfort with elevated temperature, swollen lymph glands, and red rash. All other findings appear to be normal. (*Note:* The person answering this question obtained as much background as possible about the patient.) The physician has little information on the disease and would like to know if that drug X is the most appropriate treatment.

ANSWER

Tsutsugamushi disease is an acute infectious disease seen in harvesters of hemp in Japan.[1] It is caused by *Rickettsia tsutsugamushi*. Common symptoms of the disease include fever, painful swelling of the lymph glands, a small black scab in the genital region, neck or axilla, and large dark-red papules. The disease is known by a number of other names, including akamushi disease, flood fever, inundation fever, island disease, Japanese river fever, and scrub typhus.[2-4] (*Note:* Background information presented.) The standard treatment of the disease includes either drug X or drug Y, although there are several other less effective treatments.[5-7] In the remainder of this paper, a comparison of the two major drugs will be presented. (*Note:* Clear objective for paper is presented.)

   A thorough search of the available literature was conducted. Unfortunately, there were few textbooks available on this disease. A search of MEDLINE® (1966 to present) and Embase® Drugs and Pharmacology (1980 to present) produced a number of articles that were obtained and are reviewed below. (*Note:* This documents the type of search and acts as a lead-in to the remainder of the body of the paper.)

Smith and Jones[8] performed a double-blind, randomized comparison of the effects of drug X and drug Y in patients with tsutsugamushi fever. Patients were required to be between 18 and 70 years old, and could not have any concurrent infection or disorder that would affect the immune response to the disease (e.g., neutropenia, AIDS). Twenty patients received 10 mg of drug X three times a day for 15 days. Eighteen patients received 250 mg of drug Y twice a day for 10 days. The two groups were comparable, except that the patients receiving drug X were an average of 5 years younger ($p < 0.05$). Drug X was shown to produce a cure, both in terms of symptoms and cultures in 85% of patients, whereas drug Y only produced a cure in 55.5% of patients. The difference was statistically significant ($p < 0.01$). No significant adverse effects were seen in either group. Although it appears that drug X was the better agent, it should be noted that drug Y was given at its minimally effective dose, and may have performed better in a somewhat higher dose or longer regimen. (*Note:* Evaluative comments made about the article.)

(*Note:* Other articles would be described at this point.)

Based on the literature found, it appears that drug Y is generally accepted as the better agent, except in those patients with severe renal insufficiency. Because this patient does not appear to be suffering from that problem, it is recommended that he receive a 3-week course of drug Y at a dose of 500 mg three times a day. Renal function should be monitored weekly. The patient should receive an additional week of therapy, if the symptoms have not been gone for the final week of therapy. (*Note:* This patient's situation was specifically addressed, rather than just presenting a general conclusion.)

Signature: _____ Date: March 20, 2018

Mia Q. Pharmacist, Pharm.D.

REFERENCES

(References used in answering the above question would be provided here. The citation numbers in the above paragraphs are for example only and do not refer to actual references in this example).

Appendix 12-2

Abstracts

Abstracts are a synopsis (usually 250 words or less) of the most important aspect of an article. They should be clear, concise, and complete enough for readers to have a reasonable understanding of the important portions of the article.[1] Since they are the most commonly read part of an article, they must be accurate and avoid the three most common errors: differences in information presented in the abstract and in the body of the article, information given in the abstract that was not presented in the article, and conclusions presented in the abstract that are not supported by information in the abstract.[2-4]

There are basically three types of abstracts that are seen in the literature. The first two (descriptive and informational) are somewhat traditional; however, they do not convey as much information as structured abstracts. Structured abstracts were originally designed to convey more information, and have been in use since the 1980s. The type of abstract to be used depends on the type of information and the requirements of the particular place the work is being submitted or used.

In addition to writing an abstract, some journals ask that indexing terms be submitted. Whenever possible, Medical Subject Headings (MeSH) from the National Library of Medicine should be used for the indexing terms (they may be found at https://www.nlm.nih.gov/mesh/MBrowser.html). Each of the abstracts will be discussed in more detail in the following sections.

DESCRIPTIVE ABSTRACTS

A descriptive abstract, as its name implies, simply describes the information found in an article. Few specific details are given and it is primarily used in a review article. An example of this type of abstract is as follows:

> Lists of references that should be available, depending on location of the drug information service, are presented. These lists are specific to community, hospital, long-term care facility, and academic sites. Included are general references, indexing and abstracting services, and journals. Specialty references that would be useful in specific circumstances are also presented. In addition, the equipment and software necessary to access the computerized resources is shown for the individual references.

INFORMATIONAL ABSTRACTS

Informational abstracts concisely summarize the factual information presented in a study. This type of abstract is more applicable to clinical studies.

Key points to include in an informational abstract include:

- Study design (e.g., double-blind, crossover)
- Purpose
- Number of patients and other demographic aspects
- Dosages
- Results
- Conclusions

An example of this type of abstract is as follows:

> A double-blind, randomized comparison of the effects of drug X and drug Y was performed in patients with tsutsugamushi fever, in order to determine whether either drug was superior in efficacy or safety. Twenty patients received 10 mg of drug X three times a day for 15 days. Eighteen patients received 250 mg of drug Y twice a day for 10 days. The two groups were comparable, except that the patients receiving drug X were an average of 5 years younger ($p < 0.05$). Drug X was shown to produce a cure, both in terms of symptoms and cultures in 85% of patients, whereas drug Y only produced a cure in 55.5% of patients. The difference was statistically significant ($p < 0.01$). No significant adverse effects were seen in either group. Drug X was shown to be significantly better than drug Y in the treatment of tsutsugamushi fever.

STRUCTURED ABSTRACTS

Due to perceived deficiencies in abstracts,[5] including lack of sufficient information,[6] a new type of abstract was presented in 1987[7] and later updated in 1990.[8] This structured abstract was designed to present more information about clinical studies and possibly laboratory studies, as compared to the informational abstract presented earlier.[9,10] This type of abstract is not meant for case reports, studies of tissues or animals, opinion articles, and position papers.[8] Abstracts following this standard seem to be gaining in popularity[11] and have been mandated by an influential group of journals (e.g., New England Journal of Medicine,[12] Annals of Internal Medicine,[8] JAMA: Journal of the American Medical Association,[9] BMJ,[13] Canadian Medical Association Journal,[14] CHEST[15]), sometimes in a somewhat modified form (e.g., the PICO model used by BMJ[16] and their newer, shorter print abstract[17]), although this type of abstract may not be used in the majority of articles found in popular medical journals.[18] This type of abstract has also been suggested in the pharmacy literature.[19] Although the overall acceptance and approval of this format of abstract appears to be good, there are some who disapprove.[20-22] Also, there is some data suggesting that structured abstracts do not always contain as much information as they should, if the published rules are followed,[23] and that they do not necessarily contain any more useful information than informational abstracts.[24]

It is worth noting that articles with structured abstracts are indexed with a greater number of terms in MEDLINE®, which may make it easier to find such articles in a computer search.[25]

An abstract following this procedure would contain the following subheadings and information:

- *Objective*—The main objective of the study and key secondary objectives.
- *Design*—The basic design of the study (e.g., randomized, double-blind, crossover, placebo-controlled, prospective versus retrospective) and duration of any follow-up.

- *Setting*—The location and level of clinical care available at that location (e.g., tertiary care hospital, ambulatory clinic). Also, if a single or multiple locations, nationally or globally, were involved.

- *Patients or other participants*—Description of the patients, including illnesses and key sociodemographic features and how they were selected for the study (including sampling methods such as random, volunteer, or convenient samples); it should also include the number of patients that refused to enroll in the study, proportion of the patients completing the study, and the number of patients withdrawn due to adverse effects or other reasons.

- *Intervention(s)*—A brief description of any treatment(s) or intervention(s).

- *Main outcome measure(s)*—The main study outcome measurements, as planned before data collection was begun (*a priori*); if most of the article covers other material (e.g., data or hypotheses not planned to be observed before the study was started), that should be made clear; the measurement used in the study should correspond to the outcome of interest (e.g., hemoglobin A1C for type 2 diabetes mellitus); data analysis methods should be described including appropriate level of significance, power of the study, and statistical tests used.

- *Results*—The method(s) by which patients were assessed and the main results of the study, including any blinding. Data on statistical significance (particularly confidence intervals, odds ratios, numerators, and denominators) and probability rate (*p* value, if intended for generalization to a larger population) should be mentioned. Absolute, rather than relative, differences are presented (e.g., "adverse effects were seen in 5% of patients in group A and 10% of patients in group B," rather than "Group B had twice as many adverse effects"). The response rate should be provided in survey articles.

- *Conclusion(s)*—The key conclusion(s) directly supported by the evidence presented in the study and their clinical application(s) as well as a statement regarding whether further study is necessary should be included.

An example of this type of abstract is as follows:

Study objective—To compare the safety and efficacy of drug X and drug Y in the treatment of tsutsugamushi fever.

Design—Randomized, double-blind trial

Setting—Tertiary care, military hospital located on Guam

Patients—Sequential sample of 40 young (age 20 to 37), otherwise healthy male patients with tsutsugamushi fever. Patients randomly divided into two equal groups. Two patients were removed from the group receiving drug Y, due to transfer to U.S. mainland hospitals.

Interventions—Twenty patients received 10 mg of drug X three times a day for 15 days. Eighteen patients received 250 mg of drug Y twice a day for 10 days.

Main outcome measures—Physician and patients' global assessment of disease activity; five point scale from 0 (no symptoms) to 5 (severe disability). Cure was defined as absence of organism on laboratory specimens. A level of significance was set at less than or equal to 0.05, using χ^2 test.

Results—The two groups were comparable, except that the patients receiving drug X were an average of 5 years younger ($p < 0.05$). Drug X was shown to produce a cure, both in terms of symptoms and cultures in 85% of patients, whereas drug Y only produced a cure in 55.5% of patients. The difference was statistically significant ($p < 0.01$). No significant adverse effects were seen in either group.

Conclusions—Drug X was shown to produce significantly higher cure rates than drug Y in the treatment of tsutsugamushi fever, with no difference in adverse effects. Additional trials at different doses and lengths of therapy should be performed.

A method to prepare a structured abstract for a review article differs from the first example.[26] This method would only be applicable in specific situations, where a number of similar studies were evaluated together. It would not be useful in a situation where a number of dissimilar articles dealing with the same topic were discussed (e.g., a review of all therapies for a particular disease). Such an abstract would consist of the following items:

- *Purpose*—The main objective of the review article, including information about the population tested, how they were tested, and the outcome.
- *Data sources*—A brief summary of data sources and the time periods covered.
- *Study selection*—The number of studies covered in the article and how they were selected for inclusion, with reasons for excluding other studies.
- *Data extraction*—A description of the guidelines for abstracting data and how those guidelines were applied.
- *Data synthesis*—The main results of the review and the method to obtain the results are outlined.
- *Conclusions*—Important conclusions, including applications and need for further study.

An example of this type of abstract would be as follows:

Purpose—To evaluate the effect of the antihistamine, drug X, on symptoms of allergic reactions, as determined by physicians' and patients' global symptom assessment.

Data sources—Studies published from January 1980 to December 2016 were identified by computer searches of MEDLINE® and Embase®—Drugs and Pharmacology and hand searching of bibliographies of the articles identified via the computer search.

Study selection—After applying the inclusion and exclusion criteria, 53 studies evaluating the effects of drug X in the treatment of allergies were located.

Data extraction—Descriptive data regarding the population, dosing, effects, and adverse effects were assessed, along with the study's quality.

Results of data analysis—Subjective and objective measures of effectiveness demonstrated that drug X decreased or eliminated allergy symptoms approximately 80% of the time in a variety of patient types (e.g., seasonal allergic rhinitis, perennial allergic rhinitis, anaphylaxis). The only adverse effects seen were dryness of mucous membranes and sedation, seen in approximately 5% and 2% of patients, respectively.

Conclusions—Drug X is an effective agent for the treatment of allergic reactions. It has a low incidence of typical antihistamine adverse effects. Further studies should be performed to verify the effectiveness of Drug X in comparison to other drugs commonly used for anaphylaxis.

A version of a structured abstract has also been proposed for use in describing clinical practice guidelines (see Chapter 8 for more information about such guidelines).[27] The format is as follows:

Objective—Provides the primary objective of the guideline. This must include the health problem, along with the targeted patients, providers, and settings.

Options—This includes the various clinical practice options that were considered when the guideline was formulated.

Outcomes—Presents the significant health and economic outcomes that were considered when the alternative practices were considered.

Evidence—Describes how and when the evidence was gathered, selected for use, and synthesized.

Values—Describes how values were assigned to the potential outcomes, along with who was involved in doing so.

Benefits, harms, and costs—Provides both the type and magnitude of the benefits, harms, and costs that might be expected from using the guideline.

Recommendations—Provides a summary of the key recommendations.

Validation—Describes any external validation of the guidelines that was conducted.

Sponsors—Provides a list of the people who developed, funded, and/or endorsed the guideline.

An example of this type of abstract would be as follows:

Objective—To determine the best initial therapy for allergic rhinitis. This guideline is intended for physicians and pharmacists to determine the best way to start therapy, particularly in the community.

Options—Different nonprescription medications are considered first (antihistamines, decongestants [systemic and local], cromolyn), with the place for prescription intranasal steroids in initial therapy.

Outcomes—The major outcomes evaluated are relief of symptoms, adverse effects, and direct cost to the patient.

Evidence—All randomized, controlled clinical trials published in English found in MEDLINE from 1990 to 2012 were considered. In regard to costs, the average retail cost of the medication and the cost of a physician visit (for prescription medications) were calculated, based on what therapy was used in the studies.

Values—A group of three board-certified allergy physicians and three pharmacists board certified in pharmacotherapy or ambulatory care were appointed by the American Academy of Allergy, Asthma & Immunology to review and evaluate the studies and pharmacoeconomic data. Patients were not represented.

Benefits, harms, and costs—Use of a second-generation antihistamine (e.g., loratadine, cetirizine) provides the greatest efficacy with the least cost. Decongestants may be of value in the first few days, but are contraindicated in hypertensive patients. All other therapies have less effectiveness or greater cost.

Recommendations—Patients suffering from allergies should begin therapy with a second-generation antihistamine, preferably about a week prior to anticipated allergen exposure.

If therapy cannot be started early, pseudoephedrine may be used for up to 3 days as part of initial therapy in patients without hypertension or other contraindication. If this therapy is not sufficient, patients should be evaluated by a physician and prescribed an intranasal steroid spray. *Validations*—This recommendation was reviewed by three reviewers in the normal peer-review process established by the American Academy of Allergy, Asthma & Immunology. *Sponsors*—Development of this recommendation was funded by the American Academy of Allergy, Asthma & Immunology.

REFERENCES

1. Staub NC. On writing abstracts. Physiologist. 1991;34:276-7.
2. Pitkin RM, Branagan MA. Can the accuracy of abstracts be improved by providing specific instructions? A randomized controlled trial. JAMA. 1998;280:267-9.
3. Pitkin RM, Branagan MA, Burmeister LF. Accuracy of data in abstracts of published research articles. JAMA. 1999;281:1110-11.
4. Winker MA. The need for concrete improvement in abstract quality. JAMA. 1999;281:1129-30.
5. Huth EJ. Structured abstracts for papers reporting clinical trials. Ann Intern Med. 1987;106:626-7.
6. Narine L, Yee DS, Einarson TR, Ilersich AL. Quality of abstracts of original research articles in CMAJ in 1989. CMAJ. 1991;144:449-53.
7. Ad Hoc Working Group for Critical Appraisal of the Medical Literature. A proposal for more informative abstracts of clinical articles. Ann Intern Med. 1987;106:598-604.
8. Haynes RB, Mulrow CD, Huth EJ, Altman DG, Gardner MJ. More informative abstracts revisited. Ann Intern Med. 1990;113:69-76.
9. Rennie D, Glass RM. Structuring abstracts to make them more informative. JAMA. 1991;266:116-7.
10. Haynes RB. Dissent. More informative abstracts: current status and evaluation. J Clin Epidemiol. 1993;46:595-7.
11. Ripple AM, Mork JG, Knecht LS, Humphreys BL. A retrospective cohort study of structured abstracts in MEDLINE, 1992-2006. J Med Libr Assoc 2011;99(2):160-3.
12. Relman AS. New "Information for Authors"—and readers. NEJM. 1990;323:56.
13. Lock S. Structure abstracts. Now required for all papers reporting clinical trials. BMJ. 1988;297:156.
14. Squires BP. Structured abstracts of original research and review articles. CMAJ. 1990;143:619-22.
15. Soffer A. Abstracts of clinical investigations. A new and standardized format. Chest. 1987;92:389-90.
16. New format for BMJ research articles in print. BMJ 2008;337:a2946.
17. Restructured abstracts for research in The BMJ. BMJ 2015;351:h5499.
18. Nakayama T, Hirai N, Yamazaki S, Naito M. Adoption of structured abstracts by general medical journals and format for a structured abstract. J Med Libr Assoc 2005;93(2):237-42.
19. Kane-Gill S, Olsen KM. How to write an abstract suitable for publication. Hosp Pharm. 2004;39:289-92.

20. Spitzer WO. Second thoughts. The structured sonnet. J Clin Epidemiol. 1991;44:729.

21. Heller MB. Dissent. Structured abstracts: a modest dissent. J Clin Epidemiol. 1991;44:739–40.

22. Heller MB. Structured abstracts [letter]. Ann Intern Med. 1990;113:722.

23. Froom P, Froom J. Variance and dissent: presentation. Deficiencies in structured medical abstracts. J Clin Epidemiol. 1993;46:591–4.

24. Scherer RW, Crawley B. Reporting of randomized clinical trial descriptors and use of structured abstracts. JAMA. 1998;280:269–72.

25. Harbourt AM, Knecht LS, Humphreys BL. Structured abstracts in MEDLINE®, 1989–1991. Bull Med Libr Assoc. 1995;83(2):190–5.

26. Mulrow CD, Thacker SB, Pugh JA. A proposal for more informative abstracts of review articles. Ann Intern Med. 1988;108:613–5.

27. Hayward RS, Wilson MC, Tunis SR, Bass EB, Rubin HR, Haynes RB. More informative abstracts of articles describing clinical practice guidelines. Ann Intern Med. 1993;118:731-7.

Appendix 12-3

Bibliography

Although there seems to be a different method to prepare a bibliography for every English class ever given, there is fortunately a standardized method to prepare a bibliography in medical writing. This method is used by the National Library of Medicine and has been incorporated into the Recommendations for the Conduct, Reporting, Editing, and Publication of Scholarly Work in Medical Journals[31] and published in Citing Medicine[1-3]; it has been used widely since the 1970s in both journals and other medical writing. This method will be presented here.

References in the bibliography are usually placed in the order they are first cited in the text of a document, and each reference is assigned a consecutive Arabic number. Two acceptable variations involve citing the references at the end in alphabetical order by author. In one of those cases, the citations are numbered in that order and the number appears in the text. In the other, the citation in the text includes the author's name and year (e.g., Jones 2017).[3] Those cited only in tables or figures are numbered according to the place the table or figure is identified in the text. References are not listed multiple times in the bibliography, if they are cited more than once in the text of the document. Instead, subsequent citations to the same reference use the original reference number. The reference number in the text will be the Arabic number in superscript. This number is often cited after the sentence that contains the fact being referenced. If there are several references used to prepare a specific sentence, they may be listed at the end of the sentence or throughout the sentence. Also, if the sentence is a lead-in to an abstract, the authors' names are commonly listed followed by the reference number. See the sentences below for examples.

- Drug X has been shown to cause green rash with purple spots.[2,3]
- Drug Y is useful in the treatment of hypertension,[4] congestive heart failure,[5] and arrhythmias.[6]
- Smith and Jones[7] studied the effects of...
- Brown *et al.*[9] treated...(please notice on this example, *al.* is followed by a period since it is an abbreviation, whereas *et* is a full Latin word, and there is no need for a comma after the first author's name. The term *et al.* is italicized because it is Latin)
- Brown and associates[9] treated...(this is used the same way as the previous example, but is preferred by some people over the use of *et al.*)

Before getting into the method for listing references and examples, it should be mentioned that there are a number of general rules to be followed. They are:

- Citations are often not found in conclusions of documents. The conclusions are based on the information presented, and cited, earlier in the article.

- Avoid using abstracts as references, if at all possible. Sometimes the information is only published as an abstract, so it is necessary to cite the abstract in this situation.
- Avoid using unpublished observations or personal communications as references. In the latter case, it is proper to insert references to written, but not oral, communications in parentheses in the text only and indicate that it will not be formally referenced at the end of publication. Permission must be obtained from the author for the use of this material and this should only be used if the material is not available from a public source of information. A note should be made at the end of the publication stating that permission was given.
- If reference is made to an article that has been accepted by a journal, but not yet published, the phrase Forthcoming followed by the year of planned publication should be inserted where the volume and page numbers would normally be listed. It is usually necessary to get permission to cite this type of article, since the publisher may have strict confidentiality rules, and verification of acceptance by the journal should be obtained if that is the case.
- Today the Internet is used very frequently, so it is important to use the correct citation based on where the reference was found.
- Only place a period at the end of a web address if a slash is the last character in the address.
- For items such as wikis, blogs, databases, when they are still open (people can still add something), use a hyphen with three spaces following it for date of publication. If they are closed (people can no longer add something), list the range of dates it was open.
- Do not include any headers, such as "news" or "case report" unless the table of contents of the journal indicates that is officially part of the article title.
- Cite the name of the journal that was used when that journal was published. For example, British Medical Journal became BMJ in 1988 or Annals of Pharmacotherapy at various times has been known as Drug Intelligence and Clinical Pharmacy and DICP: the Annals of Pharmacotherapy.

Examples and some general templates of the above mentioned and other types of references used in a bibliography are provided in the balance of this appendix. Please note that these should provide adequate direction in how to cite most publications. However, if detailed directions and further examples are needed, the reader is referred to Citing Medicine, which is available free on the Internet at http://nlm.nih.gov/citingmedicine.[3]

JOURNAL ARTICLES

To cite a journal article, the following information should be given:

- Last name of author(s) and initials (maximum of two) each separated by commas, with a period at the end. Please note that some publications will list only three or six authors followed by the phrase *et al*; however, according to the standard, all authors must be listed regardless of how many unless space is limited. If an author's name has a suffix, such as Jr, that is inserted at the end (e.g., Smith AB Jr), but degrees are not listed. If a study group name is included after a specific author, separate that name from the individual authors using a semicolon.
- Title of article (do not use quotation marks, capitalize only the initial word of title and proper nouns in English) followed by a period with the exception when punctuation is already at the

end of the title—for example, if a title ends with a question mark or exclamation point, use that instead of the period.

- Journal Title (abbreviated as found in the list of journals at https://www.nlm.nih.gov/archive/20130415/tsd/serials/lji.html) followed by a period. Do not italicize the journal name. If this is an Internet article, put [Internet] after the journal name. Other types of medium would similarly be indicated (e.g., [microfiche], [microfilm]).

- Date of Publication (year, month [three-letter abbreviation], and day of month [if available]) followed by a semicolon.

- Volume number (listing the issue number in parenthesis) followed by a colon.

- Page numbers (If continuous, use first and last pages separated by a hyphen. Keep page numbers concise (e.g., 561-569 should be 561-9). If separate pages, list the pages separated by a comma and a space. If a combination of continuous and separate pages, use both (e.g., 18-29, 33, 40) followed by a period. If an Internet article does not have page numbers, put the actual number of pages in square brackets, followed by p. (e.g., [20 p.]). If the article is in unpaginated format (e.g., html, xml), precede the number with the word about (e.g., [about 10 screens] or [about 15 p.]). If a journal uses an article numbering scheme for Internet articles, be sure to use that number instead of a page number.

Generally speaking, if a piece of information listed above is not given by the publisher, it is simply omitted from the citation.

A condensed version of the above information is as follows:

Author(s). Title of article. Journal Title. Date of Publication;Volume Number(Issue Number):Page Number(s).

Journal on the Internet:

Author(s). Title of article. Journal Title [Internet]. Date of Publication [Date of Update; Date of Citation]; Volume Number(Issue Number):Page Number(s) or [Length of Article]. Available from: Web Address

Example Journal Citations

Standard Journal Article

Smythe M, Hoffman J, Kizy K, Dmuchowski C. Estimating creatinine clearance in elderly patients with low serum creatinine concentrations. Am J Hosp Pharm. 1994 Jan 15;51:198–204.

Beck DE, Aceves-Blumenthal C, Carson R, Culley J, Noguchi J, Dawson K, Hotchkiss G. Factors contributing to volunteer practitioner-faculty vitality. Am J Pharm Ed. 1993 Apr;57:305–12.

Journal Article on the Internet

Robinson ET. The pharmacist as educator: implications for practice and education. Am J Pharm Ed [Internet]. 2004 Aug 5 [cited 2016 Jul 24];68(3):Article 72 [4 p.]. Available from: http://www.ajpe.org/doi/pdf/10.5688/aj680372

Nemecz G. Evening primrose. US Pharmacist [Internet]. 1998 Nov [cited 1998 Dec 10];23:[about 1 p.]. Available from: http://www.uspharmacist.com/NewLook/Docs/1998/Nov1998/EveningPrimrose.htm

Organization as Author

Task Force on Specialty Recognition of Oncology Pharmacy Practice. Executive summary of petition requesting specialty recognition of oncology pharmacy practice. Am J Hosp Pharm. 1994 Jan 15;51:219–24.

Personal Authors and Organization as Author

Wiencke K, Louka AS, Spurkland A, Vatn M; The IBSEN Study Group; Schrumpf E. Association of matrix metalloproteinase-1 and -3 promoter polymorphisms with clinical subsets of Norwegian primary sclerosing cholangitis patients. J Hepatol. 2004 Aug;41(2):209-14.

No Author Given

N.Y. court rules against Medicaid co-pay. Drug Topics. 1994 Mar;138(3):6.

Article Not in English

Translate into English and put the translation in square brackets; note that the language is stated at the end.

Antoni N. [For criticism of the erroneously called tendon- and periosteal reflex]. Acta Psychiatrica Neurologica. 1932;VII:9–19. German.

Volume with Supplement

Nayler WG. Pharmacological aspects of calcium antagonism: short term and long term benefits. Drugs. 1993 Apr;46 Suppl 2:40–7.

Issue with Supplement

Graves NM. Pharmacokinetics and interactions of antiepileptic drugs. Am J Hosp Pharm. 1993 Dec;50(12 Suppl A):S23–9.

Volume with Part

Katchen MS, Lyons TJ, Gillingham KK, Schlegel W. A case of left hypoglossal neurapraxia following G exposure in a centrifuge. Aviat Space Environ Med. 1990 Sep;61(Pt 2):837–9.

Issue with Part

Dudley MN. Maximizing patient outcomes of antiinfective therapy. Pharmacotherapy. 1993 Mar-Apr;13(2 Pt 2):29S–33S.

Issue with No Volume

Slaga TJ, Gimenez-Conti IB. An animal model for oral cancer. Monogr J Nat Cancer Instit. 1992;(13):55–60.

No Issue or Volume

Payne R. Acute exacerbation of chronic cancer pain: basic assessment and treatments of breakthrough pain. Acute Pain Sympt Manage. 1998:4–5.

Pagination in Roman Numerals

Koretz RL. Clinical nutrition. Gastroenterol Clin North Am. 1998 Jun;27(2):xi–xiii.

Expressing Type of Article (As Desired; Optional)

Goldwater SH, Chatelain F. Taking time to communicate [letter]. Am J Hosp Pharm. 1994 Feb 1;51:232, 234.

Talley CR. Reducing demand through preventive care [editorial]. Am J Hosp Pharm. 1994 Jan 1;51:55.

Saritas A, Cakir Z, Emet M, Uzkeser M, Akoz A, Acemoglu F. Factors affecting the b-type natriuretic peptide levels in stroke patients [abstract]. Ann Acad Med Singapore. 2010 May;39(5):385.

Article Containing a Retraction

Brown MD. Retraction. Am Heart J. 1986;111:623. Retraction of: Slutsky RA, Olson LK. Am Heart J. 1984;108:543–7.

Article Retracted

Slutsky RA, Olson LK. Intravascular and extravascular pulmonary fluid volumes during chronic experimental left ventricular dysfunction Am Heart J. 1984 Sep;108:543–7. Retraction in: Am Heart J. 1986 Mar;111:623.

Article with Published Erratum

Reitz MS Jr, Juo HG, Oleske J, Hoxie J, Popovic M, Read-Connole E. On the historical origins of HIV-1 (MN) and (RF) [letter]. AIDS Res Hum Retroviruses. 1992 Aug;8:1539–41. Erratum in: AIDS Res Hum Retroviruses. 1992 Aug;8:1731.

Item (e.g., Table, Figure, Box, Image, or Appendix) in Article

Hohnloser SH, Pajitnev D, Pogue J, Healey JS, Pfeffer MA, Yusuf S, Connolly SJ. Incidence of stroke in paroxysmal versus sustained atrial fibrillation in patients taking oral anticoagulation or combined antiplatelet therapy: an ACTIVE W substudy. J Am Coll Cardiol. 2007 Nov 22;50(22): 2156-61. Table 4, Incidence of stoke or non-CNS systemic embolism in patients with paroxysmal versus persistent/permanent AF treated with aspirin plus clopidogrel or OAC; p. 2159.

Unpublished Article

Malone PM. Topics in informatics. Adv Pharm. Forthcoming 2004.

BOOKS

To cite a book, which can include manuals, brochures, or fact sheets, the following information should be given:

- Last name of author(s) and a maximum of two initials for each author separated by a comma and followed by a period. Some publications will list only three authors followed by the phrase *et al.*; however, all authors should be listed unless otherwise specified by the publication or if space is limited.
- Title of book (capitalize only the initial word of title and proper nouns in English) followed by a period with the exception that punctuation is already at the end of the title—for example, if a title ends with a question mark or exclamation point, use that instead of the period.
- Edition, other than the first, followed by a period

- Place of publication (city) followed by a colon (if the location is not clear with just a city name, the state or country abbreviation may be placed in parenthesis after the city name and before the colon). If place of publication not explicitly stated, but is implied based on location of publisher then add square brackets around place of publication.
- Name of publisher followed by a semicolon
- Year of publication followed by a period

Please note: If place of publication, name of publisher, and/or year of publication cannot be found, then in square brackets, it should be stated that one or more of these are unknown (e.g. [date unknown] or [place, publisher, date unknown]).

A condensed version of the above information is as follows:

Author(s). Title of Book. Edition. Place of Publication: Publisher; Date of Publication.

Book on the Internet:

Author(s). Title of Book [Internet]. Place of Publication: Publisher; Date of Publication [Date of Update; Date of Citation]. Available from: Web Address

Example Book Citations

Standard Book

Albright RG. A basic guide to online information systems for health care professionals. Arlington (VA): Information Resource Press; 1988.

Book on the Internet

DiPiro JT, Talbert RL, Yee GC, Matzke GR, Wells BG, Posey LM, editors. Pharmacotherapy: a pathophysiologic approach [Internet]. 9th ed. New York: McGraw-Hill Education; 2014 [cited 2016 Jun 23]. Available from: http://accesspharmacy.mhmedical.com/book.aspx?bookID=689

Lexicomp online [Internet]. [place unknown]: Wolters Kluwer; 2016 [cited 2016 Jun 24]. Available from: http://online.lexi.com/lco/action/home

Editor(s) as Author

Chisholm-Burns MA, Schwinghammer TL, Wells BG, Malone PM, Kolesar JM, Dipiro JT, editors. Pharmacotherapy principles and practice. 4th ed. New York: McGraw-Hill Education; 2016.

No Specific Editor(s), Compiler, or Author Identified

Drug facts and comparisons 1999. St. Louis: Facts and Comparisons; 1998.

Organization as Author and Publisher

United States Pharmacopeial Convention, Inc. USAN and the USP dictionary of drug names. Rockville: United States Pharmacopeial Convention, Inc.; 1993.

Volumes (Same Author(s)/Editor(s))

United States Pharmacopeial Convention, Inc. USP dispensing information. 22nd ed. Vol. 2, Advice for the patient: drug information in lay language. Greenwood Village (CO): Micromedex; 2002.

If on the Internet use the following format:

Author(s). Title of Book. Volume Number, Volume Title [Internet]. Place of Publication: Publisher; Date of Publication [Date of Update, Date of Citation]. Available from: Web Address.

Ross IA. Medicinal plants of the world. Vol. 3, Chemical constituents, traditional and modern medicinal uses [Internet]. Totowa (NJ): Humana Press, Inc.; 2005 [cited 2010 Jun 23]. Available from: http://metis.findlay.edu:2080/xtf-ebc/search?keyword=pharmacy

Portion of a Book (e.g., Chapter, Table, Figure, or Appendix) with Author(s) Writing Entire Book

Bauer LA. Applied clinical pharmacokinetics. 2nd ed. New York: McGraw-Hill Education; 2008. Chapter 6, Digoxin; p. 301-55.

If on the Internet use the following format:

Author(s). Title of Book [Internet]. Edition. Place of Publication: Publisher; Date of Publication [Date of Update of Book]. Portion Number, Portion Title; [Date of Update of Portion; Date of Citation]; Page Number(s) or [Length of Portion]. Available from: Web Address

Bauer LA. Applied clinical pharmacokinetics [Internet]. 2nd ed. New York: McGraw Hill; c2008. Chapter 6, Digoxin; [cited 2010 Jun 23]; [about 20 screens]. Available from: http://accesspharmacy.mhmedical.com/content.aspx?bookid=510&sectionid=40843080

Contribution to Book (Portions of Book Written by Different Authors)

Malesker MA, Morrow LE. Fluids and electrolytes. In: Chisholm-Burns MA, Schwinghammer TL, Wells BG, Malone PM, Kolesar JM, Dipiro JT, editors. Pharmacotherapy principles and practice. 4th ed. New York: McGraw-Hill Education; 2016. p. 427-40.

If on the Internet use the following format:

Chapter Author(s). Chapter Title. In: Author(s)/Editor(s). Title of Book [Internet]. Place of Publication: Publisher; Date of Publication [Date of Citation]. Available from: Web address

Malone PM, Malone MJ. Professional writing. In: Malone PM, Kier KL, Stanovich JE, Malone MJ, editors. Drug information: a guide for pharmacists [Internet]. 5th ed. New York: McGraw-Hill Education; c2014 [cited 2016 Jun 23]. Available from: http://accesspharmacy.mhmedical.com/book.aspx?bookID=981

Unpublished Book

Malone PM, Malone MJ, Park SK, editors. Drug information: a guide for pharmacists. 6th ed. New York: McGraw-Hill Education. Forthcoming 2017.

Book on CD-ROM or DVD

Haux R, Kulikowski C. Yearbook 04 of medical informatics—towards clinical bioinformatics [CD-ROM]. Stuttgart (Germany): Schatteuer; 2004.

Video Clip, Videocast, or Podcast Associated with Book

Author(s). Title of Book [Internet]. Place of Publication: Publisher; Date of Publication [Date of Citation]. Videocast or Podcast: Length of Video. Available from: Web Address

Brunton LL, Parker KL, Murri N, Blumenthal DK, Knollmann BC, editors. Goodman and Gilman's: the pharmacological basis of therapeutics [Internet]. 11th ed. New York: McGraw-Hill Education; 2006 [cited 2010 Jun 23]. Videocast: 5 min. Available from: http://metis.findlay.edu:2209/video.aspx?file=anj_01/anj_01

OTHER MATERIAL (IN ALPHABETICAL ORDER)

Format and Example Citations

Conference Paper

Author(s) of Conference Paper. Title of Paper. In: Editors of Conference Proceedings. Conference Title; Date(s) of Conference; Conference Location. Place of Publication: Publisher; Date of Publication. Pages.

Keyserlingk E. Ethical guidelines and codes: can they be universally applicable in a multicultural world? In: Allebeck P, Jansson B, editors. Ethics in medicine:individual integrity versus demands of society. Karolinska Institute Novel Conference Series. Proceedings of the 3rd International Congress on Ethics in Medicine; 1989 Sep 13-15; Stockholm. New York: Raven Press; 1990. p. 137-49.

If on the Internet use the following format:

Author(s) of Conference Paper. Title of Paper [Internet]. In: Conference Title; Date(s) of Conference; Conference Location. Place of Publication: Publisher; Date of Publication [Date of Citation]. [Length of Paper]. Available from: Web Address

Keyserlingk E. Ethical guidelines and codes: can they be universally applicable in a multicultural world? In: Allebeck P, Jansson B, editors. Ethics in medicine: individual integrity versus demands of society. Karolinska Institute Novel Conference Series. [Internet]. Proceedings of the 3rd International Congress on Ethics in Medicine; 1989 Sep 13-15; Stockholm. New York: Raven Press; 1990 [cited 2010 Jun 23]. [about 2 p.]. Available from: http://jmp.oxfordjournals.org/cgi/issue_pdf/backmatter_pdf/13/4.pdf

Conference Proceedings

Editor(s). Book Title. Conference Title; Date(s) of Conference; Conference Location. Place of Publication: Publisher; Date of Publication.

Allebeck P, Jansson B, editors. Ethics in medicine: individual integrity versus demands of society. Karolinska Institute Novel Conference Series. Proceedings of the 3rd International Congress on Ethics in Medicine; 1989 Sep 13-15; Stockholm. New York: Raven Press; 1990.

If on the Internet use the following format:

Editor(s). Book Title [Internet]. Conference Title ; Date(s) of Conference; Conference Location. Place of Publication: Publisher; Date of Publication [Date of Citation]. [Length of Publication]. Available from: Web Address

Allebeck P, Jansson B, editors. Ethics in medicine:individual integrity versus demands of society. Karolinska Institute Novel Conference Series [Internet]. Proceedings of the 3rd International Congress on Ethics in Medicine; 1989 Sep 13-15; Stockholm. New York: Raven Press; 1990 [cited 2010 Jun 23]. 8 p. Available from: http://jmp.oxfordjournals.org/cgi/issue_pdf/backmatter_pdf/13/4.pdf

Dictionary Definition

Dictionary Name. Edition. Place of Publication: Publisher; Date of Publication. Word Being Defined; Page Number.

Stedman's medical dictionary. 27th ed. New York: Lippincott Williams & Wilkins; 2000. Asthenia; p. 158.

If on the Internet use the following format:

Dictionary Name [Internet]. Place of Publication: Publisher; Date of Publication. Word Being Defined; [Date of Citation]. Available from: Web Address

Merriam-Webster Online [Internet]. Springfield (MA): Merriam-Webster, Inc.; c2010. Blood pressure; [cited 2010 Jun 23]. Available from: http://www.merriam-webster.com/dictionary/blood%20pressure

Dissertation/Thesis

Author(s). Title [dissertation or master's thesis]. [Place of Publication]: Publisher; Date of Publication.

Wellman CO. Pain perceptions and coping strategies of school-age children and their parents: a descriptive-correlational study [dissertation]. [Omaha (NE)]: Creighton University; 1985.

If on the Internet use the following format:

Author(s). Title [dissertation or master's thesis on the Internet]. Place of Publication: Publisher; Date of Publication [Date of Citation]. Pages p. Available from: Web Address

Mil JW. Pharmaceutical care, the future of pharmacy: theory, research, and practice [dissertation on the Internet]. Groningen (Netherlands): University of Groningen; 2000 Feb 1 [cited 2010 Jun 23]. 264 p. Available from: http://dissertations.ub.rug.nl/faculties/science/2000/j.w.f.van.mil/?pLanguage=en&pFullItemRecord=ON:

Encyclopedia Entry

Author(s). Name of Encyclopedia. Place of Publication: Publisher; Date of Publication. Name of Entry; Page Number.

If on the Internet use the following format:

Author(s). Name of Encyclopedia [Internet]. Place of Publication: Publisher; Date of Publication [Date of Update; Date of Citation]. Available from: Web Address

Encyclopedia Britannica Online [Internet]. Chicago: Britannica; c2010 [cited 2010 Jun 23]. Available from: http://www.britannica.com/EBchecked/topic/569347/stroke

Legal Documents

Please consult: Harvard Law Review; Columbia Law Review; Yale Law Review. The bluebook: a uniform system of citation. 20th ed. [Cambridge (MA)]: Harvard Law Review Association; 2015.

Meeting Presentations of Paper and Poster Sessions

Author(s). Title of Paper or Poster. Paper or Poster session presented at: Conference Title; Date(s) of Conference; Conference Location.

Ciaccia V, Hinders C, Malone M, Morales R, Sanchez A. Comparison of evidence based hypertension guideline model to an alternative model. Poster session presented at: The University of Findlay Symposium for Scholarship and Creativity; 2010 Apr 13; Findlay, OH.

Newspaper Article

Author(s). Title of Article. Newspaper Title (Edition). Date of Publication; Section: Page Number (Column Number).

Fein EB. Rise in fetal tests prompts ethical debate. New York Times (National Ed.). 1994 Feb 5; Sect. A:1(col. 2).

If on the Internet use the following format:

Author(s). Title of Article. Newspaper Title [Internet]. Date of Publication [Date of Update; Date of Citation]; Section: Page Number or [Length of Article]. Available from: Web Address

Painter K. Your health: feet bear the strain of extra weight. USA Today [Internet]. 2010 Jun 20 [cited 2010 Jun 23]; Health and Behavior:[about 2 screens]. Available from: http://www.usatoday.com/news/health/painter/2010-06-21-yourhealth21_ST_N.htm

Package Insert

Package inserts are commonly cited in professional writing; however, the standards do not address the format to use. The following is a common format that is similar to those presented in this appendix.

Medication Name [package insert]. Place of Publication: Publisher; Date of Publication.

Prilosec® (omeprazole) delayed-release capsules [package insert]. Wayne, PA: Astra Merck; 1998 Jun.

If on the Internet use the following format:

Medication Name [package insert on the Internet]. Place of Publication: Publisher; Date of Publication [Date of Update; Date of Citation]. Available from: Web Address

Omeprazole [package insert on the Internet]. Bethesda (MD): U.S. National Library of Medicine; 2009 Aug [updated 2009 Dec; cited 2010 Jun 23]. Available from: http://dailymed.nlm.nih.gov/dailymed/drugInfo.cfm?id=14749

Patent

Inventor(s); Assignee. Title. Patent Country patent Country Code Patent Number. Date patent issued.

Schwartz B, inventor; New England Medical Center Hospital, Inc., assignee. Method of and solution for treating glaucoma. United States patent US 5,212,168. 1993 May 18.

Personal Communication

Normally in text citation only (e.g., Letter from or Conversation with; unreferenced, see Notes section)

Author. Letter to or Conversation with: Recipient (Recipient Affiliation). Date. Located at: Location of Letter.

In Notes section, state that permission was given to reference the letter or conversation.

Jones, Max. Letter to: Charlie Smith. 2005 Feb 14. Located at: Veterinary Medicine Division, College of Pharmacy, University of Findlay, Findlay, OH; Cabinet 1, Drawer 2, Folder 10.

Scientific or Technical Report

Author(s). Title. Place of Publication: Publisher; Date of Publication. Report No.: Report Number.

Issued by funding/sponsoring agency:

Shekelle P, Morton S, Maglione M (Southern California Evidence-Based Practice Center/RAND, Santa Monica, CA). Ephedra and ephedrine for weight loss and athletic performance enhancement: clinical efficacy and side effects. Vol 1, Evidence report and evidence tables. Rockville (MD): Agency for Healthcare Research and Quality; 2003 Mar. (Evidence report/technology assessment; no. 78). Report No.: AHRQPUB03E022. Contract No.: AHRQ-290-97-001.

Issued by performing agency:

Shekelle P, Morton S, Maglione M. Ephedra and ephedrine for weight loss and athletic performance enhancement: clinical efficacy and side effects. Vol. 1, Evidence report and evidence tables. Santa Monica: Southern California Evidence-Based Practice Center/RAND; 2003 Mar. (Evidence report/technology assessment; no. 78). Report No.: AHRQPUB03E022. Contract No.: AHRQ-290-97-001. Supported by the Agency for Healthcare Research and Quality.

If on the Internet use the following format:

Author(s). Title [Internet]. Place of Publication: Publisher; Date of Publication [Date of Citation]. Pagiation. Report No.: Report Number. Available from: Web Address

Qureshi N, Wilson B, Santaguida P, Carroll J, Allanson J, Culebro CR, Brouwers M, Raina P. Collection and use of cancer family history in primary care [Internet]. Rockville (MD): Agency for Healthcare Research and Quality; 2007 Oct [cited 2010 Jun 23]. [about 2 screens]. (Evidence reports/technology assessments no. 159) Report No.: AHRQPUB08E001. Contract No.: 290- 02-0020. Available from: http://www.ncbi.nlm.nih.gov/bookshelf/br.fcgi?book=erta159

OTHER ELECTRONIC MATERIAL (IN ALPHABETICAL ORDER)

Format and Example Citations

Part of a Blog (Only One Author)

Since this is personal communication, as above, it usually is done as an in-text citation only (posting on given date from author on given blog; unreferenced, see Notes section). In Notes section state that permission was given to reference the blog post. Otherwise can follow format below:

Author of Blog. Title of Blog [blog on the Internet] or [Internet] if the word blog is part of title of blog. Place of Publication: Publisher. Start Date of Blog- . or End Date if blog is closed- Title of Part; Date of Publication [Date of Citation]; [Length of Part]. Available from: Web Address

Please note: if a piece of information is implied, but cannot be confirmed, place that information in square brackets and if it is unknown state that in square brackets (e.g., [publisher unknown]).

Daria. Living with Cancer [blog on the Internet]. Edmonton (AB): Daria. 2008 Aug- 2011 Jan Chemo went well; 2010 Jun 12 [cited 2016 Jul 31]; [about 1 screen]. Available from: http://daria-living-withcancer.blogspot.com/.

Part of a Blog (Multiple Authors)

Since this is personal communication, as above, it usually is done as an in-text citation only (posting on given date from author on given blog; unreferenced, see Notes section). In Notes section state that permission was given to reference the blog post. Otherwise can follow format below:

Author of Comment. Title of Blog Comment. Date of Publication of Comment [Date of Citation]. In: Author of Blog. Name of Blog [blog on the Internet] or [Internet] if the word blog is part of title of blog. Place of Publication: Publisher. Date of Publication- . or End Date if blog is closed [Length of Comment]. Available from: Web Address

Please note: if a piece of information is implied, but cannot be confirmed, place that information in square brackets and if it is unknown state that in square brackets (e.g., [publisher unknown]).

Smith J. Dialysis. 2010 Jun 16 [cited 2010 Jun 16]. In: Kidney Coaching Foundation, Inc. KCF Blog and News [Internet]. Raleigh (NC): Kidney Coaching Foundation, Inc. c2005-2010- . [about 1 paragraph]. Available from: http://unckidneycenter.org/.

Database on the Internet

Title of Database [Internet]. Place of Publication: Publisher. Initial Date of Publication- (list end date if database closed) [Date of Citation]. Available from: Web Address

Please note: if a piece of information is implied, but cannot be confirmed, place that information in square brackets and if it is unknown state that in square brackets (e.g., [publisher unknown]).

PubMed [Internet]. Bethesda (MD): National Library of Medicine. 2004 - [cited 2016 Jul31]. Available from: https://www.ncbi.nlm.nih.gov/pubmed

DRUGDEX [Internet]. [place unknown]: Truven Health Analytics. c2012-2016 [cited 2016 Jul 31]. Available from: https://www.micromedexsolutions.com/home/dispatch/ssl/true

Part of a Database on the Internet (e.g., a single drug monograph out of a publication)

Title of Database [Internet]. Place of Publication: Publisher. Initial Date of Publication - (list end date if database closed). Record Identifier, Title of Part; [Date of Citation]; [Length of Part]. Available from: Web Address

Please note: if a piece of information is implied, but cannot be confirmed, place that information in square brackets and if it is unknown state that in square brackets (e.g., [publisher unknown]).

MeSH Browser [Internet]. Bethesda (MD): National Library of Medicine. 2004- . ID: D015201, Phenytoin; [cited 2004 Aug 18]; [about 670 p.]. Available from: http://www.nlm.nih.gov/mesh/MBrowser.html

DRUGDEX [Internet]. [place unknown]: Truven Health Analytics. c2012-2016. Amiodarone; [cited 2016 Jul 31]; [about 8 screens]. Available from: https://www.micromedexsolutions.com/home/dispatch/ssl/true

Electronic Mail

Since this is personal communication, as above, it usually is done as an in-text citation only (e-mail on given date from sender to recipient; unreferenced, see Notes section). In Notes section state that permission was given to reference the e-mail. Otherwise can follow format below:

Author. Title of E-mail [Internet]. Message to: Recipient(s). Date of Message [Date of Citation]. [Length of E-mail].

Malone, Patrick. Drug information textbook [Internet]. Message to: John Stanovich; Mark Malesker. 2010 Jun 14 [2010 Jun 16]. [3 paragraphs].

LISTSERV

Since this is personal communication, as above, it usually is done as an in-text citation only (posting on given date from sender to given LISTSERV; unreferenced, see Notes section). In Notes section state that permission was given from the sender to reference the e-mail. Otherwise can follow format below:

Author. Title of Message. In: Name of LISTSERV [Internet]. Place of Publication: Publisher; Date of Message [Date of Citation]. [Length of Message].

Malone PM. CAMIPR—discussion forum for medication information specialists. In: CAMIPR [Internet]. Iowa City: Consortium for the Advancement of Medication Policy and Research; 2010 May 6 [cited 2010 Jun 18]. [about 1 p.].

Video Clip, Videocast, or Podcast

Author(s). Title of Homepage [Internet]. Place of Publication: Publisher; Date of Publication of Homepage. [Video or Videocast or Podcast], Title of Video; Date of Publication of Video Clip, Videocast, or Podcast [Date of Update; Date of Citation]; [Length of Video Clip, Videocast, or Podcast]. Available from: Web Address

Gulseth MP, Messler JC. ASHP Advantage [Internet]. Bethesda (MD): American Society of Health-System Pharmacists; c2010. [Podcast], Multidisciplinary approach to identifying patients at risk for VTE; 2010 May 4 [cited 2016 Jul 31]; [45 min.]. Available from: http://www.ashpadvantage.com/podcasts/.

Website Homepage

Author(s). Title of Homepage [Internet]. Place of Publication: Publisher; Date of Publication [Date of Update; Date of Citation]. Available from: Web Address

American Society of Health-System Pharmacists [Internet]. Bethesda (MD): American Society of Health-System Pharmacists; c1997-2004 [updated 2004 Aug 18; cited 2004 Aug 18]. Available from: http://www.ashp.org/.

Part of a Website

Title of Homepage [Internet]. Place of Publication: Publisher; Date of Publication of Homepage. Title of Part; Date of Publication of Part (if different from Homepage) [Date of Update; Date of Citation]; [Length of Part]. Available from: Web Address

American Society of Health-System Pharmacists [Internet]. Bethesda (MD): American Society of Health-System Pharmacists; c1997-2004. Compounding Resource Center; [updated 2004 Aug 18; cited 2004 Aug 18]; [about 1 screen]. Available from: http://www.ashp.org/compounding

Part of a Wiki

Since this is personal communication, as above, it usually is done as an in-text citation only (posting on given date from author on given wiki; unreferenced, see Notes section). In Notes section state that permission was given from the author to reference the wiki. Otherwise can follow format below:

Author(s) of Part. Title of Part of Wiki. Date of Posting [Date of Update; Date of Citation]. In: Title of Wiki [Internet]. Place of Publication: Publisher. Start Date of Wiki- . (list end date if wiki closed) [Length of Part]. Available from: Web Address

If no author for part:

Title of Wiki [Internet]. Place of Publication: Publisher. Start Date of Wiki- . (list end date if wiki closed) Title of Part of Wiki; [Date of Update; Date of Citation]; [Length of Part]. Available from: Web Address

Please note: if a piece of information is implied, but cannot be confirmed, place that information in square brackets and if it is unknown state that in square brackets (e.g., [publisher unknown]).

Wiki Public Health [Internet]. [place unknown]: WikiPH. [date unknown]- . Health care; [updated 2007 Mar 27; cited 2010 Jun 16]; [about 2 screens]. Available from: http://wikiph.org/index.php?title=Health_care

REFERENCES

1. International Committee of Medical Journal Editors. Uniform requirements for manuscripts submitted to biomedical journals [Internet]. Philadelphia: International Committee of Medical Journal Editors; 2009 [cited 2012 May 15]. Available from: http://www.icmje.org

2. International Committee of Medical Journal Editors. Uniform requirements for manuscripts submitted to biomedical journals: sample references [Internet]. Philadelphia: International Committee of Medical Journal Editors; 2003 [updated 2011 Jul 15; cited 2012 May 15]. Available from: http://www.nlm.nih.gov/bsd/uniform_requirements.html

3. Patrias K. Citing medicine: the NLM style guide for authors, editors, and publishers [Internet]. 2nd ed. Wendling DL, technical editor. Bethesda (MD): National Library of Medicine (US); 2007 [updated 2015 Oct 2; cited 2016 Jun 24]. Available from: http://nlm.nih.gov/citingmedicine

Appendix 13–1

Pharmacy and Therapeutics Committee Procedure

This appendix includes two policy and procedure operational statements. The first is specifically written to centralize the formulary decision process for a multihospital health system: a Formulary Committee. The second, and closely related, operational statement is written as a model to function as the traditional Pharmacy and Therapeutics Committee for a Hospital's Medical Staff. Both operational statements describe the functions of their related committees based on a certain degree of autonomy. Their membership is ultimately chosen by an administrative leader as a means to best isolate the committee from organizational as well as economic influences. The decision process for each operational statement is intended to create predictability and transparency. To implement this set of operational statements, each Executive Committee of the hospitals in a multihospital system would pass the following resolution:

> The Medical Staff of Alpha Hospital delegates its Pharmacy and Therapeutic Committee responsibilities to ALPHAOMEGA HEALTH based on the policy and procedures for a "Hospital Formulary System" and a "Hospital Pharmacy and Therapeutics Committee."

The two operational statements can also be combined to reflect the traditional functions of a single hospital, medical staff-based pharmacy and therapeutics committee. Also, there may be other arrangements where the two operational statements could provide the organizational environment for a closed health system, a pharmacy benefits manager, or one of the new organizational structures created by Federal Legislation in 2004 for the new financing of drug coverage in the United States.

POLICY TITLE: HOSPITAL FORMULARY SYSTEM

I. PURPOSE

To maintain a **HOSPITAL FORMULARY** and a Formulary Committee for all ALPHAOMEGA HEALTH Hospitals as a means to enhance the quality of health care for all patients served by ALPHAOMEGA HEALTH.

II. POLICY

A. The Formulary Committee of ALPHAOMEGA HEALTH periodically evaluates its performance as a means to improve its ability to support the Vision and Mission of ALPHAOMEGA HEALTH.

B. ALPHAOMEGA HEALTH maintains one Formulary Committee and a Pharmacy and Therapeutics Committee (P&T COMMITTEE) at each ALPHAOMEGA HEALTH Hospital to implement this POLICY in accord with the applicable Medical Staff Bylaws and this POLICY.

C. The Formulary Committee of ALPHAOMEGA HEALTH maintains a standard format for a **HOSPITAL FORMULARY** that is based on the provisions of this POLICY.

D. The Formulary Committee develops and continually revises a list of therapeutic products, a **HOSPITAL FORMULARY**, that reflects the current clinical judgment of the Medical Staff of ALPHAOMEGA HEALTH Hospitals regarding the selection of the best therapeutic products for the health care of hospitalized patients. The Formulary Committee evaluates the various alternative therapeutic products available and develops the **HOSPITAL FORMULARY** based on an evaluation of each therapeutic product's indications, effectiveness, risks, patient safety, and overall impact on health care costs.

E. The Formulary Committee collaborates with the P&T Committee at each ALPHAOMEGA HEALTH Hospital to monitor compliance with the provisions of the **HOSPITAL FORMULARY**.

F. The Formulary Committee supports the quality improvement functions of ALPHAOMEGA HEALTH where necessary to improve the use of the **HOSPITAL FORMULARY**.

III. PROCEDURE

A. FORMULARY COMMITTEE DEVELOPMENT

1. The Formulary Committee recommends, when appropriate, amendments to this POLICY AND PROCEDURE to the Chief Medical Officer of ALPHAOMEGA HEALTH. After revisions to any of these proposed amendments by the Chief Medical Officer, in collaboration with the Formulary Committee, the Chief Medical Officer submits the amendments to the Executive Committee of the Medical Staff at each ALPHAOMEGA HEALTH Hospital for final approval.

2. The Officers of the Formulary Committee prepare an Annual Membership Report to the Chief Medical Officer of ALPHAOMEGA HEALTH regarding participation of its Members and any recommendations that may be important to maintain the expertise necessary for the affairs of the Formulary Committee.

3. The Officers of the Formulary Committee prepare an Annual Report and submit it to the Professional Affairs Committee of ALPHAOMEGA HEALTH for approval. As a result of this review, the Professional Affairs Committee may make recommendations to the Formulary Committee for consideration regarding its affairs or to the Chief Medical Officer regarding amendments to this POLICY AND PROCEDURE.

B. FORMULARY COMMITTEE ORGANIZATION

1. REGULAR MEMBERS

   a. MEDICAL STAFF MEMBERS

      i. Up to 16 Medical Staff members are nominated annually by the Chief Medical Officer of ALPHAOMEGA HEALTH, each President or Chief of Staff from the Medical Staff of an ALPHAOMEGA HEALTH Hospital, or the Officers of the

Formulary Committee. A Medical Staff nominee must demonstrate an active interest in evidence-based therapeutics, a willingness to be an active participant in the affairs of the Formulary Committee, and represent as a group, whenever possible, the specialties of Family Practice, Internal Medicine, Pediatrics, Obstetrics and Gynecology, Hematology and Oncology, Cardiology, Infectious Disease, Pulmonology, and General Surgery.

ii. From any Nominees, 12 to 16 are selected by the Chief Medical Officer of ALPHAOMEGA HEALTH on the basis of maintaining a reasonable balance among the following factors: hospital and outpatient-based physicians, primary care and disease-focused physicians, physician liaison to the Medical Staff Executive Committee or P&T Committee of each ALPHAOMEGA HEALTH Hospital, and a balanced representation from the Medical Staffs of the ALPHAOMEGA HEALTH Hospitals.

b. ADMINISTRATION MEMBER—The Chief Medical Officer of ALPHAOMEGA HEALTH, or designee who is a Medical Staff Member of an ALPHAOMEGA HEALTH Hospital, is a Member of the Formulary Committee.

2. SPECIAL MEMBERS AND SOURCE OF SELECTION

a. The Chief Medical Officer of ALPHAOMEGA HEALTH selects Special Members as may be needed to provide administrative or technical support for the affairs of the Formulary Committee. The Special Members include, at a minimum:

i. any pharmacist recommended by the Pharmacist in charge at a Hospital Pharmacy of ALPHAOMEGA HEALTH and

ii. at least one Registered Nurse from among the Nursing Staff of an ALPHAOMEGA HEALTH Hospital.

b. The Chairperson of the Formulary Committee selects one or more Special Members from the personnel of ALPHAOMEGA HEALTH or the Medical Staff of any ALPHAOMEGA HEALTH Hospital on a temporary basis as may be necessary for:

i. technical support for the activities of the Formulary Committee or any Ad Hoc Subcommittee of the Formulary Committee or

ii. information for the deliberations of the Formulary Committee regarding a proposal to add or delete an individual therapeutic product listed on the **HOSPITAL FORMULARY**.

3. FORMULARY COMMITTEE OFFICERS

a. The CHAIRPERSON is selected by the Chief Medical Officer of ALPHAOMEGA HEALTH from among the Regular Members of the Formulary Committee. The Chairperson:

i. manages the affairs of the Formulary Committee in a manner to

I) support the active, positive involvement of each Regular and Special Member,

II) acknowledge any conflict of interests,

III) initiate a replacement appointment of any Officer, Regular Member, or Special Member becoming inactive during a calendar year,

IV) appoint temporary Special Members, and

V) select the location for Meetings of the Formulary Committee;

  ii. prepares the Annual Membership and Self-Evaluation reports; and

  iii. appoints an Ad Hoc Committee when necessary to study decisions in greater depth or to arrive at consensus recommendations for consideration by the Formulary Committee whose membership includes

I) six or less members from the Medical Staffs of the ALPHAOMEGA HEALTH Hospitals,

II) at least one member who is a Regular Member of the Formulary Committee, and

III) the Secretary, or designee, of the Formulary Committee.

  b. The VICE CHAIRPERSON is selected by the Chief Medical Officer of ALPHAOMEGA HEALTH from the Regular Members of the Formulary Committee. The Vice Chairperson assumes the duties of the Chairperson during their absence.

  c. The SECRETARY is selected by the Chief Medical Officer of ALPHAOMEGA HEALTH from among the Regular or Special Members of the Formulary Committee. The Secretary assists the Chairperson in managing the affairs of the Formulary Committee by:

    i. preparing the minutes for each meeting of the Formulary Committee or any of its Ad Hoc Committees,

    ii. sending an Agenda to the Members prior to each meeting of the Formulary Committee,

    iii. maintaining a schedule for the annual regular review by the Formulary Committee of all therapeutic products listed on the **HOSPITAL FORMULARY**, and

    iv. coordinating the preparation of any Drug Monograph or any other report necessary for a meeting of the Formulary Committee by a Pharmacist In Charge, or designee, at an ALPHAOMEGA HEALTH Hospital.

4. TERM OF APPOINTMENT

  a. The Regular and Special Members are appointed or reappointed each January for 1 year.

  b. Each Officer is appointed or reappointed each January for 1 year.

5. VOTING

  a. Each Regular Member has one vote, and each Special Member does not have a vote.

  b. Any two Regular Members present during a Meeting of the Formulary Committee constitute a quorum.

  c. Based on attendance, the Regular Members of the Formulary Committee may delay voting, when the appropriate expertise is not available during a meeting of the Formulary Committee.

  d. A simple majority of Regular Members voting is required for any action of the Formulary Committee. Any abstention on the basis of a conflict of interests is noted in the minutes for the meeting.

6. LIAISON—A Regular or Special Member may be appointed by the Chief Medical Officer of ALPHAOMEGA HEALTH to report on the affairs of the Formulary Committee during the deliberations of any other Committee of ALPHAOMEGA HEALTH.

7. MEETINGS—The meetings of the Formulary Committee are:
    a. scheduled once a month for 1 hour or as may be planned by the Members of the Formulary Committee,
    b. attended by Regular and Special Members only, and
    c. convened at a location arranged by the Chairperson.

8. COMMITTEE PROTOCOLS—The Formulary Committee may also arrange for the:
    a. definitions applicable to the resignation and replacement of any Regular Member, Special Member, or Officer during a calendar year;
    b. management of any potential or actual conflict of interests affecting the participation of a Regular or Special Member during a meeting of the Formulary Committee;
    c. use of ALTERNATIVE MEDICATION for the health care of a patient at any ALPHAOMEGA HEALTH Hospital;
    d. information necessary to request a change in the list of therapeutic products or other information described in the **HOSPITAL FORMULARY**;
    e. contents of a DRUG MONOGRAPH that must be prepared before a therapeutic product not listed on the **HOSPITAL FORMULARY**; and
    f. management of any shortage of a therapeutic product listed in the **HOSPITAL FORMULARY** by the:
        i. timely notification of the Medical Staff at each ALPHAOMEGA HEALTH Hospital listing the specific dosage forms in limited or unavailable supply,
        ii. development of alternative strategies for a patient's health care using therapeutic products currently available on the **HOSPITAL FORMULARY** when a therapeutic product becomes either not available or in limited supply,
        iii. collaboration with the appropriate expertise within the Medical Staff of ALPHAOMEGA HEALTH Hospitals when a rationing protocol is necessary for a critical therapeutic product in limited supply, and
        iv. review of any proposal for a rationing protocol by the Ethics Council of ALPHAOMEGA HEALTH when the Formulary Committee requests assistance before final approval to ensure that the appropriate ethical standards have been considered.

C. **HOSPITAL FORMULARY FORMAT**
    1. Any therapeutic product used in the health care of a patient is eligible for the **HOSPITAL FORMULARY**. This includes samples, prescription drugs as defined by the Food and Drug Administration, herbal or other alternative therapies administered topically or enterally, nutraceuticals, nonprescription drugs, vaccines, diagnostic or contrast agents, radioactive agents, respiratory products, parenteral or enteral nutrients, blood products, intravenous solutions, and anesthetic gases. A therapeutic product may not be considered for the **HOSPITAL FORMULARY** if it would normally be considered a medical device, durable medical equipment, or implant.

2. The **HOSPITAL FORMULARY** lists the therapeutic products approved by the Formulary Committee in a format approved by the Formulary Committee. The format for the **HOSPITAL FORMULARY** reflects the recommendations of nationally recognized organizations and includes certain attributes, where appropriate, as described below.

   a. Any restricted use provision is defined by credentialing categories in use by the Medical Staffs of ALPHAOMEGA HEALTH Hospitals and be implemented when necessary to monitor or limit the use of a **HOSPITAL FORMULARY** therapeutic product known to be associated with:

      i. an increased risk of a substantial adverse patient reaction,

      ii. a highly specific therapeutic indication, or

      iii. an unusual impact on the overall cost of health care.

   b. Specific patient education provisions are added for any **HOSPITAL FORMULARY** therapeutic product known to require:

      i. special nutritional adjustments,

      ii. prevention of substantial adverse effects or noncompliance, or

      iii. unique requirements for informed consent.

   c. Continuing education provisions are added when a Medical Staff Member or qualified Hospital employee requires specialized knowledge prior to or during the administration of a given **HOSPITAL FORMULARY** therapeutic product. This is particularly applicable in the professional areas of oncology and cardiology.

   d. Special information may be added to assist the Medical Staff at each ALPHAOMEGA HEALTH HOSPITAL when necessary to improve the:

      i. level of compliance with prescribing only therapeutic products listed on the **HOSPITAL FORMULARY**,

      ii. acceptance of rational therapeutic concepts as a basis for planning health care intervention strategies, and

      iii. acceptance of therapeutic interchange strategies involving therapeutic products not listed on the **HOSPITAL FORMULARY**.

3. The Formulary Committee may establish a provision for inventory control of a **HOSPITAL FORMULARY** therapeutic product.

D. HOSPITAL FORMULARY MAINTENANCE

1. A proposal for a change in a single therapeutic product listed on the **HOSPITAL FORMULARY** requires a specific set of steps before final approval by the Formulary Committee. These steps are defined below. The Formulary Committee may make a temporary exception to this provision when necessary to improve the quality of health care to patients at an ALPHAOMEGA HEALTH Hospital.

   a. timely submission of a completed Formulary Request form to any pharmacist at an ALPHAOMEGA HEALTH Hospital by a Medical Staff member of an ALPHAOMEGA HEALTH Hospital or other professional employee of ALPHAOMEGA HEALTH,

   b. review of the Formulary Request by a pharmacist in charge, or designee, of an ALPHAOMEGA HEALTH Hospital's Pharmacy to be sure that it has been fully completed,

   c. preparation of a Drug Monograph, as may be arranged by the Secretary of the Formulary Committee if a new therapeutic product has been proposed by the Formulary Request for the **HOSPITAL FORMULARY,**

   d. preliminary review of the Formulary Request and any associated Drug Monograph by representative specialists affected by any proposed change in the **HOSPITAL FORMULARY,**

   e. initial approval or disapproval of the Formulary Request at one meeting of the Formulary Committee, followed by review for comments at each ALPHAOMEGA HEALTH Hospital's P&T Committee, before final approval or disapproval including any amendments to the Formulary Request at a subsequent meeting of the Formulary Committee.

2. The Formulary Committee annually reviews therapeutic products listed on the **HOSPITAL FORMULARY** according to a schedule of therapeutic classes as may be arranged throughout a calendar year by the Secretary of the Formulary Committee. The review of each class of therapeutic products requires a specific set of events before final approval. These steps are defined below.

   a. review of a class of therapeutic products preliminarily by the pharmacists in charge, or designees, of the ALPHAOMEGA HEALTH Hospital Pharmacies prior to a meeting of the Formulary Committee regarding the possible need to:

     i. initiate a Formulary Request for a new addition to the **HOSPITAL FORMULARY,**

     ii. deletion of a therapeutic product because of production defects, non-use, non-availability, recall, or replacement by another therapeutic product, or

     iii. a need to change information included in the **HOSPITAL FORMULARY** such as patient education, professional education, therapeutic interchange, or a restricted use provision;

   b. preliminary review of the proposed revisions to the **HOSPITAL FORMULARY** by representative specialists affected by the proposed revisions;

   c. initial approval or disapproval of the therapeutic product class review at one meeting of the Formulary Committee, followed by review for comments at each ALPHAOMEGA HEALTH Hospital's P&T Committee, before final approval or disapproval including amendments to the class review at a subsequent meeting of the Formulary Committee.

3. The Formulary Committee may authorize certain strategies by the ALPHAOMEGA HEALTH Hospital pharmacies that are necessary to offer the most appropriate therapeutic products for hospitalized patients. The Formulary Committee may authorize these special strategies when supported by its own decision and the support of each ALPHAOMEGA HEALTH Hospital's P&T Committee. Certain specific strategies to be authorized by this POLICY AND PROCEDURE are listed below.

   a. A class review of **HOSPITAL FORMULARY** therapeutic products as described above may also be initiated when there is a Formulary Request for a therapeutic product that substantially affects the inclusion or supplementary information of other therapeutic products currently listed in the **HOSPITAL FORMULARY.**

b. The pharmacist in charge, or designee, at all ALPHAOMEGA HEALTH Hospital Pharmacies arranges to prepare a preliminary or full Drug Monograph before any therapeutic product is dispensed that has not previously been ordered for a hospitalized patient at any ALPHAOMEGA HEALTH Hospital.

c. The Formulary Committee may provide for automatic therapeutic interchange between a therapeutic product that is not listed for another therapeutic product that is listed on the **HOSPITAL FORMULARY** when supported by appropriate scientific evidence and appropriately considered standards of practice.

d. The Formulary Committee may also select certain therapeutic products for the **HOSPITAL FORMULARY** that are dispensed for certain indications or any indication even if prescribed with a "Do Not Substitute" designation. The Formulary Committee uses the same process for this designation as defined above for a new change in the **HOSPITAL FORMULARY**.

E. HOSPITAL FORMULARY COMPLIANCE

1. The P&T Committee of each ALPHAOMEGA HEALTH Hospital is responsible for monitoring each Medical Staff physician's orders for a therapeutic product that is:

   a. not listed or does not have an automatic therapeutic interchange with a therapeutic product listed on the current **HOSPITAL FORMULARY**,

   b. for an indication not permitted by the **HOSPITAL FORMULARY**, or

   c. for an indication having a restricted use provision.

2. Any ALPHAOMEGA HEALTH Hospital's P&T Committee may establish a Special Formulary as a means to temporarily support the efforts of its Medical Staff in the health care of hospitalized patients having special requirements that are unique to that Hospital. The Special Formulary therapeutic products are selected using the same process defined above for a change in the **HOSPITAL FORMULARY**. For a Special Formulary, the other Committees of the Hospital's Medical Staff provide a consent process. For any therapeutic product listed on an ALPHAOMEGA HEALTH Hospital's Special Formulary for 1 year or more, continued use of the Special Formulary status for the therapeutic product requires the approval of the Formulary Committee.

3. If a P&T Committee votes to not accept a decision of the Formulary Committee, the Chairperson, or designee, of the P&T Committee is invited to a subsequent meeting of the Formulary Committee. At this Formulary Meeting, the Formulary Committee attempts to develop a strategy for resolving the conflict between the original decision of the Formulary Committee and the respective P&T Committee. In the event that a resolution is not achieved, the issue may be appealed by either Committee to the Professional Affairs Committee for a final decision within 3 months of the appeal.

F. QUALITY IMPROVEMENT

1. The Formulary Committee maintains access to the decisions of other hospital's Formulary or P&T Committees as a resource for the basis in managing difficult decisions regarding the **HOSPITAL FORMULARY**. The hospitals chosen should reflect regional as well as national locations.

2. The Formulary Committee assesses the pending availability of new therapeutic products in the future that may require the preparation of a Formulary Request and Drug Monograph.

3. The Formulary Committee monitors the possible evolution of a shortage involving the availability of a therapeutic product listed on the **HOSPITAL FORMULARY**.

4. The Formulary Committee may recommend to each P&T Committee certain quality improvement projects, such as a Drug Use Evaluations for a certain product that would reflect the health care at all ALPHAOMEGA HEALTH Hospitals.

5. The Formulary Committee monitors all black box warnings or other Advisories issued by the Food and Drug Administration or pharmaceutical manufacturing company. The Formulary Committee uses the monitoring process as a basis to collaborate with each ALPHA-OMEGA HEALTH Hospital's P&T Committee as a means to promote patient safety.

6. The Formulary Committee maintains a newsletter regarding its decisions and distribute it to each member of the Medical Staff of all ALPHAOMEGA HEALTH Hospitals.

7. The Formulary Committee collaborates with the P&T Committee at each ALPHAO-MEGA HEALTH Hospital to develop educational strategies for the ALPHAOMEGA HEALTH professional employees and each Hospital's Medical Staff that builds support for the principles and priorities used to maintain the **HOSPITAL FORMULARY**.

8. The Formulary Committee offers consultation when requested or directed by the Board of Directors of ALPHAOMEGA HEALTH, its Committees, or any other ALPHAOMEGA HEALTH Committee regarding therapeutic products in the investigation, protocols, standard order sets, or quality assessment of health care.

9. The Formulary Committee offers a means to coordinate the standardization of POLICY AND PROCEDURE's for the Pharmacy Departments of ALPHAOMEGA HEALTH Hospitals.

POLICY TITLE: HOSPITAL PHARMACY AND THERAPEUTICS COMMITTEE

I. PURPOSE

To maintain a Pharmacy and Therapeutics Committee as a means to enhance the quality of health care for all patients served by the Alpha Medical Center.

II. POLICY

A. The Pharmacy and Therapeutics Committee of Alpha Medical Center periodically evaluates its performance as a means to improve its ability to support the Vision and Mission of ALPHAOMEGA HEALTH.

B. The Alpha Medical Center maintains a Pharmacy and Therapeutics Committee (P&T Committee) to implement this POLICY in accord with the applicable Medical Staff Bylaws and this POLICY.

C. The P&T Committee may maintain a SPECIAL FORMULARY at the Alpha Medical Center based on the provisions of the Hospital Formulary System POLICY AND PROCEDURE of ALPHAOMEGA HEALTH.

D. The P&T Committee monitors compliance with the provisions of the **HOSPITAL FORMULARY.**

E. The P&T Committee supports the quality improvement functions of ALPHAOMEGA HEALTH where necessary to improve the use of the **HOSPITAL FORMULARY.**

F. The P&T Committee reviews and approves any POLICY AND PROCEDURE of the Alpha Medical Center Pharmacy.

III. PROCEDURE

A. PHARMACY AND THERAPEUTICS COMMITTEE DEVELOPMENT

1. The P&T Committee recommends, when appropriate, amendments to this POLICY AND PROCEDURE to the Administrator of Alpha Medical Center. After revisions to any of these proposed amendments by the Administrator, in collaboration with the P&T Committee, the Administrator submits the amendments to the Executive Committee of the Alpha Medical Center Medical Staff for final approval.

2. The Officers of the P&T Committee prepare an Annual Membership Report to the Administrator of the Alpha Medical Center regarding participation of its Members and any recommendations for changes in its membership that may be important to maintain the expertise necessary for the affairs of the P&T Committee.

3. The Officers of the P&T Committee prepare an Annual Report and submit it to the Executive Committee of the Alpha Medical Center Medical Staff for approval. As a result of this review, the Executive Committee may make recommendations to the P&T Committee for consideration regarding its affairs or to the Administrator regarding amendments to this POLICY AND PROCEDURE.

B. FORMULARY COMMITTEE ORGANIZATION

1. REGULAR MEMBERS AND SOURCE OF SELECTION

   a. MEDICAL STAFF MEMBERS

      i. There may be up to eight Medical Staff members nominated annually by the Administrator, or designee, of Alpha Medical Center, the President of the Medical Staff of the Alpha Medical Center, or the Officers of the P&T Committee. Any Medical Staff nominee should demonstrate an active interest in evidence-based therapeutics, a willingness to be an active participant in the affairs of the P&T Committee, and represent as a group, whenever possible, the specialties of Family Practice, Internal Medicine, Pediatrics, Obstetrics and Gynecology, Hematology and Oncology, Cardiology, Infectious Disease, Pulmonology, and General Surgery.

      ii. From any nominees, eight are selected by the Administrator, or designee, of Alpha Medical Center on the basis of maintaining a reasonable balance among the following factors: hospital and outpatient-based physicians, primary care and disease-focused physicians, physician continuity from year to year, and physician liaison to the Medical Staff Executive Committee of the Alpha Medical Center or the Formulary Committee of ALPHAOMEGA HEALTH.

   b. PHARMACY MEMBERS—The Administrator, or designee, of Alpha Medical Center selects two pharmacists and includes the Pharmacist In Charge of the Hospital's Pharmacy.

   c. NURSING SERVICE MEMBER—The Administrator, or designee, of Alpha Medical Center selects one registered nurse from the Nursing Service.

2. SPECIAL MEMBERS AND SOURCE OF SELECTION

   a. The Administrator, or designee, of Alpha Medical Center may select Special Members as needed to provide administrative or technical support for the affairs of the P&T Committee.

   b. The Chairperson of the Formulary Committee may select one or more Special Members from the personnel of the Alpha Medical Center or its Medical Staff on a temporary basis as may be necessary for:

     i. technical support for the activities of the P&T Committee or any Ad Hoc Subcommittee or

     ii. information for the deliberations of the P&T Committee regarding a proposal to add or delete an individual therapeutic product listed on the **HOSPITAL FORMULARY.**

3. P&T COMMITTEE OFFICERS AND SOURCE OF SELECTION

   a. The CHAIRPERSON is selected by the Administrator, or designee, of the Alpha Medical Center from the physician Regular Members of the P&T Committee. The Chairperson:

     i. manages the affairs of the P&T Committee in a manner to:

       I) support the active, positive involvement of each Regular and Special Member,

       II) acknowledge any conflict of interests,

       III) initiate a replacement appointment of any Officer, Regular Member, or Special Member becoming inactive during a calendar year,

       IV) appoint temporary Special Members,

       V) select the location for Meetings of the P&T Committee;

     ii. prepares the Annual Membership and Self-Evaluation reports; and

     iii. appoints an Ad Hoc Committee when necessary to study decisions in greater depth or to arrive at consensus recommendations for consideration by the P&T Committee whose membership includes

       I) six or less members from the Medical Staff of the Alpha Medical Center,

       II) at least one member who is a physician Regular Member of the P&T Committee, and

       III) the Secretary, or designee, of the P&T Committee.

   b. The VICE CHAIRPERSON is selected by the Administrator of the Alpha Medical Center from among the physician Regular Members of the P&T Committee. The Vice Chairperson assumes the duties of the Chairperson during their absence.

   c. The SECRETARY is selected by the Administrator of the Alpha Medical Center from among the Regular or Special Members of the P&T Committee. The Secretary assists the Chairperson in managing the affairs of the P&T Committee by:

     i. preparing the minutes for each meeting of the P&T Committee or any of its Ad Hoc Committees,

     ii. sending an Agenda to the Members prior to each meeting of the P&T Committee,

     iii. maintaining liaison with the other Committees of the Medical Staff,

     iv. maintaining a schedule for the annual Quality Assurance activities of the P&T Committee, and

     v. assisting in the preparation of any Drug Monograph or any other report necessary for a meeting of the Formulary Committee of ALPHAOMEGA HEALTH.

4. TERM OF APPOINTMENT
   a. The Regular and Special Members are appointed or reappointed each January for 1 year.
   b. Each Officer is appointed or reappointed each January for 1 year.
5. VOTING
   a. Each Regular Member has one vote, and each Special Member does not have a vote.
   b. Any two physician Regular Members present during a Meeting of the Formulary Committee constitute a quorum.
   c. Regular Members present at a meeting of the P&T Committee may delay voting, when the appropriate expertise is not available during a meeting of the P&T Committee.
   d. A simple majority of Regular Members voting is required for any action of the P&T Committee. Any abstention on the basis of a conflict of interests is noted in the Minutes for the meeting.
6. LIAISON—A Regular or Special Member is appointed by the Administrator to report on the affairs of the P&T Committee during the deliberations of any other Committee of the Alpha Medical Center.
7. MEETINGS—The meetings of the P&T Committee are:
   a. scheduled once a month for 1 hour or as may be planned by the Members of the P&T Committee,
   b. attended by Regular and Special Members only,
   c. convened at a location arranged by the Chairperson.
8. COMMITTEE PROTOCOLS—The P&T Committee may also arrange for the:
   a. use of definitions applicable to the resignation and replacement of any Regular Member, Special Member, or Officer during a calendar year as may be established by the Formulary Committee of ALPHAOMEGA HEALTH and
   b. management of any potential or actual conflict of interests affecting the participation of a Regular or Special Member during a meeting of the P&T Committee as may be determined by the Formulary Committee of ALPHAOMEGA HEALTH.

C. **HOSPITAL FORMULARY** DEVELOPMENT
   1. The P&T Committee reviews for comment at each meeting any therapeutic product recommended for addition or deletion to the **HOSPITAL FORMULARY** by the Formulary Committee of ALPHAOMEGA HEALTH.
   2. The P&T Committee reviews for comment at each meeting any class review of therapeutic products by the Formulary Committee of ALPHAOMEGA HEALTH and their recommendations for changes in the **HOSPITAL FORMULARY.**

D. **HOSPITAL FORMULARY COMPLIANCE**
   1. The P&T Committee monitors each Medical Staff physician's orders for a therapeutic product that is:
      a. not listed or does not have an automatic therapeutic interchange with a therapeutic product listed on the current **HOSPITAL FORMULARY**,
      b. for an indication not permitted by the **HOSPITAL FORMULARY**, or
      c. for an indication having a restricted use provision.

2. The P&T Committee may establish a Special Formulary for therapeutic products not listed on the **HOSPITAL FORMULARY** as means to temporarily support the efforts of the Medical Staff for hospitalized patients having special requirements that are unique to Alpha Medical Center. The Special Formulary therapeutic products are selected using the same process defined by the ALPHAOMEGA HEALTH Formulary Committee for the **HOSPITAL FORMULARY**. For any therapeutic product listed on Special Formulary for 1 year or more, continued use of the Special Formulary status for the therapeutic product will require the approval of the Formulary Committee.

3. If the Alpha Medical Center P&T Committee votes to not accept a decision of the Formulary Committee, the Chairperson, or designee, of the P&T Committee attends a subsequent meeting of the Formulary Committee. At this Formulary Meeting, the Formulary Committee attempts to develop a strategy for resolving the conflict between the original decision of the Formulary Committee and the P&T Committee of the Alpha Medical Center. In the event that a resolution is not achieved, the issue may be appealed by either the Formulary Committee or the Alpha Medical Center P&T Committee to the Professional Affairs Committee for a final decision within 3 months of the appeal.

E. **QUALITY IMPROVEMENT**

1. The P&T Committee regularly reviews the decisions of the ALPHAOMEGA HEALTH Formulary Committee as a means to evaluate any issues requiring the development of carefully considered implementation requirements at the Alpha Medical Center, such as the shortage of a therapeutic product.

2. The P&T Committee maintains an annually revised schedule for Drug Use Evaluations as may be established through consultation with other Medical Staff Committees.

3. The P&T Committee or an Ad Hoc Committee reviews Medication Error Reports.

4. The P&T Committee quarterly reviews Adverse Medication Reaction Reports.

5. The P&T Committee participates in the development of standard order sets as may be requested by a Member, a group of Members, or a Committee of the Medical Staff.

6. The P&T Committee prepares an annual report to the Executive Committee regarding the overall level of prescribing compliance with the **HOSPITAL FORMULARY.**

7. The P&T Committee in collaboration with the Formulary Committee monitors black box warnings or other advisories issued by the Food and Drug Administration or pharmaceutical manufacturing company. The Formulary Committee uses the monitoring process as a basis to collaborate with each P&T Committee of ALPHAOMEGA HEALTH as a means to promote patient safety.

8. The P&T Committee suggests information to the Formulary Committee for inclusion in the **HOSPITAL FORMULARY** newsletter.

9. The P&T Committee may make recommendations to the Medical Staff of Alpha Medical Center regarding the health care of hospitalized patients regarding the use of the **HOSPITAL FORMULARY** based on the outcome of certain studies undertaken by the P&T Committee. These studies exclude any direct identification of patient names or medical records.

F. **PHARMACY DEPARTMENT POLICY AND PROCEDURE**
   1. The P&T Committee periodically reviews and approves the POLICY AND PROCE-DURES of the Alpha Medical Center Pharmacy Department.
   2. The review and approval are coordinated with the operational statements of the other Pharmacy Departments of ALPHAOMEGA HEALTH Hospitals.

Appendix 13–2

Formulary Request Form

PHARMACY AND THERAPEUTICS COMMITTEE
FORMULARY ADDITION REQUEST

NOTE: Both sides of this form must be completed in order for consideration by the **Formulary Committee** at its next regularly scheduled meeting. You may submit additional information based on the outline of this **request** if more space is required. If you are not a member of the committee, you must also complete a Conflict of Interest Statement and attach it to this request.

Generic Name _____ **Brand Name** _____

Indications—Describe the FDA-approved or potential off-label uses which have prompted this **request.** _____
_____
_____
_____

Dosing—Describe the specific strength and administration form of this product necessary for this **request.** _____
_____
_____
_____

Comparative Efficacy—Describe how this agent relates to other products in terms of effectiveness. _____
_____
_____
_____

Contraindications and Warnings—Describe any substantial issues related to this product, including REMS. _____
_____
_____
_____

Adverse Effects—List any substantial issues related to this product. _____

_____

_____

Expected Outcomes—Describe how this product would substitute or add to the current **Formulary** products. _____

_____

_____

Cost of Therapy—Describe how this product would change the overall cost of medical care.

_____

_____

_____

Impact on Inpatient Care Processes—Describe any special requirements on the hospital for use of this product such as nursing/medical staff education, standards of care, discharge planning, certification, or standard order sets.

_____

_____

_____

_____

Impact on Outpatient Care Processes—Describe any special requirements on ambulatory care for use of this product such as compliance, follow-up, or monitoring.

_____

_____

_____

Other Considerations—Describe any information not applicable to the above categories (e.g., need for order set, guideline, or policy and procedure).

_____

_____

_____

Requested By—Must be a **Formulary Committee Member** or **Hospital Medical Staff Member**.

Printed Name _____

Signature _____

Response—For record keeping by the **Formulary Committee.**

    Received by a **Formulary Committee Member date** _____

    Initial **Formulary Committee** consideration **date** _____

    Final **Formulary Committee** consideration **date** _____

Action Taken_____

Notification of Medical Staff Member submitting request date _____

Appendix 13–3

P&T Committee Meeting Attributes[1–3]

I. TIMING

A. Regular—The choice is often between monthly or bimonthly. Overall, a long-term commitment to one schedule that does not vary is ideal. An atypical but practical variation might include monthly meetings except August and December, in order to adjust for times when it is difficult to get quorum, because of vacations and holidays. To support a regular meeting cycle, any cancellation on a sudden, unexpected basis must be avoided virtually without exception. Finally, a 2- to 3-year experience with a given schedule would be necessary to permit members an opportunity to work membership commitment into their own schedule.

B. Monthly work cycle—Virtually all holidays occur in association with the first or last week of any month during the calendar year. Similarly, Mondays and Fridays frequently have distractions caused by these associated weekend demands. Thus, the second or third Tuesday-Wednesday-Thursday of the calendar month are often the best choice for a regular meeting.

C. Daily work cycle—Given the character of the discussion above, the start of the morning or afternoon would be ideal for a meeting. The afternoon timing could be associated with a light lunch prior to starting the meeting.

II. MEETING ROOM CHARACTER

A. Location—A location that minimizes the travel barriers encountered by all the members of the committee is best. In a multihospital organization, this choice may not be ideal if a perception of inter-hospital territoriality would create a perception of bias in the decisions of the committee. The committee may also allow the use of teleconferencing.[4] As this becomes a more widely accepted professional tool in the future, the barriers of travel time could be eliminated as a means to incorporate a higher degree of expertise within the members of the committee.

B. Size—The room should have a rectangular table, or tables set up in a U shape if there are too many members for a single table, with chairs on all sides and enough room for additional chairs next to the walls for guests who might be attending a meeting. The room should allow a comfortable fit for a table that is large enough for the usual attendance as well as appropriate audiovisual equipment. Overall, the room or table should not be so large that the usual attendees might feel isolated and thus less engaged in the agenda of any meeting. Similarly, a full turnout would crowd the room giving greater emphasis to the character of the deliberations.

C. Seating—This can be highly defined as is seen in cases with assigned seats having a name card displayed on the table for each member. The benefits of universal identity of the members would thus be enhanced, especially if they are generally unknown to each other because of the size of an institution or hospital group. More commonly, there could be no fixed seating arrangements for a more informal tradition that could better support collaboration and open discussion. A decision by the chairperson to sit in different locations would further emphasize this approach to a seating tradition. It is also often good for pharmacy personnel to disperse themselves throughout the room to avoid a feeling of us/them in discussions.

REFERENCES

1. Doyle M, Straus D. How to make meetings work: the new interaction method. New York: Berkeley Publishing Group; 1993.
2. Nair KV, Coombs JH, Ascione FJ. Assessing the structure, activities, and functioning of P&T committees: a multisite case study. P&T. 2000;25(10):516-28.
3. Balu S, O'Connor P, Vogenberg FR. Contemporary issues affecting P&T committees. Part 2: beyond managed care. P&T. 2004;29:780-83.
4. Boedeker B. Virtual pharmacy & therapeutics meetings [Internet]. The Harry S. Truman VA Hospital experience. Columbia, MO: Harry S. Truman Memorial Veteran's Hospital; 1999 Mar [cited 2004 Jan 27]. Available from: http://www.gasnet.org/esia/1999/march/virtual.html

Appendix 13–4

Example P&T Committee Minutes*

ORGANIZATION, INC.

PHARMACY AND THERAPEUTICS COMMITTEE MEETING

January 21, 20XX

SCHEDULED AT 0700

THESE MINUTES ARE PRIVILEGED AND NOT SUBJECT TO DISCLOSURE OR LEGAL DISCOVERY PROCEEDINGS UNDER (STATUTE NUMBER)

    I. Call to order

        The members or Guests present or members absent are indicated below:

        (legal names, usually with degrees)

            The meeting was called to order by the chairperson at 7:00 AM. The physician members present represented a quorum. The minutes for the previous meeting were presented to the members. The section regarding a report of the chairperson from a discussion with the executive committee about unapproved abbreviations was specifically reviewed by the chairperson. The minutes did not describe the executive committee's request that the P&T committee quarterly forward five to eight examples of physician progress notes that reflect these two issues. The executive committee decided to have the president of the medical staff have individual contact with the medical staff members involved. A motion was made to approve the amended minutes and seconded. There being no further discussion, the motion was approved unanimously.

    II. Pharmacy and Therapeutics Committee Organizational Affairs

        A. Policy and Procedure Amendments—The chairperson submitted a draft revision of the entire policy and procedure for the P&T committee in response to new standards of TJC and previously discussed requirements for the functions of the committee. The committee reviewed the proposed draft and agreed informally to reconsider it at the next meeting after the chairperson has had a chance to meet with the Chief Medical Officer regarding any other amendments that may be necessary.

---

*Minutes listed in this appendix follow a paragraph format. Use of a table or bullet points to provide a more concise minute review is done in some places.

B. Committee Procedures
   1. Conflict of Interest Disclosure—The chairperson gave the Members the forms necessary to declare any potential or actual conflicts of interest according to the procedure established previously by the committee. The chairperson briefly reviewed this process and emphasized that conflicts of interest were only unacceptable when not acknowledged or no action is taken to resolve them during a meeting of the committee.
   2. Formulary Request format—no change
   3. Alternate Medication Use—no change
   4. Drug Monograph—no change
C. Committee membership—no action; end of year report due December 31st
D. Annual Report—Draft Report due January 5th
E. Ad hoc committees—none currently
F. Budget—reports due February, May, August, November

III. Formulary System
A. Formulary Maintenance
   1. Formulary additions/deletions
     a. IV lansoprazole (Prevacid®)—Approved Formulary
     b. Fondaparinux (Arixtra®)—Not approved—Non-formulary
     c. Escitalopram (Lexapro®)—Approved Formulary with restrictions or guidelines or policy and procedure
   2. Formulary Class Reviews
     28:04 General anesthetic agents
     72:00 Local anesthetic agents
     86:00 Smooth muscle relaxants
     24:00 Cardiovascular agents
   3. Non-formulary usage report
   4. Review of standard order sets/guidelines
     TPN order sheet

IV. Drug Use and Quality Improvement
A. Medication error report—no report
B. Adverse medication reaction report—no report
C. Drug Usage Evaluation report—no report
D. Medication recall—no report

V. Hospital Pharmacy Policies—no report

VI. Current Medication Shortages

Appendix 13–5

Chairperson Skills

I. Experience

A. KNOWLEDGE OF FORMULARY ISSUES

This occurs ideally as a result of prior experience on the committee for several years. P&T committee meetings are often associated with an individual hospital, group of hospitals, a staff model health maintenance organization, or an insurance-related pharmacy benefit management (PBM) process. A chairperson's experience in each of these areas would be ideal.

B. PROFESSIONAL PRACTICE

It could be suggested that at least 10 years is required for a pharmacist, nurse, administrator, or physician to have a sense of the overall trends evolving within health care. Within a P&T committee, the chairperson would need this background to best respond to the biases that each member might bring to the deliberations. It is beneficial if the members have had mutual experience with the chairperson at a direct patient care level.

C. LEADERSHIP

The chairperson is likely to be the most essential person for the overall success of a P&T committee. This is most directly related to the organization truism that it is nearly impossible to hold a committee responsible for anything except when a committee is acting as the ultimate authority for an organization. Thus, the value of a P&T committee is related to its ability to serve the common interests of the entire organization affected by its actions. If the costs of the P&T committee members' time are considered, the committee's activities are the result of a very expensive effort. To best utilize this expertise, a chairperson must be skilled at mobilizing these resources in a manner that bests supports the overall efforts of the organization to which it is attached. A previously demonstrated ability to create this role for a committee is the most valuable attribute for use in choosing a committee's chairperson.

II. Meeting Strategies

A. PUNCTUALITY

Given the busy schedules of the members, it is necessary to start and end on time. To open a meeting, it is best to lay out the agenda including any new additions and briefly discuss any items that will require a special discussion. Within 2 to 3 minutes, the chairperson and each member should have an understanding of the scope of the meeting ahead.

B. FAIRNESS

Often the health care process vacillates unpredictably between deductive and inductive reasoning processes. External observers are often baffled by this interplay. Related to this, it is suggested that a strict use of the *Robert's Rules of Order* for a meeting agenda may not facilitate the spontaneity for a committee's members that usually underlies their involvement in the character of health care. It is the responsibility of the chairperson to guide this process and seek out the opinions that the members have for a given issue. Also, if the knowledge necessary to make the best judgment for a given issue does not exist for a decision on the issue, it is important that the chairperson be able to facilitate a consensus that develops a means to rectify the deficiency.

C. INVOLVEMENT

Some members may not normally wish to participate spontaneously during a meeting. It is up to the chairperson to ask these members a specific question that would allow them a meaningful opportunity to participate in a given discussion. Occasionally, the chairperson might ask each member present about their opinion for a final decision being faced by the committee. This strategy should begin at one place around the table moving to each member present clockwise around the meeting room.

Appendix 13–6

Conflict of Interest Declaration

FORMULARY ADDITION REQUEST CONFLICT OF INTEREST STATEMENT

NOTE: This must be submitted along with the actual **Request** form if the person submitting the **Request** is not a member of the Formulary Committee. A copy of the Formulary Committee's Policy on Conflict of Interest Management is attached.

Generic Name _____ Trade Name _____

Substantial Involvement with a Competing Organization - ☐ Yes ☐ No

Please describe if:

1) A member of a health insurance company or another health system Pharmacy and Therapeutics Committee.
2) Another health system medical staff officer.
3) A member of a group practice primarily affiliated with another health system.

Substantial Involvement with a Company which Manufactures the Product or Competes with the Product's Company - ☐ Yes ☐ No

Please describe if:

1) Receiving financial income or support in the last 12 months of more than $100 for research, attendance at a **company** supported seminar, travel to an out-of-town meeting, or participation in a **company** sponsored speaker's bureau.
2) Receiving pharmaceutical products from the **company in** the last 12 months for personal or family use, gifts for family or personal use, or samples for use other than as a courtesy for patients.
3) Maintaining in the last 12 months a substantial ownership of stock (>10% of outstanding shares) in the **company** having >30% of its revenue from sales to **this organization**, its affiliated organizations, or another local health system.

Substantial Inside Information - ☐ Yes ☐ No

Please describe if there are other outside relationships for which involvement in this **request** may be actually or potentially perceived as affecting the decision of the committee such as:

1) Having a substantial position of authority in another organization which might affect a member of the committee for employment or medical staff privileges.

2) Disclosing information about this **request** to another organization directly or indirectly which might give **this organization**, the other organization, or the requestor an unfair advantage.

3) Receiving substantial assistance from the company or its representative which manufactures the requested product in the preparation of this **Formulary Addition Request.**

Appendix 14–1

Format for Drug Monograph

INSTITUTION NAME HEADING

Generic name: Can include other common, non-official names, for example, TPA for alteplase.

Trade brand name: If more than one, indicate company that each is from.

Manufacturer (or source of supply): Include website address

Therapeutic category: For example, thrombolytic agent for alteplase

Classification: Note—other classifications, such as the VA Class, can also be used.
- AHFS Number and Classification (if not in the book yet, see the list in the front of AHFS Drug Information book and determine the most appropriate classification)
- FDA Classification (include specific FDA website URL concerning approval)
- Status—Prescription, Nonprescription, and/or Controlled Substance Schedule (if applicable)

Similar agents: A list of common treatments used for the same indication(s).

Summary: Includes a short summary of advantages and disadvantages of the drug, particularly in relation to other drugs or treatments used for each major indication, and any other significant information. Must include indications allowed in the institution.

Recommendations: Indicate whether or not the drug should be added to the drug formulary of an institution, including specifying the indications that it is approved for use in the institution, assuming they would have patients that would be treated for illnesses where this drug might be used. Also indicate specific formulary status for the drug (i.e., uncontrolled, monitored, restricted, conditional—see ASHP guidelines) and whether the drug will replace any other product that might already be on the formulary. In addition, any information on how the drug is to be placed in any clinical guidelines. For third-party payer monographs, information will need to be included on the payment tier.

Page one of the drug monograph consists of the above information

Pharmacological Data:

- Mechanism of Action (usually brief)
- Bacterial Spectrum (if applicable)

Therapeutic Indications:

- FDA-Approved Indications (see package insert) —Clearly state which indications are FDA approved
- Potential Unlabeled Uses (list only if they are considered to be acceptable medical practice, although it is allowable to mention others that are early in investigation with a statement that the drug should not be used for them or that they require more study) —Clearly indicate they are not FDA approved
- How the drug, and similar drugs, fit into clinical guidelines.
- Clinical Comparison (abstract at least two studies; see Appendix 12-2 for more guidelines. Include human efficacy studies and, where available, studies comparing the product to standard therapy. Note: if there are other supportive studies for an indication, they can be covered briefly along with the major study covered in detail. Be sure to note any deficiencies in the studies). Also, pharmacogenomic information may need to be included here and elsewhere.

Bioavailability/Pharmacokinetics:

A table summarizing the following, in comparison to the gold standard, can be very useful.

- Absorption
- Distribution
- Metabolism
- Excretion

Dosage Forms:

- Forms and Strengths—compare to other agents (consider a table), since new products often have a limited number of dosage forms/routes as compared to established products. Purity and composition information should be included for herbal and alternative medications.
- Explain any special information needed for preparation and storage, in comparison to other products. Sometimes a product will be so difficult to prepare or have such a limited shelf-life after preparation that it is not worth stocking.

Dosage Range:

- Adults
- Children
- Elderly
- Renal or Hepatic Failure
- Special Administration Requirements
- Any anticipated problems in supplies (i.e., shortages) or restrictions in distribution (e.g., prescriber certification required)

Known Adverse Effects/Toxicities:

- Frequency and Type (a table comparing the drug to others can be a clear and concise way of expressing this information)
- Prevention of Toxicity
- Risk and Benefit Data

Special Precautions: Usually includes pregnancy and lactation.

Contraindications: List of Contraindications

Drug Interactions:

A simple one- or two-sentence statement for each—usually separate various interactions into separate short paragraphs and compare to other drugs.

- Drug-Drug
- Drug-Food
- Drug-Laboratory

Patient Safety Information:

Includes medication error information and product safety information from outside sources (e.g., ISMP, MedWatch, FDA Patient Safety News, United States Pharmacopeia Patient Safety Program)

Patient Monitoring Guidelines:

Include effectiveness, adverse effects, compliance, and other appropriate items

Patient Information:

- Name and description of the medication
- Dosage form
- Route of administration
- Duration of therapy
- Special directions and precautions
- Side effects
- Techniques for self-monitoring
- Proper storage
- Refill information
- What to do if dose is missed

Guideline/Order Set:

Guideline(s) or order set(s) needed and how operations will be effected if the drug is added to formulary

Cost Comparison:

Use AWP and institutional prices, and make sure there is a comparison with any similar products at equivalent doses—a pharmacoeconomic analysis (see Chapter 7) is the best method of comparing drugs in this section; remember to include any required concomitant therapy. Providing a spreadsheet file with information to consider different patient circumstances that can change may be helpful.

List different costs for each hospital if part of a multihospital health system (consider group purchasing organization costs, 340b program costs, retail pharmacy account costs, or other discounted pricing).

Reimbursement:

If a primarily outpatient medication, especially for an infusion center.

Date Presented to pharmacy and therapeutics committee, and name and title of the person preparing the document

References:

Follow guidelines as described in Appendix 12-3.

Appendix 14–2

Example Drug Monograph

Note: This example is based on fictional products and is condensed. It shows examples of most sections in a real drug monograph, but often does not go into all of the details (e.g., a table of adverse effects is seen, but only a couple items are listed, whereas a full drug monograph would list at least all common and/or serious reactions).

St. Anywhere Medical Center (St. AMC)
Pharmacy & Therapeutics Committee
Drug Evaluation Monograph

Generic Name:	Artiblood
Brand Name:	MegaBlood
Manufacturer:	MegaPharmics
Therapeutic Category:	Blood substitute
Classification:	AHFS 16:00 Blood Derivatives
	FDA Classification: 1A
	Status: Prescription Only
Similar Agents:	Fakered

Summary:

Artiblood is a new perfluorocarbon that has many similarities to the only other product in its class, fakered. Both products have the ability to temporarily replace the oxygen-carrying function of red blood cells in patients in whom use of whole blood or packed red blood cells is impossible due to medical or religious reasons. In general, artiblood was found to be more efficacious than fakered; however, it also has been shown to produce a greater number of adverse effects. The adverse effects are mostly gastrointestinal in nature; however, the increased INR can be a problem in some patients. Artiblood is not metabolized in the body, whereas fakered is approximately 50% metabolized to inactive components. These differences are generally not clinically significant, since the dose of either product is unlikely to need adjustment. Fakered is available in several different volume bags, allowing the dose to be matched more closely to the anticipated patient need. While the cost of fakered appears to be lower, a pharmacoeconomic analysis shows that artiblood would produce the greatest cost savings for the institution.

Recommendations:

It is recommended that artiblood be added to the Drug Formulary for use restricted to those who cannot use natural blood replacement products because of religious reasons or because suitable blood types are not available, including for use in cardiac catheterization procedures. It is not approved for use as a volume expander, except when in conjunction with the previous indications.

Pharmacologic Data:

Artiblood is a type of perfluorocarbon, similar to fakered. These products have the unique ability to freely bind with or give up oxygen, depending on the partial pressures of the gas where the product is located (i.e., in the lungs there is an abundance of oxygen, so the product adsorbs oxygen; in the tissues there is a relative deficiency of oxygen, so the product gives up the gas).[1,2] The products do not have direct immunologic properties, nor do they have the ability to aid in blood clotting, although there may be some effect on blood clotting (either interference by coating platelets or precipitation of the clotting pathway mechanism).[3]

In addition to oxygen-carrying capabilities, the products have some plasma volume expansion properties. Artiblood has a similar effect to Dextran 40,[1] whereas fakered's properties are relatively insignificant.[4] Maximum plasma volume expansion occurs within several minutes of administration and lasts for approximately 1 day in normal patients. This results in increased central venous pressure, cardiac output, stroke volume, blood pressure, urinary output, capillary perfusion, and pulse pressure. Microcirculation is improved.

Therapeutic Indications:

Indications:

Artiblood is FDA approved for the short-term replacement of the oxygen-carrying capabilities of blood in patients who cannot use normal whole blood.[1] In addition, the product has been used successfully in cardiac catheter procedures, although this use is not FDA approved.[5] There is some early research into the use of the product as a plasma expansion product, but there is not enough information to support this use.[6]

Fakered is approved only for use in cardiac catheterization,[2] although it is commonly used as a blood replacement product in patients who cannot or will not use whole blood products.[7]

Evidence-Based Clinical Guidelines:

A search of the literature was performed to identify evidence-based clinical guidelines. This included MEDLINE, Embase Drugs and Pharmacology, the National Guideline Clearinghouse website, the American College of Cardiology website, and approximately a dozen Internet search engines, however, no applicable guidelines were identified.

Clinical Studies:

Max and Sugar[6] conducted a comparison trial of artiblood (500 mL/day administered once daily to over 1 hour to 80 patients) and fakered (750 mL administered once over 90 minutes to 82 patients) in patients (18 to 80 years of age) suffering from massive blood loss (>1 L), who could not use whole blood due to religious beliefs (e.g., Jehovah's Witnesses). In the artiblood group, all patients were undergoing open-heart surgery, as were 78 of the patients in fakered group. The remainder of the fakered group consisted of gunshot patients. Patients with renal insufficiency (creatinine clearance <50 mL/min) or diagnosed with liver dysfunction were eliminated from consideration. Both groups were similar, except that the artiblood group had more smokers, which may have had an effect on oxygen requirements. Withdrawals from the artiblood group were for the following reasons: death due to failure of heart-lung machine (1 patient), noncompliance with protocol (10 patients), worsening symptoms (3 patients), and side effects (1 patient—vomiting). The authors noted that protocol compliance problems were due to inappropriate staff education and were not related to the drug itself. In the fakered group, withdrawals were due to side effects (one-patient—diarrhea, one patient—nausea, one patient—abdominal cramps) and noncompliance with protocol (two patients). The patients were assessed on the following items: oxygen and carbon dioxide content of the blood (samples drawn immediately before and after administration, and every 4 hours for 24 hours), coagulation profile of patient (drawn within 2 hours before and after administration), effect on normal blood chemistry profiles (SMA-20) (drawn within 2 hours before and after administration), and time to discontinuation of supplemental oxygen to the patient. Adverse effects were also noted. Results were analyzed using appropriate statistical methods. Artiblood was found to increase the oxygen-carrying capabilities of the blood in comparison to fakered ($p < 0.01$), although fakered did significantly improve oxygen-carrying capabilities over baseline ($p < 0.05$). While fakered had minimal effect on blood chemistry and coagulation profile, it was noted that INRs were increased in patients receiving artiblood ($p < 0.001$). Other adverse effects, mostly gastrointestinal in nature, were more common with fakered, although the symptoms typically disappeared within 2 hours of administration. Other measured characteristics seemed similar between the two groups. The authors concluded that artiblood was the superior agent, due to increased oxygen-carrying capabilities. The authors downplayed adverse effects, although the effects on INRs do appear worrisome.

[Other studies would be covered here for all likely uses within an institution.]

There were no studies found that demonstrated any effects of genome on either artiblood or fakered therapy.

Bioavailability/Pharmacokinetics[16–18]:

Absorption:

Absorption is not applicable, since these agents are administered by IV infusion.

Distribution:

Artiblood is found in the blood stream, with little being distributed to the tissues. Approximately 5% of fakered is found in the liver, with the rest being in the bloodstream.

Metabolism:

Artiblood is not metabolized in the body, whereas approximately 50% of fakered is broken down to inactive components and is excreted in the bile.

Elimination:

Artiblood has a half-life of 5 to 15 hours. It is excreted unchanged in the urine. The longer half-life is seen in patients with renal insufficiency. Since the drug is usually given as a single dose, renal insufficiency does not pose a significant problem. Fakered has a half-life of 4 to 7 hours in normal patients. Significant renal or hepatic impairment may double the half-life.

Dosage Forms:

Large Volume Parenteral:
- Artiblood—500 mL IV bags
- Fakered—500, 750, and 1000 mL IV bags

No other forms or strengths available. This product will have limited availability for the next 6 months due to the ability of the manufacturer to produce an adequate amount to satisfy demands. No problems in availability are expected after that point. Due to the restrictions on indicated uses in the institution, this is not expected to cause any difficulties and, therefore, no specific procedures are being mandated to address a possible shortage.

Dosage Range:

The normal dose of artiblood for blood replacement is 500 mL, which may be repeated once after 4 hours. Doses may be cut in half for patients weighing less than 50 kg. No dosage adjustments are necessary in renal or hepatic impairment. The product has not been tested in patients younger than 12 years of age and is not recommended in that population. No dosage adjustment is necessary in the elderly.[1]

Fakered is given in doses of 500 mL to 1 L, with a maximum daily dose of 1.5 L. The dose is adjusted based on clinical response of the patient. The product can be used in patients as young as 6 years of age; however, the initial dose is 250 mL.[2]

Known Adverse Effects/Toxicities:

The two agents are compared in the following table:

Adverse Effect	Artiblood (% of patients)	Fakered (% of patients)
Gastrointestinal		
Nausea	20	7
—	—	—

Special Precautions:

Neither drug has been studied long term, therefore, the effects are not known.

Both products are considered Pregnancy Category C. Tests in pregnant animals have shown adverse effects and no adequate, well-controlled studies have been conducted in humans. There is no information available on the excretion of the drug in human milk. Overall, when considering use in pregnant or lactating women, the physician must consider the benefits versus the risks.

Safety and effectiveness of artiblood in children have not been established, although fakered may be used in children at least 6 years old.

Contraindications:

Both agents are contraindicated in patients with hypersensitivities to the drug or any component of the dosage form.

Drug Interactions:

Drug-Drug Interactions:

Heparin—Effects of heparin or low-molecular-weight heparins may be significantly increased by either artificial blood replacement agent, although the effect by artiblood tends to be greater. There is no effect on either artiblood or fakered, although the heparin may improve circulation of the products to underperfused tissues.

[Other interactions for both drugs would be listed and compared.]

Drug-Food Interactions:

None are known or expected, since these agents are given intravenously and do not undergo entero-hepatic recirculation.

Drug-Laboratory Test Interactions:

INR—INRs can be increased by both agents, although the effect is more noticeable with artiblood.
[Other interactions for both drugs would be listed and compared.]

Patient Safety:

This product has a good patient safety profile, with relatively minor adverse effects (e.g., nausea). Since the product has no coagulation or immunologic activity, health care providers must be aware that it is only used for temporary help in oxygen-carrying capabilities. Other specific safety concerns include:

- Patients on warfarin must have a baseline INR and one each day for the 2 days following administration.
- The product has been on the market less than 6 months and information is limited.
- Product must be refrigerated until approximately 30 minutes prior to infusion.

Patient Monitoring Guidelines:

Monitor patient for objective evidence of effectiveness (e.g., oxygen content of blood and clinical effects). Obtain baseline INR and normal chemistry values, and monitor regularly. Monitor for adverse effects.

Patient Information:

In a patient receiving the product due to trauma, it is likely that he or she will not be able to be given information. In that case, provide the information to the next of kin or guardian. Inform patients that the product is an intravenous product that does not contain any blood products. The patient or family should know that he or she may receive this product once or more during the first day after surgery. The patient or family should be informed that the drug has few noticeable adverse effects other than some gastrointestinal upset; however, the physician or pharmacist should be consulted if anything unusual occurs. The patient or family should know that some blood tests will be regularly performed to exclude the possibility of adverse effects. The nurse will keep the drug refrigerated until approximately 30 minutes before infusion. Warnings about missed doses are irrelevant.

Guideline or Order Set:
None anticipated.

Cost Comparison:

General pricing information:

	AWP	Daily Dose*	St. AMC	Daily Dose*
Artiblood 500 mL	$2,500/bag	$2,500	$2,310/bag	$2,310
Fakered 500 mL	$1,000/bag	$1,000	$800/bag	$800
Fakered 750 mL	$1,500/bag	$1,500	$1,200/bag	$1,200
Fakered 1,000 mL	$2,000/bag	$2,000	$1,600/bag	$1,600

*Assume used one bag of each strength.

Pharmacoeconomic Analysis:

- *Problem Definition*—The objective of this analysis is to determine which artificial blood product should be included on the St. AMC drug formulary.
- *Perspective*—This will be from the perspective of the institution.
- *Specific treatment alternatives and outcomes*—There are two drugs to be compared, artiblood and fakered. It will be assumed that natural blood products are not an alternative, since the ability to use natural products would preclude consideration of the artificial products. The outcomes to be measured are hospital costs.
- *Pharmacoeconomic model*—A cost-benefit analysis will be performed. A cost-utility analysis would be desirable, but insufficient information is available. Note—no published pharmacoeconomic analysis is available. The following is based on information obtained from the literature concerning efficacy, adverse effects, monitoring, etc. and uses St. AMC costs, since outside prices would be irrelevant.

	Cost per Patient	Benefit-to-Cost Ratio	Net Benefit
Cost of artiblood (including administration, monitoring, adverse reactions, etc.)	$5,120	$7,430/$5,120 = 1.45:1	$7,430−$5,120=$2,310
Benefits of artiblood (money saved by early patient discharge from ICU)	$7,430		
Cost of fakered (including administration, monitoring, adverse reactions, etc.)	$4,000	$4,500/$4,000 = 1.125:1	$4,500−$4000 =$500
Benefits of fakered (money saved by early patient discharge from ICU)	$4,500		

[Note to reader—the above information is a summary of information, including averages, decision analysis, and sensitivity analysis that would be used in a pharmacoeconomic evaluation. While the details could be presented here, that may be distracting and confusing to some readers—a decision must be made as to whether all of the details will be presented. See Chapter 7 for details on how to prepare a pharmacoeconomic analysis of a drug being evaluated by the P&T committee.]

Presented by John Q. Doe, Pharm.D. to the Pharmacy and Therapeutics committee on February 30, 20XX.

REFERENCES

References would be listed in the order in which they are cited in the text—see Appendix 12-3 in Chapter 12 for format and details.

Appendix 16–1

Tools Used in Quality Assurance

FLOW CHARTS

Flow charts illustrate the steps of a process and how the steps are related to each other. They can be used to describe the process, to increase a team's knowledge of the entire process, to identify weaknesses or breakdown points in the current process, or to design a new process. An example of a flow chart outlining how adverse drug reactions might be addressed within an organization is provided below.

Flowchart: suspected adverse drug reactions

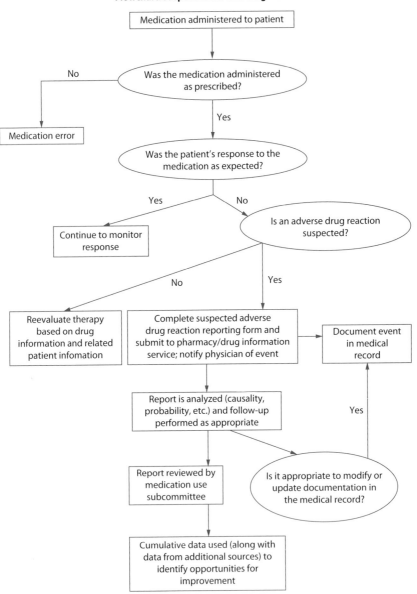

PARETO CHART

Pareto charts are vertical bar graphs with the data presented so that the bars are arranged from left to right on the horizontal axis in their order of decreasing frequency. This arrangement helps to identify which problems to address in what order. By addressing the data represented in the tallest bars (e.g., the most frequently occurring problems or contributing factors) efforts can be focused on areas where the most gain can be realized. Pareto charts are commonly used to identify issues to address, delineate potential causes of a problem, and to monitor improvements in processes. An example of a Pareto chart appears below. This example illustrates frequently occurring factors contributing to improper dose medication errors. By focusing on transcription errors as a contributing factor on which to focus quality improvement (QI) efforts, the QI team will generally gain more than by tackling the smaller bars.

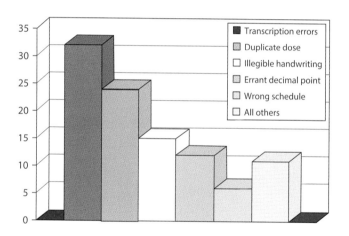

FISHBONE OR CAUSE-AND-EFFECT DIAGRAM

Fishbone or cause-and-effect diagrams represent the relationship between an outcome (represented at the head of the fish) and the possible causes of the outcome (represented as the bones of the fish). The bones of the fish should represent causes and not symptoms of the issue. Fishbone diagrams are commonly used to identify components of a process to address, delineate potential causes of a problem, or to identify practitioner groups that participate in producing an outcome and should be represented in the group addressing quality issues in the process(es). An example of a Fishbone chart is provided below.

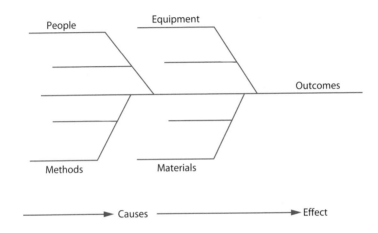

CONTROL CHARTS

Control charts are run charts or line graphs with defined allowable limits of variation. Data are plotted on the graph as they become available with new data points connected to older data by a continuous line. The *x*-axis is usually a measure of time. The control limits help to identify which variations in data are important. Control limits are statistically determined based on average ranges and sample size. Fluctuation in data points above and below the average is expected and is referred to as common variation or common cause as long as they remain between the control limits. Data points above the upper control limit or below the lower control limit are referred to as special variation or special cause. Special cause variation indicates that something different is going on outside the normal operation of the process. Also, a series of data points above or below average may indicate a trend in performance that may need to be addressed. As variability in a process is reduced by quality improvement efforts, control limits should be recalculated (and narrowed) based on ongoing data. An example of a control chart appears below. Calls from pharmacists to prescribers in response to questions or issues related to new medication orders are represented over a 6-month period. Data from the month of July indicate a significant increase in the number of calls made. A quality improvement team evaluating this data would then attempt to identify what contributed to this increase. A potential cause in many institutions might be the influx of new medical house staff into the organization each July. One potential intervention to reduce this special cause is to improve the orientation of new practitioners to the medication use process within the organization.

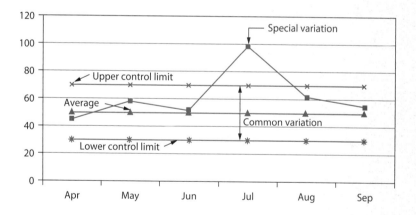

Appendix 16–2

Example of Criteria and Request for Approval

MEDICATION USE EVALUATION CRITERIA

Antiemetic Use in the Prophylaxis of Chemotherapy-induced Nausea and Vomiting

Request for Approval by Medication Use Evaluation Committee

Purpose of evaluation: The purpose of this medication use evaluation (MUE) is to evaluate the use of antiemetic therapy in the prevention of chemotherapy-induced nausea and vomiting. This agent was selected for evaluation based on its essential role in the management of this patient population, potential inappropriate use, and increased cost relative to other antiemetic agents. This class of medications has not been evaluated within the organization for at least 5 years.

Criteria: A multidisciplinary group including physicians, clinical nurse specialists, staff nurses from the oncology unit, and pharmacists developed the attached criteria. They are submitted for approval by the MUE Committee.

[The actual criteria would be listed here.]

Data Collection: Data will be collected on all patients with orders for this agent written throughout a period of approximately 30 days beginning in mid-January 20XX. A minimum of 50 cases will be reviewed. Pharmacists and clinical nurse specialists will collect data concurrently from the medical record. Patients will be identified by means of the clinical information system.

Results: Results will be presented to this Committee. Information will also be shared with the Cancer Care Committee and Health System Performance Improvement Council. Prescriber-specific results will be confidentially provided to Medical Staff Support for use in the reappointment/recredentialing process.

Appendix 16–3

Example of MUE Results

MEDICATION USE EVALUATION

Summary of Overall Results

Antiemetic: January-February 20XX

Background: This topic was selected based on high use, potential misuse, and high cost of these agents. Criteria for this evaluation were approved at the MUE Committee's December 20XX meeting. Please refer to attached criteria for additional information.

Total Patients Evaluated (All Indications for Use) = 52

ELEMENT	STANDARD	RESULTS		COMPLIANCE
PRESCRIBING				
Indication for use	95%	OVERALL RESULTS		
			Treatment/prevention of nausea/vomiting (N/F) associated with chemotherapy	100% (52/52)
			Highly emetogenic chemotherapy	46/46
			Anticipatory N/V associated with chemotherapy	6/6
DISPENSING/ADMINISTERING				
Dosing	95%	OVERALL RESULTS		71% (37/52)
			Highly emetogenic chemotherapy	31/46
			Anticipatory N/V associated with chemotherapy	6/6
MONITORING				
Adverse drug reaction(s)	≤10–25% (varies with ADR)	OVERALL RESULTS:		4% (2/52)
		Headache: 1 patient		
		Constipation: 1 patient		

continued

ELEMENT	STANDARD	RESULTS	COMPLIANCE
OUTCOME			
Prevention of nausea and emesis	95%	OVERALL RESULTS	92% (46/50)*
		Highly emetogenic chemotherapy	41/44
		Anticipatory N/V associated with chemotherapy	5/6
Chemotherapy course not interrupted	95%	OVERALL RESULTS (ALL INDICATIONS)	100% (52/52)

* Includes only patients in whom outcome was documented. Outcome was not assessed in two patients who were discharged immediately following administration of chemotherapy.

Summary of Results

Prescribing: Criteria for indication for use were met in all cases.

Dispensing/Administering: Criteria for dosing was met in 37 of 52 cases with all cases involving anticipatory nausea and vomiting meeting criteria.

In 15 cases, patients receiving the antiemetic prior to highly emetogenic chemotherapy received doses not included in the approved criteria. Five of these patients received doses based on an investigational protocol. This dose is now under consideration by the FDA for approval and preliminary results (available only in abstract form) were recently presented at the American Society of Clinical Oncology meeting. Results with the new dosing regimen have been comparable to those with the currently approved doses.

In seven cases not meeting dosing criteria, patients received a single dose prior to chemotherapy consistent with the criteria. However, an additional dose was administered 24 hours after the first dose. These orders were written by two prescribers.

Two cases did not meet dosing criteria because the dose was not adjusted based on renal dysfunction. In both cases, the estimated creatinine clearance was between 20 and 25 mL/min and nephrotoxic drugs were not being administered concurrently. In both cases, the estimated creatinine clearance increased to 30 mL/min or more by day two of the admission (probably due to rehydration of the patient). Neither patient experienced adverse effects.

One dose was not administered within the appropriate time frame. In this case, the antiemetic dose was administered just 5 minutes prior to the initiation of chemotherapy administration. The nurse administering the antiemetic documented its administration on the way to the patient's room. When she arrived, the patient was not in the room. The dose was administered after he was located, approximately 25 minutes later. The nurse did not correct the actual administration time until after the chemotherapy was administered by a second nurse.

Recommendations:
1. Add new dosing regimen to dosing criteria.
2. Send letters to prescribers giving extra dose.
3. Renal dosing was not significantly outside guidelines. Mention findings in report to be published in quality improvement newsletter but do not take prescriber specific action.

4. The dose administered late was reported via an incident report, no further action by this group is required at this time.

Monitoring: The rate of adverse drug reactions was less than that reported in the literature. This might be reflective of underreporting and underdocumenting of adverse drug events.

Recommendations:

1. The Adverse Drug Event Task Force is currently implementing a new process to improve reporting and documentation. No specific action by this group is required at this time.

Outcome: Ninety-two percent of patients did not experience nausea or vomiting. Outcome was assessable in 50 patients; two patients were discharged immediately following the administration of chemotherapy.

The patient who received his antiemetic dose just 5 minutes prior to chemotherapy experienced moderate nausea and no vomiting. Otherwise, the occurrence of nausea and vomiting was not related to problems with administration or dosing.

Recommendations:

1. Ninety-two percent success rate is acceptable based on literature; no action is necessary.

General Recommendations:

1. After approval, implement recommendations presented above.
2. Publish results in the Quality Improvement Newsletter following review by the Cancer Care Committee and the Quality Improvement Committee.
3. Perform a follow-up evaluation focusing on dosing issues.
4. Initiate planned assessment of this agent's use in postoperative nausea and vomiting as soon as possible.

Appendix 16–4

Evaluation Form for Drug Information Response

Request #   Date of Request

Response by (circle one):   DI Staff   Resident   Student

Caller (circle type):   MD   RPh   Nurse   Other:

Assessment of Search and Response to Request

	Yes	No	NA	Standard %*
1. Is requestor's demographic information complete?				100%
2. Background information is:				100%
A. Thorough				
B. Appropriate to request				
3. Is the question clearly stated?				100%
4. Search strategy/references:				100%
A. Appropriate references were used				
B. Search was sufficiently comprehensive				
C. Is search strategy clearly documented				
5. Response was:				100%
A. Appropriate for the situation				
B. Sufficient to answer the question				
C. Provided in a timely manner				
D. Integrated with available patient data				
E. Supported by appropriate materials supplied to requestor				
6. If complete response could not be provided within time frame requested, was requestor advised as to the status of their request and the anticipated delivery of the final response?				100%

* If performance falls below 90% in any category during any month, the service director will coordinate an assessment of the process and report findings and actions will be reported to the P&T committee.

Comments:

Reviewed By: _____

Appendix 17–1

Kramer Questionnaire*

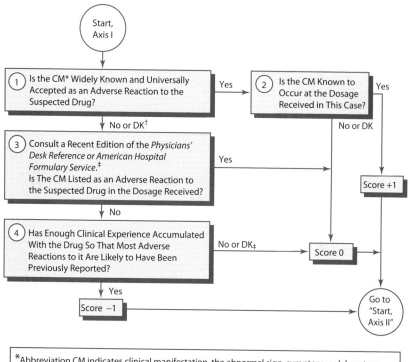

*Abbreviation CM indicates clinical manifestation, the abnormal sign, symptom, or laboratory test, or cluster of abnormal signs, symptoms, and tests, that is being considered as a possible adverse drug reaction.

† Abbreviation DK indicates do not know. This answer should be given when no data are available for the question being answered or when the quality of the data does not allow a firm "Yes" or "No" response.

‡ When these are not available, an equivalent reference source may be used.

Figure 1. Axis I. Previous general experience with drug.

*Kramer MS, Leventhal JM, Hutchinson TA, Feinstein AR. An algorithm for the operational assessment of adverse drug reaction: I. Background, descriptions, and instructions for use. JAMA. 1979; 242(7):623-32.

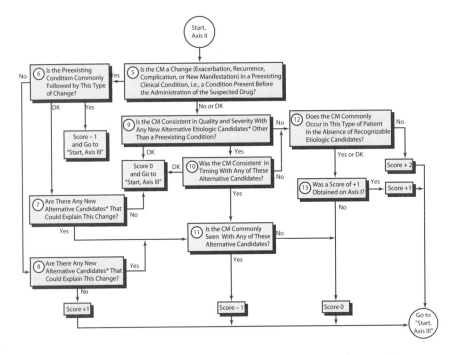

Figure 2. Axis II. Alternative etiologic candidates. For explanation of abbreviations, see Axis I.

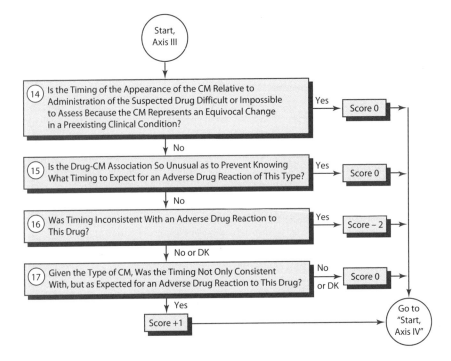

Figure 3. Axis III. Timing of events. For explanation of abbreviations, see Axis I.

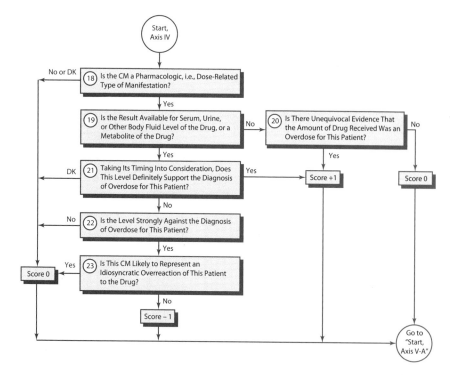

Figure 4. Axis IV. Drug levels and evidence of overdose. For explanation of abbreviations, see Axis I.

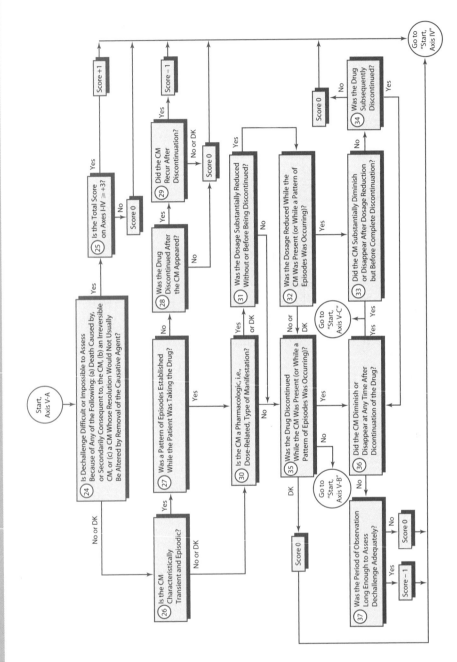

Figure 5A. Axis V-A. Dechallenge: difficult assessments. For explanation of abbreviations, see Axis I.

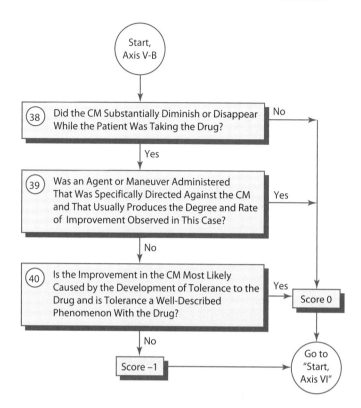

Figure 5B. Axis V-B. Dechallenge: absence of dechallenge. For explanation of abbreviation, see Axis I.

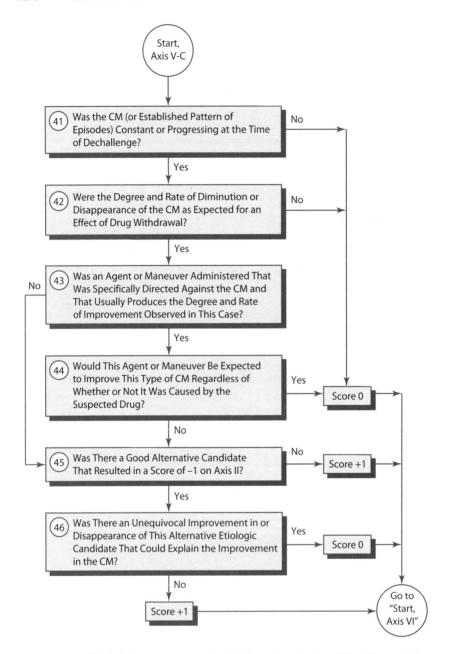

Figure 5C. Axis V-C. Dechallenge: improvement after dechallenge. For explanation of abbreviation, see Axis I.

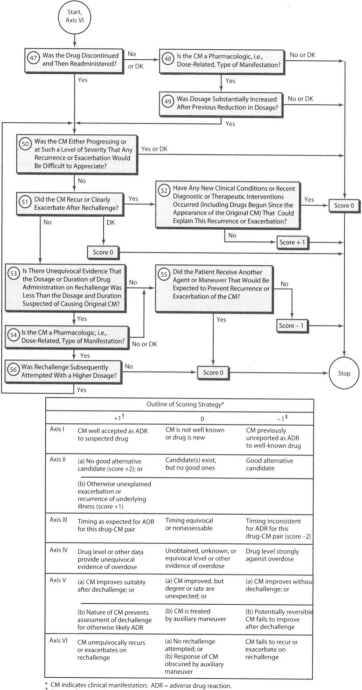

Figure 6. Axis VI. Rechallenge. For explanation of abbreviation, see Axis I.

Appendix 17–2

Naranjo Algorithm*

To assess the adverse drug reaction, please answer the following questionnaire and give the pertinent score.

	Yes	No	Don't Know	Score
1. Are there previous conclusive reports on this reaction?	+1	0	0	
2. Did the adverse event appear after the suspected drug was administered?	+2	−1	0	
3. Did the adverse reaction improve when the drug was discontinued or a specific antagonist was administered?	+1	0	0	
4. Did the adverse reaction reappear when the drug was readministered?	+2	−1	0	
5. Are there alternative causes (other than the drug) that could on their own have caused the reaction?	−1	+2	0	
6. Did the reaction reappear when a placebo was given?	−1	+1	0	
7. Was the drug detected in the blood (or other fluids) in concentrations known to be toxic?	+1	0	0	
8. Was the reaction more severe when the dose was increased, or less severe when the dose was decreased?	+1	0	0	
9. Did the patient have a similar reaction to the same or similar drugs in any previous exposure?	+1	0	0	
10. Was the adverse event confirmed by any objective evidence?	+1	0	0	
			Total Score	_____

Score Interpretation

___Definite: ≥9

___Probable: 5 to 8

___Possible: 1 to 4

___Doubtful: ≤0

---

*Naranjo CA, Busto U, Sellers EM, Sandor P, Ruiz I, Roberts EA, Janecek E, Domecq C, Greenblatt DJ. A method of estimating the probability of adverse drug reactions. Clin Pharmacol Ther. 1981;30(2):239-45.

17-3

Appendix 17–3

Jones Algorithm*

START HERE:**

```
┌─────────────────────┐          ┌─────────────────────┐
│ Does event have a   │   No     │ Causal relationship │
│ reasonable temporal │ ───────► │ considered remote.  │
│ association with    │          │                     │
│ use of the drug?    │          │                     │
└─────────────────────┘          └─────────────────────┘
        │ Yes
        ▼
┌─────────────────────┐          ┌─────────────────────┐
│ Was there a         │   No     │ Causal relationship │
│ dechallenge from    │ ───────► │ considered possible.│
│ the drug?           │          │                     │
└─────────────────────┘          └─────────────────────┘
        │ Yes
        ▼
┌─────────────────────┐          ┌─────────────────────┐
│ Did the observed    │   No     │ Causal relationship │
│ event abate upon    │ ───────► │ considered possible.│
│ dechallenge?        │          │                     │
└─────────────────────┘          └─────────────────────┘
        │ Yes
        ▼
┌─────────────────────┐   No   ┌─────────────────────┐   No   ┌─────────────────────┐
│ Was there a         │ ─────► │ Could the event be  │ ─────► │ Causal relationship │
│ rechallenge?        │        │ due to an existing  │        │ considered probable.│
│                     │        │ clinical condition? │        │                     │
└─────────────────────┘        └─────────────────────┘        └─────────────────────┘
        │ Yes                          │ Yes
        ▼                              ▼
┌─────────────────────┐   No   ┌─────────────────────┐
│ Did the reaction    │ ─────► │ Causal relationship │
│ or event reappear   │        │ considered possible.│
│ upon rechallenge?   │        │                     │
└─────────────────────┘        └─────────────────────┘
        │ Yes
        ▼
┌─────────────────────┐
│ Causal relationship │
│ considered highly   │
│ probable.           │
└─────────────────────┘
```

**Each drug is carried through independently; if >1 drug was dechallenged or rechallenged simultaneously causality for all is ≤ possible.

QUESTIONS:

1. Did the reaction follow a reasonable temporal sequence?
2. Did the patient improve after stopping the drug?
3. Did the reaction reappear on repeated exposure (rechallenge)?
4. Could the reaction be reasonably explained by the known characteristics of the patient's clinical *state*?

---

*Jones JK. Adverse drug reactions in the community health setting: approaches to recognizing, counseling, and reporting. Clin Comm Health. 1982;5(2):58-67.

Appendix 17–4

Liverpool ADR Causality Assessment Tool

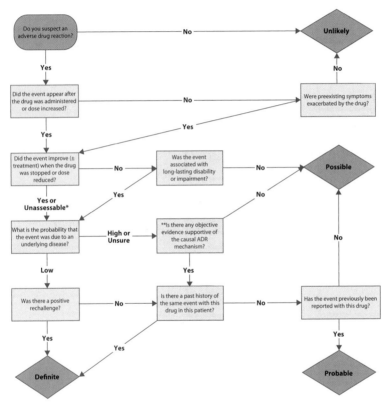

*Unassessable refers to situations where the medicine is administered on one occasion (e.g., Vaccine), the patient receives intermittent therapy (e.g., Chemotherapy), or is on medication which cannot be stopped (e.g., Immunosuppressants).

** Examples of objective evidence: positive laboratory investigation of the causal ADR mechanism (not those merely confirming the adverse reaction), supra-therapeutic drug levels, good evidence of dose-dependent relationship with toxicity in the patient.

Published with permission. Gallagher RM, Kirkham JJ, Mason JR, Bird KA, Williamson PR, Nunn AJ, Turner MA, Smyth RL, Pirmohamed M. Development and inter-rater reliability of the Liverpool Adverse Drug Reaction Causality Assessment Tool. PLoS ONE. 2011;6(12):e28096. doi:10.1371/journal.pone.0028096

Appendix 17–5

MedWatch Form

U.S. Department of Health and Human Services

MEDWATCH

The FDA Safety Information and
Adverse Event Reporting Program

For VOLUNTARY reporting of
adverse events, product problems and
product use errors

Page 1 of 3

Form Approved: OMB No. 0910-0291, Expires: 9/30/2018
See PRA statement on reverse.

FDA USE ONLY
Triage unit sequence #
FDA Rec. Date

Note: For date prompts of "dd-mmm-yyyy" please use 2-digit day, 3-letter month abbreviation, and 4-digit year; for example, 01-Jul-2015.

A. PATIENT INFORMATION

1. Patient Identifier

In Confidence

2. Age
☐ Year(s) ☐ Month(s)
☐ Week(s) ☐ Days(s)
or Date of Birth (e.g., 08 Feb 1925)

3. Sex
☐ Female
☐ Male

4. Weight
☐ lb
☐ kg

5.a. Ethnicity (Check single best answer)
☐ Hispanic/Latino
☐ Not Hispanic/Latino

5.b. Race (Check all that apply)
☐ Asian ☐ American Indian or Alaskan Native
☐ Black or African American ☐ White
☐ Native Hawaiian or Other Pacific Islander

B. ADVERSE EVENT, PRODUCT PROBLEM

1. Check all that apply
☐ Adverse Event ☐ Product Problem (e.g., defects/malfunctions)
☐ Product Use Error ☐ Problem with Different Manufacturer of Same Medicine

2. Outcome Attributed to Adverse Event (Check all that apply)
☐ Death Include date (dd-mmm-yyyy):
☐ Life-threatening ☐ Disability or Permanent Damage
☐ Hospitalization – initial or prolonged ☐ Congenital Anomaly/Birth Defects
☐ Other Serious (Important Medical Events)
☐ Required Intervention to Prevent Permanent Impairment/Damage (Devices)

3. Date of Event (dd-mmm-yyyy)

4. Date of this Report (dd-mmm-yyyy)

5. Describe Event, Problem or Product Use Error

6. Relevant Tests/Laboratory Data, Including Dates

7. Other Relevant History, Including Preexisting Medical Conditions (e.g., allergies, pregnancy, smoking and alcohol use, liver/kidney problems, etc.)

C. PRODUCT AVAILABILITY

2. Product Available for Evaluation? (Do not send product to FDA)
☐ Yes ☐ No ☐ Returned to Manufacturer on (dd-mmm-yyyy)

D. SUSPECT PRODUCTS

1. Name, Manufacturer/Compounder, Strength (from product label)

#1 – Name and Strength	#1 – NDC # or Unique ID
#1 – Manufacturer/Compounder	#1 – Lot #
#2 – Name and Strength	#2 – NDC # or Unique ID
#2 – Manufacturer/Compounder	#2 – Lot #

PLEASE TYPE OR USE BLACK INK

3. Dose or Amount | **Frequency** | **Route**
#1
#2

4. Dates of Use (From/To for each) (If unknown, give duration, or best estimate) (dd-mmm-yyyy)
#1
#2

5. Diagnosis or Reason for Use (indication)
#1
#2

6. Is the Product Compounded?
#1 ☐ Yes ☐ No
#2 ☐ Yes ☐ No

7. Is the Product Over-the-Counter?
#1 ☐ Yes ☐ No
#2 ☐ Yes ☐ No

8. Expiration Date (dd-mmm-yyyy)
#1 | #2

9. Event Abated After Use Stopped or Dose Reduced?
#1 ☐ Yes ☐ No ☐ Doesn't apply
#2 ☐ Yes ☐ No ☐ Doesn't apply

10. Event Reappeared After Reintroduction?
#1 ☐ Yes ☐ No ☐ Doesn't apply
#2 ☐ Yes ☐ No ☐ Doesn't apply

E. SUSPECT MEDICAL DEVICE

1. Brand Name

2. Common Device Name | **2b. Procode**

3. Manufacturer Name, City and State

4. Model # | **Lot #** | **5. Operator of Device**
Catalog # | Expiration Date (dd-mmm-yyyy) | ☐ Health Professional
Serial # | Unique Identifier (UDI) # | ☐ Lay User/Patient ☐ Other

6. If Implanted, Give Date (dd-mmm-yyyy) | **7. If Explanted, Give Date** (dd-mmm-yyyy)

8. Is this a single-use device that was reprocessed and reused on a patient? ☐ Yes ☐ No

9. If Yes to Item 8, Enter Name and Address of Reprocessor

F. OTHER (CONCOMITANT) MEDICAL PRODUCTS

Product names and therapy dates (Exclude treatment of event)

G. REPORTER (See confidentiality section on back)

1. Name and Address
Last Name: | First Name:
Address:
City: | State/Province/Region:
Country: | ZIP/Postal Code:
Phone #: | Email:

2. Health Professional?
☐ Yes ☐ No

3. Occupation

4. Also Reported to:
☐ Manufacturer/Compounder
☐ User Facility
☐ Distributor/Importer

5. If you do NOT want your identity disclosed to the manufacturer, please mark this box: ☐

FORM FDA 3500 (10/15) Submission of a report does not constitute an admission that medical personnel or the product caused or contributed to the event.

ADVICE ABOUT VOLUNTARY REPORTING
Detailed instructions available at: http://www.fda.gov/medwatch/report/consumer/instruct.htm

Report adverse events, product problems or product use errors with:
- Medications *(drugs or biologics)*
- Medical devices *(including in-vitro diagnostics)*
- Combination products *(medication & medical devices)*
- Human cells, tissues, and cellular and tissue-based products
- Special nutritional products *(dietary supplements, medical foods, infant formulas)*
- Cosmetics
- Food *(including beverages and ingredients added to foods)*

Report product problems - quality, performance or safety concerns such as:
- Suspected counterfeit product
- Suspected contamination
- Questionable stability
- Defective components
- Poor packaging or labeling
- Therapeutic failures (product didn't work)

Report SERIOUS adverse events. An event is serious when the patient outcome is:
- Death
- Life-threatening
- Hospitalization - initial or prolonged
- Disability or permanent damage
- Congenital anomaly/birth defect
- Required intervention to prevent permanent impairment or damage (devices)
- Other serious (important medical events)

Report even if:
- You're not certain the product caused the event
- You don't have all the details

How to report:
- Just fill in the sections that apply to your report
- Use section D for all products except medical devices
- Attach additional pages if needed
- Use a separate form for each patient
- Report either to FDA or the manufacturer *(or both)*

Other methods of reporting:
- 1-800-FDA-0178 - To FAX report
- 1-800-FDA-1088 - To report by phone
- www.fda.gov/medwatch/report.htm - To report online

If your report involves a serious adverse event with a device and it occurred in a facility outside a doctor's office, that facility may be legally required to report to FDA and/or the manufacturer. Please notify the person in that facility who would handle such reporting.

If your report involves a serious adverse event with a vaccine, call 1-800-822-7967 to report.

Confidentiality: The patient's identity is held in strict confidence by FDA and protected to the fullest extent of the law. The reporter's identity, including the identity of a self-reporter, may be shared with the manufacturer unless requested otherwise.

The information in this box applies only to requirements of the Paperwork Reduction Act of 1995

The burden time for this collection of information has been estimated to average 40 minutes per response, including the time to review instructions, search existing data sources, gather and maintain the data needed, and complete and review the collection of information. Send comments regarding this burden estimate or any other aspect of this collection of information, including suggestions for reducing this burden to:

Department of Health and Human Services	*Please DO NOT*	*OMB statement:*
Food and Drug Administration	*RETURN this form*	*"An agency may not conduct or sponsor, and a*
Office of Chief Information Officer	*to the PRA Staff e-mail*	*person is not required to respond to, a collection of*
Paperwork Reduction Act (PRA) Staff	*to the left.*	*information unless it displays a currently valid*
PRAStaff@fda.hhs.gov		*OMB control number."*

U.S. DEPARTMENT OF HEALTH AND HUMAN SERVICES
Food and Drug Administration

FORM FDA 3500 (10/15) (Back)   Please Use Address Provided Below -- Fold in Thirds, Tape and Mail

---

DEPARTMENT OF HEALTH & HUMAN SERVICES

Public Health Service
Food and Drug Administration
Rockville, MD 20857

Official Business
Penalty for Private Use $300

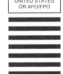

NO POSTAGE NECESSARY IF MAILED IN THE UNITED STATES OR APO/FPO

BUSINESS REPLY MAIL
FIRST CLASS MAIL PERMIT NO. 946 ROCKVILLE MD

POSTAGE WILL BE PAID BY FOOD AND DRUG ADMINISTRATION

MEDWATCH
The FDA Safety Information and Adverse Event Reporting Program
Food and Drug Administration
5600 Fishers Lane
Rockville, MD 20852-9787

U.S. Department of Health and Human Services

MEDWATCH

The FDA Safety Information and
Adverse Event Reporting Program

FORM FDA 3500 (10/15) *(continued)*

(CONTINUATION PAGE)

For **VOLUNTARY** reporting of
adverse events and product problems

Page 3 of 3

B.5. **Describe Event or Problem** *(continued)*

B.6. **Relevant Tests/Laboratory Data, Including Dates** *(continued)*

B.7. **Other Relevant History, Including Preexisting Medical Conditions** *(e.g., allergies, pregnancy, smoking and alcohol use, hepatic/renal dysfunction, etc.) (continued)*

F. **Concomitant Medical Products and Therapy Dates** *(Exclude treatment of event) (continued)*

Appendix 19–1

Policy Example: High-Alert Medications

I. PURPOSE:

This policy outlines the process for the safe use of high-alert medications.

II. DEFINITIONS:

When used in this policy these terms have the following meanings:

  A. High-alert medications: Medications that have a higher risk of causing harm when an error occurs.

  B. Independent double verification (IDV):

  1. Is performed by two staff members (as appropriate to the task, e.g., blood administration, breast milk retrieval) in the same proximity but separately, without prompting by another, as an independent cognitive task.

  2. Both professionals will dialog to confirm what was checked independently prior to administration.

  3. IDV of a medication also includes the following steps in addition to the two steps above:

  a. Performed by two professionals (e.g., nurse/pharmacist/physician [within the approved LPN scope of practice]) in the same proximity but separately, without prompting by another, as an independent cognitive task.

  b. Each professional must check: the actual prescriber's order, drug, calculation, concentration, and other information specific to the medication.

  c. Each professional performing the verification performs all calculations independently without knowledge of any prior calculations and documents the verification in the medical record.

III. POLICY:

It is the policy of the health system that:

  A. All systems and data repositories relating to medication use (medication error reports, adverse drug event reports, etc.) shall be systematically evaluated on an ongoing basis to identify those medications in the hospital formulary determined to be high-alert medications.

  B. Medications being added to the hospital formulary shall be evaluated for their high-alert potential.

  C. Medications identified as high alert shall be targeted for specific error reduction interventions.

D. The following three principles shall be followed to safeguard the use of high-alert medications:
   1. Reduce or eliminate the possibility of error (e.g., limit the number of high-alert medications on the hospital formulary; remove high-alert medications from the clinical areas).
   2. Make errors visible by detecting serious events before they reach the patient (e.g., follow the five rights and when appropriate utilize the independent double verification process).
   3. Minimize the consequences of errors (e.g., stock high-alert medications in smaller volume units of use minimizing the error effect if the medication was administered in error).
E. Engineering safety controls shall be used as appropriate.

IV. PROCEDURE:

A. The Pharmacy and Therapeutics Committee will approve all medications added to the formulary.
B. The following processes for safeguarding high-alert medication use have been implemented:
   1. Build in system redundancies (e.g., unit dose drug distribution).
   2. Use fail-safes (e.g., pumps with locking mechanisms).
   3. Reduce options (e.g., limit concentration available).
   4. Utilize engineering safety controls (e.g., oral syringes that will not fit IV tubing, computer systems that force the order of standardized products).
   5. Externalize or centralize error-prone processes (e.g., centralize IV solution preparations).
   6. Use differentiation (e.g., identify and isolate look-alike and sound-alike products, use generic names).
   7. Store medications appropriately (e.g., separate potentially dangerous drugs with similar names or similar packaging).
   8. Screen new products (e.g., inspect all new drugs and drug delivery devices for poor labeling and/or packaging).
   9. Standardize and simplify order communication (e.g., only approved abbreviations will be used, all verbal orders will be read back verbatim to the ordering physician).
   10. Limit access (e.g., high-alert medications will be securely stored).
   11. Use of constraints (e.g., pharmacy will screen all medication orders, automatic stop orders, or duration limits).
   12. Standardize or automate dosing procedures (e.g., use of standard dosing charts rather than calculating doses based on weight or renal function when appropriate).
C. When initiating any high-alert medication by any route, and for those high-alert medications administered via pump, and with all subsequent bag/syringe changes and with dose changes requiring pump adjustment, the following must occur:
   1. Independent double verification, each professional will independently:
      a. Review/verify the physician order in the medical record (i.e., on the physician's order sheet or in the clinical information system).

     b. Verify the correct medication, dose (all required dosage calculations must be done independently by each nurse), frequency/rate/titration, and route against the order.

       1) Note: After the initial IDV, ongoing titration in Level I areas is exempt from the IDV process for each continuing adjustment.

       2) Some medications require IDV of pump settings at change of shift (e.g., insulin).

       3) Additional information regarding medication-specific IDV requirements is available in the IDV Policy and Procedure.

  2. The nurse administering the medication will:

     a. Identify the patient using two acceptable identifiers.

     b. Verify the correct connection/patient access when administering the medication via an intravenous drip, trace the flow of the medication from the bag > to the pump > to the patient access, prior to hanging the medication.

     c. Document the verification.

  D. When an infusion device with prebuilt infusion parameters is used and preset infusion parameters are not available for a high-alert medication (e.g., when the medication is new and not yet added to the library), independent double verification of the medication parameters programmed into the pump must occur prior to initiation of the infusion.

V. DOCUMENTATION:

As appropriate in the medical record or clinical information system.

VI. REFERENCES:

A. Institute for Safe Medication Practices (ISMP); ISMP's list of high-alert medications. 2008.

B. Patient Care Policy and Procedure #0282, *Independent Double Verification.*

C. Patient Care Policy and Procedure #0500, *Verbal Orders.*

D. Patient Care Policy and Procedure #0700, *Abbreviations.*

E. Patient Care Policy and Procedure #0282, *IDV.*

F. Patient Care Policy and Procedure #5010, *Anticoagulant Safety.*

G. Patient Care Policy and Procedure #5020, *Chemotherapy: Oncology/Hematology.*

H. Patient Care Policy and Procedure #5070, *Electrolyte Infusions.*

I. Patient Care Policy and Procedure #5117, *Insulin Intravenous Infusions.*

J. Patient Care Policy and Procedure #5130, *Medication Administration.*

K. Patient Care Policy and Procedure #5131, *Medfusion Syringe Infusion Pump.*

L. Patient Care Policy and Procedure #5140, *Medication Use Analysis/Error Prevention.*

M. Patient Care Policy and Procedure #5150, *Moderate/Deep Sedation/Analgesia.*

VII. ATTACHMENTS:

High-Alert Medications/Classes, one page.

Source: Used by permission from Orlando Health, Orlando, FL. Available from: www.orlandohealth.com

High-Alert Medications/Classes	Safeguards, Etc.
Chemotherapy agents (all routes, includes antineoplastic, biological, immunological agents used for malignant oncology and hematology diagnoses)	Chemotherapy Policy and Procedure outlines requirements for independent double verification (IDV) of order, laboratory parameters, body surface area, medication, dose, route, frequency, etc.
	Chemotherapy order form (or electronic equivalent) required
	Only attending physicians with chemotherapy privileges may write orders
	No verbal or telephone orders allowed (except to clarify as outlined in policy)
	Only Chemo-verified RN's may administer (exceptions are made for some oral agents, refer to the Chemotherapy Policy and Procedure for details)
IV Electrolytes (i.e., potassium chloride and phosphate, concentrated sodium chloride, magnesium sulfate, calcium chloride, and calcium gluconate)	Independent double verification required (IDV not required for 1,000 mL premixed IV solutions)
	No concentrated products outside Pharmacy (*Rare exceptions exist, but only with specific safeguards*)
	Electrolyte policy provides specific administration parameters and limits
	Electrolyte replacement protocol includes dosing and monitoring parameters
	Standard concentrations/premixes
Intravenous/subcutaneous anticoagulants (i.e., heparin, lepirudin, enoxaparin, argatroban, bivalirudin—excluding flushes)	Independent double verification required
	Weight-based protocol for heparin. The prescriber must designate the specific protocol (e.g., cardiac, noncardiac) to be implemented
	Duplication warning in Clinical Information System
	Standardized order review requirements for enoxaparin and fondaparinux
	Standardized laboratory assessments for heparin, enoxaparin, and fondaparinux for treatment of deep vein thrombosis/pulmonary embolism
	Premixed heparin solutions in standard concentrations
Neuromuscular blocking agents	IDV required
	Availability limited to specific units and access limited on these units (e.g., emergency department, operating room, intensive care unit)
	Special labeling of packages
	Standard concentrations established
Insulin	IDV required (Note: verification of the insulin product is not required when insulin is supplied directly from pharmacy in patient-specific units of use [e.g., prefilled syringes versus vials])
	Floor stock limited to specific agents and Pharmacy removes unused patient-specific vials from patient care units daily
	Resources include the Insulin Infusion Policy and the IV push insulin parameters defined within policy
	Sliding scale order sets create a consistent process

continued

High-Alert Medications/Classes	Safeguards, Etc.
Anesthetic agents used outside the OR (e.g., propofol, ketamine, methohexital, etomidate, dexmedetomidine)	IDV required
	Guidelines for use and administration of propofol
	These agents have been added to the Moderate-Deep Sedation Policy with defined safeguards for use
Warfarin	IDV required
	Standard administration time to allow access to International Normalized Ratio (INR) results prior to daily dosing
	Laboratory monitoring standards and standardized order review processes
	Critical value—clinical laboratory calls with INR results >5
	Automated dispensing cabinet (ADC) inquiry—nurse is asked if he/she knows the patient's current INR as warfarin is being taken from ADC for administration to the patient
	Pharmacy monitoring of at-risk patients

20-1

Appendix 20–1

Example of a Project Charter

GOALS

The primary goal of this IV workflow improvement project is to eliminate all preventable patient harm when compounding medications. It is believed that by accomplishing the following secondary goals, significant progress toward improving patient safety will also be made:

1. Ensure correct ingredients in each compound.
2. Ensure correct quantities of admixtures in each compound.
3. Create standard compounding processes in conjunction with the electronic health record (EHR) system.
4. Ensure a retrievable historical compounding record to reference in scenarios of patient safety concern.
5. Facilitate the ability for pharmacists to remotely verify compound accuracy.
6. Facilitate compounding standards adoption.
7. Implement an automation solution that ensures the other goals are met.
8. Track and measure waste.

Through the research and selection process, Compounding Software X has been determined to be the best available automation solution for these specific needs. Within the next 12 months, the goal is to implement Software X at all hospitals throughout the health care system.

SUCCESS CRITERIA

This IV workflow improvement project will be considered a success when the following has been achieved:

	Goal	Success Criteria
1	Ensure correct ingredients in each compound.	Create a standard list of compounded products.
2	Ensure correct quantities of admixture in each compound.	Create a standard list of recipes and procedures for compounding.
3	Create standard compounding processes in conjunction with the electronic health record system.	Create a list of drugs, and all associated data points, for use in compounding.

continued

	Goal	Success Criteria
4	Ensure a retrievable historical compounding record to reference in scenarios of patient safety concern.	Develop, build, and integrate within the enterprise data warehouse repository.
5	Facilitate the ability for pharmacists to remotely verify compound accuracy.	Create a practice model, procedure, roles, and responsibilities for remote and collocated verification.
6	Facilitate compounding standards adoption.	Finalize, communicate, and enforce a benchmark percentage of compounded drugs and high-risk compounds to be created using automation technology.
7	Implement an automation solution that ensures the other goals are met.	All hospitals within the health system are using Software X for IV compounding.
8	Track and measure waste.	Finalize, communicate, and enforce a benchmark percentage of waste reduction that can be tracked and monitored using automation technology.

DELIVERABLES

The high-level deliverables for this project are as follows:

	Success Criteria		Deliverables
1	Create a standard list of compounded products.	1.1	Collaborate with facility teams to identify list of compounds to standardize.
		1.2	Create a workflow for maintenance within the hospital formulary.
		1.3	Create a workflow for maintenance of the software formulary.
		1.4	Create governance process for standard compounded products list.
2	Create a standard list of recipes and procedures for compounding.	2.1	Create a list of standard compounds and identify the piece of technology on which each solution will be created.
		2.2	Create a downtime procedure for standard compounding without the software technology.
		2.3	Standardize recipe, drug data, and process for each compound.
		2.4	Ensure new standards align with system standards and the hospital formulary.
3	Create a list of drugs, and all associated data points, for use in compounding.	3.1	Create a bidirectional interface between the electronic health record and the IV compounding software.
		3.2	Populate the database with standard compounds.
4	Develop, build, and integrate within the enterprise data warehouse repository.	4.1	Build a method to facilitate data transfer from the Software X server to the enterprise data warehouse.
		4.2	Create reporting and data analysis requirements to inform the data transfer method.
		4.3	Define storage parameters.

continued

	Success Criteria		Deliverables
5	Create a practice model, procedure, roles, and responsibilities for remote and collocated verification.	5.1	Create a workflow for collocated verification.
		5.2	Create a workflow for remote verification.
		5.3	Create a downtime procedure for remote verification.
		5.4	Create formal education for pharmacy team members.
		5.5	Create formal education for non-pharmacy team members.
6	Finalize, communicate, and enforce a benchmark percentage of compounded drugs and high-risk compounds to be created using automation technology.	6.1	Update the compounding policies, procedures, and guidelines.
7	All hospitals within the health system are using Software X for IV compounding.	7.1	Create an installation readiness matrix and assess each location for installation.
		7.2	Implement Software X at three hospitals.
8	Finalize, communicate, and enforce a benchmark percentage of waste reduction that can be tracked and monitored using automation technology.	8.1	Create reporting and data analysis requirements to inform the data extract and load.

SCOPE

In Scope: These items will be addressed by this project.	Out of Scope: These items will not be addressed by this project.
Development of batch-processing workflow with the IV compounding software	Infusion Center compounding practices
Electronic health record interface	Parenteral nutrition
IV admixtures, non-hazardous	Premixed IV medications (including minibags)
IV admixtures, hazardous	New hospitals that are planned but construction is not complete
	Oral non-sterile extemporaneous compounds

KEY STAKEHOLDERS

Name	Org./Dept./Title	Role	Contact Information
John Washington	Hospital Pharmacy Operations Director	Executive Sponsor	XXX-XXX-XXXX
Kathryn Morris	Medication Policy & Outcomes Director	Executive Sponsor	XXX-XXX-XXXX
Robert Henry	Pharmacy Automation and Technology Manager	Project Owner	XXX-XXX-XXXX
Eliot Cogan	Drug Information Manager	Subject Matter Expert	XXX-XXX-XXXX
Natalie Smyth	Project Manager	Project Manager	XXX-XXX-XXXX
Emily Garfield	Automation and Technology Pharmacy Technician	Subject Matter Expert	XXX-XXX-XXXX
Michael Kline	National Strategic Accounts Manager, Software Company X	Software X account representative	XXX-XXX-XXXX

PROJECT BUDGET

Funds have been secured to implement the IV workflow at each hospital. As with most new technology, there are significant upfront costs for both the software and hardware ($10,000 per workstation). When fully implemented, the annual maintenance fees will be $75,000 per year with an unlimited number of workstations within the health care system. Projections have identified the need for 50 workstations for the enterprise. In this regard, the annual maintenance fees will be approximately $1,500 per workstation per year. In contrast, the request for proposal (RFP) from the company not selected was listed as $15,500 per workstation per year until the organization reached 50 workstations, and then the cost dropped to $9,000 per workstation per year. At full capacity the annual maintenance for the selected product is significantly less than the competitor. The company has also agreed to price protection in the contract. The hardware costs include scales, bar code scanners, cameras, monitors, and a keyboard (specifically designed to be in a cleanroom).

Contract Funding

Purchase Costs	Year #1	Year #2	Each Additional Year
Service fees or license fees	$400,000		
Implementation	$175,000		
Training costs	$25,000		
Hardware	$800,000		
Maintenance fees		$75,000	$75,000
Total cost	**$1,400,000**	**$75,000**	**$75,000**

Hardware Funding Per Facility

Hospital	No. of Workstations	Cost per Workstation	Hardware Cost
Hospital 1	5	$10,000	$50,000
Hospital 2	8	$10,000	$80,000
Hospital 3	4	$10,000	$40,000
Total hardware costs year # 1			$170,000

CONSTRAINTS, ASSUMPTIONS, RISKS, AND DEPENDENCIES

Constraints

- The initial project scope will not encompass all compounded products. The expansion of the system to include all compounded products will happen during optimization.
- An installation readiness assessment will be conducted for each installation site at every location. Each site must meet the readiness criteria for installation to begin.

Assumptions

- Use of a software solution during IV compounding is not currently a standard practice at the hospitals. The assumption is that staff will adopt this practice to accommodate the project and mitigate patient risk in compounding.

Risks

- Installation of power and data was not factored into the original budget. Hospitals will need to fund the construction required to pull power and data.
- If approved for a site, augmenting the barrier isolators will require contract labor, the cost of which was not included in the original budget.

20-2

Appendix 20–2

Stakeholder Matrix—IV Compounding Software Project

Name	Position	Role	Contact Information	Requirements	Expectations	Classification
Stakeholder's name	*Position in the organization*	*The function they perform on the project*	*Communication and correspondence information*	*High-level needs or wants for the project/product*	*High-level expectations from the project/product*	*See classification table below*
John Washington	Hospital Pharmacy Operations Director	Primary Executive Sponsor	Weekly meetings	Improved IV workflow	Patient safety improvement and operational efficiency	C
Kathryn Morris	Medication Policy and Outcomes Director	Secondary Executive Sponsor	Weekly e-mail	Formulary and recipe standardization	System-wide standardization and improved patient safety	C
Robert Henry	Pharmacy Automation and Technology Manager	Project Owner	Weekly meetings	Implementation system wide	Patient safety improvement and operational efficiency	D
Gregory Smith	Drug Information Specialist	Project participant	Weekly meetings	Formulary and recipe validation and standardization	System-wide standardization and improved patient safety	D
Dean Kipling	Inpatient Pharmacy Operations Manager	Interested in project	Monthly e-mail	Improved IV workflow	Improved patient safety and operational efficiency	B

*A = monitor; B = keep informed; C = keep satisfied; D = manage closely/key stakeholder.

Appendix 20-3

Example PESTLE Analysis—IV Compounding Software Project

Categories	Factors	What Does It Affect?	Probability of Impact (Rate 1–5)*	Severity of Impact (Rate 1–5)*	Score (Add Previous Two Columns)	Potential Responses	Who Will Monitor This Factor?
1 Political	Pharmacy Services	Hospital leadership reorganization may result in Key Stakeholders changes to include Central Entities hospital representation. This may ultimately impact the priorities of the project.	3	2	5	Prioritize the project as requested	Project owner
2 Economic	Unplanned Funding	Completing the facility work required to prepare an installation site for implementation may require leaders from that location to acquire additional funding. The facility work (including running data and power, adding data switches, buying biosafety cabinets, and/or remodeling clean rooms) was not budgeted in the original project cost estimates.	4	5	9	Inquire with Central Entities if they could support funding for the site(s)	Project owner
5 Social	Front-line staff response	The successful completion of this project is dependent upon a significant amount of standardization. Front-line staff will likely have a variety of responses to the new technology, application permissions, and compounding recipes as well as the new governance process.	4	3	7	Develop a communication plan outlining benefits to patient safety	Project owner

Appendix 20–4

Example Work Breakdown Structure (WBS)—IV Compounding Software Project

WBS ID	Action Item	Predecessor	Individual Responsible	Start Date	Effort	Duration
1.0	**Create governance process for identifying and managing system standard compounded products**		**Robert Henry**		**9 days**	**9 days**
1.1	Determine, document, and communicate that pharmacy team members throughout the system need to participate on this committee	—	Robert Henry		1 day	1 day
1.2	Determine, document, and communicate the frequency with which this committee needs to meet	—	Robert Henry		1 day	1 day
1.3	Determine, document, and communicate the decisions, rights, and reporting structure for this new committee	—	Robert Henry		1 day	1 day
1.4	Determine, document, and communicate a system leader for this committee	—	Robert Henry		1 day	1 day
1.5	Develop and document a committee charter	—	Robert Henry		5 days	5 days
2.0	**Create system standards for compounded products**		**Eliot Cogan**		**24 days**	**184 days**
2.1	**Identify initial compounds to standardize**		**Eliot Cogan**		**5 days**	**92 days**
2.1.1	Create a criteria matrix for compounds that can and will be created using the IV software	—	Robert Henry		1 day	1 day
2.1.2	Review inventory provided by Pharmacy Informatics team of all compounds created throughout system	—	Eliot Cogan		1 day	1 day
2.1.3	Assess all compounds created throughout system against criteria matrix	2.1.1	Eliot Cogan		1 day	30 days
2.1.4	Committee will approve and document compounding opportunities	2.1.3	Eliot Cogan		1 day	30 days

continued

WBS ID	Action Item	Predecessor	Individual Responsible	Start Date	Effort	Duration
2.1.5	Request feedback and elaboration from hospital pharmacies on the compounds they are creating (as needed)	2.1.4	Eliot Cogan		1 day	30 days
2.2	**Create a standard list of recipes and procedures for compounding**		**Eliot Cogan**		**19 days**	**92 days**
2.2.1	Review inventory provided by Pharmacy Informatics team of all compound recipes created throughout system	—	Eliot Cogan		1 day	1 day
2.2.2	Evaluate tertiary and primary references to validate compounds and associated information (i.e., beyond use date); verify that best practice aligns with system formulary	2.1.3	Eliot Cogan		15 days	50 days
2.2.3	Committee will review and approve best practice for each compound	2.2.2	Eliot Cogan		2 days	40 days
2.2.4	Record and communicate best practice for each compound	2.2.3	Eliot Cogan		1 day	1 day

Appendix 21–1

Investigational New Drug Application

Next Page	Export Data	Import Data	Reset Form

DEPARTMENT OF HEALTH AND HUMAN SERVICES
Food and Drug Administration

INVESTIGATIONAL NEW DRUG APPLICATION (IND)
(Title 21, Code of Federal Regulations (CFR) Part 312)

Form Approved: OMB No. 0910-0014
Expiration Date: February 28, 2019
See PRA Statement on page 3.

NOTE: No drug/biologic may be shipped or clinical investigation begun until an IND for that investigation is in effect (21 CFR 312.40)

1. Name of Sponsor	2. Date of Submission *(mm/dd/yyyy)*

3. Sponsor Address

Address 1 *(Street address, P.O. box, company name c/o)*

Address 2 *(Apartment, suite, unit, building, floor, etc.)*

City	State/Province/Region
Country	ZIP or Postal Code

4. Telephone Number *(Include country code if applicable and area code)*

5. Name(s) of Drug *(Include all available names: Trade, Generic, Chemical, or Code)*

[Continuation Page for #5]

6. IND Number *(If previously assigned)*

7. (Proposed) Indication for Use

Is this indication for a rare disease (prevalence <200,000 in U.S.)? ☐ Yes ☐ No

Does this product have an FDA Orphan Designation for this indication? ☐ Yes ☐ No

If yes, provide the Orphan Designation number for this indication: [Continuation Page for #7]

8. Phase(s) of Clinical Investigation to be conducted ☐ Phase 1 ☐ Phase 2 ☐ Phase 3 ☐ Other *(Specify):* ___

9. List numbers of all Investigational New Drug Applications (21 CFR Part 312), New Drug Applications (21 CFR Part 314), Drug Master Files (21 CFR Part 314.420), and Biologics License Applications (21 CFR Part 601) referred to in this application.

10. IND submission should be consecutively numbered. The initial IND should be numbered "Serial number: 0000." The next submission (e.g., amendment, report, or correspondence) should be numbered "Serial Number: 0001." Subsequent submissions should be numbered consecutively in the order in which they are submitted.

Serial Number

___ ___ ___ ___

11. This submission contains the following *(Select all that apply)*

☐ Initial Investigational New Drug Application (IND)
☐ Request For Reactivation Or Reinstatement
☐ Development Safety Update Report (DSUR)

☐ Response to Clinical Hold
☐ Annual Report
☐ Other *(Specify):* ___

☐ Response To FDA Request For Information
☐ General Correspondence

Protocol Amendment(s)	Information Amendment(s)	Request for	IND Safety Report(s)
☐ New Protocol ☐ Human Factors Protocol	☐ Chemistry/Microbiology	☐ Meeting	☐ Initial Written Report
☐ Change in Protocol	☐ Pharmacology/Toxicology	☐ Proprietary Name Review	☐ Follow-up to a Written Report
☐ New Investigator	☐ Clinical/Safety ☐ Statistics	☐ Special Protocol Assessment	
☐ PMR/PMC Protocol	☐ Clinical Pharmacology	☐ Formal Dispute Resolution	

12. Select the following only if applicable. *(Justification statement must be submitted with application for any items selected below. Refer to the cited CFR section for further information.)*

Expanded Access Use, 21 CFR 312.300

☐ Emergency Research Exception From Informed Consent Requirements, 21 CFR 312.23 (f)
☐ Charge Request, 21 CFR 312.8

☐ Individual Patient, Non-Emergency 21 CFR 312.310
☐ Individual Patient, Emergency 21 CFR 312.310(d)

☐ Intermediate Size Patient Population, 21 CFR 312.315
☐ Treatment IND or Protocol, 21 CFR 312.320

For FDA Use Only

CBER/DCC Receipt Stamp	DDR Receipt Stamp	Division Assignment
		IND Number Assigned

FORM FDA 1571 (3/17)　　　Page 1 of 3　　　PSC Publishing Services (301) 443-6740　EF

| Previous Page | Next Page |

13. Contents of Application – This application contains the following items *(Select all that apply)*

- [ ] 1. Form FDA 1571 *(21 CFR 312.23(a)(1))*
- [ ] 2. Table of Contents *(21 CFR 312.23(a)(2))*
- [ ] 3. Introductory statement *(21 CFR 312.23(a)(3))*
- [ ] 4. General Investigational plan *(21 CFR 312.23(a)(3))*
- [ ] 5. Investigator's brochure *(21 CFR 312.23(a)(5))*
- [ ] 6. Protocol(s) *(21 CFR 312.23(a)(6))*
  - [ ] a. Study protocol(s) *(21 CFR 312.23(a)(6))*
  - [ ] b. Investigator data *(21 CFR 312.23(a)(6)(iii)(b))* or completed Form(s) FDA 1572
  - [ ] c. Facilities data *(21 CFR 312.23(a)(6)(iii)(b))* or completed Form(s) FDA 1572

6. Protocol(s) *(Continued)*
- [ ] d. Institutional Review Board data (21 CFR 312.23(a)(6)(iii) (b)) or completed Form(s) FDA 1572
- [ ] 7. Chemistry, manufacturing, and control data *(21 CFR 312.23(a)(7))*
  - [ ] Environmental assessment or claim for exclusion *(21 CFR 312.23(a)(7)(iv)(e))*
- [ ] 8. Pharmacology and toxicology data (21 CFR 312.23(a)(8))
- [ ] 9. Previous human experience *(21 CFR 312.23(a)(9))*
- [ ] 10. Additional information *(21 CFR 312.23(a)(10))*
- [ ] 11. Biosimilar User Fee Cover Sheet *(Form FDA 3792)*
- [ ] 12. Clinical Trials Certification of Compliance *(Form FDA 3674)*

14. Is any part of the clinical study to be conducted by a contract research organization? [ ] Yes [ ] No

If Yes, will any sponsor obligations be transferred to the contract research organization? [ ] Yes [ ] No

If Yes, provide a statement containing the name and address of the contract research organization, identification of the clinical study, and a listing of the obligations transferred *(use continuation page)*.

| Continuation Page for #14 |

15. Name and Title of the person responsible for monitoring the conduct and progress of the clinical investigations

16. Name(s) and Title(s) of the person(s) responsible for review and evaluation of information relevant to the safety of the drug

I agree not to begin clinical investigations until 30 days after FDA's receipt of the IND unless I receive earlier notification by FDA that the studies may begin. I also agree not to begin or continue clinical investigations covered by the IND if those studies are placed on clinical hold or financial hold. I agree that an Institutional Review Board (IRB) that complies with the requirements set forth in 21 CFR Part 56 will be responsible for initial and continuing review and approval of each of the studies in the proposed clinical investigation. I agree to conduct the investigation in accordance with all other applicable regulatory requirements.

17. Name of Sponsor or Sponsor's Authorized Representative

18. Telephone Number *(Include country code if applicable and area code)*

19. Facsimile (FAX) Number *(Include country code if applicable and area code)*

20. Address

Address 1 *(Street address, P.O. box, company name c/o)*

Address 2 *(Apartment, suite, unit, building, floor, etc.)*

City

State/Province/Region

Country

ZIP or Postal Code

21. Email Address

22. Date of Sponsor's Signature *(mm/dd/yyyy)*

23. Name of Countersigner

24. Address of Countersigner

Address 1 *(Street address, P.O. box, company name c/o)*

Address 2 *(Apartment, suite, unit, building, floor, etc.)*

City

State/Province/Region

Country
United States of America

ZIP or Postal Code

25. Email Address

WARNING : A willfully false statement is a criminal offense (U.S.C. Title 18, Sec. 1001).

26. Signature of Sponsor or Sponsor's Authorized Representative

| Sign |

27. Signature of Countersigner

| Sign |

The information below applies only to requirements of the Paperwork Reduction Act of 1995.

The burden time for this collection of information is estimated to average 100 hours per response, including the time to review instructions, search existing data sources, gather and maintain the data needed and complete and review the collection of information. Send comments regarding this burden estimate or any other aspect of this information collection, including suggestions for reducing this burden to the address to the right:

"An agency may not conduct or sponsor, and a person is not required to respond to, a collection of information unless it displays a currently valid OMB number."

Department of Health and Human Services
Food and Drug Administration
Office of Operations
Paperwork Reduction Act (PRA) Staff
PRAStaff@fda.hhs.gov

Please do NOT send your completed form to this PRA Staff email address.

Appendix 21–2

Statement of Investigator

DEPARTMENT OF HEALTH AND HUMAN SERVICES FOOD AND DRUG ADMINISTRATION **STATEMENT OF INVESTIGATOR** *(TITLE 21, CODE OF FEDERAL REGULATIONS (CFR) PART 312)* (See instructions on reverse side.)	Form Approved: OMB No. 0910-0014 Expiration Date: April 30, 2015 *See OMB Statement on Reverse.* NOTE: No investigator may participate in an investigation until he/she provides the sponsor with a completed, signed Statement of Investigator, Form FDA 1572 (21 CFR 312.53(c)).

1. NAME AND ADDRESS OF INVESTIGATOR

Name of Principal Investigator

Address 1		Address 2	
City	State/Province/Region	Country	ZIP or Postal Code

2. EDUCATION, TRAINING, AND EXPERIENCE THAT QUALIFY THE INVESTIGATOR AS AN EXPERT IN THE CLINICAL INVESTIGATION OF THE DRUG FOR THE USE UNDER INVESTIGATION. ONE OF THE FOLLOWING IS PROVIDED *(Select one of the following.)*

☐ Curriculum Vitae   ☐ Other Statement of Qualifications

3. NAME AND ADDRESS OF ANY MEDICAL SCHOOL, HOSPITAL, OR OTHER RESEARCH FACILITY WHERE THE CLINICAL INVESTIGATION(S) WILL BE CONDUCTED

CONTINUATION PAGE for Item 3

Name of Medical School, Hospital, or Other Research Facility

Address 1		Address 2	
City	State/Province/Region	Country	ZIP or Postal Code

4. NAME AND ADDRESS OF ANY CLINICAL LABORATORY FACILITIES TO BE USED IN THE STUDY

CONTINUATION PAGE for Item 4

Name of Clinical Laboratory Facility

Address 1		Address 2	
City	State/Province/Region	Country	ZIP or Postal Code

5. NAME AND ADDRESS OF THE INSTITUTIONAL REVIEW BOARD (IRB) THAT IS RESPONSIBLE FOR REVIEW AND APPROVAL OF THE STUDY(IES)

CONTINUATION PAGE for Item 5

Name of IRB

Address 1		Address 2	
City	State/Province/Region	Country	ZIP or Postal Code

6. NAMES OF SUBINVESTIGATORS *(If not applicable, enter "None")*

CONTINUATION PAGE – for Item 6

7. NAME AND CODE NUMBER, IF ANY, OF THE PROTOCOL(S) IN THE IND FOR THE STUDY(IES) TO BE CONDUCTED BY THE INVESTIGATOR

FORM FDA 1572 (7/13)   PREVIOUS EDITION IS OBSOLETE.   Page 1 of

PSC Publishing Services (301) 443-6740   EF

8. PROVIDE THE FOLLOWING CLINICAL PROTOCOL INFORMATION. *(Select **one** of the following.)*

☐ For Phase 1 investigations, a general outline of the planned investigation including the estimated duration of the study and the maximum number of subjects that will be involved.

☐ For Phase 2 or 3 investigations, an outline of the study protocol including an approximation of the number of subjects to be treated with the drug and the number to be employed as controls, if any; the clinical uses to be investigated; characteristics of subjects by age, sex, and condition; the kind of clinical observations and laboratory tests to be conducted; the estimated duration of the study; and copies or a description of case report forms to be used.

9. COMMITMENTS

I agree to conduct the study(ies) in accordance with the relevant, current protocol(s) and will only make changes in a protocol after notifying the sponsor, except when necessary to protect the safety, rights, or welfare of subjects.

I agree to personally conduct or supervise the described investigation(s).

I agree to inform any patients, or any persons used as controls, that the drugs are being used for investigational purposes and I will ensure that the requirements relating to obtaining informed consent in 21 CFR Part 50 and institutional review board (IRB) review and approval in 21 CFR Part 56 are met.

I agree to report to the sponsor adverse experiences that occur in the course of the investigation(s) in accordance with 21 CFR 312.64. I have read and understand the information in the investigator's brochure, including the potential risks and side effects of the drug.

I agree to ensure that all associates, colleagues, and employees assisting in the conduct of the study(ies) are informed about their obligations in meeting the above commitments.

I agree to maintain adequate and accurate records in accordance with 21 CFR 312.62 and to make those records available for inspection in accordance with 21 CFR 312.68.

I will ensure that an IRB that complies with the requirements of 21 CFR Part 56 will be responsible for the initial and continuing review and approval of the clinical investigation. I also agree to promptly report to the IRB all changes in the research activity and all unanticipated problems involving risks to human subjects or others. Additionally, I will not make any changes in the research without IRB approval, except where necessary to eliminate apparent immediate hazards to human subjects.

I agree to comply with all other requirements regarding the obligations of clinical investigators and all other pertinent requirements in 21 CFR Part 312.

INSTRUCTIONS FOR COMPLETING FORM FDA 1572
STATEMENT OF INVESTIGATOR

1. Complete all sections. Provide a separate page if additional space is needed.

2. Provide curriculum vitae or other statement of qualifications as described in Section 2.

3. Provide protocol outline as described in Section 8.

4. Sign and date below.

5. FORWARD THE COMPLETED FORM AND OTHER DOCUMENTS BEING PROVIDED TO THE SPONSOR. The sponsor will incorporate this information along with other technical data into an Investigational New Drug Application (IND). INVESTIGATORS SHOULD NOT SEND THIS FORM DIRECTLY TO THE FOOD AND DRUG ADMINISTRATION.

10. DATE *(mm/dd/yyyy)*	11. SIGNATURE OF INVESTIGATOR	Sign

(**WARNING**: A willfully false statement is a criminal offense. U.S.C. Title 18, Sec. 1001.)

The information below applies only to requirements of the Paperwork Reduction Act of 1995.

The burden time for this collection of information is estimated to average 100 hours per response, including the time to review instructions, search existing data sources, gather and maintain the data needed and complete and review the collection of information. Send comments regarding this burden estimate or any other aspect of this information collection, including suggestions for reducing this burden to the address to the right:

Department of Health and Human Services
Food and Drug Administration
Office of Chief Information Officer
Paperwork Reduction Act (PRA) Staff
PRAStaff@fda.hhs.gov

"An agency may not conduct or sponsor, and a person is not required to respond to, a collection of information unless it displays a currently valid OMB number."

DO NOT SEND YOUR COMPLETED FORM TO THIS PRA STAFF EMAIL ADDRESS.

Appendix 21–3

Protocol Medication Economic Analysis

Date:
Protocol title:
Study chairperson:

Hospital Cost Analysis

Drug	Hospital Cost per Cycle*	Number of Cycles	Total Cost per Patient	Number of Patients	Total Protocol Cost	Annual Cost
Primary Therapy						
Supportive Care						

*When applicable, doses calculated on 1.7 m^2 or 70 kg at initial dose level and costs include infusion fluids, administration sets, and tubing.

Patient Charge Analysis

Drug	Patient Charge per Cycle*	Number of Cycles	Total Charge per Patient	Number of Patients	Total Patient Billing
Primary Therapy					
Supportive Care					

*When applicable, charges include infusion fluids, administration sets, and tubing.

Reimbursement Risk

Drug	FDA Labeled	Compendium

Comments

Summary
_____
_____

Appendix 21-4

Investigational Drug Accountability Record

Form approved
OMB No. 0925-0240
Expires: 6/30/91

National Institutes of Health National Cancer Institute			PAGE NO. _____					
			CONTROL RECORD ☐					
Investigational Drug Accountability Record			SATELLITE RECORD ☐					
Name of Institution			Protocol No. (NCI)					
Drug Name, Dose Form and Strength								
Protocol Title			Dispensing Area					
Investigatior								

Line No.	Date	Patient's Initials	Patient's I.D. Number	Dose	Quantity Dispensed or Received	Balance Forward / Balance	Manufacturer and Lot No.	Recorder's Initials
1.								
2.								
3.								
4.								
5.								
6.								
7.								
8.								
9.								
10.								
11.								
12.								
13.								
14.								
15.								
16.								
17.								
18.								
19.								
20.								
21.								
22.								
23.								
24.								

NIH-2564
9-85

Appendix 22–1

Response Letter Drug A—Incidence of Yellow Stripes

DRUG A—Adverse Event—Yellow Stripes

Dear Dr. Smith,

Thank you for your inquiry. The following information is provided in response to your question regarding the use of DRUG A® and the incidence of yellow stripes appearing on the skin.

Please note that the information provided is not intended to advocate the use of our product in any manner other than as described in the enclosed full prescribing information.

INDICATION(S)

DRUG A® is indicated for the relief of moderate to severe hiccups in patients 18 years of age or older.[1]

PRESCRIBING INFORMATION

Please refer to the following sections of the enclosed Full Prescribing Information that are relevant to your inquiry: ADVERSE REACTIONS, WARNINGS, PRECAUTIONS.[1]

LITERATURE SEARCH RESULTS

A literature search of MEDLINE databases (and other resources) pertaining to the incidence of yellow stripes appearing on the skin associated with the use of DRUG A® was conducted through May 2016.

CLINICAL STUDIES

In phase III efficacy and safety studies of DRUG A® for the relief of moderate to severe hiccups, yellow stripes appearing on patients skin was reported in 7% of patients (see Table 1).[2]

TABLE 1. INCIDENCE OF YELLOW STRIPES APPEARING ON SKIN[2]

Adverse Event	DRUG A®	Placebo
Yellow stripes on skin	7%	7%

In a 12-month long-term safety study, the incidence of yellow stripes appearing on the skin was evaluated. DRUG A® users reported yellow stripes on their skin with an incidence rate of 9% (see Table 2).[3]

TABLE 2.   INCIDENCE OF YELLOW STRIPES APPEARING ON SKIN—LONG-TERM STUDY[3]

Adverse Event	DRUG A®	Placebo
Yellow stripes on skin	9%	8%

Multiple case reports were identified reporting yellow stripes appearing on patient's skin.

In a report by Jones and associates,[4] a 90-year-old woman suffering from severe hiccups reported yellow stripes appearing on the skin within 4 days of starting treatment. She was treated with DRUG FIX-IT® and her yellow stripes resolved immediately.

In a report by Jones and associates,[5] a 20-year-old man suffering from moderate hiccups reported yellow stripes on his skin within 2 minutes of starting treatment. The patient did not seek treatment, continued taking DRUG A®, and the yellow stripes resolved.

ADVERSE EVENT REPORTING

Please see the enclosed Prescribing Information for the complete safety and drug interaction information on our product. In order to monitor the safety of our products, we encourage clinicians to report adverse events by calling 1-800-555-9999 from 9 AM to 9 PM Mountain Time, Monday through Sunday. Adverse events may also be reported to the FDA MedWatch program by phone (1-800-FDA-1088), fax (1-800-FDA-0178), or e-mail (http://www.fda.gov/medwatch). To view a description of ongoing clinical trials for our products, please visit www.clinicaltrials.gov.

REFERENCES

1. DRUG A® [package insert]. Awesome Drugs R Us, Inc. Any Town, USA; 2016.
2. Jones Z, Smith Y, Miller T. Efficacy and safety of DRUG A® in the treatment of hiccups. JAHA. 2009;6542:735-46.
3. Jones Y, Davis C, Rodriguez J. Long-term safety of the use of DRUG A® in severe hiccups. JAHA. 2009; 6543:887-96.
4. Jones A, Haines R, Lane K. 90-year old woman with yellow stripes. Hiccup Central. 2009;78(4):232-5.
5. Jones B, Owens C, Cooper S. 20-year-old male with resolved yellow stripes. Hiccup Central. 2010;83(3):196-9.

Glossary

340b program   A program created by the U.S. government and managed by the Health Resources and Services Administration that requires drug manufacturers to provide significant discounts to qualifying health organizations for outpatient medications.

a priori   Determining specific study criteria prior to study initiation.

absolute risk reduction   The difference in the percentage of subjects developing the adverse event in the control group versus subjects in the intervention group. Also refers to the number of subjects spared the adverse event by taking the intervention compared to the control.

abstracting   A literature cataloging activity that includes a brief description (or abstract) of the information provided by the article or resource cited.

abstracting service   A database that provides abstracts and citations for journal articles.

abstracts   A synopsis (usually of 250 words or less) of the most important aspect(s) of an article.

academia   Pertaining to a college, school, or other educational institution.

academic detailing   A process by which a health care educator visits physicians to provide 15- to 20-minute educational intervention on specific topics. Information provided is based on prescribing patterns and evidence-based medicine.

Accountable Care Organization (ACO)   A collaborative group of hospitals, doctors, and other providers of health care who coordinate their patient care efforts for Medicare patients. An emphasis is placed on minimizing duplication of effort and on preventing medical errors, in particular, for the chronically ill.

ACO   See accountable care organization.

action-guides   A term coined by Beauchamp and Childress to refer to a hierarchical approach to analysis of an ethical issue when forming particular judgments about the issue.

active control   A standard therapy or procedure (but not a placebo) used in a study to determine the difference in effect produced by the study intervention.

active pharmaceutical ingredient   The active portion of a medication, sometimes known as the "raw material" or API.

adaptive clinical trial   A trial design, also known as group sequential design, that allows adaptation of various components such as inclusion/exclusion criteria, dosing, efficacy outcomes, and duration of trial based on continuously emerging knowledge throughout the study.

ADC   See automated dispensing cabinets.

ADE   See adverse drug event.

adjunctive therapy   A therapy (e.g., medication, exercise, diet) that all subjects within a study receive; since all subjects are receiving, it is not considered a study bias because the effect of this therapy occurs among all subjects within the study.

ADR   See adverse drug reaction.

adverse drug event (ADE)   An injury from a medicine or lack of intended medicine. An ADE refers to all adverse drug reactions (ADRs), including allergic or idiosyncratic reactions, as well as medication errors that result in harm to a patient.

adverse drug event (ADE) monitoring   Computer programs that use electronic data and predetermined rules to identify when an ADE may have occurred or is about to occur.

adverse drug event (ADE) trigger tool   An augmented chart review method that uses automated systems to identify alerts or triggers to efficiently identify patients with potential ADEs. The triggers are cues that a patient may have experienced an error and/or adverse event. When these triggers are identified, it is suspected that the patient may have experienced a medication error. The patient's chart is reviewed for evidence of error and/or level of harm and data are collected and collated to determine potential common causes.

adverse drug reaction (ADR)   Defined broadly, any unexpected, unintended, undesired, or excessive response to a medicine. Many national and international organizations, including the U.S. Food and Drug Administration (FDA) and World Health Organization, as well as individual facilities or institutions, have their own definitions of what constitutes an adverse drug reaction. Several of these are discussed in Chapter 17.

Agenda for Change   An initiative adopted by the JCAHO in 1986 intended to improve standards by focusing on key functions of quality of care, to monitor the performance of health care organizations using indicators, to improve the relevance and quality of the survey process, and to enhance the accuracy and value of JCAHO accreditation.

aggregate indicators   Provide a summary of the frequency, or timeliness, of a process by aggregating numerous cases.

aggregator   A piece of software that is used to automatically collect information from RSS and weblog sites, which allows the user to look at material from many of those sites at one time and in one place.

AGREE II instrument   See Appraisal of Guidelines for Research and Evaluation II instrument.

AHFS   American Hospital Formulary Service.

alert fatigue   A situation in which a provider ignores or overrides clinical decision support system (CDSS) messages.

alpha value   Criterion for rejecting the null hypothesis. It is the upper bound of the Type I error rate. A value (usually 0.05) that is set prior to the beginning of a study and in which the p-value is compared at the end of the study to determine if statistical difference is present in the outcome being measured. A p-value less than alpha (e.g., $0.001 < 0.05$) is interpreted as a statistical difference was determined between the intervention and control groups of a study. Also is the amount of error the researchers are willing to accept that a false-positive result is identified between the study intervention and control groups (e.g., alpha of 0.05 is up to a 5% chance of a false-positive result).

alternative hypothesis   See research hypothesis.

alternative medicine   An approach to health care outside conventional medicine. Alternative medicine refers to using a non-mainstream approach in place of conventional medicine.

American Hospital Formulary System (AHFS) classification   A classification that can be found in the *AHFS Drug Information* reference book, published by the American Society of Health-Systems Pharmacists. It groups agents by use and/or drug class into specific numbered categories (e.g., 24:32.04 Angiotensin-Converting Enzyme Inhibitors).

analysis   The critical assessment of the nature, merit, and significance of individual elements, ideas, or factors. Functionally, it involves separating the information into its isolated parts so that each can be critically assessed. Analysis requires thoughtful review and evaluation of the quality and overall weight of available evidence.

analytic research   Quantitative research conducted in a controlled environment to determine cause and effect relationships.

ancillary therapy   A therapy (e.g., medication, exercise, diet) that is disproportional in use among the subjects in the groups within a study and has an effect on the outcome being measured; this can lead to a difference in effect between the groups, which can bias the study results.

antibiotic use review (AUR)   Retrospective evaluation of antibiotic use. Usually quantitative and limited to identifying patterns of use.

application service provider   See software as a service.

Appraisal of Guidelines for Research and Evaluation (AGREE) II instrument   A structured instrument to assess guideline quality, provide a methodological strategy for guideline development and inform what information and how information ought to be reported in guidelines.

article proposal   A letter asking the publisher whether he or she would be interested in possibly publishing something on a particular topic written by the person(s) who are inquiring.

ASP   See software as a service.

aspect of care   A term used in quality assurance programs to indicate the title that describes the area being evaluated.

assay sensitivity   If non-inferiority is established for the test drug, further concluding that the test drug is effective can only be made if the reference drug's efficacy has been confirmed with high-quality clinical trials against placebo.

assumption of the risk   A defense in the law of torts, which bars a plaintiff from recovery against a negligent party if the defendant can demonstrate that the plaintiff voluntarily and knowingly assumed the risks at issue inherent to the dangerous activity in which he or she was participating at the time of his or her injury.

attributable risk   A statistical technique used in follow-up studies to determine the risk associated with exposure to a certain factor on disease state development. Attributable risk estimates the number of disease cases per number of exposures to the factor. This is primarily used in cohort studies and is considered an epidemiological term.

AUR   See antibiotic use review.

automated dispensing cabinets (ADCs)   Automated devices with a range of functions. Core capabilities include medication storage and retrieval for administration to patients, especially in patient care areas, as well as audit trails of cabinet access. Other functions can include medication charging and automated inventory management.

autonomy   Autonomy is the personal rule that is free from both controlling interferences by others and from personal limitations that prevent meaningful choice. Autonomous individuals act intentionally, with understanding, and without controlling influences.

avatar   A movable three-dimensional image used to represent somebody in cyberspace.

bar code verification   The use of bar code scanning to ensure that the correct drug, strength, and dosage form were dispensed in the drug selection process and to ensure that the five basic patient rights (i.e., right patient, right drug, right dose, right route, right time) are followed at the point of care.

beneficence   A basic principle of consequentialist theory that expresses the duty to promote good.

Berkson's Bias   A type of selection bias noted in case-control studies and is produced when the probability of hospitalization of cases and controls differ. This probability can be increased based on the specific exposure being studied and increases the chance of hospital admission.

beta   The probability of a false negative result in a study.

bias   An intentional or unintentional systematic error in the way a study is designed, conducted, analyzed, or reported.

bibliography   A list of references, usually seen at the end of a piece of professional writing.

biocreep (also known as placebo creep)   A situation that can exist that complicates using an active control to confirm efficacy, as is done with an noninferiority trial. Biocreep is the phenomenon where a somewhat inferior test drug is chosen as the reference drug for a future generation of noninferiority trials.

Bioequivalence studies   Research that evaluates whether products are similar in rate and extent of absorption.

biologics license applications (BLA)   A biologics license application is a submission that contains specific information on the manufacturing processes, chemistry, pharmacology, clinical pharmacology, and the medical effects of the biologic product. It is a request for permission to introduce, or deliver for introduction, a biologic product into interstate commerce.

BLA   See biologics license applications.

Black Letter Rules   Principles of law that are known generally to all and are free from doubt and ambiguity. Also known as hornbook law, since they are in a format that would probably be enunciated in a hornbook.

blinding   Study technique used in research to reduce bias by having the study subjects and/or investigators not know which group the study subjects are assigned.

blog   See weblog.

body area network (BAN)   A multi-device, interconnected computer system carried on a person. Sometimes referred to as a wearable computer.

CAM   See complementary and alternative medicine.

case report   A descriptive record of a single individual (case report) in which the possibility of an association between an observed effect and a specific intervention or exposure is described (often an unexpected complication of treatment or procedure) based on detailed clinical evaluation and history of the individual.

case series   A grouping of records (case studies or case reports) that documents a practitioner's experiences, thoughts, or observations related to the care of multiple patients with similar medical situations.

case study   A record of descriptive research that documents a practitioner's experiences, thoughts, or observations related to the care of a single patient. Not useful to test a hypothesis but can serve to generate pilot information to design future controlled trials.

case-control study   A retrospective trial design (often using medical charts or cases) strictly based on the observation of a group of people that have experienced a similar outcome. The study is used to determine the possible exposure these patients have had that would lead to this known outcome.

categorical variable   A variable measured on a nominal or ordinal scale.

CBA   See cost-benefit analysis.

CCA   See cost-consequence analysis.

CD-ROM   See compact disc-read only memory.

CDSS   See clinical decision support systems.

CEA   See cost-effectiveness analysis.

central limit theorem   States when equally sized samples are drawn from a non-normal distribution, the plotted mean values from each sample will approximate a normal distribution as long as the non-normality was not due to outliers.

CER   See cost-effectiveness ratio.

CHI   See consumer health information.

civil liability   Negligent acts and/or omissions, other than breach of contract, normally independent of moral obligations for which a remedy can be provided in a court of law. This form of liability is imposed under civil laws and processes, not criminal law. For example, a person injured in someone's home can bring suit under civil liability law.

clinical decision support systems (CDSS)   Computer programs that augment clinical decision making by combining referential information with patient-specific information to prevent negative actions and update providers of patient status.

clinical investigation   Any experiment in which a drug is administered or dispensed to one or more human subjects. An experiment is any use of a drug (except for the use of a marketed drug) in the course of medical practice. Although there are many other definitions, this is the FDA's definition and would seem the appropriate one to use given the nature of this topic. Note that the FDA does not regulate the practice of medicine and prescribers are (as far as the agency is concerned) free to use any marketed drug for off-label use.

clinical practice guidelines   Recommendations for optimizing patient care developed by systematically reviewing evidence and assessing the benefits and harms of health care interventions.

clinical response letters   Written correspondence that contains company approved content in response to an unsolicited request for medical information.

Clinical Safety Officer (CSO)   Also known as the Regulatory Management Officer (RMO). This will be the sponsor's Food and Drug Administration contact person. Generally the CSO/RMO assigned to a drug's investigational new drug application will also be assigned to the new drug application.

clinical significance   The clinical importance of data generated in a study, irrespective of statistical results. Usually refers to the application of study results into clinical practice. Also, can be called clinical meaningfulness.

clinically significant   A result large enough to cause an effect on an efficacy outcome measure that noticeably changes a patient's condition.

closed formulary   A drug formulary that restricts the drugs available within an institution or available under a third-party plan.

CMA   See cost-minimization analysis.

coauthor   Any individual who writes a portion of an article, chapter, book, etc. This includes individuals other than the primary author whose name is normally listed first on a publication.

cohort study   A prospective trial design strictly based on the observation of a group of people that experience a known exposure over time. The study is used to determine outcomes to this exposure.

COI   See conflict of interest.

commercial IND   An IND for which the sponsor is usually either a corporate entity or one of the institutes of the National Institutes of Health (NIH). In addition, CDER may designate other INDs as commercial, if it is clear that the sponsor intends the product to be commercialized at a later date.

community rule   See locality rule.

Compact Disc-Read Only Memory (CD-ROM)   A storage and retrieval system for large quantities of computerized data. Modern computers usually can not only read the data on these disks, but usually can write new data to disks designed to accept that new data.

comparative negligence   The allocation of responsibility for damages incurred between the plaintiff and defendant, based on the relative negligence of the two.

complementary and alternative medicine (CAM)   An approach to health care outside conventional medicine. Complementary medicine, also known as integrative medicine, refers to using a non-mainstream approach *together with* conventional medicine. Alternative medicine refers to using a non-mainstream approach *in place of* conventional medicine.

compliance   A measure of how well instructions are followed. In a study, compliance refers to how well a patient follows instructions for medication administration and how well the investigator follows the study protocol.

computer network   An interconnection of computers and computer-related devices (e.g., printers, modems) that allows the devices to interchange data, electronic mail, programs, and other files. In addition, a network allows sharing of peripheral devices, such as printers, modems, fax boards, etc. Normally, this interconnection is via a dedicated wiring system (other than telephone/modem communication); however, wireless connections are becoming common.

computer-based clinical decision support systems   See clinical decision support systems.

computerized provider order entry (CPOE)   A process allowing medical provider instructions to be electronically entered for the treatment of patients who are under a provider's care.

concurrent indicator   An indicator used in any quality assurance program that determines whether quality is acceptable while an action is being taken or care is being given.

concurrent negligence   The wrongful acts or omissions of two or more persons acting independently, but causing the same injury.

confidence interval   Range calculated for a study result in which the true value for the population exists; the percentage association with the range (e.g., 95%) indicates the confidence in which the true population value is within the range. For instance, the investigators are 95% confident that the mean blood pressure lowering effect of the medication for the population is between -8 and -12 mm Hg for the 95% confidence interval of (-8 to -12 mm Hg).

confidentiality   A moral rule, related to the principle of autonomy, which specifically addresses the individual client's right to give or refuse consent relative to release of privileged information.

conflict of interest (COI)   A situation in which the interests of an investigator conflicts with the study purpose, design, and/or result interpretation. An investigator may be a stockholder of and/or speaker for a pharmaceutical company; the study may be designed to produce favorable results and/or these be interpreted or promoted with a bias to use the study intervention.

confounder   A difference between the two groups within a study that can directly alter the difference in effect between the intervention and control group.

consent   A moral rule related to the principle of autonomy which states that the client has a right to be informed and to freely choose a course of action.

consequential damages   Also called special damages; damages claimed and/or awarded in a lawsuit which were caused as a direct foreseeable result of wrongdoing. Consequential damages occur with injury or harm that does not ensue directly and immediately from the act of a party, but only from some of the results of such act, and that is compensable by a monetary award after a judgment has been rendered in a lawsuit.

consequentialist   An ethical theory which holds that the rightness or wrongness of decisions or actions is determined by the total of good that is achieved or harm that is prevented.

constancy assumption   That historical studies and a new noninferiority study should be as identical as possible regarding important characteristics.

consumer health information (CHI)   Information actively sought by the patient in response to their need for more information about their health. Information is not individualized for a specific patient but rather general health information.

content filter   A term used to limit a search to specific things, such as specific drugs or disease states.

continuous indicators   Provide a simple count, or time estimate, related to a process (e.g., average turnaround time on medication orders).

continuous quality improvement (CQI)   The term given to the methodologies used in the process of total quality management. Efforts to improve quality are part of each participant's responsibilities on an ongoing basis.

continuous variable   A variable measured on an interval or ratio scale.

contract research organization (CRO)   An individual or organization that assumes one or more of the obligations of the sponsor through an independent contractual agreement.

control group   The group of test animals or humans that receive a placebo (a dosage that does not contain active medicine) or active (a dosage that does contain active medicine) treatment. For most preclinical and clinical trials, the FDA will require that this group receive placebo (commonly referred to as the placebo control). However, some studies may have an active control, which generally consists of an available (standard of care) treatment modality. An active control may, with the concurrence of the FDA, be used in studies where it would be considered unethical to use a placebo. A historical control is one in which a group of previous patients is compared with a matched set of patients receiving the new therapy. A historical control might be used in cases where the disease is consistently fatal (i.e., acquired immunodeficiency syndrome [AIDS]). (Refer to Chapter 4 for additional information on control groups.)

controlled clinical trial   Research design that prospectively and directly compares plus measures and quantify differences in outcome between an intervention and control. This is the best study design to determine a cause-and-effect relationship between an item under investigation and an outcome.

controls A treatment (placebo, active, historical) used for comparison in a study to measure a difference in effect against an investigational agent. The investigator usually wishes to determine superiority of a new treatment over the control in terms of efficacy and safety.

co-payment Payment made by an individual who has health insurance at the time the service is received to offset the cost of care. Co-payments may vary depending on the service rendered.

cost-benefit analysis study (CBA) A study where monetary value is given for both costs and benefits associated with a drug or service. The results are expressed as a ratio (benefit-to-cost), and the ratio is used to determine the economic value of the drug or service.

cost-consequence analysis (CCA) An informal variant of a cost-effectiveness analysis (CEA). The costs and various outcomes are listed but no evaluations are conducted.

cost-effectiveness analysis (CEA) A study where the cost of a drug or service is compared to its therapeutic impact. Cost-effectiveness studies determine the relative efficiency of various drugs or services in achieving desired therapeutic outcomes.

cost-effectiveness ratio (CER) The CER is the ratio of resources used per unit of clinical benefit, and implies that this calculation has been made in relation to doing nothing or no treatment.

cost-effectiveness study See cost-effectiveness analysis.

cost-minimization analysis (CMA) A study that compares costs of drugs or services that have been determined to have equivalent therapeutic outcomes.

cost-utility analysis (CUA) A study that relates therapeutic outcomes to both costs of drugs or services and patient preferences, and measures cost per unit of utility. Utility is the amount of satisfaction obtained from a drug or service.

counterfeit drugs Medications that do not contain the correct active ingredient or the correct amount.

covenant An ethical covenant in medical ethics suggests an implicit contract between client and health care provider that broadly describes the relationship involved whenever a health care service is provided, including the provision of information. Within this contract the service recipient has a right to competently provided service, as well as respectful treatment. The service recipient also has an obligation to provide needed information to the provider in a respectful manner.

coverage error Form of bias occurring when the sample population actually surveyed does not coincide with the target population intended for the survey.

coverage rules Criteria for specific drugs determined by the health plan in conjunction with the pharmacy and therapeutics committee that is used to determine if a prescription is covered. Criteria are based on evidence-based medicine.

CPOE See computerized provider order entry.

CQI See continuous quality improvement.

criteria Definitions of safe and effective use of medications used to assess components of the medication use process that are endorsed by the organization within which they are to be applied. Criteria summarize an organization's definition of appropriate or acceptable use of the medication.

critical appraisal The process of systematically and critically evaluating a scientific study for relevance and value within a specific context.

crossover study   A study where each subject receives all study treatments, and endpoints during the various treatments are compared.

cross-sectional   Data that is measured one time.

cross-sectional study   A trial design involving data collection only once on members of the study population that represents a snapshot in time. These members are not required to be studied all at once, but each member can be studied at a different time. The key is that the data collected represents a specific period in time.

CUA   See cost-utility analysis.

Current Good Manufacturing Practices (cGMPs)   Regulations enforced by the FDA to assure proper design, monitoring, and control of manufacturing processes and facilities.

cybermedicine   A concept broader than telemedicine that includes the marketing, relationship creation, advice, prescribing, and selling pharmaceuticals and devices in cyberspace.

Dear Health Care Provider letter   A letter from a manufacturer to highlight critical information for health care providers about new or updated information about a medication.

dechallenge   In relation to adverse drug reactions, this occurs when the drug is taken away and the patient is monitored to determine whether the adverse drug reaction (ADR) abates or decreases in intensity.

decision analysis   A tool that can help visualize a pharmacoeconomic analysis. It is the application of an analytical method for systematically comparing different decision options. Decision analysis graphically displays choices and performs the calculations needed to compare these options.

deep pocket   Practical consideration that involves the naming of additional co-defendants in personal injury lawsuits to provide assurance to the plaintiff that there will be sufficient assets to pay the judgment.

degrees of freedom   The number of data points that are free to vary.

deliverable   Term used in project management referring to a tangible component produced in order to achieve predefined success criteria.

delta   The amount of difference that the investigators wish to detect between intervention and control groups in a study.

deontological   An ethical theory that seeks to establish what is a right or wrong decision or action on the basis of prioritizing specific recognized ethical rules or principles.

descriptive statistics   Statistics that describe data such as medians, modes, and standard deviations.

detailing   Promotions made directly from pharmaceutical industry to health care professionals, generally in one-on-one or small-group meetings.

diagnostic review bias   Occurs when the reference test results are not definitive and the study test results affect or influence how the final diagnosis is established.

DIC   See drug information center.

dichotomous variable   A variable that has two mutually exclusive categories.

digital video disk (DVD)   Also known as digital versatile disk. A disk that physically resembles a CD-ROM, but allows the storage of much larger amounts of data. It requires a special reading/writing device in a computer, although this device may also be combined with that used for

CD-ROMs. DVDs have been used to a large extent to store and replay movies; however, it is now being used on computers to store large amounts of computer data, particularly large multimedia files.

direct medical costs   One of four categories of costs in pharmacoeconomic studies. These are the medically related inputs used directly in providing the treatment.

direct nonmedical costs   One of four categories of costs in pharmacoeconomic studies. These are costs directly associated with treatment, but are not medical in nature. Examples include travel, food, and lodging to get to a place of treatment.

DIS   See drug information service.

discount rate   A term from finance which approximates the cost of capital by taking into account both the projected inflation rate and the interest rates of borrowed money, and then estimates the time value of money.

drug class review   A drug evaluation monograph comparing all products in a particular class of drugs. It is used to determine what products will be available for use.

drug evaluation monograph   A structured document covering all aspects of a particular drug product or class of drugs. It compares similar agents and is used to determine which products will be available for use.

drug formularies   See formulary.

drug formulary system   See formulary system.

drug informatics   A technologically advanced version of drug information. This often denotes the electronic management of drug information.

drug information   Facts or advice on drugs (including chemicals that have medicinal, performance-enhancing, or intoxicating effects) regarding a specific patient or a group of patients, based on the most current and accurate evidence.

drug information center (DIC)   A physical location where pharmacists have the resources (e.g., books, journals, computer systems) to provide drug information. This area is generally staffed by a pharmacist specializing in drug information, but may be used by a variety of the pharmacy staff or other individuals.

drug information service   A professional service providing drug information. This service is normally located in a drug information center.

drug interaction   The U.S. Food and Drug Administration defines this as "a pharmacologic response that cannot be explained by the action of a simple drug, but is due to two or more drugs acting simultaneously."

drug master file (DMF)   A submission to the U.S. Food and Drug Administration that may be used to provide confidential detailed information about facilities, processes, or articles used in the manufacturing, processing, packaging, and storing of one or more human drugs.

drug product   The final dosage form prepared from the drug substance.

drug promotion   Information provided by pharmaceutical industry through advertising, detailing, and other printed material intended to increase sales of a medication.

drug substance   An active ingredient that is intended to furnish pharmacological activity or other direct effect in the diagnosis, cure, mitigation, treatment, or prevention of disease or to affect the structure or any function of the human body. Bulk compound from which the drug product is prepared.

drug use evaluation (DUE) Concurrent evaluation of prescribing and outcome only. Multidisciplinary involvement.

drug use review (DUR) A program related to outpatient pharmacy services designed to educate physicians and pharmacists in identifying and reducing the frequency and patters of fraud, abuse, gross overuse, or inappropriate or medically unnecessary care. DUR is typically retrospective in nature and utilizes claims data as its primary source of information.

DUE See drug usage evaluation.

due care See reasonable care.

DUR See drug use review.

duty A moral or legal obligation.

EBM See evidence-based medicine.

editorial A commentary usually written by an expert that describes a study's strengths and limitations plus the application of the study results into practice. This is published in the same journal issue as the study, but not all studies have an accompanying editorial.

electronic mail (e-mail) Brief messages sent from one computer to another, similar in use to interoffice memos. This serves as a quick, informal method of written communication. Also, e-mail may be used to send other items, such as word processing files, graphics, video, etc. to others.

electronic medication administration record (eMAR) An electronic version of the traditional medication administration record. It supports patient safety by incorporating clinical decision support and bar coded medication administration. It also enables real-time documentation and billing of medication administration.

electronic prescribing (e-prescribing) Prescription entered by a prescriber directly into an electronic format using agreed-upon standards that is securely transmitted to the pharmacy that the patient chooses. Faxes and printed prescriptions are not e-prescriptions.

e-mail See electronic mail.

eMAR See electronic medication administration record.

endpoint A parameter measured in a clinical study. The primary endpoint is the major variable analyzed and reflects the main objective of the study. Secondary endpoints are additional variables of interest monitored during clinical studies.

endpoint, primary An outcome measured by the study investigators that quantifies the difference in effect between the intervention and control of the clinical trial. The results of this outcome measurement are used to answer the primary study objective. This outcome also is used by the study investigators to determine other study methods (e.g., sample size, statistical tests, duration, dose, patient type to enroll).

endpoint, secondary An outcome measured by the study investigators that quantifies the difference in effect between the intervention and control of the clinical trial, but not considered the focus of the study. The results of this outcome measurement are used to answer secondary study objectives. For example, a study compares a statin to placebo to determine if the statin can reduce the risk of having a stroke (primary endpoint); change in LDL-C levels also are compared between the two groups (secondary endpoint).

e-prescribing See electronic prescribing.

error, type I Rejecting the null hypothesis instead of failing-to-reject (i.e., accepting) the null hypothesis; also known as a false-positive result or alpha-error; chance is the reason for this to occur.

error, type II   Failing-to-reject (i.e., accepting) the null hypothesis instead of rejecting the null hypothesis; also known as a false-negative result or beta-error; chance or small sample size are reasons for this to occur.

ethical theories   Integrated bodies of principles and rules that may include mediating rules that govern cases of conflicts.

ethics   The philosophical inquiry of the moral dimensions of human conduct. An ethical issue involves judgments between right and wrong human conduct or praiseworthy and blameworthy human character.

evidence-based medicine (EBM)   A philosophy of practice and an approach to decision making in the clinical care of patients that involves making individual patient care decisions based on the best currently available evidence.

exclusion criteria   Characteristics of subjects defined prior to starting the study that are used as parameters to disqualify subjects from enrolling into the study (e.g., patients with cancer, lactating females, patients receiving corticosteroid therapy).

exculpatory clause   An exculpatory clause is part of an agreement which relieves one party from liability. It is a provision in a contract which stipulates: (1) one party is relieved of any blame or liability arising from the other party's wrongdoing, or (2) one party (usually the one that drafted the agreement) is freed of all liability arising out of performance of that contract. An exculpatory clause will not be enforced when the party protected by the clause intentionally causes harm or engages in acts of reckless, wanton, or gross negligence or when found to be unreasonable under the particular circumstances (e.g., a restaurant checks a person's coat but the ticket states they are not responsible for loss or damage).

exploratory research   Research of a qualitative nature in which the investigators examines an unknown area to generate hypotheses.

extemporaneous compounding   The practice of compounding prescriptions from a list of several ingredients—usually performed by a pharmacist.

external validity   See validity, external.

failure mode and effects analysis (FMEA)   FMEA is a structured proactive method of evaluating a process to identify the gaps—how the process might fail. The process includes identification of the likelihood of each of the failures along with its relative impact to the patient. This provides a prioritization of action plans to drive improvement and reduce the likelihood of failure.

fair balance   A quality of drug promotions where similar attention is given to safety risks (e.g., contraindications, precautions/warnings, adverse effects) and efficacy benefits.

false negatives   Individuals with the disease that were incorrectly identified as being disease-free by the test.

false positives   Individuals without the disease that were incorrectly identified as having the disease by the test.

FDA   See Food and Drug Administration.

FDA Form 483   A report issued after an inspection if investigators observe any violations of the Food Drug and Cosmetic Act and other FDA acts.

FDS   See formulary decision supports.

fellowship   A directed, highly individualized postgraduate training program designed to prepare the participant to function as an independent investigator. The purpose of fellowship training programs is to develop competency and expertise in the scientific research process, including hypothesis generation and development, study design, protocol development, grantsmanship, study coordination, data collection, analysis and interpretation, technical skills development, presentation of results, and manuscript preparation and publication. A fellowship candidate is expected to possess appropriate practice skills relevant to the knowledge area of the fellowship. Such skills may be obtained through prior practice experience or completion of a residency program.

fidelity A principle of moral duty in deontological theory that addresses the responsibility to be trustworthy and keep promises.

file transfer protocol (FTP) A method to transfer of files from one computer to another.

FMEA See failure mode and effects analysis.

follow-up study A study where subjects exposed to a factor and those not exposed to the factor are followed forward in time and compared to determine the factor's influence on disease state development. Also called a cohort study.

Food and Drug Administration (FDA) The agency of the U.S. government that is responsible for ensuring the safety and efficacy of all drugs on the market.

Forest plot Preferred method to display the results from a meta-analysis, and includes the 95% confidence intervals for the primary efficacy outcome for each study included in the meta-analysis with the overall resulting 95% CI for the meta-analysis.

formulary A continually revised list of medications that are readily available for use within an institution or from a third-party payer (e.g., insurance company, government) that reflects the current clinical judgment of the medical staff or the payer. Restrictions on this list may be placed that indicate certain drugs will not be reimbursed by insurance, or will only be reimbursed if several other alternatives are tried first.

formulary decision supports (FDS) Program (often software) used to enhance compliance with formulary by guiding the prescriber to preferred formulary drugs over those considered nonformulary.

formulary system A method used to develop a drug formulary. It is sometimes even thought of as a philosophy.

Funnel plot A scatter plot of treatment effect versus sample size of studies included in a meta-analysis. They are used to assist in detecting potential publication bias which is a form of selection bias based on the magnitude, direction, or statistical significance of the study results.

futility Stopping a trial because of recognition of the inability of that study to achieve its objectives.

galley proofs A copy of a written work as it is to be published. The purpose of this document is to allow the author(s) to make a final check to ensure everything is correct before actual publication. This is sometimes referred to as page proofs.

Gantt chart Project management tool used to provide a visual progression and overall timeline for a project.

GCP See good clinical practice.

gender bias Showing favoritism or discrimination toward a selected gender.

Good Clinical Practice (GCP) A standard for the design, conduct, monitoring, analyses, and reporting of clinical trials that provides assurance that the results are credible and accurate, and that the rights of study subjects are protected.

GRADE   See Grading of Recommendations, Assessment, Development, and Evaluation system.

Grading of Recommendations, Assessment, Development, and Evaluation (GRADE) system   A standardized system for grading evidence quality and the strength of recommendations in clinical practice guidelines.

gray literature   Documents provided in limited numbers outside the formal channels of publication and distribution. The concern with these documents is that they may include inaccurate information (not completely correct information), misinformation (incorrect information), and disinformation (false information deliberately provided in order to influence opinions) that can confound the meta-analysis results.

group purchasing organization (GPO)   An organization that assists health care providers or organizations by aggregating purchase volume to negotiate cost savings from suppliers.

guideline   Document that provides suggestions or advice for a particular activity. Guidelines are evidence-based recommendations, but should not replace professional judgement.

Health 2.0   The utilization of health care related tools provided by Web 2.0.

health applications (apps)   Software for devices designed to manage various aspects of health for the specific user.

health equity   Attainment of the highest level of health for all people. Achieving health equity requires valuing everyone equally with focused and ongoing societal efforts to address avoidable inequalities, historical and contemporary injustices, and the elimination of health and health care disparities.

Health Insurance Portability and Accountability Act of 1996   Commonly referred to as HIPAA, this act includes privacy restrictions for electronic health records.

health literacy   The capability of patients to read or hear health information, understand it, and then act upon the information.

Health Maintenance Organization (HMO)   Form of health insurance whereby the member prepays a premium for the HMO's health services which generally include inpatient and outpatient care.

Health Plan Employer Data and Information Set (HEDIS)   A set of performance measures used to compare managed health care plans.

health product information   Identified by Project Destiny as a service area where pharmacists augment patient's health care by providing information to patients based on information from prescription history, patient profiles, and purchases.

health-related quality of life (HR-QOL or HRQL)   The value assigned to the duration of a patient's life when altered by various impairments, functional states, perceptions, and social opportunities that have been modified by disease, injury, treatment, and social policy.

help-seeking advertisement   A type of direct to consumer advertisement that describes a disease or condition but does not recommend or suggest a treatment medication.

heterogeneity   Noted in meta-analyses, this describes a situation where there are differences in the way the studies being included in the meta-analysis were conducted. Ideally, all studies included should be identical in design and the way they are conducted (same medication doses used, same patient inclusion/exclusion criteria, same outcome measurements, same duration, etc.). There can be different degrees of heterogeneity; however, if there are significant variations in true effects underlying the studies, then the meta-analysis results are in question.

HIPAA See Health Insurance Portability and Accountability Act of 1996.

Hippocratic Oath A central ethical tradition of Western medicine that is committed to producing good for one's patient and protecting that patient from harm. There is a special emphasis placed on the responsibility of the medical professional to the specific patient.

historical data Data used in research that was collected prior to the decision to conduct the study (e.g., medical records, insurance information, Medicaid databases).

Historical Evidence of Sensitivity to Drug Effects (HESDE) In non-inferiority trials, this concept applies to appropriately designed and conducted past trials using the reference drug and regularly exhibiting the reference drug to be superior to placebo.

HMO See health maintenance organization.

homogeneity Describes the properties or characteristics of a dataset, or several datasets regarding their similarity.

homogenicity tests Tests used when conducting a meta-analysis to determine the similarity of studies whose results were combined for the analysis.

homoscedasticity In correlation and regression, the variability around the best fit line of the linear relationship is constant across all data points.

HRQL See health-related quality of life.

HR-QOL See health-related quality of life.

http (hypertext transfer protocol) A method by which information is encoded and transmitted on the World Wide Web.

https A secure form of http used to transmit confidential information, such as credit card numbers.

hyperlink Also called a link; is a word, group of words, or image that can be clicked on to jump (link) to another place within the same document or to an entirely different document. When the cursor is moved over a link in a website, the arrow will turn into a little hand. Hyperlinks are the most essential ingredient of all hypertext systems, including the Internet.

hypothesis The researchers' assumptions regarding probable study results. The research hypothesis or alternative hypothesis (H_A) is the expectations of the researchers in terms of study results. The null hypothesis (H_O) is the no-difference hypothesis, which assumes equality among study treatments. The null hypothesis is the basis for all statistical tests and must be rejected in order to accept the research hypothesis.

ICER See incremental cost-effectiveness ratio.

IDE See investigational device exemption.

impact factor The number of times a journal is cited in the literature relative to its number of publications within the same timeframe; used to determine the relative prestige of a journal.

in vitro Experiments conducted using components of an organism that have been isolated from their usual biological surroundings. These types of experiments are also referred to as "test tube experiments."

in vivo Experiments conducted in living organisms in their intact state.

incidence rate Measures the probability that a healthy person will develop a disease within a specified period of time. It is the number of new cases of disease in the population over a specific time period.

inclusion criteria   Characteristics of subjects defined prior to starting the study that are used as parameters to enroll participants into the study (e.g., males and females between 50 and 75 years of age with a prior myocardial infarction).

incremental cost-effectiveness ratio (ICER)   The ratio of the change in costs to incremental benefits of a therapeutic intervention or treatment.

incremental cost-utility ratio   See marginal (or incremental) cost-utility ratio.

IND   See investigational new drug application.

INDA   See investigational new drug application.

independent data monitoring committee   A group of experts that are independent of the ongoing clinical study they are monitoring. This group looks at the blinded data being generated by the study to determine if changes or adjustments should be made about how the study is being conducted.

indexing   A literature cataloging activity that consists of providing bibliographic citation information (e.g., title, author, and citation of the article).

indexing service   A searchable database of biomedical journal citations.

indicator   A statement of a measurable item in the area being evaluated which signals whether the area being evaluated is or is not of sufficient quality. It can focus on structure, process, or outcomes.

indicator drug   A drug that, when prescribed, may offer evidence that an adverse effect to a drug may have occurred. Pharmacists can then investigate further to determine whether there really was an adverse effect.

indirect medical costs   One of four categories of costs in pharmacoeconomic studies. Indirect costs involve costs that result from the loss of productivity due to illness or death.

inference engine   Also known as the reasoning engine, this forms the brain of the clinical decision support system, working to link patient-specific information with information in the knowledge base. It evaluates the available information and determines what to present to the user.

inferential statistics   Statistics (i.e., parametric and nonparametric tests) that determine the statistical importance of differences between groups and allow conclusions to be drawn from the data.

informatics specialist   An individual that has advanced medication information skills with a keen understanding of computer and information technology.

information therapy   Evidence-based patient education and/or medical information presented at an appropriate time to most effectively assist the patient in making a specific health decision or change in their behavior.

informed consent   The document signed by a subject, or the subject's representative, entering into a trial that informs him or her of his or her rights as a research subject, plus potential benefits and risks of the trial. This document indicates that the person is willing to participate in the study.

inherent drug risks   Are unique to the drug and usually identified in the package insert, but do not include probable or common side effects.

injunction   A judicial remedy issued in order to prohibit a party from doing or continuing to do a certain activity.

institutional review board (IRB)   A group of individuals from various disciplines (e.g., laypeople, physicians, pharmacists, nurses, clergy) who evaluate protocols for clinical studies to assess risks to the research participants and benefits to society, along with the ethical implications of the study protocol. Approval by a local IRB (i.e., an IRB located in the community in which the study is to be conducted) is necessary prior to initiation of a clinical study involving patients.

intangible costs   One of four categories of costs in pharmacoeconomic studies. Includes such items as the costs of pain, suffering, anxiety, or fatigue that occur because of an illness or the treatment of an illness.

intelligent infusion pumps (smart pumps)   Infusion pumps containing software designed to help eliminate pump programming errors.

intention-to-treat (ITT)   Study design technique used to include results of all subjects in the final analysis even when the subject does not complete the entire study.

interim analysis   Evaluation of data at specified time points before scheduled termination or completion of a study.

internal validity   Refers to how well an experiment is done, especially whether it avoids confounding factors that could affect the results.

Internet   A worldwide computer network.

interoperability   The ability of disparate computer systems to exchange information in a manner that allows the information to be used meaningfully.

interval data   Data in which each measurement has an equal distance between points, but an arbitrary zero (e.g., temperature in Fahrenheit).

interval scale   A scale of measurement that has rank-ordered data with meaningful distance between two ranks, but no natural zero.

interventional study   A study where the investigator introduces a factor and examines the factor's influence on certain variables or outcomes.

intranet   A computer network with restricted access, as within a health system.

Inverse Variance Test   A statistical test commonly used to combine continuous data in meta-analyses.

Investigational Device Exemption (IDE)   An approved IDE means that the IRB (and FDA for significant risk devices) has approved the sponsor's study application and all requirements under 21CFR812 are met. It allows the use of a device in a clinical investigation to collect safety and effectiveness data.

Investigational New Drug   A drug, antibiotic, or biological that is used in a clinical investigation. The label of an investigational drug must bear the statement: "Caution: New Drug-Limited by Federal (or United States) law to investigational use."

Investigational New Drug Application (IND or INDA)   The application by the study sponsor to the FDA to begin clinical trials in humans.

investigator   The individual responsible for initiating the clinical trial at the study site. This individual must treat the patients, assure that the protocol is followed, evaluate responses and adverse reactions, solve problems as they arise, and assure proper conduct of the study.

IRB   See institutional review board.

JCAHO   Joint Commission on Accreditation of Healthcare Organizations. See The Joint Commission.

joint and several liability   Refers to the sharing of liabilities among a group of people collectively and also individually. If the defendants are "jointly and severally" liable, the injured party may sue some or all of the defendants together, or each one separately, and may collect equal or unequal amounts from each.

journal club   A group of individuals who meet on a regular basis to discuss and critically evaluate the biomedical literature.

Just Culture   A term coined by David Marx, which is a structured accountability model that supports patient safety and a learning culture. It is intended to balance recognition and understanding of system contribution to errors with an understanding of human error concepts in order to facilitate an accountability process that is valued by leadership and staff. When applied consistently and fairly, it is also a proactive approach to identifying gaps in system processes.

justice   A concept that relates to fairness and tendering what is due, resource allocation, and providing that to which the individual is entitled.

key opinion leaders   Health professionals considered to be experts in their area by their peers. Key opinion leaders are often highly regarded for their expertise in publications, speaking engagements, and influential value in the medical community.

kurtosis   Refers to how flat or peaked the curve appears. A curve with a flat or board top is referred to as platykurtic while a peaked distribution is described as leptokurtic.

language bias   Occurs when only specific articles are included in a review or study that are published in a specific language such as the review author's native language. The issue is that potentially important articles are eliminated from the review.

law   Involves written rules set by the whole society, or its representatives, that address the responsibilities of that society's members.

Learned Intermediary Doctrine   A doctrine of products liability law and personal injury law; the manufacturer of a prescription drug fulfills its duty to warn of potentially harmful effects of the drug by informing the prescribing physician and is not also obligated to warn the user. The prescribing physician acts as a learned intermediary between manufacturer and consumer and has the primary responsibility of warning patients of the hazards of prescribed pharmaceutical products. This doctrine is an exception to the rule that one who markets goods must warn foreseeable ultimate users of dangers inherent in their products.

letter to the editor   A written piece to the editor of a medical journal or other publication expressing opinions or concerns of the reader.

level of evidence   A scale used to categorize the overall quality of a specific clinical trial. The reliability of the results can be inferred from the category given a trial.

life table methods   In the context of cohort study life tables, data are collected by following patients throughout their lives or a specific duration of their life and then compiled into tables for such uses as survival or mortality analyses comparing exposed to nonexposed situations.

listserver   A service offered by some e-mail systems that allows a member of the listserver to send an e-mail message to one particular Internet address where it will be sent to all members of the listserver. This acts as a dynamic distribution list for e-mail messages.

local area network (LAN)   A group of computers connected in a way that they may share data, programs, and/or equipment over a small geographic area (e.g., building, department).

locality rule   Legal doctrine created in the latter part of the nineteenth century that stated that the local defendant practitioner would have his or her standard of performance evaluated in light of the performance of other peers in the same or similar communities. Also known as community rule.

logical operator   A term such as AND, OR, NOT, NEAR, or WITH that can be used in searching a computer database. See the chapter 3 on electronic information management for more detailed information.

logit   See log-odds.

log-odds   A linear transformation of probability. That is, probability is bounded between 0 and 1, log-odds transform probability to a continuous scale ranging from $-\infty$ to $+\infty$. The log-odds become the dependent variable in logistic regression.

longitudinal   Data that is measured repeatedly over time.

macro   Level of decision-making that sets policy for the health system, as a standard established for an entire profession, or through government as law/regulation for the society as a whole.

mail service drug program   Program that provides free home delivery for up to a 90-day supply of maintenance prescription drugs.

mainframe computer   A large centralized computer that is used via computer terminals or other devices. This term is becoming blurred as smaller computer systems gain greater capabilities.

major statement   Used in broadcast (TV or radio) advertisements for prescription medications in which the drug's most important risks are verbally presented.

managed care organization (MCO)   Health care provider who contracts with participating providers to provide a variety of services to enrolled members.

Mantel-Haenszel Test   A statistical test commonly used to combine categorical data in meta-analyses.

marginal (or incremental) cost-utility ratio   The gain in a benefit from an increase, or loss from a decrease, in a good or service, such as the QALY. Calculated to estimate the added cost for an added benefit, not calculated when the added benefit comes at a lower cost.

marginal cost-effectiveness ratio   The additional cost of one unit expansion of a single intervention.

matching   A statistical technique which is used to evaluate the effect of a treatment by comparing the treated and the non-treated units in an observational study such as case-controlled studies. The goal is to identify a non-treated patient with similar observable characteristics for every treated patient (cases and controls are similar) so treatment effect can be measured more accurately.

material issue of fact   Genuine issue of material fact is a legal term often used as the basis for a motion for summary judgment. A summary judgment is proper if there is no genuine issue of material fact and the movant is entitled to a judgment as a matter of law. Such a motion will be granted if the party making the motion proves there is no genuine issue of material fact to be decided. When the moving party makes a prima facie showing that no genuine issue of material fact exists, the burden shifts to the nonmoving party to rebut the showing by presenting substantial evidence creating a genuine issue.

MCO   See managed care organization.

mean   The arithmetic average of a set of numbers.

meaningful Use   A set of standards defined by the CMS as the use of certified EHR technology to (1) improve quality, safety, and efficiency, (2) engage patients and their families, (3) improve care coordination, as well as public and population health, and (4) maintain privacy and security of PHI.

measurement error   Occurs when the collection of data is influenced by the interviewer or when the survey item itself is unclear from the respondent's point of view.

measures of association   Calculation and interpretation of nominal study results using relative risk (RR), relative risk reduction (RRR), absolute risk reduction (ARR), and numbers needed to treat (NNT).

median   The absolute middle value of a set of number.

medical executive committee   A committee that acts as the administrative body of a medical staff in an institution. It is responsible for overseeing all aspects of care within the institution. This committee may be known by other names at specific institutions.

Medical Literature Analysis and Retrieval System (MedLARS)   The computerized information retrieval system at the National Library of Medicine.

Medical Subject Heading (MeSH terms)   A set of specific medical words that the National Library of Medicine uses to define or categorize a topic for the purpose of indexing articles in PubMed.

medication error   Any preventable event that may cause or lead to inappropriate medication use or patient harm while the medication is in the control of the health care professional, patient, or consumer. Such events may be related to professional practice, health care products, procedures, and systems, including prescribing; order communication; product labeling, packaging, and nomenclature; compounding; dispensing; distribution; administration; education; monitoring; and use.

medication guides   Information for drug and biological products that FDA determines pose a serious and significant public health concern requiring the distribution of FDA-approved patient medication information that is necessary for patients' safe and effective use of the drug products.

medication information   Facts or advice on medicines regarding a specific patient or a group of patients.

medication misadventure   Any iatrogenic hazard or incident associated with medications that is an inherent risk when medication therapy is indicated; is created through either omission or commission by the administration of a medicine or medicines during which a patient may be harmed, with effects ranging from mild discomfort to fatality; may be attributable to error (human or system, or both), immunologic response, or idiosyncratic response; is always unexpected or undesirable to the patient and the health professional; and whose outcome may or may not be independent of the preexisting pathology or disease process. It includes adverse drug events (ADEs), adverse drug reactions (ADRs), and medication errors.

medication therapy management   Medication therapy management is a distinct service or group of services that optimizes drug therapy with the intent of improved therapeutic outcomes for individual patients.

Medication Tier Status   An indication, usually designated by the payer for prescriptions, as to whether a medication is a preferred agent within its class (i.e., first tier), second choice (second tier), third choice (third tier), or not covered. Each "tier" is generally associated with decreasing payment from the payer and increasing patient responsibility for the cost of the drug, with "not covered" (or non-formulary) being entirely the patient's responsibility to pay.

medication usage patterns   Trends and patterns of drug use. Often influenced by reimbursement decisions and formularies of insurance companies, Medicare and Medicaid, direct-to-consumer-advertising, etc.

medication use evaluation (MUE)   A part of the overall performance improvement program within institutional settings that provides in-depth assessment of the medication use process including prescribing, transcribing, dispensing, administering, monitoring, and outcome. Multidisciplinary involvement. Prior to 1986, this function was commonly referred to as drug use (or usage) evaluation (DUR).

MedLARS   See Medical Literature Analysis and Retrieval System.

MedWatch   FDA's safety information and adverse event reporting program either by health care professionals or patients.

meso Level of decision making variably described as occurring at the institutional/organizational level or at community/regional levels of health care.

meta-analysis Results of previously conducted similar clinical trials are combined, statistically analyzed, and new data are created for interpretation. Meta-analyses are especially useful when previous studies are inconclusive or controversial. They are also useful where sample size of multiple similar studies are too small to detect a statistically significant difference, but combining them will provide adequate sample size to meet a set power.

micro Level of health care-related decision making, which involves decisions made at the individual professional–patient level of health care.

middle technical style A writing style used by professionals addressing professionals in other fields. It tends to be formal and avoids use of the first person (e.g., I, us). Technical jargon is avoided in this writing style.

mobile apps Software applications intended for use on mobile platforms, or web-based software applications tailored to mobile platforms, but executed on a server.

mode The most frequently occurring data point in a set of numbers.

modified systematic approach A seven-step approach to answering drug information requests that includes (1) secure demographics of requestor, (2) obtain background information, (3) determine and categorize ultimate question, (4) develop strategy and conduct search, (5) perform evaluation, analysis, and synthesis, (6) formulate and provide response, and (7) conduct follow-up and documentation.

morbidity Detrimental consequences (other than death) related to a treatment, exposure, or disease state.

MTM See medication therapy management.

MUE See medication use evaluation.

multicollinearity Two or more variables that have extremely high correlations (e.g., >0.90) indicating that they are redundant or that they are measuring the same construct.

narrative review See nonsystematic review.

narrow therapeutic index Used to describe a drug with small differences in dose or blood concentration that may lead to dose and blood concentration dependent serious therapeutic failures or adverse drug reactions.

National Committee for Quality Assurance (NCQA) An organization dedicated to assessing and reporting on the quality of managed care plans; it surveys and accredits managed care organizations much like The Joint Commission accredits hospitals.

National Patient Safety Goals (NPSGs) Program established and updated by The Joint Commission to assist health care organizations to address safety concerns related to patient safety.

NCQA See National Committee for Quality Assurance.

negative formulary A drug formulary that starts out with every marketed drug product and specifically eliminates products that are considered inferior, unnecessary, unsafe, too expensive, etc.

negligence Failure to exercise that degree of care that a person of ordinary prudence or a reasonable person would exercise under the same circumstances. Elements of a negligence case include (1) duty breached, (2) damages, (3) direct causation, and (4) defenses absent.

negligent misrepresentation Occurs when the defendant carelessly makes a representation or statement without reasonable basis to believe it to be true. The burden of proof that is required passes to the person who made the statement who must prove that the statement was either not one of fact but opinion and that he or she had reasonable ground to believe and did believe that the facts represented were true.

network analysis   Also known as multiple treatment comparison or mixed treatment meta-analysis. A network meta-analysis simultaneously compares and ranks a "network" of treatments in which subsets have been compared in individual studies.

New Drug Application (NDA)   The application to the FDA requesting approval to market a new drug for human use. The NDA contains data supporting the safety and efficacy of the drug for its intended use.

New Molecular Entity (NME)   A compound that can be patented and has not been previously marketed in the United States in any form.

NME   See new molecular entity.

N-of-1 trial   A study design similar to a crossover study design conducted in a single patient who receives treatments in pairs (one period of the experimental therapy and one period of either alternative treatment or placebo) in random order.

nominal data   Data that is categorical (e.g., yes/no; male/female).

nominal scale   A scale of measurement that places data into mutually exclusive categories without reference to rank order.

non-inferiority   Any difference shown in a non-inferiority design trial between two treatments is small enough to conclude the test drug has an effect not too much smaller (no worse) than the active control or reference drug.

non-inferiority margin   A prespecified amount of effect used to show that the test drug's treatment effect is not worse than the reference drug by more than this specific degree.

noninherent drug risks   Created by the particular drug in combination with some extrinsic factor that the pharmacist should reasonably know about.

nonmaleficence   A basic principle of consequentialist theory which encompasses the duty to do no harm.

nonparametric tests   Statistical tests that do not assume a conditional normal distribution.

non-pharmacologic   Treatment options focusing on a holistic approach to patient care (e.g., nutrition- and exercise-related interventions).

Nonpublic unsolicited requests   Unsolicited requests that are directed privately to a firm using a one-on-one communication approach.

nonresponse bias   Can result in surveys where the answers of respondents differ from the potential answers of those who did not answer.

nonresponse error   Occurs when a significant number of subjects in a sample do not respond to the survey.

non-systematic review   A review article that summarizes previously conducted research, but does not provide a description of the systematic methods used to identify the research included in the article. Also called a narrative review.

NPSG   See National Patient Safety Goals.

null hypothesis   Statement of no difference in outcome between the intervention and control; created before the beginning of a study. This statement is either rejected or failed-to-be-rejected (i.e., accepted) at the end of the study based upon the p value compared to the alpha value.

number needed to treat (NNT)   A measure used to determine the effectiveness of an intervention. This measure states the average number of patients who need to be treated with the intervention to prevent one additional negative outcome such as a myocardial infarction. The higher the value, the less effective is the intervention. NNT is calculated as the reciprocal of absolute risk reduction.

OBRA '90   See Omnibus Reconciliation Act of 1990.

observational study   A study where the investigator analyzes naturally occurring events.

observer bias   Tendency for observer/investigator to consciously or unconsciously distort what they see and record as the effect in a clinical trial situation. In other words, seeing what they expect to see.

odds ratios   A statistical technique used in case-control studies to determine the risk of exposure to a factor on development of a certain characteristic or disease state. A measure of association between an exposure and an outcome. This ratio represents the chances that an outcome will occur given a particular exposure compared to the chances of the outcome occurring in the absence of that exposure. Odds ratios estimate relative risk.

off-label   The use of a drug for indications, dosage forms or regimens, or other use parameter not stated in the product labeling approved by the FDA. Information that originates from sources (e.g., clinical studies, case reports) outside of the FDA-approved prescription drug labeling.

omission negligence   Consulting the correct source, but failure to locate the correct answer(s) when providing information.

Omnibus Reconciliation Act of 1990 (OBRA '90)   A statute (Public Law 101-508) focused on drug benefits provided under Medicaid. The statute requires pharmacists to conduct drug utilization review (DUR) including prescription screening, patient counseling, and documentation of interventions.

omnibus test   A statistical test of an overall difference. That is, the test indicates if at least one difference or relationship is statistically significant.

one-tailed test   A hypothesis that makes claim to the direction of the difference or relationship.

online   The process of connecting to a remote computer via modem or network.

open formulary   A formulary that allows any marketed drug to be ordered in an institution or under a third-party plan. Can be considered an oxymoron.

operation   Term used in project management to define routine, day-to-day activities without a clear beginning and end.

ordinal scale   A scale of measurement that has rank order, but makes no reference to the distance between ranks.

ordinary care   See reasonable care.

ORYX™   A JCAHO initiative to mandate the use of performance measurement tools to monitor outcomes and to integrate this data into the accreditation process.

outcome indicators   Quality assurance indicators that review whether the final desired result was obtained from whatever action was being reviewed.

outcomes   A change in a patient's health status (e.g., recovery, death, disability, disease, discomfort, dissatisfaction) that can be attributed to the care provided.

outcomes research   An attempt to identify, measure, and evaluate the end results of health care services. It may include not only clinical and economic consequences, but also outcomes, such as patient health status and satisfaction with their health care. A systematic investigation which seeks to provide evidence about which interventions are best for certain types of patients and under certain circumstances.

overview   A general term for a summary of the literature. Includes nonsystematic (narrative), systematic (qualitative), and quantitative (meta-analyses) reviews.

p-value   The probability of obtaining a test statistic as large or larger than the one actually obtained, conditional on the null hypothesis being true. It is the remaining area under a given probability distribution. Statistical value calculated based upon the study results; when this number is less than the alpha value, it is interpreted as the probability of rejecting a true null hypothesis or the probability of chance being the reason that a difference in the results between the two groups was calculated.

P&T committee   See pharmacy and therapeutics committee.

page proofs   See galley proofs.

pair-wise analysis   The pair-wise approach is the traditional method to compile a meta-analysis by synthesizing the results of different trials to obtain an overall estimate of the treatment effect of one intervention relative to the control.

parallel forms   Alternatively worded survey items placed throughout a survey used to increase reliability of survey research.

parallel study   A study where two or more groups receive different treatments and the outcomes are compared.

parameter negligence   Failure to consult the correct source in providing information.

parametric tests   Statistical tests that assume a conditional normal distribution.

parenteral admixtures   Solutions containing drug products for intravenous administration.

participatory medicine   A new model of cooperative health care where patients no longer play a passive part when it comes to their health but an active role alongside the health care provider.

Patient Centered Medical Home (PCMH)   Team-based health care delivery led by a physician or other primary care provider, but including multiple other types of providers, such as pharmacists, to optimize patient outcomes.

Patient education   Written or verbal drug information through a planned activity initiated by a health care provider with the goal of changing patient behavior, improve adherence, and ultimately improve health.

Patient pocket formulary   Pocket-sized drug formulary listing top therapeutic drug classes, preferred products within those classes, cost index for the products, and other pertinent information.

Patient Safety Organizations (PSOs)   The Patient Safety and Quality Improvement Act of 2005 (Patient Safety Act) authorized the creation of a nationwide network of PSOs to improve safety and quality through the collection and analysis of data on patient events.

patient-by-treatment interaction   Describes the variation in response to therapy due to the heterogeneity of multiple patients' individual characteristics. This heterogeneity can be reduced somewhat with inclusion and exclusion criteria. The best method to minimize patient-by-treatment interaction is to use the patient as their own control such as in a crossover trial design.

PBM   See pharmacy benefit management companies.

PCMH   See patient-centered medical home.

peer review   A quality assurance program that centers on the evaluation of specific individuals by other similar professionals. Also, the process where a group of experts review a manuscript for accuracy and appropriateness for publication in a biomedical journal.

performance indicators   Items used to measure quality as part of the check function of quality improvement. The indicators typically focus on the process or outcomes of a care system, although they can also focus on structure.

per-protocol   Study design technique to analyze the study results of only those subjects who completed the entire duration of the study.

personal health records (PHRs)   Health 2.0 applications that provide the patient increased opportunity to participate in the collection, maintenance, and sharing of their personal health-related information through a web-based environment.

perspective   A pharmacoeconomic term that describes whose costs (such as the insurer, or the patient) are relevant based on the purpose of the study.

PESTLE   A type of external environment analysis used in project management that encompasses political, economic, social, technological, legal, and environmental factors that may influence a project.

PGY1 residency   See postgraduate year one residency.

PGY2 residency   See postgraduate year two residency.

pharmaceutical care   The responsible provision of drug therapy for the purpose of achieving definite outcomes that improve a patient's quality of life.

pharmacoeconomics   The description and analysis of the costs of drug therapy to health care systems and society—it identifies, measures, and compares the costs and consequences of pharmaceutical products and services.

pharmacoepidemiologic trials   A type of trial that combines clinical pharmacology and epidemiology design concepts to study the use of and the effects of drugs in large number of people.

pharmacovigilance   The process of preventing and detecting adverse effects from medications.

pharmacy and therapeutics (P&T) committee   An interdisciplinary group in an institution or company that oversees any and/or all aspects of drug therapy for that institution or company. In hospitals, it is usually a subcommittee of the medical staff. May be known by a variety of similar names, such as pharmacy and formulary committee, drug and therapeutics committee (DTC), or formulary committee.

pharmacy benefit design   Contract that specifies the level of coverage and types of pharmaceutical services available to the health plan member.

pharmacy benefit management (PBM) companies   Organizations that manage pharmaceutical benefits for managed care organizations, medical providers, or employers.

pharmacy informatics   A subspecialty of clinical informatics focusing on the management and integration of medication-related data, information, and knowledge across systems that support the medication use process. Focuses on the use of information, information systems, and automation technology to ensure safe and effective medication usage.

pharmacy informatics specialist   An individual who has advanced drug information skills with a keen understanding of computer and information technology.

pharmacy network   Select pharmacies and pharmacy chains where members of a health plan have to go to get their prescriptions filled usually at a lower cost.

PHI   See protected health information.

PHRs   See personal health records.

pivotal trial   Clinical trial which provides the data that serves as the basis of FDA approval or guideline recommendations.

placebo   A pharmaceutical preparation that does not contain a pharmacologically active ingredient, but is otherwise identical to the active drug preparation in terms of appearance, taste, and smell.

placebo creep   See biocreep.

placebo effect   A phenomenon where the patient has a perceived or actual improvement in their medical condition after receiving placebo treatment.

poison information   A specialized area of drug information. By definition, it is the provision of information on the toxic effects of an extensive range of chemicals, as well as plant and animal exposures.

poison information center   A place that specializes in research, management, and dissemination of toxicity information. A physician usually directs it, although a pharmacist directs many on a day-to-day basis. Often, pharmacists and nurses provide staffing of these centers.

policy   Document that ensures consistency, establishes expectations, and sets minimum standards. Policies change infrequently and address the "what," "who," and "why," laying the foundation for a procedure.

popular technical style   A writing style used by professionals addressing laypeople. This is less formal than writing addressed to professionals.

population   Every individual in the entire universe with the characteristics or disease states under investigation. Since entire populations are generally very large, a sample representative of the population is usually selected for an investigation.

portfolio   Term used in project management to define various programs, projects, and operations aimed at meeting an overall strategic objective.

positive formulary   A drug formulary that starts out with no drug products and specifically adds products, after appropriate evaluation, that are needed by the institution or company.

post hoc   In clinical trial design, this distinguishes something that is done after the study is completed.

postgraduate year one (PGY1) residency   An organized, directed, accredited program that builds upon knowledge, skills, attitudes, and abilities gained from an accredited professional pharmacy degree program. The first-year residency program enhances general competencies in managing medication use systems and supports optimal medication therapy outcomes for patients with a broad range of disease states.

postgraduate year two (PGY2) residency An organized, directed, accredited program that builds upon the competencies established in postgraduate year one of residency training. The second-year residency program is focused on a specific area of practice. The PGY-2 program increases the resident's depth of knowledge, skills, attitudes, and abilities to raise the resident's level of expertise in medication therapy management and clinical leadership in the area of focus. In those practice areas where board certification exists, graduates are prepared to pursue such certification.

postmarketing surveillance The process of continually monitoring and reviewing suspected adverse reactions associated with medications once they reach the market and are available to the public. Legislation mandates this activity for pharmaceutical manufacturers and the U.S. Food and Drug Administration (FDA), but health care providers can also participate by reporting adverse drug events, adverse drug reactions, and medication errors to the FDA and other regulatory bodies.

postmarketing surveillance study A study designed to examine drug use and frequency of side effects following approval by the Food and Drug Administration (FDA).

power The ability of a study to detect a difference between a study intervention and control if a difference exists. Usual minimum target value is 80%; power increases by increasing sample size, which also decreases the probability of a Type II or beta error.

power analysis A statistical procedure conducted by the investigators to determine a sample size for the trial.

practice document General term referring collectively to a policy, procedure, guideline, or other similar document.

preferred drug product Specific drug product within a specific therapeutic class selected as the most appropriate to treat a specific disease or condition as determined by the pharmacy and therapeutics committee.

preferred therapeutic class Specific drug class selected as the most appropriate to treat a specific disease or condition as determined by the pharmacy and therapeutics committee.

prescribability The ability of a drug to be prescribed for the first time.

prevalence Measures the number of people in the population who have the disease at a given time.

prima facie A fact presumed to be true unless it is disproved. That is, evidence that is sufficient to raise a presumption of fact or to establish the fact in question unless rebutted.

primary author The author listed first on a publication. Sometimes referred to as the "first author."

primary endpoint See endpoint, primary.

primary literature/resource A literature that contains an original information such as a clinical trial protocol, case reports, trial data, dissertation, and descriptive reports.

principles In ethical analysis, a principle is relatively broad and fundamental in scope, and guides ethical decision making or actions.

prior authorization Authorization from the health plan or pharmacy benefit manager in conjunction with the pharmacy and therapeutics committee for specified medications or specified quantities of medications. Request is reviewed against preestablished criteria which are based on evidence-based medicine.

privacy A rule within the principle of autonomy, more generally relating to the right of the individual to control his or her own affairs without interference from or knowledge of outside parties.

probabilistic sensitivity analysis   A sensitivity analysis allows one to determine how the results of an analysis would change when these best guesses or assumptions are varied over a relevant range of values. In cost-effectiveness analysis, probability distributions are created for each factor about which there is uncertainty. By simulating the results of random samplings from these distributions, it enables judgments to be formed about the decisions in relation to each factor.

procedure   Document that outlines the steps of specific actions to be taken to achieve an objective or implement a policy. Procedures focus on the "how" and are more flexible and subject to change.

process   Refers to the set of activities that occur between patient and provider, encompassing the services and products that are provided to patients and the manner in which the services are provided.

process change   Making a change to routine process. It may be through changes in policy or procedures, implementation of new services, acquisition of new equipment, changes in staffing, generation of regular notifications, or other methods. It is used to correct practice when quality assurance/drug usage evaluation/medication usage evaluation shows a deficiency.

process indicators   Quality assurance indicators based on the presence or absence of policies and procedures. These assume that if policies and procedures are appropriate they will be effective and be properly performed.

process mapping   A workflow diagram that provides a clear and consistent understanding of the steps and/or parallel processes required to accomplish a task. This is a process undertaken in many industries as an approach to developing standardized work as part of process improvement. It generally identifies variations within a process that may contribute to excess waste or risk.

product claim advertisement   A type of direct to consumer advertisement that includes the name of the medication, the indication, and a balanced overview of the risks and benefits.

product label   The information affixed to the product and used to identify the contents.

product labeling   Product information including prescribing information.

professional ethics   Rules of conduct or standards by which a particular group in society regulates its actions and sets standards for its members.

professional writing   Any written communication prepared in the fulfillment of the practice of a profession.

program   Term used in project management to describe a group of related projects that are managed in a coordinated way. Programs have their own goals and objectives that ultimately support the main strategic objective of a portfolio.

programmatic research   Research focused on the impact and economic value of programs and services provided by pharmacists in community and institutional settings.

project   Finite endeavors with a distinct beginning and end, which are also progressively elaborate.

project charter   Project management tool guidepost used to outline the scope, goals and success criteria, final deliverables, stakeholders, budgets, quality assessments, and constraints of a project.

project constraints   Term used to describe factors that could limit or constrain a project; constraints typically include the scope, time, and available resources (funding, personnel, etc.).

project management   A discipline or science that is goal-oriented, organized, detailed, and has built-in accountability.

prospective indicator An indicator used in any quality assurance program that determines whether quality is acceptable before an action is taken or care is given.

prospective study A study where data are collected forward in time from date of study initiation.

protected health information (PHI) A term under the HIPAA Privacy Rule, which refers to individually identifiable health information which can be linked to a particular person. Specifically, this information can relate to the individual's past, present, or future physical or mental health or condition; the provision of health care to the individual; or the past, present, or future payment for the provision of health care to the individual. Common identifiers of health information include names, social security numbers, addresses, and birth dates.

protopathic bias When a treatment for the first symptoms of a disease or other outcome appears to cause the outcome. In this case, the first symptoms of the outcome of interest are the reason for the treatment under study and not the outcome itself. For instance, early symptoms of pancreatic cancer can be the symptoms of diabetes since beta cells are being destroyed by the cancer.

proximate cause Cause which immediately precedes and produces the effect, as distinguished from the remote or intervening cause.

PSO See Patient Safety Organizations.

public unsolicited requests An unsolicited request made in a public form, whether directed to a firm specifically or to a forum at large.

publication bias A form of selection bias where publication of studies is based on the magnitude, direction, or statistical significance of the results.

pure technical style A writing style used by professionals addressing other professionals in the same field. It tends to be formal and avoids use of the first person (e.g., I, us). Technical jargon can be used in this writing style.

push technology A method by which information is actively sent to users' computers with little, if any, effort required by the user. The information may be displayed as a screen saver or the computer may in some way let the user know that the information is available to be displayed (e.g., pop-up notification).

QALY See quality-adjusted life years.

QR (Quick Response) codes A type of two-dimensional bar code that provides more information than is possible with a standard UPC bar code. It is increasingly common to find these codes on advertisements or items available for purchase, where the code can be scanned by an application on a smartphone to provide referral to a website where further information may be found on something of interest.

qualitative systematic review See meta-analysis or systematic review.

quality Project management term that refers to how good the end result or accomplishment is. Quality is often thought of as a function of time, scope, and resources.

quality assessment and assurance committee A committee found in long-term care facilities to evaluate quality of care, including drug usage evaluation.

quality assurance Activities that prevent deficiencies along the process.

quality control Activities that ensure the value of the final product/deliverable.

quality measure When this term is used in health care, it is used to indicate methods of quantifying the type of care a patient received (indicators may include details about processes and organization structure, overall patient outcomes, and even patients' perceptions of the quality of the care received). Metric tools with specifications to assess the performance of individual clinicians, care entities (hospitals, nursing homes, home care agencies, etc.), and health insurance plans.

quality of life An evaluation of a patient's living situation based on the patient's environment, family life, financial situation, education, and health. It is used in quality assurance programs when developing indicators. In some cases, quality-of-life aspects will take precedence over the absolute best treatment. For example, a quick cure to a disease state may not be as desirable when it costs so much that a family is bankrupted in the process.

quality-adjusted life years (QALY) A health-utility measure combining quality and quantity of life, as determined by some valuations process.

quantitative systematic review See meta-analysis.

quantity limits Set quantity of drug that can be prescribed that is set by the health plan in conjunction with the pharmacy and therapeutics committee that is usually based on FDA prescribing guidelines.

random error See sampling error.

randomization Process used in a study in which all subjects enrolled in the study have an equal opportunity to be in any of the study groups. This is used to reduce bias, enable the groups to be as similar as possible at baseline, and is required to validate certain statistical tests.

randomized clinical trial See controlled clinical trial.

range The difference between the highest data value and the lowest data value.

rate-based indicators Usually measure the proportion of activities, or patients, that conform to a desired standard (e.g., the proportion of stat orders that are dispensed within 15 minutes).

ratio data Rank ordered data in which each measurement has a meaningful equal distance between points and also an absolute/natural zero (e.g., temperature in Kelvin).

ratio scale A scale of measurement that has rank ordered data with meaningful distance between ranks and a natural zero.

RCA See root cause analysis.

reasonable or due care Also called ordinary care; conduct that an ordinarily prudent or reasonable person would normally exercise in a particular situation to avoid harm to another, taking the circumstances into account. The concept of due care is used as a test of liability for negligence and usually made on a case-by-case basis where each juror has to determine what a reasonable man or woman would do.

reasoning engine See inference engine.

rechallenge In relation to adverse drug reactions, this occurs when the drug is discontinued and, after the adverse drug reactions (ADR) abates, the patient is given the same medication in an attempt to elicit the response again.

referee An expert in a particular area who reviews a written document to determine whether it is appropriate for publication.

refereed publication A publication in which the editors have experts in the appropriate field review items submitted for possible publication to determine whether those items are of suitable quality.

regulatory project manager (RPM)   This will be the sponsor's primary FDA contact person. Each application that is submitted is assigned a regulatory project manager (RPM). Contact information for the RPM is provided in the letter sent to the applicant acknowledging receipt of the application. If the RPM is changed during the course of the review, the applicant is notified by the new RPM.

relative risk   A statistical technique used in follow-up studies to determine the risk associated with exposure to a certain factor on disease state development. Relative risk estimates how many times greater the risk of disease state development is in patients exposed to a certain factor compared to those who are not exposed.

reminder advertisement   A type of direct-to-consumer advertisement that provides a medication's name but does not include or imply the medication's indication.

REMS   See Risk Evaluation and Mitigation Strategy.

requirements matrix   A project management tool used to align the requirements of a project with the goals in the charter.

research hypothesis (also known as the alternative hypothesis or hypothesis, H_a)   A difference between the therapy under investigation and the control.

residual value   The difference between the model predicted dependent variable and the actual dependent variable value.

Respondeat Superior   Refers to the proposition that the employer is responsible for the negligent acts of its agents or employees.

response bias   See measurement error.

Restatement (Second) of Torts   "An attempt by the American Law Institute to present an orderly statement of the general common law of the United States, including in that term not only the law developed solely by judicial decision, but also the law that has grown from the application by the courts of statutes..." It takes into account other factors, such as the modern trend of the law according to influential jurisdictions and well-thought out opinions.

retrospective indicator   An indicator used in any quality assurance program that determines whether quality was acceptable after an action was taken or care was given.

retrospective study   A study that analyzes historical data (e.g., previously collected data such as medical records or insurance information).

Risk Evaluation and Mitigation Strategy (REMS)   A risk management plan required by the FDA that goes beyond requirements in the drug prescribing information to manage serious risks associated with a drug.

Risk Minimization Action Plans (RiskMAPs)   A strategic safety program designed to meet specific goals and objectives in minimizing known risks of a product while preserving its benefits.

RiskMAPs   See Risk Minimization Action Plans.

robustness   The ability of the statistical test to produce correct test statistics and parameter estimates in the presence of assumption violations.

root cause analysis (RCA)   In response to a sentinel or serious event, the expectation of The Joint Commission is that the organization will conduct a timely, thorough, and credible analysis to determine root causes of the event, develop and implement an action plan to reduce the risk of recurrence, and monitor the effectiveness of the plan and its implementation.

RPM   See regulatory project manager.

RSS   This acronym has multiple meanings, but is usually defined as Really Simple Syndication. It is a method by which an aggregator program collects information from websites and weblogs (blog), which is then displayed as a collation. This allows individuals to monitor new or additional information on the Internet without having to use a browser to go to multiple websites.

rule   In ethical analysis, a rule guides ethical decision making or actions, but is relatively specific in context and restricted in scope.

rules engines   Computer programs, similar to ADE monitoring systems, with built-in, logic rules designed to aid in monitoring specific aspects of patient care.

run-in phase   A short duration of patient assessment but prior to being enrolling into the study. Various reasons exist for this phase and include assessment of medication compliance, meeting an inclusion criteria (e.g., LDL-C less than 130 mg/dL), and allowing for medication wash-out.

SaaS   See software as a service.

sample   A group of subjects, taken from the population, who are enrolled in a study; these individuals should represent the population in order for the study results to be extrapolated to the population.

sample frame   A term describing the population that will actually be drawn from to make up the survey sample.

sampling error   Refers to the difference between the estimate derived from a sample survey and the true value that would result if a census of the entire target population were taken under the same conditions.

scope   Project management term that refers to the amount of work that is to be done, as well as what the project will and will not entail.

secondary endpoint   See endpoint, secondary.

secondary literature/resource   A literature mainly in the form of searchable database that enables location and retrieval of primary or tertiary resources. This category of resources is similar to an old cataloging system.

selection bias   Study subjects who meet the study inclusion/exclusion criteria but are not randomized into either the intervention or control (i.e., excluded from the study).

SEM   See standard error of the mean.

sensitivity   The probability an individual with a disease will have a positive test result.

sensitivity analysis   Tests that are undertaken to determine the influence of various criteria or conditions on study results. Sensitivity analyses are commonly used in meta-analyses and pharmacoeconomic research.

sentinel event   The Joint Commission defines a sentinel event as an unexpected occurrence involving death or serious physical or psychological injury, or the risk thereof. Serious injury specifically includes loss of limb or function. The phrase "or the risk thereof" includes any process variation for which a recurrence would carry a significant chance of a serious adverse outcome. Such events are called "sentinel" because they signal the need for immediate investigation and response.

sentinel indicators   Reflect the occurrence of a serious event that requires further investigation (e.g., adverse drug-related event, death).

skewness   The measure of symmetry of a curve.

smart pumps   See intelligent infusion pumps.

smartphone   A cellular device that has Internet capabilities and supports various software functions.

social media   Form of electronic communication allowing interactions with users to share information, messages, and other various forms of content. Consists of social networking sites, content-sharing sites, and blogs.

software as a service (SaaS)/application service provider (ASP)   A computing model in which an organization's data and software are hosted by an off-site vendor who is responsible for maintaining data storage as well as the equipment on which it is stored.

special protocol assessment   A statement from the U.S. Food and Drug Administration that an uninitiated or ongoing Phase III trial's design, clinical endpoints, and statistical analyses are adequate for FDA approval.

specificity   The probability an individual without a disease will have a negative test result.

sponsor   An organization (or individual) who takes responsibility for and initiates a clinical investigation. The sponsor may be an individual or pharmaceutical company, government agency, academic institution, private organization, or other organization.

sponsor-investigator   An individual who both initiates and conducts a clinical investigation (i.e., submits the IND and directly supervises administration of the drug as well as other investigator responsibilities).

stability study   A study designed to determine the stability of drugs in various preparations.

stakeholder   Term used in project management to describe anyone who is involved in, interested in, or affected by a project.

stakeholder matrix   Project management tool used to identify stakeholders, as well as their involvement, expectations, interest, and engagement for a given project.

standard   A term used in quality assurance program that indicates how often an indicator must be complied with. The level of compliance will be set at either 0% (i.e., never done) or 100% (i.e., always done). A threshold, which allows compliance of between 0% and 100%, has sometimes been used instead of a standard.

standard deviation   (1) A measurement of the range of data values (i.e., variability) around the mean. (2) The measure of the average amount by which each observation in a series of data points differs from the mean. In other words, how far away is each data point from the mean (dispersion or variability) or the average deviation from the mean.

standard error of the mean (SEM)   Estimates the variability between sample means when multiple samples are taken from the same population. The standard error of the mean estimates the variability between samples whereas the standard deviation measures the variability within a single sample.

standard gamble   One method used in measuring health preferences. Each subject is offered two alternatives. Alternative one is treatment with two possible outcomes: either the return to normal health or immediate death. Alternative two is the certain outcome of a chronic disease state for life. The probability of dying is varied until the subject is indifferent between alternative one and alternative two. Used to assess his or her QALY estimate.

statistic   A measurement that describes part of a sample.

statistical significance   The impact of a study in terms of the outcome of statistical tests conducted on the data. A study is said to be statistically significant when statistical tests demonstrate a difference between treatment groups.

statute   Written law enacted by a legislature other than that of a municipality.

step therapy   Prescribing guidelines set by the health plan in conjunction with the pharmacy and therapeutics committee that specify which drugs should be prescribed first before more expensive drugs will be covered. Guidelines are based on evidence-based medicine.

stratification   An advanced type of randomization to produce study groups as similar as possible; considers baseline demographic information of the subjects selected for the study.

strict liability   Also called absolute liability; the legal responsibility for damages, or injury, even if the person was not at fault or negligent. Strict liability has been applied to certain activities, such as holding employers absolutely liable for the torts of their employees, but it is most commonly associated with claims for injuries resulting from defectively manufactured or designed products. A successful plaintiff need only show that the product was in fact defective in design or manufacture, rendering it unreasonably dangerous and the cause of injury.

structure   Refers to the characteristics of providers, the tools and resources at their disposal, and the physical or organizational settings in which they work.

structure indicators   Quality assurance indicators based on the presence or absence of items, such as staffing patterns, available space, equipment, resources, or administrative organization.

study objective   A brief statement of the goals and purpose of a research study.

subgroup analysis   Evaluation of study results within a subset of subjects enrolled in the study according to specific demographic (e.g., age, gender, disease state).

subject   An individual who participates in a clinical investigation either as the recipient of the investigational drug or as a member of the control group.

success criteria   Term used in project management to describe quantifiable measures that indicate when a project goal has been accomplished.

summary judgment   A party moving (applying) for summary judgment is attempting to avoid the time and expense of a trial when the outcome is obvious. A party may also move for summary judgment in order to eliminate the risk of losing at trial, and possibly avoid having to go through discovery (i.e., by moving at the outset of discovery), by demonstrating to the judge, via sworn statements and documentary evidence, that there are no material factual issues remaining to be tried. If there's nothing for the factfinder to decide, then the moving party asks rhetorically, why have a trial? A dispute over a material fact (see above) upon which the outcome of a legal case may rely, and which therefore must be decided by a judge or jury; a dispute which precludes summary judgment.

surrogate endpoint   An effect that can be easily measured to correlate an outcome that is more difficult and/or time-consuming to measure (e.g., lowering LDL-C levels [measured effect] should result in reducing cardiovascular events [predicted outcome] such as myocardial infarction, stroke, or death).

survey instrument   Questionnaire used for the survey.

survey research   Research where responses to questions asked of subjects are analyzed to determine the incidence, distribution, and relationships of sociological and psychological variables.

switchability   The ability to exchange one drug for another.

SWOT   A type of internal environment analysis used in project management that encompasses strengths, weaknesses, opportunities, and threats.

symposium   A meeting focused on a particular topic.

synthesis   The careful, systematic, and orderly process of integrating varied and diverse elements, ideas, or factors into a coherent response. This process relies not only on the type and quality of the data gathered, but also on how the data are organized, viewed, and evaluated. Synthesis, as it relates to pharmacotherapy, involves the careful integration of critical information about the patient, disease, and medication along with pertinent background information to arrive at a judgment or conclusion.

systematic review   A summary of previously conducted studies where the research to be included in the review is systematically identified; however, the results are not statistically combined as would occur with a quantitative systematic review or meta-analysis. Also called a qualitative systematic review.

target drug program   A program that evaluates the use of a medication or group of medications on an ongoing basis. Within these programs, interventions are usually made at the time of discovery based on established criteria or guidelines.

target population   The entire group a researcher is interested in because this is the population that the findings of the survey are meant to generalize and the researcher wishes to make inferences and draw conclusions.

telemedicine   The use of telecommunications and interactive video technology to provide health care services to patients who are at a distance.

telnet   A program for microcomputers that causes the computer to mimic a dumb terminal, so that it can run programs on other computers (usually minicomputers or mainframes) over the Internet or other computer networks.

Ten Major Considerations   Ten items identified to evaluate a clinical trial article that if any single item is considered a limitation, the reliability of the entire article is questionable and the results deemed possibly unreliable.

teratogenicity   Toxicity of drugs to the unborn fetus.

tertiary literature/resource   A literature that reviews, summarizes, compares, and reports what has already been published as primary literature. This includes systematic reviews and meta-analyses as well as clinical practice guidelines.

The Joint Commission (TJC)   Organization that accredits health care organizations and programs in the United States.

third-party payer   Organization that pays for or underwrites coverage for health care expenses for another entity.

third-party plan   A method of reimbursement for medical care in which neither the care provider nor the patient is charged. Third-party payers include insurance, health maintenance organizations, and government entities.

threshold   A term used in quality assurance program that indicates how often an indicator must be complied with. Unlike standards, thresholds can be set at any level of compliance from 0% to 100%.

tiered copayment benefit   A pharmacy benefit design that encourages patients to use generic and formulary drugs, by requiring the patient to pay progressively higher copayments for brand name and non-formulary drugs.

time trade-off   A method for measuring health preferences. The subject is offered two alternatives. Alternative one is a certain disease state for a specific length of time t, the life expectancy for a person with the disease, then death. Alternative two is being healthy for time x, which is less than t. Time x is varied until the respondent is indifferent between the two alternatives. The proportion of the number of years of life a person is willing to give up (t − x) to have his or her remaining years (x) of life in a healthy state is used to assess his or her QALY estimate.

TJC   See The Joint Commission.

tort liability   Civil wrongs recognized by law as grounds for a lawsuit.

total quality management (TQM)   A management concept dealing with the implementation of continuous quality improvement.

TQM   See total quality management.

treatment effect   A mean difference in the outcome measure over time between two drugs (i.e., drug − placebo or test drug − reference drug).

treatment order effect   A situation where the order in which patients receive the treatment in a trial (generally a crossover design) affects the results of that trial.

treatment-by-time interaction   Chance that the effects associated with each treatment might vary over time.

trohoc study   See case-control study.

true experiment   A study where researchers apply a treatment and determine its effects on subjects.

true negatives   Individuals without the disease that were correctly identified as being disease-free by the test.

true positives   Individuals with the disease that were correctly identified as diseased by the test.

two-tailed test   A hypothesis that does not claim a direction of the difference or relationship.

type I error   Falsely rejecting the null hypothesis when, in fact, the null hypothesis is true.

type II error   Failing to reject the null hypothesis when, in fact, the null hypothesis is false.

unexpected drug reaction   The Food and Drug Administration defines this as "one that is not listed in the current labeling for the drug as having been reported or associated with the use of the drug. This includes an ADR that may be symptomatically or pathophysiologically related to an ADR listed in the labeling but may differ from the labeled ADR because of greater severity or specificity (e.g., abnormal liver function vs. hepatic necrosis)."

uniform resource locator (URL)   An Internet address (e.g., http://druginfo.creighton.edu).

unsolicited requests   Requests initiated by persons or entities that are completely independent of the relevant firm.

USENET news   A large number of discussion groups that are replicated in numerous places on Internet. Users can read items posted on a topic and can contribute their own items to be posted.

validity   The truthfulness of study results. Internal validity refers to the extent to which the study results reflect what actually happened in the study (i.e., appropriate and sound study methods). External validity is the degree to which the study results can be applied to patients routinely encountered in clinical practice.

validity filter A type of term or limit used to narrow a search to only the highest quality studies, such as randomized controlled trial or double-blind.

validity, external Quality of the study design that allows the result to be applied into practice. Study results are meaningful to practitioners and can be used for patient care.

validity, internal Quality of the study design that produces accurate results. Strong study design should translate into reliable results.

value Has been assigned many definitions, but within health care, it usually reflects the ratio of quality and costs (value = quality/cost).

variables Factors (characteristics that are being observed or measured) that are the focus of a study. The independent variable (e.g., treatment) causes change in the dependent variable (e.g., outcome).

variance A measurement of the range of data values (i.e., variability) about the mean. Variance is the square of the standard deviation.

veracity This term addresses the obligation to truth telling or honesty.

vicarious liability Also called imputed liability or imputed negligence; the doctrine that attaches responsibility upon one person for the failure of another, with whom the person has a special relationship (such as parent and child, employer and employee, husband and wife, or owner of vehicle and driver), to exercise such care as a reasonably prudent person would use under similar circumstances. Ordinarily, the independent negligence of one person is not imputable to another person.

virtual private network (VPN) A method to connect computers over a distance, for example, over the Internet, that allows secure transmission of confidential data.

warning letter An official message from the FDA to a pharmaceutical manufacturer, identifying rule violations such as not following cGMP.

warranty An assurance by one party to a contract of the existence of a fact upon which the other party may rely, intended to relieve the promisee of any duty to ascertain the fact for himself or herself. Amounts to a promise to indemnify the promisee for any loss if the fact warranted proves untrue. Warranties may be express (made overtly) or implied (by implication).

Web 2.0 Simply refers to those applications of the Internet that are interactive and social, allowing for collaboration and interactivity among patients, caregivers, and providers.

web browser A computer program used to access information on the World Wide Web. The most popular programs are Microsoft Internet Explorer or Edge, Google Chrome, and Mozilla Firefox.

web portal A website that acts as an interface to the Internet for users. Many Internet search engines are considered to be web portals. A variation on this, the enterprise portal, can also be used by an institution to help guide employees to necessary information within the institution or out on the Internet.

weblog (also known as blog) This is a public website where a person maintains a journal that is open to viewers.

website A group of web pages that will provide information to the person requesting that information. These pages are generally grouped under one main Internet address (URL).

wide area network (WAN) A group of computers connected in a way that they may share data, programs, and/or equipment over a distance (e.g., connection between computers owned by an institution that are scattered in clinics around a city).

wikis Websites which allow its users to add, modify, or delete its content via a web browser usually using a simplified markup language or a rich-text editor. Wikis are powered by wiki software, are created collaboratively, and can be community websites and intranets, for example. Some permit control over different functions (levels of access). For example, editing rights may permit changing, adding, or removing material. Others may permit access without enforcing access control.

work breakdown structure Project management tool used to identify and collate tasks needed to complete a deliverable.

World Wide Web (WWW) Computers connected to the Internet that provide a graphical interface to a variety of information that is available as text, pictures, sounds, databases, and other electronic files. Generally accessed using a web browser, such as Google Chrome.

XHTML—Extensible HTML A combination of HTML and Extensible Markup Language.

XML—Extensible Markup Language A superset of HTML that provides information on the content of a web page, presentation of the information (how it looks), and semantics (what it means). This is designed to make it easier to find more relevant information using search engines.

z-score The distance a data point is from its variable's mean in standard deviation units.

Answers for Case Studies

Chapter 3

CASE STUDY 3-1

Common side effects would be included in all major compendia (e.g., Micromedex® 2.0, Clinical Pharmacology, or Facts & Comparisons) which would be a good initial search. In addition, some of the adverse effect specific resources (e.g., Meyler's Side Effects of Drugs) would be appropriate to consult for less common side effects.

CASE STUDY 3-2

- There are a variety of resources that could be consulted for this information including the text Drugs in Pregnancy and Lactation or some of the major compendia (possibly, Micromedex® 2.0 or Clinical Pharmacology).
- The resources classify levofloxacin as an agent with unknown safety, but likely to be safe.
- In order to best answer this question, the requestor should determine if the disease state has other treatment options which have more data available and if the infant is receiving any formula supplementation.

CASE STUDY 3-3

- The student might start a search for general information in a toxicology text such as Goldfrank's Toxicologic Emergencies. That could be followed with a search in Micromedex® 2.0 to find some general toxicology information; specifically the POISINDEX component of that resource would provide comprehensive information on this topic.
- The student would do best to search using the generic name of the medication, in this case using chlorpheniramine.

CASE STUDY 3-4

In a case you are not familiar with a term, a general Internet search might be a good start to help streamline your search. An Internet search shows that AMDUCA stands for Animal Medicinal Drug Use Clarification Act of 1994. Knowing that the term refers to a specific piece of legislation, you would be prompted to consider searching the American Veterinarian Medical Association web page or Food and Drug Administration web page.

CASE STUDY 3-5

- Since this would be an off-label use, there may be less data in the tertiary resources. In this case it is likely more efficient to do a search in the secondary resources. Medline is a good place to start.
- Initially conducting a search with no restrictions/limits ensures that valuable information is not missed.
- If the initial search yields a significant number of results, then a restriction to human clinical trials would be beneficial. When conducting this search, it is important to realize that the term female sexual arousal disorder has changed over time, so maybe a more general search for female sexual dysfunctions will give more responses. In addition, searching for the specific drug sildenafil will yield useful data, but expanding the search using the class of drugs will provide more data.

CASE STUDY 3-6

Since the patient specifically provided you the news venue, going directly to the NBC web page would be an excellent start. Since content changes quickly on news pages, possibly a general Internet search might be needed if the story was run a while back.

CASE STUDY 3-7

- Tertiary resources could provide a good overview on how a treatment might work in a large patient population, appropriate dosing, as well as provide a quick summary of safety data. The disadvantage is the lag time from when the information is updated until it is published, so recently discovered safety or efficacy information might not be included in that type of resource.
- Primary literature would provide very timely information, but in a case like this, the volume of primary literature can be overwhelming and makes it difficult to navigate.

Chapter 4

CASE STUDY 4-1[1]

- The use of ezetimibe is technically considered ancillary therapy, as not all subjects in the study received the extra therapy option, just those needing additional assistance reducing LDL levels. However, the significance of the use of the ezetimibe is lessened because participants from both treatment arms of the study were eligible to receive the ancillary ezetimibe therapy if needed. It would be important for the reader of this study to look at the results of the study and determine if a disproportionate number of subjects in one of the treatment arms received the ancillary ezetimibe therapy. As the reader can see, there was a greater than twofold increase in subjects receiving ancillary ezetimibe in the placebo group versus the intervention group. This finding should be taken into context when evaluating other attributes of the study.
- The purpose of a run-in phase is to assess for toxicity and/or tolerability of investigational drug therapies in study subjects. In studies that utilize novel drugs or potentially toxic medications the use of a run-in phase is an excellent control mechanism to help ensure patient safety. Subjects who do not tolerate the therapy are excluded from the study. Run-in phases can also be conducted to determine subject adherence to medication therapy. Those subjects who are not adherent to a medication at a predetermined rate will be excluded from the study. While common, results of studies that utilize run-in phases to control for adherence should be closely examined, particularly

in the instance where results of the study are statistically analyzed using the intention-to-treat (ITT) method, as this could artificially inflate performance of the intervention therapy compared to the intended "real-world" perspective when used in the general population.

- The ITT principle is a way of viewing data for analysis. This analytical method includes the data points (i.e., endpoints) of everyone who is included in the study protocol. Thus, this method of analysis gives the reader a "worst case scenario" viewpoint on medication therapy performance in the general population. ITT analysis is desired in a controlled clinical trial designed to determine superiority of one treatment versus another. The fact that a medication therapy can generate significant outcomes in a worst case scenario implies that the medication is durable and can generate significant results even though some patients may not be as adherent to their medication therapy as they should be. Alternatively, the per-protocol (PP) analysis only utilized the data points (i.e., endpoints) of subjects who complete the study "per the protocol." This method of analysis can be viewed as a "best case scenario" approach to viewing study results. PP data are helpful in studies that have high rates of attrition, as the ITT data set may contribute to artificial worsening of drug outcome data.

- A composite endpoint is an endpoint type where several event occurrences can qualify as attainment of the composite primary endpoint. This type of endpoint is usually reserved for studies that analyze health events that are negative or undesired and associated with one another on a pathophysiological basis (e.g., cardiovascular death, myocardial infarction, stroke). Utilization of composite endpoints makes it easier for a subject to attain the primary endpoint because the study investigators are not having to wait on a subject to experience one health event, but rather, one of several associated health events. Use of composite endpoints can be beneficial in terms of shortening the duration of a study. Some disadvantages of the practice of utilizing a composite endpoint is that a disproportionate number of subjects may experience one of the qualifying endpoints over other endpoints, which could cloud the interpretation of the results. It is important for the reader to closely analyze outcome rates within studies that utilize composite endpoints to ensure that the distribution of event rates among qualifying events is somewhat matched and if not, that any statistically significant differences between individual outcome rates receive comment in the discussion section of the article.

CASE STUDY 4–2

- Yes, any study enrolling human subjects requires IRB approval. This is especially true since this clinical trial includes children, who represent a protected group of individuals, who may be at increased risk due to participation in the clinical trial. The IRB approval is needed to protect the enrolled subjects.

- The type of data being evaluated for the primary endpoint is nominal data, which is represented by an endpoint that is "yes/no" or dichotomous in nature. For the study under consideration, the endpoint of incidence of clinical cure falls into this category. Either someone is cured or they are not cured.

  A benefit of endpoints that are nominal in nature is that they represent an objective outcome and are driven by clinical events (e.g., occurrence of "event x" or no occurrence of "event x"). With nominal endpoints there is no ranking or scaling of endpoint results or any ability to influence outcomes by personal perception or opinion. Furthermore, nominal endpoints are useful from the standpoint that measures of association (i.e., RR, ARR, RRR, NNT) can be conducted. Thus, such endpoints are very good for comparing objective outcomes between treatments.

- Mode is the appropriate measure of central tendency to present nominal data. The mode is the most frequently occurring observation in the data set.

- $p = 0.52$ indicates that there is a 52% probability for a false positive conclusion (i.e., Type 1 error) with respect to the primary endpoint result. The p-value of 0.52 is greater than the predetermined alpha value of 0.05 (i.e., 5%) which indicates that the primary endpoint result is not statistically significant and leads the investigators to fail-to-reject the null hypothesis.

- The point estimate of −2.6% represents a between-group difference in cure rates of 2.6% in favor of clindamycin in this sample and the investigators are 95% confident that the true between-group difference in cure rates in the general population ranges between -10.2% in favor of clindamycin and $+4.9$ in favor of TMP-SMX. The value of equality (zero) is contained in this range, indicating lack of statistical significance and, therefore no possibility for clinical significance. Investigators must fail to reject the null hypothesis that there is no difference in cure rates for uncomplicated skin infections with cellulitis, abscesses >5 cm in diameter, or both in adults and children in the outpatient setting between TMP-SMX and clindamycin.

CASE STUDY 4–3[2,3]

- Double-dummy blinding is a sophisticated blinding scheme that is utilized in select situations. Double-dummy means that both the intervention and control arm receive "dummy" doses of the opposing therapy. Use in the case of this study was necessary in order to conceal therapies, as this study used therapies that utilize different dosing schedules (i.e., adjusted-dose warfarin scheduling is customized to the patient based upon his/her INR values).

  Double-dummy blinding is also utilized in situations where medications in different study arms may be in different dosage forms (e.g., transdermal fentanyl versus oral morphine for the treatment of chronic pain). If possible, utilization of a double-dummy approach in a trial that has an active control is desired and increases the internal validity of the study by reducing the potential for confounding due to subjects being able to identify their assigned therapy.

- RR high-dose edoxaban versus warfarin $= 1.18\%/1.5\% = 0.78$

  This quotient value is less than 1, indicating a protective benefit conferred to the recipient of edoxaban 60 mg versus dose-adjusted warfarin for the prevention of stroke or systemic embolism within the given study sample. In other words, the quotient value of 0.78 could be utilized to indicate that use of edoxaban 60 mg is associated with 78% of the risk of stroke or systemic embolization that is associated with adjusted-dose warfarin.

- RRR $= 1 -$ RR $= 1 - 0.78 = 0.22 = 22\%$

  This value indicates that 22% of baseline risk of the occurrence of stroke or systemic embolization is removed by receiving edoxaban 60 mg versus dose-adjusted warfarin. This result indicates that edoxaban 60 mg reduces stroke or systemic embolization risk versus dose-adjusted warfarin.

- ARR $= \%C - \%I = 1.5\% - 1.18\% = 0.32\%$

  This value indicates that 0.32% of subjects were spared from experiencing stroke or systemic embolization by receiving edoxaban 60 mg versus dose-adjusted warfarin. This result indicates that edoxaban 60 mg reduces stroke or systemic embolization risk versus dose-adjusted warfarin.

- NNT $= 1/$ARR (in decimal format) $= 1/0.0032 = 312$

  This result indicates that the investigators would have to treat 312 patients for the median trial follow-up period (2.8 years) to prevent one primary endpoint occurrence that otherwise would with receipt of warfarin. This value is not an ideal value as lower NNT values are preferred, with 1 being the best possible NNT value, inferring a 100% effectiveness rate with respect to the primary endpoint.

- The HR for stroke or systemic embolism in this sample is 1.13 and the investigators are 97.5% confident that the true HR in the general population lies between 0.96 and 1.34. The value of equality (one) is contained in this range, indicating lack of statistical significance and, therefore no possibility for clinical significance. Investigators must fail to reject the null hypothesis with respect to the comparison of low-dose edoxaban and warfarin in the context of the primary endpoint.

REFERENCES

1. AIM-HIGH Investigators, Boden WE, Probstfield JL, Anderson T, Chaitman BR, Desvignes-Nickens P, Koprowicz K, McBride R, Teo K, Weintraub W. Niacin in patients with low HDL cholesterol levels receiving intensive statin therapy. N Engl J Med. 2011 Dec 15;365(24):2255-67. doi: 10.1056/NEJMoa1107579.

2. Giugliano RP, Ruff CT, Braunwald E, Murphy SA, Wiviott SD, Halperin JL, Waldo AL, Ezekowitz MD, Weitz JI, Špinar J, Ruzyllo W, Ruda M, Koretsune Y, Betcher J, Shi M, Grip LT, Patel SP,

Patel I, Hanyok JJ, Mercuri M, Antman EM; ENGAGEAF-TIMI 48 Investigators. Edoxaban versus warfarin in patients with atrial fibrillation. N Engl J Med. 2013 Nov 28;369(22):2093-104.
3. Thursz MR, Richardson P, Allison M, Austin A, Bowers M, Day CP, Downs N, Gleeson D, MacGilchrist A, Grant A, Hood S, Masson S, McCune A, Mellor J, O'Grady J, Patch D, Ratcliffe I, Roderick P, Stanton L, Vergis N, Wright M, Ryder S, Forrest EH; STOPAH Trial. Prednisolone or pentoxifylline for alcoholic hepatitis. N Engl J Med. 2015 Apr 23;372(17):1619-28. doi: 10.1056/NEJMoa1412278.

Chapter 5

CASE STUDY 5–1

- Null hypothesis: The mean treatment difference (change in VAS from baseline to end of study for each product) and 95% CI associated with that treatment difference fail to exhibit non-inferiority for transdermal buprenorphine compared to sustained release tramadol regarding pain control. In other words, the study results would be inconclusive.

  Alternative hypothesis: The mean treatment difference (change in VAS from baseline to end of study for each product) and 95% CI associated with that treatment difference exhibit non-inferiority for transdermal buprenorphine compared to sustained release tramadol regarding pain control.
- How was the NI margin determined? Did the investigators set the NI margin prior to the study being conducted? Did the investigators confirm sustained-release tramadol efficacy against placebo which is referred to as assay sensitivity? Were historical trials and this NI study as identical as possible regarding important characteristics (referred to as "constancy assumption")?
- Yes, both an ITT and PP analyses were used. Comparison between the two would have shown any concerns that the ITT approach "diluted" the results to show non-inferiority. Smaller observed treatment effects can result with an ITT analysis since patients did not necessarily complete the duration of the trial and experience the maximum effect of transdermal buprenorphine. Using just an ITT analysis with an NI trial design can significantly increase the risk of falsely claiming non-inferiority. The FDA recommends performing both ITT and PP analyses and checking to see if there are significant differences between the results. An explanation as to why there was a significant difference is expected.
- See Figure 5-1. The conclusion would be that transdermal buprenorphine is non-inferior to sustained-release tramadol regarding alleviation of moderate to severe musculoskeletal pain.
- See Figure 5-1. This result of the study would be inconclusive that transdermal buprenorphine is non-inferior to sustained-release tramadol regarding alleviation of moderate-to-severe musculoskeletal pain since the 95% CI crosses over the NI margin instead of being located completely on one side "non-inferior" or the other side "inferior" of the NI margin.
- Performing a superiority analysis after non-inferiority has been established is acceptable and appropriate. The investigators should have stated the plan to test for superiority if non-inferiority was the result *a priori*. It is generally not acceptable or appropriate to seek the conclusion of non-inferiority from a failed superiority trial.

CASE STUDY 5–2

- Observation studies provide no guarantee that the two groups have similar characteristics with the exception of being in the same observational cohort study. The women consuming four or more cups of coffee may be made up of healthier subjects than the group of women that consumed less than one cup of coffee per day.

- Other factors (some not even known at this time) not controlled by this observational study may be playing the important "protective" role in those women that had an associated reduction in endometrial cancer risk. This might include health of immune system, genetic familial effects, and exposure to other factors that may be causing the cancer. There are many other confounding factors that can be identified.
- The outcome should be measured the same way and at the same frequency for both groups. Adequate follow-up should be determined.
- No cause-effect relationship can be determined with an observational study such as this cohort study.

CASE STUDY 5-3

- The quality of the meta-analysis depends on the quality of the individual studies used to develop the meta-analysis in addition to the homogeneity of the studies as a whole.
- Publication bias is a form of selection bias where publication of studies is based on the magnitude, direction, or statistical significance of the results. It is documented that researchers are more likely to publish studies that demonstrate positive effects of drugs.

  Yes, the investigators utilized a technique called funnel plot to identify the potential existence of publication bias. A funnel plot is a scatter plot of treatment effect versus study size. If this plot shows an inverted symmetrical funnel, publication bias is probably not present. An asymmetrical funnel plot indicates the possibility that publication bias is present (see Figure 5-5).

- Same primary outcome measure used, similar participant attrition, same study design, differences in intervention duration, and equivalent doses of statins between trials.
- The authors used a Forest plot to provide the results of this meta-analysis because the reader can easily visualize the similarities and differences noted between studies and a confidence interval is included which provides additional information about the variability of the results for individual studies.

CASE STUDY 5-4

Proprietary content of active ingredients prevents you from knowing for sure that any of the other products contain the same amount, more, or less than the product that provided this evidence. Also, specific plant parts utilized in a study are important to consider. If a trial evaluated the use of an herb's root, but the product about which a practitioner is searching for information contains the herb's leaves and flowers, the results cannot be extrapolated. Unfortunately, not knowing the amount or exact part of the pelargonium plant used for the study prevents us from using this evidence for making evidence-based clinical decisions for our patients.

- The majority of dietary supplement trials are conducted in Europe and Asia. Appropriateness of generalizability of results to a practitioner's own patient population must always be considered, just as with standard drug trials.
- Probably not with this trial although it might take longer than 7 days to completely alleviate the symptoms of acute bronchitis so this would need to be taken into consideration. In this study, we saw clear clinical improvement in the patients receiving pelargonium.
- Small subject population is a common flaw with dietary supplement trials. This study utilized a reasonable number of patients to have some comfort with external validity. Also, the number of patients was adequate to meet power and show a difference between treatment groups. In addition, adverse reactions or drug interactions can be overlooked in smaller groups versus a larger one. This could be a reason why no adverse drug effects were noted.

Chapter 6

CASE STUDY 6–1

- The population of interest is patients who are undergoing total knee replacement. However, these results would only generalize to patients who have similar background characteristics to the patients seen by this practice.
- A stratified random sample was taken based on the convenience of the surgeons' practice.
- Yes. Patients were randomized to medication group.
- The DV is hemoglobin. It is measured on a continuous (ratio) scale. Yes, it is measured repeatedly on two occasions.
- The IV is medication group; it is nominal and has two levels—TXA versus EACA.
- Yes, there are a number of patient and surgeon characteristics that could be potential confounders. For example, a patient's surgery time, tourniquet time, transfusion requirements, or the volume of total knee replacement surgeries completed by each surgeon. You will likely come up with others as there is never a shortage of confounding variables in human subjects research.
- This would be the correct descriptive statistics only if the hemoglobin values followed some normal distribution.

CASE STUDY 6–2

- This is an adaptive design given there are two planned interim analyses.
- Statistical power of 80% indicates that there is an 80% probability of detecting a 10% mean difference in hemoglobin between groups, given that it actually exists.
- A two-tailed hypothesis is appropriate because the surgeon did not specify that TXA would consistently have better blood-sparing effects than EACA, or vice versa. The surgeon does not care so much about which medication is better, he cared more about the medications being not different.
- The mixed between-within ANOVA model would answer whether the two groups changed differently from pre-op to post-op. This does not test the surgeon's hypothesis because he was concerned only with postoperative differences, not change across hemoglobin measures.
- No, controlling for biological sex and weight would be wholly redundant. Specifically, you would not expect there to be any differences in biological sex and weight because these variables were already addressed using the stratified sampling design.
- No, small p-values provide no information about the size of the difference or whether the difference is clinically meaningful. Further, small p-values do not provide any information about how likely the results are to replicate. In isolation, a p-value is not enough to stop a clinical trial (or any study for that matter). Aside from p-values, the surgeon should present the mean difference, an estimate of effect size for the difference (e.g., Cohen's d), and a 95% confidence interval around the size of the difference.

Chapter 8

CASE STUDY 8–1

Establish transparency. According to the Institute of Medicine steps, the clinical practice guidelines evaluated appear to consider transparency from the beginning of their development. Look to see if the details and steps of guideline development can easily be replicated or followed throughout. Look for any conflicts of interest or bias, such as funding, if it exists it should be publicly available.

Consider whether the specific disease conditions for which the clinical practice guidelines are being evaluated possess the maximum potential for benefit from implementation of a clinical practice guideline. Do the conditions have a high prevalence, high frequencies or severities, availability of high-quality evidence supporting reduction in morbidity and mortality with treatments, feasibilities of guideline implementation, potential cost-effectiveness, evidence that current practices are not optimal, evidence of practice variations, and availability of personnel, expertise, and resources to implement the practice guidelines.

Management of conflict of interest. Before selecting the clinical practice guidelines, think about how the guideline panel managed conflicts of interest. Determine whether the individuals considered for membership on each panel were asked to declare in writing potential conflicts of interest. These conflicts of interest not only may have included financial conflicts, but also possibly intellectual conflicts, institutional conflicts, and patient-public activities.

How the multidisciplinary guideline development group was established. Determine if when clinical practice guidelines are developed, they should consist of a multidisciplinary process. Look to see if patients were involved, since patient involvement is critical in the formulation and prioritization of questions addressed by the guidelines. Additionally, look to see if member of the panel have expertise in the content area.

Consideration of whether a systematic search for evidence was conducted. As a health care practitioner, recognize that conducting a systemic review of available literature is important. Recognize that before a clinical practice guideline is developed, the clinical questions to be addressed must be defined. Consider if study screening selection criteria was determined before any systematic search was conducted. See if the clinical practice guideline states how studies were appraised and the body of evidence was synthesized.

Consider how studies were selected. This evaluation includes types of published or unpublished research that were considered. Look to see if the panel included evidence from previous guidelines, meta-analyses, systematic reviews, randomized, controlled trials, observational studies, diagnostic studies, economic studies, and qualitative studies.

Evaluate if specialized database searched were performed. Furthermore, determine whether available bibliographic resources were used. Citations listed in published bibliographies, textbooks, and identified literature should have been reviewed in the identification of evidence not produced from database searches. Remember that search terms should be easily identifiable from clinical questions addressed by the clinical practice guideline.

The guideline development panels should have appraised individual studies in efforts to identify issues that exist in studies for potential inclusion such as with trial design or potential biases that would affect internal or external validity. Consider whether details of trial design, sample size, statistical power, selection bias, inclusion/exclusion criteria, choice of control group, randomization methods, comparability of groups, definition of exposure or intervention, definition of outcome measures, accuracy and appropriateness of outcome measures, attrition rates, data collection methods, methods of statistical analysis confounding variables, unique study population characteristics, and adequacy of blinding were provided.

Consider how the information was summarized to develop conclusions. Look for clinical practice guidelines formatted to consider individual studies, consistency of results between studies, scope of evidence, and size of treatment effects.

CASE STUDY 8–2

In consideration of how the clinical questions addressed were defined, remember that a process or format of framing questions addressed by clinical practice guidelines is critical. Describe this to your health care system administrators and explain that guideline development groups use such formats as PICO to frame the clinical question of focus. The "P" stands for patients or problems which are being considered. The "I" represents the treatment intervention to be considered and the "C" stands for comparison or alternatives compared to the intervention. The "O" stands for the outcome of focus and greatest importance to patients. Examples of outcomes of focus include mortality, morbidity, complications, physical function, quality of life, costs, and other outcomes.

CASE STUDY 8–3

The seven categories of guideline implementation barriers that limit or restrict complete prescriber adherence include lack of awareness, familiarization, agreement, self-efficacy (disbelief that the guideline recommendations could be performed), outcome expectancy (disbelief that expected outcomes would occur), and motivation to change current practice (inertia of present practice). External barriers such as patient resistance, patient embarrassment, lack of reminder system, cost to patient, and lack of time also exist.

CASE STUDY 8–4

Importance of establishing plans for updating the guideline. Recognize the importance of establishing plans for updating the guideline. In review of a clinical practice guideline, explain that the publication date and dates of systematic reviews used should be clear. It is important to have a plan to update a guideline identify new technology or evidence that may affect the guideline. A review interval to update a guideline should always be established. The duration of the interval is dependent on the topic and existence of ongoing studies. A plan also should be made regarding the expiry of a guideline.

Chapter 9

CASE STUDY 9–1

Many practitioners find article discussions more interesting when they can relate the information to a previous or current patient care scenario. One method may be to solicit topics from staff to gather opinions for interesting topics. Additionally, articles should be sent out in advance of the discussion so that participants have the opportunity to review and come prepared. If feasible, providing snacks or food has been shown to lead to increased participation.

CASE STUDY 9–2

Inviting a drug information specialist or another clinician with advanced training in this area can help address issues relating to study design and methodology. Inclusion of a content expert in the condition that is being studied can help provide greater clinical context and insight.

CASE STUDY 9–3

It is possible to host an asynchronous online journal club, where participants post their critiques online via an online forum at their availability.

Chapter 10

CASE STUDY 10-1

- Factors that favor finding the pharmacist liable for negligence:
  - Pharmacist is a specialist (e.g., BCACP)
  - Anticoagulation pharmacist
  - Reasonable pharmacist should know that an INR of 5.2 in a patient on warfarin places the patient at increased bleeding risk.
  - Reasonable pharmacist would question the use of the two medications together and document same. For example, enoxaparin may be used for bridging anticoagulation when initiating warfarin but the INR of 5.2 would not indicate warfarin initiation.
- No. While combining these two drugs may increase the risk of serious or life-threatening bleeding complications, enoxaparin and warfarin may be used together to treat acute deep vein thrombosis with or without pulmonary embolism. However, where the pharmacist possesses special knowledge of the patient's condition, there is a responsibility to the patient to clarify the order.
  - If there is any protocol or guideline used at the clinic which was not followed.
  - If there was no follow-up or documentation of the rationale for the combination.
- Yes. The courts would hold a specialist to a higher standard. The fact that the pharmacist is the anticoagulation clinic pharmacist and is board certified places this individual into a higher liability category.

  If there was a collaborative practice agreement, it would be seen as a voluntary undertaking to provide expanded services to the physician and patient.
- All three would be liable—the pharmacist, physician, and the clinic under the theory of *respondeat superior* for actions of employee.

CASE STUDY 10-2

- The pharmacist fell below the standard of care. A health system pharmacist has access to the patient's renal function tests. Dispensing metformin without checking renal function falls below the standard. Not following a pharmacy department policy which requires both checking and documenting the patient's creatinine clearance prior to dispensing metformin also falls below the standard of care.

  Looking at the elements of negligence: (1) duty was breached; (2) damages resulted; (3) the damages would seem to be directly caused by the breach of the duty; and (4) defenses to not checking the renal function or following the policy are absent.

CASE STUDY 10-3

- Several activities occurring in this case violate the copyright law.
  - Mere listing of all drugs which should not be crushed—derived from published references.
  - Not classroom use.
  - Permission must be obtained to use material that is paraphrased, abridged, or condensed. However, a new table created from data that is copyrighted would probably not require permission in this case. Copy work is informational.
  - Unless the reference was government material, permission must be obtained. A four-pronged test is used to determine 'fair use'—the nature of the work; the amount copied; commercial use; and effect on the market would all be considered.
  - You take several direct sentences without providing a source reference. One of the references is out of print. One factor in copying infringement is the amount copied. Even though only several sentences were copied, there is no minimal amount or threshold quantity standard where fair use would be presumed.

The fact that some of the material is out of print does not mean the material is in the public domain. Out of print does not necessarily mean out of copyright. The rights revert to the author, and the underlying copyright remains unaffected.

CASE STUDY 10-4

- HIPAA prohibits:
    - The pharmacist sharing PHI and diagnosis in an area where it was easily overheard by others.
    - PHI faxed to a fax machine in an unsecured area where many people have access.
- Safeguards:
    - Private area for discussing patient information
    - Fax machine should be in a private and secure location
    - Reasonable steps which may include: programming, testing, and double-checking numbers; using a fax cover sheet with an erroneous transmission statement; and checking confirmations.

Chapter 11

CASE STUDY 11-1

- Assessment of whether this drug information request constitutes a potential ethical dilemma:
    1. What does it mean to you if confronting an ethical dilemma for such judgments of right or wrong to be ultimate/fundamental?
    2. How do you interpret what it means for an ethical issue to be universal, in your own words?
    3. Who are the various parties whose welfare could be impacted by the resolution to this situation, if indeed it does constitute an ethical dilemma?
- Background information to obtain to clarify this information request:
    - What are facts of this case that you will want to learn more about before reaching a determination of whether it is indeed an ethical dilemma?
    - Considering who is affected is really a continuation of item 3 above defining an ethical dilemma. However, it may help you further to consider specific people involved in the case at hand—the study subject, the family members of the study subject, and the study team.
- Given that a specific patient's welfare must be addressed, this case certainly involves a micro level of ethical decision making; however, as is often the case with ethical dilemmas, it might be argued that there are also meso level decision-making issues to be considered—What standards and policies does the organization have to address in informing study subjects of IGFs?
- Refer to the listing of rules and principles provided in the chapter—Which if any seem to have relevance to this case? For example, how do you think the principles of "Confidentiality" and "Privacy" impact this case?
- Remember that rules often apply best to more narrow cases, and may be reasonably limited in some circumstances to meet the demands of more fundamental ethical principles. Decisions about competing principles will often rely on the decision maker's priorities relative to primacy of anticipated good/bad consequences of the action (for the individual only? how about for society?) versus for instance certain core beliefs about fundamental rights (e.g., deontological principle prioritizing "respect for persons").
- What kinds of standards, policies, or procedures might be useful to help the study team with ethical decision making?

Refer to the article *Management and return of incidental genomic findings in clinical trials* by C. Ayuso et al. for further information regarding IGF during clinical trials.[1]

CASE STUDY 11-2

- Assessment of whether this drug information request constitutes a potential ethical dilemma:
  1. What does it mean to you if confronting an ethical dilemma for such judgments of right or wrong to be ultimate/fundamental?
  2. How do you interpret what it means for an ethical issue to be universal, in your own words?
  3. Who are the various parties whose welfare could be impacted by the resolution to this situation, if indeed it does constitute an ethical dilemma?
- Background information to obtain to clarify this information request:
  - What are facts of this case that you will want to learn more about before reaching a determination of whether it is indeed an ethical dilemma? (For example: What is the clinical condition of the patient in question? and What standards or patient care commitments has your institution established for addressing patient pain issues?)
  - Considering who is affected is really a continuation of item 3 above defining an ethical dilemma. However, it may help you further to consider specific people involved in the case at hand—the patient himself; the supervising physician; the various other staff and trainees who must try to meet this patient's needs under the circumstances at hand, and may learn to address future patients' needs based on their experience; family members of the patient who will observe their loved ones suffering; the future patients who will be treated in similar or different ways based on the accumulating experience from this case.
  - What cultural perspectives might be at work for the prescribing physician (imagine for instance an older practitioner, or one trained in a particular perspective relative to standards of pain control). Likewise, what is the culture in the case environment relative to lines of authority, or freedom to question authority, or approaches to patient rights?
- Given that a specific patient's welfare must be addressed, this case certainly involves a micro level of ethical decision making; however, as is often the case with ethical dilemmas, it might be argued that there are also meso level decision-making issues to be considered—What standards is the organization held to in meeting the pain control needs of its patients? What policies are there established within the organization regarding supervision/accountability of practitioners charged with patient care relative to specified standards?
- Refer to the listing of rules and principles provided in the chapter—Which if any seem to have relevance to this case?
- Remember that rules often apply best to more narrow cases, and may be reasonably limited in some circumstances to meet the demands of more fundamental ethical principles. Decisions about competing principles will often rely on the decision makers' priorities relative to primacy of anticipated good/bad consequences of the action (for the individual only? how about for society?) versus for instance certain core beliefs about fundamental rights (e.g., deontological principle prioritizing "respect for persons").
- What kinds of standards, policies, or procedures might be useful to this nurse specialist, both to aid in her ethical decision making and to provide support in her dealings with the prescriber and other involved staff as well as the patient/family?

Refer to the article *Ethical dilemmas: controversies in pain management* by Janet Brown to read the analysis of a similar case.[2]

REFERENCES

1. Ayuso C, Millan JM, Dal-Re R. Management and return of incidental genomic findings in clinical trials. Pharmacogenomics J. 2015;15:1-5.
2. Brown J. Ethical dilemmas: controversies in pain management. Adv Nurse Pract. 1997:69-72.

CASE STUDY 11-3

- First recognize and understand the meaning of these characteristics as they apply to this specific case. However, final determination of whether they apply will require the reader to first address other steps of analysis below.
- There are a number of important factual questions that Dr. Levine is honor bound to address before deciding on any ethical dimensions of this case:
  - Examples: What is the drug in question? How available is it, other than relative to cost?
  - What is the level of evidence supporting or refuting the agent's efficacy and safety when used for the requested purpose?
    - At a macro level of decision making, cost-effectiveness is often deemed another appropriate factor to consider in recommendations for use at a population level.
    - However, the pharmacy and therapeutics committee will need to assess the safety and efficacy of the medication in question.
  - How do the formulary management policies instruct the pharmacy and therapeutics committee regarding making formulary considerations?
- Certainly the professional must address this dilemma at a meso level. His/her decision making may be improved if he/she also thinks about what his or her responsibility is to the individual patients who will undoubtedly be impacted by the decision, as well as overall macro (system or societal) level consequences of policies established by this and similar organizations.
- How do you think the principles of "Veracity" or "Fidelity" might apply to this case? How do you think Justice Theory might speak in favor of or in opposition to restrictions?
- Please imagine a specific product and case in order to personally decide how you would prioritize the various pertinent rules and principles in order to make a decision in such a case as this. Do you think that you would be justified in simply acting on the orders from your job supervisor, regardless of the factual circumstances and possible ethical issues of the case?
- Organizational strategies that might best prepare this pharmacist to most effectively respond to ethical dilemmas:
  - What organization policies or standards do you think should be established in health care systems to support ethical decision making pertinent to cases such as this one?
  - Do you think there are laws or regulations that should be in place at the governmental level to guide health care systems in providing ethical service to their patients? If so, what measures do you think could be useful?

Chapter 12

CASE STUDY 12-1

- Since the topic is known, it is possible to skip the first step listed in this chapter. You will need to find out if anyone else is to work with you (e.g., perhaps someone very involved with the use of that agent) and get that person involved, if only as a reviewer. Also, it is known where it will be published—in the policy and procedure section of the institutional intranet. So, the next thing to do is probably review the format of policies and procedures in the institution to determine what needs to written. As a part of this, determine that it needs to be written in the middle technical style, since it is being aimed at a variety of health care practitioners (e.g., pharmacist, physician, nurse). Then, it is necessary to do research into the topic.
- First, organize the material. This can be done in conjunction with preparation of an outline of the order in which the material needs to be covered. That outline can be done on a word processor and

serve as the template for the document. In many cases, the way the institution lays out its policy and procedure documents can serve as a good part of the outline. Perhaps even a preexisting template can be used as the outline. Then proceed to write the material. At this stage, simply make sure everything necessary is recorded in the document. The document can be written in order of the topics, or each individual section may be written separately, in whatever order is easiest. Also, remember to cite material as the document is written, preferably using the endnote feature in the word processor. Besides being appropriate to give credit, it is also useful for the future when someone may have to come back to revise the document after several years and may not otherwise be able to tell the origin of some of the information.

- Some would say to just present it to the pharmacy and therapeutics committee, but there are a couple of things that need to be done first. To start, the author should reread the document and edit the document. Then, get others who have expertise in the area to read and edit the document. These others should include one or more representatives from each group affected by the document (e.g., pharmacist, physician, nurse). An effort must be made to make sure the document is in a logical order, covers all aspects of the topic, and is understandable. Then incorporate any necessary revisions. This process may need to be done several times (e.g., some chapters in this book went through a dozen versions before being submitted to the publisher). Sometimes, there will even be a pre-meeting of key members of a committee to look over things briefly in order to make sure everything is appropriately addressed.

CASE STUDY 12–2

First, clarify who the website is addressing—the audience. It will be different for patients versus other health care practitioners. Sometimes it will be both groups. Then, in relationship to the above, determine what information or features need to be on the website. It may simply be a reference site, but also may provide much more information and communication. Then determine what equipment (e.g., computer hardware and software) and budget are available to prepare the website.

CASE STUDY 12–3

First, be sure to prepare slides on something that is compatible with the program used at the meeting. Then determine what information needs to be on the slides. Generally, assume that each slide should be shown for a minute or two. Each slide should be kept simple, with a maximum of five bullet points and five words per bullet point, so that attendees can concentrate on the message. Also, remember that the speaker is not to read directly from the slides, but use them just as a jumping off spot for the presentation and to organize thoughts. In addition, be sure to make them look attractive and professional. Graphics may help, as long as they do not make the slide too busy.

Chapter 13

CASE STUDY 13–1

- A local P&T committee can be more restrictive than the system on an already existing restriction. A new restriction would be outside the realm of a local P&T committee (e.g., system restricts to infectious diseases and now the local level wants to add emergency medicine to the restriction criteria). If a proposed restriction is simply further restricting the medication (e.g., system restricts to infectious diseases and now the local level wants to further restrict to two ID physicians), this would be appropriate.

- Yes. This would be more restrictive than the system level guidance. In some systems, you cannot remove a drug locally, but you can refuse to stock it, which has the same effect.
- The medication needs to be removed from local formulary.

CASE STUDY 13-2

- Non-formulary request form.
- All proton pump inhibitors (esomeprazole, lansoprazole, dexlansoprazole, omeprazole, pantoprazole, rabeprazole) are generally considered therapeutically equivalent. While there are many examples of published interchange protocols (both inpatient and outpatient), there may be a given patient who may have a better tolerability and response for one product over another.
- Most inpatient hospitals have preprinted or preprogrammed orders for preapproved therapeutic interchanges. This form has been approved by the P&T committee. The pharmacist has been granted the responsibility to automatically fill the order with the equivalent dose of pantoprazole. Once the form is completed, it becomes part of the medical record (electronic or paper). If an interchange is chosen for a medication that is not on the preapproved therapeutic interchange list, then a new order must be written for the alternative agent.
- You can tell the physician the process for filling out the formulary request form.

CASE STUDY 13-3

- Physicians, pharmacists, nurses, students, and administrators affiliated with the health system.
- Newsletters, announcements at meetings, intranet communication, e-mail messages, personal communication, or even posting alerts in specific areas of the hospital.
- Current inventory, expected length of shortage, alternative agents available.
- In the case of furosemide, other loop diuretics are available alternatives. You may find it necessary to restrict the remaining inventory to specific hospital units or for a specific diagnosis. You may emphasize that during the shortage, oral furosemide should be used whenever possible. It would be wise to produce a comparative chart for equivalent dosing and route of administration for alternative loop diuretics (bumetanide, furosemide, or torsemide). This comparison chart can be sent along with the message regarding the shortage.

CASE STUDY 13-4

- See Appendix 13-4 for an example of routine agenda items. Review the minutes from the previous meeting. Add agenda items based upon the meeting minutes such as follow-up information or new agenda items that came from discussion. Verify agenda with Director of Pharmacy and P&T Committee Chair.
- You would need to know some background on the formulary application, who requested it and for what application. You would need to be familiar with similar agents within category (if applicable) for comparable indications, dosing, cost, etc. It is not unreasonable to have several communications with the person requesting the new medication or other specialists who may have insight into formulary justification.

  The summary page should include the following: generic name, trade name, indications, clinical pharmacology, pharmacokinetics, adverse reactions, drug interactions, dosing, product availability and storage, drug safety/REMS, pricing, conclusion, and references, with appropriate comparisons to other similar agents.
- Pertinent discussions and final voting results are included for documentation about committee decisions.
- Intranet communication, e-mails, newsletters, personal communication, dissemination through appropriate meetings.

- Once a formulary change has been made (e.g., add a new medication to formulary), the following items should be updated. Additional items may be added depending on the institution.
  - ○ Computerized order entry system
  - ○ Smart pumps
  - ○ Order sets (paper or electronic)
  - ○ Guidelines and policy and procedures
  - ○ Education for all involved
  - ○ Formulary management system (e.g., Lexicomp, Micromedex)
- Monitoring of safety issues from the FDA and completing either an annual class review or MUE are common follow-up evaluations of a formulary change.

Chapter 14

CASE STUDY 14–1

- Steps to add this drug to the formulary:
  - ○ Review non-formulary utilization and indications for use.
  - ○ Review utilization of similar agents in the therapeutic class (if applicable) that are on the formulary.
  - ○ Seek input from the appropriate specialists who would have knowledge of the product or recommendations for formulary status.
  - ○ Review available literature to evaluate clinical evidence.
  - ○ Consider discussions with pharmacists at other hospitals.
  - ○ Determine financial implications of product addition by reviewing cost information with purchasing agent and contract information from the wholesaler and manufacturer.
  - ○ Prepare a drug monograph.
- Essential elements of a medication monograph:
  - ○ Generic name (trade name)
  - ○ Approval rating
  - ○ Therapeutic class
  - ○ Sound/Look-alike
  - ○ Indications/Place in therapy
  - ○ Adverse effects
  - ○ Drug interactions
  - ○ Recommended monitoring
  - ○ Dosing
  - ○ Product availability and storage
  - ○ Drug safety/REMS
  - ○ Comparative pricing information/Pharmacoeconomic analysis
  - ○ Operational considerations
  - ○ Formulary implications/Conclusion/Recommendation
  - ○ References
- Sources of information to develop a complete, evidence-based, medication monograph:
  - ○ Current published clinical studies and abstracts
  - ○ Non-published data or data awaiting publication (contact manufacturer)
  - ○ Current package labeling
  - ○ Obtaining a formulary kit from the manufacturer may be helpful for double checking information, but this should not be the primary reference source for your monograph
  - ○ Check current evidence-based clinical guidelines

CASE STUDY 14-2

- Each of the following would be necessary, with comparison to other similar products. Essentially, it will be a quick comparison of the major similarities and differences, which can be fit on a single page.
  - Generic name and trade name
  - Indications
  - Clinical pharmacology
  - Pharmacokinetics
  - Adverse reactions
  - Drug interactions
  - Dosing
  - Product availability and storage
  - Drug safety/REMS
  - Evidence-based clinical guidelines
  - Recommendation
- The following information should be included:
  - All of the previous mentioned items
  - Defined tier status for copayments
  - Restrictions—such as prior approvals
  - REMS
  - Outpatient medication acquisition cost and if covered by Medicare or other key local pharmacy benefits management organizations
- Different types of formulary status recommendations:
  - Added for uncontrolled use by the entire medical staff.
  - Added for monitored use—No restrictions placed on use, but the drug will be monitored via a quality assurance study (e.g., drug usage evaluation and medication usage evaluation) to determine appropriateness of use. This is a tie-in to the institution's quality assurance/drug usage evaluation process. Please note: this category does not mean that the patient is monitored, since that is necessary for every drug. It means that the quality and appropriateness of how the drug is used is monitored.
  - Added with restrictions—The drug is added to the drug formulary, but there are restrictions on who may prescribe it and/or how it may be used (e.g., specific indications, certain physicians or physician groups, and certain policies to be followed).
  - Conditional—Available for use by the entire medical staff for a finite period of time.
  - Not added/deleted from formulary. The product can be ordered as a non-formulary product, but will not be routinely stocked in the pharmacy. Non-formulary products may take up to 24 hours or longer to obtain.
  - Therapeutic interchange.

CASE STUDY 14-3

1. The financial components of this medication in a complex health system with different medication pricing can best be calculated with a spreadsheet program and one method of calculating this is summarized in the below table:

	Vial Cost	Cost per Patient	Medicare Payment	Patient Charge	Private Insurance Payment	Medicare Margin	Private Insurance Margin	Blended Margin
GPO price	$10,000	$30,000	$28,500	$60,000	$31,800	−$1,500	$1,800	$150
340b price	$9,000	$27,000	$28,500	$60,000	$31,800	$1,500	$4,800	$3,150

	Patients	Doses	Total Spend	Total Charges	Total Margin
GPO price	63	28	$52,920,000	$105,840,000	$264,600
340b price	7	28	$5,292,000	$11,760,000	$617,400
Total	70		$58,212,000	$117,600,000	$882,000

The cost impact of adding this medication to formulary given the high cost of the medication, the number of patients predicted to need the medication, and the number of doses they would receive is significant. This medication has the potential to add up to $58,212,000 of total drug expenses to the health system.

2. Reimbursement varies significantly between Medicare and private insurers. For this medication, the health system will on average lose $1,500 per Medicare patient at hospital buying the drug at GPO pricing and will make $1,500 on Medicare patients at 340b pricing. For private insurances, hospital with GPO pricing will make $1,800 and hospitals with 340b pricing will make $3,150 in margin. The total impact of adding this medication could be up to a positive net margin of $882,000.

3. Medication pricing is dynamic. Medicare reimbursement changes quarterly for medications and there is a trend toward payment reform and even bundled pricing which may change the way pharmacies are reimbursed for medications.

Hospitals that evaluate the price of a medication and note that reimbursement is less than cost, resulting in a net loss for the medication, must evaluate their medication pricing and evaluate contracting opportunities to lower the acquisition cost of the drug.

Chapter 15

CASE STUDY 15-1

- Check both the ASHP and FDA drug shortage websites. Also check with the purchasing agents at your organization.

CASE STUDY 15-2

- Determine the clinical impact of the shortage—this is a potentially lifesaving drug and for some infections, there may not be clear alternatives. Contact the infectious diseases clinicians or the antimicrobial committee within the institution to get their management suggestions. Potential actions could include restricting the product for approval from infectious diseases or contacting the ethics committee and pharmacy and therapeutics committee to determine and approve a rationing strategy.

CASE STUDY 15-3

- Both substitutes pose patient-safety risks, but the most concerning is the dopamine substitution. Using a four times lower strength product will affect smart pumps and may not be appropriate for patients who are fluid-restricted. Without changes to the ordering system and smart pump libraries, patients could be given subtherapeutic doses of the medication. The heparin vials also pose potential risks. The clean room will have to prepare bags of heparin during a shortage of premixed bags. This will pose operational challenges and may also affect IV workflow technology. Convene a team to work through the management challenges that both of these shortages pose.

Chapter 16

CASE STUDY 16–1

Steps to assess medication reconciliation:
- Identify an appropriate sampling strategy to review medication reconciliation at admission.
- Include necessary demographic data elements to collect for each patient record reviewed (gender, age groups, race/ethnicity, preferred language, payer, other).
- Develop a data dictionary specifying each data element and where to locate the information in the patient record so that each reviewer will obtain consistent results.
- Conduct the review by nursing staff and the consultant pharmacist.
- Summarize the results in aggregate and by demographic subgroups.
- If differences are found, investigate possible causes.

CASE STUDY 16–2

Possible responses include:
- Staff do not know that the medication should be infused over 60 minutes.
- The medication label does not provide infusion-time directions to the nurse administering the medication.
- Nurses are not using the smart features of the infusion pumps that would default to the appropriate infusion rate for a 60-minute infusion.
- Staff are rushed and opt to infuse medications more rapidly in order to get everything done.

CASE STUDY 16–3

Possible responses include:
- Physicians (surgeons, medicine/family medicine, infectious disease specialists)
- Nurses from the perioperative areas, inpatient units, and home care areas
- Pharmacists
- Discharge planners/case managers who help to plan for discharge and arrange home care

CASE STUDY 16–4

- Search the medical literature.
- Ask practitioners with experience/expertise in this area.
- Consult professional organizations and their published best practices (pharmacy, nursing, medical).
- Identify any prior evaluations of this topic with the organization.
- Post an inquiry on professional LISTSERV.

Chapter 17

CASE STUDY 17-1

- There was no dechallenge in this case; the patient has been taking the product continuously for about 4 weeks.
- Although there was not a formal dechallenge and rechallenge, the patient reports taking the product again after his symptoms subside. His symptoms reappear each time.
- Yes. The patient's symptoms are always preceded by administration of the drug, and they disappear soon afterward.
- Yes, the patient's symptoms are consistent with the known pharmacology of *XL Fit*. The product contains synephrine, which has stimulant effects. The pharmacology of synephrine is similar to its isomer, phenylephrine.
- Using clinical judgment, you can determine that the product is likely responsible for the side effects described. This is supported by the fact that the symptoms occurred after ingestion of the product, that the symptoms recurred following rechallenge, and that the symptoms are consistent with the known pharmacology of the ingredients contained in the product. You could also complete one of the algorithms discussed above in order to assess the likelihood that this reaction was caused by *XL Fit*.

CASE STUDY 17-2

- There are several options for reporting the reaction to the FDA. You can report this ADR to the FDA through the Department of Health and Human Services' online Safety Reporting Portal. Because this ADR involved a nonprescription natural supplement product, you also have the option of reporting the reaction through a third-party system like Natural MedWatch, or directly to the product's manufacturer or distributor. These entities will forward your ADR report to the FDA.
- Your patient can report the ADR through the Department of Health and Human Services' online Safety Reporting Portal.

Chapter 18

CASE STUDY 18-1

- Advantages and disadvantages of including multiple cases in the root cause analysis process:
  - Combining cases of similar types provides a larger volume of information from which to extract potential causes common to many events. For example, reviewing one case and making major system changes may in fact miss the most common factor that is causing the events. The power of multiple cases increases the chance that the frequent causative reasons are identified, which can then be addressed.
  - One disadvantage is that each case that is included in an aggregate RCA[1,2] requires adequate investigation in order to understand the causes and therefore takes more time. All the cases are then reviewed in aggregate to determine those most common causes.

CASE STUDY 18–2

This is a much debated topic. While eliminating errors seems like our goal, it is important to understand and remember that it is not possible to eliminate all human errors. Humans err many times per day and fortunately, most of the time there is no consequence. Forgetting to attach an attachment to an e-mail or putting the milk in the pantry is embarrassing, but not life-threatening. Understanding human error concepts is important in developing systems and barriers that will prevent a human error from reaching a patient. These barriers may include technology checking systems, pharmacist review of medications prior to administration, double check, focusing techniques, checklists, or time outs. The goal is to work to reduce and eliminate events of harm by instituting reliable barriers to errors, building in layers designed to catch these errors, improving monitoring strategies such that an error can be detected rapidly, all of which are meant to reduce the potential harm to a patient. Quality improvement work should focus on knowing how humans commonly err in a process in order to develop both prevention and identification strategies. Defining and avoiding preventable harm may provide the most clarity and feel to be an achievable goal.

- Questions you would like to ask the pharmacist involved in the error as part of an interview:
  - It is important to ask staff to provide a description of the situation as they remember it, without leading questions. It is also very important to interview staff early to prevent unintentional alterations to the story based on fading memory or hearing other discussions related to the event.
  - Ask the pharmacist to describe what happened and what they remember.
  - Ask the pharmacist what they do if/when they realize an error has occurred. What resources are they aware of to identify what patient they may have entered the orders on in error—many computer systems have a searching function that enables a report that identifies all patients on a given drug.
  - Ask other pharmacists what their process is when interrupted to assure they are entering orders on the correct patient.
- Classification of error as human-error only, system-error only, or a combination of both:
  - It depends on the information that is gathered during interviews and observation of the usual process. If there exists the opportunity to devise a no-interruption zone for order entry (in which telephone calls are received by other staff), then this is a system opportunity. It is a human error in that it was not an intentional action and the system set up the pharmacist to potentially fail. It is likely considered a combination of both human error and system contributing cause.

CASE STUDY 18–3

- System issues that contributed to the error:
  - The nurse had more patients than the recommended nurse:patient ratio.
  - The drug label had the volume first and the drug listed second, yet the infusion pump requires programming the drug first and the volume second, setting up the nurse to program it incorrectly.
- Your reaction as manager of the unit:
  - Were the actions as intended? Did the nurse intentionally program the pump incorrectly? No.
  - Was the person under the influence of unauthorized substances? No.
  - Did he or she knowingly violate a safe operating procedure? There was not a required double check and pump programming was taught to all staff upon institution of the new pumps. She did override a warning that the rate was just over the maximum rate. Upon further inquiry, she asked her charge nurse about the situation, who recommended she override the warning and continue with the rate. She did not make a conscious choice to skip steps within the process or subvert the process.
  - Do they pass the substitution test described above? When this was discussed with several other nurses, two of the three noted that they had made a similar error and/or caught

a similar error. Would others have made the same decisions and, if so, less likely to be culpable? If not, were there deficiencies in training or experience? The training must be carefully considered. Providing didactic information without practice or competency testing is not the most appropriate method of teaching staff. Adequate practice is needed to develop good habits and skill-based actions. What is the role of the charge nurse and her recommendation to continue despite the warning? Further inquiry should include asking if she reviewed the programming prior to her recommendation.

- ○ Does the individual have a history of unsafe acts? This is the first error of this type that has been identified for this nurse. If not, again less likely to be culpable.

- Identifying potential system fixes:
  - ○ The label design should match the entry in the pump if at all possible. Rearranging or increasing the visibility of the required information for programming is another option.
  - ○ Providing adequate staffing ratios to decrease the risk of competing priorities with multiple patients is appropriate. The charge nurse had taken several patients of her own and was rushed in her review of the concern.
  - ○ Lack of an independent check means that we shouldn't criticize either nurse for not doing a double check if it's not required, however, it could have been used to slow both nurses down and validate accurate pump programming.

CASE STUDY 18-4

- Identifying system or process issues:
  - ○ The epidural medication was brought into the patient's room before there was an order, at the request of the anesthesiologists. They wanted to have everything ready when the patient and team decided it was time for the epidural. This increases the risk of inadvertent administration due to availability.
  - ○ The nurse had not placed an identification band on the patient which is required for use of the medication bar code scanning process. Part of this was because of the lack of immediate availability of labels in the patient's room or upon admission, requiring the nurse to go searching for the identification band. A contributing factor was found to be a prior tolerance of not using the bar code scanning on this unit.
  - ○ The nurse did not use the bar code scanning technology to verify the medication prior to administration. This would have detected the error prior to administration to the patient if used correctly. This was partly due to the lack of patient identification band and a unit tolerance to inconsistent use of this technology. This unit experienced a difficult implementation with this process which was ineffective at times leading nurses to skip the process.
  - ○ The nurse picked up the wrong medication, didn't closely read the label, and prepared the incorrect medication. Contributing factors to this human error include the similar bag size and look of the two medications, a rushed nature, and a low suspicion of risk—never having experienced an error or problem in the treatment of a laboring mother in this manner. This nurse was fatigued due to her work schedule and distracted, both of which increase the risk of a human error.
- Read the related article cited below to identify additional information about the case. Lead a discussion related to system errors and their impact on health care professionals' behaviors and the potential impact to patients.

  Smetzer J, Baker C, Byrne FD, Cohen MR. Shaping systems for better behavioral choices: lessons learned from a fatal medication error. Jt Comm J Qual Patient Saf. 2010 Apr;36(4):152-63.

- Key elements to successful implementation of new technology include the need for processes to support: engagement and buy-in into the implementation requiring change management techniques, standardization of processes prior to implementation, effective education and training that is timed in close proximity to implementation, technological and emotional support at go-live, efficient methods of feedback about problems with closed-loop communication back to the reporting individual, and development and adaptation of optimization process post-go-live for continued improvement. There are likely many others that can be identified but these are key processes.

- In a world of competing priorities, it is important to set expectations and standard work for key processes. Perhaps as important is how organizations monitor for compliance and opportunities to improve standard work, to be followed by accountability actions. Throughput and financial pressures may be perceived as more important than safety. If someone has a concern that needs to be raised and it's perceived that working toward a resolution is too time consuming or is met with resistance by others, this important clarifying action may not occur. Supporting and provide positive feedback for prioritizing these behaviors is one strategy to build the culture of "Safety First." All professionals should be included and mentored in these expectations. It is critical that a "stop-the-line" process be supported by administrative and physician leadership to avoid significant events.

- Confirmation bias is a phenomenon in which humans are programmed into patterns of recognition which may lead to inappropriate assumptions based on those patterns. One example is color-coding. This can be an effective technique for recognition purposes, however there is no guarantee that there is only one "pink-capped drug." For example, if furosemide injectable was always in the pink cap and a generic heparin manufacturer starts to utilize a pink cap, human behavior may lead to a tragic error. Bar code scanning is designed to prevent these types of assumptions. However, assuring that the technology functions reliably and the culture supports the technology to include accountability measures are appropriate are critical to the use of the scanning process.

REFERENCES

1. Using aggregate root cause analysis to improve patient safety. Jt Comm J Qual Patient Saf. 2003 Aug;29(8):434-39.
2. Using aggregate root cause analysis to reduce falls. Jt Comm J Qual Patient Saf. 2005 Jan;31(1):21-31.

Chapter 19

CASE STUDY 19–1

- Steps used to approach this assignment:
  - Collect information on the background related to this formulary decision.
  - If unfamiliar with the role and development of an automatic therapeutic interchange, engage in background readings to help understand this type of policy, including the strengths and limitations.
  - Determine what the standard format/template will be for policies.
  - Conduct a systematic search to determine comparative dosing, safety profiles, and cost considerations.
  - Review the information gathered in your search and consider this information in the context of the needs of the health system.
  - Solicit input from colleagues in similar institutions or professional organizations for sample policies.
  - Prepare a draft policy that is specific, yet succinct, and well referenced.

- ○ An automatic therapeutic interchange should include specific guidance on how non-formulary agents will be converted to the formulary agents and should include all potential medications, all usual prescribed regimens (i.e., drug, dose, route, frequency) with an equally specific regimen for the formulary agent.
  - ○ Convene a group of stakeholders and solicit input on the policy.
- A variety of resources can be used in this process. As discussed in Chapter 3, an appropriate search should begin with tertiary references and should progress to secondary resources and eventually to primary literature in this scenario. The safety and efficacy of the proton pump inhibitors is well documented in the tertiary literature and resources such as Micromedex®, AHFS® Drug Information, and textbooks (e.g., Pharmacotherapy Principles and Practice) are a good starting point for understanding a comparison of the agents with respect to clinical efficacy, safety profile, and dosing and administration considerations, in addition to other parameters. Following a thorough search of the tertiary literature, in this case, it is appropriate to conduct a literature search in a secondary database (e.g., PubMed) to identify primary literature that supports a conversion from one agent to another. Adequate clinical trials should be collected and evaluated to assess the appropriateness of such a therapeutic interchange policy. Ideally, comparative head-to-head studies would be available to draw conclusion about comparative efficacy and safety. Finally, cost should be obtained directly from the pharmacy department regarding institution-specific pricing to develop a cost comparison for the conversion to the formulary agent.
- Once the information is collected from tertiary and primary resources, a thorough evaluation should be conducted. This will involve a critical assessment of the literature in the context of the needs of the organization.
- Stakeholder and identifying key stakeholders for this policy are defined as follows:
  - ○ A stakeholder is an individual who has a vested interest in the matter and policy in question.
  - ○ For the policy on a proton pump inhibitor automatic therapeutic interchange, the key stakeholders would be physicians in the specialties of gastroenterology, internal medicine, and critical care medicine. This policy would affect the pharmacy department and clinical pharmacists practicing in these specialties as well.
  - ○ Once a draft policy is developed, it should be presented to key stakeholders for review and input prior to its presentation for approval by a pharmacy and therapeutics committee or medical director. This can be accomplished in several ways. Perhaps a formal meeting of the stakeholders could be convened (e.g., expert panel) or individual discussions and dissemination of the draft could be handled by the pharmacist responsible for drafting the policy.

Chapter 20

CASE STUDY 20-1

- Before undertaking this assignment, it would be helpful to clarify and narrow the project goal and scope. For example, is the purpose to reevaluate all tumor necrosis factor (TNF) inhibitor products on the market, or just focus on the newer infliximab biosimilar? Similarly, is the ultimate goal of the formulary evaluation to reduce variation in prescribing patterns or to simply ensure that the existing formulary-preferred products are appropriate? It would also be useful to understand any previous work that has been done on this project, such as when the last time a class review was conducted. Additionally, it would be important to understand the urgency of this project and where it ranks in the overall priorities for your department.

- Recall that success criteria are quantifiable measures that define when the goal is accomplished, whereas a deliverable is a tangible component that is produced to achieve the success criteria. With this current project, one success criteria might be that a decision is voted upon by the hospital pharmacy and therapeutics committee. A corresponding deliverable might be to develop an evidence-based class review with a formulary recommendation that the committee can use. Another success criterion might be to reduce utilization of non-formulary TNF inhibitors. A corresponding deliverable may include a standardized order form or therapeutic interchange to better ensure utilization of formulary products.
- Stakeholders may vary greatly depending on the size and scope of an organization. For this specific example, some stakeholders may include adult and pediatric physicians (specifically in the specialties of rheumatology and gastroenterology); adult and pediatric clinical pharmacy specialists (specifically in the specialties of rheumatology and gastroenterology); nursing; informatics personnel (if an electronic medical record system is used); and drug sourcing or contracting personnel.
- Potential constraints may include limited time to dedicate to the project due to existing patient care responsibilities; poor access to key physician stakeholders that prevents the gathering of timely input; and functionality limitations within an electronic health record system that may prevent using medication management strategies, such as automatic therapeutic interchanges.
- Major tasks that would inform the project timeline may include gathering primary and tertiary literature, synthesizing the evidence you identified, gathering input from stakeholders, undertaking contract negotiations, presenting recommendations to the pharmacy and therapeutics committee, and implementing final decisions (e.g., updating technology systems with any changes). It may also be reasonable to break down the project further by dividing work on the evidence review into sections (e.g., complete the background and FDA-indications section one day, then complete the adverse effects section another day, etc.).

Chapter 21

CASE STUDY 21–1

- Yes, the product is going to be used in a different patient population and be infused using a different route of administration. In both cases the risk profile is higher for the new usage and as such submission of a new IND is going to be required.

  The company may select to work with Dr. Smith's data to further develop the product, develop an appropriate protocol, and submit the IND to the FDA.

  Alternatively, the company may select to simply support Dr. Smith as he develops a protocol and IND for submission. In that case the company will provide Dr. Smith with a letter of cross reference for his use in supporting his IND application.

CASE STUDY 21–2

- A well-researched comparison of the risks of liver metastases as compared to the risks of cirrhosis will be needed to justify further development of this product using this route of administration. In addition, submission of an REMS will be crucial.
- Appropriate components of the REMS:
  - Letters to health care providers
  - Patient medication guide
  - Patient registry to track enrollment of patients receiving the drug via this route of administration
  - Patient monitoring of liver function tests

CASE STUDY 21-3

- The IRB is likely to determine that not only must this risk be included in the consent form, but that if the purpose of the new studies is to obtain further information about this risk, that must be explained to the subjects as part of the consent form.
- Children are considered a special population in clinical research. 45CFR46 specifies criteria for the evaluation of risk as compared to benefit when research is conducted in children. In this case it is likely that an IRB would still consider this study to be approvable since the product holds the promise of potential benefit to the patient in addition to the known risks. In children prior to the age of legal majority (as defined by state law), their guardians are responsible for making health care decisions for them. In some situations the agreement of one guardian is sufficient; however, if the IRB has determined that there is risk to the child and no direct benefit to them, the agreement of both guardians is required. In addition, the agreement of the child (referred to as assent) is also required.
- At the point at which a child reaches the age of majority, they must provide their own consent to participate in the study.

Chapter 22

CASE STUDY 22-1

- Employees should prepare standard operating procedure (SOP) documents to ensure consistency between work by various functions.
- Amazing Drugs LP should educate employees on the sNDA submission process as well as other FDA regulations and guidance documents.
- Regulatory affairs professionals ensure submission of information to FDA is complete and accurate. Medical information HPs work to create standard responses and respond to unsolicited requests.
- Amazing Drugs LP should consider developing a publications group to communicate scientific information in the medical literature. They should also create an outcomes research and managed markets group to evaluate the real-world outcomes, patient reported outcomes, and health care utilization with the new product.

CASE STUDY 22-2

- Medical education would review grants for educational programming.
- Medical information and marketing will be involved in approving marketing materials.
- Medical science liaisons and medical information will engage in scientific exchange.

CASE STUDY 22-3

- The medical information department at Amazing Drugs LP should search the medical literature for any studies comparing their product to other compounds. They should evaluate the literature and create a standard response letter with the information.
- Amazing Drugs LP should anticipate receiving safety questions regarding the adverse events that occur with STRIPES®.

CASE STUDY 22-4

- Amazing Drugs LP must obtain information regarding the adverse event and collect required information about the event. Then they are required to submit a Form 3500A to FDA regarding the adverse event reports.

CASE STUDY 22-5

- Safety information is communicated using various tools including drug safety communication, social media, e-mail, labeling updates, and medication guides, among others.

CASE STUDY 22-6

- The SPOTS® manufacturer may want to submit additional or detailed safety data regarding this risk and adverse event.

CASE STUDY 22-7

- The manufacturers are allowed to market these products until September 6, 2017; however, after this date, these OTC products must not be marketed or sold. Manufacturers must reformulate their product to abide by FDA OTC regulations. More information is available at http://www.fda.gov/NewsEvents/Newsroom/PressAnnouncements/ucm517478.htm.
- This final rule does not apply to antibacterial products used by health professionals in health care settings. The pharmacy does not need to discard these products.
- The patient may feel or think that the antibacterial wash is more effective than other methods, however a good alternative is using soap and water to wash hands. A hand sanitizer (≥60% alcohol) is an adequate alternative if soap and water are not available. Additional information is available at http://www.cdc.gov/handwashing/.
- The safety with long-term daily use of these products and effectiveness have not been demonstrated and manufacturers did not provide the necessary information. The FDA regulates over-the-counter products utilizing OTC monographs and the new drug application process.
- Antibacterial washes containing chloroxylenol, benzalkonium chloride, and benzethonium chloride may be marketed for 1 additional year, as FDA deferred rulemaking for these ingredients for 1 year based on industry comments and to allow for data collection.

Chapter 23

CASE STUDY 23-1

- A help-seeking advertisement should include a product's brand and generic name. The advertisement should encourage patients to get their medication refilled.
- The help-seeking advertisement should not include images or references to the product's indication or make dosing recommendations.

CASE STUDY 23-2

- It is very important to have a clear conflict of interest policy in place. This policy and procedure should guide who may meet with pharmaceutical industry, how often individuals should meet with industry representatives, what topics are discussed, and what types of information and/or items may be exchanged. It is also wise to have a system in place to track and document these visits. Finally, it is also beneficial to complete a training session or course regarding best practices for industry interactions.

- Prior to the visit, it is recommended to determine what medications will be discussed, either by directly asking the representative or reviewing their portfolio. Key evidence-based information from resources such as the prescription drug labeling will be used. It is also helpful to conduct a primary literature search and ensure you are up-to-date with current clinical literature regarding the medications.
- Be polite and professional but also use active listening skills to detect use of flawed logic (e.g., appeal to authority, red herring).

CASE STUDY 23-3

- Health care professionals should critically analyze all information presented at these programs for accuracy, reliability, and potential violations.
- Common violations likely to occur in this setting include presenting inadequate risk information and minimizing risks, exaggerating benefits, presenting off-label or unapproved information, and making false or deceiving comparisons with other medications.
- Health care professionals can report advertising violations to the FDA through the Bad Ad program via e-mail BadAd@FDA.gov or by phone 855-RX-BADAD (855-792-2323).

CASE STUDY 23-4

- Some type of needs assessment should be done prior to launching an academic detailing programing. Possible sources of data include review of prescribing practices, patient demographics, financial data, and survey of health care professionals and/or patients.
- Materials used in academic detailing should be developed using an evidence-based approach; they should draw from tertiary resources and primarily literature. One organization that may provide validated materials is NaRCAD. Academic institutions may also serve as valuable partners. You could also consider networking with SCORxE or iDiS.
- The advantage of a one-on-one approach is that it may facilitate a more meaningful discussion as well as allow for privacy of the prescriber. However, a group approach has the advantage of potentially reaching a larger audience. Either approach could be considered depending on the scope and goals of the program.
- Metrics should be specific to the intervention targets and actionable. For example, if a program was designed to promote evidence-based use of antihypertensives, prescribing patterns could be monitored with the goal of observing increased adherence to an institutional guideline. If increasing use of generic medications was a goal, prescription data could also be monitored to ensure effectiveness. Finally, humanistic data may also be collected in the form of prescriber and/or patient survey.

Chapter 24

CASE STUDY 24-1

Accurate, reputable treatment guidelines may be quickly found in sources such as National Guidelines Clearinghouse (NCG), PubMed®, as well as through links from the websites of the American Society of Health-System Pharmacists (ASHP) at https://www.ashp.org/Pharmacy-Practice/Policy-Positions-and-Guidelines or from the American Pharmacists Association.™ The professional organizations such as the American Academy of Dermatology (www.aad.org) or the American Academy of Family Physicians (www.aafp.org) also have published clinical guidelines and recommendations on their websites.

CASE STUDY 24–2

- Drug information questions that PP has either requested or implied:
    - What is meant by the term "not on formulary"?
    - What *is* covered on this patient's prescription formulary?
- *Dr. Collins* might begin to answer each of these questions as follows:
    - "Not on formulary" means that a medication is not listed in a prescription drug plan as being paid for or being provided at a discounted rate through a prescription insurance plan.
    - Prescription formulary coverage information may be determined in a variety of ways, including visiting http://medicare.gov for Medicare recipients, by typing prescription insurance provider + formulary + the calendar year you desire (e.g., 2016) in an Internet search engine, searching select drug information databases such as Epocrates® or Lexicomp®, or within e-prescribing platform formulary decision support systems.
- Reputable databases with information geared specifically toward the patient, and with materials that have been reviewed and placed at 8th grade reading level or below include Clinical Pharmacology®, Facts & Comparisons eAnswers®, Lexicomp®, and Micromedex®.
- Clinical Pharmacology®, Facts & Comparisons eAnswers®, and Lexicomp® each contain patient-oriented materials in both English and Spanish. In addition, the Lexicomp® database includes medication leaflets in up to 19 additional languages, and Micromedex®'s Patient Connect Suite includes medication information in up to 15 languages geared toward the patient (although the reading level for the additional languages in Lexicomp® and Micromedex® is not specified).

CASE STUDY 24–3

- It is most important to advise a patient or caregiver to avoid flushing a medication down a toilet or pouring it down a drain. Patients should be informed that certain pharmacies will now take back medications for disposal; the program is voluntary for pharmacies. Patients can mail their unused prescription medications in or they can place them in a pharmacy-maintained collection container or one found at several law-enforcement agencies. Consumers should also be encouraged to take advantage of medication take-back collection days. If none are available, methods for safe personal disposal of medications, including syringes, can be found on the Institute for Safe Medical Practice (ISMP) website, http://www.ismp.org, as well as the Pharmacist's Letter website, http://www.pharmacistsletter.com. A very small number of drugs may be flushed (due to the potential risk of inappropriate exposure), and these are listed online at http://www.fda.gov/downloads/Drugs/ResourcesForYou/Consumers/BuyingUsingMedicineSafely/EnsuringSafeUseofMedicine/SafeDisposalofMedicines/UCM337803.pdf as well as in Table 24-1 of this chapter.
- While multiple governmental initiatives exist to promote the safe and appropriate disposal of unused, unwanted, and/or expired medications (e.g., The White House Office of National Drug Control Policy), these are not enforceable laws on the consumer.

CASE STUDY 24–4

- Examples of such quality indicators include, but are not limited to, efficiency (resource use), structure, process, intermediate outcomes, long-term outcomes, and patient centeredness. Newer measures may include those focused on medication-related patient safety (e.g., detecting/preventing medication errors and adverse drug reactions).

- Yes, it is, and it falls under the quality measure related to patient centeredness.
- Yes; the U.S. Department of Health and Human Services, as part of the Accountable Care Organization model, has specified and published 33 required quality measures that are evaluated to determine payment structure for patient care networks (including ambulatory care settings).

Chapter 25

CASE STUDY 25-1

- As a pharmacist in a busy pharmacy, it is important to triage the problems in front of you. In this situation, you have multiple things going on and you are the only pharmacist on duty. It is up to you to decide what takes priority. This patient may be making decisions about her health based solely on information found online. If the patient follows through on her plan to stop taking the carbamazepine she will be at risk of being harmed. This should make her your top priority.

  The patient in this particular case is actually seeking input from you in her attempt to have a dialogue about quitting her medication. You would be negligent in your duties if you did not choose to counsel the patient on the pros and cons of obtaining health information online, the danger of stopping an anticonvulsant medication abruptly, and the risk of potential seizure recurrence.

  As a pharmacist, you have a professional obligation to engage with your patients and provide them with the education and tools to obtain the best health care possible. Patients are increasingly using alternative sources beyond health care providers for advice and/or counseling, which makes it vital that pharmacists initiate even difficult conversations.

- First, the patient should be encouraged to continue to take an active role in her own health care. Patient empowerment has many positives for health outcomes. On the flipside, it is important to make the patient aware that when taking her health care into her own hands there can be negative consequences as well. It is crucial that she involves a health care practitioner if she decides to change her therapy in anyway.

  Second, agree with your patient that there are a lot of good places to find health information out there but that it is really important they identify quality websites from which to obtain that information. Even then, every individual is different and the information they find on these websites may not necessarily be patient-specific or applicable to his or her situation. For example, the patient in this case is making a decision to discontinue her anticonvulsant medication based on other patients' opinions of the medication. These other patients quite possibly have an entirely different health situation. Encourage the patient to take these concerns to her primary care practitioner so that they may have a discussion on whether or not what she found online is relevant to her situation.

  Third, you review suggestions for determining a quality health information website, thereby ensuring she is obtaining information from reputable sources and bringing information to discuss with her health care practitioner that has value. In this specific case, you are extremely busy and unable to meet now so you should arrange a time to call the patient or make an appointment for her to come back in to discuss her plans.

Our role as health care practitioners is to support the patient and their beliefs. Show respect and the desire to collaborate with them and you will gain their trust. If you trivialize what they bring to you and insist that the health care practitioner is the expert and the one who knows best, you may damage the relationship with the patient beyond repair.

- Safety first. If the patient has made up her mind that there is no stopping her from discontinuing her carbamazepine immediately, advising her how to do so safely becomes your number one priority. First, direct the patient to see her primary care provider as soon as possible. Together they can work out a plan of action to taper her off the medication and possibly get her started on something she feels more comfortable taking.

If you sense the patient will not consult her physician, it is important to counsel her on possible withdrawal symptoms she may experience as well as the consequences of quitting her medication all at once without tapering. Also arrange a follow-up time after your initial discussion to evaluate the control of her disease state and how well she tolerated stopping the medication.

CASE STUDY 25–2

- The first question that should come to mind as a health care professional is whether or not the patient has discussed the use of this particular app with his primary care provider. Although the tracking of health data to assist in the management of a disease state can be extremely helpful for the patient, it can become dangerous when an app is making clinical recommendations about treating a condition (i.e., adjusting insulin dosage) without the supervision of a health care professional.

Second, it is important to confirm the patient's diabetes truly has been under control over the past few months. Although the patient sings the app's praises because of the positive difference he feels in terms of his disease state since downloading it, you want to verify that his blood glucose levels are well controlled. Taking a look at the patient's chart and A1C can better help you determine whether or not the app has been harmful or helpful. It is also necessary to redirect the patient back to their primary care provider in order to ensure both the health care professional and patient are on the same page in regards to how the disease state is being managed. Encouraging communication between these two health care partners creates a perfect opportunity for patient and physician to discuss the mobile software and whether or not it will be a part of their treatment plan going forward.

Finally, you should ask more questions about the particular app in question. Was it developed by a credible source? Are clinical recommendations based on evidence? Is the app capable of tailoring a recommendation to a specific patient? The answers to these questions and others may help you better guide the patient in whether the app is a reliable one or in some cases FDA approved as a medical device to use in managing a disease state.

- In this particular scenario, it seems the patient has not just dipped his toes into the mobile health arena but has jumped head first. The app he describes using puts him, the patient, in a position to be very reliant on a device to make therapeutic decisions that his physician would normally make. While it seems the application does factor in patient-specific data when making its decisions, without the supervision of a clinician, this is risky territory.

The single best piece of advice you can give a patient who is interested or has been using mobile health apps is to always check with a health care professional before making any changes to their prescribed medication regimen. Use of mobile health software by a patient wanting to get more involved in their health should never be discouraged; in fact, the benefits seen in patients who use apps to keep track of health and fitness progress, find health information, and to stay connected with others in their health situation are infinite. The danger lies when patients start using apps as a sole resource to diagnose, manage their disease state, adjust their medication regimens, etc. Smartphone apps with these types of capabilities should be used in conjunction with a physician. In some cases, they may be medically prescribed.

CASE STUDY 25–3

In general, there are five key areas that are important to consider when evaluating a new mobile health app: credibility, accuracy, whether or not it is evidence-based, ease-of-use, and health literacy. There are several questions under each key area that are important to ask yourself as a reviewer of an app.

- Credibility of app
    Are credentials of the app suitable?
    Are authors/publishers clearly listed?
    Are there advertisements?
    Is the organization that developed the app reputable?
    Are there disclaimers of content?
- Accuracy of information
    Is it peer reviewed?
    Is the information current and/or frequently updated?
    Are recent and reputable guidelines used to support recommendations made?
    Are references cited?
- Evidence-based medicine
    Are recommendations evidence based?
    Do recommendations target a specific audience or are they general in nature?
    Are opinion statements clearly marked?
    Are users directed to a health care professional before making changes to health care routine?
- Ease-of-use
    Does the app fit to the screen?
    Is the setup of the app well designed and organized?
    Is the app easily navigated?
    Does the app have a search function?
    Is there a main menu that helps clearly lay content out?
- Health literacy
    Is medical jargon used easy for the lay reader to understand?
    Is font and setup of app easy to read?
    Does the app gear information for the consumer?

Unfortunately, even after thoroughly reviewing a mobile health app using the five key areas there still may be some questions as to whether or not the app is capable of making therapeutic decisions for a patient. In these instances, it may be best to suggest contacting the developer of the software to better determine how their particular app arrives at therapeutic decisions.

Chapter 26

CASE STUDY 26–1

- Computerized provider order entry (CPOE) systems allow medical provider instructions to be electronically entered for the treatment of patients who are under the provider's direct care in an acute care facility. This may include medication orders as well as orders for tests, procedures, and consultations. Electronic prescribing (e-prescribing) systems allow medical providers to electronically enter and transmit a prescription for a medication, which is then verified and processed in an electronic format at an outpatient or community pharmacy.

- It can be a long and difficult process to integrate CPOE into a complex medical environment, which often requires ongoing changes to system design in order to adequately fit the CPOE system to the unique care setting. Beyond the technical challenges of CPOE implementation, changes in workflow can often be the greatest barrier to successful implementation.
- Clinical decision support systems (CDSS) are computer programs that augment clinical decision making by combining referential information with patient-specific information. CDSS can provide alerts and messages in CPOE and e-prescribing systems that ultimately improve the safety, quality, efficiency, and cost-effectiveness of care.
- CPOE and e-prescribing systems may introduce new types of errors. For inexperienced users, order entry and therefore communication may be slower. CDSS-based alerts and warnings that appear too often may lead to alert fatigue for providers.

CASE STUDY 26-2

- Whereas providers are on the data entry end of these systems, which occurs at the prescribing stage of the medication use process, pharmacists are on the receiving end and interact with these systems at the order-verification stage of the medication use process. Once the order for a medication enters the pharmacy computer system through one of these systems, the pharmacist assesses the appropriateness of the order and addresses any issues or discrepancies before filling the order.
- Bar code medication administration (BCMA) systems are used in the hospital setting at the administration stage of the medication use process. The purpose of a BCMA system is to ensure that the six rights of medication administration are followed by electronically validating and documenting medications at the point of care.
- Clinical surveillance systems are used to actively monitor patients. Rules are built to identify potential problems. These rules, if met, then prompt medical providers to follow-up with or reevaluate the patient.

CASE STUDY 26-3

- The medication use process is a cyclical process in which various interconnected parts—people, systems, procedures, and policies—work together to achieve the common goal of safe and effective medication therapy. The five stages of the medication use process as well as the technologies used at each stage are as follows:
  - ○ **Order entry (prescribing)**—computerized provider order entry, clinical decision support systems
  - ○ **Order verification (transcribing)**—clinical decision support systems
  - ○ **Dispensing**—automated dispensing cabinets, carousel cabinets, robotic cart filling systems, sterile compounding devices
  - ○ **Administration**—bar code medication administration, electronic medication administration record, intelligent infusion pumps, medication event monitoring systems (MEMS)
  - ○ **Monitoring**—clinical surveillance systems, clinical documentation systems

CASE STUDY 26-4

- Journal of Medical Internet Research, Journal of Participatory Medicine
- Initially, Facebook can be used to provide general information about services offered, to showcase the expertise of staff, and to provide basic health and medical information. As the institution's comfort with the technology grows, Facebook can be used for online question and answer sessions, to host videos of highly advanced procedures, and to provide patient perspectives on their experiences at the facility. Twitter can also be used to send the latest news about significant additions to the medical staff, to inform followers about upcoming clinical education classes, and to highlight the acquisition of high-tech tools for patient care. As resources become available and as patients

express interest, Twitter may also be used for targeted messaging to remind patients of activities that encourage healthy behaviors. Ultimately, the information that is shared on Facebook, Twitter, or any other medium should address the needs of the institution's patients. The best way to find out what information patients want to receive or access electronically is to ask them. Additionally, the hospital could start a patient-focused blog. Topics covered could be informed by patient input and feedback. The hospital could also recommend vetted PHRs for patient use on the blog site.

- The hospital could utilize the IoT for indoor navigation, allowing patients and visitors to use their smartphones to navigate to desired locations within the hospital. The IoT could also be used to keep track of devices, personnel, and patients.

CASE STUDY 26-5

- Electronic health records (EHRs) contain information related to a patient's care and are meant to be used by health practitioners. EHRs are maintained by health care organizations, whereas personal health records (PHRs) are maintained by patients themselves.
- The Office of the National Coordinator for Health Information Technology
- The Centers for Medicare and Medicaid Services
- There are three stages of Meaningful Use, focused on: (1) capturing patient data and sharing that data with either the patient or other health care providers, (2) advanced clinical processes, and (3) improved patient outcomes.
- There are many barriers to EHR implementation. Primary barriers cited in the literature include costs related to EHR implementation and use, lack of physician support, and perceived or actual difficulty meeting the Meaningful Use criteria.

Chapter 27

CASE STUDY 27-1

Instructional methods to teach drug information include didactic lectures, small group learning, Internet-based learning including online course management programs (e.g., Blackboard, Joule), audience response systems, YouTube, online blogs, tweets, and wikis. Literature evaluation is often taught in a stand-alone course placed in the second professional year. Other options include embedding within a drug information and teaching within laboratory-based courses.

CASE STUDY 27-2

Individuals with expertise in drug information may work in many different roles beyond that of drug information specialist, including medication safety pharmacist, informatics pharmacist, medication policy pharmacist, regulatory pharmacist, and medical writer/editor. These individuals may practice in a variety of settings including hospital, community, industry, government, medical publishing company, and schools of pharmacy. The recommended training for drug information specialists is completion of a postgraduate year one residency followed by a postgraduate year two drug information residency program.

Answers for Self-Assessment Questions

Chapter 1

1. c	6. d	11. a
2. e	7. e	12. d
3. e	8. c	13. e
4. c	9. e	14. b
5. e	10. a	15. b

Chapter 2

1. c	6. d	11. b
2. d	7. b	12. d
3. b	8. a	13. a
4. a	9. d	14. d
5. a	10. c	15. c

Chapter 3

1. c	6. b	11. b
2. a	7. a	12. c
3. c	8. b	13. b
4. d	9. a	14. a
5. c	10. a	15. b

Chapter 4

1. d	6. b	11. b
2. a	7. c	12. a
3. c	8. c	13. a
4. e	9. e	14. e
5. c	10. e	15. e

Chapter 5

1. b	6. b	11. d
2. b	7. d	12. c
3. c	8. a	13. d
4. a	9. d	14. c
5. d	10. d	15. b

Chapter 6

1. b	6. b	11. b
2. a	7. d	12. c
3. a	8. a	13. b
4. c	9. a	14. d
5. d	10. d	15. a

Chapter 7

1. d	6. d	11. b
2. c	7. a	12. a
3. c	8. d	13. b
4. c	9. a	14. a
5. b	10. c	15. c

Chapter 8

1. e	6. c	11. e
2. c	7. b	12. e
3. d	8. d	13. c
4. d	9. b	14. a
5. e	10. e	15. b

Chapter 9

1. b	6. a	11. a
2. d	7. a	12. c
3. a	8. d	13. a
4. b	9. b	14. a
5. d	10. b	15. b

Chapter 10

1. c	6. e	11. c
2. d	7. c	12. d
3. b	8. e	13. b
4. d	9. c	14. e
5. d	10. c	15. e

Chapter 11

1. a, c, and d	6. b, c, and d	11. b and d
2. a	7. c	12. d
3. a, b, c	8. a	13. a
4. b	9. b, c, and d	14. c
5. d	10. a, b, and d	15. a

Chapter 12

1. e	6. b	11. b
2. e	7. b	12. b
3. a	8. a	13. b
4. e	9. a	14. d
5. b	10. a	15. b

Chapter 13

1. a	6. d	11. a
2. a	7. d	12. b
3. e	8. a	13. c
4. c	9. d	14. b
5. a	10. a	15. d

Chapter 14

1. a	6. d	11. b
2. a	7. d	12. a
3. a	8. a	13. b
4. e	9. a	14. d
5. a	10. a	15. b

Chapter 15

1. d	6. b	11. c
2. c	7. a	12. d
3. d	8. b	13. a
4. a	9. d	14. a
5. c	10. a	15. c

Chapter 16

1. d	6. c	11. d
2. d	7. d	12. c
3. d	8. e	13. b
4. e	9. e	14. d
5. a	10. b	15. c

Chapter 17

1. d	6. e	11. d
2. d	7. a	12. e
3. a	8. d	13. a
4. d	9. e	14. b
5. c	10. a	15. b

Chapter 18

1. c	6. b	11. a
2. c	7. b	12. d
3. c	8. a	13. b
4. d	9. d	14. a
5. c	10. a	15. c

Chapter 19

1. c	6. e	11. b
2. d	7. b	12. e
3. b	8. b	13. a
4. e	9. e	14. b
5. e	10. d	

Chapter 20

1. c	6. e	11. a
2. b	7. a	12. c
3. d	8. d	13. e
4. e	9. c	14. a
5. b	10. a	15. b

Chapter 21

1. a	6. c	11. c
2. b	7. c	12. b
3. c	8. b	13. a
4. d	9. a	14. b
5. d	10. c	15. c

Chapter 22

1. c	6. e	11. b
2. a	7. a	12. d
3. d	8. c	13. a
4. c	9. b	14. c
5. e	10. c	15. d

Chapter 23

1. b	6. b	11. a
2. a	7. a	12. d
3. b	8. d	13. c
4. a	9. b	14. b
5. b	10. c	15. a

Chapter 24

1. b	6. c	11. b
2. e	7. e	12. a
3. c	8. c	13. b
4. a	9. b	14. b
5. d	10. d	15. a

Chapter 25

1. e	6. e	11. c
2. e	7. b	12. d
3. d	8. e	13. b
4. e	9. d	14. e
5. e	10. b	15. a

Chapter 26

1. b	6. d	11. a
2. e	7. d	12. e
3. c	8. e	13. a
4. c	9. d	14. c
5. e	10. e	15. c

Chapter 27

1. b	6. d	11. d
2. d	7. e	12. a
3. a	8. d	13. e
4. d	9. d	14. e
5. d	10. d	15. b

Index

Ancillary therapies, 160–161
ANCOVA. *See* Analysis of covariance
AND, Boolean operator, 88–89
Anesthesia, 645
Angie's List, 1091t
Angina pectoris, 132
Angiotensin-converting enzyme (ACE)
   inhibitor, 167, 725, 826
Animal Poison Control Center, 85
Annals of Pharmacotherapy, 120
ANOVA. *See* Analysis of variance
Antacids, 619, 673, 674
Antibiotics, 721, 780
Anticancer agents, 15
Anticoagulation
   enoxaparin, 141, 419, 493
   warfarin, 169–170, 419, 453, 493,
      683, 684
Anticoagulation subcommittee, 657
Antidiarrheal agents, 825t, 866t
Antifibrinolytics medications,
   314–315
Antihypertensive therapies, 144, 165, 174,
   209, 210, 211, 985, 1042
Anti-inflammatories, 1042
Anti-Kickback Statute, 523, 539–542
Antimicrobial/infectious disease
   subcommittee, 657
Antineoplastics, 721
Antithrombotic Therapy Guidelines, 453
AoA. *See* Administration on Aging
APhA. *See* American Pharmacists
   Association
Apixaban (Eliquis), 1022
APM. *See* Alternative Payment Model
Appeals to authority, 1038t
Appeals to pity, 1038t
APPEs. *See* Advanced pharmacy practice
   experiences
Application service provider (ASP), 1130
Applications (apps), 5, 11–12, 65–66,
   498–499, 1096, 1099
Applied Biopharmaceutics and
   Pharmacokinetics, 76
Applied Clinical Pharmacokinetics, 76
Applied Therapeutics (Koda-Kimnle and
   Young's), 81
Appraisal of Guidelines for Research and
   Evaluation (AGREE) collaboration,
   458–459
ARI, 171t
Aristotle, 558
ARR. *See* Absolute risk reduction
ARRA. *See* American Recovery and
   Reinvestment Act
ART. *See* Adverse Reaction Tracking (ART)
   database

Article proposals, 597, 598f
ASHP. *See* American Society of Health-
   System Pharmacists
Asimov, Isaac, 608
ASP. *See* Application service provider
ASPCA. *See* American Society for
   the Prevention of Cruelty to
   Animals
Aspirin, 129, 159, 495, 780, 782
*Association of American Publishers v. New
   York University*, 528
Association of Clinical Research
   Professionals (ACRP), 994t
Association tests
   nonparametric tests
      logistic regression, 376–380
      Spearman rank-order correlation
         coefficient, 375–376
      survival analysis, 380–389, 382f,
         383f386f, 386f
   parametric tests
      multiple linear regression, 337, 338,
         372–373, 374–375, 376
      Pearson's product-moment correlation,
         368f, 3669
      simple linear regression, 335,
         369–373
Asthma, 309, 780
Atenolol, 350–351
Atomoxetine, 75
Atorvastatin, 36, 126–127, 133, 142, 150, 158,
   165, 172, 1022
Atrial fibrillation, 169, 447, 779t, 780
Atropine, 825t, 866t
ATSDR. *See* Agency for Toxic Substances
   and Disease Registry
Attention deficit/hyperactivity disorder
   (ADHD), 75, 88, 89
Attributable risk, 279
Attrition, in clinical trials,
   155–157, 317
Audience
   of newsletters and websites, 615
   for professional writing, 600
Authors
   coauthors, 598–600
   primary, 599
Autism, Childhood Autism Spectrum Test,
   353–354
Automated dispensing cabinets (ADCs),
   1118–1119, 1129
Autonomy, 562, 569
Average (mean), 147–148, 295–296
Average wholesale price (AWP), 734
AVMA. *See* American Veterinary Medical
   Association
AWP. *See* Average wholesale price

S